BIOCHEMICAL

and

PHYSIOLOGICAL

ASPECTS

of HUMAN

NUTRITION

Martha H. Stipanuk, PhD

Professor
Division of Nutritional Sciences
Cornell University
Ithaca, New York

W.B. Saunders Company
A Division of Harcourt Brace & Company
Philadelphia London Toronto Montreal Sydney Tokyo

W.B. SAUNDERS COMPANY
A Division of Harcourt Brace & Company

The Curtis Center
Independence Square West
Philadelphia, Pennsylvania 19106

Library of Congress Cataloging-in-Publication Data

Biochemical and physiological aspects of human nutrition / Martha H. Stipanuk.

p.   cm.

ISBN 0–7216–4452–X

1. Nutrition.   2. Metabolism.   3. Biochemistry.   I. Stipanuk, Martha H.

QP141.B57   2000

612.3'9—dc21   98-13993

BIOCHEMICAL AND PHYSIOLOGICAL ASPECTS OF HUMAN NUTRITION   ISBN 0–7216–4452–X

Printed in the United States of America.

Last digit is the print number: 9   8   7   6   5   4   3   2   1

To my students and colleagues in the Division of Nutritional Sciences at Cornell University, 1977–1999, and to the two former directors of the Division of Nutritional Sciences, Malden C. Nesheim and Cutberto Garza.

Sharing the study of nutrition with you has been challenging, productive, and fun. I have been blessed to have had so many expert scientists and caring people as supportive colleagues and to have had so many capable students eager to learn along with me.

Contributors

◆ ◆

Roy D. Baynes, MD, PhD
Professor of Medicine and Oncology, Charles Martin Professor of Cancer Research, and Director, Bone Marrow Transplantation, Barbara Ann Karmands Cancer Institute, Wayne State University, Detroit, Michigan
Iron

Ching K. Chow, PhD
Professor, Department of Nutrition and Food Science, University of Kentucky, Lexington, Kentucky
Vitamin E

Karen D. Crissinger, MD, PhD
Associate Professor of Pediatrics, Vanderbilt Pediatric Gastroenterology, Vanderbilt University School of Medicine, Nashville, Tennessee
Overview of Digestion and Absorption; Digestion and Absorption of Lipids

Rushad Daruwala, PhD
Postdoctoral Fellow, Molecular and Clinical Nutrition Section, National Institute of Diabetes and Digestive and Kidney Diseases, National Institutes of Health, Bethesda, Maryland
Vitamin C

Mary J. DeLong, PhD
Associate Professor, Department of Environmental Health Sciences, Emory University; Director of Laboratories, Rollins School of Public Health, Emory University, Atlanta, Georgia
Detoxification and Protective Functions of Nutrients

Dominick P. DePaola, DDS, PhD
Professor, Department of Oral Health Epidemiology and Policy, Harvard Medical School/Harvard School of Dental Medicine; President and Chief Executive Officer, Forsyth Dental Center, Boston, Massachusetts
Diet and Oral Disease

Christopher J. Fielding, PhD
Professor of Physiology and Neider Professor of Cardiovascular Physiology, Cardiovascular Research Institute, University of California San Francisco, San Francisco, California
Lipoprotein Synthesis, Transport, and Metabolism

James C. Fleet, PhD
Assistant Professor, Department of Nutrition and Food Service Systems, University of North Carolina at Greensboro, Greensboro, North Carolina
Zinc, Copper, and Manganese

Hedley C. Freake, PhD
Associate Professor, Department of Nutritional Sciences, University of Connecticut, Storrs, Connecticut
Iodine

Malcolm F. Fuller, PhD, ScD
Visiting Scientist, Massachusetts Institute of Technology, Boston, Massachusetts
Protein and Amino Acid Requirements

Peter J. Garlick, PhD

Professor in Surgery, State University of New York at Stony Brook, Stony Brook, New York

Protein Synthesis and Degradation

Henry N. Ginsberg, MD

Professor of Medicine, Columbia University College of Physicians and Surgeons, New York, New York

Nutrition, Lipids, and Cardiovascular Disease

Alan G. Goodridge, PhD

Dean, College of Biological Sciences, Ohio State University, Columbus, Ohio

Lipid Metabolism—Synthesis and Oxidation; Regulation of Fuel Utilization

Gary M. Gray, MD

Professor and Director, Digestive Disease Center, Department of Gastroenterology, Stanford University School of Medicine, Stanford, California

Digestion and Absorption of Carbohydrate

James O. Hill, PhD

Director, Clinical Nutrition Research Center, Center for Human Nutrition, University of Colorado Health Science Center, Denver, Colorado

Cellular and Whole-Animal Energetics; Control of Energy Balance; Disturbances of Energy Balance

Michael F. Holick, PhD, MD

Professor of Medicine, Dermatology, and Physiology, Boston University School of Medicine; Chief, Endocrinology, Nutrition, Diabetes, Boston Medical Center, Boston, Massachusetts

Vitamin D

Dean P. Jones, PhD

Professor of Biochemistry and Winship Cancer Center, Emory University School of Medicine, Atlanta, Georgia

Detoxification and Protective Functions of Nutrients

Wahida Karmally, MS, RD

Associate Research Scientist and Director of Nutrition, The Irving Center for Clinical Research, Columbia University, New York, New York

Nutrition, Lipids, and Cardiovascular Disease

Taru Kosonen, PhD

Clinical Research Associate, Leiras Dy, Clinical Research, Helsinki, Finland

Structure and Properties of Proteins and Amino Acids

Adamandia W. Kriketos, PhD

Postdoctoral Fellow, Metabolism Research Program, Garvan Institute of Medical Research, Darlinghurst, Sydney, Australia

Cellular and Whole-Animal Energetics; Control of Energy Balance; Disturbances of Energy Balance

Mark Levine, MD

Chief, Molecular and Clinical Nutrition Section, and Senior Staff Physician, National Institute of Diabetes and Digestive and Kidney Diseases, Bethesda, Maryland

Vitamin C

Betty A. Lewis, PhD

Associate Professor, Division of Nutritional Sciences, Cornell University, Ithaca, New York

Structure and Properties of Carbohydrates

Joanne R. Lupton, PhD

Professor, Department of Animal Sciences, Texas A&M University, College Station, Texas

Dietary Fiber

Donald B. McCormick, PhD

F. E. Callaway Professor of Biochemistry, Department of Biochemistry, Emory University, Atlanta, Georgia

Niacin, Riboflavin, and Thiamin

Mary M. McGrane, PhD

Associate Professor, Departments of Nutritional Sciences and Molecular Cell Biology, University of Connecticut, Storrs, Connecticut

Carbohydrate Metabolism—Synthesis and Oxidation

Margaret A. McNurlan, PhD

Assistant Professor, Department of Surgery, State University of New York at Stony Brook, Stony Brook, New York

Protein Synthesis and Degradation

Forrest H. Nielsen, PhD

Center Director and Research Nutritionist, United States Department of Agriculture, Agricultural Research Service, Grand Forks Human Nutrition Research Center, Grand Forks, North Dakota

The Ultratrace Elements

Noa Noy, PhD

Associate Professor, Division of Nutritional Sciences, Cornell University, Ithaca, New York

Vitamin A

Jae B. Park, PhD

Research Biochemist, Phytonutrients Laboratory, Beltsville Human Nutrition Research Center, United States Department of Agriculture, Beltsville, Maryland

Vitamin C

John C. Peters, PhD

Associate Director, Regulatory and Clinical Development, The Procter & Gamble Company, Cincinnati, Ohio

Cellular and Whole-Animal Energetics; Control of Energy Balance; Disturbances of Energy Balance

Robert B. Rucker, PhD

Professor of Nutrition and Biological Chemistry, Department of Nutrition, University of California–Davis, Davis, California

Structure and Properties of Proteins and Amino Acids

Robert K. Rude, MD

Professor of Medicine, Department of Medicine, University of Southern California, Los Angeles, California

Magnesium

Steven C. Rumsey, PhD

Research Scientist, Meade Johnson Nutritionals, Evanston, Illinois

Vitamin C

Charles F. Schachtele, PhD

Associate Dean for Research and Professor of Oral Sciences, University of Minnesota School of Dentistry, Minneapolis, Minnesota

Diet and Oral Disease

Barry Shane, PhD

Professor, Department of Nutritional Sciences, University of California–Berkeley, Berkeley, California

Folate, Vitamin B_{12}, and Vitamin B_6

Hwai-Ping Sheng, PhD

Associate Professor, Faculty of Medicine, Department of Physiology, The University of Hong Kong, Hong Kong

Sodium, Chloride, and Potassium; Body Fluids and Water Balance

Donald M. Small, MD

Chairman, Department of Biophysics, Boston University School of Medicine; Visiting Physician, Boston Medical Center, Boston, Massachusetts

Structure and Properties of Lipids

Arthur A. Spector, MD

University of Iowa Foundation Distinguished Professor, Departments of Biochemistry and Internal Medicine, University of Iowa, College of Medicine, Iowa City, Iowa

Lipid Metabolism: Essential Fatty Acids

Christina M. Stark, MS, RD, CN

Nutrition Specialist, Division of Nutritional Sciences, Cornell University, Ithaca, New York

Translating Biochemical and Physiological Requirements into Practice

Bruce R. Stevens, PhD

Professor of Physiology, Department of Physiology, College of Medicine, University of Florida, Gainesville, Florida

Digestion and Absorption of Protein

Martha H. Stipanuk, PhD
Professor, Division of Nutritional Sciences, Cornell University, Ithaca, New York
Amino Acid Metabolism; Iron

Hei Sook Sul, PhD
Professor, Department of Nutritional Sciences, University of California–Berkeley, Berkeley, California
Lipid Metabolism—Synthesis and Oxidation

Roger A. Sunde, PhD
Professor of Nutritional Sciences and Biochemistry, University of Missouri, Columbia, Missouri
Selenium

John W. Suttie, PhD
Professor, Department of Biochemistry, University of Wisconsin–Madison, Madison, Wisconsin
Vitamin K

Lawrence Sweetman, PhD
Professor, Institute of Biomedical Studies, Baylor University, Waco; Director, Mass Spectrometry Laboratory, Institute of Metabolic Disease, Baylor University Medical Center, Dallas, Texas
Pantothenic Acid and Biotin

Patrick Tso, PhD
Professor of Pathology, Department of Pathology, University of Cincinnati College of Medicine, Cincinnati, Ohio
Overview of Digestion and Absorption; Digestion and Absorption of Lipids

Nancy D. Turner, PhD, CNS
Research Assistant Professor, Department of Animal Science, Texas A&M University, College Station, Texas
Dietary Fiber

Anton J. M. Wagenmakers, PhD
Department of Human Biology, University of Limburg, Maastricht, The Netherlands
Fuel Utilization by Skeletal Muscle During Rest and During Exercise

Yaohui Wang, MD
Senior Staff Fellow, Molecular and Clinical Nutrition Section, National Institute of Diabetes and Digestive and Kidney Disease, National Institutes of Health, Bethesda, Maryland
Vitamin C

Malcolm Watford, DPhil
Associate Professor, Department of Nutritional Sciences, Cook College, Rutgers University, New Brunswick, New Jersey
Amino Acid Metabolism; Regulation of Fuel Utilization

Gary M. Whitford, PhD, DMD
Regents' Professor, Department of Oral Biology and Maxillofacial Pathology, School of Dentistry, Medical College of Georgia, Augusta, Georgia
Fluoride

Richard J. Wood, PhD
Associate Professor, School of Nutrition Science and Policy, Tufts University; Chief, Mineral Bioavailability Laboratory, United States Department of Agriculture Human Nutrition Research Center on Aging, Boston, Massachusetts
Calcium and Phosphorus

Reviewers

Sharon Akabas, PhD
Adjunct Assistant Professor, Institute of Human Nutrition and Teachers College, Columbia University, New York, New York

James W. Bawden, DDS, PhD, MS
Professor, Department of Pediatric Dentistry, University of North Carolina, Chapel Hill, North Carolina

Wayne E. Billon, PhD, RD, LD
Associate Professor, School of Family and Consumer Services, The University of Southern Mississippi, Hattiesburg, Mississippi

William S. Blaner, PhD
Associate Professor of Nutritional Medicine, Columbia University College of Physicians and Surgeons, New York, New York

Carmen Boyd, MS, LPC, RD
Instructor, Biomedical Sciences Department, Southwest Missouri State University, Springfield, Missouri

John T. Brosman, PhD
Professor and Chair, Department of Biochemistry, Memorial University of Newfoundland, St. John's, Newfoundland, Canada

Margaret C. Craig-Schmidt, PhD
Associate Professor, Department of Nutrition and Food Sciences, Auburn University, Auburn, Alabama

Robert DiSilvestro, PhD
Associate Professor, Department of Human Nutrition, Ohio State University, Columbus, Ohio

Kent L. Erickson, PhD
Professor and Chair, Department of Cell Biology and Human Anatomy, School of Medicine, University of California–Davis, Davis, California

Thomas O. Frommel, PhD
Assistant Professor of Medicine and Molecular and Cellular Biochemistry, Loyola University Medical Center, Maywood, Illinois

Ralph Green, MD
Professor and Chair, Department of Pathology, University of California–Davis, Medical Center, Sacramento, California

R. Jean Hine, PhD
Associate Professor, University of Arkansas for Medical Sciences, Little Rock, Arkansas

Anil K. Jaiswal, PhD
Associate Member, Department of Pharmacology, Fox Chase Cancer Center, Philadelphia, Pennsylvania

Jay Kandiah, PhD, RD, CD
Associate Professor, Department of Family and Consumer Sciences, Ball State University, Muncie, Indiana

Penny M. Kris-Etherton, PhD, RD
Professor, Department of Nutrition, Pennsylvania State University, University Park, Pennsylvania

Shiu-Ming Kuo, PhD
Associate Professor, Nutrition Program, State University of New York at Buffalo, Buffalo, New York

Edith Lerner, PhD
Associate Professor, Department of Nutrition, School of Medicine, Case Western Reserve University, Cleveland, Ohio

Lawrence J. Machlin, PhD
Consultant, Nutrition Research and Information
Inc., Livingston, New Jersey

Suzanne Martin, PhD, RD
College of the Ozarks, Point Lookout, Missouri

Dwight E. Matthews, PhD
Professor, Department of Medicine, University of
Vermont College of Medicine, Burlington, Vermont

Charles C. McCormick, PhD
Associate Professor, Division of Nutritional
Sciences, Cornell University, Ithaca, New York

Sohrab Mobarhan, MD
Associate Chief of Gastroenterology, Director of
Clinical Nutrition Unit, Loyola University Medical
Center, Maywood, Illinois

Donald M. Mock, MD, PhD
Professor, University of Arkansas for Medical
Sciences, Little Rock, Arkansas and Arkansas
Children's Hospital, Little Rock, Arkansas

Kris S. Morey, PhD
Professor, California Polytechnic State University,
San Luis Obispo, California

Linda C. Nebeling, PhD, MPH, RD
Cancer Prevention Fellow, Division of Cancer
Prevention and Control, National Cancer Institute,
Bethesda, Maryland

Susan A. Nitzke, PhD, RD
Associate Professor, Department of Nutritional
Sciences, University of Wisconsin–Madison,
Madison, Wisconsin

David E. Ong, PhD
Professor of Biochemistry, Department of
Biochemistry, Vanderbilt University, Nashville,
Tennessee

Annette L. Pedersen, MS, RD, LD, CDE
Director, Diabetics Program, Notre Dame College,
Cleveland, Ohio

John Thomas Pinto, PhD
Director, Nutrition Research Laboratory, Memorial
Sloan-Kettering Cancer Center, New York, New
York; and Associate Professor of Biochemistry,
Cornell University Medical College, Ithaca, New
York

Marsha H. Read, PhD, RD
Professor, Department of Nutrition, University of
Nevada, Reno, Reno, Nevada

Clifford J. Rosen, MD
Executive Director, St. Joseph Hospital Maine
Center for Osteoporosis Research and Education,
Bangor, Maine

John C. Saari, PhD
Professor of Ophthalmology and Biochemistry,
University of Washington School of Medicine,
Seattle, Washington

Patricia Sanders, MS, MBA, RD, LD
Texas A&M University–Kingsville, Kingsville, Texas

Howerde E. Sauberlich, PhD
Professor and Director, Department of Nutritional
Sciences, University of Alabama at Birmingham,
Birmingham, Alabama

Nancy I. Sheard, ScD, RD
Associate Professor, Departments of Nutritional
Sciences and Medicine, University of Vermont,
Burlington, Vermont

Kathryn Silliman, PhD, RD
Assistant Professor, Department of Biological
Sciences, California State University, Chico,
California

Silke Vogel, PhD
Post-doctoral Research Scientist, Department of
Medicine, Columbia University, New York, New
York

Stella L. Volpe, PhD
Assistant Professor, Department of Nutrition,
University of Massachusetts, Amherst,
Massachusetts

Barry Wolf, MD, PhD
Professor, Departments of Human Genetics,
Pediatrics, Biochemistry and Molecular
Biophysics, Medical College of Virginia, Virginia
Commonwealth University, Richmond, Virginia

Preface

◆ ◆

Biochemical and Physiological Aspects of Human Nutrition represents the collective efforts over the past several years of numerous researchers and teachers in the field of nutrition. We saw a need for a book that covers the biological bases of human nutrition, specifically in a human context and at a level that encompasses the molecular, cellular, tissue, and whole-body levels. Our goal was to produce a book that will serve both as a textbook and as a reference book for students and professionals in various areas of nutrition, biological sciences, and medicine.

To accomplish these objectives, chapters have been written by investigators with expertise in specific areas. We have made an effort to be up-to-date and to identify areas of active research and controversy. At the same time, efforts have been made to ensure the consistency of content and approach that is needed for a book intended to introduce the subject to those who are new to the field.

The study of human nutrition integrates many disciplines, and knowledge and understanding of each of these basic disciplines are essential to the understanding of nutrition. This book is intended for upper-level undergraduate students, graduate students, and professionals who have completed studies in organic chemistry, biochemistry, molecular biology, and physiology. Hence, topics are covered at an advanced level. Nevertheless, an effort has been made to present material in a manner that allows a reader who is unfamiliar with a particular topic to obtain a clear, concise, and thorough understanding of the essential concepts. Particular attention has been given to the design of figures and choice of tabular material to ensure that illustrations and tables clarify, extend, and enrich the text.

The text consists of six units that encompass a traditional coverage of nutrients by classification (carbohydrates, proteins, lipids, vitamins, minerals) but that also allow for discussion of the integrated metabolism and utilization of these nutrients. The macronutrients or energy-yielding nutrients (carbohydrates, proteins, and lipids) are discussed in Units I through IV. Unit I provides an overview of the structure and properties of the macronutrients. The digestion and absorption of the macronutrients are discussed in Unit II, and the metabolism of the macronutrients is the topic of Unit III. Finally, the relation of these macronutrients to energy is discussed in Unit IV. The depth and breadth of coverage given to the macronutrients make this text somewhat unique among advanced nutrition texts. The vitamins are discussed in Unit V. The B vitamins have been grouped and discussed in a manner that facilitates an understanding of their functions in macronutrient metabolism. The unique functions of vitamins C, K, E, A, and D are described in individual chapters. The minerals are the subject of Unit VI; those with well-characterized nutritional or health-related roles are discussed in detail.

The final section, Unit VII, on nutrition, diet, and health, includes six chapters on selected health- and nutrition-related topics: body fluids and water balance; carbohydrates and oral disease; fuel needs of muscle during exercise; detoxification and protective functions of nutrients; lipids and cardiovascular disease; and translating biochemical and physiological requirements into practice. Another significant health-related topic, obesity, is discussed in Chapter 19 of Unit IV.

The reader may wish to read some of the chapters in Unit VII along with other related units (i.e., Chapter 37 along with Chapter 30; Chapter 38 along with Unit II; and Chapters 39 and 40 along with Unit III).

The text is designed so it can easily be used for a comprehensive advanced nutrition and metabolism course in which all nutrients are covered. Alternatively, sections of the text could easily be used for courses that focus specifically on the macronutrients, the vitamins, or the minerals.

Each chapter begins with an outline and, when appropriate, a listing of common abbreviations. The text includes many new figures drawn for this book. Illustrations have been carefully selected to enhance the text and designed to provide insight and to facilitate understanding. References to the research literature and recommended readings are provided for each chapter. Also included within the text are a number of nutrition insights, clinical correlations, life cycle considerations, and food sources/recommended intakes; these have been incorporated to demonstrate the relevance of the text material to practical nutritional considerations in both health and disease.

A separate instructor's manual is available that provides supplemental information to accompany each chapter of the text. The *Instructor's Manual* provides responses to "Thinking Critically" questions from the text. Also included are many additional questions suitable for either exams or problem sets. Summaries of selected research articles that can be used for focused reading assignments or discussions are provided; these may be used to enhance and extend the text material and to reinforce the integration of content across chapters.

MARTHA H. STIPANUK

Acknowledgments

◆ ◆

Malden Nesheim, former director of the Division of Nutritional Sciences at Cornell University, is perhaps most responsible for this book because my involvement in teaching this subject came as a result of his "invitation" to join him in co-teaching "Physiological and Biochemical Bases of Human Nutrition" in 1986. I have been both teaching this course and continuing to study and learn along with my students ever since. This book also would not have been possible were it not for the support of Cutberto Garza, director of the Division of Nutritional Sciences from 1988 to 1998, who provided the support and flexibility I needed to accomplish this task. The extremely capable and motivated students I have taught at Cornell have been a delight. Teaching them and watching their excitement as they "put together" their studies of chemistry and biology in the context of human nutrition have been a privilege and a stimulus to this work. Thanks are also due to my many teachers and mentors over the years. Although all cannot be mentioned, several of my undergraduate advisors and teachers at the University of Kentucky played particularly noteworthy roles: Doris Tichenor challenged me to reach higher than I thought important at the time, Linda Chen provided my first laboratory research opportunity, and L. V. Packett encouraged me to attend Cornell University for graduate study. Also deserving of special thanks is N. J. Benevenga of the University of Wisconsin–Madison, for the persistent questions and training in the ways of scientific thought during my PhD work and for modeling a life devoted to research that was balanced with family, friends, and fun.

This project would never have been started were it not for the persistence of Daniel Ruth, formerly of the W. B. Saunders Company, who was convinced I should undertake the effort of developing this book. It would never have been completed were it not for the equally persistent efforts over a longer course of time of Maura Connor, former Senior Editor for the W. B. Saunders Company, and Elena Mauceri, Publishing Consultant, to set deadlines and ensure that the process kept moving forward. The support and efforts of Wynette Kommer, Freelance Copy Editor, Shelley Hampton, Production Manager, Tina Rebane, Copy Editor, Victoria Legnini, Assistant Developmental Editor, and Amelia Cullinan, former Editorial Assistant, who capably worked on various aspects of the publication process, are greatly appreciated.

My deep appreciation goes to each of the contributors to *Biochemical and Physiological Aspects of Human Nutrition* as well as to the many individuals who served as reviewers of chapters. The target was "to obtain the best" when both authors and reviewers were selected, and the text is much enriched by the contributions of so many talented researchers and teachers. The commitment of the chapter contributors to education and sharing of knowledge was clear from the willingness of these busy individuals to accept the challenge and commit the time and effort required to see their chapters through the entire process. Their willingness to respond to queries, to discuss and resolve apparent differences of opinion among authors, and to allow the editorial flexibility needed to turn individual chapters into a coherent and integrated text was superb.

During the time I worked on this book, my colleagues in the Division of Nutritional Sciences at Cornell University supported my efforts in many ways, especially by serving as sources of expertise. They were gracious in providing answers to my almost endless questions about potential contributors, interpretations of research, and accuracy of statements and wording. Special thanks go to Andre Bensadoun, J. Thomas Brenna, Patricia Cassano, Jean-Pierre Habicht, Michael Kazarinoff, Betty Lewis, Charles McCormick, Noa Noy, Robert Parker, Kathleen Rasmussen, Christina Stark, Patrick Stover, and Virginia Utermohlen, who each handled more than their share of these queries. Donald McCormick of Emory University and Malcolm Watford of Rutgers University, also provided insights on many issues related to the vitamin and metabolism chapters, respectively. Much gratitude is also due to Beth Burlew, who willingly used her computer graphic skills to generate the preliminary drawings for many of the figures. I also wish to especially acknowledge the superb efforts of Lawrence Hirschberger, Deborah Bella, Young Hye Kwon, and Jun Ohta in capably keeping my research program moving forward during the course of my work on this book; I could always count on them to display generosity and good humor in coping with the consequences of my demanding schedule.

Last, but not least, I acknowledge the love, encouragement, and support I have had from my family members, especially my husband, children, and parents, during the course of editing this book as well as over the longer course of my education and career. As always, they brought balance, perspective, and purpose, as well as joy and laughter, into my life.

Martha H. Stipanuk

Contents

◆ ◆

UNIT **II**

Digestion and Absorption of the Macronutrients

UNIT **III**

Metabolism of the Macronutrients

UNIT **V**

The Vitamins

UNIT **VI**

The Minerals

Structure and Properties of the Macronutrients

◆◆◆◆◆◆◆◆◆◆◆◆◆◆◆◆◆◆◆◆◆◆◆◆◆◆◆◆◆◆◆◆◆◆◆◆◆◆

Nutrition may be defined simply as the utilization of foods by living organisms for normal growth, reproduction, and maintenance of health. The compounds that are classed as nutrients include water, carbohydrates, proteins or amino acids, lipids, vitamins, and minerals. These nutrients make up living tissues whether they be plant, animal, or microbial tissues. Thus, these nutrients are obtained by intake of food and are then used by the human body to build and maintain its own tissues.

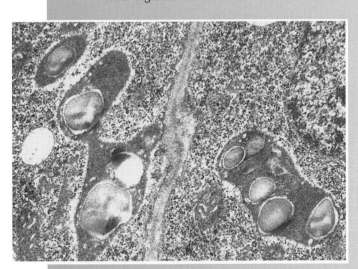

The organic macronutrients are carbon compounds synthesized by living organisms. They include carbohydrates, proteins or amino acids, and lipids. In the individual chapters in this unit on the structure and properties of the organic macronutrients, specific compounds in each class are described both from the viewpoint of dietary macronutrients and of organic compounds formed in the human body during metabolism of carbohydrates, proteins and amino acids, and lipids. The fourth group of organic nutrients, the vitamins, are micronutrients and are considered in Unit V. Organic macronutrients are required in large amounts and are sources of energy for the body.

Like all organic compounds, proteins, carbohydrates, and lipids are made up largely of six elements: hydrogen, oxygen, carbon, and nitrogen along with some phosphorus and sulfur. These six relatively small elements with atomic weights ≤ 32 make up the structure of proteins, carbohydrates, lipids, and vitamins as well as nucleic acids and intermediates of metabolism. If water (H_2O), which makes

Electron micrograph of starch granules in plant cells; courtesy of Cornell Integrated Microscopy Center, Cornell University, Ithaca, NY.

up about 63% of the human body, is not considered, carbon, oxygen, hydrogen, and nitrogen (in organic compounds) make up 88.5% of the "dry weight" of the human body; these elements are present in about 11 kg of protein, 10 kg of fat and 0.6 kg of carbohydrate (mainly glycogen) in a 65-kg adult man.

The ability of carbon to form carbon-to-carbon bonds, extended carbon chains, and cyclic compounds permits the formation of a myriad of organic compounds; the structure of a number of these are considered in this unit. In organic molecules, the atoms of carbon, hydrogen, oxygen, phosphorus, and sulfur are held together by covalent bonds, which are formed when two atoms share a pair of outer orbital electrons. Each covalent bond of every molecule represents a small amount of stored energy, allowing organic molecules to serve as a source of energy to the body. Units II, III, and IV describe the processes involved in the assimilation of dietary organic macronutrients, how these are used by the body for growth and maintenance via synthesis of the structural and functional components of the human body, and how these macronutrients are used as fuels with conversion of excess substrate to stored fuels for subsequent use.

◆ ◆

Martha H. Stipanuk

CHAPTER **1**

◆ ◆

Structure and Properties of Carbohydrates

Betty A. Lewis, Ph.D.

O U T L I N E

CLASSIFICATION, STRUCTURES, AND NOMENCLATURE OF THE MONOSACCHARIDES

Carbohydrates are the most abundant organic components in most fruits, vegetables, legumes, and cereal grains, and they provide texture and flavor in many processed foods. They are the major energy source for humans by digestion and absorption in the small intestine and, to a lesser extent, by microbial fermentation in the large intestine. Glucose is an essential energy source for humans; some types of cells such as red blood cells are not able to use other fuels. Glucose for the body's use may be derived from dietary starch, sucrose, and lactose; from glycogen stores in the body; or from synthesis in vivo from gluconeogenic precursors such as amino acid carbon skeletons. Glucose also serves as a precursor for synthesis of all other carbohydrates that are found as covalently bound constituents of glycoproteins, glycolipids, and proteoglycans in the body. These complex biomolecules are important components of body fluids, matrix tissues, membranes, and cell surfaces.

Classification

Carbohydrates are defined as polyhydroxy aldehydes (the aldoses) and ketones (the ketoses) or derivatives of these sugars. This definition emphasizes the hydrophilic nature of most carbohydrates and allows inclusion of sugar alcohols (alditols), sugar acids (uronic, aldonic, and aldaric acids), glycosides, and polymerized products (oligosaccharides and polysaccharides) among the classes of carbohydrates. The hydroxyl groups of carbohydrates may be modified by substitution with other groups to give esters and ethers or replaced to give deoxy and amino sugars. Carbohydrates are also covalently bound to many proteins and lipids. These glycoconjugates include the glycoproteins, proteoglycans, and glycolipids.

Aldoses and ketoses are monosaccharides (also called sugars). Monosaccharides are further classified by the number of carbon atoms in their structures (the trioses, tetroses, pentoses, hexoses, heptoses, octoses, and nonoses), by their stereochemistry (D or L),

and by the degree to which they may be polymerized (disaccharides, oligosaccharides, and polysaccharides). The nutritionally important glucose is a D-aldohexose monosaccharide.

Structures of the Aldoses and Ketoses

D-Aldoses are related to D-glyceraldehyde as can be illustrated by their chemical synthesis from D-glyceraldehyde (Fig. 1–1). L-Aldoses are similarly related to L-glyceraldehyde. In this synthetic scheme, a nucleophilic cyanide ion (:CN) adds to the carbonyl double bond (C-1) of glyceraldehyde, giving two cyanohydrin products. Selective reduction and hydrolysis of the CN group to an aldehyde completes the conversion of the triose D-glyceraldehyde to the pair of aldotetroses having a new chiral carbon at C-2. A chiral carbon atom is one that is bonded to four different groups. Accordingly, this reaction scheme lengthens the carbon chain from the carbonyl end, giving two new aldoses whose last three carbons derive from glyceraldehyde. Thus, the configuration of the hydroxyl on the highest numbered chiral carbon of an aldose or ketose determines D or L status. For a D-sugar, this hydroxyl is to the right of the carbon chain in the Fischer formula. Each cycle of the synthesis creates a new chiral center at carbon 2 and a pair of stereoisomers. Accordingly, there are two tetroses, four pentoses, and eight hexoses in the D- (Fig. 1–1) and also in the L-series; not all of these occur commonly in nature. L-Sugars are mirror images of the D-sugars, with the configuration of all chiral carbons reversed (e.g., D-glucose and L-glucose). Sugars that vary in their configuration at only one carbon are epimers. Thus, glucose and galactose are C-4 epimers, and enzymes that catalyze this conversion are epimerases.

In the common ketoses (Fig. 1–2), the carbonyl group is usually at carbon 2, but other ketoses occur as well. A few ketoses, such as fructose, are known by their trivial names, but others are named systematically with the suffix "-ulose" denoting a ketose sugar. In this nomenclature, a group of up to four consecutive chiral carbons is named after the aldose (triose, tetrose, pentose, or hexose) possessing this chiral group, and the number

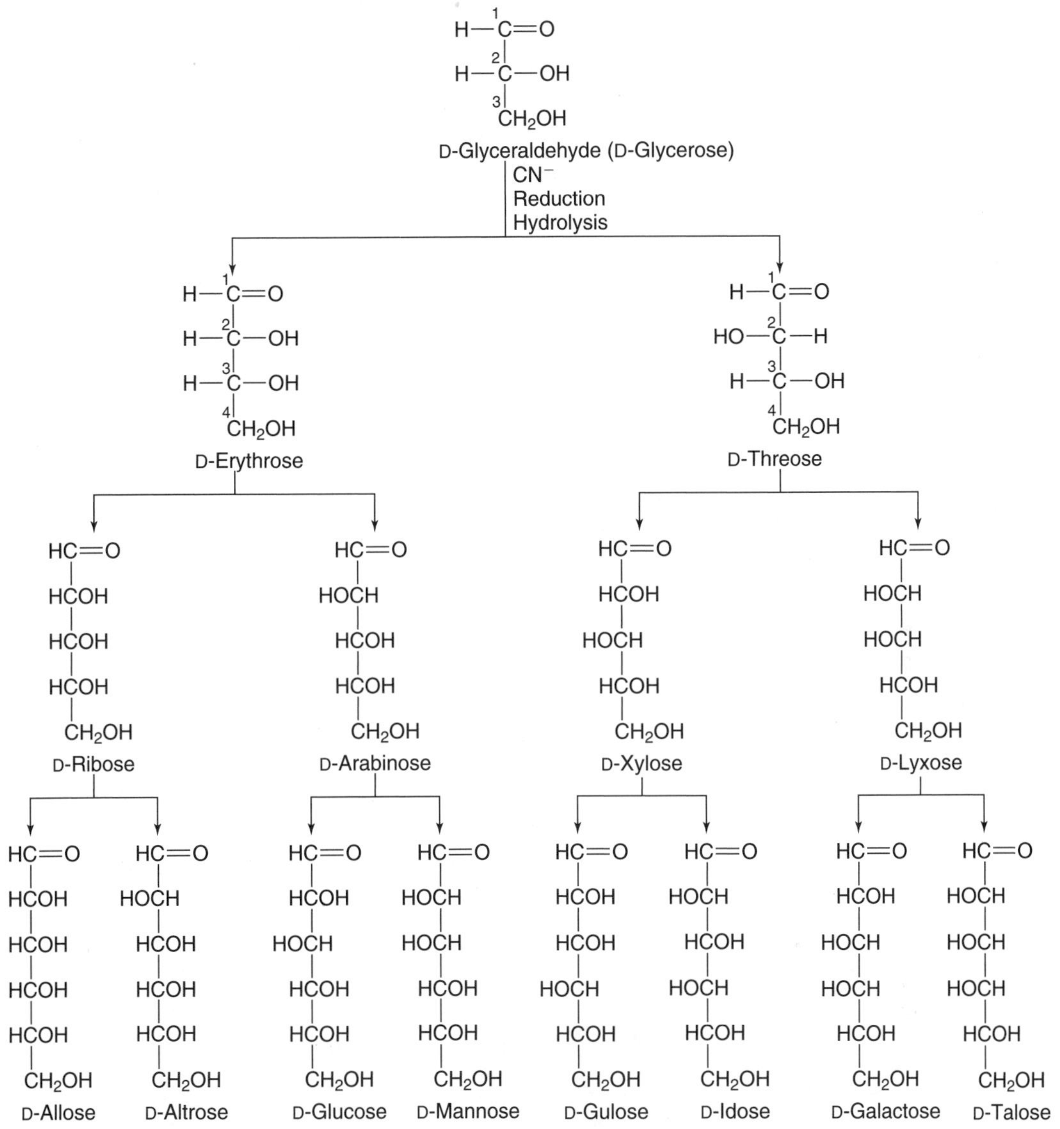

Figure 1–1. Structures of the D-aldoses (tetroses, pentoses and hexoses), showing their derivation from D-glyceraldehyde by chemical synthesis. At each application of this reaction scheme, the :CN anion adds to the carbonyl carbon, lengthening the carbon chain by one carbon and creating a new chiral center at C-2 and a new pair of isomers. Reduction and hydrolysis of the :CN group restore the aldehyde function.

of carbon atoms is designated also. D-Fructose is the most common ketose, and its systematic name is D-*arabino*-hexulose, showing that the three chiral carbons in D-fructose have the same configuration as those in D-arabinose. Frequently, the names ribulose and xylulose are used for the two ketopentoses. Their correct systematic names, however, are D-*erythro*-pentulose and D-*threo*-pentulose, respectively, showing that they have only two chiral carbons.

Although the common monosaccharides are pentoses and hexoses, sugars with more than six carbon atoms also occur naturally. Some have trivial names, but most sugars having more than six carbons and possessing four or more chiral carbons are named systematically, as described above for the ketoses. Sedoheptulose (D-*altro*-heptulose), a seven-carbon sugar, and the other ketoses shown in Figure 1–2 are involved as phosphorylated intermediates in carbohydrate metabolism. N-Acetyl-

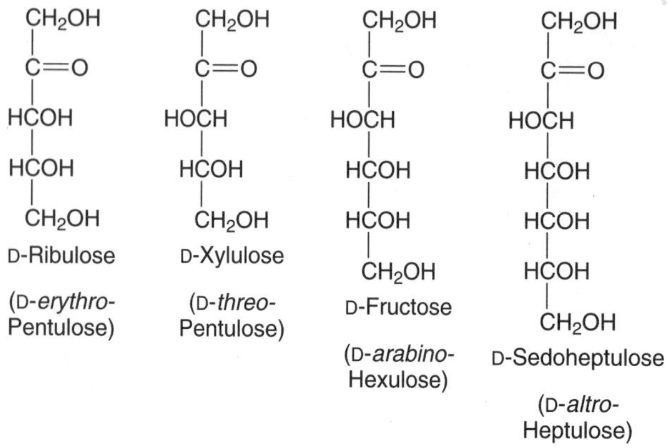

CH$_2$OH
|
C=O
|
HCOH
|
HCOH
|
CH$_2$OH

D-Ribulose

(D-*erythro*-
Pentulose)

CH$_2$OH
|
C=O
|
HOCH
|
HCOH
|
CH$_2$OH

D-Xylulose

(D-*threo*-
Pentulose)

CH$_2$OH
|
C=O
|
HOCH
|
HCOH
|
HCOH
|
CH$_2$OH

D-Fructose

(D-*arabino*-
Hexulose)

CH$_2$OH
|
C=O
|
HOCH
|
HCOH
|
HCOH
|
HCOH
|
CH$_2$OH

D-Sedoheptulose

(D-*altro*-
Heptulose)

Figure 1–2. Physiologically important ketoses and their common names. Systematic names are shown in parentheses.

neuraminic acid, a nine-carbon acidic ketose, is an important signaling epitope in glycoproteins.

The abbreviations or symbols for the sugars usually consist of the first three letters of their names (Table 1–1). Glucose (Glc) and some ketoses are exceptions to this rule.

Cyclic and Conformational Structures

Aldoses and ketoses are more stable in their five- or six-membered cyclic hemiacetal form than in acyclic form. Cyclization of an aldose

TABLE 1–1
Abbreviated Names for Some Common Carbohydrates *

Name	Abbreviation
Arabinose	Ara
Fructose	Fru
Fucose	Fuc
Galactose	Gal
Galacturonic acid	GalA
N-Acetylgalactosamine	GalNAc
Glucose	Glc
Glucuronic acid	GlcA
N-Acetylglucosamine	GlcNAc
Iduronic acid	IdoA
Mannose	Man
N-Acetylneuraminic acid	Neu5Ac
Rhamnose	Rha
Xylose	Xyl

*Abbreviations for di-, oligo-, and polysaccharides often add D- or L- to indicate the enantiomeric form, *p* or *f* to indicate the pyranose or furanose ring form, α- or β- to indicate the stereochemistry of the glycosidic linkage, and carbon numbers to indicate the carbon atoms that are *O*-linked by the glycosidic bond. The designation is often omitted for the more common D-enantiomers and *p*-ring form.

occurs via an intramolecular reaction of the nucleophilic hydroxyl group on C-4 or C-5 (C—O—) with the C-1 aldehyde (Fig. 1–3). This spontaneous reaction transforms the carbonyl carbon (C-1 of an aldose) into a chiral carbon (the anomeric carbon), giving new isomers: the α- and β-anomers of both the furanose and pyranose ring forms. The same type of cyclization reaction occurs with the ketoses in which the C-5 or C-6 hydroxyl group (C—O—) reacts with the C-2 ketose carbonyl. In the Fischer formula, the hemiacetal (anomeric) —OH of the α-anomer is on the same side of the carbon chain as the D designator oxygen (C5—O of a hexose). In aqueous solution, the acyclic and cyclic isomers are in equilibrium, with the most energetically stable isomers predominating. For most aldoses, the six-membered pyranose ring is more stable than the five-membered furanose ring. However, some sugars, including arabinose, ribose, and fructose, frequently occur in the furanose ring form in disaccharides, oligosaccharides, and polymers. The equilibrium nature of the hemiacetal reaction dictates that all hydroxyls and the carbonyl group can undergo reactions, i.e., the sugar can react in acyclic or in ring form.

Sugar ring structures are depicted in several ways, as shown for glucose and fructose (Fig. 1–4). The Fischer projection formula is based on the convention that the carbons are either in the plane of the paper or in back of the plane (never in front). The Haworth formula was introduced as a more realistic depiction of the bond lengths in the cyclic sugars. Hydroxyl groups on the right of the

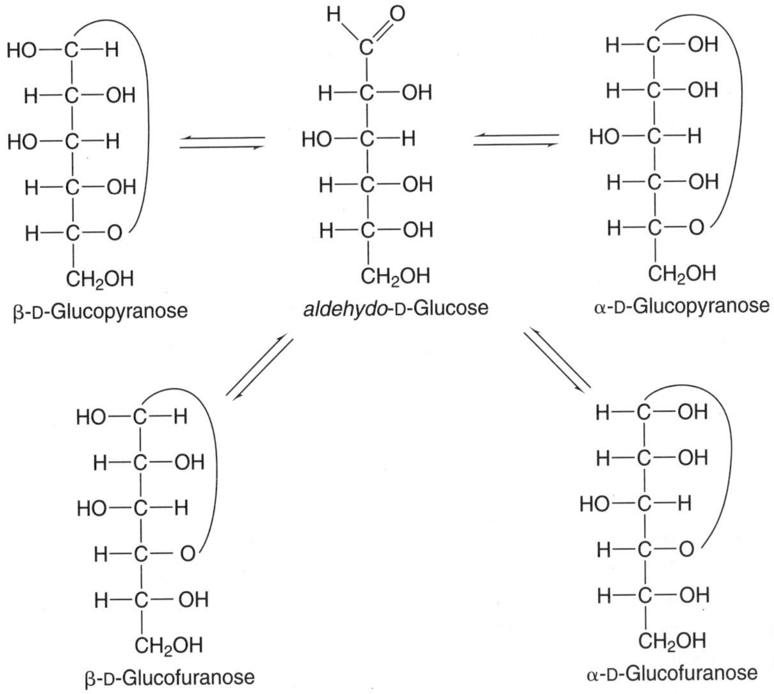

Figure 1–3. The equilibrium mixture of cyclic anomeric and acyclic forms of D-glucose in aqueous solution.

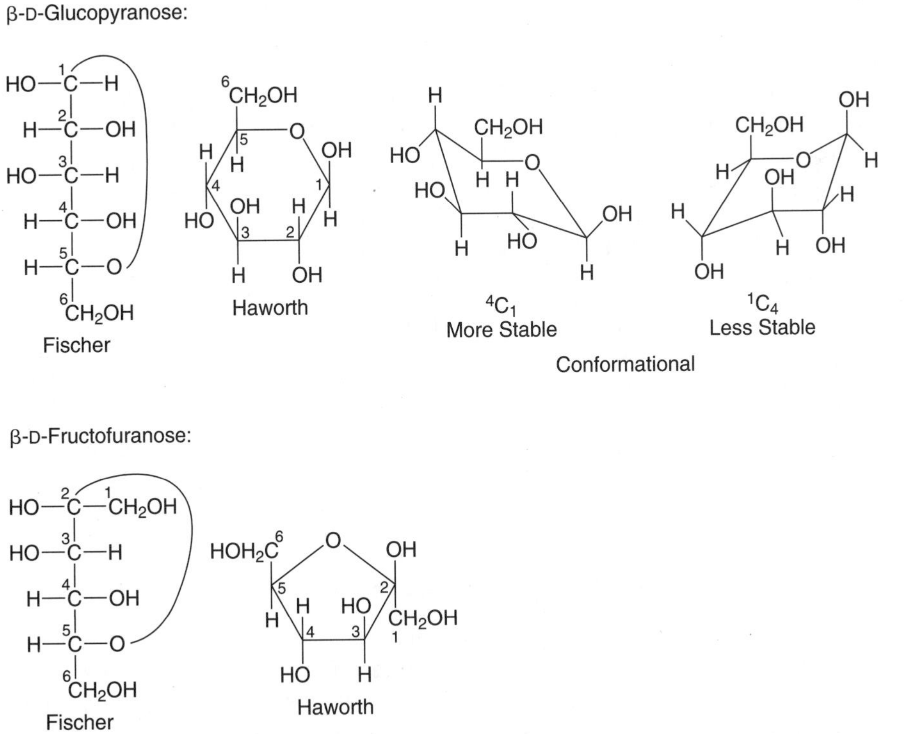

β-D-Glucopyranose:

β-D-Fructofuranose:

Figure 1–4. Representations of the cyclic structures of β-D-glucopyranose and β-D-fructofuranose. The chair conformations are designated "C" with the superscript number on the left, indicating the number of the sugar carbon that lies above the plane, and with the subscript number on the right, indicating the number of the sugar carbon that lies below the plane. The other three ring carbons and the ring oxygen lie within the plane.

carbon chain in the Fischer projection are below the plane of the ring in the Haworth formula. The exocyclic group (the —CH_2OH group of aldohexopyranoses, for example) is placed above or below the plane in the Haworth formula, depending on the origin of the ring oxygen (C-4 or C-5 for glucofuranose or pyranose, respectively, and C-5 for fructofuranose). If the ring connects from an oxygen on the right of the carbon chain in the Fischer structure, then the exocyclic group is above the plane in the Haworth structure.

Because five- and six-membered rings are not planar, the conformational formula is preferred for showing spatial relationships, such as in enzyme-catalyzed reactions where fit of substrate to enzyme binding site is important. In chair conformations, carbons 2, 3, 5, and the ring oxygen are planar, and carbons 1 and 4 are out of the plane and on opposite sides of the plane. The orientations of the hydroxyls are axial or equatorial. Pyranose sugars assume a chair conformation based in part on maximizing the number of large groups (—OH and —CH_2OH) at equatorial positions, which are less sterically hindered than are axial positions. Thus, the $^4C_1$ conformation, in which C-4 is above and C-1 is below the plane, is preferred (lower energy) for α- and β-D-glucopyranose and most of the other aldohexoses.

CHEMICAL REACTIVITY OF THE MONOSACCHARIDES

Sugars are relatively stable when pure and dry. In solution, they undergo the reactions of alcohols, aldehydes, and ketones by enzymatic and chemical catalysis.

General Reactivity of Sugars

Aldoses are reducing agents, and their carbonyl group is simultaneously oxidized to a carboxyl during the reduction. Ketoses are not good reducing agents because simultaneous oxidation of the carbonyl would require carbon chain cleavage. However, they isomerize to aldoses in an alkaline reducing test and therefore test positive. Formerly glucose in urine was analyzed by reducing sugar assay,

but more specific methods are now available. In vivo oxidation of the aldehyde group of glucose is catalyzed enzymatically by a dehydrogenase giving the lactone (an intramolecular ester of the carboxylic acid), as in the conversion of glucose 6-phosphate to 6-phosphoglucono-δ-lactone in the pentose phosphate pathway of metabolism (see Chapter 9, Fig. 9–19).

The carbonyl group of aldoses and ketoses is readily reduced to an alcohol by chemical catalysis, giving an alditol from an aldose or an epimeric pair of alditols from a ketose. These alditols, absent the carbonyl group, are more stable than the aldoses and ketoses, and they are not reducing agents. Aldehyde reductases catalyze a similar reduction in vivo—for example, in conversion of glucose to sorbitol (glucitol). The carbon proton adjacent to the carbonyl (i.e., the α-carbon proton) in aldoses is acidic and easily abstracted in basic solution, leading to epimerization of the aldoses at C-2 as well as isomerization to ketoses. Thus, glucose is epimerized to mannose and isomerized to fructose. Similar reactions occur in carbohydrate metabolism, as seen in the phosphoglucose isomerase-catalyzed conversion of glucose 6-phosphate to fructose 6-phosphate (see Chapter 9, Fig. 9–3). Similar reactions occur with ketoses. Hydroxyl groups of carbohydrates are readily converted into a variety of esters, but the phosphate esters of the monosaccharides are particularly important as intermediates in metabolism. Sugar phosphates are also components of biological polymers. This is illustrated by the nucleic acids that have ribose and 2-deoxyribose phosphates as key constituents. Other derivatives of hydroxyls, including ethers, are also important in modification of monosaccharides in living systems and contribute to the diversity of carbohydrate structure.

Formation of Glycosidic Linkages

Sugars react intermolecularly with alcohols under appropriate catalysis, forming α- and β-glycosides as shown in Figure 1–5 for the acid-catalyzed synthesis of methyl α-D-glucopyranoside. The alcohol may be aliphatic, aromatic, or another sugar. When properly activated, sugars react with each other to form specific

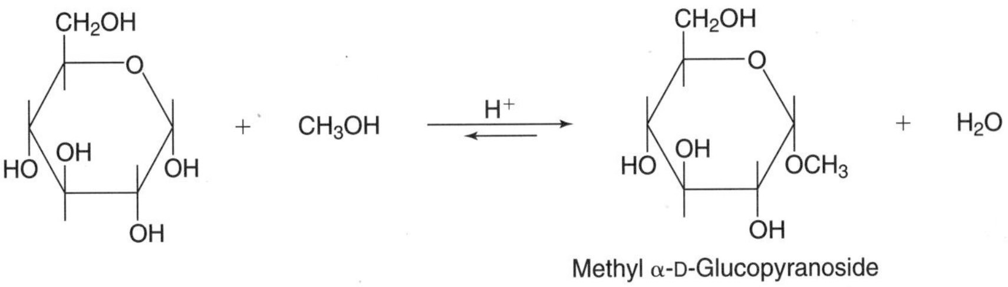

Figure 1–5. *Reactions of sugars with alcohols. Acid-catalyzed synthesis of the glycoside methyl α-D-glucopyranoside. This reaction is reversible. The glycosidic bond is hydrolyzed by cleavage between the anomeric carbon of the glucosyl group and the oxygen of the bond.*

oligosaccharides and polysaccharides. Thus, the sugar units in oligosaccharides and polysaccharides are linked by *O*-glycosidic bonds. Sugars also react with amines or thiols to give *N*- or *S*-glycosides, respectively. Thus, β-D-ribose and 2-deoxy-β-D-ribose in nucleic acids are bonded to purines and pyrimidines by *N*-glycosidic bonds. In uridine diphosphate (UDP)-glucose, the β-D-ribose is linked to uracil by an *N*-glycosidic bond, and the α-D-glucose and β-D-ribose units are each ester-linked to phosphate, as shown in Figure 1–6. The sugar nucleotides are used extensively in vivo for enzymatic synthesis of carbohydrates, including lactose and glycogen. In glycoproteins, the oligosaccharide chains are linked to the β-carboxamide nitrogen of asparagine (an *N*-glycosidic bond) or to the hydroxyl of serine/threonine (an *O*-glycosidic bond). Plants use the glycosidic bond extensively in synthesizing different glycosides, many of

which are physiologically active. Various hydroxylated compounds are glycosylated in the liver and excreted as glucuronic acid glycosides (β-D-glucuronides), which is a major means of detoxification and excretion.

Glycosides are more stable than aldoses and ketoses in several respects. The carbonyl/hemiacetal carbon is protected from base-catalyzed reactions and from reduction and oxidation. The pyranose and furanose ring structures and the anomeric configuration are also stabilized and do not undergo the interconversions shown in Figure 1–3. However, the glycosidic bonds can be hydrolyzed by acid or enzyme catalysis releasing the free sugar and alcohol. Glycosidases, which catalyze hydrolysis of glycosides, have high specificity for the sugar and the anomeric linkage (α or β) but lower specificity for the alcohol unit (the aglycone).

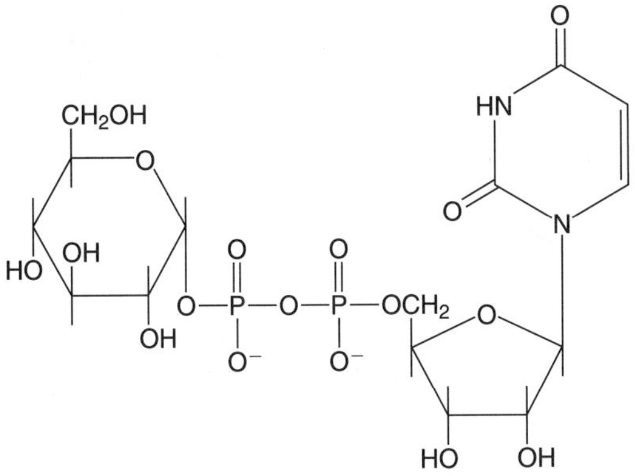

The Maillard Reaction of Reducing Sugars with Amines

Aldoses and ketoses react with aliphatic primary and secondary amines (including amino acids and proteins) to form *N*-glycosides, which readily dehydrate to the respective Schiff base by the Maillard reaction, as shown in Figure 1–7 (reactions i and ii). The aldose Schiff base spontaneously undergoes an Amadori rearrangement at C-1 and C-2, giving a substituted 1-amino-1-deoxyketose (reaction iii); a ketose Schiff base will rearrange to a substituted 2-amino-2-deoxyaldose. These sugar amines undergo additional very complex reactions, leading to highly reactive dicarbonyls (such as 3-deoxy-D-glucosone), cross-linking of proteins (as in reaction iv), fluorescent compounds and brown pig-

Figure 1–6. *The structure of uridine diphosphate (UDP)-glucose (UDPG), an activated form of glucose and an intermediate in the synthesis of glycogen in vivo. In this structure, β-D-ribose is linked to the amine uracil by an N-glycosidic bond, and the α-D-glucose unit is esterified to phosphate.*

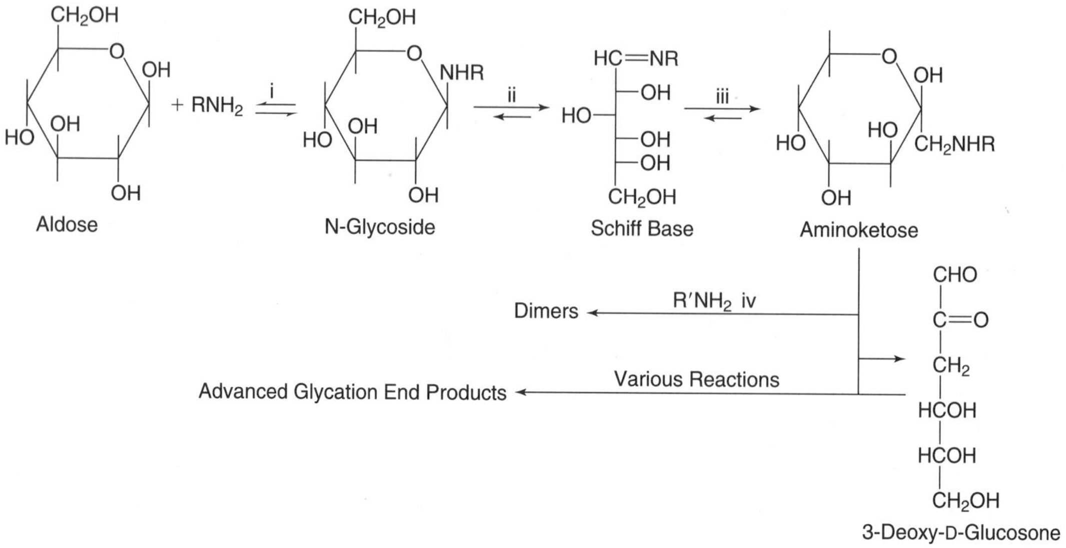

Figure 1–7. *Initiation of the Maillard reaction of amines with aldoses. The aminoketose undergoes various reactions, including conversion to a highly reactive dicarbonyl compound (3-deoxy-D-glucosone). When the amino group is from a protein, the reaction may result in cross-linked proteins.*

ments, and to low molecular weight compounds, some of which are useful flavoring agents. The Maillard and subsequent reactions occur in food systems such as powdered or evaporated milk during processing or storage, giving off-white colors and decreasing the nutritive value of the proteins. Loss of lysine accounts for only part of the decrease in nutritive value. Although the Maillard complex of reactions has been extensively studied, the reactions are understood only in part. Realization that these reactions occur under physiological conditions in vivo has come more recently, and this is now an active area of research (Baynes and Monnier, 1989; Brownlee, 1995). The reaction of glucose with hemoglobin was discovered first. Plasma glucose reacts with hemoglobins via the Maillard reaction, and the modified protein, detected by gel electrophoresis, is an indicator of plasma glucose levels in diabetics over the life span of the erythrocytes. The term *glycated* protein is used to distinguish these Maillard-derived, carbohydrate-modified proteins from true *glycosylated* proteins (glycoproteins).

OTHER CLASSES OF CARBOHYDRATES

Monosaccharides or monosaccharide residues may be modified or derived in several ways. Carbonyl groups can be reduced or oxidized, and terminal —CH_2OH groups can be oxidized. Hydroxyl groups on any of the carbons are subject to various modifications.

Alditols

The alditols (polyols) (Fig. 1–8), which occur naturally in plants and other organisms, are reduction products of aldoses and ketoses in which the carbonyl has been reduced to an alcohol. Reduction of ketoses, however, gives an epimeric pair of alditols unless the reaction is enzyme catalyzed and therefore stereospecific. The alditols, like the sugars, are soluble in water and vary in degree of sweetness. Xylitol, the sweetest, approaches the sweet-

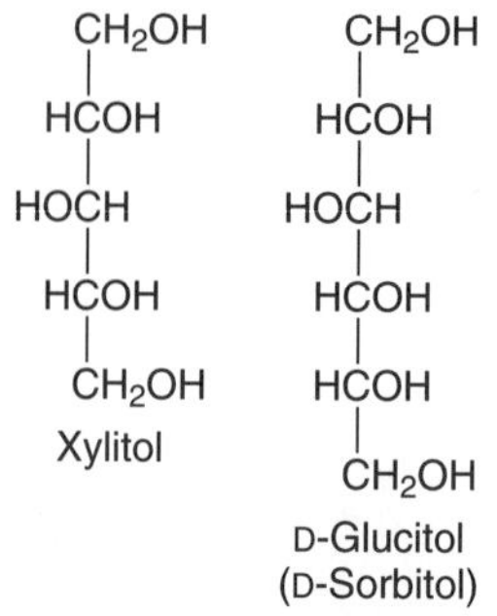

Figure 1–8. *Structures of the common sugar alcohols (alditols) xylitol and D-glucitol.*

CLINICAL CORRELATION

Sugar-Protein Reactions in Diabetes and Aging

The Maillard/Amadori reactions of sugars with amino acids and proteins lead to a cascade of reactions. Products of these reactions are referred to as advanced glycation end products. These reaction end products have been observed in collagen-rich tissues in vivo and in vitro, and they are associated with stiffening of artery walls, lung tissue, and joints and with other aging symptoms. Considerable evidence links hyperglycemia with increased formation of these end products; these products accumulate in the blood vessel wall proteins and may contribute to vascular complications of diabetes. Glycation of lens proteins increases somewhat with aging, but it is accelerated in diabetes. Incubation of lens proteins with glucose or glucose 6-phosphate in vitro results in changes in the lens proteins that mimic most of those observed with age- and cataract-related changes in the lens. Drug-induced inhibition of the reactions leading to these end products in diabetic animals prevented various diabetes-inducible pathologies of arteries, kidneys, nerves, and retina.

---

ness of sucrose. Because the alditols do not have a carbonyl group, they are considerably less reactive than the sugars. They do not undergo base-catalyzed reactions of epimerization and isomerization, the formation of glycosides (unless they are participating as the "alcohol"), or the Maillard reaction. Alditols share the same hydrophilic character as the sugars and are used in products as humectants to prevent excessive drying. D-Glucitol (D-sorbitol) and xylitol are not readily metabolized by oral bacteria and are used in chewing gums and candies for this noncariogenic characteristic. Both D-glucitol and xylitol are passively absorbed in the small intestine and metabolized in the liver. Excessive amounts of alditols passing into the colon may induce diarrhea owing to osmotic action. (Note that xylitol, although it has three chiral carbons, is a symmetrical molecule and does not possess optical activity.)

Glycuronic, Glyconic, and Glycaric Acids

The uronic acids are weak sugar acids that have a carboxyl group (—COOH) instead of the terminal —CH$_2$OH (Fig. 1–9). D-Glucuronic acid is an important constituent of glycosaminoglycans in mammalian systems, and its C-5 epimer, L-iduronic acid, is present to a lesser extent. Glucuronic acid (and its 4-O-methyl ether), D-galacturonic acid, D-mannuronic acid, and the less common L-guluronic

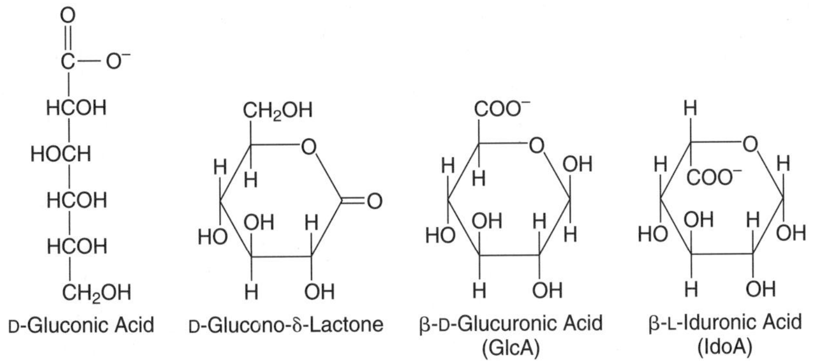

Figure 1–9. *Carboxylic acid derivatives of D-glucose and L-idose. D-Gluconic acid is shown along with its 1,5-lactone, an intramolecular ester. D-Glucuronic and L-iduronic acids are shown as their β anomers; uronic acids are important constituents of glycosaminoglycans. The acids are shown in their anionic forms (gluconate, glucuronate, and iduronate).*

acid are constituents of the nondigestible polysaccharides of plants and algae, which contribute to dietary fiber. Glycaric acids are dicarboxylic acids in which both terminal groups of the aldose have been oxidized to carboxyls. They are much less common than the glycuronic acids. Glyconic acids are oxidation products of the aldoses in which C-1 has been oxidized to a carboxyl group. Glyconic acids lactonize easily to the neutral cyclic lactones.

Deoxy and Amino Sugars

Several common sugars lack the complete complement of hydroxyl groups; examples of these are shown in Figure 1–10. Deoxy sugars, in which a hydroxyl group is replaced by a hydrogen, include 2-deoxy-D-ribose, L-fucose (6-deoxy-L-galactose), and L-rhamnose (6-deoxy-L-mannose). L-Fucose is a constituent of many glycoproteins and serves as a signaling epitope for physiological events—for example, in the inflammatory response. The presence of fucose in crucial oligosaccharides of cell surface glycoproteins is required for recruitment of leukocytes to sites of inflammation and injury. L-Rhamnose occurs in plant polysaccharides, and 2-deoxy-D-ribose is the sugar constituent of deoxynucleic acids.

In the common amino sugars, the C-2 hydroxyl group is replaced by an amino group. These common amino sugars are D-glucosamine (2-amino-2-deoxy-D-glucose) and D-galactosamine (2-amino-2-deoxy-D-galactose), which usually occur as the N-acetyl derivatives (N-acetyl-D-glucosamine and N-acetyl-D-galactosamine). They are constituents of glycosaminoglycans and of many glycoproteins. Glycoproteins may also contain the sialic acids, which are N-acyl derivatives of neuraminic acid, a unique nine-carbon amino deoxy keto sugar acid. Although the amino group of neuraminic acid is frequently acetylated in sialic acids, other acyl groups may be present in sialic acids. N-Acetylneuraminic acid is also an important biological signaling epitope of glycoproteins. One role it seems to play is protection of circulating plasma proteins from degradation by proteases. Chemically, neuraminic acid is very sensitive to acid degradation, and its glycosidic linkage in glycoproteins and gangliosides is very easily hydrolyzed.

DISACCHARIDES AND OLIGOSACCHARIDES AND THEIR PROPERTIES

Oligosaccharides are composed of monosaccharides covalently linked by glycosidic bonds. They are either reducing or nonreducing. An oligosaccharide terminating with a residue that has an unsubstituted anomeric —OH is reducing. Reducing oligosaccharides undergo all the chemical reactions of the aldose sugars, including reduction, oxidation,

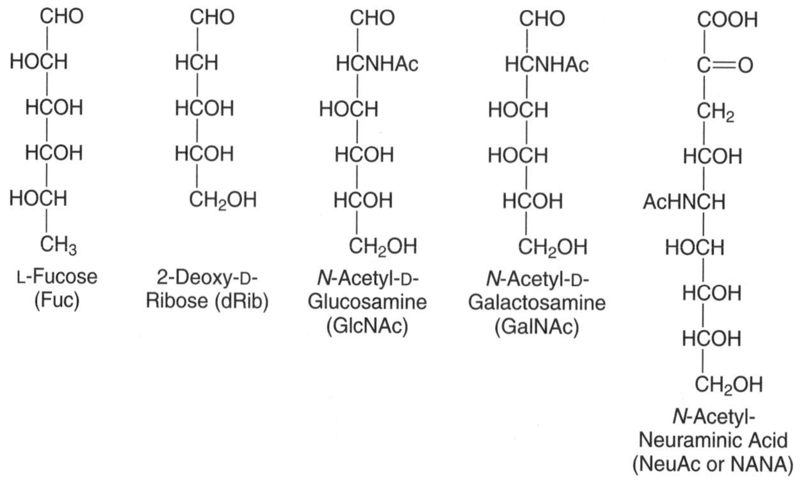

Figure 1–10. *Examples of deoxy and amino sugars that are constituents of important biological compounds such as DNA, glycoproteins, and glycoconjugates.*

and base-catalyzed epimerization and isomerization at their reducing end. Oligosaccharides are readily hydrolyzed to their constituent sugars by acid or enzyme catalysis, with the enzymes showing strong specificity for the sugar units and their anomeric linkage. As a result of this specificity, humans digest primarily two types of oligosaccharides: those containing α-D-glucose or β-D-galactose at the nonreducing end. The structures of the three major dietary disaccharides (sucrose, lactose, and maltose) are shown in Figure 1–11.

Sucrose (table sugar), a nonreducing disaccharide, is composed of α-D-glucopyranosyl and β-D-fructofuranosyl units covalently linked through the anomeric carbon of each sugar unit to form α-D-glucopyranosyl-(1→2)-β-D-fructofuranoside. Sucrose is widely distributed in plants and produced commercially from sugar cane and sugar beets. It is easily hydrolyzed to glucose and fructose in acid solution and rapidly digested by sucrase, an α-glucosidase of the intestinal villi. Sucrose is the major caloric sweetener for commercial or home use.

Lactose (β-D-galactopyranosyl-(1→4)-D-glucopyranose, milk sugar) is synthesized in the mammary glands of mammals. The concentration in milk varies with species and constitutes about 4 g/100 mL of bovine milk compared with 6.4 g/100 mL of human milk (Newburg and Neubauer, 1995). Lactose has about one third the sweetness of sucrose. It is readily digested to glucose and galactose by a β-galactosidase (lactase) of the intestinal villi. Lactose is a reducing disaccharide and therefore susceptible to reactions of the glucose carbonyl group, including the Maillard reaction. Alkaline isomerization of lactose gives lactulose, in which the glucose unit has been isomerized to fructose. This isomerization also occurs to some extent during heating of milk. Lactulose is not digested or absorbed in the body, and it appears to promote growth of *Bifidobacterium* and *Lactobacillus* species in the colon. Colonization by these bacteria is effective in preventing acute diarrhea. Production of short-chain fatty acids from the lactulose and dietary fiber polysaccharides leads to a decrease in colonic pH and limits potential growth of pathogenic bacteria. Lactulose is also used as a therapeutic agent in the treatment of hepatic encephalopathy.

Only small amounts of maltose (α-D-glu-

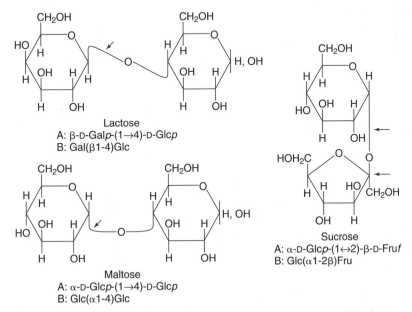

Figure 1–11. *Reducing (lactose and maltose) and nonreducing (sucrose) disaccharides. The free anomeric —OH of the glucosyl unit of lactose and of maltose indicates the reducing nature of these disaccharides. In sucrose, both anomeric carbons are involved in the glycosidic bond, and sucrose is nonreducing. The small arrows point to the glycosidic bonds. Two abbreviated structural notations are shown for these disaccharides. Notation A defines the complete structure, whereas B assumes the more common ring form and D-configuration for each sugar unit.*

NUTRITION INSIGHT

Nutritional Consequences of Sucrose Polyester Fat Replacer

The low cost and purity of sucrose make it an appealing starting material for chemical modification into other useful products, such as the fat replacer sucrose polyester. Although the trivial name implies a polymer, olestra is only a modified disaccharide. Sucrose polyester (olestra, Olean) is a mixture of the hexa-, hepta-, and octa-esters of sucrose obtained by esterification with natural long-chain fatty acids. Esterification of at least six of the eight hydroxyls of sucrose renders it stable to lipase action, and therefore it is not digested and not absorbed. The water-insoluble hydrophobic character of olestra gives it oily laxative properties, a potential problem if it is consumed in excessive amounts. Olestra is excreted intact without any metabolism by the colonic microflora.

A small fraction of dietary fat-soluble vitamins (A, D, E, and K) is excreted along with the olestra because of mutual solubility. Supplemental vitamins are recommended when this is a concern. The more water-soluble vitamins are not partitioned into the olestra and are not lost. Several types of beneficial phytochemicals have been evaluated also, but only members of the lipophilic phytosterols and carotenoids show losses via excretion with olestra. Olestra showed no toxicity in human and animal studies. Because olestra has organoleptic and functional properties similar to those of natural fats and oils as well as good heat stability, it offers advantages over other fat replacers for certain foods.

copyranosyl-(1→4)-D-glucopyranose) are consumed as such in the diet. Maltose occurs naturally in the seeds of starch-producing plants, and small amounts are used in processed foods. Isomaltose (α-D-glucopyranosyl-(1→6)-D-glucopyranose) probably does not occur naturally. Both maltose and isomaltose are formed by acidic hydrolysis of starch; isomaltose results from the structural branch points of amylopectin. α,α-Trehalose (α-D-glucopyranosyl-(1↔1)-α-D-glucopyranoside) is a nonreducing disaccharide found in fungi (particularly in young mushrooms), yeasts, and insects.

These three α-linked glucose disaccharides are readily digested by intestinal α-glucosidases (glucoamylase, sucrase/α-dextrinase, and trehalase). Digestion of starch by α-amylases in the lumen of the gastrointestinal tract yields maltose, maltotriose, and α-dextrins containing the isomaltose moiety; glucoamylase and sucrase/α-dextrinase also complete the digestion of these products. It is curious that trehalase has persisted in the brush border of the human small intestine, because trehalose is a rather insignificant dietary disaccharide. Digestion of carbohydrates is discussed in detail in Chapter 5.

Raffinose and stachyose are oligosaccha-rides carrying an α-D-galactopyranosyl and an α-D-galactopyranosyl-(1↔6)-α-D-galactopyranosyl unit, respectively, attached to C-6 of the glucose unit of sucrose. They occur in relatively large amounts in soybeans, lentils, and other legume seeds. Because humans do not have a digestive α-galactosidase, these oligosaccharides pass into the lower gut to be metabolized by the anaerobic bacteria. Excessive flatulence may result from fermentation of these oligosaccharides, as well as of pectic polysaccharides.

POLYSACCHARIDES OF NUTRITIONAL IMPORTANCE

Polysaccharides are polymers composed of sugars linked by glycosidic bonds and varying in size from about 20 to over 10^7 sugar units (degree of polymerization). Because of the multiple hydroxyl groups in monosaccharides, which serve as linkage sites for glycosidic bonds, there is opportunity for great structural diversity in polysaccharides. The structural diversity includes molecular size, kinds and proportions of sugars, ring size (furanose or pyranose), anomeric configuration (α or β), and linkage site of the glycosidic bonds, as well as the sequence of sugars and linkages and the presence of noncarbohydrate components.

General Characteristics

Polysaccharides may be linear or branched, and branched polysaccharides exhibit various branching modes that range from branches consisting of a single sugar unit to longer branches carrying other branches, as illustrated in Figure 1–12. In heteropolysaccharides composed of more than one kind of sugar, the sugar units may be linked in alternating sequence or in blocks of various length in which one sugar repeats itself. The physical properties of polysaccharides depend highly on their chemical and conformational structures. In general, polysaccharides that are highly branched are water soluble, whereas linear polysaccharides tend to be insoluble. However, linear polysaccharides possessing structural irregularities that hinder intermolecular hydrogen bonding may be soluble and give viscous solutions. Hyaluronic acid, a linear polysaccharide with two different sugars in alternating sequence, shows this mucilaginous characteristic. In contrast, glycogen, which is highly branched and very soluble, gives relatively nonviscous solutions. Many different polysaccharide structures are represented in the plant kingdom, whereas only a few have been identified in vertebrates. Bacteria synthesize many unusual sugars, which greatly increases the diversity of their polysaccharide antigens.

Polysaccharides are designated either by a trivial name, such as starch and glycogen, or by a systematic name constructed from the constituent sugar names and the suffix "an." Thus, $(1{\rightarrow}4)$-β-D-glucan is the systematic name for cellulose.

Digestible Polysaccharides

Starch and glycogen are digestible polysaccharides of glucose. Starch is found in plant cells, in both linear and branched forms. Glycogen has a highly branched structure and is found in animal tissues, particularly muscle and liver.

Starch. Starch is one of the most abundant polysaccharides in plants, where it is stored in the seeds, tubers, roots, and some fruits. It is composed of two families of polymers, a mostly linear amylose [$(1{\rightarrow}4)$-α-D-glucan] and the branched amylopectin [$(1{\rightarrow}4)$-α-D-glucan with branches linked to C-6]. Starches from different sources vary in structure, but typically amylopectin has an average chain length between branch points of 20 to 25 glucose units. Typical starches contain 20% to 30% amylose and 70% to 80% amylopectin; however, high amylopectin (waxy corn, 98% amylopectin) and high amylose starches are also available. Starches for food processing are produced from many sources. The most important sources are corn (regular, waxy, and high amylose), potato, rice, tapioca, and wheat. The physical properties and, to some extent, the digestibility of the starches vary with their fine structure and reflect their source.

Amylose and amylopectin molecules are laid down during biosynthesis in highly organized particles called granules. The hydrogen-

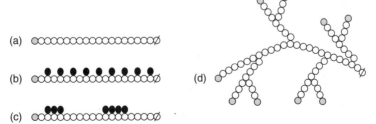

Figure 1–12. *A cartoon illustrating branching structures of polysaccharides. (a) Linear polysaccharide. Circles represent sugar units linked by glycosidic bonds. (b) Alternating branches consisting of a single sugar unit, ●; (c) blocks of consecutive single sugar unit branches, ●; (d) ramified structure (branches on branches). Nonreducing end, ●; reducing end, ∅; one sugar of a sequence of sugar units, ○.*

bonded structure of the starch components renders the granules insoluble in water below about 55°C. Above this temperature the granule imbibes water, swells, and eventually undergoes fragmentation, releasing the amylopectin and amylose. The swollen granules are responsible for the high viscosity of partially gelatinized starch dispersions. Pure amylose and amylopectin have limited solubility in water, and there is a tendency for the amylose chains, and to a lesser extent the amylopectin branches, to aggregate through hydrogen bonding and become insoluble in cold water. This can occur in processed foods, causing resistance to α-amylase digestion.

Hydrated (gelatinized) starch is readily hydrolyzed by the various amylases, whereas the native starch granule is more resistant to enzymatic digestion. Gelatinized starch is hydrolyzed to glucose in the gastrointestinal tract by the combined action of salivary and pancreatic α-amylase and the intestinal mucosal α-glucosidases (glucoamylase, sucrase/

α-dextrinase). The α-amylases, which cleave the (α1→4)-linkages only, catalyze hydrolysis of starch to maltose, maltotriose, and maltotetraose and to oligosaccharides called α-limit dextrins, composed of a minimum of four glucose units and including an (α1→6)-linked branch point. These disaccharides and oligosaccharides are then converted to glucose by the α-glucosidases. Figure 1–13 shows a fragment of the amylopectin structure and the (1→4)- and (1→6)-α-glucosidic linkages that can be hydrolyzed by human digestive enzymes. The human upper digestive tract does not possess an endogenous (1→4)-β-D-glucanase, and therefore cellulose, with its β-linkage, is not digestible.

Glycogen. Glycogen, like starch amylopectin, is a (1→4)-α-D-glucan with branches on branches that are (α1→6)-linked. The average length of the (1→4)-linked chain between branch points is 10 to 14 glucose units. Because of this increased branching compared

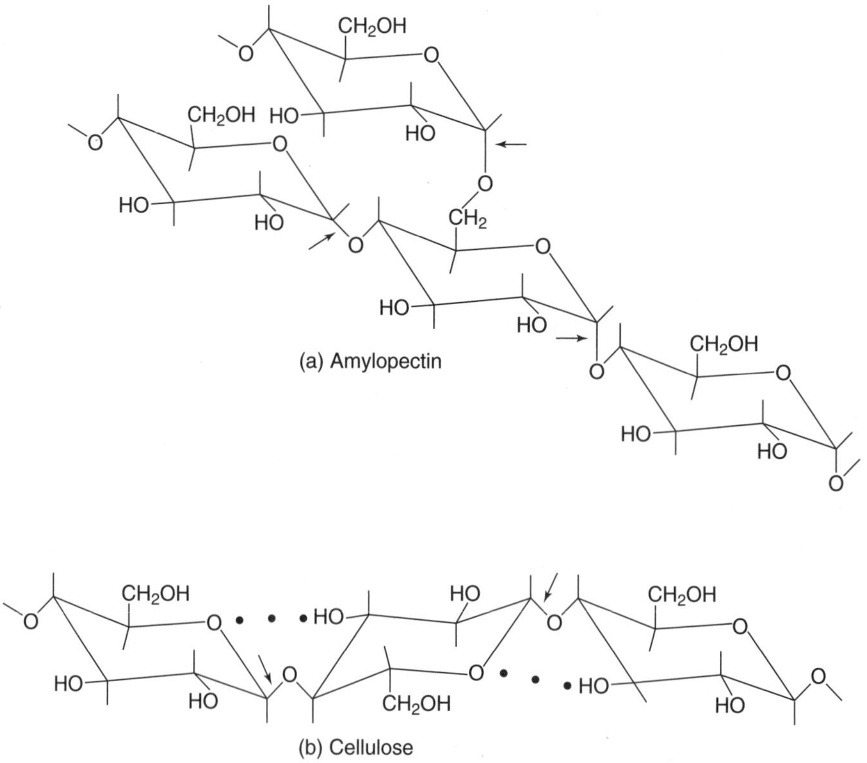

(a) Amylopectin

(b) Cellulose

Figure 1–13. (a) A segment of starch amylopectin structure showing the α-D-glucosidic bonds and the branch points. Glycogen has a similar structure. (b) The conformational structure of cellulose shows that alternate β-D-glucosyl units are flipped 180°, giving a flat, ribbon-like structure stabilized by hydrogen bonds (● ● ●). The glucosidic bonds are indicated by the small arrows.

with amylopectin, glycogen is readily soluble in cold water and gives solutions of relatively low viscosity, which facilitate its use as a readily available endogenous energy source. The branching pattern interferes with intra- and intermolecular hydrogen bonding of the glycogen chains, thus permitting rapid solvation and easy access to the enzymes. A low viscosity facilitates diffusion of the substrate to the enzymes and diffusion of the products away from the active sites of the enzymes.

Glycogen is present in most animal tissues, with the highest content in liver and skeletal muscle. It may constitute up to 10% (wet weight) of the human liver. Mammalian tissue levels of glycogen are highly variable and affected by factors such as nutritional status and time of day. Glycogen has a high molecular mass, in the range of 10^6 to 10^9 Da.

By electron microscopy, glycogen appears as uniform spherical particles and higher molecular weight aggregates of these particles (β and α particles, respectively). The α-particles are composed of a few β-particle carbohydrate chains covalently linked to protein, which is aggregated by disulfide linkages.

Nondigestible Plant Polysaccharides

Polysaccharides represent the major components of plant cell walls and interstitial spaces.

Plants also synthesize storage polysaccharides other than starch, including galactomannans, the $(1\rightarrow3)(1\rightarrow4)$-$\beta$-D-glucans of cereal grains, and the fructans of grasses and some tubers. All of these nonstarch polysaccharides as well as those added during food processing constitute dietary fiber (Table 1–2).

Cellulose is a linear $(1\rightarrow4)$-β-D-glucan with a flat, ribbon-like conformation in which alternate glucose units are flipped 180°, and hydrogen bonded intramolecularly (Fig. 1–13). These ribbon-like chains are aligned in parallel arrays called microfibrils in which the chains are strongly hydrogen bonded to each other. The microfibrils are similarly packed together into strong fibers, which are very insoluble and which provide rigidity to the plant cell wall. Associated with cellulose in the cell wall are several other insoluble polysaccharides, the hemicelluloses. These include the xyloglucans, which have a cellulose-like backbone with α-D-xylose units linked to C-6 of the glucosyl unit, and arabinoxylans, in which the $(1\rightarrow4)$-β-D-xylan chain has α-L-arabinofuranose and D-glucuronic acid branches at C-2 or C-3.

Pectic polysaccharides [$(1\rightarrow4)$-α-D-galacturonan with occasional α-L-rhamnose units] and other associated polysaccharides (galactans and arabinans) are present in the cell

---

TABLE 1–2
Nondigestible Food Polysaccharides of Plant, Algal, and Bacterial Origin

Polysaccharide	Main Chain or Repeat Unit*	Branches, Other Substituents*
Plants		
Cellulose	-Glc(β1–4)Glc-	none
Arabinoxylan	-Xyl(β1–4)Xyl-	L-Ara$f$(α1–2 or 1–3)-
Xyloglucan	-Glc(β1–4)Glc-	Xyl(α1–6)-β-Gal-; α-L-Ara$f$ or α-L-Fuc linked to Xyl
Pectin	-[GalA(α1–4)]$_n$GalA(α1–2)L-Rha(α1–4)-	Gal- and L-Ara$f$-; methyl ester of GalA
Cereal β-glucan	-[Glc(β1–4)]$_n$Glc(β1–3)-	none
Galactomannan	-Man(β1–4)Man-	Gal(α1–6)-
Arabinogalactan	-Gal(β1–4)Gal-	L-Ara$f$(α1–5)L-Ara$f$-
Algae		
Alginic acid	-[ManA(β1–4)]$_n$[L-GulA(α1–4)]$_n$-	none
Carrageenan	-[Gal(β1–4)3,6-anhydroGal(α1–3)]-	-SO$_3^-$ at C–4, C–2†
Bacteria		
Xanthan gum	-Glc(β1–4)Glc‡	4,6-Pyr-Man(β1–4)GlcA(β1–2)Man(α1–3)-
		Pyr = pyruvic acid CH$_3$CCOO$^-$ at C-4 and C-6 of Man /\\

*Sugars are D in pyranose form unless indicated otherwise.
†The substituent group replaces the proton of the —OH of a sugar unit in the main chain.
‡Alternating glucose units are substituted at C-3 by the trisaccharide branch. The nonreducing terminal Man carries a pyruvic acid substituent, and the other Man is substituted at C-6 by an acetyl group.

walls of immature plant tissues and in the interstitial spaces. Native pectic galacturonan in the plant tissue is relatively insoluble, but isolated commercial pectin is soluble in hot water. Calcium ions form complexes with the galacturonic acid units of pectin, cross-linking the chains into a gel network. This is thought to account partially for the insolubility of native pectin in the plant tissue. The calcium-pectin complex is also the basis for dietary low-sugar, low-calorie fruit jams and jellies, whereas jellies prepared without calcium require a high sugar content to form a gel structure. More comprehensive descriptions of the structures and properties of the polysaccharides constituting dietary fiber, and their organization in the plant tissue, are provided in the reviews by Carpita (1990) and Selvendran (1984).

Natural and Modified Polysaccharides for Use in Processed Foods

Several natural polysaccharides are used in processed foods for their functional properties. These natural polysaccharides include starches from several sources, guar and locust bean galactomannans, alginic acid and carrageenan from seaweed, and xanthan gum. Polysaccharides are also modified physically and chemically to enhance their functionality (Table 1–3). Starch and cellulose are alkylated or esterified to convert a very small proportion of the hydroxyls into ethers or esters for increased solubility. Starches are also subjected to partial acid or enzymatic hydrolysis,

resulting in starch dextrins and maltodextrins with improved solubility. Starch dextrins also are produced by a process that promotes alteration of the structure, including new linkages, increased branching, and some decrease in size. Maltodextrins are much smaller, in the oligosaccharide range, but without other structural alterations. For most modified starch products the enhanced solubility should lead to faster digestion by α-amylases. The high-amylose starches are an exception, because they tend to be more crystalline and less readily digested. In general, the modified starches are digestible and caloric, whereas the other polysaccharides added to foods contribute to dietary fiber.

GLYCOCONJUGATES OF PHYSIOLOGICAL INTEREST

Conjugates of sugars and oligosaccharides play essential physiological roles. These glycoconjugates include the glycosaminoglycans and proteoglycans, the glycoproteins, and the glycolipids.

Glycosaminoglycans

Glycosaminoglycans (Table 1–4) are linear polysaccharides that have a disaccharide repeat unit composed of a hexosamine and a uronic acid. They are constituents of the extracellular spaces of mammalian tissues and vary in molecular weight and in fine structure. Many are sulfated and thus more highly

TABLE 1–3
Modified Polysaccharides Added to Processed Foods

Polysaccharide	Modifying Group or Treatment*	Product
Starch	$-COCH_3$	Starch acetate (ester)
	$-CH_2CHOHCH_3$	Hydroxypropyl starch (ether)
	$-PO_2^-$	Phosphate cross-linked starch (diester)
	Acid, heat	Dextrins
	Water, heat	Cold-water-soluble starch
Cellulose	$-CH_2COOH$	Carboxymethylcellulose (CMC)
	$-CH_2CHOHCH_3$	Hydroxypropylcellulose
	$-CH_3$	Methylcellulose
	Acid, heat	Microcrystalline cellulose

*The modifying group replaces the proton of one of the three free hydroxyls of the glucose units at a degree of substitution usually less than 1 per 10 glucose units.

TABLE 1–4

Structural Repeating Units of the Glycosaminoglycans, Showing Sulfation Patterns and Structural Variation *

Glycosaminoglycan	Repeat Unit†
Hyaluronan	$[\text{-GlcNAc}(\beta1\text{–}4)\text{GlcA}(\beta1\text{–}3)\text{-}]_n$
Chondroitin 4-sulfate and 6-sulfate	$[\text{-GalNAc}(\beta1\text{–}4)\text{GlcA}(\beta1\text{–}3)\text{-}]_n$ 4 (or 6) | SO_3^-
Dermatan sulfate	$[\text{-GalNAc}(\beta1\text{–}4)\text{L-IdoA}(\alpha1\text{–}3)\text{-}]_n$ 4 2 | | SO_3^- R R = H or SO_3^- and $[\text{-GalNAc}(\beta1\text{–}4)\text{GlcA}(\beta1\text{–}3)\text{-}]_n$ 4 (or 6) | SO_3^-
Keratan sulfate	$[\text{-Gal}(\beta1\text{–}4)\text{GlcNAc}(\beta1\text{–}3)\text{-}]_n$ 6 6 | | R R R = H or SO_3^-
Heparan sulfate and heparin	$[\text{-GlcNR}(\alpha1\text{–}4)\text{GlcA}(\beta1\text{–}4)\text{-}]_n$ 6 R = Ac or SO_3^- | R' R' = H or SO_3^- and $[\text{-GlcNAc}(\alpha1\text{–}4)\text{L-IdoA}(\alpha1\text{–}4)\text{-}]_n$ 2 | R R = H or SO_3^-

*With the exception of hyaluronan and keratan sulfate, the glycosaminoglycans are glycosidically linked to a protein chain by the sequence -4GlcA(β1–3)Gal(β1–3)Gal(β1–4)Xyl(β1–3)L-serine. Keratan sulfate is glycosidically linked to the *N*- or *O*-linked oligosaccharides of some glycoproteins. Sugars are D unless noted as L. Hyaluronan is not covalently linked to proteins.

†R in the abbreviated structure format refers to the proton of an —OH or an —NH₂ group or a substitution for the proton. —SO_3^- replaces the proton of the —OH group.

charged. Most glycosaminoglycans are covalently bound to proteins, and the resulting proteoglycans vary considerably in the number and types of bound glycan chains.

Hyaluronic acid (hyaluronan) is a negatively charged, soluble, high-molecular-weight, linear glycan composed of D-glucuronic acid and *N*-acetyl-D-glucosamine. It is found in the extracellular matrix, especially in soft connective tissue. Unlike most glycosaminoglycans, it is not covalently linked to protein but binds physically to receptor proteins on many different cells. Hyaluronic acid is noted for its ability to form highly viscous solutions, and some of its clinical applications depend on this rheology. The viscosity stems from the extended helical conformation, high molecular weight, and network of aggregated chains. Thus, hyaluronic acid may have a role in water and protein homeostasis in the intercellular matrix. Interaction between hyaluronic acid and its cell receptors is involved in cell locomotion and migration, as shown for lymphocytes. It may also be important in development and cell differentiation. Hyaluronic acid is synthesized by transfer of sugar units from their nucleotide diphosphate-derivatives to the reducing end of the growing hyaluronic acid chain. This is in contrast to the usual mode of chain lengthening of oligo- and polysaccharides, which involves addition of sugar units to the nonreducing end of the growing chain.

Chondroitin sulfate has a disaccharide repeat unit of D-glucuronic acid and N-acetyl-D-galactosamine with sulfate ester groups at C-2 of glucuronic acid and C-4 or C-6 of the galactosamine. This sulfation adds sequence heterogeneity, defined by the amount and positions of the sulfate esters along the chain. The large number of ionized sulfate groups and the weaker carboxyl groups assures that this large polysaccharide will attract counter cations and water for osmotic balance and hydration of the polysaccharide.

Dermatan sulfate is synthesized from chondroitin sulfate by intracellular C-5 epimerization of some of the D-glucuronic acid units to L-iduronic acid. The consequence of this is not only creation of a new uronic acid, but also of another element of structural diversity relative to the proportion and sequence of each acid. The other major differences between dermatan sulfate and chondroitin sulfate reside in the number of sulfate groups and their positions.

Heparin and heparan sulfate have disaccharide repeat units of D-glucuronic acid and D-glucosamine with some L-iduronic acid. The glucosamine units may be N-acetylated or N-sulfated, and all sugar residues may be O-sulfated. Heparin is more extensively epimerized, whereas heparan sulfate chains vary widely in extent of epimerization and sulfation, with some chains having little iduronic acid or sulfate. Heparin has a high proportion of N-sulfates and total sulfate, as well as more iduronic acid. Heparin is found predominantly as a component of mast cell granule proteoglycan, whereas heparan sulfate is linked to many cell surface proteins and matrix proteoglycans. Lipoprotein lipase in the capillaries of muscle and adipose tissue is closely associated with a heparan sulfate proteoglycan.

Keratan sulfate, composed of alternating D-galactose and N-acetyl-D-glucosamine units, lacks a uronic acid constituent, but it is heavily sulfated. The N-acetyl-D-glucosamine units carry sulfate groups at C-6, and some of the galactose units are sulfated also at C-6.

Proteoglycans

Proteoglycans are large, macromolecular components of the extracellular matrices of most eukaryotic cells, where they have many functions. Their size and complexity vary. A proteoglycan may carry more than one covalently linked glycosaminoglycan as well as N- and O-linked oligosaccharides attached to the core protein. Heparan sulfate/heparin proteoglycans contain at least one heparin sulfate chain, and usually O- and N-linked oligosaccharides in addition. The proteoglycans containing chondroitin sulfate, dermatan sulfate, and heparan sulfate frequently share a common oligosaccharide-linkage region by which they are attached to the protein (see footnote, Table 1–4). Keratan sulfate, however, may be O-linked to the protein, as in cartilage, or N-linked, as in cornea.

Glycoproteins

Many proteins carry covalently linked oligosaccharides as minor components. The number and size of the oligosaccharide chains vary. The N-linked oligosaccharides tend to have a common core and are β-glycosidically linked from the N-acetyl-D-glucosamine unit to the nitrogen of the β-carboxamide of asparagine (Fig. 1–14). Mucin-type glycoproteins have an α-D-galactosyl unit O-linked to the hydroxyl group of serine or threonine. Collagen is unique in that the carbohydrate chains are O-linked to the C-5 of 5-hydroxylysine. The carbohydrate moieties of glycoproteins may play a role in stabilization of the proteins to denaturation and may be involved in protein folding in addition to other specific biological roles.

Glycolipids

Glycolipids are widespread in nature but only as minor components of the lipid fraction and usually associated with proteins. The common glycolipids of mammalian systems include cerebrosides and gangliosides, which are glycosyl (glucosyl or galactosyl) derivatives of sphingolipids (Table 1–5). These glycosphingolipids contain a base such as sphingosine, which has an 18-carbon monounsaturated chain substituted with two hydroxyl groups and an amine group. The amine nitrogen of the sphingosine unit is acylated with a long-chain (C_{14} to C_{26}) fatty acid. A carbohydrate

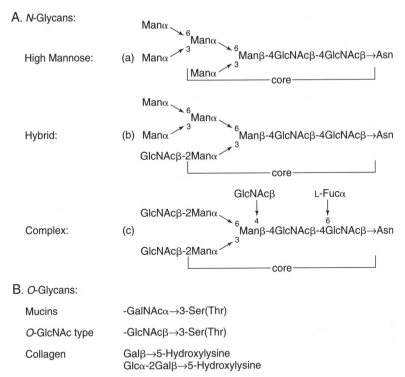

A. *N*-Glycans:

B. *O*-Glycans:

Mucins	-GalNAcα→3-Ser(Thr)
O-GlcNAc type	-GlcNAcβ→3-Ser(Thr)
Collagen	Galβ→5-Hydroxylysine Glcα-2Galβ→5-Hydroxylysine

Figure 1–14. *Structural variations in oligosaccharide chains of glycoproteins and their attachment site in the protein. (A) A core of 5 sugar units, common to all three types of N-linked glycans, is linked to asparagine (Asn). High-mannose N-glycans contain up to 9 mannose units in addition to N-acetylglucosamine. Other sugars, including galactose and sialic acid, also may be linked to the nonreducing ends of the antennary (branch) chains in the complex N-glycans. (B) O-Linked oligosaccharides in the mucins and O-GlcNAc type in glycoproteins may be extended at the nonreducing end by addition of N-acetylglucosamine, galactose, L-fucose, and sialic acid. Sugars are D-enantiomers unless noted otherwise.*

unit (usually glucose or galactose) is glycosidically attached to the *N*-acylsphingosine (ceramide) at its C-1 hydroxyl group to form a cerebroside (monoglycosylceramide). The sugar unit of a cerebroside may also be sulfated to form a sulfatide. Cerebrosides are neutral glycosphingolipids, whereas sulfatides are acidic glycosphingolipids. Large amounts of galactocerebroside and galactocerebroside 3-sulfate are found in the brain.

Additional sugar residues (usually glu-cose, galactose, L-fucose, or *N*-acetylgalactosamine) are attached to cerebrosides (usually to glucosylceramide) to form globosides and gangliosides. Neutral ceramide oligosaccharides (globosides) and acidic, sialic acid–containing ceramide oligosaccharides (gangliosides) are also sphingoglycolipids. Globosides are ceramides with two or more neutral sugar residues. The neutral diglycosylceramide, called lactosylceramide, is the precursor of other globosides and of ganglio-

---

TABLE 1–5

The Major Neutral and Acidic Glycolipids of Bovine and Human Milk

Neutral Glycolipid	Acidic Glycolipid
Gal(β1–1)Cer Glc(β1–1)Cer Gal(β1–4)Glc(β1–1)Cer	Neu5Ac(α2–3)Gal(β1–4)Glc(β1–1)Cer Neu5Ac(α2–8)Neu5Ac(α2–3)Gal(β1–4)Glc(β1–1)Cer

Cer, Ceramide, HOCH$_2$-C(H)(NHR)-C(H)(OH)-CH=CH-C$_{13}$H$_{27}$ with R representing a long-chain acyl group.

sides; lactosylceramide is also found in the membrane of red blood cells. Tetraglycosylceramides ("aminoglycolipids") are globosides that contain an additional sugar (i.e., galactose) and an N-acetylhexosamine unit (i.e., N-acetylgalactosamine); these compounds frequently show blood group activity.

Gangliosides are formed by the addition of sialic acid (N-acetylneuraminic acid) to diglycosylceramide; additional sugar residues such as galactose, N-acetylgalactosamine, and N-acetylglucosamine may also be added to form a variety of gangliosides, many containing branches formed by the addition of one or two sialic acid units to the linear portion of the oligosaccharide chain. Gangliosides are found on the surface membranes of most cells, and they make up about 6% of total brain lipids. Gangliosides are most highly concentrated in the ganglion cells of the central nervous system.

Aberrant glycosylation expressed in glycosphingolipids in tumor cells is strongly implicated as an essential mechanism in tumor progression. Abnormal accumulation of specific glycosphingolipids in specific cancers has been correlated with altered cell-cell or cell-substratum interactions, and reagents that block glycosylation have been shown to inhibit tumor cell metastasis.

Plants and microorganisms synthesize several simple glycolipids, which include fatty acid esters of the sugars and glycosides of diglycerides, hydroxy fatty acids, and myo-inositol phospholipids. Highly complex lipopolysaccharides of cell walls of gram-negative bacteria are both antigens and endotoxins. The lipopolysaccharides (also called "endotoxins") are composed of three domains: the terminal carbohydrate chain, which defines the O-specific antigenicity; the lipid A, which has the endotoxin activity; and an oligosaccharide core, which is sandwiched between. These endotoxins cause some types of food poisoning (e.g., salmonellosis).

REFERENCES

Baynes, J. W. and Monnier, V. M. (eds.) (1989) The Maillard Reaction in Aging, Diabetes, and Nutrition. Alan R. Liss, New York.
Brownlee, M. (1995) Advanced protein glycosylation in diabetes and aging. Annu Rev Med 46:223–234.
Carpita, N. C. (1990) The chemical structure of the cell walls of higher plants. In: Dietary Fiber: Chemistry, Physiology, and Health Effects (Kritchevsky, D., Bonfield, C. and Anderson, J. W., eds.), pp. 15–30. Plenum Press, New York.
Newburg, D. S. and Neubauer, S. H. (1995) Carbohydrates in milk. Analysis, quantities and significance. In: Handbook of Milk Composition (Jensen, R. G., ed.), pp. 273–349. Academic Press, San Diego, CA.
Selvendran, R. R. (1984) The plant cell wall as a source of dietary fiber: Chemistry and structure. Am J Clin Nutr 39:320–337.

RECOMMENDED READINGS

Chaplin, M. F. and Kennedy, J. F. (eds.) (1994) Carbohydrate Analysis: A Practical Approach, 2nd ed. Oxford University Press, London.
Fukuda, M. (1994) Cell surface carbohydrates: Cell-type specific expression. In: Molecular Glycobiology (Fukuda, M. and Hindsgaul, O, eds.), pp. 1–52. Oxford University Press, London.
Lowe, J. B. (1994) Carbohydrate recognition in cell-cell interaction. In: Molecular Glycobiology (Fukuda, M. and Hindsgaul, O., eds.), pp. 163–205. Oxford University Press, London.
Pigman, W. and Horton, J. (eds.) (1970, 1972) The Carbohydrates: Chemistry and Biochemistry, vol. IA, IIA, IB, IIB. Academic Press, New York.
Varki, A. and Marth, J. (1995) Oligosaccharides in vertebrate development. Semin Dev Biol 6:127–138.

◆ ◆

CHAPTER 2

Structure and Properties of Proteins and Amino Acids

Robert B. Rucker, Ph.D., and Taru Kosonen, Ph.D.

O U T L I N E

AMINO ACIDS

An understanding of the chemical and structural features of amino acids, peptides, and proteins is essential from a number of perspectives. For nutritionists, there is the need to appreciate the essential nature of amino acids and the dietary aspects of peptides and proteins as nutrients. There is also the obvious importance of amino acids, peptides, and proteins as informational and regulatory molecules. This chapter focuses on the chemical characteristics of amino acids and their role in defining properties of peptides and proteins. The diverse nature of amino acids is the basis for the ability of organisms to adapt to environments that differ substantially in polarity, water content, temperature, and pressure. Emphasis is given to the chemical modifications that allow amino acids, peptides, and proteins to perform specific functions, such as acting as catalysts and regulatory molecules (Branden and Tooze, 1991; Darby, 1993).

General Features

All peptides and proteins, regardless of their origin, are constructed from a set of about 20 common amino acids that are covalently linked together, usually in a linear sequence (Davies, 1985). The structures and selected chemical features of the most common amino acids are given in Table 2–1. Amino acids have distinctive side chains that give each amino acid a characteristic size and shape, and properties that dictate solubility and electrochemical characteristics. With such diverse building blocks, it should be easy to visualize that peptides and proteins can be designed for complex activities (Darby, 1993).

The first chemical description of an amino acid appeared in 1806. The last of the common amino acids to be described was threonine in 1938. The names for amino acids largely are derived from Greek terms. For example, the designation glycine is derived from the Greek *glykos* (sweet), because glycine has a sweet taste.

Although each amino acid is unique, the chemical properties of amino acids do have a number of common features. As the term amino acid implies, each contains an amino group and an acid moiety, a carboxylic acid group. Both of these functional moieties are bonded directly to a central carbon atom designated as the α-carbon (Fig. 2–1). Except for glycine, the α-carbon for each of the amino acids has four different functional groups bonded to it: an amino group, a carboxylic acid group, hydrogen, and a "side chain" or "R" group.

The presence of these four different functional groups creates what is called a chiral center. A chiral center exists when an arrangement around a given molecule cannot be superimposed. For all the amino acids (with the exception of glycine), there are two nonsuperimposable, mirror-image forms. These two forms are referred to as stereoisomers, designated as L- and D-isomers. This terminology comes from the Latin, *laevus* and *dexter*, and the Greek, *levo* and *dextro*, meaning left and right, respectively. That is, the use of the designation L or D in combination with the given name of an amino acid infers a specific spatial configuration around the amino acid's α-carbon. Although there are other systems of assigning stereochemistry (e.g., the RS system used in organic chemistry), the L and D designations remain in common usage for most amino acids.

Molecules with a chiral center are optically active. The presence of a chiral center causes the rotation of plane-polarized light.

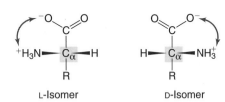

Figure 2–1. *General structure for the α-amino acids. Stereoisomers are shown in their L and D forms. Note the position of the α-carbon. The four valences of carbon result in chemical bonds that may be viewed as an equilateral tetrahedron. When a carbon atom has four different substituents, two distinct spatial arrangements are possible. Fisher projections are used to depict the L and D isomers. In a Fisher projection, bonds pointing horizontally are viewed as coming out of the plane on which they are depicted, whereas those pointing vertically go below the plane. A zwitterion is also depicted, wherein the arrows designate the potential balance and interaction between the positive (+) charge of the amino group and the negative (-) charge of the carboxylate group.*

TABLE 2–1
Common Amino Acids

Neutral R Groups

	Alanine	Valine	Proline	Leucine	Isoleucine
Amino Acid	Alanine	Valine	Proline	Leucine	Isoleucine
Abbreviation	Ala, A	Val, V	Pro, P	Leu, L	Ile, I
Molecular Weight	89	117	115	131	131
Occurrence (%)[a]	9–10	6–7	4–5	7–8	4–5
pK_a					
–COOH	2.34	2.32	1.99	2.36	2.36
–NH$_2$	9.69	9.62	10.6	9.68	9.68
–RH	—	—	—	—	—
pI	6.01	5.97	6.48	5.98	6.02
Hydropathy Index (kcal/mol)[b] and [Solubility in H$_2$O (g/100 mL) at 25°C]	0.5 [16.7]	1.5 [8.3]	−3.3 [162]	1.8 [2.4]	2.5 [4.1]
Nutritional Essentiality[c]	—	*	—	*	*

Aromatic R Groups / Acidic R Groups

	Phenylalanine	Tyrosine	Tryptophan	Aspartate	Glutamate
Amino Acid	Phenylalanine	Tyrosine	Tryptophan	Aspartate	Glutamate
Abbreviation	Phe, F	Tyr, Y	Trp, W	Asp, D	Glu, E
Molecular Weight	165	181	204	133	147
Occurrence (%)[a]	3–4	3–4	1–1.5	5–6	6–7
pK_a					
–COOH	1.83	2.20	2.38	2.09	2.19
–NH$_2$	9.13	10.07	9.39	9.82	9.67
–RH	—	9.11 (–OH)	—	3.86 (–COOH)	4.25 (–COOH)
pI	5.48	5.66	5.89	2.77	3.22
Hydropathy Index (kcal/mol)[b] and [Solubility in H$_2$O (g/100 mL) at 25°C]	2.5 [2.96]	2.3 [0.045]	3.4 [1.14]	−7.4 [0.5]	−9.4 [0.84]
Nutritional Essentiality[c]	*	†	*	—	—

Table continued on following page

The direction and magnitude differ among the various amino acids. Furthermore, optical rotation of amino acids is dependent on other factors, such as pH (the hydrogen ion concentration) and the degree of ionization of the carboxylic acid or amine group(s). Optical rotation may also be influenced by the nature of the solvent in which the amino acid is dissolved.

In proteins and peptides, amino acids are found almost exclusively in the L form, although occasionally D-amino acids are found in bacterial proteins and peptides (Davies, 1985). This has a number of important connotations and underscores the importance of appreciating properties of compounds that contain chiral centers. For example, that proteins are constructed largely of L-amino acids

TABLE 2–1
Common Amino Acids Continued

Positively Charged R Groups

Amino Acid	Lysine	Arginine	Histidine
Abbreviation	Lys, K	Arg, R	His, H
Molecular Weight	146	174	154
Occurrence (%)[a]	7	4–5	2
pK$_a$			
−COOH	2.18	2.17	1.82
−NH$_2$	8.95	9.04	9.17
−RH	10.53 (−NH$_2$)	12.48 (−NH=CH−NH$_2$)	6.0 (imidazole ring)
pI	9.74	10.76	7.59
Hydropathy Index (kcal/mol)[b] and [Solubility in H$_2$O (g/100 mL) at 25°C]	−4.2 [freely soluble]	−11.2 [freely soluble]	0.5 [15]
Nutritional Essentiality[c]	*	†	*

Polar, Uncharged R groups

Amino Acid	Glycine	Serine	Threonine	Cysteine	Methionine	Asparagine	Glutamine
Abbreviation	Gly, G	Ser, S	Thr, T	Cys, C	Met, M	Asn, D	Gln, Q
Molecular Weight	75	105	119	121	149	132	146
Occurrence (%)[a]	7–8	7–8	6	1–2	3–4	4–5	3–4
pK$_a$							
−COOH	2.34	2.21	2.63	1.71	2.28	2.04	2.17
−NH$_2$	9.60	9.15	10.43	10.78	9.31	9.82	9.13
−RH				8.33 (−SH)			
pI	5.97	5.68	5.87	5.07	6	5.41	5.65
Hydropathy Index (kcal/mol)[b] and [Solubility in H$_2$O (g/100 mL) at 25°C]	0 [25]	−0.3 [freely soluble]	0.4 [freely soluble]	−2.8 [freely soluble]	1.3 [18]	−0.2 [3.4]	−0.3 [4.7]
Nutritional Essentiality[c]	†	—	*	†	*	—	—

[a]Distribution, expressed as a percentage of the total amino acids found in common proteins.

[b]The hydropathy index combines measures of hydrophobicity and hydrophilicity and is used to predict which amino acids will most likely be found in an aqueous environment (− values) or a nonpolar environment (+ values). Hydrophobicities are usually measured by estimating the distribution of the amino acid between a nonpolar solvent and water. Note that hydrophobicity does not relate directly to solubility in water, because a number of factors related to the orientation of the R group and its configuration (see value for proline) can directly influence how the amino acid interacts with water.

[c]The designation (*) indicates that higher order animals have a nutritional requirement for the amino acid. The designation (—) indicates that in most instances the amino acid is sufficiently synthesized at critical periods in growth or development. The designation (†) implies that for some animals there may be a conditional need; i.e., sufficient quantities may not be synthesized. For example, in the rapidly growing and feathering chick, there is a conditional need for glycine, an amino acid abundant in connective tissue proteins and feathers (i.e., glycine is not synthesized in sufficient amounts).

indicates that reactions involving amino acids are highly stereospecific. The metabolic pathways for amino acid synthesis create predominantly amino acids in their L form. Moreover, the biological machinery required for protein assembly recognizes L-amino acids almost exclusively (Davies, 1985).

Regarding other important properties, purified amino acids are colorless and nonvolatile crystalline solids in the physiological pH range. Decomposition usually requires temperatures above 200°C. In aqueous solutions, amino acids are easily ionized. An amino group and carboxyl group bonded to a common carbon atom result in a zwitterion, a term used to designate a dipolar, chemical structure with both a positive and negative charge (see Fig. 2–1). Although the zwitterion portion of an amino acid is water soluble in the physiological pH range, it is ionically neutral because the positive charge of the amino group cancels out the negative charge associated with the carboxylate group. The zwitterionic character causes amino acids to be held together by electrostatic forces in a crystalline lattice (i.e., analogous to the crystalline lattice of sodium chloride and other salt crystals). In this regard, the high decomposition temperature is related to the zwitterionic characteristics of amino acids and their ability to form crystalline lattices.

Amino Acid Side Chains

Other properties of amino acids are dictated by their side chains, referred to as R groups (Rucker and Wold, 1988; Rucker and McGee, 1993). A given R group often confers novel chemical properties to an amino acid. Consequently, amino acids can be classified based on the chemical properties of their respective R groups. Some amino acids are soluble in water, but the relative degree of solubility is modulated by the nature of the R group and its relative polarity or hydropathy (i.e., the tendency to interact with a polar or nonpolar solvent or environment). This property of amino acid R groups can vary widely from totally nonpolar or hydrophobic (water insoluble) to polar or hydrophilic (water soluble).

Examples of non-polar or hydrophobic R groups are those that consist of multiple car-bon units, such as the side chains of leucine, valine, proline, or isoleucine. In this group of amino acids, proline deserves special comment because the R group is joined both at the α-carbon and amino group to form a ring of connected carbon atoms. For this reason, proline is referred to as a secondary amino acid or imino acid. Its α-carbon lacks a hydrogen, but remains a chiral center because the hydrogen is replaced by a cyclic group. The cyclization also renders proline more rigid, with no ability to rotate easily around the α-carbon. The presence of proline in a polypeptide segment can reduce peptide chain flexibility (Hamaguchi, 1992; Konig, 1993).

The amino acids that have aromatic structures have R groups with positive hydropathic values. The aromatic amino acids are phenylalanine, tyrosine, and tryptophan. Aromatic side chains contribute specific optical properties to proteins, such as the ability to absorb light in the ultraviolet range.

Aspartate and glutamate are examples of polar amino acids that contain a net negative charge because the R group contains a carboxylate group. In contrast, lysine, arginine, and histidine are examples of polar amino acids with functional groups capable of forming positive changes depending on the pH of the medium in which they are dissolved. Lysine, arginine, and histidine have side chains that contain amino, guanidino, or imidazole groups.

There are also amino acids that have polar characteristics with uncharged R groups, such as threonine, serine, cysteine, asparagine, glutamine, and methionine. The polarity of threonine and serine are properties contributed by the oxygen of their hydroxyl groups. The polarity of cysteine and methionine is related to the presence of sulfur in the form of a thiol or methylthio group, respectively. The polarity of asparagine and glutamine is caused by the presence of the nitrogen- and oxygen-containing carboxamide group.

Modifications of Amino Acid Side Chains

The characteristics of some amino acids may be directly affected by enzymatic and nonenzymatic modifications of the R group. Indeed, hundreds of compounds found in nature are derived from the common 20 amino acids that are commonly found in proteins (Rucker and McGee, 1993). Such modifications can occur as co- or posttranslational modifications following incorporation of the amino acid into protein. Posttranslational protein modifications and their importance are discussed later in this chapter. However, it is important at this point to appreciate that specific amino acid modifications are often introduced to modulate or modify a given chemical property. Posttranslational modifications can extend the structures and properties of amino acids in proteins beyond those of the 20 or 21 (including selenocysteine) amino acids coded for in DNA/RNA and incorporated during protein translation.

Specific chemical properties can be modified subtly or dynamically by posttranslational modification. For example, consider the net change in charge (0 to 2−) that occurs when a seryl residue (as a part of a peptide sequence) is phosphorylated at its hydroxyl group (Fig. 2–2). Other examples of posttranslational modifications of amino acid R groups in proteins include the methylation of lysyl and histidyl residues, the hydroxylation of pro-

lyl and lysyl residues, and the carboxylation of glutamyl residues (Fig. 2–3). These types of modifications of R groups are essential in defining the structural and functional properties of proteins.

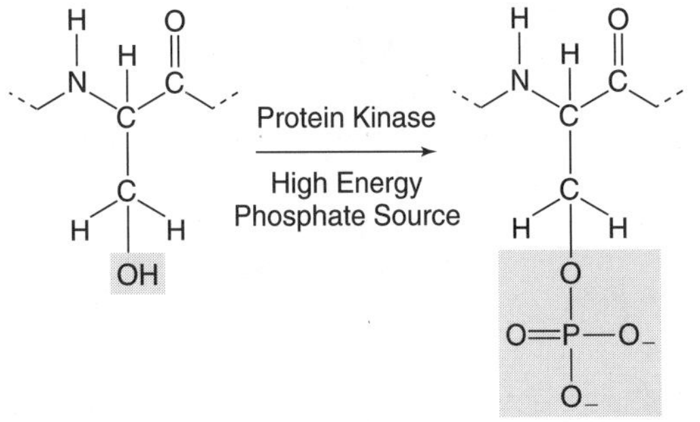

A number of other amino acids are derived from metabolism of the common amino acids found in proteins. Many of these amino acids are discussed in Chapter 11. Amino acids, such as ornithine, citrulline, taurine, homocysteine, and certain biogenic amine compounds (e.g., dopamine, serotonin, and histamine) are derived from distinct metabolic pathways. Careful attention should also be given to the description of thyroxine synthesis and release as outlined in Chapter 33 and to selenocysteine synthesis as described in Chapter 34. The production of thyroxine results from a complex series of events in which several steps are excellent examples of posttranslational protein modifications. The synthesis of selenocysteine occurs cotranslationally in conjunction with transfer RNA (tRNA) using seryl-tRNAs specific for the uracil-guanine-adenine (UGA) codon as substrate.

The Acid and Base Characteristics of Amino Acids

When an amino acid is titrated (i.e., exposed to an acid or base), the resulting reactions can be described by a titration curve. The shape of this curve is influenced by the types and number of the functional groups capable of reacting with or exchanging a hydrogen ion. In an amino acid such as alanine, there are two titratable groups (Fig. 2–4). At a low pH (i.e., a high hydrogen ion concentration), both the amino group and the carboxylic acid group of alanine are protonated. As a result, alanine is positively charged and migrates toward the negative pole in an electrical field. If a base is added (to decrease the concentration of hydrogen ions or, alternatively, to increase the concentration of hydroxyl ions), the carboxylic acid group and then the amino group lose their protons. At the midpoint of this process when the carboxylate group is unprotonated and negatively charged and the amino group is still protonated and positively charged, alanine is neutral. The addition of

Figure 2–2. *The modification of peptidyl serine to peptidyl phosphoserine. Some amino acids undergo chemical modifications that significantly alter their original properties. This example emphasizes how adding a substituent such as a phosphate group can alter electrochemical properties and net charge. The reaction depicted is important to many metabolic pathways in which protein phosphorylation causes either activation or inhibition of enzymatic activity. A seryl residue in given enzymes and regulatory proteins is often the site of modification. The high-energy phosphate source is most often adenosine triphosphate (ATP). There are a number of different protein kinases, each with specificity for the enzyme or regulatory protein targeted for regulation.*

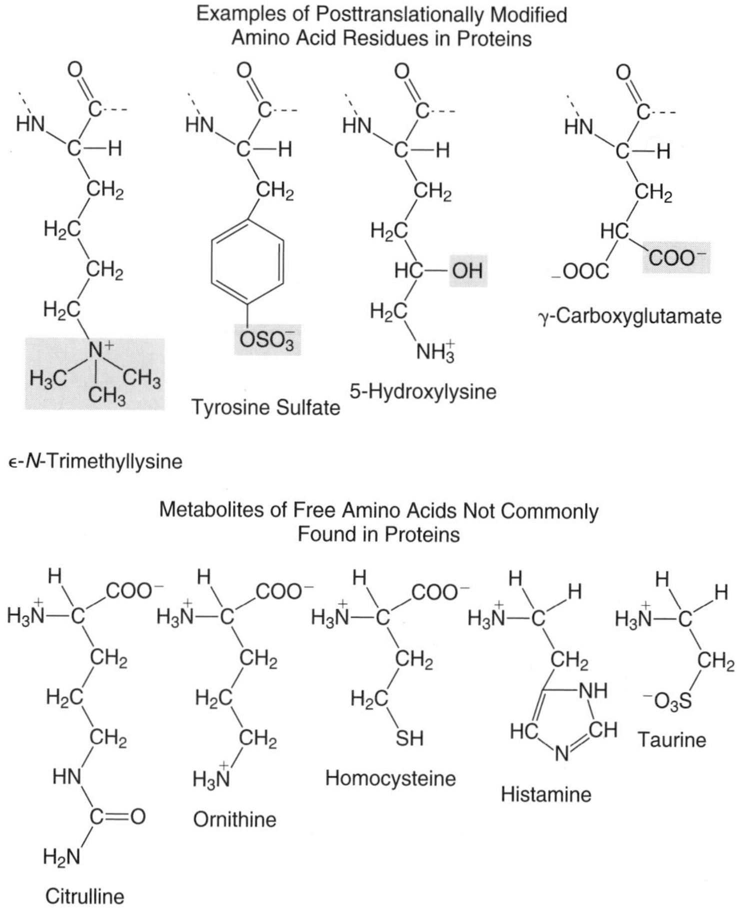

Examples of Posttranslationally Modified Amino Acid Residues in Proteins

ε-N-Trimethyllysine

Tyrosine Sulfate

5-Hydroxylysine

γ-Carboxyglutamate

Metabolites of Free Amino Acids Not Commonly Found in Proteins

Citrulline

Ornithine

Homocysteine

Histamine

Taurine

Figure 2–3. *Examples of posttranslationally modified and less conventional amino acids. (A), Some of the modifications are the result of specific enzymatic reactions wherein the amino acid to be modified is first incorporated into a given peptide or protein and then altered by an enzyme-catalyzed reaction. Examples of the products of a methylation (ε-N-trimethyllysine residue formation), sulfation (tyrosine sulfate residue formation), hydroxylation (5-hydroxylysine residue formation), and a γ-carboxylation (γ-carboxyglutamate residue formation) are shown. (B), The structures for citrulline, ornithine, homocysteine, histamine, and taurine are shown. These amino acids and related compounds are derived from amino acids, but in contrast to the amino acids shown in A, these amino acids and amino acid-derived products are produced in a step-wise fashion in metabolic pathways. Arginine and glutamate are precursors of citrulline and ornithine. Homocysteine is the demethylation product of methionine. Histamine is formed by decarboxylation of histidine. Taurine is formed by oxidative catabolism of cysteine. It is the free amino acid rather than an amino acid residue in a protein that is substrate for the metabolic pathways that produce these amino acids and amino acid derivatives.*

more base eventually causes the amino group to lose its proton, and alanine becomes negatively charged because of the loss of the positively charged amino group. Compare the titration curve for alanine to the more complex titration curve for histidine, which contains three titratable functional groups (Fig. 2–4).

As is the case with organic acids and amine compounds, amino acid titration curves can be described by constants called pK_as that help to define characteristics of the associated titratable groups. A pK_a is the nega-

tive log of the dissociation constant K_a for an acid. When the associated (protonated) and dissociated (nonprotonated) species are present in equal concentrations, the pK_a is equal to the pH. The pK_as of carboxylic acid groups are relatively low, usually around 2 to 4. Amino groups have pK_as that are relatively high, usually 9 to 11 (see Table 2–1). Accordingly, the classification of an amino acid as acidic or basic depends on the pK_a of a titratable group on its side chain (Darby, 1993).

Why is it important to have a knowledge

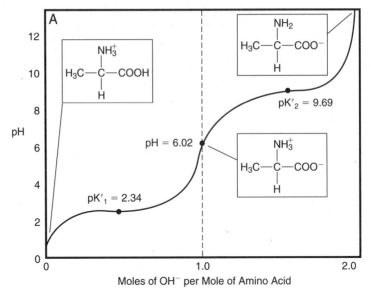

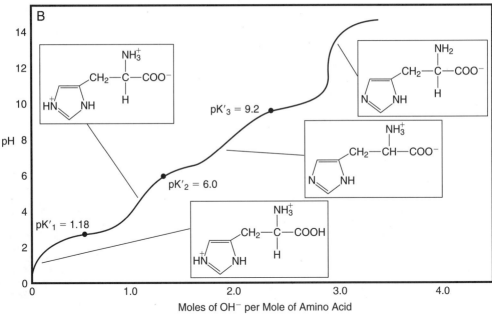

Figure 2–4. *Titration curves for alanine* (A) *and histidine* (B). *The pH equivalent to the isoelectric point (see text) for alanine is shown as the midpoint between the two pKₐs.*

of the titration characteristics? First, inter- and intramolecular ionic interactions are very important to protein structure. For example, if it is essential for a protein to be electrically or ionically neutral to function, then the protein must be designed with a combination of amino acids that result in a zero net charge. Cell communication, as articulated through specific proteins, is often dependent on the ionic characteristics of given amino acids.

Amino acids and proteins also have the ability to act as buffers because of their acid and base characteristics.

Information about the ionic properties of proteins also has a practical significance. When a protein is titrated to the point that corresponds to neutrality (i.e., to a pH where a protein has no net charge), this pH is referred to as the isoelectric point (p*I*) of the protein. Many proteins are insoluble at their isoelectric points. Thus, protein isolation and concentration can sometimes be achieved by adjusting the pH. A good example is the isolation of the major milk protein fractions, casein and whey (Darby, 1993).

PEPTIDES

Amino acids are covalently joined by peptide bonds. Peptide bond formation is endergonic with a free energy change of about 20 kJ/mol (~4.8 kcal/mol) at physiological pH (Fig. 2–5). A positive free energy change of this magnitude means that combining an amino group of one amino acid with the carboxyl group of another does not occur spontaneously to any appreciable extent (Davies, 1985). Consequently, peptide synthesis requires both energy and specialized mechanisms (see Chapter 10).

PROTEINS

Levels of Protein Structure

It should now be apparent that altering the charge and hydrophobic or hydrophilic nature of amino acids, as well as the length of polypeptide chains, can influence their function. The numerous combinations of amino acids give rise to possibilities that dictate the size and shape of proteins. Small proteins contain 50 to 100 amino acids. The upper limit in size for a protein is ~5000 amino acid residues. For example, apolipoprotein B has a single polypeptide chain with a molecular weight of 513 kDa corresponding to about 5000 amino acid residues. In addition, many proteins are made of multiple subunits. In some structural proteins the subunits are often covalently cross-linked into larger complexes that have molecular masses in the millions of daltons. (Note that a dalton is the mass of a hydrogen atom. Protein and peptide molecu-

NUTRITION INSIGHT

Use of Milk Proteins in Other Foods

Milk proteins are a heterogeneous mixture that includes two main groups of protein, casein and whey or serum protein. Within these two classes of proteins are six major subclasses: α_1-casein, α_{s2}-casein, β-casein, κ-casein, β-lactoglobulin, and α-lactalbumin. In addition, a number of other proteins are present, such as serum albumin, immunoglobulins, and lactoferrin.

Casein is used in a number of food preparations. Casein may be precipitated from the whey by acidification to its isoelectric point, ~ pH 6.0. This phenomenon is easily demonstrated by adding lemon to tea or coffee that contains milk or cream. The serum protein or whey fractions remain in solution.

The separation of casein from whey is important in that both protein classes have novel properties. Casein in the presence of lipids can form micellar structures ranging in size from 30 to 300 nm. Micellar structures are responsible for the opaqueness of milk. The ability to form micelles is useful, because a number of hydrophobic substances can be incorporated into casein micelles. The whey fraction in milk is also used in the preparation of fabricated foods. Whey proteins are hydrophilic and may be added to beverages to increase the protein content. Furthermore, whey proteins are highly water binding because of their hydrophilicity, which makes them well suited for addition to soups, gravies, and salad dressings. The knowledge that one can separate these two important milk fractions by acid precipitation is very useful. The separated forms differ in solubility, viscosity, and utility as thickening agents. Whey is ideally suited for increasing viscosity and thickening, whereas casein is an excellent choice when emulsification is needed to add flavoring agents. Moreover, under certain processing conditions, whey or whey/casein mixtures can be formed into hydrophobic micelles. Hydrophobic micellar structures can be designed to have oily characteristics for use as fat substitutes. An example is Simplesse.

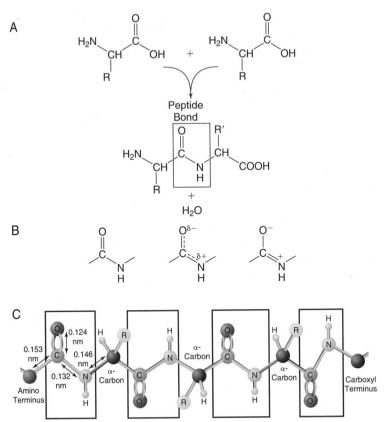

Figure 2–5. *Formation of a peptide bond (A). The α-amino group of one amino acid displaces the hydroxyl of the carboxyl group in another. Although amino acids are good nucleophiles, the hydroxyl group is a poor leaving group. Therefore, the reaction is endergonic with a free energy of change of about 20 kJ or ~80-90 kcal/mol. As shown in B, the peptide bond is capable of resonance and charge separation. As indicated in C, the oxygen and nitrogen of the amide bond lie in a plane, which contributes to peptide bond stabilization. The hydrogen of the amino group is usually trans to the oxygen in the peptide backbone. Note that the bond length between the oxygen and carbon originating from the carboxyl group is 0.124 nm, which is typical of a C=O double bond. The nitrogen that is attached to the C=O forming the peptide bond also has a relatively short bond length (0.132 nm), indicating some double bond character. This causes an electric dipole. Because each bond has some double bond character, there is also restricted rotation. However, the nitrogen to α-carbon bond is 0.146 nm, which is typical of a single bond. Around this bond rotation can occur, unless it is hindered by the presence of a large R group or the presence of a prolyl residue.*

lar masses are often reported as daltons [Da] or kilodaltons [kDa].)

Protein structure is complex. Consequently, it is described at a number of different levels (Branden and Tooze, 1991; Darby, 1993). The first level is the linear sequence of amino acids. The term *primary structure* is used to delineate this one-dimensional linear sequence of amino acids. The amino acid sequence of a peptide or protein can be determined by sequencing the amino acids along the linear polypeptide chain. Alternatively, the sequence may be inferred from the corresponding nucleotide sequence of the protein's gene or messenger RNA (mRNA).

Considerable information may be inferred from knowing the primary structure. Many sequences act as specific signals for certain protein modifications that impact biological regulation. Examples include: (1) the sequences asn-x-ser and asn-x-thr, which are commonly associated as sites for *N*-linked glycosylation in proteins (i.e., the addition of sugars at specified sites along the polypeptide chain); (2) the sequence arg-gly-asp-ser, which corresponds to a cell surface-binding domain in certain proteins (e.g., fibronectin) that allows a protein to bind to a cell's surface; and (3) the sequence lys-asp-glu-leu, which is one of several signals important for the vectoral movement of soluble proteins within the endoplasmic reticulum (ER). The use of x in the first example indicates that virtually any amino acid can be substituted for x without affecting the functional significance of the sequence when it appears in a protein. When a given amino acid sequence is commonly associated with a function, the sequence is often designated as a consensus sequence, particularly if the sequence is found in a di-

verse array of animal, plant, or bacterial cells and is consistently associated with a specific property or function.

Additional information that may be obtained from a primary sequence is an indication of regions of hydrophobicity and hydrophilicity. A hydropathy plot is given in Figure 2–6. Hydropathy plots are useful in defining regions in a polypeptide or clusters of amino acids that differ in their polar or non-polar

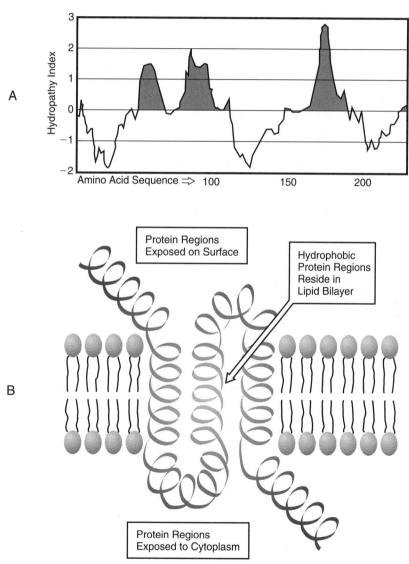

Figure 2–6. A hydropathy plot. Hydrophobic regions are usually found in the interior of proteins, whereas hydrophilic regions are likely to interact with aqueous or ionic environments. See Table 2–1 for hydropathic indices for given amino acids. A hydropathy plot (A) identifies regions of a polypeptide chain that contain amino acids that are predominantly hydrophobic (shaded) or, in contrast, hydrophilic in nature. The example shown could apply to a transmembrane protein (B). Transmembrane proteins often cross the lipid bilayers of cell membranes. The hydrophobic regions are associated with the interior, whereas the hydrophilic regions may extend into the cytoplasmic compartment or toward the exterior of the cell.

characteristics. Protein folding is dependent on the location of hydrophobic and hydrophilic amino acids within a given segment or domain in a polypeptide chain. Moreover, hydropathy characteristics are important for the insertion of protein polypeptide sequences into cell membranes or for creation of networks of proteins that function in transmembrane communication (Hamaguchi, 1992).

Secondary structure refers to the spatial arrangement of atoms around the backbone of a given polypeptide chain. Amino acid R groups can influence this type of orientation. For example, large, bulky groups prevent rotation around the backbone and fix given conformations into place. As noted previously, in amino acids such as proline, rotation is prohibited because of an imine bond. In addition, electrostatic attractions and repulsions between amino acid residues, interactions between the amino acids at the ends of the helix, and the electric dipole inherent to the peptide backbone contribute to secondary beta structures. When polypeptide chains are arranged in long strands or sheets (e.g., β-sheets), the consequence is often a fibrous protein (Nesloney and Kelly, 1996). In contrast, globular proteins are folded in spirals or globular shapes and coils. In the polypeptides that form fibrous proteins, a common feature is segmental repeats of amino acids whose side chains restrict free rotation around the polypeptide backbone. In contrast, in α-helical structures, the polypeptide chains are enriched in amino acids with freer rotation around the polypeptide chain. However, many different types of segmental polypeptidyl structures may exist in a single protein. Indeed, most proteins contain segments that have the characteristics of both α-helical and β-sheet structures (Fig. 2–7).

Tertiary structure is used to describe the three-dimensional arrangements of amino acids within the entire protein (Darby, 1993). Another term, *quaternary structure*, is used to describe complex arrangements of tertiary structures (e.g., arrangement of subunits). Tertiary structures may also accommodate specific prosthetic groups. The term prosthetic group is used to describe a unique moiety or defined chemical structure that confers a specific function or additional property to a given protein. Prosthetic groups may be covalently or non-covalently linked to the proteins they serve. Examples of prosthetic groups include the heme group in hemoglobin and myoglobin and enzyme cofactors such as lipoic acid and pyridoxal 5′-phosphate.

How Protein Conformations Are Stabilized

Most protein conformations are stabilized by relatively weak interactions. Some examples of the types of interactions that stabilize proteins are given in Table 2–2. The difference in free energy between folded and unfolded states in typical proteins is in the range of 20 to 70 kJ/mol (5 to 17 kcal/mol). To put the value of 20 to 70 kJ/mol into perspective, the amount of energy needed to break covalent bonds is ~350 kJ/mol (83 kcal/mol) for C–C bonds and ~410 kJ/mol (98 kcal/mol) for C–H bonds. Although many conformations are possible, a large number of weak interactions can result in a degree of stabilization.

The stability of a given conformation is dictated by the entropy term associated with the energy relationships important to the folding and unfolding of the polypeptide chain. When stabilization occurs, it is the result of the sum total of the hydrophobic and ionic interactions of the various amino acid side chains. In particular, hydrophobic interactions are important for protein–protein interactions and tertiary structure in large proteins. As proteins become smaller in size, it often becomes difficult to accommodate or appropriately place hydrophobic residues. It is for this reason that many small proteins are held together by covalent bonds, usually disulfide linkages. When such covalent bonds are formed, they impose restrictions on folding (Hamaguchi, 1992).

The process of folding and unfolding of proteins is dynamic. For most proteins, this process results from a sequential series of events that takes place in a programmed manner. When a protein is folded so that it is functional, the process is referred to as naturation (Branden and Tooze, 1991). When unfolding or inappropriate folding occurs and results in a dysfunctional state, the process is

·····Met-Tyr-Lys-Gly-Gly-Pro-Leu-Ile-Arg·····

Primary Structure

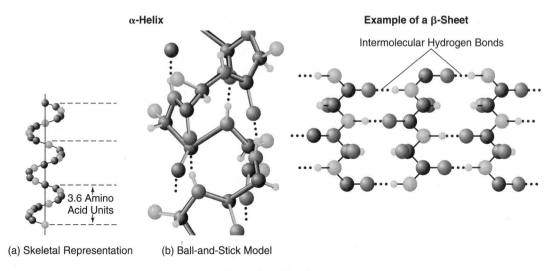

α-Helix

Example of a β-Sheet

Intermolecular Hydrogen Bonds

3.6 Amino
Acid Units

(a) Skeletal Representation   (b) Ball-and-Stick Model

Secondary Structure

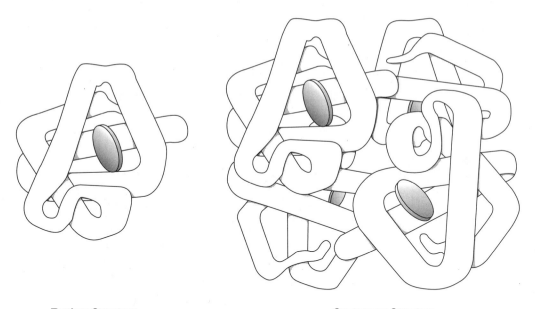

Tertiary Structure   **Quaternary Structure**

Figure 2–7. *Levels of structure in proteins. The primary structure consists of a sequence of amino acids with secondary structures that often exist as α-helices or as β-sheets. These structures combine to make complex tertiary structures, which may serve as a subunit that eventually forms the quaternary structure of multimeric proteins. The example is a representation of the tertiary and quaternary structure of hemoglobin. The heme molecules are shown within the folds.*

referred to as denaturation. Most commonly, proteins are denatured by (1) substances that disrupt associated water structures, (2) heat, and/or (3) extremes in the acid or base balance. Disruption of water organization by a denaturant (e.g., urea) influences the secondary or tertiary structure of proteins. Extremes of heat denature proteins, because vibrational energy within the protein molecule is altered. An increase in vibrational energy, when exces-

NUTRITION INSIGHT

Vitamin and Mineral Prosthetic Groups Give Color to Certain Holoproteins

When some prosthetic groups associate with proteins, they often lend color to the protein as a functional property. A good example is the addition of flavin adenine dinucleotide (FAD) or flavin mononucleotide (FMN) to the apoprotein subunits that form into flavoproteins. Flavoproteins appear yellow. Prosthetic groups that contain iron, such as heme, give proteins colors that range from brown to bright red, depending on the oxidation state of the iron-containing heme moiety. As an example, the amount of myoglobin in muscle tissue imparts to meat varying amounts of color. White poultry meat contains relatively small amounts of myoglobin and heme (0.1 to 0.4 mg/g), whereas dark poultry meat often contains five to six times that amount of myoglobin. Veal and pork contain 2 to 7 mg of myoglobin per gram, and beef usually contains 10 mg or more of myoglobin per gram. The globins of myoglobin and hemoglobin are colorless; yet when they are complexed with heme through coordinate and synergistic histidyl residue interactions, red to pink colors are imparted.

Oxymyoglobin is usually red-pink in color, whereas deoxygenated myoglobin is purple-red. Denaturation of meat protein by cooking can cause dissociation of heme and the formation of protein, iron, and imidazole (from histidine) complexes that are brown to tan in color. When a prosthetic group imparts color to a protein, it is referred to as a chromophore.

sive, disrupts tertiary structures. Extremes of acid–base balance or pH cause denaturation by interfering with the organization of water or by altering the redox state of proteins. Finally, chemical modifications that change amino acid R groups can have dramatic effects on protein structure. For example, introducing a reducing agent such as mercaptoethanol ($HS—CH_2—CH_2—OH$) can disrupt disulfide bond formation, which in turn can cause the opening of associated polypeptide chains.

NUTRITIONAL INFLUENCES ON PROTEIN STRUCTURE AND ASSEMBLY FUNCTION

There are a number of co- and posttranslational steps that depend on optimal nutrition and where protein structure or assembly is influenced when nutrition is suboptimal (Rucker and McGee, 1993). In particular, nutritional deficiencies may affect steps important to the co- and posttranslational processing of

TABLE 2–2
Forces that Stabilize Protein Structures

Type of Bond or Force	Description
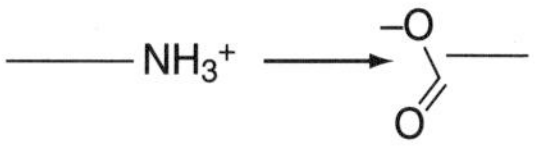 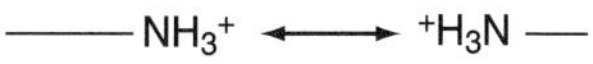 **Ionic bond**	Charged complexes that are capable of creating very strong interactions depending on the dielectric constant

Attractive Forces

——— NH_3^+ ——→ $\overset{-O}{\underset{O}{\diagdown}}$ —

Repulsive Forces

——— NH_3^+ ←——→ ^+H_3N —

Hydrogen bond 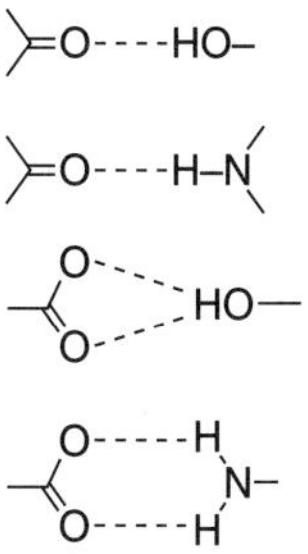	Noncovalent bonds that result from the association of hydrogen with atoms that are electronegative

$\diagup{=}O{-}{-}{-}{-}HO{-}$

$\diagup{=}O{-}{-}{-}{-}H{-}N\diagup$

$\overset{O\cdots}{\underset{O\diagup}{\diagdown}}\cdots HO{-}$

$\overset{O{-}{-}{-}{-}H}{\underset{O{-}{-}{-}{-}H}{\diagdown}}\diagdown N{-}$

Hydrophobic interactions 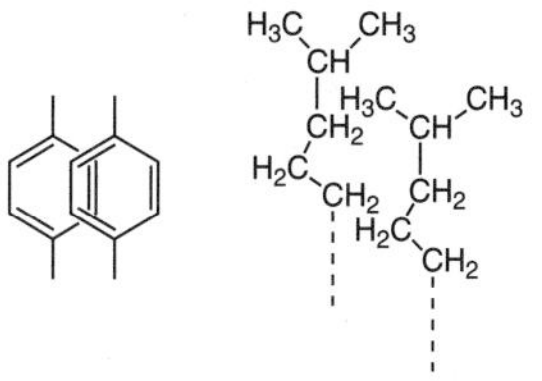	Hydrocarbons in an aqueous medium force associations between adjacent hydrocarbon moieties; the energy required for the process comes from the reorganization of the surrounding water structure

van der Waals interactions	Weak electrostatic attractions

proteins, because many of the enzymatic proteins involved in protein modifications require metals or vitamin-derived cofactors to function properly. A cotranslational event occurs coincident with the actual translation (synthesis) of a protein. A posttranslational modification occurs after the protein has been synthesized. Posttranslational modifications of proteins usually occur in the Golgi or post-Golgi sites associated with the smooth ER or secretory vesicles. It is important to appreciate that (1) posttranslational modifications extend the range of chemical properties of the common amino acids within protein and (2) posttranslational protein modifications are as important to protein production as are any of the transcriptional and translational events that initiate polypeptide synthesis. That is, a defect at any of the steps in the process of protein assembly or modification can result in a dysfunctional product.

Most protein modifications can be placed in one of three broad categories: (1) modifications that involve peptide bond cleavage and formation, (2) those that involve the amino- or carboxy-terminal amino acid, and (3) those that involve specific amino acid side chains. Modifications in the first category may already be familiar. Activation of many peptide hormones and conversion of zymogens to active enzymes are examples of the first category (Konig, 1993). For example, trypsinogen and other protease zymogens are converted to active proteinases by hydrolysis of a specific peptide bond to release an N-terminal segment. Formation of the hormone insulin

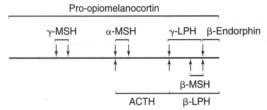

Figure 2–8. *Examples of peptide hormone formation. Bioactive peptides can arise by several mechanisms. As an example, the production of α-, β-, and γ-melanocyte-stimulating hormones (MSH), adrenocorticotrophic hormone (ACTH), β-endorphin, and β- and γ-lipotropin (LPH) are shown in A. The peptides arise from the cleavage of peptide bonds in the protein pro-opiomelanocortin, which acts as a precursor. Arrows indicate sites where enzyme proteinases cleave specific peptide bonds to give rise to the designated peptides.*

from its precursor polypeptide, proinsulin, occurs by proteolytic excision of an internal segment, leaving two polypeptide chains attached by disulfide bonds. Other examples are shown in Figure 2–8. The precursor polypeptide pro-opiomelanocortin produced by the pituitary gland can be cleaved to yield seven different polypeptide hormones. The size of peptide hormones may be quite small

(e.g., thyrotropin-releasing factor is only a tripeptide) or relatively large (e.g., glucagon contains 29 amino acids and insulin contains 51 amino acid residues).

The second major type of modification, N- or C-terminus modifications, are important in (1) directing proteins to specific compartments within the cell, (2) protecting the amino- and carboxy-terminal sequences from proteolysis, and (3) selective activation of enzymes and hormones. For example, amidation of the carboxy-termini of many hormones (e.g., calcitonin) is essential for activity.

The third major type of modification, R group or side chain modifications, provide chemical features important for cellular compartmentalization and trafficking, receptor binding, regulatory signaling, prosthetic group addition or formation, protein cross-linking, and the creation of novel chemical sites such as those important to metal binding. Table 2–3 lists some examples of chemical modifications of side chains of amino acid residues in proteins that are common targets for the modifications.

As signals for compartmentalization, typi-

TABLE 2–3
Examples of Modifications Involving Amino Acid Side Chains

Selected Functions	Process or Example	Commonly Targeted Amino Acids in Proteins
Compartmentalization, receptor binding	Acylations	Asn, Cys, Gln, Lys, Ser
	Acetylations	Ala, Arg, Gly, His, Lys
	Glycosylations	Asn, Cys, Gln, Hyp, Lys, Ser, The, Tyr
Regulatory signaling	Acetylations	Lys
	Adenylylations	Tyr
	ADP-ribosylations	Cys, Glu, Arg, Lys, Ser
	Methylations	Arg, Asp, Glu, His, Lys, Ser, The
	Phosphorylations	His, Lys, Ser, The, Tyr
	Ubiquitin addition	Arg, Tyr
	Sulfations	Tyr
Prosthetic group additions or formation	Biotinylations	Lys
	Flavin (FAD and FMN) additions	Cys, His
	Phosphopantetheine addition	Ser
	Pyridoxal phosphate addition	Lys
	Retinal addition	Lys
Protein cross-linking	Allysine and dehydronorleucine formation	Lys
	Cystine formation	Cys
	Glutamyllysine formation	Gln, Lys
Other	Carboxylations	Asp, Glu
	Halogen addition (iodine)	Tyr
	Hydroxylations	Asp, Lys, Pro
	Nonenzymatic glycosylations	Arg, Lys
	Sulfoxide formation	Met
	Glutamylation	Glu

NUTRITION INSIGHT

Niacin and Polyribosylation of Histone Proteins

Pellagra is a well known deficiency disease that results from an insufficient intake of niacin and tryptophan (see Chapter 20). Niacin is a precursor for nicotinamide adenine dinucleotide (NAD) synthesis. The amount of NAD in cells is very much dependent on the amount of niacin, which is either made from tryptophan-related pathways or present in the diet as a vitamin. One of the functions of NAD is as a substrate for mono- and polyribosylation reactions.

Polyribosylations change the surface property and structural conformation of some proteins (e.g., histones that are found in the nucleus of cells). Ribosylation reactions are important in many of the complex steps in enzyme regulation and also for DNA repair. In this regard, it is important to note that the skin lesions associated with pellagra may be due to the inability to carry out normal DNA repair because of an inability to alter histone structure as influenced by polyribosylation reactions.

cal reactions involve acylations, acetylations, and glycosylations. Acylation, the attachment of a long-chain fatty acid, provides lipophilic handles that facilitate the vectorial movement of protein from one compartment to another and that create specific sites to enhance attachments and compartmentalization within cells as well. There are also enzymes in post-translational pathways that modify lysyl, cysteinyl, and glutamyl residues in specific proteins that may be influenced by changes in nutritional status.

Moreover, the formation or incorporation of various prosthetic groups in proteins can occur as posttranslational protein modifications. The addition of a given prosthetic group may be essential to the creation of an enzymatic or functional active site (e.g., the addition of biotin, one of the flavocoenzymes, heme, or a metal such as iron or copper). See Chapters 20, 22, 31, and 32 for more discussion of these prosthetic groups and the proteins that contain them.

For stabilization of protein structures, it is often essential to cross-link specific polypeptide chains together (Fig. 2–9). For structural proteins such as collagen and elastin, the formation of interchain cross-links facilitates the

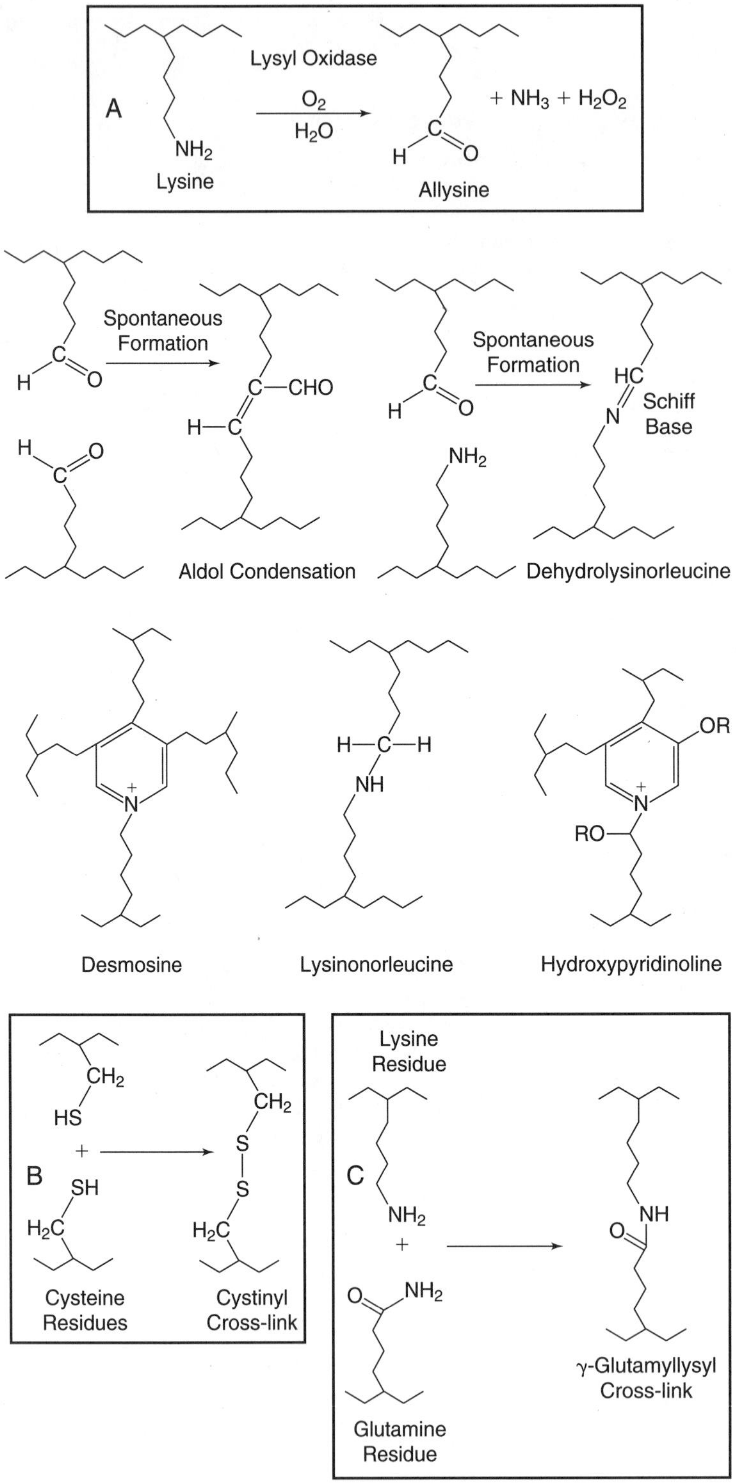

Figure 2-9. *Amino acids that function to cross-link polypeptide chains. Examples include the lysine-derived cross-links (A), cystine formation from cysteine (B), and cross-links derived from the enzyme-catalyzed condensation of lysyl and glutaminyl residues (C). For the reactions shown in A, the first step is the oxidation and deamination of specific lysyl residues in proteins, such as elastin and collagen to form residues of allysine. The next steps occur nonenzymatically. Two examples are shown. An aldol condensation product is formed from condensation of two peptide-bound allysine residues. Peptidyl dehydrolysinonorleucine occurs as a product of the Schiff-base reaction. Peptidyl allysine on a polypeptide chain reacts with peptidyl lysine on an adjacent polypeptide chain to cause cross-linking of the two chains. These products may condense further to form even more complex cross-linking amino acids, such as desmosine, which is found in the structural protein elastin, or hydroxypyridinoline, which occurs in collagen. For hydroxypyridinoline, hydroxylysine residues (see Fig. 2-3) serve as lysine-derived precursors. Note that the R depicted as a part of the hydroxypyridinoline structure can also be the site for glycosylation. As shown in B, the formation of peptidyl cystine cross-links from peptidyl cysteine oxidation is also a common strategy for cross-linking or joining protein polypeptide chains together. C, The cross-linking amino acid residue, γ-glutamyllysine. The formation of this cross-linking amino acid is catalyzed by a transaminase, and γ-glutamyllysyl residues are present in the proteins fibrin and keratin.*

NUTRITION INSIGHT

Vitamin C and Connective Tissue Protein Synthesis

The nutritional deficiency disease scurvy has a dynamic and important impact on connective tissue and extracellular matrix integrity. With respect to extracellular matrix stability, ascorbic acid serves as a cofactor for lysyl and prolyl hydroxylases. A decrease in prolyl and lysyl hydroxylase activity causes a net decrease in the production of hydroxyprolyl and hydroxylysyl residues in collagen and related proteins. Collagen is a protein that constitutes one third of the total protein in the body and is the major protein in the extracellular matrix of the connective tissue. Under-hydroxylated collagen polypeptide chains do not associate properly and often are more susceptible to degradation than normal forms of collagen; this is an underlying factor in many of the lesions associated with scurvy. (Pro, proline; Hypro, hydroxyproline.)

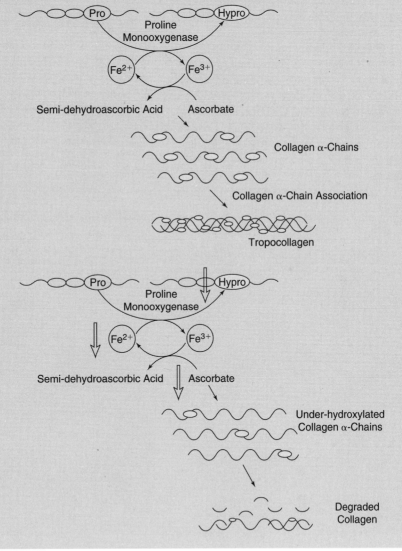

formation of fibers and protein complexes, whose molecular masses can range into the millions of daltons (Reiser et al., 1992). The formation of interchain cross-links also renders collagen and elastin resistant to the action of many proteinases so that these proteins can exist in a proteinase-enriched environment without significant damage or alteration.

As mechanisms for the involvement of nutrition in protein modifications, specific nutrient deficiencies can cause decreases in given enzymatic activities or catalytic functions, particularly if the nutrient serves as a cofactor for the activity or catalytic function. Caloric restrictions or excesses may also alter the synthesis or degradation of amino acids and other components important to amino acid, peptide, or protein modification.

Much of the regulation and metabolism discussed in subsequent chapters is largely the result of events that depend on posttranscriptional/posttranslational modifications of proteins. Transcription, translation, and the movement of substances into, through, and out of given cells are all dependent on changes in proteins brought about by enzymatic and nonenzymatic chemical modifications.

In subsequent chapters, when the actions of specific nutrients are described, continually ask how the action or role of the nutrient may be related to some aspect of protein structure or amino acid modification.

REFERENCES

Branden, C. and Tooze, J. (eds.) (1991) *Introduction to Protein Structure.* Garland, New York

Darby, N. J. (1993) *Protein Structure.* IRL Press/Oxford University Press, Oxford.

Davies, J. S. (1985) *Amino Acids and Peptides.* Chapman and Hall, New York.

Hamaguchi, K. (1992) *The Protein Molecule: Conformation, Stability, and Folding.* Japan Scientific Societies Press, Tokyo; Springer-Verlag, New York.

Konig, W. S. (1993) *Peptide and Protein Hormones: Structure, Regulation, Activity. A Reference Manual.* Weinheim VCH, New York.

Nesloney, C. L. and Kelly, J. W. (1996) Progress towards understanding beta-sheet structure. Bioorg Med Chem 4:739–766.

Reiser, K., McCormick, R. J. and Rucker, R. B. (1992) Enzymatic and non-enzymatic cross-linking of collagen and elastin. FASEB J 6:2439–2449.

Rucker, R. B. and McGee, C. (1993) Chemical modifications of proteins in vivo: Selected examples important to cellular regulation. J Nutr 123:977–990.

Rucker, R. B. and Wold, F. (1988) Cofactors in and as post-translational protein modifications. FASEB J 2:2252–2261.

RECOMMENDED READINGS

Branden, C. and Tooze, J. (eds.) (1991) *Introduction to Protein Structure.* Garland, New York.

Karplus, M. and McCammon, J. A. (1986) The dynamics of proteins. Sci Am 254:42–51.

◆ ◆

CHAPTER 3

Structure and Properties of Lipids

Donald M. Small, M.D.

O U T L I N E

C O M M O N   A B B R E V I A T I O N S

CMC (critical micellar concentration)
DHA (docosahexaenoic acid)
EPA (eicosapentaenoic acid)
PC (phosphatidylcholine)
PE (phosphatidylethanolamine)
PG (phosphatidylglycerol)
PI (phosphatidylinositol)
PS (phosphatidylserine)

LIPIDS AND THEIR FUNCTIONS

Lipids are one of the four major classes of biologically essential organic molecules found in all living organisms (the other classes are proteins, carbohydrates, and nucleic acids). A broad range of compounds are included in this class, based on their solubility characteristics. Lipids contain a substantial contiguous portion of aliphatic or aromatic hydrocarbon and have intermediate gram molecular weights that range between 100 and 5000. Included are hydrocarbons, steroids, soaps, detergents, and more complex molecules such as waxes, triacylglycerols (fats and oils), phospholipids, sphingolipids, fat-soluble vitamins, and lipopolysaccharides.

The major lipids are classified chemically in Table 3–1. They function as barriers, receptors, antigens, sensors, electrical insulators, biological detergents, membrane anchors for proteins, and, last but not least, a major energy source. Phospholipids play a critical role in maintaining the integrity of all living things, plant and animal, because they form the barrier separating the living cell from the extracellular environment. This barrier is called the cell or plasma membrane. It consists of a continuous bilayer of phospholipids into which other lipids, such as cholesterol and glycosphingolipids, are inserted. Into this lipid bilayer, protein channels, transporters, receptors, structural pillars such as integrins, and other functional elements are inserted to give the plasma membrane its unique characteristics. The fatty acid composition of the phospholipids and the cholesterol content regulate the fluidity and perhaps the thickness of the membrane. More cholesterol and saturated or *trans*-unsaturated fatty acyl groups in phospholipids and glycosphingolipids tend to stiffen the membrane. Glycosphingolipids are present only on the external surface of the plasma membrane. They act as receptors for toxins (e.g., ganglioside GM_1 is the receptor for cholera toxin) and probably as antigens to mark the cell as being of a certain type.

Phospholipids also form membranes, or barriers, between compartments of the cell (e.g., the membranes of the nucleus, the mitochondria, the endoplasmic reticulum (ER), the Golgi apparatus, secretory vesicles, and

TABLE 3–1
A Chemical Classification of Lipids *

   I. Hydrocarbons (normal, branched, saturated, unsaturated, cyclic, aromatic)
  II. Substituted hydrocarbons
    A. Alcohols
    B. Aldehydes
    C. Fatty acids, soaps, acid-soaps
    D. Amines
 III. Waxes and other simple esters of fatty acids
 IV. Fats and most oils (esters of fatty acids with glycerol)
    A. Triacylglycerols
    B. Diacylglycerols
    C. Monoacylglycerols
  V. Glycerophospholipids (diacyl; *O*-alkyl, acyl; di-*O*-alkyl)
    A. Phosphatidic acid
    B. Choline glycerophospholipids
    C. Ethanolamine glycerophospholipids
    D. Serine glycerophospholipids
    E. Inositol glycerophospholipids
    F. Phosphatidylglycerols
    G. Lysoglycerophospholipids
 VI. Glycoglycerolipids (including sulfates)
VII. Sphingolipids
    A. Sphingosine
    B. Ceramide
    C. Sphingomyelin
    D. Glycosphingolipids [ceramide monohexosides (cerebrosides), ceramide monohexoside sulfates, ceramide polyhexosides]
    E. Sialoglycosphingolipids (gangliosides)
VIII. Steroids (sterols, bile acids, digitonin and other cardiac glycosides, sex and adrenal hormones)
 IX. Other lipids [vitamins (A, D, E, K), eicosanoids, acyl CoA, acylcarnitine, glycosyl phosphatidylinositols, lipopolysaccharides, ubiquinone, dolichols]

*The chemical classification of lipids given in this table is necessarily incomplete and somewhat arbitrary. It progresses from hydrocarbons to more complex chemical structures. Simple esters and glycerol esters yield, on hydrolysis, the alcohol and/or glycerol and fatty acid. The major membrane lipids, glycerophospholipids, yield fatty acid (or alcohol), glycerol, phosphate, and the appropriate base (choline, ethanolamine, etc.). Sphingolipids yield the base sphingosine and a fatty acid on hydrolysis.

From Small, D. M. and Zoeller, R. A. (1991) Lipids. In: Encyclopedia of Human Biology, Vol. 4, pp. 725–748. Academic Press, Inc., Orlando, Florida.

peroxisomes). Phospholipids by themselves form very strong bilayers, which are effective barriers and do not let most molecules, including water and ions, cross readily. Each membrane must have specific proteins bound to or inserted through the membranes to allow certain molecules to pass or be transported from one side to the other. These protein assemblies are often called pores, channels, or transporters. They transport very large molecules such as RNA through the nuclear pores and medium-sized molecules such as proteins through the ER. Small ions [e.g., hydrogen (H^+), sodium (Na^+), potassium (K^+), and calcium (Ca^{2+})] and water are also carried by transporters. There are many such transporters, and they often have receptors for a specific molecule associated with them. These receptors bind the molecule and pass it to the transporter, which moves it across the cell membrane. It is widely believed that the function of these receptors and channels is affected by the type of membrane lipids in which they reside. However, firm proof of this hypothesis in vivo is lacking (Edidin, 1997).

Fats, oils, and waxes are stored in cytoplasmic droplets and represent a major source of cellular energy. An average human being in metabolic balance may easily ingest and absorb 100 g of fat in a day. The 900 kcal derived from burning this fat would represent 35% to 45% of the total energy consumed. Components of fats (i.e., fatty acids, fatty alcohols, and glycerol) are used as building blocks for membranes during growth, maintenance, and repair. Many hormones are lipids. The steroid hormones (cortisol, estrogens, progesterones, and androgens), derived from cholesterol, and prostaglandins and leukotrienes, derived from polyunsaturated fatty acids, are examples. Low concentrations of these molecules affect important physiological changes. Cholesterol has recently been found to be essential in embryogenesis, and an absolute deficiency of this sterol leads to severe and often fatal defects (Porter et al., 1996; Salen et al., 1996). Other lipids act as regulators of intracellular processes (e.g., diacylglycerol, sphingosine, ceramides, and platelet-activating factor). Some lipids are secreted and act as pheromones that attract or repel other organisms. In higher animals, lipids are transported to and from cells in the form of small (10 to 10,000 nm diameter) aggregates called lipoproteins. Lipids in the brain, spinal cord, and nerves are ordered in a way that permits the transmission of electrical impulses without short-circuiting between nerves or tracts. Lipids also play a role in many diseases that afflict humans (e.g., atherosclerosis, obesity, gallstone disease, Reye's syndrome, the familial lipidoses such as Tay-Sachs disease, Niemann-Pick disease, and Gaucher's disease, and the familial lipoproteinemias).

Most lipids, including most fatty acid building blocks of complex glycero- or sphingolipids, can be made by cells. However, in humans, certain fatty acids cannot be synthesized de novo and must be ingested. These are called the essential fatty acids, and if they are not ingested, deficiencies will occur. Two key types of essential fatty acids are known, one having a cis double bond at the 3rd carbon from the methyl end and the other a cis double bond at the 6th carbon counting from the terminal methyl group. These are called the omega 3 (ω3) and omega 6 (ω6) series of fatty acids (Nestlé Nutrition Workshop, 1992). These essential fatty acids are discussed in detail in Chapter 15. The ω3 series is present in some plant oils as α-linolenic acid (Table 3–2). This 18 carbon fatty acid with 3 cis double bonds can be elongated and further unsaturated to form the 20-carbon eicosapentaenoic acid (EPA) and then converted to the 22-carbon acid docosahexaenoic acid (DHA). EPA and DHA are found in high amounts in some fish oils. These fatty acids become acyl groups on some phospholipids. DHA is very enriched in parts of the brain and retina and appears essential for proper neural function and vision. The ω6 series is widely found in plant oils as linoleic and γ-linolenic acids (Table 3–2). They are elongated and further unsaturated to arachidonic acid (C20:4ω6), which is essential for the formation of prostaglandins and leukotrienes.

Essential fatty acid deficiency can occur in premature infants, children, and adults deprived of adequate ω3 and/or ω6 fatty acids as can occur in individuals with large resections of the intestine, fat malabsorption syndromes, or inadequate dietary intake. Adults need some fat (perhaps 30 to 50 g/day) and must have an adequate supply of essential fatty acids (a few grams a day), but average fat intake is much higher than this, perhaps 100 to 110 g/day in the United States and other westernized countries. Excess intake of cholesterol and fat, especially saturated fat, contributes greatly to obesity, atherosclerosis, diabetes, gallstone disease, and perhaps cancer.

TABLE 3–2

Names, Formulas, and Selected Properties of Some Common Fatty Acids

Fatty Acid	Chemical Name	Δ Formula*	ω Formula†	MW	Melting Point (°C)	Solubility μmol/L (25°C)
Saturated						
Lauric (D)	Dodecanoic acid	12.0	—	200.31	44.2	11.5
Myristic (M)	Tetradecanoic acid	14.0	—	228.36	54.4	0.79
Palmitic (P)	Hexadecanoic acid	16.0	—	256.42	62.9	0.12
Stearic (S)	Octadecanoic acid	18.0	—	284.47	69.6	(18×10^{-3})‡
Arachidic	Eicosanoic acid	20.0	—	312.52	75.4	(27×10^{-4})‡
Behenic	Docosanoic acid	22.0	—	340.57	80.0	
Lignoceric	Tetracosanoic acid	24.0	—	368.62	84.2	
Monounsaturated						
Myristoleic	cis-9-Tetradecenoic acid	14.1 9c	14:1ω5	226.34		
Palmitoleic	cis-9-Hexadecenoic acid	16.1 9c	16:1ω7	254.40	0.5	(2.00)‡
Oleic (O)	cis-9-Octadecenoic acid	18.1 9c	18:1ω9	282.45	13.4α; 16.3β	(0.30)‡
Elaidic (E)	trans-9-Octadecenoic acid	18.1 9t	18:1ω9 (trans)	282.45	46.5	(45×10^{-3})‡
cis-Vaccenic	cis-11-Octadecenoic acid	18.1 11c	18:1ω7	282.45	14.5	
Petroselinic	cis-6-Octadecenoic acid	18.6 6c	18:1ω12	282.45	30	
Erucic (Er)	cis-13-Docosenoic acid	22.1 13c	22:1ω9	348.55	34.7	(7×10^{-3})‡
Polyunsaturated						
Linoleic (L)	all cis-9,12-Octadecadienoic acid	18.2 9c12c	18:2ω6	280.44	−5	
γ-Linolenic	all cis-6,9,12-Octadecatrienoic acid	18.3 6c9c12c	18:3ω6	278.44		
Linolenic (Ln)	all cis-9,12,15-Octadecatrienoic acid	18.3 9c12c15c	18:3ω3	278.44	−10 (−11.3)	
ETA§	all cis-5,8,11-Eicosatrienoic acid	20.3 5c8c11c	20:3ω9			
Arachidonic (A)	all cis-5,8,11,14-Eicosatetraenoic acid	20.4 5c8c11c14c	20:4ω6	304.5	−49.5	
EPA‖	all cis-5,8,11,14,17-Eicosapentaenoic acid	20.5 5c8c11c14c17c	20:5ω3	302.5		
DHA‖	all cis-4,7,10,13,16,19-Docosahexaenoic acid	22.6 4c7c10c13c16c19c	22:6ω3	328.5		

*Formulas are shown as the number of carbon atoms followed by the number of double bonds. The position of each double bond is indicated by the lower of the numbers of the two doubly bonded carbon atoms, counting from the carboxyl carbon and specified as to cis (c) or trans (t) configuration. Thus, oleic (cis-9-octadecenoic) acid is 18.1 9c.

†The number of the carbon atoms starts from the methyl end, and the location of the first (or only) double bond is indicated by a single number as a suffix preceded by "ω". Oleic acid is therefore designated as c18:1ω9, which informs the reader that the most distal double bond is 9 carbons from the methyl terminus. It is assumed that unless otherwise specified, all multiple double bonds in polyunsaturated fatty acids have the 1,4 relation to each other.

‡Extrapolated from solubility of shorter-chain acids.

§ETA, eicosatrienoic acid, an acid that accumulates in essential fatty acid deficiency.

‖Found in marine animals in high concentration. EPA, eicosapentaenoic acid; DHA, docosahexaenoic acid.

From Small, D. M. and Zoeller, R. A. (1991) Lipids. In: Encyclopedia of Human Biology, Vol. 4, pp. 725–748. Academic Press, Inc, Orlando, Florida.

THE CHEMICAL CLASSES OF LIPIDS

As summarized in Table 3–1, lipids include many types of compounds: hydrocarbons, steroids, soaps, detergents, and more complex molecules such as waxes, triacylglycerols (fats and oils), phospholipids, sphingolipids, fat-soluble vitamins, and lipopolysaccharides.

Hydrocarbons

Hydrocarbons contain only hydrogen and carbon. They may be saturated or unsaturated, branched or unbranched, cyclic or aliphatic, or they may exhibit a combination of these characteristics. The polyisoprenoids are a major source of hydrocarbons of biological origin (Ness and McKean, 1977). For example, a group of 40-carbon polyenoic compounds (phytoene, phytofluenes, lycopene, etc.), composed of isoprene units:

$$CH_3$$
$$|$$
$$(-CH_2-C=CH-CH_2-)$$

is synthesized from mevalonic acid in plant cells to produce the carotenoids (Fig. 3–1). These complex hydrocarbons are ingested by animals, and some proportion is taken up into the gut cells. One of these, β-carotene, is oxidatively cleaved in the center to produce vitamin A, a 20-carbon polyisoprenoid alcohol, as discussed in Chapter 26. In animals, a similar pathway from mevalonic acid leads to the formation of ubiquinone (coenzyme Q), farnesyl (15 carbons) and geronylgeronyl (20 carbons) moieties, and the 30-carbon polyisoprenoid squalene (Fig. 3–1), which undergoes cyclization and oxidation to form steroids.

Dolichols are also derived through the isoprenoid synthetic pathway and consist of 15 to 19 isoprene units (75 to 90 carbon atoms), with phosphate esterified to the terminal alcohol group. They are found in the ER and Golgi membranes and function as anchors for oligosaccharide chains being synthesized in the lumen of these organelles. Their organization within these membranes is not known. These 75- to 95-Å-long molecules are either buried in the center of the bilayer, or they fold back and forth within the membrane three or four times, or their hydrophobic parts must be shielded by hydrophobic domains of proteins on either the cytosolic or luminal surface. The hydroxyl group of dolichol, which is usually esterified to phosphate, appears to be on the cytosolic side (outside) of the ER or Golgi apparatus, and to this a large number of sugars (up to 14) are attached by specific transferases. The oligosaccharide chain is then translocated en bloc to protein in the lumen during the posttranslational glycosylation process. Little is known about the physical properties of the dolichol phosphates and the dolichol glycophosphates.

The fat-soluble vitamins A, E, and K are also derived through modifications in the isoprenoid pathway. Vitamin D, which is derived from a sterol, contains isoprene units. These lipophilic molecules are found largely associated with lipid membranes or bound to specific carrier proteins.

Substituted Hydrocarbons

Alcohols ($R-CH_2OH$), aldehydes ($R-CHO$), acids ($R-COOH$), and amines ($R-CH_2NH_2$) are examples of substituted hydrocarbons.

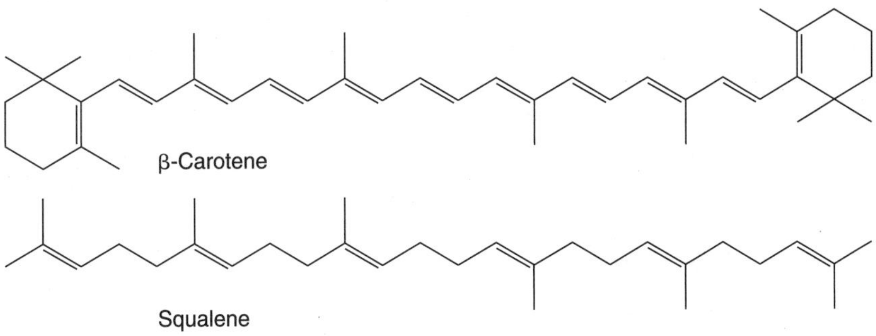

Figure 3–1. Line models of β-carotene and squalene, showing the similarity of their structures.

Such molecules are usually found in low (usually micromolar) concentrations in cells, as they are rapidly metabolized. Fatty acids are the most abundant of the substituted hydrocarbons. The plasma concentration is about 0.5 to 1.0 mmol/L with about 99% bound to albumin. Fatty acids have the potential to reach high local concentrations during fat catabolism. For instance, during lipolysis of chylomicron or very low density lipoprotein (VLDL) triacylglycerols by plasma lipoprotein lipase, free fatty acids are liberated. Sites of high lipolytic activity (e.g., the capillary beds in adipose tissue, muscle, and heart) may see very high concentrations of the fatty acids. In certain disease states (e.g., diabetic ketoacidosis, nephrotic syndrome, hypertriglyceridemia, and hyperthyroidism), the concentration of plasma fatty acids rises; this results in an elevation of the fatty acid to albumin ratio and facilitates greater partitioning of the fatty acids to plasma lipoproteins and to cell membranes, which may possibly cause local damage (Cistola et al., 1986).

The major saturated fatty acids in higher animals are palmitic (16 carbons) and stearic (18 carbons), followed by smaller amounts of 12-, 14-, and 20-carbon fatty acids (Table 3–2). The major monounsaturated fatty acids are oleic acid (18:1ω9), which has 18 carbon atoms and a *cis* double bond at carbon 9; vaccenic acid (18:1ω7), which has the double bond at carbon 11 (numbering from the carboxyl end); and palmitoleic acid, (16:1ω7), which has a *cis* double bond at carbon 9. The major polyunsaturated fatty acids in plasma and tissues are linoleic (C18:2ω6), arachidonic (C20:4ω6), eicosapentaenoic (EPA; C20:5ω3), and docosahexaenoic (DHA; C22:6ω3). In polyunsaturated fatty acids, the double bonds are usually three carbons apart ($-CH_2-CH=CH-CH_2-CH=CH-CH_2-$). Arachidonic acid is shown in Figure 3–2. Abbreviated nomenclature for fatty acids, numbering carbons from either the carboxyl (Δ system) or from the terminal methyl (ω system) end, is shown in Table 3–2.

Fatty acids are essential building blocks for membrane lipids. The essential fatty acids linoleic (C18:2ω6), arachidonic (C20:4ω6), EPA (C20:5ω3), and DHA (C22:6ω3) are necessary for proper growth and membrane function. Arachidonic acid, which is derived from linoleic acid by chain elongation and desaturation, is a major precursor of eicosanoids such as prostaglandins, prostacyclins, thromboxanes, and leukotrienes.

Recently it has been shown that some proteins are covalently linked to fatty acids. The reactions show high specificity for certain fatty acids. For instance, myristic acid (C14:0) is specifically attached to the amino group of the N-terminal glycine by an amide bond in a number of proteins, including the oncogenic viral Src protein, calcineurin, and recoverin (Johnson et al., 1994). Viral Src protein is oncogenic only when it is myristoylated; calcineurin and recoverin are Ca^{2+}-sensing proteins in the brain and retina, respectively. The myristoyl group acts as a switch when Ca^{2+} binds to the protein and allows the protein to anchor to a membrane to start a cascade of reactions (Ames et al., 1996). Palmitic acid (16:0) is covalently bound to many proteins at cysteinyl residues along the peptide chain through *S*-palmitoyl cysteine esters. These palmitates may anchor proteins such as caveolin to membranes. Many proteins are also linked to the polyisoprenoid alcohols farnesol (15 carbons) and geronylgeronol (20 carbons) as thioesters (Zhang and Casey 1996). These covalent linkages are essential for proper function of such mammalian proteins as nuclear lamin, a structural protein of the nuclear membrane, and Ras, guanosine triphosphate (GTP)-binding proteins that play a crucial role in signaling pathways essential to cell differentiation and growth.

Waxes, Esters, and Ethers

Waxes are long-chained, rather nonpolar compounds found on the surfaces of plants and animals (Hamilton, 1995). Some waxes are

CH₃(CH₂)₄(CH=CHCH₂)₄(CH₂)₂COOH

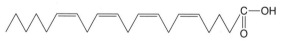

Figure 3–2. Arachidonic acid (all-cis-5,8,11,14-eicosatetraenoic acid).

straight-chained, branched, or unsaturated hydrocarbons, but many are esters of long-chain alcohols, $R'–CH_2OH$, and long-chain fatty acids, $R–COOH$, (e.g., $R–COOCH_2–R'$). These saturated long-chain waxes tend to be solids at ambient temperature.

Plankton and higher members of the aquatic food chain, including coral, mollusks, fish, sharks, and even whales, store large quantities of waxes. Waxes are also present in human skin lipids, beans, seeds, and leaves, serving to make the outer surface nonwettable. Ethers ($R–CH_2OCH_2–R'$) are also present in skin lipids, forming a barrier against water loss (Elias, 1991). Waxes of long-chain alcohols and acids are nonpolar molecules. They accumulate in intracellular droplets or on surfaces of leaves or skin and have almost no solubility in cellular membranes.

Acylglycerols and Fats

Many complex lipids have a backbone of glycerol, a 3-carbon polyalcohol. When a substitution is made at one end of the glycerol molecule, the 2-carbon becomes optically active, as, for instance, in glycerophosphate. The standard nomenclature used is the *sn* terminology. A single substitution of octadecanoic acid to form an ester bond, e.g., at the 1-position of glycerol, produces 1-octadecanoyl-*sn*-glycerol (Fig. 3–3). When two fatty acids are reacted with glycerol to form ester bonds, a diacylglycerol or diglyceride is formed (e.g., 1,3-diacyl-*sn*-glycerol or 1,2-diacyl-*sn*-glycerol). Diacylglycerols are biochemical intermediates in many lipolytic reactions, are critical building blocks used in the synthesis of more complex phospholipids and triacylglycerols, and

are second messengers for some membrane-triggered reactions.

A triacylglycerol or triglyceride is formed when all three hydroxyls of glycerol form ester bonds with fatty acids. If all three fatty acids are the same, the triacylglycerol is called a simple triacylglycerol (e.g., triolein). If one of the fatty acids is different, it becomes a complex triacylglycerol. The properties of glycerides (e.g., melting point) depend greatly on the fatty acid chains involved. Triacylglycerols are the major storage lipids of plants and higher animals. Both plant oils (olive, corn, safflower) and animal fats (lard, suet, tallow) are nearly pure mixtures of complex triacylglycerols. Trace amounts of sterols, vitamins, free fatty acids, carotenoids, and other fat-soluble molecules can also be present in fats. In animals, adipose tissue is the main source of fat, but skeletal muscle, heart, liver, skin, and bone marrow often contain appreciable amounts of triacylglycerols in intracellular oil droplets.

A single meal often contains dietary fat from a variety of sources (dairy, meat, vegetable). These mix with digestive secretions in the stomach and small intestine and undergo digestion and absorption (Carey et al., 1983; Patton, 1981). It is surprising that absorption from the lumen is generally quite efficient, and only about 4% of the ingested fat escapes into the feces (Carey et al., 1983). However, absorption of specific, highly saturated fats may be less efficient.

Vegetable oils, margarine, meat fats, butter, and other dietary fats are each composed of hundreds of different complex triacylglycerols, and most of these have not been analyzed completely. The general structure of a triacyl-

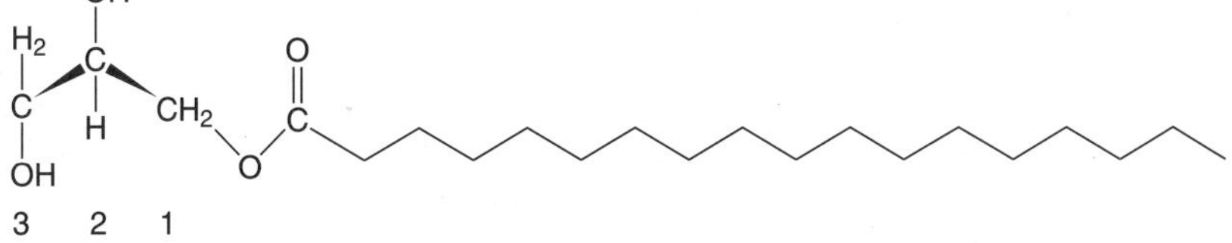

1-Octadecanoyl-*sn*-Glycerol
(D-α-Monostearin)

Figure 3–3. Line model of a monoacylglycerol, showing the stereospecificity of the glycerol conformation. With the glycerol carbon in the 2 (middle) position in the plane of the page and carbons 1 and 3 behind the plane of the page, if the –OH on carbon 2 points up then the carbon on the right is designated carbon 1 and the one on the left, carbon 3. Glycerol carbon numbers are shown below the glycerol structure.

glycerol is shown in Figure 3–4. The three R groups stand for different acyl groups. Using the International Union of Pure and Applied Chemistry/International Union of Biochemistry (IUPAC-IUB) nomenclature (Commission on Biochemical Nomenclature, 1968) with the carbon in the central (secondary) position in the plane of the page and the primary or end carbons behind the plane of the page, if the hydroxyl group on the midcarbon is drawn to the left, then the top carbon becomes *sn*-1, the midcarbon becomes *sn*-2, and the bottom carbon becomes *sn*-3. If the groups at the 1 and 3 positions are different (e.g., as shown for the different acyl groups in Figure 3–4), then the molecule has an asymmetrical carbon at the 2 position, and the optical isomers (enantiomers) 1R′-2R″-, 3R‴-*sn*-glycerol and 1R‴-, 2R″-, 3R′-*sn*-glycerol are possible.

The triacylglycerol composition of oils, fats, and lipoproteins is usually reported as the total overall fatty acid composition of the triacylglycerol mixture. This information is easily obtained (Bailey, 1950; Consumer and Food Economics Institute, 1976–1990; Gunstone et al., 1994; Kuksis, 1978; Sonntag, 1979) and is valuable because it tells us which major fatty acids are esterified to the glycerol; however, it does not tell us their position on glycerol or how many specific triacylglycerol species are present in a given sample (Small, 1991). If the sample is treated with pancreatic lipase to cleave the fatty acids in the primary 1 and 3 positions of each triacylglycerol to produce two fatty acids and a 2-monoacylglycerol, and if these in turn are analyzed, then we learn globally which fatty acids are in the 2 position and in the 1 and 3 positions. This procedure does not distinguish between the 1 and 3 positions or reveal which primary fatty acids were linked to which monoacylglycerol. In theory, the number of triacylglycerols (N) that could be present in a sample having n different fatty acids is n^3 (Farines et al., 1988).

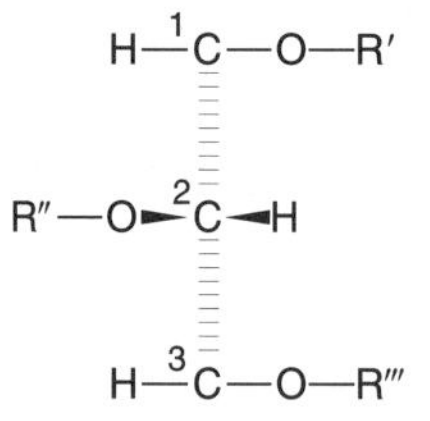

For example, if a sample of fat had 10 different fatty acids, the possible number of individual triacylglycerols would be $10^3 = 1000$. This includes positional isomers and enantiomers—that is, optical isomers in which a specific fatty acid is either at the *sn*-1 or *sn*-3 position. If one simply considers racemic mixtures in which the 1 and 3 positions can be interchanged, then $N = (n^3 + n^2)/2$. If one considers only the fatty acid combinations on the three positions and ignores positional isomers, then $N = (n^3 + n^2 + 2n)/6$. Thus, if a specific sample contains only three different fatty acids (e.g., R′, R″, R‴), then the total number of isomers, including positional isomers and enantiomers, would be 27. If we exclude optical isomers, there would be 18, and if we exclude positional isomers, there would be 7. Considering that many dietary fats and oils often have 10 or more major fatty acids, the number of potential individual triacylglycerols becomes enormous. In fact, butterfat has both short- and long-chain fatty acids as well as many unsaturated ones (Breckinridge, 1978) and, therefore, probably consists of thousands of individual stereospecific triacylglycerols. For this reason even cow's milk fat has not been completely analyzed (Myher et al., 1988).

In a careful search of the literature (Small, 1991), the major triacylglycerols found in a variety of natural fats and oils were identified and are listed in Table 3–3. Most of these have not been fully analyzed, and the specific stereoisomers are generally not reported. In some examples positional isomers are indicated, and in a few rare cases the optical isomers are given (i.e., mustard seed oil; Myher et al., 1979). The melting point (MP) (or range of melting) of the fat is also given. Fats with a high content of saturated long-chain fats have high MPs. Butter, lard, and

Figure 3–4. *The Commission on Biochemical Nomenclature (1968) has recommended nomenclature for substituted glycerides—e.g., the phosphoglycerides. With the carbon in the 2 (middle) position in the plane of the page and carbons 1 and 3 behind the plane of the page, if the –OH on carbon 2 of the glycerol is drawn to the left, then the top carbon is designated carbon 1 and the bottom carbon becomes 3. A triacylglycerol with myristic acid on position 1, oleic acid on position 2, and palmitic acid on position 3 would be described as sn-glycerol-1-myristate-2-oleate-3-palmitate, or simply as sn-MOP.*

TABLE 3–3
Composition and Melting of Some Natural Fats and Oils*

Fat or Oil	Melting Point (°C)†	Major Triacylglycerols
Butterfat	37 to 38	PPB‡ PPC‡ POP‡
Horse fat		OOO POO LOO
Lard	46 to 49	SPO‡ OPL‡ OPO‡
Tallow (beef)	40	POO POP POS
Cocoa butter	28 to 36	POS SOS POP
Coconut oil	24 to 27	DDD CDD CDM
Palm kernel oil	24 to 29	DDD MOD ODO
Almond oil		OOO OLO OLL
Corn oil	−14	LLL LOL LLP
Cottonseed oil	5 to 11	PLL POL LLL
Egg triglycerides		POO PLO POS
Grapeseed oil	8	LLL OLL POL
Hazelnut oil		OOO OLO POO
Olive oil	−7	OOO OOP OLO
Palm oil	30 to 36	POP POO POL
Peanut oil	−8 to +12	OOL POL OLL
Rice bran oil		PLO OOL POO
Safflower oil	−15	LLL LLO LLP
Soybean oil	−14	LLL LLO LLP
Sunflower oil	−17	LLL OLL LOO
Walnut oil		LLL OLL PLL
Rapeseed oil (low Er)	5	OOO LOO OOLn
Linseed oil	−17	LnLnLn LnLnL LnLnO
Rapeseed oil (high Er)		ErOEr ErLEr ErLnEr
Mustard seed oil§		ErOEr‡ ErLEr‡ OOEr‡

*Abbreviations used for acyl chains in the triacylglycerols: B = C-4:0 (butyric), C = C-10:0 (capric), D = C-12:0 (dodecanoic), M = C-14:0 (myristic), P = C-16:0 (palmitic), S = C-18:0 (stearic), O = C-18:1 (*cis*) (oleic), E = C-18:1 (*trans*) (elaidic), L = C-18:2 (linoleic), Ln = C-18:3 (linolenic), G = C-20:1 (gogoleic), Er = C-22:1 (erucic).

†The melting points or ranges of melting of these fats and oils are taken from references reported in Small (1991).

‡Specific triacylglycerols estimated from stereospecific fatty acid analyses, as in 1S,2P,3O-*sn*-glycerol.

§The stereospecific composition of the eight most prevalent triacylglycerols of mustard seed oil, which comprise 40% of the total, is ErOEr = 8.2%, ErLEr = 6.8%, OOEr = 5.9%, ErLnEr = 5.3%, OLEr = 4.9%. OLnEr = 3.8%, GOEr = 3.3%, and GLEr = 2.7%.

From Small, D. M. (1991) The effects of glyceride structure on absorption and metabolism. Annu Rev Nutr 11:413–434. Used with permission, from the Annual Review of Nutrition, Volume 11 © 1991 by Annual Reviews.

tallow, all animal fats, have MPs at or above body temperature (37°C). Excess intake of high-melting fats has been shown to increase plasma concentrations of beta lipoproteins (LDL, VLDL) (Grundy, 1991). The concentrations of these lipoproteins are raised by ingestion of high amounts of saturated fat (>30 g intake per day). This "bad fat" increases the risk of cardiovascular disease, such as stroke and heart attack, and dietary intake of saturated fats by adults should be limited to 20 to 30 g/day (less than 10% of total calories).

Glycerophospholipids

Glycerophospholipids have a phosphate at the 3 position of glycerol and acyl or alkyl groups on at least one (usually both) of the other glycerol carbons. The phosphate esterified to the *sn*-3-glycerol may be free (phosphatidic acid) or esterified to other small molecules (Fig. 3–5) to form phosphatidylcholine (PC, lecithin), phosphatidylethanolamine (PE), phosphatidylserine (PS), phosphatidylglycerol (PG), or phosphatidylinositol (PI). All these phospholipids have two acyl chains esterified to the glycerol but different head groups, some carrying a net negative charge (PS, PI, PG) and some zwitterionic (PC, PE) at pH 7. The net charge is due to ionization of the phosphate and of the amino alcohols. In some cases alkyl chains are linked to the glycerol moiety by ether bonds (–C–O–C–). One ether-linked phospholipid, platelet-activating factor (hexadecyl, 2-acetyl-*sn*-glycerol-3-phosphocholine) causes marked vasoactivity. Plasmalogens have a vinyl ether –C–O–C=C–, and these may act as antioxidants.

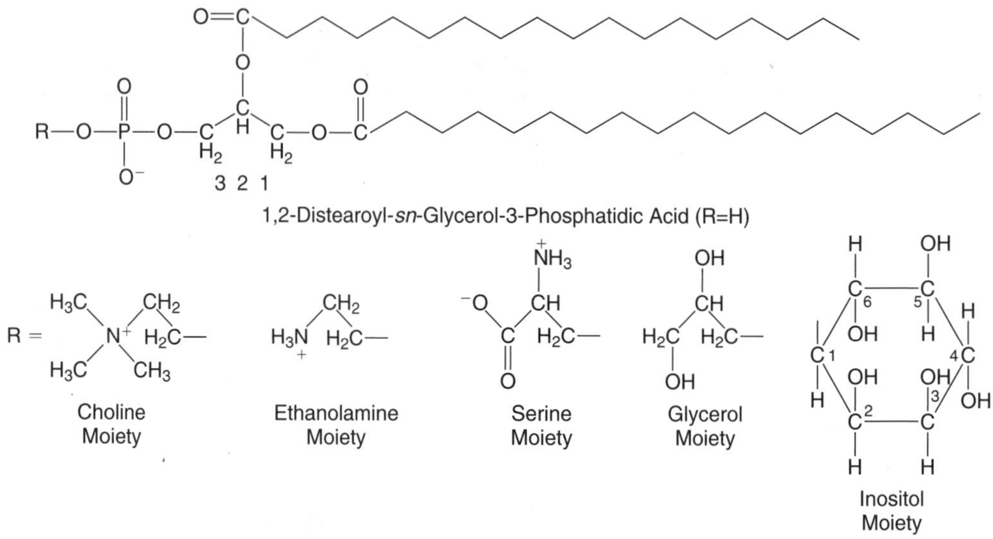

Figure 3–5. *Line models of some phospholipids. If R= hydrogen, the compound is the phosphatidic acid as indicated. If the polar moieties shown below are substituted at R, the compound is the corresponding phosphatidyl-R (i.e., if R is choline, the compound is phosphatidylcholine).*

When one of the acyl groups of a glycerolphospholipid is removed, a phospholipid with a single hydrocarbon chain is formed; this is called a "lyso" compound. Lysophospholipids are detergents because of their strong water-soluble head group and their lipid-soluble hydrocarbon chain. A rare genetic deficiency of the enzyme lecithin:cholesterol acyltransferase (LCAT), which transfers the fatty acid on the *sn*-2 position of lecithin (PC) to cholesterol to form a cholesterol ester and lysolecithin, has been described. Deficiency of this enzyme results in accumulation of lecithin (PC) and free cholesterol in plasma lipoproteins. Most phospholipids are part of the main structure of membranes but some, such as PS and PI, may have more specific functions. PS seems to be a marker for apoptotic cells, and PI plays a role in generating two second messengers, inositol triphosphate (IP_3) and diacylglycerol, at the membrane surface. Glucosyl phosphatidylinositols are a recently described class of lipid moieties that are attached to certain proteins (Englund, 1993) and act as membrane anchors for the protein (e.g., alkaline phosphatase). Such proteins may be released from the membranes by phospholipase C, which hydrolyzes the PI, leaving diacylglycerol in the membrane.

Sphingolipids

Sphingolipids (Bell et al., 1993) are formed by the addition of fatty acids to the base sphingosine. Ceramide is formed when a fatty acid is linked to sphingosine through an amide bond at the 2 position. Substituted ceramides are important constituents of skin lipids (Elias, 1991). (See Chapter 15 for the role of essential fatty acid in skin ceramides.) Elevated ceramide concentrations have been found in a disorder characterized by the inability of lysosomes to catabolize ceramide, known as Farber's disease. When ceramide is esterified with phosphocholine, sphingomyelin is formed. When sphingomyelin catabolic enzymes are absent, sphingomyelins accumulate in tissue, giving rise to Niemann-Pick disease.

Sphingosine can react with sugars to form psychosine, in which a monosaccharide is linked to the 1 carbon of sphingosine. When a monosaccharide is linked to the one position of a ceramide, a cerebroside such as galactocerebroside is formed (Fig. 3–6). Different sugars may be added to form a variety of neutral glycosphingolipids. Complex-charged glycocerebrosides, called gangliosides, are formed when sialic acid (negatively charged) is added to the sugars. Gangliosides in low

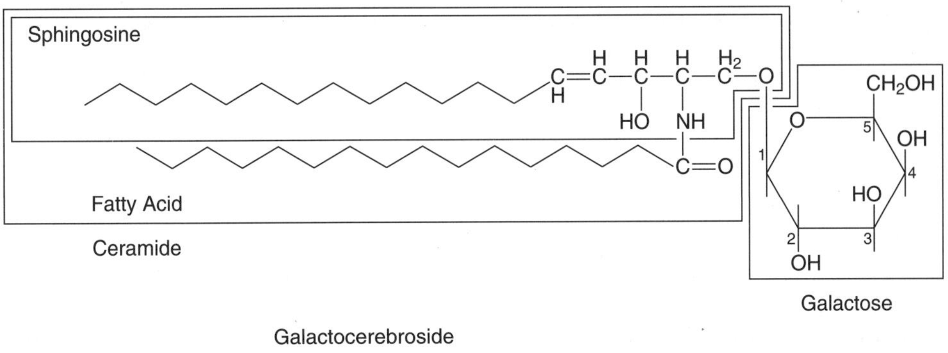

Figure 3–6. *Line model of a cerebroside. Sphingosine is D-erythro-2-amino-4-octadecene-1,3-diol. The ceramide shown is 2-stearoyl sphingosine, and the galactocerebroside is 1-galactosyl ceramide. The fatty acid is attached to sphingosine through an amide bond.*

concentration are firmly anchored to the outer surfaces of many plasma membranes and appear to act as both antigens and receptors for certain toxins, antibodies, and lectins. Specific enzymes are necessary for the catabolism of each of these glycolipids; when an enzyme is either absent or defective, the non-metabolized glycolipid molecule accumulates, resulting in a lipid storage disease.

Sphingolipid precursors or breakdown products such as sphingosine and ceramide may have important roles as cellular second messengers (Hannun, 1996). Sphingomyelin may also have a role in the intracellular movement of cholesterol.

Steroids

Steroids (Gunstone et al., 1994; Hamilton, 1995) are defined as "all those substances that are structurally related to the sterols and bile acids to the extent of possessing the characteristic perhydro-1,2-cyclopentano-phenanthrene ring system." This polycyclic structure, consisting of four linked rings, is illustrated in the structure of cholesterol (Fig. 3–7), a molecule that may modulate membrane fluidity, permeability, fusibility, and thickness. Although cholesterol appears in low amounts in some primitive animals such as sponges, it is the predominant sterol in higher animals. Steroid hormones (i.e., testosterone, androgens, estrogens, progesterones, cortisol, cortisone, aldosterone, and vitamin D hormone) are formed from cholesterol. These molecules exert major effects in regulating metabolism in higher ani-

mals. Plant sterols are present in vegetable oils. Normally, plant sterols are not absorbed by the intestine of humans, as discussed in Chapter 7. However, a rare genetic condition that permits their absorption leads to β-sitosterolemia, a disease in which large amounts of plant sterols are deposited in the body tissues. More complex molecules with a steroid nucleus, such as digitalis, are also found in plants. Digitalis is a strong stimulant for heart contractions and has been used for centuries to combat heart failure.

Cholesteryl esters are formed from fatty acids and cholesterol. These interesting molecules are often stored in organs, such as the adrenal gland and the corpus luteum of the ovary, where they serve as precursors for steroidal hormones. They also accumulate in certain disorders (e.g., cholesteryl ester storage disease, atherosclerosis, familial hypercholesterolemia, and Tangier disease). Cholesteryl esters form liquid crystals, which have been identified by polarizing microscopy in living tissues (Small, 1988; Waugh and Small, 1984).

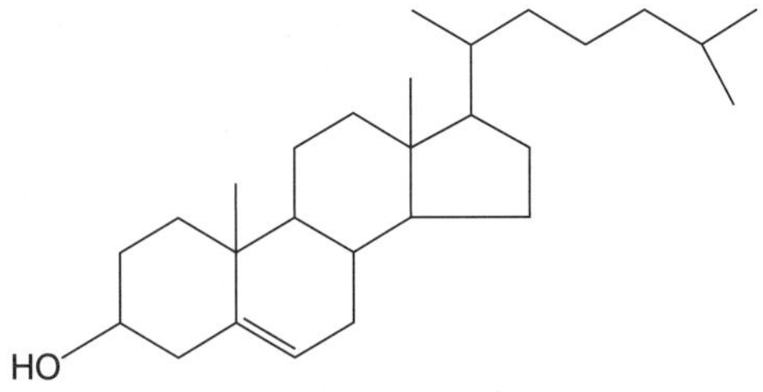

Cholest-5-en-3β-ol
(Cholesterol)

Figure 3–7. *Line drawing of cholesterol (cholest-5-en-3β-ol).*

Bile acids (Nair and Kritchesky 1971; Cabral and Small, 1989) are formed by degrading the terminal side chain of cholesterol from 27 carbon atoms to 24 carbon atoms and by adding hydroxyl (–OH) groups to various positions in the ring. Thus, bile acids such as cholic and chenodeoxycholic acids are formed (Fig. 3–8). The alkali metal salts of hydroxylated bile acids conjugated with taurine or glycine are natural detergents synthesized in the liver and secreted into bile. They solubilize phospholipid and cholesterol in the bile of higher animals, thus permitting secretion of cholesterol into the gut. The excretion of both cholesterol and bile acids is the major way cholesterol is removed from the body.

Bile salts also aid in the digestion and absorption of fat and fat-soluble vitamins in the intestine (Carey et al., 1983). Bile salt deficiency caused by intestinal pathology [e.g., mutant ileal bile acid transporter (Oelkers et al, 1997), celiac disease, tropical sprue, bacterial overgrowth, or ileal resection] can cause fat malabsorption and malnutrition. This problem is especially serious in children, in whom growth may be impaired. Bile acid deficiency may also lead to cholesterol gallstone formation, because bile salt is required for cholesterol solubilization in bile. Abnormal bile acid metabolism is associated with accumulation of cholestanol (the saturated analog of cholesterol) in the disease cerebrotendinous xanthomatosis.

Other Lipids

Eicosanoids are oxygenated fatty acids principally derived from the 20-carbon fatty acids, arachidonic acid, eicosatrienoic acid, and eicosapentaenoic acid (see Table 3–2). These oxygenated derivatives are present in low concentration, are chemically unstable, have a very short lifetime, and act as autocoids to influence contractility, membrane permeability, and many other cellular functions.

Acyl coenzyme A and acylcarnitine are key intermediates in fatty acid metabolism; they are usually present in low concentrations, but under certain conditions they may accumulate and disrupt cellular functions. Cytidine diphosphate-diacylglycerol (CDP-DAG) is an intermediate in phospholipid synthesis and probably partitions into membranes.

Lipopolysaccharides (endotoxin) are a large class of bacterial glycolipids, present in the outer leaf of the outer membrane of gram-negative organisms, that are complex in nature and may act in higher animals as toxins,

Bile Acid	R_1	R_2	R_3
Lithodeoxycholic	αOH	H	H
Deoxycholic	αOH	H	αOH
Chenodeoxycholic	αOH	αOH	H
Ursodeoxycholic	αOH	βOH	H
Cholic	αOH	αOH	αOH
Ursocholic	αOH	βOH	αOH

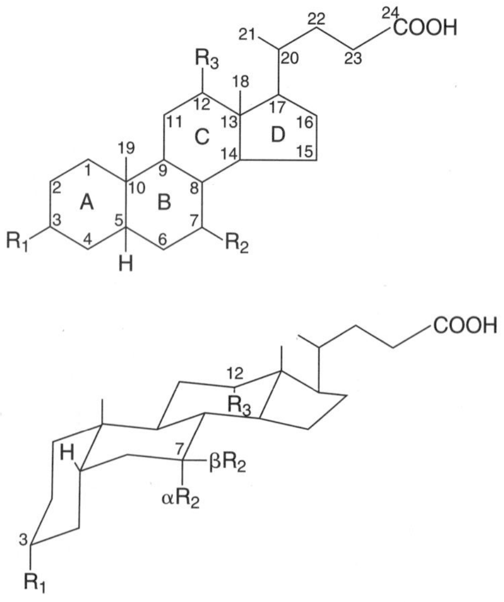

Figure 3–8. *Molecular structure of common bile acids, showing the common steroid ring and side chain structure. The location and orientation of hydroxyl group(s) are given for each bile acid.*

activators of phagocytic cells, transforming factors, and mutagens.

THE GENERAL PROPERTIES OF LIPIDS

The physical properties of lipids (see Small, 1986, for in-depth review), coupled with the reactivity of their substituent groups, determine the biological properties of lipids. The aliphatic hydrocarbon chain is an important constituent of many lipid molecules. A knowledge of the properties of the hydrocarbon chain is fundamental to understanding the behavior of any given lipid class, because there are striking similarities between chain packing in normal alkanes and chain packing in more complex aliphatic lipids. Most lipids, because of their hydrocarbon chains, are elongated molecules that align along their long axis and pack in layers more or less perpendicular to their molecular axis. X-ray diffraction has been extensively used to study the structure of the hydrocarbon chain, the packing between chains, and the crystalline and liquid crystalline packing of lipid molecules. The hydrocarbon chain, in its rigid, most stable crystalline state, forms a zigzag, all-*trans* arrangement from carbon to carbon (Fig. 3–9). The distance between carbons is about 1.533 Å, similar to the carbon-carbon distance in the diamond. The carbon-carbon bond angle slightly varies but approximates

112°. Thus, the distance between every other carbon atom is 2.54 Å, and the increment along the chain for each carbon atom is 1.27 Å.

Packing of Lipids in the Solid State

Crystalline hydrocarbons and the hydrocarbon chains of more complex lipids pack into two distinct classes of subcells. The first class is characterized by dense, tightly packed chains in which there is specific chain-chain interaction. In the second class, the chains are more loosely packed, and specific chain-chain interaction is weakened because of partial rotation of the chain and/or of its methylene (–CH$_2$–) groups. The tightly packed class includes lipids packed in orthorhombic, triclinic, or monoclinic subcells, which are important in such food products as chocolate but probably do not occur in vivo. The second class, with more loosely packed chains aligned hexagonally, may occur as microdomains in membrane subcells and may occasionally be present in pathological deposits in living organisms (Edidin, 1997).

The Liquid Crystalline State of Lipids

In nature, lipid aggregates are not usually crystalline but rather are found as liquid crystal-like arrays. The liquid crystal state (Small, 1986) is the fourth state of matter (the others

*Figure 3–9. Line and space-filling models of the hydrocarbon chain in its most stable zigzag, all-*trans* conformation. Carbon-carbon distances and bond angles are given. Projections down the chain are shown on the right. The space-filling models show the outlines of the minimal van der Waals radii, i.e., they show the shape of the chain. Carbon atoms are black and hydrogen atoms are white. Projections down the chain show the lumps and grooves formed by the chain and that the chain is a little wider in the direction vertical to the page than in that horizontal to the page. (Modified from Small, D. M. [1986] The Physical Chemistry of Lipids from Alkanes to Phospholipids. Handbook of Lipid Research, vol. 4. Plenum Press, New York.)*

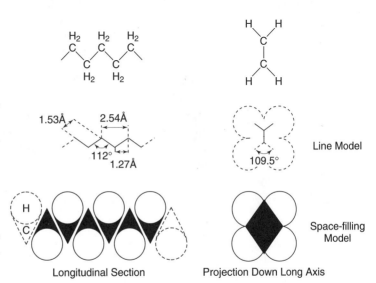

being gas, liquid, and solid), and it has properties of both crystals and liquids. This intermediate state combines both order and fluidity and thus is particularly suited to cellular function, especially the formation of membranes and other ordered structures such as retinal rods and cones, myelin, and chloroplasts. At least four factors can induce liquid crystalline formation in a particular lipid: temperature, pressure, magnetic field, and electrostatic field. Furthermore, certain molecules may be induced to form liquid crystals by the addition of water.

Many biological lipids form liquid crystals. For instance, when heated, cholesteryl esters, phospholipids, soaps (Na or K salts of long-chain fatty acids, e.g., K$^+$-stearate), and glycosphingolipids transform from crystals to liquid crystals. Hydration causes most phospholipids, monoacylglycerols, sphingosine, and glycosphingolipids to form hydrated liquid crystals at body temperature, and thus liquid crystals are the predominant state of these lipids in vivo. Fatty acids (RCOOH) exist only in low pH (<6), whereas Na and K acyl carboxylates (soaps) exist only at high pH (>8). At neutral pH, fatty acids exist as "acid-soaps," which are composed of 1 acid and 1 soap [e.g., K$^+$H$^+$ (RCOO$^-$)$_2$]. These compounds form liquid crystals in water.

Liquid crystals formed by lipids have been classified and are illustrated in Fig. 3–10 depending on their degree of long-range order as determined by x-ray diffraction (Small, 1986). Liquid crystals that have three-dimensional (3D) long-range order pack in a cubic lattice (Fig. 3–10, upper left) and could be considered crystalline. However, because the chain packing is liquid (melted), they are classified as liquid crystals. Lipids that form cubic crystals (the viscous isotropic state) include hydrated soaps, hydrated monoacylglycerols, and some hydrated phospholipids. Cubic structures of phospholipids may be efficient structures in which to store intracellular membrane phospholipids. Two-dimensional liquid crystals are ordered in either rectangular or hexagonal 2D lattices. The rectangular lattice is also called the "ribbon-like structure," in which finite bundles of polar head groups pack in ribbons of infinite length. Hexagonal 2D liquid crystalline states are composed of long rods or cylinders packed in a hexagonal array. When no or little water is present, the polar parts of the molecules align (with small amounts of water if present) to form the cores of the rods, and the liquid hydrocarbon chains are the continuous matrix. This is called the "Hex II phase." Lipids forming Hex II phases include some anhydrous soaps, dry and hydrated phospholipids, and acid-soaps. Hex II phospholipid phases have been implicated as intermediate structures in cellular membrane fusion processes.

In higher water concentration, particularly when the polar group tends to interact strongly with water and the hydrocarbon part is a single chain, a hexagonal phase forms in which the hydrocarbon chains form the center of the rod and the polar groups are on the exterior of the rod, with water as the continuous matrix (Fig. 3–10, upper right). Lipids forming this so-called Hex I phase include many micelle-forming molecules, such as sphingosine-HCl, hydrated soaps, detergents, and some lysophosphatides.

Lamellar liquid crystals (also called smectic liquid crystals) are ordered in one dimension (1D), i.e., the only order is the stacking between the lamellae. In 1D liquid crystals, the acyl chains may be either crystalline (gel state) or liquid. In the gel state, the chains are packed in a hexagonal lattice. Molecules that form the gel state include hydrated K, rubidium (Rb), and cesium (Cs), soaps, and many phospholipids, especially the lung surfactant dipalmitoyl PC. Dipalmitoyl PC forms a bilayered gel (Fig. 3–10, lower left), whereas K, Rb, and Cs soaps, lyso PC, and platelet-activating factor form interdigitated gels. Thus one polar group covers two chains in both types of gel (Fig. 3–10). Phospholipids with one short-chain and one long-chain fatty acid form an interdigitated "1 per 3" structure in which the short chains from two opposing phospholipids lie end to end (Fig. 3–10), and one polar group covers 3 chains. When the chains are melted (liquid), the state is called Lα; synonyms are lamellar liquid crystalline and smectic A. The lamellar liquid crystalline phase (Lα) is formed by hydrated soaps, acid-soaps, phospholipids, monoacylglycerols, and glycosphingolipids, and it is the progenitor of all membrane structure.

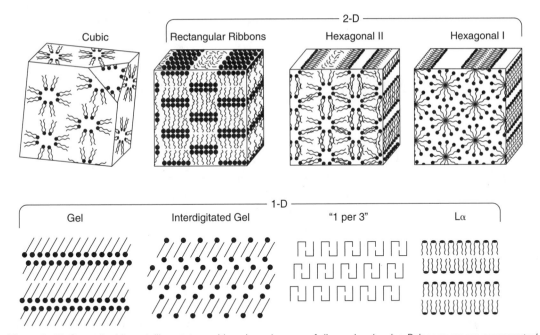

Figure 3–10. *Some liquid crystalline states, with various degrees of dimensional order. Polar groups are represented by dots, the hydrocarbon chains by wriggles or lines, and water by blank areas.*

The three-dimensional cubic phase unit cell formed by egg lecithin at low hydration is centered cubic. The structure consists of rigid rods of finite length, all identical and crystallographically equivalent, joined three-by-three to form two interwoven three-dimensional networks. The hydrocarbon chains are fluid.

Liquid crystals with two-dimensional (2D) order may be rectangular or hexagonal. The 2D centered rectangular phase of the anhydrous Na soaps has the loci of the polar groups arranged in infinitely long ribbons of finite width. The two hexagonal phases have the loci of the polar groups arranged in infinitely long rods packed hexagonally. Hexagonal II is the water-in-oil type observed in low water-phospholipid systems and in the anhydrous soaps of divalent cations. Hexagonal I is the oil-in-water type observed in lipid-water systems containing monovalent soaps, lysolecithin, or aliphatic detergents.

Lameller systems are generally one-dimensional. However, if the chains are packed in a 2D hexagonal array, 2D order is perpendicular to the chain axis. These lamellar systems, called "gels," are ordered. Lamellae may be fully or partially interdigitated layers or bilayers. Transitions between interdigitated layers and bilayers change the lamellar thickness greatly, and such transitions may have a biological role.

(From Small, D. M. and Zoeller, R. A. [1991] Lipids. In: Encyclopedia of Human Biology, Vol. 4, pp. 725–748. Academic Press, Inc., Orlando, Florida).

Liquid crystals that have no long-range periodic order are ordered liquids (nematic and cholesteric) but have been called liquid crystals because of their birefringence. They have no true x-ray diffraction and show only x-ray scattering that corresponds to their molecular length. These observations indicate that many rod-shaped lipids lie side by side but not in strict layers like the lamellar liquid crystals. The particular lipids that exhibit this kind of liquid crystalline behavior are generally steryl esters and, in particular, cholesteryl esters.

The Liquid State—Melts, Solutions and Suspensions

The general properties of liquids, including fluidity, cohesiveness, relative incompressibility, and rapid molecular motions, are characteristic of melted lipids. Because only a 10% to 20% change in volume occurs when a lipid melts from a solid, some short-range order must remain in the liquid. It has been shown that many molten lipids form nonideal liquids consisting of clusters of a few hundred molecules, aligned along their long axes, separated by more disordered molecules. These clusters may act as nucleating centers for the formation of more ordered liquids or liquid crystals (Small, 1986). In mixtures of different lipids, some domain separation of individual lipids may occur in the liquid state.

Fluidity, which is defined as the reciprocal of viscosity, and diffusivity in liquid and liquid crystal systems are directly proportional to the free volume of the molecule (i.e., that volume above the minimum volume at zero fluidity). The free volume is a function of the temperature, and thus fluidity increases with temperature (Small, 1986).

The solubility of different types of lipids in aqueous systems is quite variable, extending from virtually insoluble (large hydrocarbons, triacylglycerols) to very soluble (soaps and detergents). The solubility of fatty acids is quite low (see Table 3–2). The solubility is less at temperatures below the MP than above it, and at any given temperature solubility decreases as the length of the hydrocarbon chain increases (i.e., the longer the chain or the larger the hydrophobic moiety, the lower the solubility). Some of the more polar lipids (e.g., K and Na soaps; detergents such as sodium dodecyl sulfate, commonly called SDS; and bile salts) form optically clear aqueous solutions in which the apparent solubility may

be as high as 60 g/100 g of solution. These lipids, in fact, have a low monomer solubility but spontaneously form small aggregates of molecules called micelles when their true (monomer) solubility is exceeded. These solutions are called micellar solutions.

A micellar solution is a thermodynamically stable system formed spontaneously in water above a critical concentration and temperature (Fig. 3–11). The solution contains small aggregates (micelles) whose molecules are in rapid equilibrium with a low concentration of monomers. This low concentration of monomers is, in fact, the true solubility of the lipid and is called the critical micellar concentration (CMC). Above the CMC, the excess lipid forms micelles. Micellar solutions can solubilize other less soluble lipids to form mixed micelles. Micelles are spherical structures, about 2 molecular lengths in diameter

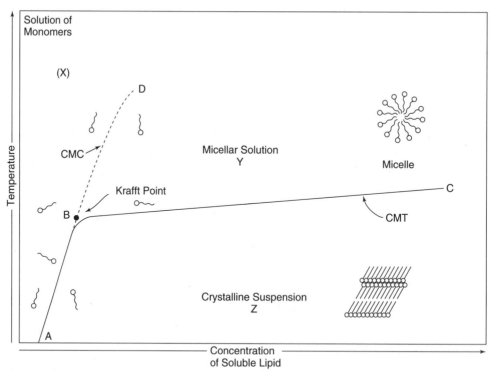

Figure 3–11. Behavior of soluble lipids at high-water concentration as a function of temperature and concentration. The temperature is plotted on the ordinate and increasing concentrations of soluble lipid (amphiphile) on the abscissa. Micelles occur only in region Y. In this region the amphiphile is above a concentration indicated by the curve BD and above a temperature indicated by BC. BD is the critical micellar concentration (CMC). Thus, the CMC varies along BD with the temperature. The solution must also be above a certain temperature (BC), which indicates the transition temperature from the crystalline state to a micellar solution. This temperature is called the critical micellar temperature (CMT). The point B at which the CMC and CMT curves meet is termed the Krafft point. It can be considered a triple point and indicates the CMT at the CMC. (From Small, D. M. [1986] The Physical Chemistry of Lipids from ·Alkanes to Phospholipids. Handbook of Lipid Research, vol. 4. Plenum Press, New York.)

in pure water, but when salt is added they often enlarge and assume cylindrical or discoid shapes. Bile salts allow formation of mixed micellar solutions in bile and in intestinal contents during fat absorption. Such solutions are necessary for the proper digestion and absorption of fat and fat-soluble vitamins.

Lipids may also be suspended in aqueous systems. Insoluble lipids such as triacylglycerols or cholesteryl esters can be made to form relatively stable suspensions (emulsions) of lipid in water by adding an emulsifier such as a phospholipid. For instance, emulsions containing particles with a core of triacylglycerol and a surface layer of an emulsifier such as PC can be formed in vitro by agitation. Plasma lipoproteins are similar lipid particles formed in vivo in intestinal enterocytes or hepatocytes and modified in plasma by enzymes and transfer factors (Small, 1992). (See Chapters 7 and 14 for further discussion of lipoproteins.)

Determinants of Lipid Melting

Lipid melting is the melt (solid to liquid) of the aliphatic chains, illustrated, for instance, by melting butter or animal fat. It is affected by chain length, polar substitution, or double bonds and is illustrated in Figure 3–12, in which the chain-melting transition (crystal to liquid chain) is shown for lipids with increasing chain length and for a variety of molecules having different substituents. Note that as the chain length increases, the melting temperature rises. Double bonds, triple bonds, methylene branches, and halide substitutions at the end of the chain decrease the melting temperature, but polar substituents, particularly those that can form hydrogen bonds or ionic bonds, increase the melting transition. The order of increasing melting temperatures for a given chain length is as follows: 1 olefins<alkanes<ethyl esters<normal alcohols<carboxylic or fatty acids<triacylglycerols<1,2 diacylglycerols=3 monoacylglycerols<dry PC. Interaction of water with the polar groups decreases the melting transition (see anhydrous and hydrated PC in Fig. 3–12).

Surface Behavior of Lipids at the Water Interface

Lipids accumulate at air/water or oil/water interfaces. The interaction of a specific lipid with an aqueous interface depends on the hydrophilic-lipophilic balance of the lipid (i.e., the relative strengths of the hydrocarbon and water-seeking parts). Thus, when a drop of pure lipid contacts a water surface of limited area, one of three events will occur: (1) a very lipophilic lipid, like mineral oil, cholesteryl oleate, or oleoyl palmitate (a wax ester), will simply sit on the water as an intact droplet or lens; (2) a more hydrophilic lipid, like triolein or oleoyl alcohol, will spread to form a continuous insoluble monolayer of molecules in equilibrium with the remainder of the droplet; or (3) a highly hydrophilic lipid, like K oleate or Na cholate (a bile salt), will spread to form an unstable film from which molecules desorb into the water. Lipids are found in almost all interfaces between cellular compartments. Between two aqueous compartments within a cell, a membrane bilayer is present. Between fat and aqueous compartments in the cytoplasm (e.g., a fat droplet in a fat cell) or plasma (e.g., a lipoprotein particle), a phospholipid monolayer forms the interface.

Lipid Classification Based on Physical Interaction with Water

Because most known biological systems are aqueous systems, a classification based on the behavior of lipid in water and at aqueous interfaces (Table 3–4) is given to help one predict how certain classes of lipids will assemble and distribute in cells. This classification generally applies to lipids with melted chains. Nonpolar lipids are water insoluble, do not spread at an air/water interface, have extremely limited solubility in membranes (less than 3% by weight of total membrane lipids), and will usually be found in intracellular droplets. These lipids are highly soluble in organic solvents like hexane (C_6H_{14}) and chloroform ($CHCl_3$). All other lipids are amphiphiles (i.e., they have affinity for both oil and water). The interaction with water (or hydrocarbons) is determined by the nature of the polar group (water-soluble) and the mass of the hydrocarbon part.

Class I polar lipids have a weak polar group compared with the hydrocarbon mass. They are virtually insoluble in water but

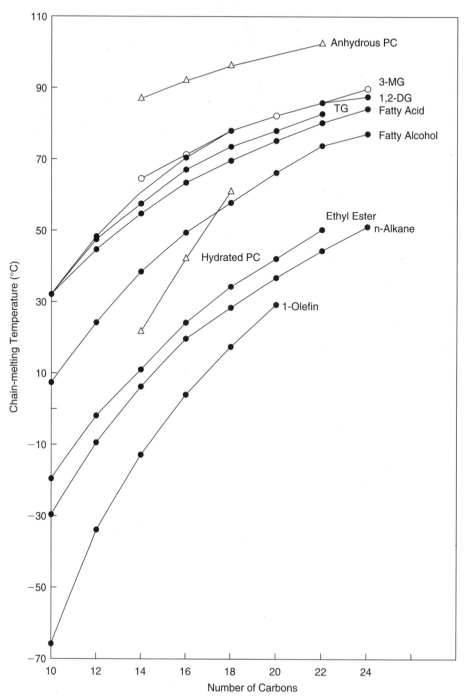

Figure 3–12. *Effects of polar substituents on melting of the hydrocarbon chain for a variety of lipids. The major chain-melting transition (i.e., to liquid chain) temperatures for a variety of lipids are plotted against the number of carbons in the aliphatic chain. The stronger the interactions of the polar groups with each other, the higher the melting point (MP). This is illustrated by the difference between fatty acids, which can form hydrogen bonds between the carboxyl groups, and ethyl esters of fatty acids, which cannot. The MP of the hydrogen-bonded fatty acids is 30 to 40° C higher. Note that the melting transitions increase in temperature with increasing hydrocarbon chain length, even in water. The presence of water, however, lowers the chain transition when compared with the dry lipid, as shown for phosphatidylcholine (PC). DG, diacylglycerol; MG, monoacylglycerol; TG, Triacylglycerol.*

TABLE 3–4
Classification of Biologically Active Lipids

Class	Surface Properties*	Bulk Properties	Examples
Nonpolar	Will not spread to form monolayer	Insoluble	Long-chain, saturated or unsaturated, branched or unbranched, aliphatic hydrocarbons with or without aromatic groups (e.g., dodecane, octadecane, hexadecane, paraffin oil, phytane, pristane, carotene, lycopene, gadusene, squalene) Large aromatic hydrocarbons (e.g., cholestane, benzopyrenes, coprostane, benzophenanthrocenes) Esters and ethers in which both components are large, hydrophobic lipids (e.g., steryl esters of long-chain fatty acids, waxes of long-chain fatty acids, and long-chain normal monoalcohols, ethers of long-chain alcohols, steryl ethers, long-chain triethers of glycerol)
Polar Class I: Insoluble, nonswelling amphiphiles	Spreads to form stable monolayer	Insoluble, or solubility very low	Triglycerides, diglycerides, long-chain protonated fatty acids, long-chain normal alcohols, long-chain normal amines, long-chain aldehydes, phytols, retinols, vitamin A, vitamin K, vitamin E, cholesterol, desmosterol, sitosterol, vitamin D, un-ionized phosphatidic acid, sterol esters of very short-chain acids, waxes in which either acid or alcohol moiety is less than 4 carbon atoms long (e.g., methyl oleate)
Class II: Insoluble swelling amiphiphilic lipids	Spreads to form stable monolayer	Insoluble but swells in water to form lyotropic liquid crystals	Phosphatidylcholine, phosphatidylethanolamine, phosphatidyl inositol, sphingomyelin, cardiolipid, plasmalogens, ionized phosphatidic acid, cerebrosides, phosphatidylserine, monoglycerides, acid soaps, α-hydroxy fatty acids, monoethers of glycerol, mixtures of phospholipids and glycolipids extracted from cell membranes or cellular organelles (glycolipids and plant sulfolipids)
Class IIIA: Soluble amphiphiles with lyotropic mesomorphism*	Spreads but forms unstable monolayer because of solubility in aqueous substrate	Soluble, forms micelles above a critical micellar concentration; at low water concentrations forms liquid crystals	Sodium and potassium salts of long-chain fatty acids, many of the ordinary anionic, cationic, and nonionic detergents, lysolecithin, palmitoyl and oleoyl coenzyme A and other long-chain thioesters of coenzyme A, gangliosides, sulfocerebrosides
Class IIIB: Soluble amphiphiles, no lyotropic mesomorphism	Spreads but forms unstable monolayer due to solubility in aqueous substrate	Forms micelles but not liquid crystals	Bile salts, sulfated bile alcohols, sodium salts of fusidic acid, rosin soaps, phenanthrene sulfonic acid, penicillins, phenothiazines

*Lyotropic mesomorphism means the formation of liquid crystals on interaction with water.

From Small, D. M. (1986) The Physical Chemistry of Lipids from Alkanes to Phospholipids. Handbook of Lipid Research, vol. 4. Plenum Press, New York.

spread to form stable monolayers. That is, they have a surface solubility. They have limited solubility in membranes, and they partition between membranes and intracellular lipid droplets. Cholesterol and free protonated long-chain fatty acids are good examples. The partition coefficient (K_p) of cholesterol between membranes and oils [K_p = % (w/w) in membranes/% (w/w) in oil] varies from about 6 in membranes versus cholesteryl ester oil to 22 in membranes versus triacylglycerol oil (Miller and Small, 1987). Thus on a weight basis, much more cholesterol distributes to membranes than to oils. For fatty acids such as oleic acid, the K_p between membranes and oils is about 12.

Class II lipids have more balanced polar and hydrocarbon parts and are the "membrane formers." They are insoluble in water and in oil and seek out the interface between oil and water; thus, they are good emulsifiers. When no water-oil interface is present, they form bilayers.

Class III lipids have a very strong polar moiety relative to the hydrophobic region, have measurable monomer solubility, and form micelles. They also partition into membranes and can be disruptive to membranes. They are oil insoluble, are not found in fat droplets, and are not readily soluble in hexane and chloroform. They are soluble in polar solvents like methanol (CH_3OH) or ethanol (CH_3CH_2OH).

PROPERTIES OF DIETARY FATS AND OILS AND THEIR PRODUCTS: DIACYLGLYCEROLS, MONOACYLGLYCEROLS, AND FATTY ACIDS

Physical properties of dietary triacylglycerols and their hydrolysis products affect the digestion and absorption of dietary lipids and thus have important physiological implications.

Melting and Crystallization of Acylglycerols, Fatty Acids, and Acid-Soaps

The melting and crystallization temperatures for a variety of triacylglycerols, diacylglycer-ols, and monoacylglycerols that are present during fat metabolism have been reported (Small, 1991). The MPs of many individual dietary triacylglycerols are above body temperature. The pure saturated triacylglycerols tristearin (MP 73.1°C) and tripalmitin (MP 66.4°C) are not well absorbed. Pancreatic lipase will not hydrolyze them, and they pass through the gut unhydrolyzed and unabsorbed, still in solid form. Dietary fat is nevertheless well absorbed. Some food fats that are partly solid at body temperature, such as lard and tallow, are digested and absorbed. So why are the fats with high MPs such as lard well absorbed? Although foods contain some simple saturated triacylglycerols, most fat is a mixture of complex triacylglycerols (see Table 3–3), and MPs of mixed fats are very broad. Beef fat starts to melt at about 25°C and finishes melting at 55 to 60°C. At 37°C, most of the fat is melted. Therefore, it is a good substrate for intestinal and gastric lipases.

Once hydrolysis of fat or oil begins in the stomach by action of gastric lipase, fatty acids are released. Long-chain saturated fatty acids also have quite high MPs (Fig. 3–13); for instance, the MPs for myristic, palmitic, and stearic acids are 54, 63, and 70°C, respectively. In addition, they are poorly soluble. For instance, the solubility of palmitic acid at 25°C is 3×10^{-5} g/L (10 nmol/L) (Small, 1986). In the stomach, the pH is low (1.5 to 3), and fatty acids are protonated (RCOOH). However, at the pH of the duodenum (5.5 to 7.5), the fatty acid would be rapidly converted into hydrated acid-soaps [e.g., $H^+K^+(RCOO^-)_2$] (Cistola et al., 1986; Small, 1986). Like protonated fatty acids, these compounds are almost insoluble in aqueous media, but the melting temperatures for acid-soaps are about 10°C lower than for the corresponding acids (Fig. 3–13). For instance, the melting temperatures for hydrated K acid-soaps are 43°C (myristic), 51°C (palmitic), and 61°C (stearic) (Cistola et al., 1986). It should be noted here that alkali metal soaps of fatty acids (K^+RCOO^-) do not form until the pH is quite high, more than 8.5. Therefore, the form of most fatty acids at biological pH (5.5 to 8) is the acid-soap and at pH lower than 5, the protonated acid. The commonly held concept that fatty acids are biological detergents is incorrect. Sodium and

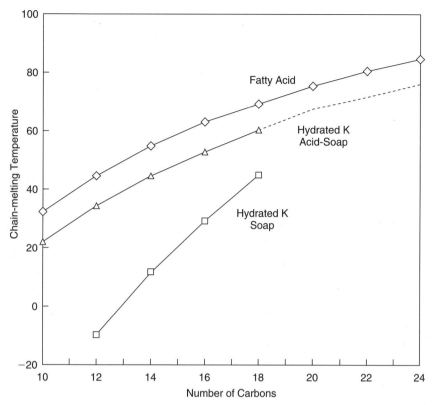

Figure 3–13. *The melting point of saturated fatty acids (RCOOH), acid-soaps [e.g., $H^+K^+(RCOO^-)_2$], and potassium soaps (K^+RCOO^-) plotted against the number of carbon atoms in the molecule. R stands for $CH_3–(CH_2)_n–CH_2–$.*

K soaps of fatty acids are detergents, but because they do not form except at high pH, they do not exist in vivo under most circumstances.

Thus when 1 mol of dietary fat is hydrolyzed by intestinal lipases, the products are 2 mol of fatty acid and 1 mol of 2-monoacylglycerol. If the fatty acids released are unsaturated or medium-chain (less than 14 carbon-) saturated fatty acids, they are above their MPs and can be solubilized by bile salts and moved to the intestinal brush border membrane where they are absorbed. However, if the fatty acids released by the lipase have a high content of long-chain (18 to 24 carbon-) saturated fatty acids, which are below their MPs, they form a solid precipitate that is not solubilized well by bile acids and thus are poorly absorbed (Redgrave et al., 1988; Small, 1991). This effect of MP on solubility appears to be a factor in certain "low-calorie" structured fats.

Fatty acids may also be malabsorbed if they are hydrolyzed from glycerides in a high calcium environment. Calcium intake correlates with the fecal loss of fatty acids. The probable reason for this is that with an adequately high concentration of calcium ions, fatty acids will react to form calcium soaps, $Ca^{2+}(RCOO^-)_2$, which have very high MPs (>200°C), precipitate in the intestine, and pass out in the feces (Carey et al., 1983).

Saturated diacylglycerols also have high MPs (e.g., dipalmitin, 70.1°C; distearin, 77.2°C), which are not affected by hydration. These saturated diacylglycerols are class I polar amphiphiles (see Table 3–4) and partition mainly into the surface of fat droplets, lipoproteins, and membranes. As surface constituents of fat droplets, they might interfere with lipolysis of intestinal fat or of chylomicrons in the plasma. Monoacylglycerols in the hydrated state have considerably lower melting temperatures than in the dry state (about 25°C lower). However, even in water, the longer-chain saturated monoacylglycerols, such as

NUTRITION INSIGHT

Structured Triglycerides

Recently the synthesis of "structured triglycerides" (Babayan, 1982) has become a popular method for reducing the caloric values of triglycerides (triacylglycerols). Structured triglycerides may be produced in mass amounts either by mixing short-chain fatty acids with a long-chain triglyceride and transesterifying or by mixing together 2 or more relatively pure triglycerides of chosen composition and then transesterifying and isolating particular classes of triglycerides. For instance, very long-chain triglycerides may be transesterified with medium-chain triglycerides to produce a series of triglycerides that have 1 very long-chain fatty acid and 2 medium-chain fatty acids (e.g., dioctanoyl, behenoyl glycerol). These triglycerides, called "caprenin," have melting characteristics (MP ~32°C) similar to those of chocolate, but because a large proportion of the very long-chain fatty acid is malabsorbed and the medium-chain fatty acids have less caloric value, the overall caloric value per molecule is considerably (50% to 60%) less than that of cocoa butter.

Similarly, triglycerides containing 2 molecules of very short acids, such as acetate, propionate, or butyrate, and 1 molecule of a long-chain fatty acid have been synthesized, and these generally form oils. Other structured triglycerides include those made with medium-chain and essential fatty acids, such as linoleic, linolenic, EPA, and DHA. These may be useful in infant formulas and for treating patients with severe debilitation and essential fatty acid deficiencies (Jensen et al., 1994). Procedures for synthesis and definition of the physical and biochemical characteristics of structured triglycerides have been described, and it is likely that some will become included into our food sources and others used in therapy.

2-monostearin, could be crystalline at body temperature, and these could potentially segregate into partially crystalline structures on the surfaces of fat globules in the intestine or of lipoproteins in plasma. If such monoacylglycerols accumulate in high enough quantities, this could slow lipolysis. Monoacylglycerols accumulate sufficiently in normal lipolysis for this to occur (Boyle et al., 1995).

Effects of Positions of Fatty Acids in Mixed-Chain Triacylglycerols upon Their Absorption from the Intestine

It has been known for some time that the stereospecific position of fatty acids on triacylglycerols can alter the availability of the component fatty acids for absorption from the small intestine in both rats and in humans (Small, 1991). Filer et al. (1969) gave newborn infants a formula that contained either lard, which has an abundance of palmitate in the 2 position (see Table 3–3), or randomized lard, in which palmitate was randomly distributed to all positions. Ninety-five percent of all the fatty acids was absorbed from natural lard,

but only 72% was absorbed from the randomized lard. In the randomized lard, both palmitic and stearic acids were malabsorbed, 58% and 40%, respectively. Similar observations were made in studies with cocoa butter and randomized cocoa butter (Kritchevsky, 1988). The principal triacylglycerols in cocoa butter are SOS, POP and SOP (O, oleoyl, P, palmitoyl, and S, stearoyl), and absorption of the saturated stearate and palmitate is somewhat low. After randomizing the fatty acids, the saturated acids appear more in the 2 position, and absorption is improved. These studies appear to indicate that if the saturated fatty acid is in the 2 position, it is more likely to be absorbed than if it is in the 1 or 3 position.

In studies in rats with OSO and OOS, as shown in Figure 3–14, about 94% of the stearate in OSO was absorbed, whereas only about 62% of the stearate in OOS was absorbed (Redgrave et al., 1988). When intestinal enzymes hydrolyze 1 mol of OSO, they produce 1 mol of 2-monostearin and 2 mol of oleic acid. The MP of hydrated 2-monostearin is close to the body temperature of rats (39°C), and it can be solubilized by bile salts and

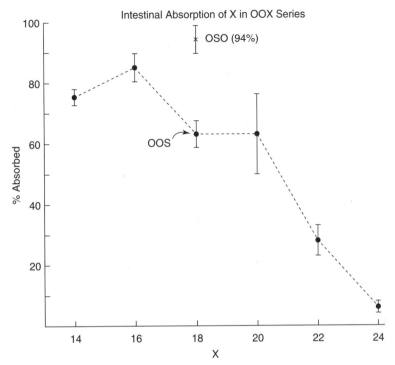

Figure 3–14. *Absorption of the saturated fatty acid in the* sn *3 position (X refers to the chain length) of 1,2 dioleoyl, 3 acyl-sn-glycerols (the OOX series). OSO is 1-oleoyl, 2-steroyl, 3-oleoyl-glycerol. As the chain lengthens from 16 to 24 carbons, there is a sharp decline in the absorption of the saturated fatty acid. Oleate absorption was greater than 90% for all of the triacylglycerols. (Based on data of Redgrave, T.G., Kodali, D. R. and Small, D. M. [1988]. The effect of triacyl-sn-glycerol structure on the metabolism of chylomicrons and triacylglycerol-rich emulsions in the rat. J Biol Chem 263:5118–5123.)*

thus be absorbed. However, hydrolysis of OOS gives a mole of stearic acid or its acid-soap; these products have MPs above 50°C (see Fig. 3–13) and therefore solidify and are poorly absorbed.

If the fatty acid in the 1 or 3 position has a high MP and consequently its acid-soap has a high MP, then it is unlikely to be readily absorbed. This is shown in Figure 3–14, which illustrates the absorption and incorporation of fatty acids into lipids in chylomicrons in rats fed a series of stereospecific triacylglycerols containing oleic acid in the 1 and 2 positions and a saturated fatty acid in the 3 position. These 1,2-dioleoyl, 3 acyl-*sn*-glycerols all have melting points below body temperature (Fig. 3–15) and are oils in the intestine. After hydrolysis, the MP of the fatty acid-soaps (see Fig. 3–13) and the absorption of the fatty acid liberated from the *sn*-3 position depend on chain length. Absorption of myristate (C14) and palmitate (C16) is quite good at about

80%, but the absorption of stearate (C18) falls to 62% and that of C22 and C24 (behenic and lignoceric acids) falls precipitously so that only about 6% of the lignoceric acid released from 1,2-dioleoyl-3-lignoceroyl-*sn*-glycerol is absorbed (Redgrave et al., 1988). Because the MP of the acid-soaps of these long-chain saturated fatty acids (see Fig. 3–13) is very high (greater than 65°C), they probably precipitate in the intestine and are lost in the feces.

Polymorphism of Fats and Oils

The relatively simple chemical structures of the fatty acids esterified to glycerol gives rise to very complicated physical properties of solid triacylglycerols. The capacity of a single molecular species to form several different solid crystalline forms (polymorphism) is a characteristic of glycerides and especially of triacylglycerols. This arises because there are many possible orientations of the chains in

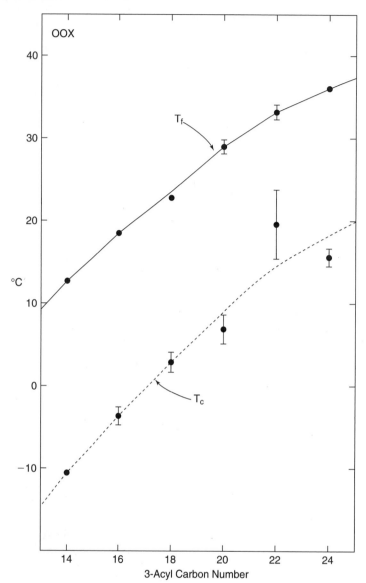

Figure 3–15. Melting and crystallization points (T_f, T_c) of 1,2-dioleoyl, 3-acyl-sn-glycerols (OOX series). The MPs are all below body temperature. The melting and crystallization points of OSO for comparison with those of OOS are 25.2°C and − 7°C. (Based on data of Fahey, D., Small, D. M., Atkinson, D., Kodali, D., and Redgrave, T. [1985]. Structure and polymorphism of 1,2-dioleoyl-3-acyl-sn-glycerols, three- and six-layered structures. Biochemistry 24:3757–3764.)

layers, which may vary in tilt from the basal plane; for instance, structures may organize into bilayered structures (two layers of chains), trilayered structures, or even more complicated structures with six layers (Fahey et al., 1985; Small, 1986; Kodali et al., 1989). The chains themselves may pack in a variety of different subcells, generally classified as β, β′, and α. The combination of different layers, different angles of tilt, and different chain packing can give rise to many different crystalline forms in the same triacylglycerol.

A rather simple case is illustrated by 1,3-dioleoyl-2-stearoyl-glycerol (OSO), a component of lard and butterfat, shown in Figure 3–16 (Kodali et al., 1987). The stablest form of this symmetrical triacylglycerol is the β phase (Small, 1991). It is a trilayer (three layers of chains) that repeats every 65 Å. It melts at 25°C to a liquid oil. On rapid cooling of the liquid, an α phase, which is a bilayered phase with hexagonal packed chains, is formed. This can convert to another bilayered phase with β′ chain packing at − 7°C. The β′ phase transforms to the β phase at 11°C. Many other triacylglycerols have more complicated polymorphisms, and natural mixtures of triacylglycerols such as oils and fats may exist as a combination of polymorphic forms and stoichiometric ratios of molecules in the same crystal. It is striking, however, that many natural fats and oils behave in a general way like a single species of triacylglycerol in that they show the different polymorphic forms of α,

β′, and β. These properties are important in producing palatable and attractive foods. Polymorphic transitions from β′ to β forms that produce white films on chocolate or grainy textures in shortenings are rather unacceptable.

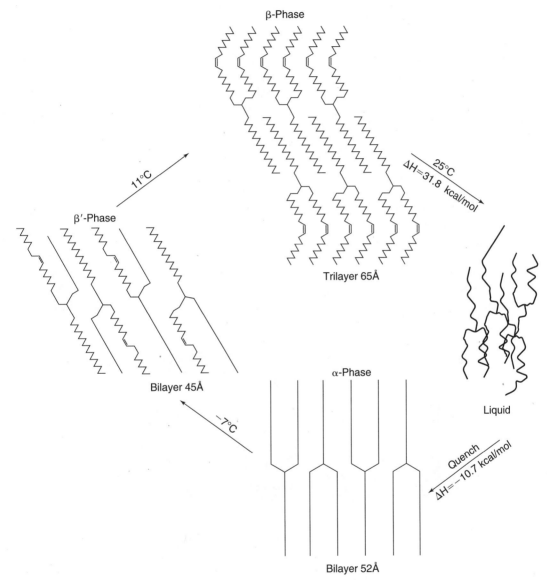

Figure 3–16. *Polymorphic forms of 1,3-dioleoyl-2-stearoyl-sn-glycerol (OSO), a common component of pork fat. The MP is given above the arrow, and the enthalpy of the transition is given in kcal/mol below the arrow. The ⋀⋀⋀⋀⋀ lines indicate the zigzag shown in Figure 3–9. In β packing, the most stable form, the chains are all parallel. In β′ packing, every other chain is twisted 90° to the next, so that ⋀⋀⋀⋀⋀ and _____ alternate. In the α-phase, all the chains are packed in a loose hexagonal chain packing, and all are drawn as _____. In the melt, the chains have movement and are drawn as squiggly lines ⋀⋁⋁. The most stable structure, β, melts at 25°C and is a trilayer (3 layers of chains): 2 layers of oleates with the 9 to 10 double bond and a separate layer of stearates (middle layer). All other structures are bilayers (two layers). (From Kodali, D. R. Atkinson, D., Redgrave, T. G. and Small, D. M. [1987]. Structure and polymorphism of 18-carbon fatty acyl triacylglycerols: Effect of unsaturation and substitution in the 2-position. J Lipid Res 28:403–413.)*

The Surface Orientation of Different Triacylglycerols at the Water Interface

Lipolytic enzymes work at water/lipid interfaces of intestinal fat emulsions, plasma lipoproteins, and membranes. Thus the interfacial conformation of triacylglycerols must be recognized by lipases so that they can react with the ester bond and water to effect hydrolysis.

Triacylglycerols have a different conformation at an aqueous/oil interface than in the bulk liquid. In bulk liquid, triacylglycerols have "tuning fork" conformation, with one chain pointing in one direction and the other two chains pointing in the opposite direction (Fig. 3–17). In general, at an aqueous interface, when the three fatty acid chains are long, all three ester groups protrude into the aqueous phase, and the three chains point upward in the oil (Fig. 3–17). The area of a triacylglycerol at the interface in the expanded liquid state is about 100 to 120 Å² per molecule. When the surface becomes solid—that is, when the molecules freeze on the surface—the molecule occupies about 60 Å², which is about 20 Å² per acyl chain, the area occupied by a crystalline solid. At a condensed liquid surface such as might occur

between a fat droplet and water, an interfacial area of ~75 Å² is found. Lipolytic enzyme activity tends to be lowest when the interfacial substrate is in the crystalline state and highest when the substrate is in the liquid condensed state. As surface triacylglycerols are hydrolyzed, the products (fatty acids and 2-monoacylglycerols) are removed, and other triacylglycerol molecules move from the bulk liquid to the interface.

In butterfat, one chain is quite short (2 to 6 carbons). In this case, only the 2 long chains lie pointing up from the water into the oil while the short chain is submerged in the aqueous milieu, as shown in Figure 3–17 (Fahey and Small, 1986). This may be an important factor in the rapid hydrolysis of the short chains of fats that have short chains (such as butyric acid) at the *sn*-3 position. When one chain is a medium-chain fatty acid of 8 to 11 carbons, it cannot enter the water because it is too hydrophobic; it points into the oil phase and causes the melting of the two other longer-chain fatty acids by creating a partial void (due to its shortness), thus depressing the MP (Fahey and Small, 1988). This can be seen in the depression of the surface

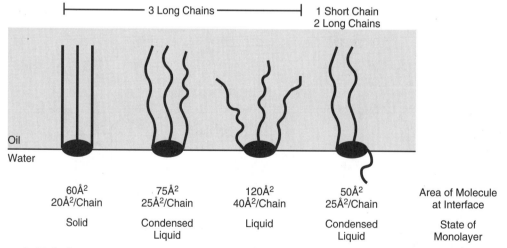

3 Long Chains			1 Short Chain 2 Long Chains
60Å² 20Å²/Chain	75Å² 25Å²/Chain	120Å² 40Å²/Chain	50Å² 25Å²/Chain	Area of Molecule at Interface
Solid	Condensed Liquid	Liquid	Condensed Liquid	State of Monolayer

Figure 3–17. *Surface orientation of long and of long- and short-chain triacylglycerols, as found in dairy fat. All three ester bonds are anchored in the water interface. The short chains (e.g., butyric, hexanoic) are in the water phase, whereas the long-chain fatty acyl chains all point into the oil phase. When the chains crystallize at the surface, they form a rigid 2D solid monolayer that is tightly packed in a small area (20 Å²/hydrocarbon chain). If the temperature is raised, the solid monolayer will melt to a condensed liquid, and at higher temperatures or lower surface pressures to an extended liquid. These interfaces are potentially present in any fat/water system (e.g., fat globules in adipose tissue, fat in the stomach and intestine, and fat in lipoprotein particles in plasma). These interfaces are probably the substrates for many lipases (Small, 1997). Note that these conformations are quite different from those in the bulk liquid phase (see Fig. 3–16).*

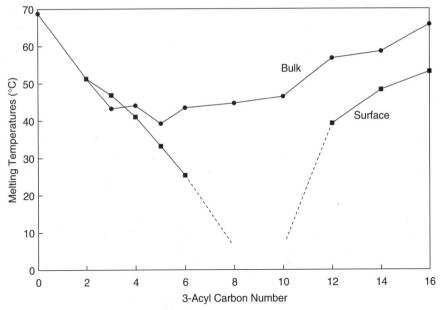

Figure 3–18. *Surface and bulk MPs of 1,2 dipalmitoyl, 3 acyl-sn-glycerols. Bulk MPs were determined for the most stable crystalline forms (●). As the chain at the 3-position lengthens to about 5 carbons, the MP falls. It then remains at about 40 to 50°C until the chain reaches 12 carbons, where the MP rises again. Melting of the triacylglycerol/water interface (■) is different. When the chain reaches 5 or greater, the surface MP becomes low and is below 5°C for the 8- and 10-carbon acids. This is due to the void left in the surface when shorter and longer chains stand side-by-side.*

MP compared with the bulk value in the series of 1,2-dipalmitoyl-3-acyl-*sn*-glycerols, as depicted in Figure 3–18.

Using ^{13}C-enriched triolein, it was shown by nuclear magnetic resonance (NMR) that the same interfacial conformation (3 chains side-by-side with all ester groups at the aqueous interface) occurs in a monolayer of phospholipid in which a few molecules of triacylglycerol are imbedded (Hamilton and Small, 1981; Hamilton et al., 1983). The solubility of triacylglycerol in phospholipid monolayers is about 3% (3 mol triacylglycerol/100 mol total lipid). The orientation shows that the 1,3 ester groups are slightly more deeply embedded in the water layer than the *sn*-2 ester group, but all three are exposed to the aqueous phase, and the 3 acyl chains lie side by side, parallel to the chains of the phospholipid. Thus in fat emulsions, membranes, or lipoproteins, triacylglycerol can have an interfacial orientation in which lipolytic enzymes will have ready access to the 1 and 3 ester linkages of triacylglycerol, which are the sites of hydrolysis of triacylglycerols by the gut and plasma lipases.

REFERENCES

Ames, J. B., Tanaka, T., Stryer, L. and Ikura, M. (1996) Portrait of a myristoyl switch protein. Curr Opin Struct Biol 6:432–438.

Babayan, V. K. (1982) Medium-chain triglycerides and structured lipids. Lipids 22:417–420.

Bailey, A. E. (1950) Melting and Solidification of Pure Compounds; Melting and Solidification of Fats, pp. 117–237. Interscience, New York.

Bell, R. M., Hunnun, Y. A. and Merrill, A. H. Jr., eds. (1993) Sphingolipids. Part A: Functions and Breakdown Products. Part B: Regulation and Function of Metabolism. *In*: Adv Lipid Res (Havel, R. J. and Small, D. M., Series eds.), Vols. 25 and 26. Academic Press, New York.

Boyle, E., Small, D. M., Gantz, D., Hamilton, J. A. and Berman, J. B. (1995) Monoacylglycerols alter both the lipid composition and molecular mobility of phosphatidylcholine bilayers: ^{13}C NMR evidence of dynamic lipid remodeling. J Lipid Res 37:764–772.

Breckenridge, W. C. (1978) Stereospecific analysis of triacylglycerols. In: Handbook of Lipid Research; Fatty Acids, and Glycerides (Kuksis, A., ed.), Vol. 1, pp. 197–232. Plenum Press, New York.

Cabral, D. J. and Small, D. M. (1989) The physical chemistry of bile. In: Handbook of Physiology (Schultz, S. G., Forte, J. G. and Rauner, B. B., eds.), Sec. 6, Vol. III, pp. 621–662. American Physiological Soc., Waverly Press, Baltimore.

Carey, M. C., Small, D. M. and Bliss, C. M. (1983) Lipid digestion and absorption. Annu Rev Physiol 45:651–677.

Cistola, D. P., Atkinson, D., Hamilton, J. A. and Small, D.

M. (1986) Phase behavior and bilayer properties of fatty acids: Hydrated 1:1 acid soaps. Biochemistry 25:2804–2812.

Commission on Biochemical Nomenclature (CBN) of the International Union of Pure and Applied Chemistry/International Union of Biochemistry (1968) The nomenclature of lipids. Chem Phys Lipids 2:156.

Consumer and Food Economics Institute (U. S.) (1976–1990) Composition of Foods: Raw, Processed, Prepared. Agriculture Handbook No. 8. Agricultural Research Service, U. S. Department of Agriculture, Washington, D. C.

Edidin, M. (1997) Lipid microdomains in cell surface membranes. Curr Opin Struct Biol 7:528–532.

Elias, P. M., ed. (1991) Skin Lipids; Advances in Lipid Research (Havel, R. J. amd Small, D. M., eds.), Vol. 24. Academic Press, New York.

Englund, P. T. (1993) The structure and biosynthesis of glycosyl phosphatidylinositol. Annu Rev Biochem 62:121–138.

Fahey, D., Small, D. M., Atkinson, D., Kodali, D. and Redgrave, T. (1985) Structure and polymorphism of 1,2-dioleoyl-3-acyl-*sn*-glycerols, three- and six-layered structures. Biochemistry 24:3757–3764.

Fahey, D. and Small, D. M. (1986) Surface properties of 1,2-dipalmitoyl-3-acyl-*sn*-glycerols. Biochemistry 25:4468–4472.

Fahey, D. and Small, D. M. (1988) Phase behavior of monolayers of 1,2-dipalmitoyl-3-long chain-*sn*-glycerols. Langmuir 4:589–594.

Farines, M., Soulier, R. and Soulier, J. (1988) Analysis of the triglycerides of some vegetable oils. J Chem Ed 65:464–466.

Filer, L. J., Jr., Mattson, F. H. and Fomon, S. J. (1969) Triglyceride configuration and fat absorption by the human infant. J Nutr 99:293–298.

Grundy, S. M. (1991) The role of low density lipoproteins in the development of coronary artery atherosclerosis. In: Plasma Lipoproteins in Coronary Artery Disease (Kreisberg, J. I. and Segrest, J. P., eds.), pp. 93–124. Blackwell Scientific Publishing Ltd., Oxford Press, New York.

Gunstone, F. D., Harwood, J. L. and Padley, F. B. (1994) The Lipid Handbook, 2nd ed. Chapman and Hall, London.

Hamilton, R. J. (1995) Waxes: Chemistry, Molecular Biology, and Functions, Vol. 6 in the Oily Press Lipid Library. The Oily Press, Ltd., Dundee, Scotland.

Hamilton, J. A. and Small, D. M. (1981) Solubilization and localization of triolein in phosphatidylcholine bilayers: A ^{13}C NMR study. Proc Natl Acad Sci USA 78:6878–6882.

Hamilton, J. A., Miller, K. W. and Small, D. M. (1983) Solubilization of triolein and cholesteryl oleate in egg phosphatidylcholine vesicles. J Biol Chem 258:12821–12826.

Hannun, Y. A. (1996) Functions of ceramide in coordinating cellular responses to stress. Science 274:1855–1859.

Jensen, G. L., McGarvey, N., Taraszewski, R., Wixson, S. K., Seidner, D. L., Pai, T., Yeh, Y. Y., Lee, T. W. and DeMichele, S. J. (1994) Lymphatic absorption of enterally fed structured triacylglycerol vs. physical mix in a canine model. Am J Clin Nutr 60:518–524.

Johnson, D. R., Bhatnagar, R. S., Knoll, L. J. and Gordon, J. I. (1994) Genetic and biochemical studies of protein N-myristoylation. Annu Rev Biochem 63:869–914.

Kodali, D. R., Atkinson, D., Redgrave, T. G. and Small, D. M. (1987) Structure and polymorphism of 18-carbon fatty acyl triacylglycerols: Effect of unsaturation and substitution in the 2-position. J Lipid Res 28:403–413.

Kodali, D. R., Atkinson, D. and Small, D. M. (1989) Molecular packing in triacyl-sn-glycerols: Influences of acyl

chain length and unsaturation. J Dispersion Sci Technol 10:393–440.

Kritchevsky, D. (1988) Effects of triglyceride structure on lipid metabolism. Nutr Rev 46:177–181.

Kuksis, A. (1978) Fatty Acids and Glycerides. In: Handbook of Lipid Research, Vol. 1. Plenum Press, New York.

Miller, K. W. and Small, D. M. (1987) Structure of triglyceride-rich lipoproteins: An analysis of core and surface phases. In: New Comprehensive Biochemistry (Gotts, A. M., ed.), Vol. 14: Plasma Lipoproteins, pp. 1–75. Elsevier Science Publishing (Biomedical Division), New York.

Myher, J. J., Kuksis, A. and Marai, L. (1988) Identification of the more complex triacylglycerols in bovine milk fat by gas chromatography–mass spectrometry using polar capillary columns. J Chromatogr 452:93–118.

Myher, J. J., Kuksis, A., Vasdev, S. C. and Kako, K. J. (1979) Acylglycerol structure of mustard seed oil and of cardiac lipids of rats during dietary lipidosis. Can J Biochem 57:1315–1327.

Nair, R. P. and Kritchevsky, D., eds. (1971) The Bile Acids: Chemistry, Physiology, and Metabolism. Plenum Press, New York.

Ness, W. R. and McKean, M. L. (1977) Biochemistry of Steroids and Other Isopentenoids. University Park Press, Baltimore.

Nestlé Nutrition Workshop (1992) Polyunsaturated Fatty Acids in Human Nutrition (Bracco, U. and Deckelbaum, R. J., eds). Raven Press, New York.

Oelkers, P., Kirby, L. C., Heubi, J. E. and Dawson. P. A. (1997) Primary bile acid malabsorption caused by mutations in the ileal sodium-dependent bile acid transporter gene (9SLC10A2). J Clin Invest 99:1880–1887.

Patton, J.S. (1981) Gastrointestinal lipid digestion. In: Physiology of the Gastrointestinal Tract (Johnson, L. R., ed.), pp. 1123–1146. Raven Press, New York.

Porter, J. A., Young, K. E. and Beachy, P. A. (1996) Cholesterol modification of hedgehog signaling proteins in animal development. Science 274:255–259.

Redgrave, T. G., Kodali, D. R. and Small, D. M. (1988) The effect of triacyl-*sn*-glycerol structure on the metabolism of chylomicrons and triacylglycerol-rich emulsions in the rat. J Biol Chem 263:5118–5123.

Salen, G., Shefer, S., Batta, A. K., Tint, G. S., Xu, G., Honda, A., Irons, M. and Elias, E. R. (1996) Abnormal cholesterol biosynthesis in the Smith-Lemli-Opitz syndrome. J Lipid Res 37:1169–1180.

Small, D. M. and Zoeller R. A. (1991) Lipids. In: Encyclopedia of Human Biology, Vol. 4, pp. 725–748. Academic Press, New York.

Small, D. M. (1991) The effects of glyceride structure on absorption and metabolism. Annu Rev Nutr 11:413–434.

Small, D. M. (1992) Structure and metabolism of the plasma lipoprotein. In: Plasma Lipoproteins in Coronary Artery Disease. (Kreisberg, J. I. and Segrest, J. P., eds.), pp. 57–85. Blackwell Scientific Publishing, Ltd., Oxford Press, New York.

Small, D. M. (1988) Progression and regression of atherosclerotic lesions: Insights from lipid physical biochemistry. Arteriosclerosis 8:103–129.

Small, D. M. (1986) The Physical Chemistry of Lipids from Alkanes to Phospholipids. Handbook of Lipid Research Series (Hanahan, D., ed.), Vol. 4. Plenum Press, New York.

Small, D. M. (1977) Liquid crystals in living and dying systems. J Colloid Interface Sci 58:581–602.

Small, D. M. (1997) Physical behaviors of lipase substrates. Methods Enzymol 286:153–167.

Sonntag, N. O. V. (1979) Composition and characteristics

of individual fats and oils. In: Bailey's Industrial Oil and Fat Products (Swern, D., ed.), Vol. 1, pp. 289–478. John Wiley & Sons, New York.

Waugh, D. A. and Small, D. M. (1984) Methods in laboratory investigation. Identification and detection of in situ cellular and regional differences of lipid composition and class in lipid-rich tissue using hot stage polarizing light microscopy. Lab Invest 51:702–714.

Zhang, F. L. and Casey, P.J. (1996) Protein prenylation: Molecular mechanisms and functional consequences. Annu Rev Biochem 65:241–269.

RECOMMENDED READINGS

Small, D. M. and Zoeller, R. A. (1991) Lipids. In: Encyclopedia of Human Biology, Vol. 4, pp. 725–748. Academic Press, Inc., New York.

Small, D. M. (1991) The effects of glyceride structure on absorption and metabolism. Annu Rev Nutr 11:413–434.

Small, D. M. (1992) Structure and metabolism of the plasma lipoprotein. In: Plasma Lipoproteins in Coronary Artery Disease. (Kreisberg, and Segrest, eds.), pp. 57–85. Blackwell Scientific Publishing, Ltd., Oxford Press, New York.

Digestion and Absorption of the Macronutrients

◆ ◆

Some of the earliest investigations of biochemical and physiological events involved the study of the digestive fluids and processes. In 1822, William Beaumont, an American physician, studied gastric juice obtained from a gastric fistula that remained in a patient who had recovered from a gunshot wound. This led to the discovery that hydrochloric acid was secreted into the stomach. In 1836, the German anatomist and physiologist Theodor Schwann described the ability of

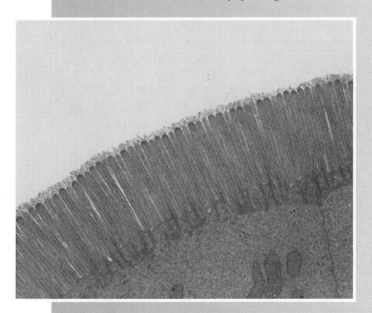

gastric juice to break down albumin. This was the first recognition of the enzymatic breakdown of food, and Schwann coined the word "pepsin" from the Greek *pepsis* (digestion) to describe this new factor in gastric juice. In 1899–1902, in the laboratory of the Russian physiologist Ivan Pavlov, the observation that an intestinal factor was required for activation of pancreatic proteases was first made; Pavlov named this factor enterokinase. These processes are understood in much more detail today, and research is continuing to provide new insights into digestive and particularly absorptive processes.

The average American diet contains approximately 15% protein, 60% carbohydrate, and 25% fat by weight. Because fat has a higher caloric density than does protein or carbohydrate, typical diets provide about 11%, 46%, and 43% of total energy needs in the form of protein, carbohydrate, and fat, respectively, with the average diet containing relatively more fat and less complex carbohydrate than is generally recommended by nutritionists. In addition to handling the digestion and

Electron micrograph of the brush border membrane of an enterocyte; from Poley, J. R. (1988) Loss of the glycocalyx of enterocytes in small intestine. J Pediatr Gastroenterol Nutr 7:388.

absorption of nutrients provided by the diet, the digestive system must also process endogenous proteins (~70 g/day) and endogenous lipids (~25 g/day, mainly from bile), which are secreted into the lumen of the digestive tract in the salivary, gastric, pancreatic, biliary, and intestinal secretions or are components of the epithelial cells cast off into the lumen of the gastrointestinal tract.

Digestion largely involves the processes of enzymatic breakdown of these complex macronutrients to their smaller units (e.g., digestion of polysaccharides such as starch to monosaccharides such as glucose). Absorption of these smaller molecules across the epithelial cell layer of the intestinal mucosa into the interstitial fluid allows them to enter the blood or lymph for circulation to the rest of the body. Release and absorption of vitamins and minerals are also essential, and these processes are described in Units V and VI.

The gastrointestinal tract can be considered as a tubular structure extending from the mouth to the anus, and the contents in the lumen of the gastrointestinal tract can be considered as "outside" the cellular tissues of the body. Uptake of nutrients into the circulatory systems (blood and lymph), which supply the cellular tissues of the body with nutrients, depends upon the efficiency with which complex nutrients are broken down to smaller components that can be transported across the epithelial cells; upon the transporters located in the brush border (luminal) membrane of the mucosal epithelial cells (enterocytes), which allow their uptake from the luminal contents; upon further hydrolysis (e.g., peptide hydrolysis to amino acids) or processing (e.g., triacylglycerol synthesis and formation of chylomicrons) within the enterocytes; and upon transport out of the enterocyte across the contra-luminal or basolateral membrane into the interstitial fluid. From the interstitial fluid, products of digestion and absorption enter either the capillaries (and hence the portal blood) or the lacteals (and hence the lymph and ultimately the blood). The processes involved in the entrance of nutrients into the body circulation are discussed in this unit, and the subsequent utilization of these absorbed nutrients by body tissues is discussed in Unit III.

Certain dietary components, especially complex carbohydrates from plant cell walls, are not hydrolyzed by enzymes of the human digestive system and pass into the large intestine undigested. Some of these undigestible residues may be fermented by colonic bacteria to form short-chain fatty acids and gases, whereas others add directly to the mass of the stool or are used by the colonic bacteria for their own growth. The short-chain fatty acids may cross the colonic epithelium by diffusion, enter the portal blood, and be used as a fuel by tissues. The undigestible components of plant cells are called dietary fiber; fiber is not an essential nutrient, but it is considered to have physiological and health benefits and to be an important component of healthy diets.

♦ ♦

Martha H. Stipanuk

CHAPTER 4

◆ ◆

Overview of Digestion and Absorption

Patrick Tso, Ph.D., and Karen Crissinger, Ph.D.

OUTLINE

DIGESTION AND ABSORPTION IN THE GASTROINTESTINAL TRACT

Most foodstuffs are ingested in forms that are unavailable to the body and must be broken down into smaller molecules before they can be absorbed into the body fluids. The gastrointestinal tract is the system that carries out the functions of digestion and absorption. The gastrointestinal tract extends from the mouth to the anus (Fig. 4–1) and consists of a tubular structure with openings for the entry of secretions from the salivary glands, the liver, and the pancreas. The gastrointestinal system includes the mouth, stomach, small intestine, and large intestine, as well as accessory organs (salivary glands, pancreas, liver, and gallbladder) that provide essential secretions. The major function of the gastrointestinal tract is to digest complex molecules in foods and to absorb simple nutrients, including monosaccharides, monoacylglycerols, fatty acids, amino acids, vitamins, minerals, and water. It also serves as a barrier to the entry of bacteria into the body and contains specialized cells that secrete mucus, fluids, some digestive enzymes, intrinsic factor, and some peptide hormones.

Digestion is defined as the chemical breakdown of food by enzymes secreted into the lumen of the gastrointestinal tract by glandular cells in the mouth, chief cells in the stomach, and the exocrine cells of the pancreas, and by enzymes in the brush border (luminal) membrane and in the cytoplasm of mucosal cells of the small intestine. As such, digestion occurs prior to the entrance of nutrients into the interstitial fluid and hence into the circulatory system by which nutrients are carried to all cells of the body.

Absorption is the movement of nutrients, including water and electrolytes, across the mucosal cells into the interstitial fluid, from which they enter the blood or lymph. Processes involved in absorption include diffusion, facilitated diffusion, active transport (primary and secondary), solvent drag, and endocytosis. Most substances pass from the intestinal lumen into the mucosal cells and then out of the mucosal cells to the extracellular fluid, and the processes responsible for movement across the luminal or brush border membrane are often quite different from those responsible for movement across the basolateral or contraluminal cell membranes to the interstitial fluid. Once nutrients have exited from the intestinal absorptive cells into the interstitial fluid, they either enter the capillaries (into the blood) or lacteals (into the lymph). Water and some other molecules may be taken up by paracellular movement between cells.

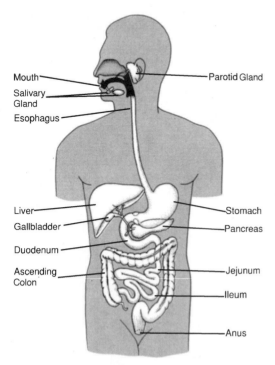

Mouth
Salivary Gland
Esophagus
Parotid Gland
Liver
Gallbladder
Duodenum
Ascending Colon
Stomach
Pancreas
Jejunum
Ileum
Anus

Figure 4–1. *Gross anatomy of the gastrointestinal system. (From Guyton, A. C. and Hall, J. E. [1997] Human Physiology and Mechanisms of Disease, 6th ed. W. B. Saunders, Philadelphia.)*

THE MOUTH

Chewing involves the cutting as well as grinding of food by the teeth. The process of chewing not only ensures that the bolus of food is crushed into smaller particles but also allows the mixing of saliva with food. As food is mixed with saliva, salivary amylase may begin the digestion of starch, and more importantly, the bolus of food is lubricated to facilitate swallowing.

Saliva has many functions, including digestion of nutrients, antibacterial activity (due to the presence of thiocyanate, lactoferrin, and lysozyme), moistening of the mouth to facilitate speech and swallowing, and buffering. The salivary glands secrete α-amylase, which is active within the food bolus until it is inactivated by the acidic secretions of the stomach. Secretion of saliva is under neural control. In some species, lingual lipase is secreted by glands in the tongue, and this enzyme is most active in the acidic environment of the gastric lumen. Secretion of lingual lipase is insignificant in humans, but humans do secrete a gastric lipase that has similar acid lipase activity (Abrams et al., 1988; Moreau et al., 1988).

Swallowing is a highly coordinated process, and the lower esophageal sphincter relaxes following swallowing to allow the entry of food into the stomach. Otherwise, the lower esophageal sphincter is closed to prevent the reflux of stomach acid into the esophagus. During pregnancy, the lower esophageal sphincter may not be as contracted as usual, and this may allow the reflux of acid into the esophagus to give the feeling of "heartburn."

THE STOMACH

The major functions of the stomach are to store food and to process the swallowed food in a preliminary fashion for delivery into the small intestine. Upon entry of food into the stomach, the stomach muscles relax. This phenomenon is called adaptive relaxation. While in the stomach, the food undergoes substantial physical and chemical modifications. Although the stomach is not an important absorptive organ, some water and lipid-soluble substances are absorbed by the stomach. For instance, ethanol and short- and medium-chain fatty acids are absorbed rapidly.

The gastric mucosa of the stomach contains many deep glands made up of chief cells, parietal cells, and mucous cells. The mixed secretions of these cells is known as gastric juice. Gastric juice contains mucin, inorganic salts, hydrochloric acid (HCl), and digestive enzymes or zymogens (gastric lipase and pepsinogens/pepsins). The parietal cells are the source of gastric HCl, with secretion of H^+ being driven by a membrane H^+, K^+-

ATPase. The gastric acidity that favors the denaturation (unfolding) of proteins, is necessary for activation of pepsinogen to pepsin and for the proteolytic activity of pepsin, and destroys many microorganisms that entered the gastrointestinal tract via the oral cavity. The parietal cells also secrete intrinsic factor, a glycoprotein that is required for vitamin B_{12} absorption. The neck mucous cells secrete bicarbonate and mucus. The chief cells of the gastric glands secrete pepsinogens and gastric lipase. Stimulation of gastric secretions depends on neural, endocrine, and paracrine mechanisms. Protein in food is a potent stimulant of gastrin release into the blood stream by endocrine cells of the stomach, but vagal stimulation, calcium ions (Ca^{2+}), and alkalinization of the antrum of the stomach also promote gastrin release. Gastrin stimulates gastic HCl and pepsinogen secretion, and gastrin secretion is inhibited by acid within the lumen of the antrum.

Pepsins begin the process of protein digestion in the stomach by cleaving the protein into large peptide fragments and some free amino acids. Gastric lipase hydrolyzes triacylglycerol in the acidic medium to form predominantly diacylglycerol and free fatty acid. Some products of fat hydrolysis may play a role in beginning the emulsification of lipids in the stomach contents.

Peristaltic contractions of the distal stomach propel the stomach contents toward the pylorus (located between the stomach and the duodenum) (Fig. 4–2). The pylorus is composed of a thickened band of circular muscle. Although it has been called the "pyloric sphincter," it does not function as a true sphincter because there is not a zone of high pressure in the pyloric region. Rather, it contracts in opposition to an approaching peristalsis. As the contractions reach the terminal antrum, the pylorus closes. This results in the grinding of solids to form finer particles. In addition, the acidic chyme (semifluid mass of partially digested food) that cannot pass forward through the opening of the pylorus will be retropelled into the body of the stomach. The retropulsion of the chyme results not only in the mixing of chyme but also in dispersion of oil droplets into very fine emulsion particles. The dispersion of oil droplets

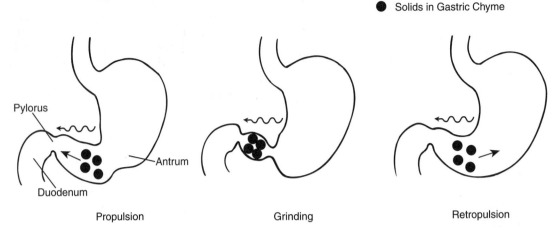

↶∿∿ Direction of Antral Peristaltic Wave
● Solids in Gastric Chyme

Pylorus

Antrum

Duodenum

Propulsion   Grinding   Retropulsion

Figure 4–2. *A diagram showing the consequences of antral peristalsis. (Modified from Kelly, K. A. [1981] Motility of the stomach and gastroduodenal junction. In: Physiology of the Gastrointestinal Tract [Johnson, L. R., ed.], Vol. 1, p. 400. Raven Press, New York.)*

greatly facilitates the subsequent digestion of lipids in the small intestine, because pancreatic lipase acts at the water/lipid interface, and emulsification significantly increases this surface area. Only liquids and small particles in chyme are allowed to pass into the duodenum because of the small opening that results from the contraction of the pyloric sphincter.

Gastric motility and secretion are regulated by both neural and humoral mechanisms. The gastrointestinal hormone that stimulates gastric motility as well as gastric acid secretion is gastrin. The neural stimulation of gastric acid secretion and gastric motility is via the vagus nerve. The stomach regulates the amount of food presented to the duodenum so as not to exceed the absorptive capacity of the small intestine. This occurs largely as a result of the actions of hormones such as gastric inhibitory peptide and cholecystokinin, which are released by the small intestine in response to the presence of digesta and which inhibit gastric motility, gastric emptying, and gastric secretion.

THE SMALL INTESTINE

Most of the digestion and uptake of nutrients takes place in the small intestine, and the small intestine is uniquely adapted to accommodate these processes. The small intestine is quite long and is often divided into three sections. The first section is the duodenum, which is about 1 foot long and ends at the ligament of Treitz; this section receives the chyme from the stomach and secretions from the liver or gallbladder and the pancreas. The remainder (about 9 feet) of the small intestine consists of the jejunum (the upper 40% below the duodenum) and the ileum (the lower 60%).

Anatomy

Figure 4–3 shows the general organization of the intestinal wall. Four distinct strata can be identified: mucosa, submucosa, muscularis propria, and serosa. The mucosa itself is composed of four layers: a surface layer of epithelial cells, a layer of basement membrane, the lamina propria (containing connective tissue, blood vessels, lymphatic vessels, nerves, and various types of cells such as lymphocytes, macrophages, and mast cells), and lastly the muscularis mucosa (containing smooth muscle cells). Next to the mucosa is the submucosa, which is composed of connective tissues, blood vessels, and lymphatic vessels. The third stratum of the small intestine is the muscularis propria, which consists of a layer of circular muscle followed by a layer of neurons (myenteric plexus) and lastly by a layer of longitudinal muscle. The outermost stratum

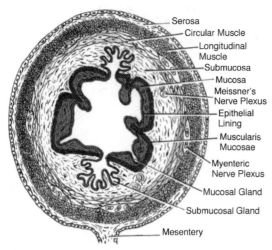

Figure 4–3. *General organization of the intestinal wall. (From Guyton, A. C. and Hall, J. E. [1997] Human Physiology and Mechanisms of Disease, 6th ed. W. B. Saunders, Philadelphia.)*

of the small intestine is called the serosa, composed of a layer of mesothelial cells. This general structural organization is preserved throughout the gastrointestinal tract in the stomach and the large intestine, but the small intestine has some additional adaptations that greatly increase its surface area.

To facilitate the surface digestion and absorption of nutrients, the small intestine is anatomically adapted to enhance greatly the epithelial digestive and absorptive surface, as illustrated in Figure 4–4. The small intestine has a surface area of approximately $200\,m^2$ due to folds of the mucosa, villi or finger-like projections of the mucosa, and the microvillar structure of the luminal or brush border membrane of the absorptive cells that make up the surface layer of the villi. Altogether, these adaptations of mucosal structure increase the surface area of the small intestine to 600 times the surface area of a cylinder of the same diameter.

The epithelial absorptive cells that have a brush border apical membrane are called enterocytes. The surface layer of the mucosa also contains a few goblet or mucus-secreting cells, some epithelial M cells that are associated with underlying lymphoid cells, and some intraepithelial lymphocytes; these cells can be recognized microscopically as not having a brush border apical membrane. The

epithelial cells are connected to each other by tight junctions and by desmosomes to form a mechanical seal that prevents mixing of the interstitial fluid with luminal contents.

An important characteristic of the gastrointestinal tract is that it continuously renews the cells lining its surface. Enterocytes lining the intestinal surface have an average life span of about 72 hours once they enter the villus from the crypt (simple glandular tubes at the base of the villus). The crypts contain proliferative units that provide the various types of cells for the gastrointestinal tract. These cells migrate up from the crypts to the tips of the villi and, soon thereafter, are sloughed off into the intestinal lumen, where they may undergo digestion. Cells in the crypts secrete a fluid called succus entericus, which contains water and electrolytes. As the epithelial cells proliferate and migrate up the villus, the activity of mucosal digestive enzymes and the capacity to absorb nutrients increases, whereas the capacity to secrete succus entericus decreases.

A single enterocyte is represented by Figure 4–5. The brush border membrane with its microvillar projections can be observed. The brush border membrane contains many embedded glycoproteins that extend from the membrane into the lumen. The carbohydrate side chains of these membrane glycoproteins make up a glycocalyx next to the brush border membrane itself; this glycocalyx acts to "trap water" and to form an "unstirred water layer" near the absorptive surface. Many of these glycoproteins are digestive enzymes, which will be discussed in more detail in Chapters 5 and 6. Because this fluid layer next to the epithelial cell surface is poorly mixed, the major mechanism for solute movement across the unstirred water layer is diffusion down the concentration gradient.

Digestion

Digestion in the small intestine is brought about by enzymes secreted by the pancreas, by enzymes located on the luminal membranes of the enterocytes lining the small intestine, and by enzymes within the enterocytes. As the acidic chyme from the stomach enters the duodenum, the acid stimulates the enteroendocrine S cells (special endocrine

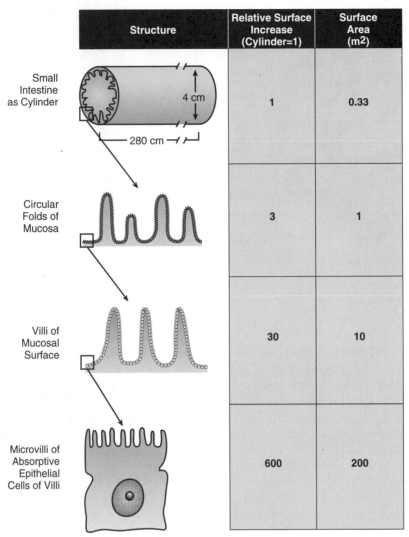

Structure	Relative Surface Increase (Cylinder=1)	Surface Area (m2)
Small Intestine as Cylinder	1	0.33
Circular Folds of Mucosa	3	1
Villi of Mucosal Surface	30	10
Microvilli of Absorptive Epithelial Cells of Villi	600	200

Figure 4–4. The small intestinal mucosal surface is amplified by specialized features of the mucosa. (From Waldeck, F. [1983] Functions of the gastrointestinal canal. In: Human Physiology [Schmidt, R. F. and Thews, G., eds.], p. 602. Springer-Verlag, New York.)

cells in the duodenum) to release a gastrointestinal hormone called secretin, which stimulates the pancreatic acinar cells (cells involved in the secretion of water, electrolytes, and enzymes) to secrete a bicarbonate-rich pancreatic secretion that has an alkaline pH of about 8. As expected, the highest densities of S cells are found in the duodenum and jejunum and the lowest densities are found in the ileum.

The presence of partially hydrolyzed fat (fatty acids) and protein (amino acids and peptides) in the chyme that enters the duodenum, as well as the acidic pH of the chyme, stimulates enteroendocrine I cells in the upper small intestine to release the hormone cholecystokinin (also known as pancreozymin), which causes discharge of zymogen granules from the pancreatic acinar cells and the secretion of an enzyme/zymogen-rich pancreatic juice. The pancreatic secretion contains pancreatic α-amylase, lipases (pancreatic lipase and cholesterol esterase), prophospholipase A_2, nucleolytic enzymes (ribonuclease and deoxyribonuclease), several proenzymes for proteolytic enzymes (trypsinogen, chymotrypsinogen, proelastase, and procarboxypeptidases), and a nonen-

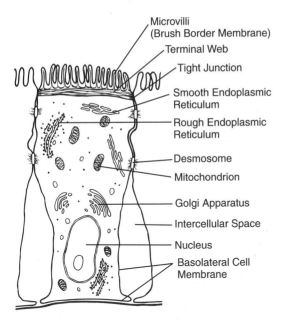

Figure 4–5. *Ultrastructure of a small intestinal epithelial cell (enterocyte).*

Microvilli (Brush Border Membrane)
Terminal Web
Tight Junction
Smooth Endoplasmic Reticulum
Rough Endoplasmic Reticulum
Desmosome
Mitochondrion
Golgi Apparatus
Intercellular Space
Nucleus
Basolateral Cell Membrane

pancreatic juice in the upper duodenum facilitates digestion of nutrients by pancreatic enzymes.

The liver secretes bile into the bile duct that empties into the duodenum. Between meals, the duodenal opening of this duct is closed and bile flows into the gallbladder, a saccular organ attached to the hepatic bile duct that serves to store and concentrate bile. The hormones released by the upper small intestine stimulate biliary flow. Secretin stimulates bile secretion by the liver, and cholecystokinin stimulates gallbladder contraction and the release of bile from the gallbladder into the intestine. Bile is an alkaline solution containing electrolytes, pigments, bile salts, and other substances. The pancreatic duct joins with the hepatic bile duct to form the common bile duct just prior to entering the duodenum, so the bile mixes with pancreatic secretions before they enter the duodenum. Bile salts play an important role in the normal digestion and absorption of lipids, as is discussed in more detail in Chapter 7.

Although the digestion of most nutrients in the small intestine is extensively carried out by enzymes secreted by the pancreas,

zyme proprotein called procolipase. Pancreatic enzymes are most active in the neutral pH range, and the rapid neutralization of the acid in the chyme by the bicarbonate in the

CLINICAL CORRELATION

Pancreatic Insufficiency and Malabsorption in Cystic Fibrosis

Cystic fibrosis is a fatal autosomal recessive genetic disorder with an incidence of approximately 1 in 2500 live white births. It is a systemic disorder that is caused by a dysfunction of the mucus-producing exocrine cells of the pancreas, bronchi, liver, and intestine. Symptoms of malabsorption and chronic pulmonary disease should suggest the diagnosis. However, infants and children with the disorder often present only with pancreatic insufficiency or with chronic pulmonary disease without apparent intestinal symptoms.

Diagnosis of the disease is based on the following tests:

(1) an abnormal sweat test with greater than 60 mEq/L of chloride;

(2) the presence of chronic pulmonary obstruction; and

(3) pancreatic insufficiency with evidence of steatorrhea, the presence of undigested protein in the stool, and the presence of very low concentrations of pancreatic enzymes in duodenal aspirates.

Pancreatic insufficiency can be remedied by pancreatic enzyme replacement therapy.

Using molecular biological techniques, the gene causing cystic fibrosis was cloned in 1989 (Riordan et al., 1989). The protein product called cystic fibrosis transmembrane conductance regulator (CFTR) has been conclusively demonstrated to be a 3',5'-cyclic adenosine monophosphate (cAMP)–regulated chloride channel (Breuer et al., 1992).

enzymes located at the brush border membrane of enterocytes are responsible for the completion of this process to release molecules that can be transported across the brush border membrane. Several α-glucosidases, a β-galactosidase, and several peptidases are present; these enzymes are necessary for futher digestion of oligosaccharide and peptide products of luminal hydrolysis, as well as of dietary disaccharides and other compounds. These brush border enzymes are called ectoenzymes because they are located outside the cell (i.e., on the luminal side of the membrane). In general, the hydrophobic domain of the protein is anchored to the lipid bilayer of the brush border membrane, and the bulk of the protein, including the active site domain, is exposed to the external environment.

Di- and tripeptides may be taken up by the intestinal epithelial cells, and they are further hydrolyzed to form free amino acids by intracellular peptidases. The enterocytes contain peptidases that actively catalyze the hydrolysis of these small peptides to free amino acids, as is discussed in Chapter 6. Also present in the intestinal epithelial cells are enzymes that are involved in the assimilation of lipid digestion products to form triacylglycerols, cholesteryl esters, and phospholipids for incorporation into chylomicrons. This subject is discussed in detail in Chapter 7.

Small Intestinal Motility

Small intestinal motility is uniquely adapted to facilitate both digestion and uptake of nutrients by the small intestine. The rate of digestion is dependent on the exposure of nutrients to the enzymes in the lumen of the small intestine. Consequently, a major function of intestinal motility is to ensure thorough mixing of intestinal contents. Thorough mixing of the intestinal contents also ensures the efficient digestion and uptake of nutrients by the small intestinal epithelial cells. Mixing is achieved by the presence of slow waves of contractions, followed by relaxation of different segments of the small intestine (called segmentation). Another function of the contractile activity of the small intestine is to ensure the slow migration of chyme away from the duodenum and toward the large intestine while allowing adequate time for the digestion and absorption of intestinal contents. The aboral gradient in the frequency of the slow waves along the small intestine, with about 12 cycles/min in the duodenum and a gradual decrease to about 9 cycles/min in the ileum, ensures that the chyme moves slowly from a region of higher contractile frequency to a region of lower contractile frequency.

Absorption

For nutrients to be absorbed, they must move across the mucosal cells (enterocytes) that comprise a barrier between the lumen of the gastrointestinal tract and the interstitial fluid on the other side of the mucosal cell layer. Transport processes are involved in the uptake of nutrients by the brush border or luminal membrane and also in the release of nutrients across the basolateral membrane into the extracellular fluid.

The uptake of nutrients and electrolytes by the intestinal epithelial cells is usually mediated by one of four general mechanisms. The first mechanism is mediated transport. Many compounds require a specific carrier or membrane transport protein for uptake. These carriers are located in the cell membrane. Mediated transport systems may be uniports (move only one compound), symports (move two compounds together), or antiports (exchangers that move one substance in and a different substance out of the cell).

Mediated transport systems may be passive or active. Passive transport by a carrier is also called facilitated diffusion, because passive transport, like diffusion, is down the electrochemical gradient from an area of high concentration to an area of low concentration. It can be bidirectional, allowing for an equalization of the concentration of a substance on both sides of the membrane. Examples of passive mediated transport are the Na^+-independent hexose transporters, such as GLUT5, which transports fructose across the brush border membrane into the enterocyte, and GLUT2, which transports glucose, galactose, and fructose out of the enterocyte across the basolateral membrane.

Active mediated transport involves energy expenditure, and these systems can be unidirectional and concentrative. Energy is supplied via ATP hydrolysis, but the energy requirement may be primary or secondary. For example, sodium (Na^+) and potassium (K^+) concentrations in cells are maintained by the Na^+,K^+-ATPase, which pumps Na^+ out of cells and K^+ into cells (against their concentration gradients) at the expense of ATP hydrolysis; this is primary active transport of Na^+ and K^+ by an antiport. The stoichiometry of the Na^+,K^+-ATPase reaction is 1 mol of ATP hydrolysis coupled to the outward pumping of 3 mol of Na^+ and the simultaneous inward pumping of 2 mol of K^+, which generates a low Na^+ concentration in the cytosol, and an electrical potential of about -60 mV in the cytosol relative to the extracellular fluid. On the other hand, the cotransport of Na^+ and glucose and of H^+ and dipeptides is by secondary active transport processes. In these processes the energy is directly derived from a concentration gradient or an electrical potential across the membrane rather than the chemical energy of a covalent bond change, such as ATP hydrolysis. Gradients may be established by ATP hydrolysis, as seen in the case of the Na^+,K^+-ATPase. For example, the Na^+-glucose transporter SGLT1 can concentrate glucose (against its concentration gradient) due to the cotransport of Na^+ down its electrochemical gradient. Thus, it is the low intracellular Na^+ concentration and the negative electrical potential, which are maintained by the Na^+,K^+-ATPase pump, that provide the "force" for glucose uptake. SGLT1 provides an example of secondary active transport by a symport.

Mediated transport allows uptake of nutrients and other compounds to be site-specific, because only the segment of the small intestine that expresses the carrier protein is capable of taking up the substrate. The advantage of expressing the transporters in a specific segment of the small intestine is illustrated by the concentrative reuptake of bile salts by a Na^+-bile acid cotransport system in the brush border membrane of enterocytes in the lower portion of the ileum. By delaying the uptake of bile salts by the small intestine until they reach the lower ileum, the presence of adequate bile salts in the lumen of the small intestine for efficient lipid digestion is ensured.

A second mechanism for the uptake of nutrients and electrolytes by the small intestinal epithelial cells is passive diffusion. This is especially true for water, many lipid-soluble molecules such as short-chain fatty acids, and for gases such as H_2 or CO_2 because they can diffuse through the lipid bilayer of the epithelial cell membranes. These substances diffuse across membranes in both directions, with net movement occurring down the concentration gradient. Uptake of substances by diffusion may also occur in the stomach and large intestine.

A third mechanism for uptake of some large molecules is pinocytosis. Receptor-mediated endocytosis may be responsible for uptake of some proteins as well as of any smaller molecules that are trapped within the endocytic vesicle. Similarly, molecules may be transported out of cells by exocytosis. Chylomicrons are exported from the enterocytes by exocytosis across the basolateral membrane.

The fourth mechanism for uptake of nutrients or of water and electrolytes by the small intestine is the paracellular pathway, which involves passage between cells through tight junctions. Osmolality plays an important role in the absorption of water and electrolytes by the small intestine via this process. The osmolality of the plasma is about 300 mOsm. When a hypotonic meal is ingested, water is rapidly absorbed by the duodenum and the jejunum paracellularly (between the cells) through the tight junctions. The tight junctions (pores between intestinal epithelial cells) of the duodenum and the jejunum have a larger diameter (8 Å) than those existing in the ileum (4 Å). The absorption of water facilitates the absorption of electrolytes by the small intestine (called solvent drag). When a hypertonic meal is ingested, water is drawn into the lumen. The accumulation of water in the lumen and the absorption of ions and nutrients by the small intestine brings the luminal contents to isotonicity. As shown in Figure 4–6, the proximal small intestine plays an important role in the absorption of water from a hypotonic meal, whereas the distal small intestine plays a more important role in the

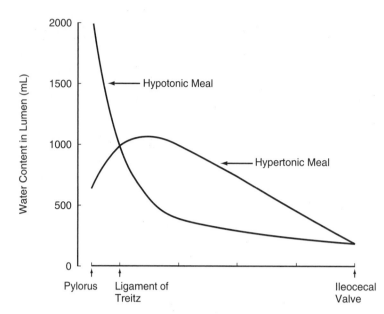

Figure 4–6. *Water content in lumen along the small intestine after a hypotonic (steak) meal and a hypertonic (doughnut and milk) meal. (Adapted from Fordtran, J. S. and Ingelfinger, F. J. [1968]. Absorption of water, electrolytes, and sugars from the human gut. In: Alimentary Canal. III: Intestinal Absorption [Code, C.F. and Heidel W., eds.], pp. 1457–1490. Williams and Wilkins, Baltimore.)*

absorption of water and electrolytes following a hypotonic meal.

Pancreatic and biliary secretions enter the upper duodenum via the sphincter of Oddi, and luminal digestion may occur throughout the duodenum and jejunum. Although the entire small intestine is capable of absorbing nutrients, the jejunum is by far the major site for the uptake of nutrients, and the absorption of most nutrients is complete before the chyme reaches the ileum. If nutrients are still present in the chyme that reaches the ileum, the physiological phenomenon called "ileal brake" may occur; this phenomenon refers to the observation that the presence of nutrients, especially long-chain fatty acids, in the ileum is a potent stimulus for slowing the emptying of chyme from the stomach as well as for reducing intestinal motility. The gastrointestinal hormone peptide YY has been implicated as a potential candidate for inducing the "ileal brake response."

Bile Acids and the Enterohepatic Circulation

The liver plays an important role in the digestion and uptake of lipids by the gastrointestinal tract because of its role in bile acid synthesis and secretion. Primary bile acids, cholic acid and chenodeoxycholic acid, are synthesized from cholesterol in the liver. The liver also conjugates bile acids with either taurine or glycine to form more polar compounds. The ionizable sulfonate group of taurine or the ionizable carboxyl group of glycine has a lower pKa than the carboxyl group of the unconjugated bile acid, and conjugated bile acids exist as negatively charged sulfonate or carboxylate ions. The ratio of glycine to taurine conjugates in adult human bile is about 3:1. Because bile contains significant amounts of Na^+ and K^+ and has an alkaline pH, the bile acids and their conjugates exist in bile in a salt form and are called bile salts. The terms bile acid and bile salt may be used interchangeably. The bile salts also solubilize some cholesterol in the bile and allow cholesterol to be transported from the liver to the intestine.

Conjugated bile acids exhibit detergent properties; at neutral pH values above their pKas (i.e., above pH 1.5 to 3.7) and at concentrations above 2 to 5 mmol/L, they reversibly form aggregates called micelles. Emulsification of dietary fat to increase the surface area between the lipid and aqueous phase; the digestion of cholesteryl esters, phospholipids and monoglycerides; and the solubilization and absorption of products of lipid digestion are facilitated by bile salts due to their ability to act as detergents and to form micelles.

Bile salts are recovered by the body via passive diffusion along the entire small intestine and via receptor-mediated transport in the lower ileum. The recirculation of compounds such as bile salts between the small intestine and the liver is called the enterohepatic circulation. The enterohepatic circulation of bile salts is extremely efficient, with only about 1% of the bile salts being lost via the feces per pass through the intestine. The body pool of bile salts (about 4 g) is cycled through the intestine about 12 times per day (depending on the frequency of meal intake); a loss of 1% (0.05 g) per pass results in a loss of about 0.5 g of bile salts per day via the feces. This loss is compensated for by daily synthesis of an equivalent amount of bile salts by the liver. Despite the synthesis of only about 0.5 g of bile salts/day by the liver, as much as 50 g of bile salts enter the small intestinal lumen each day to participate in the digestion and uptake of lipids. The loss of a small percentage of the bile salts in the feces with each pass through the intestinal tract represents the major route for excretion of cholesterol from the body.

A portion of the primary bile acids in the intestine may be metabolized by intestinal bacteria, leading to deconjugation and 7α-dehydroxylation to produce secondary bile acids; deoxycholate is produced from cholate, and lithocholate is produced from chenodeoxycholate. These secondary bile acids, especially deoxycholate, may be reabsorbed and participate in the enterohepatic circulation along with the primary bile acids.

METABOLISM OF NUTRIENTS IN THE ENTEROCYTES

Following the uptake of digestion products into the small intestinal epithelial cells, nutrients are either assimilated into the portal blood or the lymphatic vessels for export to other parts of the body or they are utilized by the cells themselves. Because the small intestinal epithelial cells are metabolically very active and are continuously being renewed, nutrients supplied by the arterial circulation or taken up from the intestinal lumen are necessary for maintenance of the structural and functional integrity of the small intestinal mucosa. The small intestine particularly uses glutamine as a fuel, as is discussed further in Chapters 6 and 11, and glutamine also stimulates the proliferation of enterocytes. Fasting causes atrophy of the small intestinal mucosa, and this atrophy can be reversed by feeding certain amino acids such as glutamine.

Within the enterocytes, most of the products of fat digestion, particularly the monoacylglycerols and long-chain fatty acids, are reesterified to form triacylglycerols, incorporated into chylomicrons, and exported. Chylomicrons also transport cholesteryl esters, phospholipids, and fat-soluble vitamins. Chylomicrons are too large to enter the pores of the capillaries, but they can pass through the large fenestrations of the lacteals and be transported by the lymphatic system. The lymphatic vessels ultimately empty into the venous circulation (by way of the thoracic duct) prior to the point where blood enters the heart.

TRANSPORT OF NUTRIENTS IN THE CIRCULATION

Nutrients that are absorbed from the gastrointestinal tract are subsequently transported either via the portal circulation or the lymphatic system. Most of the water-soluble nutrients (amino acids, monosaccharides, glycerol, short-chain fatty acids, electrolytes, and water-soluble vitamins) are transported predominantly by the portal route. These nutrients enter the capillaries that feed into the portal vein, which carries the venous blood draining from the splanchnic bed to the liver. The liver is unusual in that its major blood supply is the venous portal blood, with the hepatic artery supplying only about one quarter of the liver's blood flow.

The lymphatic system in the gastrointestinal tract plays a pivotal role in the transport of lipophilic (lipid-soluble) substances. A substance transported by the lymphatic system will enter the blood just before it goes to the heart and will then circulate throughout the body in the arterial blood, whereas those substances transported in the portal blood will first pass through the liver, where they may be taken up and metabolized by the hepatocytes or returned to the venous circulation via the hepatic vein. This distinction between lymphatic versus portal transport is of great importance to the pharmaceutical industry for targeting the delivery of drugs. The lymphatic system also, of course, plays an important role in maintaining the fluid balance in the body by acting as a drainage system to return excess fluid and proteins from tissue space into the circulatory system. Although many of the molecules carried by the portal circulation can also be carried by the lymphatic circulation, the portal blood flow is many times higher than lymphatic flow, so transport by the lymphatic circulation is only of minor significance, compared with the portal circulation, for transport of most water-soluble compounds.

REGULATION OF DIGESTION AND ABSORPTION

The digestion and absorption of nutrients are both neurally and hormonally regulated. The regulation of digestive and absorptive processes involves a number of levels. In terms of the digestive process, regulation involves the modification of the rate of delivery of chyme to the small intestine for digestion, the release of gastric secretions, the release and composition of pancreatic secretions, and the release of biliary secretions. The regulation of the absorptive process involves the absorptive surface area as well as the expression of certain transporter molecules located in the brush border membrane.

Neural Control

The gastrointestinal tract is innervated both by an intrinsic as well as an extrinsic nervous system. The intrinsic nervous system is responsible for much of the neural regulation of gastrointestinal motility and function, but it is influenced by the extrinsic nervous system, mainly the parasympathetic nervous system and to a lesser degree the sympathetic nervous system. The entire gastrointestinal tract is innervated by the vagal (parasympathetic) afferent nerve fibers (afferent refers to the fact that they are carrying information away from the gastrointestinal tract to the central nervous system). The vagal afferent system plays an important role in the regulation of gastrointestinal functions. The gastrointestinal tract is also innervated by vagal efferents (efferent refers to the fact that they are carrying information from the central nervous system to the gastrointestinal tract).

A good example of the neural control of gastrointestinal function is the regulation of salivary secretion. Salivary secretion by the salivary glands is almost exclusively controlled by neural signals. This is quite different from gastric and pancreatic secretions, which are under both neural and hormonal controls. The parasympathetic nervous system is the most important physiological regulator of salivary secretion. Smell, sight, taste, and tactile stimuli excite the salivary nuclei in the central nervous system, which, in turn, increase the parasympathetic activity innervating the salivary glands. As a result of parasympathetic activation, salivary secretion can increase by as much as six- to eight-fold. Although the salivary glands are also innervated by the sympathetic nervous system, the sympathetic system seems to play a minor role in the regulation of salivary secretion.

A neural mechanism is involved in the increase in gastric emptying induced by gastric distention of the stomach and in the inhibition of gastric emptying induced by the presence of a hypertonic meal in the duodenum. Neural mechanisms are also involved in the regulation of pancreatic exocrine secretion. For instance, gastric distention stimulates acetylcholine release by vagal impulses, and this, in turn, stimulates the secretion of pancreatic juice that is rich in enzymes. Vagal impulses are also involved in the release of acetylcholine in response to the presence of fat and protein digestion products in the small intestinal lumen; this, likewise, stimulates the release of an enzyme-rich pancreatic secretion.

Gastrointestinal Hormones

Gastrointestinal hormones are intimately involved in the coordinated release of secretions into the duodenum, in maintenance of the integrity and cellular homeostasis of the gastrointestinal tract, and in regulation of the motility of the gastrointestinal tract. Gut regulatory peptides are involved in a wide range of processes, and in many cases their functions overlap.

Gastrin. Gastrin is a hormone produced by the antrum of the stomach. Its major role in the gastrointestinal tract is the stimulation of gastric acid and pepsinogen secretion and gastric motility. Gastrin also plays an important role in the proliferation of gastric mucosal cells, in particular the acid-secreting mucosa of the stomach. Gastrin is released by the gastrin (G) cells in the antrum in the presence of protein in the gastric lumen. Gastric release by the G cells is inhibited by acidification of the gastric lumen below pH 3. This feedback mechanism regulates the amount of gastrin released (and therefore the amount of acid secreted) in response to a meal. The circulating level of gastrin in neonates is significantly elevated compared with that of adults, and this higher level is sustained for days after birth (Christie, 1981; Euler et al., 1978). This may be due to an elevated luminal pH, because gastric acid production does not approach adult levels until an infant is about 3 months of age (Christie, 1981; Grand et al., 1976). Another possible explanation for higher levels of gastrin in neonates is that the high protein and calcium content of a milk diet stimulates gastrin release (Lichtenberger, 1984). Gastrin may contribute to both the maturation of gastrointestinal function and the acceleration of mucosal growth during the newborn period (Lucas et al., 1981).

Secretin. Secretin was the first gastrointestinal hormone discovered. Secretin is secreted by the S cells of the duodenum. Secretion by these S cells is markedly stimulated by the acidification of the duodenal lumen. The major function of secretin in the gastrointestinal tract is the stimulation of pancreatic bicarbonate secretion, which neutralizes acidic chyme and promotes intestinal digestion by pancreatic enzymes. Secretin may inhibit gastric emptying. Plasma secretin levels are higher in neonates than in adults (Lucas et al., 1980). Because secretin is considered to be a major factor in triggering the release of bicarbonate-rich secretion from the pancreas, the higher levels of circulating secretin in the neonate may be of considerable importance in muco-sal protection during the newborn period. It is notable that the postnatal surge of secretin, unlike that of the other alimentary hormones, occurs even in the absence of feeding (Lucas et al., 1982).

Cholecystokinin. Cholecystokinin is a gastrointestinal hormone secreted by the I enteroendocrine cells of the duodenum and the jejunum, as well as by the neurons in the brain and the gastrointestinal tract. Cholecystokinin is responsible for postprandial pancreatic enzyme secretion and gallbladder contraction (Liddle et al., 1985; O'Rourke et al., 1990). Cholecystokinin is released in response to the presence of fat or protein in the small intestine (Liddle et al., 1985). In addition to its secretory effects, cholecystokinin can stimulate hyperplasia and hypertrophy of the pancreas (Peterson et al., 1978).

Somatostatin. Somatostatin has been found in neurons throughout the brain and spinal cord and in the D cells of the gastrointestinal tract. Somatostatin possesses powerful inhibitory effects on endogenous hormone release (growth hormone, thyroid-stimulating hormone, gastrin, glucagon, gastric inhibitory polypeptide, insulin, motilin, neurotensin, pancreatic polypeptide, secretin, calcitonin, and renin) and on gastrointestinal secretion (gastric acid, pepsin, pancreatic exocrine secretions, and small intestinal secretions). It is interesting that, in the human fetus and neonate, somatostatin is the second most abundant hormone after insulin in the pancreas, but a rapid reversal occurs in maturity so that somatostatin takes fourth place in abundance in the adult pancreas, after insulin, pancreatic polypeptide, and glucagon.

Other Peptides. In addition to those just discussed, other peptides of possible gastrointestinal significance include epidermal growth factor, transforming growth factor, insulin-like growth factor, hepatocyte growth factor, pancreatic glucagon, enteroglucagon, pancreatic polypeptide, gastric inhibitory polypeptide, motilin, vasoactive intestinal polypeptide, bombesin, neurotensin, substance P, leucine enkephalin, methionine enkephalin, and peptide YY. Detailed discussion of the numerous effects of these peptides is beyond the scope of this chapter.

DEVELOPMENTAL ASPECTS OF GASTROINTESTINAL PHYSIOLOGY

The development of peptic activity in the stomach is complete at birth, with term infants having pepsin levels (units per milligram of protein) similar to those of older children and adults (DiPalma et al., 1991). Premature infants weighing 1000 g have approximately half the peptic activity of term infants (Adamson et al., 1988). Gastric lipase activity is low in premature infants younger than 26 weeks of gestation, but it increases from 26 to 35 weeks of gestation (Hamosh et al., 1981; Lee et al., 1993) and is similar to adult levels at birth (DiPalma et al., 1991).

Pancreatic secretory function is immature in the neonate. Although trypsin, lipase, and amylase are found in the duodenum of premature infants at 32 weeks of gestation, the concentrations of these enzymes are lower in premature infants than in term infants (Zoppi et al., 1972). During the neonatal period, pancreatic enzymes do not develop in parallel with each other; trypsin appears in greatest quantity relative to adult levels first, followed by chymotrypsin, carboxypeptidase, lipase, and then amylase (Lebenthal and Lee, 1980).

Fat malabsorption does not pose a major problem in premature and term infants despite the immature pancreatic secretion, presumably because of the action of gastric lipases as well as lipases present in milk (Hamosh and Burns, 1977; DeNigris et al., 1988; Moreau et al., 1988). In contrast to digestion of fat, however, the digestion of complex carbohydrates and starches varies (De Vizia et al., 1975). In term infants, blood glucose levels fail to rise in response to starch ingestion, and the duodenal hydrolysis of amylopectin is low (Auricchio et al., 1967). Nevertheless, formulas containing glucose polymers and corn syrup solids are generally well tolerated and support growth in infants. Salivary amylase is present early in gestation and presumably contributes to the digestion of glucose polymers (Cicco et al., 1981). Moreover, negligible amounts of carbohydrate are found in the stools of infants, presumably as a result of bacterial fermentation in the colon (Shulman et al., 1983).

Most of the luminal protein hydrolysis occurs in the duodenum and jejunum and is dependent on the presence of enterokinase (an intestinal enzyme) as well as pancreatic proteases. Enterokinase initiates the process of protein digestion by the activation of trypsinogen (see Chapter 6). Activity levels of enterokinase at birth are 25% of those at 1 year, and 10% of adult levels, and increase thereafter until adult levels are reached by approximately 4 years of age. The relative deficiency of enterokinase activity, however, is not rate-limiting for protein digestion in infants.

The activity of lactase, a brush border β-galactosidase, increases at 14 weeks of gestation but then remains at 30% of the newborn level until birth (Antonowicz and Lebenthal, 1977; Raul et al., 1986). Peak lactase activity is found during early postnatal life. Within the first few years of life, lactase activity decreases to the adult level (one tenth that at birth in most adults; see Chapter 5). In contrast, sucrase-α-dextrinase activity rises steadily, but at variable rates; 70% of the adult level is achieved at 34 weeks of gestation, and adult levels are achieved at birth (Raul et al., 1986). Glucoamylase (maltase) and trehalase activities have been detected at 13 weeks of gestation. Most of the activities of the brush border peptidases (peptidyl dipeptidase, aminopeptidase, dipeptidylpeptidase IV, and γ-glutamyl hydrolase) are present at 8 weeks of gestation.

Bile acid metabolism is immature in premature and term infants relative to that in adults. The rate of bile acid synthesis increases throughout gestation and with increasing postnatal age (Heubi et al., 1982; Watkins et al., 1975). The bile acid pool size in premature and term infants is about 3% to 4% and 10%, respectively, that of adults (Watkins et al., 1975). The pool size increases, however, with increasing postnatal age. The concentration of bile acids in the duodenum of premature infants is less than that found in term infants and adults, and a critical micellar concentration of bile acids, sufficient to maintain adequate dispersion of the products of fat digestion, may not be achieved in premature infants (Watkins et al., 1975).

The enterohepatic pathway of bile acid absorption is also immature in the human infant. Taurine-conjugated bile acids are passively absorbed by the fetal gut (Lester et al.,

1977); active ileal transport begins after birth (de Belle et al., 1979). It is likely that the immaturity of bile acid synthesis, secretion, metabolism, and enterohepatic circulation contributes to the presence of steatorrhea in premature infants.

THE LARGE INTESTINE AND THE ROLE OF COLONIC BACTERIA

The residues from digestion and absorption in the small intestine pass through the ileocecal valve into the large intestine. The colon or large intestine is larger in diameter than the small intestine; it has no villi but has colonic glands that secrete mucus. The large intestine serves two general functions: The ascending colon is the location where most fermentation occurs, and the descending colon provides for water and electrolyte absorption and stool formation. It takes about 4 h for the first part of a test meal to reach the upper large intestine, and all the undigested portion from a meal enters the large intestine within about 8 h of eating. In contrast, transport through the large intestine is much slower, and it may take more than a week to recover all residues from a given meal in the feces.

Carbohydrates that are not absorbed in the small intestine, as well as the carbohydrate components of mucus, are transformed into acetic, propionic, and butyric acids by bacteria within the lumen of the colon. The short-chain fatty acids produced by carbohydrate fermentation account for over 50% of the total anion content of human feces. Luminal bicarbonate neutralizes a significant fraction of the acid load generated by production of these volatile short-chain fatty acids, resulting in the formation of carbon dioxide and water. The human large intestine absorbs significant quantities of short-chain fatty acids, primarily by diffusion. Once absorbed, the fatty acids either are metabolized to ketone bodies by the colonic epithelium or are transported via the portal vein to other tissues where they can be used as an energy source. Although the nutritional importance of short-chain fatty acid absorption remains uncertain for humans, it is well recognized that some ruminants obtain 70% of their energy requirements from short-chain fatty acids produced and absorbed in the forestomach.

A variety of bacteria in the colon produce hydrogen gas, methane, and carbon dioxide through metabolism (fermentation) of unabsorbed polysaccharides and other food residues. Other bacteria consume gases produced by the bacterial gas producers. The degree of flatus passed is determined by the balance of bacterial gas production versus gas consumption.

Colonic microbes also have enzymes that can metabolize long-chain fatty acids. Up to 25% of total fecal fatty acids are hydroxylated by bacteria in the colon. Hydroxylated fatty acids such as hydroxystearic acid (a product of microbial hydration of oleic acid) can exert a profound influence on colonic electrolyte and water transport. These substances inhibit net absorption of water and electrolytes by the colon and induce net secretion (and diarrhea) at high luminal concentrations. Almost all the cholesterol entering the colon is excreted in feces. A small proportion of the cholesterol is metabolized by colonic bacteria to coprostanol and coprostanone, both of which are poorly soluble and unavailable for absorption.

The small fraction of bile acids that are not reabsorbed in the ileum enter the colon, where they are extensively metabolized by the microflora. The number of bile acid metabolites produced by colonic bacteria is enormous. The degradative reactions produce products that are more lipid-soluble than the substrates, facilitating their passive absorption in the colon. It is estimated that the equivalent of 50 mg/day of bile acids are passively absorbed in the human colon, primarily as microbial degradation products. Both fat and fiber sequester bile acids and their metabolites in the lumen of the colon and thereby interfere with their absorption.

Approximately 25% of the urea synthesized in the liver reaches the gastrointestinal tract by diffusion from the blood. Bacterial urease in the colon converts it to ammonia, and the ammonia diffuses readily across the colonic mucosa and enters the portal venous blood and returns to the liver, where it is used for resynthesis of urea. The absorption of ammonia from the colon is believed to contribute to the raised blood ammonia levels of patients with liver disease in whom portal-systemic shunting (the flow of blood from the gastrointestinal tract to the circulation with bypass of the liver) may occur.

REFERENCES

Abrams, C. K., Hamosh, M., Lee, T. C., Ansher, A. F., Collen, M. J., Lewis, J. H., Benjamin, S. B. and Hamosh, P. (1988) Gastric lipase: Localization in the human stomach. Gastroenterology 95: 1460–1464.

Adamson, I., Esangbedo, A., Okolo, A. A. and Omene, J. A. (1988) Pepsin and its multiple forms in early life. Biol Neonate 53:267–273.

Antonowicz, I. and Lebenthal, E. (1977) Developmental pattern of small intestinal enterokinase and disaccharidase activities in the human fetus. Gastroenterology 72:1299–1303.

Auricchio, S., Della-Pietra, D. and Vegnente, A. (1967) Studies on intestinal digestion of starch in man: II. Intestinal hydrolysis of amylopectin in infants and children. Pediatrics 39:853–862.

Breuer, W., Kartner, N., Riordan, J. R. and Cabantchik, Z. I. (1992) Induction of expression of the cystic fibrosis transmembrane conductance regulator. J Biol Chem 267:10465–10469.

Christie, D. L. (1981) Development of gastric function during the first month of life. In: Textbook of Gastroenterology and Nutrition in Infancy (Lebenthal, E., ed.), pp. 109–120. New York, Raven Press.

Cicco, R., Holzman, I. R., Brown, D. R. and Becker, D. J. (1981) Glucose polymer tolerance in premature infants. Pediatrics 67:498–501.

de Belle, R. C., Vaupshas, V., Vitullo, B. B., Haber, L. R., Shaffer, E., Mackie, G. G., Owen, H., Little, J. M. and Lester, R. (1979) Intestinal absorption of bile salts: Immature development in the neonate. J Pediatr 94:472–476.

DeNigris, S. J., Hamosh, M., Kasbekar, D. K., Lee, T. C. and Hamosh, P. (1988) Lingual and gastric lipases: Species differences in origin of prepancreatic digestive lipases and in the localization of gastric lipases. Biochim Biophys Acta 959:38–45.

De Vizia, B., Ciccimarra, F., De Cicco, N. and Auricchio, S. (1975) Digestibility of starches in infants and children. J Pediatr 86:50–55.

DiPalma, J. A., Kirk, C. L., Hamosh, M., Colon, A. R., Benjamin, S. B. and Hamosh, P. (1991) Lipase and pepsin activity in gastric mucosa of infants, children, and adults. Gastroenterology 101:116–121.

Euler, A. R., Ament, M. E. and Walsh, J. H. (1978) Human newborn hypergastrinemia: An investigation of prenatal and perinatal factors and their effects on gastrin. Pediatr Res 12:652–654.

Grand, R. J., Watkins, J. B. and Torti, F. M. (1976) Development of the human gastrointestinal tract. Gastroenterology 70:790–810.

Hamosh, M. and Burns, W. A. (1977) Lipolytic activity of human lingual glands. Lab Invest 37:603–608.

Hamosh, M., Scanlon, J. W., Ganot, D., Likel, M., Scanlon, K. B. and Hamosh, P. (1981) Fat digestion in the newborn: Characterization of lipase in gastric aspirates of premature and term infants. J Clin Invest 67:838–846.

Heubi, J. E., Balistreri, W. F. and Suchy, F. J. (1982) Bile salt metabolism in the first year of life. J Lab Clin Med 100:127–136.

Lebenthal, E. and Lee, P. C. (1980) Development of functional responses in human exocrine pancreas. Pediatrics 66:556–560.

Lee, P.-C., Borysewicz, R., Struve, M., Raab, K. and Werlin, S. L. (1993) Development of lipolytic activity in gastric aspirates from premature infants. J Pediatr Gastroenterol Nutr 17:291–297.

Lester, R., Smallwood, R. A., Little, J. M., Brown, A. S., Piasecki, G. J. and Jackson, B. T. (1977) Fetal bile salt metabolism: The intestinal absorption of bile salt. J Clin Invest 59:1009–1016.

Lichtenberger, L. (1984) A search for the origin of neonatal hypergastrinemia. J Pediatr Gastroenterol Nutr 3:161–166.

Liddle, R., Goldfine, I., Rosen, M., Taplitz, R. A. and Williams, J. A. (1985) Cholecystokinin bioactivity in human plasma: Molecular forms, responses to feeding, and relationship to gallbladder contraction. J Clin Invest 75:1144–1152.

Lucas, A., Adrian, T. E., Bloom, S. R., and Aynsley-Green, A. (1980) Plasma secretin in neonates. Acta Pediatr Scand 69:205–210.

Lucas, A., Aynsley-Green, A. and Bloom, S. R. (1981) Gut hormones and the first meals. Clin Sci 60:349–353.

Lucas, A., Bloom, S. R. and Aynsley-Green, A. (1982) Postnatal surges in plasma gut hormones in term and preterm infants. Biol Neonate 41:63–67.

Moreau, H., Laugier, R. Gargouri, Y., Ferrato, F. and Verger, R. (1988) Human preduodenal lipase is entirely of gastric fundic origin. Gastroenterology 95:1221–1226.

O'Rourke, M. F., Reidelberger, R. D. and Solomon, T. E. (1990) Effect of CCK antagonist L 364718 on meal-induced pancreatic secretion in rats. Am J Physiol 258:G179–G184.

Peterson, H., Solomon, T. and Grossman, M. (1978) Effect of chronic pentagastrin, cholecystokinin, and secretin on pancreas of rats. Am J Physiol 234:E286–E293.

Raul, F., Lacroix, B. and Aprahamian, M. (1986) Longitudinal distribution of brush border hydrolases and morphological maturation in the intestine of the preterm infant. Early Hum Dev 13:225–234.

Riordan, J. R., Rommens, J. M., Keren, B., Alon, N., Rozmahel, R., Grzelczak, Z., Zielenski, J., Lok, S., Plavsic, N., Chou, J. L., Drumm, M. L., Iannuzzi, M. C., Collins, F. S. and Tsui, L.-C. (1989) Identification of the cystic fibrosis gene: Cloning and characterization of complementary DNA. Science 245:1066–1073.

Shulman, R. J., Wong, W. W., Irving, C. S., Nichols, B. L. and Klein, P. D. (1983) Utilization of dietary cereal by young infants. J Pediatr 103:23–28.

Watkins, J. B., Szczepanik, P., Gould, J. B., Klein, P. and Lester, R. (1975) Bile salt metabolism in the human premature infant. Gastroenterology 69:706–713.

Zoppi, G., Andreotti, G., Pajno-Ferrara, F., Njai, D. M. and Gaburro, D. (1972) Exocrine pancreas function in premature and full-term infants. Pediatr Res 6:880–886.

RECOMMENDED READINGS

Davenport, H. W. (1978) A Digest of Digestion, 2nd ed. Year Book Medical Publishers, Inc., Chicago.

Hobsley, M. (1982) Disorders of the Digestive System. University Park Press, Baltimore.

Johnson, L. R., ed. (1994) Physiology of the Gastrointestinal Tract, 3rd ed., Vols. 1 and 2. Raven Press, New York.

CHAPTER **5**

◆ ◆

Digestion and Absorption of Carbohydrate

Gary M. Gray, M.D.

OUTLINE

CARBOHYDRATE COMPONENTS OF THE HUMAN DIET

A variety of simple and complex carbohydrates are present in human diets. The digestible carbohydrates are important sources of energy for the body, and their digestion and absorption are the focus of this chapter. The complex nondigestible carbohydrates from plant foods are the major components of dietary fiber. These nondigestible carbohydrates are discussed in detail in Chapter 8.

Digestible Carbohydrates

Carbohydrates are relatively inexpensive and readily assimilated nutrients that have comprised an increasingly higher fraction of the Western diet in recent years. Most of the ingested carbohydrates are polymers, oligomers, or dimers of hexoses (i.e., glucose, galactose, and fructose), and these are digested efficiently as they travel down the small intestine by processes involving enzymatic cleavage of the oxygen bridge, called a glycosidic bond, between the hexose units. Final transport across the intestine is reserved for the released free hexoses. The processes of enzymatic digestion predominantly occur (1) within the lumen of the initial segment of the small intestine, the duodenum, under the influence of secreted pancreatic amylase, and (2) through hydrolysis on the intestinal surface membrane by the abundant constituent oligosaccharidases of the columnar epithelial enterocytes lining the small intestine.

About 300 g (1200 kcal) of carbohydrates are ingested daily in the Western diet. The fate of the major dietary carbohydrates within the small intestine is shown in Table 5–1. Although the starches are quantitatively the predominant carbohydrate type, refined table sugar (sucrose) and lactose from milk products are important dietary disaccharides. Although lactose is a major carbohydrate in the diets of infants, consumption of lactose declines during later childhood and adolescence as milk makes up a smaller portion of the diet. Additional commercially processed carbohydrates are often consumed in prepared sweetened drinks and desserts. These include corn syrup, which is a partially hydrolyzed starch preparation consisting of glucosyl oligosaccharides joined by α-1,4 and α-1,6 links (commonly referred to as maltodextrins), and invert sugar, which is a mixture of glucose and fructose commonly produced by acid-hydrolysis of sucrose. Free fructose is a more potent sweetener than the parent sucrose itself, and concentrated invert sugar preparations can be readily incorporated into confections.

Nondigestible Carbohydrates

In addition to the readily assimilated carbohydrates, nondigestible carbohydrates are of nutritional concern, especially because of the emphasis on possible health benefits of a high-fiber diet. Mammals have no digestive capacity for certain oligosaccharides with α-galactosidic linkages (raffinose and stachyose) that are constituents of some legumes, particularly the kidney-shaped beans. Dietary fiber includes polysaccharide components that are homopolymers of glucosyl units connected by β-glycosidic linkages (e.g., cellulose and β-glucans), as well as various heteropolysaccharides (e.g., hemicelluloses, pectic substances, gums and mucilages, and algal polysaccharides) that contain a variety of sugar residues and types of linkages. Because mam-

TABLE 5–1
Digestion of Dietary Carbohydrate

Food Source	% of Carbohydrate	Luminal Hydrolysis	Intestinal Hydrolysis
Starches (amylose, amylopectin)	60–70	→ Maltose and maltotriose and α-dextrins	→ Glucose
Lactose	0–10	None	→ Glucose and galactose
Sucrose	30	None	→ Glucose and fructose

malian pancreatic secretions and integral intestinal carbohydrases are incapable of cleaving the β-linked glucosyl and α-linked galactosyl bonds, these polysaccharides and oligosaccharides cannot be digested by the intestinal machinery. Instead, they remain intact and may have local effects on intestinal transport as they travel to lower levels of the ileum and to the colon where the resident bacteria then cleave and modify them extensively to short-chain fatty acids, hydrogen gas, carbon dioxide, and methane.

Dietary fiber does produce a great increase in the osmotically active particles in the lower small intestine and colon, resulting in an increase in the stool water output, but some of the potential osmotic excess is compensated for by colonic absorption of the short-chain fatty acids generated by bacteria (see Chapter 8 for more discussion of dietary fiber).

SITES AND MECHANISMS OF DIGESTION OF CARBOHYDRATES

Carbohydrate digestion occurs by enzymatic cleavage of bonds between adjacent units, leading to the release of small oligosaccharides, disaccharides, and monosaccharides. Starch digestion begins with the action of secreted α-amylase in the lumen of the gastrointestinal tract and is completed by the action of three α-glucosidases that are associated with the brush border membrane of the intestinal mucosal cells. Dietary disaccharides are hydrolyzed by α-glucosidases or the β-galactosidase associated with the brush border membrane of the enterocytes.

Luminal Digestion of the Starches by α-Amylase

Production and secretion of amylase are restricted to the salivary and pancreatic exocrine glands. The high concentrations of amylase achieved within the duodenal lumen greatly exceed those required for cleavage of the bonds joining the glucose components of the starches. The amylase gene is transcribed under the influence of cell-specific nuclear factors, particularly pancreatic transcription factor 1 and a group of several hepatocyte-type nuclear factors (Cockell et al., 1995). The presence of ingested carbohydrate in the intestinal lumen (Tsai et al., 1994) and the direct action of the hormone cholecystokinin (CCK) on the exocrine pancreas (Chen et al., 1993) augment the transcription of amylase mRNA, leading to enhanced amylase synthesis. The α-amylases are secreted as soluble proteins via the salivary and pancreatic ducts.

Food starches are present in grains and legumes in association with proteins, many of which are hydrophobic and hence hinder the luminal interaction of the secreted polar α-amylases with the polysaccharide within the interior of the starch granule. Fortunately, physical processing of grains such as cracking, milling, and heating at 100° C for several minutes changes the physical relationship of starch to the accompanying protein, making it more available to the water-soluble α-amylase. Also, nondigestible polysaccharides (e.g., cellulose, hemicellulose, and pectin) may interfere with the efficiency of the amylase–starch interaction by hindering the physical interaction of amylase with its substrate.

Refined starches are hydrolyzed efficiently, even in exocrine pancreatic insufficiency, despite the fact that α-amylase concentrations are reduced to only 10% of normal (Fogel and Gray, 1973). However, various inhibitory factors retard the digestion of starch in grains and legumes, even when pancreatic amylase secretion is normal. Hence, depending upon the physical availability of starch in the food preparation, a small proportion (1% to 10%) of the ingested starch may escape α-amylase action; this residual starch passes into the colon to be subjected to bacterial action, as described earlier for the nondigestible carbohydrates.

Although amylase is secreted in large quantities via the pancreatic ducts into the intestinal lumen and appears to act primarily in the polar milieu of the luminal contents, some of the secreted enzyme does adhere to intestinal mucosal membrane at the outer brush border surface. This has been proposed to provide a topographic advantage by virtue of the release of the glucosyl oligosaccharide products at the lumen–membrane interface, where final digestion can be catalyzed by integral brush border enzymes. However, the great majority of the starch component of grains or legumes establishes contact with the α-amylases within the polar bulk phase of the intestinal luminal milieu. Indeed, the cleavage to the final oligosaccharide products occurs by the time the meal reaches the duodenal-jejunal junction (Fogel and Gray, 1973).

Digestion begins in the mouth by salivary α-amylase, but this ceases abruptly after passage of the contents to the acid milieu of the stomach, because of the neutral pH requirement of the amylase. Although the α-amylase protein is labile in acid, the presence of starch in the meal protects the enzyme from gastric degradation (Rosenblum et al., 1988), and salivary amylase may pass with the meal into the duodenum where it may complement pancreatic α-amylase in continuing the cleavage of the starches. In newborn infants, particularly when birth is premature, the passed salivary amylase may play a functional role in the duodenum, because pancreatic amylase levels are low in the early neonatal period in the premature infant. However, the relatively low concentration of luminal pancreatic amylase in neonates has prompted pediatricians and nutritionists to recommend withholding starch from the diet until the baby is about 6 months of age.

It is important to consider the structure of the principal dietary starches, because amylase has specificity for only the α-1,4-linked straight chain regions of the glucosyl polysaccharides, and the most abundant food starches also have the α-1,6-branching links. The simplest starch is the linear and unbranched amylose, which is a polymer of α-1,4-linked glucosyl units (~600 glucose residues per molecule).

α-Amylase has maximal specificity for the interior links, and its active site binds five consecutive glucosyl residues at specific subsites and cleaves between the second and third subsites, as shown in Figure 5–1, to form two smaller polymers. Sequential cleavage eventually leads to the production of a pentasaccharide that binds with high affinity at all five of the amylase subsites. The pentasaccharide will be hydrolyzed at the penultimate linkage from the reducing end of the pentasaccharide to release the trisaccharide malto-

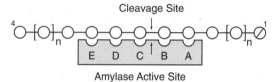

Cleavage Site

Amylase Active Site

Figure 5–1. Model of the active site of α-amylase. Five α-1,4-linked glucose units indicated as ◯ are shown positioned in subsites A through E, with the reducing end glucosyl residue indicated as ⊘. Each designated subsite has the appropriate conformation to accept an α-1,4-linked glucosyl residue; the glucosyl residues of amylose are shown in the figure with the 1-C (potential reducing carbon) on the right and the 4-C on the left. The cleavage site is between subsites B and C. Preference is for the interior of the α-1,4-linked linear chain of the starch molecule. Maximal affinity (lowest K_m) and cleavage rate (V_{max} or K_{cat}) occur when all subsites are occupied with glucose units. n, variable number of glucose residues in amylose; when amylopectin is the substrate, the portions of the starch in brackets also contain branches created by α-1,6 links of glucose residues, as shown in Figure 5–2.

triose and the disaccharide maltose. Products smaller than the pentasaccharide, being unable to bind at all subsites, have very low affinity for the amylase active site; hence, productive cleavage of these smaller oligosaccharides is markedly hampered. Thus the sequential actions of amylase promote the release of maltotriose and maltose as the main final products of luminal digestion of amylose.

Amylopectin is a more complex form of starch, representing about 80% of dietary polysaccharide. Figure 5–2 depicts the action of α-amylase on amylopectin to yield the final oligosaccharide products within the distal duodenal lumen. Although its linear segments

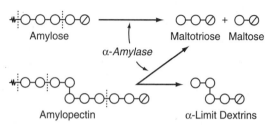

Figure 5–2. Action of salivary and pancreatic α-amylases on linear (amylose) and branched (amylopectin) forms of starch. ◯, glucose units; ⊘, reducing end glucose unit; horizontal links denote α-1,4 linkages; vertical links indicate α-1,6 linkages. (From Gray, G. M. [1981] Carbohydrate absorption and malabsorption. In: Physiology of the Gastrointestinal Tract [Johnson, L. R., ed.], pp. 1063–1072. Lippincott-Raven Publishers, Philadelphia.)

are similar to those for amylose, amylopectin is branched by virtue of α-1,6 links positioned approximately every 25 glucosyl residues along the chain. Glycogen, though a minor dietary carbohydrate, has a structure analogous to that of amylopectin. α-Amylase is unable to cleave the α-1,6 branching link, and the structural angulation created by this linkage inhibits the enzyme from attacking some of the adjacent α-1,4 links. As a consequence, in addition to the linear maltose and maltotriose, branched oligosaccharides called α-limit dextrins (or α-dextrins) are also final products of amylopectin hydrolysis by α-amylase. α-Dextrins composed of an average of 5 to 6 glucose units (mass, 800 to 1000 Da) represent nearly one third the mass of the final breakdown products of amylopectin. The intraluminal hydrolysis of both amylose and amylopectin to their final oligosaccharide products proceeds efficiently, usually providing sufficient products at the intestinal surface membrane to support optimal surface digestion of the glucosyl oligosaccharides by the constituent brush border oligosaccharidases.

Digestion on the Outer Luminal Intestinal Surface by Integral Oligosaccharidases

The brush border membranes of the small intestinal enterocytes that cover the villous projections of the small intestine are replete with a group of special glycoprotein hydrolases that are responsible for the last stage of hydrolysis of the oligosaccharide and disaccharide products released by luminal α-amylase action. These integral carbohydrases of the enterocyte also cleave the two other major nutrient carbohydrates: the disaccharides sucrose and lactose.

Oligosaccharidases with the appropriate characteristics to catalyze the final cleavage of dietary oligosaccharides are expressed only in the enterocyte and are processed in the endoplasmic reticulum (ER) and Golgi membranes, with final vectorial transport to the intestinal brush border surface. The N-terminal hydrophobic segment of the oligosaccharidase, called the signal sequence, directs the synthesizing ribosome to the ER, where carbohydrate chains are synthesized as a unit and added to the protein backbone at the side-chain amide group of selected asparaginyl residues. The N-glycosylated intermediate is then vectorially transferred via vesicles to the Golgi apparatus, where maturation of the N-linked carbohydrate chains occurs. The mechanism of the final transport from Golgi to the brush border membrane is not yet defined, but there appears to be a process involving transport vesicles that ensures preferential movement to the apical (brush border) membrane.

The oligosaccharidases also possess a hydrophobic amino acid sequence at either the amino or carboxyl terminus to promote anchoring in the brush border. Their orientation is such that at least 95% of the oligosaccharidase domains, including the active catalytic site, are exterior to the brush border membrane and available for efficient cleavage of the luminal substrates. The oligosaccharidases are acquired during the fetal period prior to birth, and newborn infants have a full complement of these enzymes.

As shown in Table 5–2, several α-glucosidases recognize the α-type oxygen bridge that is below the plane of the glucosyl ring structure. These are sucrase, α-dextrinase, and glucoamylase. In contrast, no glycosidases are capable of catalyzing cleavage of the β-linked polymers of glucose that make up cellulose, the major type of fiber. The brush border membrane α-glucosidases all display specificity for the α-1,4 bond between the nonreducing terminal glucose unit and the penultimate glucose to which it is attached. The functional difference among these enzymes is the degree of their specificity for a particular substrate or glycosidic linkage at the nonreducing terminus, as illustrated in Figure 5–3, and this provides the basis for the enzyme nomenclature. The specificity of the enzymes can be estimated from the affinity or K_m values for the various substrates and from the cleavage efficiency or the maximal hydrolytic rate (V_{max} or K_{cat}).

Although its specificity extends to the trisaccharide maltotriose and the disaccharide maltose, glucoamylase has high specificity for the α-1,4 link at the nonreducing terminus of straight chain glucosyl oligosaccharides, particularly those containing 4 to 9 glucose units.

TABLE 5–2
Intestinal Surface Membrane Oligosaccharidases

Enzyme	Principal Substrate	K_m (mmol/L)	K_{cat}* (sec^{-1})
α-Glucosidases			
Sucrase	Sucrose	18	120
	Malto-oligosaccharides (α-1,4 links only)	3	110
α-Dextrinase	α-Dextrins (α-1,4 and α-1,6 links)	2–4	20–45
		1	120
Glucoamylase	Malto-oligosaccharides	1–4	50–65
	α-Dextrins (α-1,4 links only)	1	30–40
Trehalase	Trehalose	3	20
β-Galactosidase			
Lactase	Lactose	2	40

*K_{cat} is the maximal hydrolytic rate, expressed as millimoles of substrate hydrolyzed per millimole of enzyme per second.

Sucrase displays high efficiency for the α-1,4 links of the smallest glucosyl oligosaccharides, which are maltose and maltotriose, and hence is an efficient maltase, but its unique capacity to cleave the α-1,β-2 link between the glucose and fructose units of sucrose [α-D-glucopyranosyl (1→2) β-D-fructofuranoside] provides the basis for its name. Similarly, α-dextrinase has appreciable specificity for the α-1,4 links in the oligosaccharide products of starch digestion, but its maximal and unique specificity is for the α-1,6 branching link of the α-dextrins. Because of its α-1,6 specificity and the use of the α-1,6 disaccharide isomaltose as substrate, α-dextrinase is commonly called isomaltase. However, because isomaltose is not a substrate produced by α-amylase

action on amylopectin, the α-dextrinase designation is preferred.

Glucoamylase, α-dextrinase, and sucrase work in a complementary manner to cleave the bonds in the α-dextrins in sequence from the nonreducing end to release free glucose units. As shown in Figure 5–3, at each step in the process one or more of these enzymes has high specificity for the α-glucosyl link closest to the nonreducing end of certain of the oligosaccharide products. These glucosidases produce free glucose for the final transport into the enterocyte.

Sucrase–α-dextrinase is initially synthesized and assembled as a single glycoprotein in association with ER and Golgi membranes, transferred preferentially to the brush border

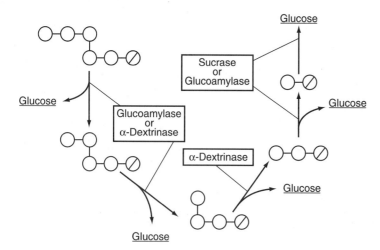

Figure 5–3. Concerted action of intestinal surface membrane oligosaccharidases on a typical α-dextrin final product of amylopectin digestion. The active hydrolases for each removal of a glucose residue from the nonreducing terminus is shown in the boxed area. Note that only the α-dextrinase is capable of removing the α-1,6-linked glucose "stub" from the intermediate tetrasaccharide substrate (bottom of figure). (From Gray, G. M. [1981] Carbohydrate absorption and malabsorption. In: Physiology of the Gastrointestinal Tract [Johnson, L. R., ed.], pp. 1063–1072. Lippincott-Raven Publishers, Philadelphia.)

(apical) membrane, and cleaved by luminal trypsin to sucrase and α-dextrinase subunits, which then recombine noncovalently so that the sucrase as well as the α-dextrinase remains anchored to the surface membrane by the hydrophobic amino-terminal segment of the original protein (Shapiro et al., 1991). This mechanism of intracellular assembly, brush border membrane insertion, cleavage, and reassociation of sucrase and α-dextrinase is diagrammed in Figure 5–4. The other oligosaccharidases are assembled analogously, though they are not structurally modified after arriving at the brush border surface.

α,α-Trehalose [α-D-glucopyranosyl (1→1) α-D-glucopyranoside] is a disaccharide containing two glucose units linked α-1,α-1. Trehalose is present in insects and mushrooms, and brush border trehalase cleaves this sugar to free glucose. Only small amounts of trehalose are found in typical Western diets.

There is a single β-glycosidase at the enterocyte brush border surface; this is a β-galactosidase that has high specificity for lactose [β-D-galactopyranosyl (1→4) D-glucopyranose]. Although uniformly present at birth and crucial for cleavage of lactose in maternal milk, lactase decreases appreciably either in young childhood (about ages 3 to 5 years) or in adolescence (ages 14 to 18 years) in most of the world's population groups. Lactase does remain at high neonatal levels in most Caucasians of Northern European origin, but adult deficiency of this enzyme still occurs in approximately 5% to 20% of Caucasian adults. Table 5–3 shows the prevalence of adult lactase deficiency, now commonly referred to as hypolactasia, in various populations of the world.

ABSORPTION OF HEXOSES BY THE ENTEROCYTE: MECHANISMS AND REGULATION

The oligosaccharides of two or more six-carbon monosaccharide units cannot be transported intact across the intestinal membrane barrier but instead must be hydrolyzed by the oligosaccharidases and disaccharidases, as detailed. An appreciable increase in our understanding of the final hexose transport by the intestinal enterocyte has occurred in the last few years. Because the intestine is lined

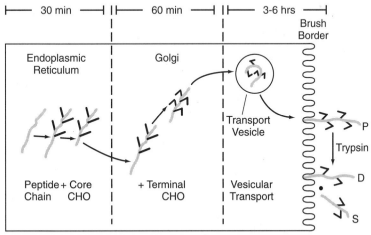

Figure 5–4. Diagram of the synthesis, membrane-associated modification, surface membrane insertion, and modification by luminal trypsin of sucrase–α-dextrinase in the intestinal enterocyte. The precursor sucrase–α-dextrinase (P) is (1) synthesized in association with ribosomes on the endoplasmic reticulum, (2) glycosylated by addition of carbohydrate chains (CHO) consisting of chains of complex hexose units attached to asparagine residues via N-glycosidic linkages while in the interior of the endoplasmic reticulum, (3) transferred via vesicles to the Golgi apparatus, where additional terminal hexose units are added, and then (4) vectorially transported to the apical (brush border) membrane where it remains anchored by the amino terminus of the precursor P. Luminal pancreatic trypsin cleaves the P glycoprotein to components containing the sucrase (S) and α-dextrinase (D) active sites. These subunits recombine at the outer brush border membrane where they catalyze the surface hydrolysis of sucrose and the α-dextrin oligosaccharide end products of luminal starch digestion. The time sequence indicates the residence time in various cellular compartments as determined for the intact rat model.

TABLE 5–3

Prevalence of Hypolactasia in Healthy Populations *

Group	% Lactase-Deficient[†]
North American (White)	5–20
North American (Black)	70–75
African Bantu	50
Puerto Rican	21
Danish	3
Asians	
Filipino	95
Indian	55
Thai	97
Chinese	87
Eskimo (Greenland)	88
Nigerian	
Yoruba	99
Fulani	58
Israeli Jews[‡]	61
Israeli Arabs	81
Mexican	74

*Based on work of numerous authors; see Gray (1983) for primary references.

†Lactase activity below 1.0 U/g tissue or 15 U/g protein, or blood glucose rises of less than 20 mg/100 mL after ingestion of 50 g of lactose, accompanied by abdominal symptoms and diarrhea. One International Unit of enzyme activity is 1 μmol/min at 37° C.

‡Includes Ashkenazi, Sephardi, Iraquis, Yemenite, and Oriental groups with deficiency rates of 44% to 84%.

Modified from Gray, G. M. (1983) Intestinal disaccharidase deficiencies and glucose-galactose malabsorption. In: Metabolic Basis of Inherited Disease (Stanbury, J. B., Wyngaarden, J. B., Fredrickson, D. S., Goldstein, J. L. and Brown, M. S., eds.), 5th ed., pp. 1729–1742. McGraw-Hill, New York. Used with permission of The McGraw-Hill Companies.

with a single layer of columnar cells that are attached by tight junctions, making it impermeable to even small solute molecules, it is necessary for one or more transporters or carriers to promote entry and exit from the enterocyte. Several mechanisms operate in concert to regulate the movement of the hexoses across the enterocyte layer for delivery to the capillaries within the core of the villi. The enterocyte's specialized processes are restricted to uptake and movement of the released hexose monosaccharides, and specific hexose transporters have been identified and characterized.

Hexose Transporters

As diagrammed in Figure 5–5, distinct transporters work in a coordinated manner in a sequential two-step process to support the ef-

ficient uptake of hexoses from the intestinal lumen across the brush border, followed by exit from the basolateral membrane of the enterocyte. Glucose and galactose, which are hexose isomers differing only by the position of the hydroxyl and hydrogen attached at the fourth carbon in the ring structure, both utilize the same sodium glucose transporter, SGLT1. This is a specialized high-affinity aldohexose and Na^+ co-transport protein, which is expressed at high abundance in the brush border membrane of the intestinal enterocyte and which supports the binding and transport into the cell of 2 Na^+ ions and 1 molecule of glucose or galactose. The amino-terminal segment of SGLT1 protrudes into the extracellular luminal milieu, and its sequence then extends as a series of strategically positioned hydrophobic stretches that traverse the apical enterocyte membrane a total of 14 times, the last 2 of which are separated by a large, charged intracellular loop. The carboxyl terminus of SGLT1 culminates in a carboxyl-terminal domain, with its final extension projecting from the brush border into the lumen (Turk et al., 1996).

SGLT1 is a high-affinity transporter (K_t, 0.5 mmol/L for glucose and 5 mmol/L for Na^+), indicating that it is capable of supporting half-maximal transport rates at only 8 mg/100 mL (0.4 mmol/L) of glucose, one tenth of the extracellular glucose concentration, and at a Na^+ level less than one twentieth of that in body fluids (Panayotova-Heiermann et al., 1996). The entry step into the enterocyte that is facilitated by SGLT1 is complemented by an exit mechanism provided by the relatively low affinity of the glucose transport protein GLUT2 at the basolateral membrane (for glucose, K_t ~11 mmol/L, 200 mg/100 mL, which is comparable to peak postprandial plasma glucose concentrations). Thus glucose or galactose accumulates in the enterocyte to exit down a glucose or galactose concentration gradient into the extracellular milieu beneath the enterocyte layer, from which it can enter the capillary beds of the portal system.

After glucose or galactose and its Na^+ partners have entered the enterocyte, they are released and go their separate ways. The Na^+ exits from the enterocyte via the Na^+,K^+-ATPase in the basolateral membrane, an

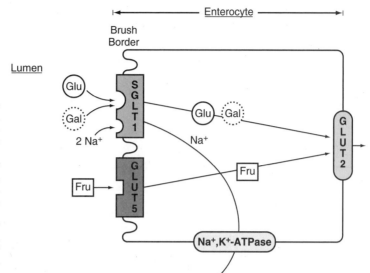

Figure 5–5. *Hexose transport by the enterocyte occurs by membrane carrier proteins. Designations and positions in the brush border or basolateral membrane are shown. Energy is provided by the exit of Na+ via the Na+,K+-ATPase. Glucose (Glu) and galactose (Gal), being closely related structurally, share the glucose transporter (SGLT1). Fructose (Fru) enters via GLUT5. All three hexoses exit via the high-capacity GLUT2 in the basolateral membrane. See text for elaboration.*

energy-utilizing process that promotes glucose or galactose and Na+ co-entry down the Na+ concentration gradient maintained by the Na+,K+-ATPase. The glucose achieves relatively high intracellular concentrations to drive the low-affinity, high-capacity GLUT2 hexose transporter in the basolateral membrane, thereby facilitating the exit of glucose and galactose from the enterocyte for diffusion into the underlying capillaries (Mueckler, 1994; Olson and Pessin, 1996).

A third principal hexose is fructose, which has a structure that is distinctly different from that of glucose or galactose. Fructose is released by the brush border membrane digestion of sucrose, which makes up a significant portion of Western diets. An increasingly important carbohydrate nutrient, fructose is now incorporated as a potent sweetener in many commercially prepared breakfast and dessert products. Fructose has its own transport mechanism, a facilitated diffusion process supported by GLUT5, a brush border membrane protein that efficiently accommodates luminal fructose and functions independently of Na+. Like glucose and galactose, fructose exits from the enterocyte primarily via the GLUT2 transporter of the basolateral membrane. Some GLUT5 transporters also appear to be localized to the basolateral membrane, where they may complement the GLUT2 mechanism for exit of fructose from the enterocyte (Blakemore et al., 1995).

The regulation of the enterocyte hexose transport systems is complex, and much new information has come forth in the last few years. The mRNA abundance of all three major hexose transporters displays a diurnal variation with a marked increase just prior to feeding. Based on studies in rats, intraluminal glucose released from the luminal and surface digestion of ingested poly- and oligosaccharides increases the mRNA abundance of both SGLT1 and GLUT2 (Corpe and Burant, 1996). That this luminal effect is due to the hexose structure itself rather than to a metabolic product such as phosphorylated glucose is indicated by the fact that the nonmetabolizable 3-O-methylglucose is also capable of augmenting the mRNA levels of these apical and basolateral transporters. Similarly, the presence of sucrose or fructose in the intestinal lumen produces a specific and abrupt increase in the GLUT5 mRNA that is responsible for the synthesis of the fructose transporter (Shu et al., 1997).

Cyclic AMP augments the expression of both SGLT1 and GLUT5 proteins by activation of protein kinases, but the final mechanisms appear to differ between these two transporters. In the case of SGLT1, the protein kinase activation increases the quantity and transport capacity by virtue of transfer of SGLT1 units from the intracellular compartment to the apical membrane (Hirsch et al., 1996). In contrast, protein kinase activation stabilizes the

NUTRITION INSIGHT

Primary and Secondary Hypolactasia

In lactose-producing mammals, a characteristic developmental pattern of lactase activity has been observed. Lactase activity is high in the neonatal and suckling period, declines after the species-specific weaning phase, and remains low in adult animals. A decline in intestinal lactase activity during childhood, or sometimes during the second decade of life, also occurs in the majority of the world's human population and should be considered phylogenetically normal. Most adults have primary adult-type hypolactasia with intestinal lactase activities or lactose digestion capacities that are about 5% to 10% of the levels observed in newborn infants within the same population. Individuals with primary adult-type hypolactasia are homozygous for a recessive autosomal allele that causes the physiological postweaning decline of lactase activity; this gene is regulatory and no differences in the lactase gene or protein are observed.

Some adults, however, have lactase activity that is not much lower than that of normal infants in the same population—in particular, individuals whose ancestry traces to Central and Northern Europeans or some nomadic, milk-consuming populations in the arid zones of North Africa and Arabia. Adults with high lactase activity are either heterozygous or homozygous for a dominant allele that prevents the normal decline of lactase activity.

Secondary disaccharidase deficiencies often occur in children with active celiac disease or cow's milk protein intolerance or in patients with infectious diarrheas. These conditions affect numerous brush border proteins. Of the intestinal mucosal glycosidases, lactase activity is usually the most severely affected. Treatment of the primary problem alleviates the secondary hypolactasia caused by damage to the brush border enzymes of the intestinal mucosa.

Another cause of low lactase activity is congenital lactase deficiency, which has an autosomal recessive mode of inheritance. The lactase gene is affected in this case, and the gene product is absent or defective. Infants with this inborn error develop diarrhea within the first day or days of life. Infants with congenital lactase deficiency can be treated effectively with lactose-free diets. This type of primary lactase deficiency is very rare.

Lactose intolerance due to lactase deficiency is a cause of gastrointestinal complaints such as abdominal distention, audible bowel activity, nausea and an osmotic diarrhea, irritable bowel syndrome, and recurrent abdominal pain. Diagnosis of lactose intolerance is based on observation of the clinical effects of dietary withdrawal and subsequent reintroduction of lactose, on measurement of the rise in blood glucose or breath hydrogen following an oral dose of lactose (usually 50 g in an adult), or on assay of lactase in a jejunal biopsy specimen. Subjects with high lactase activity can completely digest the usual test dose of lactose and have a significant rise in blood glucose concentration within 30 minutes following lactose administration; because lactose is digested and does not reach the colon, colonic fermentation and hydrogen excretion in the breath are not observed.

mRNA for GLUT5, resulting in enhanced GLUT5 protein expression.

The common mechanism of enhancement of the hexose transporters appears to be an induction of their gene transcription by the particular transportable substrate itself. But, whether the augmentation of the particular mRNA is induced by the hexose substrate itself as it enters the cell, or whether a second messenger is required, is not yet known.

Enhancement of Water Absorption by Glucose Transport via SGLT1

The absorption of NaCl and solutes is known to be accompanied by the movement of water, presumably by virtue of the osmotic gradient produced by absorption of the electrolytes and of solutes such as amino acids and monosaccharides. Although the exact mechanisms involved are still being worked out and appear

NUTRITION INSIGHT

Primary and Secondary Hypolactasia *(Continued)*

On the other hand, the lactose digestion capacity of individuals with low lactase activity is usually exceeded by a single dose of 50 g of lactose, and these individuals show only a small increase or no increase in blood glucose concentration. The undigested lactose reaches the colon where it is fermented by colonic bacteria, with some of the hydrogen (H_2) produced in this process being absorbed and then excreted in the expired air. Additionally, the osmotic effects of undigested lactose, the acidification of the colonic contents by the short-chain fatty acids produced by lactose fermentation, and the large amounts of gas formed during lactose fermentation cause the symptoms of lactose intolerance, such as flatulence, bloating, abdominal distention, and diarrhea. Despite these symptoms, upon ingestion of a 50-g dose of lactose, most adults with primary hypolactasia can tolerate at least 1 cup of milk per day with no symptoms.

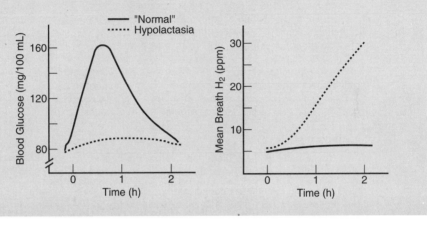

Digestion and absorption of dietary carbohydrate may be affected by a number of factors, but the rate-limiting step in the overall assimilation is usually a step in luminal hydrolysis, intestinal surface hydrolysis, or monosaccharide transport. The initial factor involved in carbohydrate processing is the rate of chewing and residence time in the mouth that would allow interaction of the starch component with salivary amylase. This is usually a relatively short period, and the meal is then exposed to the low pH of the stomach, which stops the action of the salivary α-amylase. The stomach acts principally as a reservoir, and

to involve both transcellular and paracellular movement, there is evidence that SGLT1 serves as a major enhancer of water absorption. A study of injection of SGLT1 mRNA into oocytes from *Xenopus* (a genus of clawed frogs) has extended the information on the quantitative interaction of water and glucose movement. Based on documentation of water movement induced by expression of the glucose/Na$^+$ co-transporter in a *Xenopus* oocyte system, 260 molecules of water accompany the transport of 2 Na$^+$ and a single glucose molecule by SGLT1 (Loo et al., 1996). This amounts to nearly 3 liters of water accompanying 100 g (or 400 kcal) of glucose absorbed. Based on this calculation, the transport of the usual quantity of glucose-containing nutrients consumed daily could support water absorption of several liters by the human intestine. Although this might seem rather amazing, approximately 9 to 11 liters of fluid are reabsorbed daily by the human

gastrointestinal tract, and the osmotic effects of glucose and amino acids are used routinely in oral rehydration therapy.

FACTORS INFLUENCING CARBOHYDRATE ASSIMILATION

CLINICAL CORRELATION

Glucose and Galactose Malabsorption

Carbohydrate intolerance is a rare but very serious hereditary disorder. Cases due to lack of digestive enzyme (e.g., primary sucrase–α-dextrinase deficiency) and to impaired hexose transport (i.e., primary glucose–galactose malabsorption) have been reported. Based on experience in a Boston hospital, it was estimated that glucose–galactose malabsorption accounted for about 2% of the patients with protracted diarrhea of infancy (Lloyd-Still et al., 1988).

In two reported cases of carbohydrate intolerance, the infants developed diarrhea soon after birth, and reducing sugars and an acid pH were present in the stools. Intestinal biopsy tissue from the infants showed normal villi with normal disaccharidase values. Monosaccharide load tests showed a normal rise in blood glucose in response to a fructose load, which was tolerated well, in contrast to a flat glucose curve in response to a glucose load, which was accompanied by marked abdominal distention, profuse diarrhea, and reducing sugars in the stools. Thus, these two patients were diagnosed as having glucose–galactose malabsorption.

Although a sucrose- and lactose-free formula with fructose was fed to these two patients, diarrhea and the excretion of reducing sugars in the stool continued. This was due to a small amount of tapioca starch (2.5 g/100 mL of formula, which supplied >12.5 g of starch per day for these patients) in the "sugar-free" formula that was being used. Rigid exclusion of all carbohydrates and sugars except for fructose resulted in cessation of diarrhea and elimination of sugars from the stools.

Thinking Critically

1. These patients were diagnosed before the hexose transporters had been identified. Which hexose transport protein was probably lacking in these patients?

2. If the plasma glucose concentration had been monitored in these two patients following a load dose of sucrose, would a rise in plasma glucose have been observed? following a load dose of lactose?

3. How would you expect the findings (carbohydrate tolerance, the glucose load test results, and the intestinal biopsy results) to differ in a case of secondary disaccharidase deficiency due to infective gastroenteritis (i.e., rotavirus infection)?

---

the rate of gastric emptying depends upon the nutrient composition of the meal. For instance, fat, nondigestible carbohydrate (dietary fiber), and high osmolality such as that present in concentrated desserts sweetened with sucrose all will retard gastric emptying, thereby slowing the rate of overall carbohydrate assimilation.

Despite these factors, the intraluminal digestion of the starches in the small intestine is a highly efficient process that is restricted only by the physical state of the starch itself, as noted earlier. There is considerable variation in intestinal motility, depending upon the nutrient type and consequent differences in transit time through the small intestine, which may alter the rate of carbohydrate assimilation. However, in the absence of an intestinal

or pancreatic disease, the effect of intestinal motility on the overall assimilation of nutrients does not appear to cause any significant malabsorption. Other than the physical condition of the carbohydrate nutrient, particularly for starch, the most important factor affecting the rate of carbohydrate assimilation is usually the rate-limiting step in enzymatic hydrolysis or transport of the nutrient.

Rate-Limiting Steps in Carbohydrate Assimilation

The overall assimilation of digestible dietary carbohydrate nutrients is very efficient. For instance, at least ten times as much intestinal amylase is secreted in response to a meal as is required for optimal intraluminal digestion of starch to the final oligosaccharide products (Fogel and Gray, 1973). Although a small percentage of starch escapes α-amylase action, this is related to the polysaccharide's physical state rather than to a limiting quantity of amylase. Similarly, the digestion of the oligo- and disaccharides on the intestinal brush border surface while the substrate is still within the lumen is highly efficient and usually yields more than sufficient concentrations of monosaccharides for the glucose–galactose and fructose transporters. However, in contrast, lactase activity in jejunal biopsies from lactose-tolerant adults is relatively lower than that of the other oligosaccharidases. Notably, the lower limit for intestinal lactase activity in adults who retain the capacity to digest lactose is only one third that of sucrase. Because of this, lactose digestive capacity, even in individuals who retain high lactase activity throughout adulthood, is relatively limited compared with that for other digestive processes. As estimated from human intestinal studies, the intestinal hydrolysis of lactose in lactose-tolerant subjects is the rate-limiting step in the overall assimilation of lactose (Gray and Santiago, 1966). In essence, the lactase activity at the intestinal brush border is insufficient to catalyze the release of optimal quantities of glucose and galactose for the terminal transport step across the enterocyte, and the membrane hydrolysis of lactose becomes the slowest process for its overall assimilation.

Quantitative comparison of equivalent amounts of lactose versus glucose plus galactose revealed that the assimilation of hexoses was only about half as rapid from lactose as when equivalent amounts of its component monosaccharides were fed. In contrast, absorption of monosaccharide components from starch or sucrose was as rapid as was absorption of hexoses from equivalent amounts of glucose or glucose plus fructose.

Discrete Genetic Defects in Carbohydrate Digestive or Absorptive Processes

The processes of starch and oligosaccharide digestion and final monosaccharide transport are usually very efficient, enabling total assimilation of ingested starch and disaccharides. Indeed, the great majority of starch is digested within the duodenal lumen followed by hydrolysis of the starch-derived oligosaccharides at the lumen–enterocyte interface and uptake of the released monosaccharides by hexose transport within the proximal half of the small intestine. Under normal conditions, the ileum has some capacity to digest and absorb carbohydrates, but this is appreciably reduced compared with the jejunum. In the case of extensive jejunal disease or surgical removal of the upper intestine, the ileum can adapt appreciably and assume an important role in carbohydrate digestion and absorption.

Altered assimilation can occur at any stage of the digestive-absorptive processes. For instance, reduction in secretion of amylase from the pancreas in duct obstruction caused by chronic pancreatitis or cancer can cause amylase insufficiency and consequent starch maldigestion in the duodenum. Diseases of the small intestine, such as celiac sprue (gluten-sensitive enteropathy) or extensive inflammatory bowel disease (Crohn's disease), may reduce the number of functioning enterocytes to cause generalized oligosaccharidase deficiency and insufficient hexose transport. Failure of carbohydrate assimilation in disease states produces an osmotic diarrhea.

A defect in a single specific process essential for carbohydrate digestion or transport may also occur. Figure 5–6 depicts the consequences when lactase is appreciably reduced or absent from the enterocyte apical membrane surface. A defect of other oligosaccharidases or of a required transporter will produce the same pathophysiological alterations. When carbohydrate remains undigested or unabsorbed within the intestinal lumen, it is processed within the lower ileum and colon by resident bacteria to smaller 2- to 4-carbon compounds in the form of short-chain fatty acids, which increase the intraluminal osmolality and produce retention of water. In addition, methane, carbon dioxide, and hydrogen gases are released.

These effects produce an increase in the quantity of fluid and gas in the lower small intestine and colon, manifested by symptoms of abdominal bloating and cramping discomfort, audible bowel sounds, and a watery,

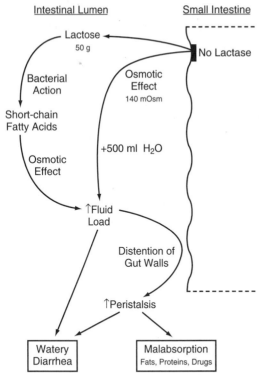

Figure 5–6. *Pathogenesis of the carbohydrate malabsorption syndrome. Maldigestion of lactose allows bacteria to produce fragments, thereby increasing osmolar forces, producing increased ileal and colonic water, and augmenting peristalsis of the gut and secondary malabsorption of other nutrients. A block in any oligosaccharidase or hexose transporter would result in the same pathophysiological events. (Modified from Gray, G. M. [1983] Intestinal disaccharidase deficiencies and glucose-galactose malabsorption. In: Metabolic Basis of Inherited Disease [Stanbury, J. B., Wyngaarden, J. B., Fredrickson, D. S., Goldstein, J. L., and Brown, M. S. eds.], 5th ed., pp. 1729–1742. Blakiston Division, McGraw-Hill, New York. With permission of The McGraw-Hill Companies.)*

foamy diarrhea. In small children, unmetabolized carbohydrate may be passed in stools, and more severe symptoms, including vomiting, may develop.

The most common cause of the carbohydrate malabsorption syndrome is the hypolactasia that can develop in young children any time from shortly after weaning until the early teenage years. This occurs in a high proportion of the world's population groups because of reduction in lactase expression at the enterocyte brush border surface (see Table 5–3), and lactose intolerance must be considered to be the normal condition of most healthy adults worldwide. Even among Caucasians of

Northern European heritage, hypolactasia develops in 5% to 20% of adult individuals. The cause of hypolactasia appears to be complex, and no defect in the cDNA sequence has been identified. Instead, one or more regulatory changes are likely to produce the developmental reduction in expression. Whereas in many patients a relatively low abundance of lactase mRNA points to a reduction in lactase gene transcription (Lloyd et al., 1992; Escher et al., 1992), others with hypolactasia have mRNA levels sufficient for normal expression of lactase, suggesting that a posttranscriptional or posttranslational event may be paramount (Rossi et al., 1997).

A lack of other carbohydrate digestive and transport processes is found much less commonly than hypolactasia, but discrete genetic defects have been identified that produce clinical symptoms. These include sucrase–α-dextrinase (S-D) deficiency, glucoamylase deficiency, glucose-galactose malabsorption, and isolated fructose malabsorption. Sucrase-α-dextrinase is involved in digestion of both starch and sucrose. S-D deficiency, observed in as high as 10% of the Greenland Eskimo population (McNair et al., 1972) but much less commonly in most regions of the world (~0.2% of North Americans), is due to a failure of accumulation of S-D protein in the enterocyte (Gray et al., 1976). Recently, an altered S-D structure was shown to be produced by a single nucleotide substitution, producing a discrete amino acid change (Gln[1098]→Pro) and yielding an S-D product that can neither be properly glycosylated nor transferred from the intracellular membranes to the brush border surface (Ouwendijk et al., 1996). Consequently, the altered S-D protein is degraded within the enterocyte interior. Starch intolerance may also develop secondary to a reduced capacity to digest the α-1,4 links of the oligosaccharide products because of glucoamylase deficiency. This has been noted in approximately 1% of children who have chronic diarrhea (Lebenthal et al., 1994), but the molecular defect has not been defined.

Although a rare entity, a defect in hexose transport may lead to severe malabsorption, manifested by symptoms of abdominal rumbling, bloating, cramping pain, and a watery diarrhea produced by the incremental increase in osmotic force of the retained hexose and the products of its fermentation by colonic bacteria. Glucose–galactose malabsorption is usually identified in infancy and may be fatal unless all dietary carbohydrate is eliminated from the diet (Meeuwisse and Dahlqvist, 1968). Patients with this discrete defect can absorb the fructose component of sucrose. However, neither sucrose nor commercially processed monosaccharide mixtures produced from sucrose, which contain the offending glucose as well as the absorbable fructose, will be tolerated by patients with glucose–galactose malabsorption.

Recently, glucose–galactose malabsorption has been found in some probands (original persons presenting with the hereditary condition, who serve as the basis for a genetic study) to be due to missense mutations of SGLT1 that produce single amino acid changes (Leu^{147}→Arg or Cys^{355}→Ser) (Martin et al., 1997). Either of these substitutions produces a mutant SGLT1 protein that cannot be processed properly in the ER or Golgi and that consequently remains within the enterocyte's interior rather than being transferred to the brush border. The absence of SGLT1 at the enterocyte surface results in loss of the capacity to internalize glucose or galactose. In contrast to the defect discovered for glucose–galactose malabsorption, fructose malabsorption does not appear to be accounted for by expression of a mutant GLUT5 protein (Wasserman et al., 1996).

Therapy of Carbohydrate Malassimilation

Although carbohydrates are a relatively inexpensive source of calories, they are not essential for overall nutrition. Therefore, the main approach to therapy when a specific carbohydrate maldigestive or malabsorptive defect is identified is the elimination of the particular offending nutrient carbohydrate from the diet. Thus, for individuals with hypolactasia, it is often necessary to avoid dairy products, the main source of lactose. But because milk products are an excellent source of nutrients, it is often beneficial to add a lactose-hydrolyzing enzyme to the dairy products, such as β-galactosidase purified from microorganisms,

to promote digestion of the lactose (Lin et al., 1993). Fermented milk products may be acceptable owing to their lower lactose content. Recently, the sucrose-hydrolyzing enzyme from yeast has been shown to be usable as an enzyme supplement in patients with sucrase–α-dextrinase deficiency (Treem et al., 1993).

REFERENCES

Blakemore, S. J., Aledo, J. C., James, J., Campbell, F. C., Lucocq, J. M., and Hundal, H. S. (1995) The GLUT5 hexose transporter is also localized to the basolateral membrane of the human jejunum. Biochem J 309:7–12.

Chen, D., Andersson, K., Iovanna, J. L., Dagorn, J. C., and Hakanson, R. (1993) Effects of hypercholecystokinemia produced by pancreaticobiliary diversion on pancreatic growth and enzyme mRNA levels in starved rats. Scand J Gastroenterol 28:311–314.

Cockell, M., Stolarczyk, D., Frutiger, S., Hughes, G. J., Hagenbuchle, O., and Wellauer, P. K. (1995) Binding sites for hepatocyte nuclear factor 3 beta or 3 gamma and pancreas transcription factor 1 are required for efficient expression of the gene encoding pancreatic alpha-amylase. Mol Cell Biol 15:1933–1941.

Corpe, C. P., and Burant, C. F. (1996) Hexose transporter expression in rat small intestine: Effect of diet on diurnal variations. Am J Physiol 271:G211–G216.

Escher, J. C., de Koning, N. D., van Engen, C. G., Arora, S., Buller, H. A., Montgomery, R. K., and Grand, R. J. (1992) Molecular basis of lactase levels in adult humans. J Clin Invest 89:480–483.

Fogel, M. R., and Gray, G. M. (1973) Starch hydrolysis in man: An intraluminal process not requiring membrane digestion. J Appl Physiol 35:263–267.

Gray, G. M., and Santiago, N. A. (1966) Disaccharide absorption in normal and diseased human intestine. Gastroenterology 51:489–498.

Gray, G. M., Townley, R. R. W., and Conklin, K. A. (1976) Sucrase-isomaltase deficiency: Absence of an inactive enzyme variant. N Engl J Med 294:750–753.

Hirsch, J. R., Loo, D. D. F., and Wright, E. M. (1996) Regulation of Na$^+$/glucose cotransporter expression by protein kinases in *Xenopus laevis* oocytes. J Biol Chem 271:14740–14746.

Lebenthal, E., Khin-Maung, U., Zheng, B. Y., Lu, R. B., and Lerner, A. (1994) Small intestinal glucoamylase deficiency and starch malabsorption: A newly recognized alpha-glucosidase deficiency in children. J Pediatr 124:541–546.

Lin, M. Y., Dipalma, J. A., Martini, M. C., Gross, C. J., Harlander, S. K., and Savaiano, D. A. (1993) Comparative effects of exogenous lactase (beta-galactosidase) preparations on in vivo lactose digestion. Dig Dis Sci 38:2022–2027.

Lloyd, M., Mevissen, G., Fischer, M., Olsen, W., Goodspeed, D., Genini, M., Boll, W., Semenza, G., and Mantei, N. (1992) Regulation of intestinal lactase in adult hypolactasia. J Clin Invest 89:524–529.

Lloyd-Still, J. D., Listernick, R., and Buentello, G. (1988) Complex carbohydrate intolerance: Diagnostic pitfalls and approach to management. J Pediatr 112:709–713.

Loo, D. D. F., Zeuthen, T., Chandy, G., and Wright, E. M. (1996) Cotransport of water by Na$^+$/glucose cotransporter. Proc Nat Acad Sci USA 93:13367–13370.

Martin, M. G., Lostao, M. P., Turk, E., Lam, J., Kreman, M., and Wright, E. M. (1997) Compound missense mutations in the sodium/D-glucose cotransporter result in trafficking defects. Gastroenterology 112:1206–1212.

McNair, A., Gudmand-Hoyer, E., Jarnum, S., Orrild, L. (1972) Sucrose malabsorption in Greenland. Br Med J 2:19–21.

Meeuwisse, G. W., and Dahlqvist, A. (1968) Glucose-galactose malabsorption. A study with biopsy of the small intestinal mucosa. Acta Paediatr Scand 57:273–280.

Mueckler, M. (1994) Facilitative glucose transporters. Eur J Biochem 219:713–725.

Olson, A. L., and Pessin, J. E. (1996) Structure, function, and regulation of the mammalian facilitative glucose transporter gene family. Annu Rev Nutr 16:235–256.

Ouwendijk, J., Moolenaar, C. E. C., Peters, W. J., Hollenberg, C. P., Ginsel, L. A., Fransen, J. A. M. and Naim, H. Y. (1996) Congenital sucrase-isomaltase deficiency. Identification of a glutamine-to-proline substitution that leads to a transport block of sucrase-isomaltase in a pre-Golgi compartment. J Clin Invest 97:633–641.

Panayotova-Heiermann, M., Loo, D. D., Kong, C. T., Lever, J. E., and Wright, E. M. (1996) Sugar binding to Na$^+$/glucose cotransporters is determined by the carboxyl-terminal half of the protein. J Biol Chem 271:10029–10034.

Rosenblum, J. L., Darwin, C. L., and Alpers, D. H. (1988) Starch and glucose oligosaccharides protect salivary-type amylase activity at acid pH. Am J Physiol 254:G775–G780.

Rossi, M., Maiuri, L., Fusco, M. I., Salvati, V. M., Fuccio, A., Auricchio, S., Mantei, N., Zecca, L., Gloor, S. M., and Semenza, G. (1997) Lactase persistence versus decline in human adults: Multifactorial events are involved in down-regulation after weaning. Gastroenterology 112:1506–1514.

Shapiro, G. L., Bulow, S. D., Conklin, K. A., Scheving, L. A., and Gray, G. M. (1991) Post-insertional processing of brush border sucrase-α-dextrinase precursor to authentic subunits: Multiple step cleavage by trypsin. Am J Physiol 261:G847–G857.

Shu, R., David, E. S., and Ferraris, R. P. (1997) Dietary fructose enhances intestinal fructose transport and GLUT5 expression in weaning rats. Am J Physiol 272:G446–G453.

Treem, W. R., Ahsan, N., Sullivan, B., Rossi, T., Holmes, R., Fitzgerald, J., Proujansky, R., and Hyams, J. (1993) Evaluation of liquid yeast-derived sucrase enzyme replacement in patients with sucrase-isomaltase deficiency. Gastroenterology 105:1061–1068.

Tsai, A., Cowan, M. R., Johnson, D. G., and Brannon, P. M. (1994) Regulation of pancreatic amylase and lipase gene expression by diet and insulin in diabetic rats. Am J Physiol 267:G575–G583.

Turk, E., Kerner, C. J., Lostao, M. P., and Wright, E. M. (1996) Membrane topology of the human Na$^+$/glucose cotransporter SGLT1. J Biol Chem 271:1925–1934.

Wasserman, D., Hoekstra, J. H., Tolia, V., Taylor, C. J., Kirschner, B. S., Takeda, J., Bell, G. I., Taub, R., and Rand, E. B. (1996) Molecular analysis of the fructose transporter gene (GLUT5) in isolated fructose malabsorption. J Clin Invest 98:2398–2402.

RECOMMENDED READINGS

Lee, M. F., and Krasinski, S. D. (1998) Human adult-onset lactase decline: An update. Nutr Rev 56:1–8.

McDonald, R. B. (1995) Influence of dietary sucrose on biological aging. Am J Clin Nutr 62 (Suppl. 1):284S–292S.

Rings, E. H., Grand, R. J., and Buller, H. A. (1994) Lactose intolerance and lactase deficiency in children. Curr Opin Pediatr 6:562–567.

CHAPTER **6**

◆ ◆

Digestion and Absorption of Protein

Bruce R. Stevens, Ph.D.

O U T L I N E

DIGESTION OF PROTEIN IN THE GASTROINTESTINAL TRACT

The body requires nutritional protein to be broken down initially into small peptide fragments and amino acids within the stomach and small intestinal lumen. The digestion and absorption process ultimately supplies the circulating blood with free amino acids. In the absorptive state, amino acids are transported via the portal blood from the small intestine to the liver, with subsequent transport to other organs.

The Recommended Dietary Allowance (RDA) for protein is 0.8 g dietary protein per kg body weight, or 56 g for a 70-kg adult. The typical daily Western diet can supply over 100 g of protein, which is rapidly and efficiently digested and absorbed. Besides dietary protein, the body digests an additional 50 to 100 g of endogenous protein that is secreted into or sloughed into the lumen of the gastrointestinal tract. These sources include saliva, gastric juice, pancreatic enzymes and other secretions, sloughed intestinal cells, and proteins that leak into the intestinal lumen from the blood. Most of this mixture of exogenous and endogenous proteins (150 to 200 g per day) is efficiently digested and absorbed (as free amino acids and di- and tripeptides) with daily fecal losses from the gastrointestinal tract of only about 1.6 g of nitrogen (equivalent to 10 g of protein). The nitrogen excreted in the feces primarily represents endogenous or dietary nitrogen that was not absorbed from the small intestine and was used in the large intestine by the microflora for growth and, hence, is present in the feces as part of the bacterial mass.

An overall concept diagram of the major events of protein digestion and absorption is presented in Figure 6–1. The normal events of digestion and absorption are grouped into phases corresponding to physiological events. The major phases covered in this chapter primarily involve:

1. Gastric hydrolysis of peptide linkages in the protein
2. Digestion of protein to smaller peptides by action of pancreatic proteases, which are secreted as zymogens and activated in the lumen of the small intestine where they then carry out digestion
3. Hydrolysis of peptide linkages in oligo-peptides by brush border (apical) membrane peptidases and transport of amino acids and di- and tripeptides across the brush border membrane of the absorptive enterocytes
4. Further digestion of di- and tripeptides by cytoplasmic peptidases in the enterocyte
5. Metabolism of some amino acids within the enterocyte
6. Transport of amino acids across the basolateral membrane of the enterocyte into the interstitial fluid from which the amino acids enter the venous capillaries and hence the portal blood

Under various metabolic demands, the requirement for daily protein can increase by a factor of over two- to threefold. Such conditions exist, for example, in burn patients, lactating mothers, growing infants and adolescents, and cancer patients. Responding to dietary content and metabolic demands, the cells and tissues of the gastrointestinal tract adaptively regulate the digestive and absorptive processes. In addition to normal gastrointestinal physiology and biochemistry, this chapter covers some of the major pathophysiological mechanisms associated with protein digestion and absorption.

THE GASTRIC PHASE: DENATURATION AND INITIAL HYDROLYSIS OF PROTEINS

Protein digestion begins with modest processing by the stomach. Here, gastric hydrochloric acid (HCl) and pepsins partially denature and hydrolyze proteins. The stomach plays a minor role in the overall digestion process and primarily serves to prepare polypeptides for the main events of digestion and absorption that take place within the small intestine. Indeed, complete protein assimilation occurs even after surgical removal of the stomach.

When food is present in the stomach or if the appropriate vagal cholinergic efferents

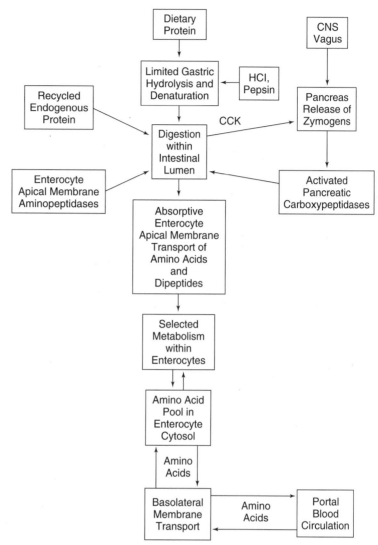

Figure 6–1. Overall "concept" diagram of the normal events of protein digestion and absorption.

are activated, the gastric chief cells secrete inactive pepsinogens into the stomach lumen. Several isozymes of pepsinogen are released, and each is converted to an active pepsin isozyme by cleavage of a peptide from the amino terminus. Activation spontaneously occurs below pH 5 by an intramolecular process that involves proteolytic cleavage of a highly basic amino terminal precursor segment. In the zymogen, the active site of pepsin is blocked by interaction of basic residues in the precursor segment with carboxylate side chains and with the pair of aspartyl residues at the active site. These salt bridges are broken as the carboxylates become protonated at the acidic pH of the gastric contents; this exposes

the catalytic site and results in hydrolysis of the peptide bond between the precursor segment and the pepsin moiety. After this autoactivation process forms some pepsin, activation of pepsinogen by active pepsin (autocatalysis) also occurs.

Pepsins are chemically categorized as endopeptidases because they attack peptide bonds within the polypeptide chain. Their catalytic mechanism involves two carboxylic acid groups at the active site of the enzyme, so pepsins are classified as carboxyl proteases. Most digestive enzymes are relatively permissive in the range of substrates they will accept, and the pepsins partially hydrolyze a broad variety of proteins to large peptide fragments and some free amino acids. Pepsins show a preference for hydrolysis of internal peptide bonds that involve the carboxyl groups of tyrosyl, phenylalanyl, or tryptophanyl residues and that do not involve a linkage to the imino nitrogen of proline.

SMALL INTESTINAL LUMINAL PHASE: ACTIVATION AND ACTION OF PANCREATIC PROTEOLYTIC ENYZMES

Following partial hydrolysis of protein in the stomach, the polypeptides and amino acids enter the lumen of the proximal small intestine where they stimulate the mucosal cells to release the hormone cholecystokinin (CCK) into the circulation. CCK subsequently reaches the pancreas, whereupon it binds to the acinar cells and stimulates the secretion of a variety of inactive precursor digestive enzymes called zymogens. Zymogens are delivered to the small intestinal lumen by way of the pancreatic duct. In addition to CCK stimulation, stomach distension or the sight and smell of food invoke parasympathetic cholinergic vagal nerve efferents, which in turn stimulate the exocrine pancreatic acinar cells to release zymogens.

Based on work that originated in the Russian laboratory of I. P. Pavlov in the late 1890s, research has established that protein digestion follows a multi-step conversion of inactive zymogens to their active states within the lumen of the small intestine. The current understanding of the entire sequence covered in this section is summarized in Figure 6–2.

Pancreatic Zymogens and Their Activation Cascade

The pancreatic zymogens are released directly into the intestinal lumen via the pancreatic duct and the common bile duct. The major zymogens are trypsinogen, proelastase, chymotrypsinogen, procarboxypeptidase A, and procarboxypeptidase B. The initial step of the activation cascade is catalyzed by enterokinase (enteropeptidase), which is bound to the brush border (apical) membranes of epithelial cells of the mucosa that lines the proximal small intestine (duodenum/upper jejunum).

Enterokinase's importance is emphasized by the fact that congenital deficiency of this enzyme leads to life-threatening malabsorption of nitrogen. Human enterokinase is structurally organized as a heavily glycosylated dimer attached to membranes of cells lining the

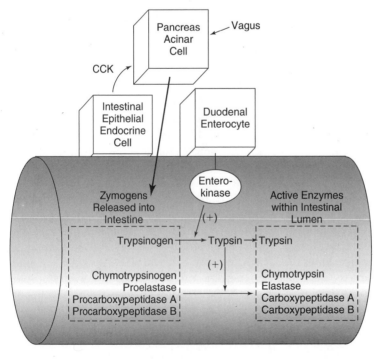

Figure 6–2. *Cascade activation of pancreatic zymogens within the small intestinal lumen.*

upper intestine. It is a member of the serine protease family of enzymes. The partial complementary DNA (cDNA) sequence for human enterokinase indicates that the active dimer is derived from a single-chain precursor (Kitamoto et al., 1995). In this sense, biosynthesis of the nascent enterokinase precursor may actually be considered the true "first" step of the cascade, with the implication that a proenterokinase activator is yet to be discovered!

Intestinal enterokinase cleaves an amino terminal octapeptide from human trypsinogen, thereby forming the activated trypsin enzyme within the intestinal lumen. The specificity of enterokinase for trypsinogin is high; the scissile (to be cleaved) peptide bond in trypsinogen involves a lysyl residue that contributes the carboxyl group and an isoleucyl residue that contributes the amino group to the linkage. Specificity of trypsinogen as the substrate for enterokinase depends on the peptide sequence Asp-Asp-Asp-Asp-Lys that contains four acidic aspartyl residues adjacent to the lysyl residue of the scissile peptide bond.

Trypsin, which is also a member of the serine protease family but with very different specificity than enterokinase, then activates the other zymogens (chymotrypsinogen, proelastase, and carboxypeptidase A and B, as well as procolipase and prophospholipase A_2, which are required for lipid digestion) by cleaving off selected peptide sequences. The net result of this cascade is a pool of activated proteases within the lumen. Proteolysis is facilitated by the secretion of pancreatic bicarbonate into the intestinal lumen; the bicarbonate titrates the gastric acid in the chyme to pH 6 to 7, which is optimal for activity of pancreatic proteases.

It was formerly thought that once some trypsin was formed from trypsinogen by enterokinase, the active trypsin could act on trypsinogen as substrate in an autocatalytic process. Although both trypsin and enterokinase cleave at scissile bonds that involve a basic (lysyl or arginyl) residue attached to an isoleucyl residue, the aspartyl-rich sequence in the activation peptide segment of trypsinogen inhibits the ability of trypsin to accept trypsinogen as a substrate. Thus, enterokinase

in the small intestine is essential for activation of trypsin and the activation cascade.

A benefit of synthesis of proteolytic enzymes as zymogens with the activation cascade occurring in the intestinal lumen is the prevention of proteolytic digestion and tissue damage within the pancreas and pancreatic duct. In addition to this protective mechanism, pancreatic juice normally contains a small peptide that acts as a trypsin inhibitor to prevent any small amount of trypsin prematurely formed within the pancreatic cells or pancreatic ducts from catalyzing proteolysis.

Pancreatic Digestive Enzymes

The pancreatic enzymes can be divided into two general types—serine proteases and carboxypeptidases. Trypsin, chymotrypsin, and elastase are all endopeptidases of the serine protease class. They are categorized as endopeptidases because they hydrolyze internal peptide bonds within the polypeptide. They are classified as serine proteases because of their catalytic mechanism, which involves a seryl residue in the catalytic site. Serine proteases, including those involved in the blood-clotting cascade, as discussed in Chapter 24, are normally synthesized in inactive zymogen or proenzyme form. Each of these serine proteases catalyzes the hydrolysis of peptide (amide) bonds, but with different selectivities or preferences for the side chains flanking the scissile peptide bond. The site of hydrolysis in the polypeptide substrate is flanked by approximately four amino acid residues in both directions that can bind to the enzyme and impact on the reactivity of the peptide bond hydrolyzed; the hydrolyzable bond is designated $P_1-P'_1$ and adjacent amino acids are numbered P_2, P_3, and P_4 toward the amino terminus and P'_2, P'_3, and P'_4 toward the carboxy-terminus. Trypsin is most likely to cleave peptide bonds with a positively charged residue (arginine or lysine) at the P_1 site (contributing the carboxyl group to the peptide bond); chymotrypsin prefers bonds in which large hydrophobic amino acid residues such as tryptophan, phenylalanine, tyrosine, methionine, or leucine are at the P_1 site; and elastase preferentially cleaves peptide bonds that have a small neutral residue such as alanine,

NUTRITION INSIGHT

Trypsin Inhibitors

Small molecular weight proteins or polypeptides that act as protease inhibitors are naturally produced by cells in both animals and plants. In particular, pulses (peas, beans, and lentils) and cereals (wheat, buckwheat, rice bran) contain trypsin inhibitors that can lower the nutritional quality of their proteins. These trypsin inhibitors can be inactivated to a large extent by wet heating or removed by processing techniques used during protein concentration and isolation (e.g., soy protein). Soybean trypsin inhibitors have been studied widely. Although these are inactivated by heating, animals sometimes ingest large amounts of these inhibitors by consuming raw soybeans.

The pancreas, intestinal cells, liver, and other tissues also synthesize a certain amount of trypsin inhibitors. For example, human pancreatic secretory trypsin inhibitor is secreted from pancreatic acinar cells into the pancreatic duct along with the zymogen precursors of the proteolytic digestive enzymes. The possibility that some symptoms observed in diseases such as acute pancreatitis or gastric ulcer are due to an absence of normal synthesis/secretion of these inhibitors is under active investigation. The therapeutic use of trypsin inhibitors to treat pancreatitis and other inflammatory conditions is also being tested in animal models.

Thinking Critically

1. Why would the presence of trypsin inhibitors in a food decrease the nutritional quality of its protein? Explain.

2. Feeding of raw soybean flour or soybean trypsin inhibitor results in an increase in the amounts of secretory products (presumably due to an increase in protein synthesis) within the acinar cells and in enhanced protein secretion by the pancreas. Why might this occur?

3. Why might a lack of endogenous trypsin inhibitor result in acute pancreatitis? Why might therapeutic administration of trypsin inhibitor alleviate ulceration or inflammation of tissues?

---

serine, glycine, or valine at the P_1 site. Proline at the P'_1 site inhibits cleavage by all three serine proteases. The rate at which particular bonds are cleaved also varies with the identities of the amino acid residues in the adjacent positions ($P_2 - P_4$ and $P'_2 - P'_4$).

The second group of proteolytic enzymes secreted by the pancreas, the carboxypeptidases, are exopeptidases that cleave off one amino acid at a time from the carboxy- or C-terminus. Exopeptidases can attack the oligopeptides formed by the endopeptidases to sequentially cleave off free amino acids, leaving a mixture of free amino acids and small peptides of two to eight residues. Carboxypeptidases A and B are both metalloenzymes that require Zn^{2+} at the active site where it functions as a Lewis acid. (See Chapter 32 for a discussion of zinc metalloenzymes.) Carboxypeptidase B preferentially cleaves C-terminal lysine or arginine residues of peptides, and carboxypeptidase A selectively hydrolyzes most C-terminal amino acids except proline, lysine, and arginine, with a preference for valine, leucine, isoleucine, and alanine. Carboxypeptidase A and B do not readily cleave C-terminal amino acids that are linked to a prolyl residue.

These pancreatic enzymes act as a team within the small intestinal lumen to hydrolyze many of the peptide bonds in proteins, resulting in efficient digestion of protein to small peptides (two to eight residues) and free amino acids.

SMALL INTESTINAL MUCOSAL PHASE: BRUSH BORDER AND CYTOSOLIC PEPTIDASES

The products of pancreatic hydrolysis are free amino acids, tri- and dipeptides, and larger peptide fragments called oligopeptides. The free amino acids, dipeptides, and tripeptides are transported across the absorptive epithelial cell apical membrane by specific carriers, as described below. Most larger oligopeptides are not transported, but must be further hydrolyzed by epithelial brush border membrane-bound enzymes.

With one known exception, the peptidases in the brush border membrane of the enterocyte are all categorized chemically as aminopeptidases, meaning that they hydrolyze amino acids one at a time from the amino or N-terminus. These enzymes also show specificities or preferences for the amino acid residues and peptide sequences that they hydrolyze. The apical membrane possesses a single known carboxypeptidase, which is peptidyl dipeptidase. Both the aminopeptidases and the carboxypeptidase are classified as exopeptidases.

The enterocyte membrane–bound peptidases are dimers that extend into the lumen about 15 nm from the membrane surface. One subunit is anchored to the membrane, and the other subunit participates in the hydrolytic activity. A variety of membrane-bound aminopeptidases exist, each having a different preference for specific residues involved in the amide bonds that they hydrolyze. Some examples include aminopeptidase A, aminopeptidase N, proline iminopeptidase, and dipeptidylpeptidase IV.

For the tri- and dipeptides that are transported into the enterocyte, additional cytosolic aminopeptidases act within the absorptive epithelial cells to complete the process of hydrolyzing proteins and peptides to free amino acids. Most protein nitrogen exits the basolateral membrane to the portal blood as free amino acids. As explained later in this chapter, a small fraction ($< 1\%$) of undigested luminal protein and peptides may enter the portal blood intact.

ABSORPTION OF FREE AMINO ACIDS AND SMALL PEPTIDES

The products of digestion—free amino acids and small peptides—are absorbed from the lumen by a variety of transport mechanisms.

Free amino acid absorption mechanisms are presented first, followed by a discussion of small peptide absorption.

Amino Acid Transport Systems in the Brush Border and Basolateral Membranes

The L-stereoisomers of free amino acids in the intestinal lumen move across the brush border membrane of villous absorptive enterocytes, are pooled within the enterocyte, and then finally exit the enterocyte via the basolateral membranes. Following basolateral membrane transport to the interstitial fluid, the amino acids are transported into mucosal capillaries and eventually reach the portal circulation. The intestine is 95% to 99% efficient in extracting the essential and nonessential amino acids from the lumen. This occurs largely due to the activity of brush border (apical) and basolateral membrane transporter systems that serve specific substrates. (These basolateral membrane transporters can also serve to take up amino acids, particularly glutamine, from the arterial circulation.)

The known transport systems for each membrane of an absorptive enterocyte are summarized in Figure 6–3 (Stevens, 1992; Mailliard et al., 1995). Note that many of the brush border (apical) membrane pathways are different from those found in the basolateral membrane. The amino acid transport systems are cataloged by letter abbreviations. Each system prefers specific amino acid substrates. Many amino acid transporters are activated by sodium (Na^+) ions, and these systems are designated with capital letter abbreviations. Transporters designated with lower case letters represent Na^+-independent systems. One exception to this designation system is amino acid transport system L, which is Na^+-independent. Some of the membrane carriers or regulatory subunits have been cloned and localized to specific genes.

Sodium-dependent system B is the primary pathway by which the neutral amino acids cross the brush border membrane (Pan and Stevens, 1995b; Stevens, 1992). A protein composed of 541 amino acids responsible for system B transport activity has been cloned, and the messenger RNA (mRNA) coding for

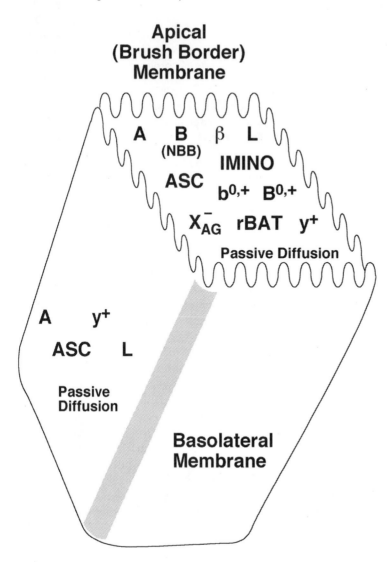

Figure 6–3. *Membrane transport systems of absorptive enterocytes. Each system, denoted by code letters (Stevens, 1992; Mailliard et al., 1995), serves L-amino acids with specific structural features. rBAT not a transporter per se, but is likely a regulatory or structural subunit that binds to other subunits of transport system $b^{0,+}$. Based on Stevens, B. R. (1992) Amino Acid Transport in Intestine. In: Mammalian Amino Acid Transport: Mechanisms and Control, (Kilberg, M. S. and Haussinger, D., eds.), pp. 149–164, Plenum, New York; and Mailliard, M. E., Stevens, B. R. and Mann, G. E. (1995) Amino acid transport by small intestinal, hepatic, and pancreatic epithelia. Gastroenterology 108:888–910. Redrawn from Stevens (1992) with permission of Plenum Publishing Corp.*

this transport protein has been identified in human intestinal cell lines (Kekuda et al., 1996). Systems A and ASC serve the neutral amino acids at the basolateral membrane, with some activity reported in the apical surface. The IMINO system is restricted to transporting proline and the imino acids. System X_{AG}^{-} is a Na^{+}-dependent system that serves the anionic substrates aspartate and glutamate.

Enterocyte membranes possess Na^{+}-independent systems denoted y^{+}, $b^{0,+}$, and L (Pan and Stevens, 1995a; Mailliard et al., 1995). System y^{+} serves the cationic substrates arginine, lysine, and ornithine, and is the expression product of human gene *ATRC1* located on chromosome 13 at 13q12-q14. There are two cDNA clones for isoforms of system y^{+},

designated as CAT-1 and CAT-2 (cationic amino acid transporter). System $b^{0,+}$ is a Na^{+}-independent transporter serving both cationic and neutral amino acids. Although $b^{0,+}$ itself has not been cloned, a cloned polypeptide subunit denoted rBAT may be associated with $b^{0,+}$ activity. The rBAT (related to $b^{0,+}$ amino acid transporter) gene has been identified on human chromosome 2. In the brush border membrane, a Cl^{-}-dependent and Na^{+}-dependent variant of $b^{0,+}$, denoted system $B^{0,+}$, serves cationic amino acids, taurine, β-alanine, and several of the neutral amino acids. System L is a Na^{+}-independent transport system that handles large hydrophobic or branched substrates such as leucine, isoleucine, valine, phenylalanine, and tyrosine. (See

Chapter 11 for more discussion of amino acid transport systems.)

Experimental evidence suggests that the mechanism of Na^+-dependent amino acid active transport occurs as shown in Figure 6–4 (Stevens et al., 1990). This model depicts a single transporter molecule arranged as a tetramer of subunits embedded in the epithelial cell plasma membrane. The subunits are organized to form a gated pore that spans the plasma membrane of absorptive epithelial cells. In the process of nutrient absorption, Na^+ ions within the intestinal lumen activate amino acid uptake by attaching to a binding site on the transporter. The transporter then selectively binds an amino acid molecule. The transporter molecule subsequently catalyzes the coupled movement of both Na^+ and amino acid across the membrane and into the enterocyte cytoplasm (Stevens, 1992).

The continual extraction of nutrients from the intestinal lumen results in a pooling of Na^+ and amino acids within the enterocyte. In the absorptive state, these nutrients subsequently exit the enterocyte to the interstitial fluid via the basolateral membranes. In the postabsorptive state, basolateral membrane transporters can supply enterocytes with amino acids from the blood. In both states the Na^+ electrochemical potential gradient is continually maintained by the Na^+/K^+-ATPase pump in the basolateral membrane. It is the Na^+ electrochemical potential that energizes the (secondary or coupled) active transport of amino acids (Gerencser and Stevens, 1994). The absorption of positively charged cationic amino acids via Na^+-independent transport systems y^+ and $b^{0,+}$ is driven by the amino acid chemical gradient plus the negative electrical potential across the enterocyte mem-

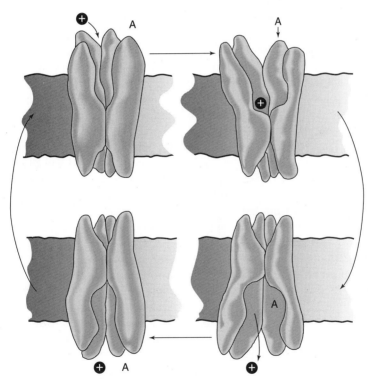

Figure 6–4. *Model of Na^+-coupled L-amino acid transport in intestinal cell plasma membranes. In this model, the transporter is a tetramer made of four subunit monomers. The sequence of transport events is depicted by the four drawings of the transporter. Extracellular sodium ions (circled "+") first bind to a specific extracellular binding site of the tetramer. This results in a conformational shift that subsequently permits an L-amino acid molecule (A) to bind. The loaded transporter then moves Na^+ and amino acid together across the plasma membrane into the enterocyte cytoplasm. In the final step, the transporter releases Na^+ and the amino acid and reverts back to the initial conformation, ready for another cycle of binding and transporting. From Stevens, B. R., Fernandez, A., Hirayama, B., Wright, E. M. and Kempner, E. S. (1990) Intestinal brush border membrane Na^+/glucose cotransporter functions in situ as a homotetramer. Proc Natl Acad Sci USA 87:1456–1460. Used with permission of the author.*

brane. The chemical gradient of neutral amino acids is the sole driving force for absorption via transport system L.

Regulation of Intestinal Absorption of Amino Acids

From the perspective of the whole body, the intestinal capacity to absorb nutrients must not be the rate-limiting step that governs whole-body intermediary metabolism of amino acids. Therefore, one of the major roles of the gastrointestinal tract is to maintain a net positive flow of nutrient nitrogen in the direction of diet-to-organism. To do this, the small intestine is able to adaptively upregulate its capacity for amino acid absorption.

As the dietary protein content and physiological state of the body changes over a period of days, the intestine adaptively regulates its capacity to absorb amino acids. The adaptations occur both at the mucosal tissue level and absorptive enterocyte cellular level. Acting on the mucosa, various factors can nonspecifically change the absorptive surface area of the intestine. For example, in animal models, mucosal hyperplasia occurs in response to corticosteroids and peptide growth factors or in response to hyperphagia associated with diabetes, hyperthyroidism, neoplasia, pregnancy and lactation, or accelerated growth.

Furthermore, in response to specific peptides and amino acids within the intestinal lumen, individual enterocytes upregulate the de novo biosynthesis of aminopeptidases and specific membrane transporters (Stevens, 1992; Pan and Stevens, 1995a). Exposure to a single amino acid substrate species can upregulate expression of its own membrane transporter by two- to tenfold, following a 10- to 24-hour lag period. In intestinal cell kinetic studies performed in vitro, the lag period was sensitive to the protein synthesis inhibitors actinomycin D or cycloheximide (Pan and Stevens, 1995b). This means that the induction of transport involves de novo synthesis and membrane expression of either new transporter molecules or their regulatory subunits. Interestingly, animal studies have shown that consumption of diets supplemented with individual amino acids can activate the uptake

of substrates that may be unrelated to the transporter used by the activator itself. In mice, for example, aspartate stimulates the absorption of acidic as well as basic amino acids, and orally fed arginine (but not lysine) induces aspartate uptake (Ferraris and Diamond, 1989). This pattern of interaction between substrates and transporter induction suggests that independent regulatory proteins may be involved in a common regulatory process, although the mechanism is unknown. The regulation of neutral amino acid uptake via system B occurs by a mechanism involving enterocyte protein kinase C phosphorylation sites (Pan and Stevens, 1995b).

With the concerted effects of both individual cell upregulation and general mucosal hyperplasia, the small intestine can increase its absorptive capacity by a factor of two- to 20-fold compared to the constitutive fasting level. Absorption is generally greatest in the jejunal region, and transport is upregulated to a greater extent within the jejunual mucosa than in the duodenum or ileum. The concept of regional upregulation of amino acid absorption is shown in Figure 6–5.

Intestinal downregulation of amino acid transport is essentially a return to the constitutive baseline absorptive capacity that occurs in the absence of stimulating agent. The down-regulation occurs over a period of several days, because the absorptive cells with enhanced transport capacity are gradually sloughed off from the villus tip into the lumen and are replaced with cells possessing only constitutive transport activity (Stevens, 1992). In the absence of luminal feeding, as in the case of total parenteral nutrition (TPN), the absorptive capacity of the intestine may become severely reduced as intestinal atrophy gradually occurs. This phenomenon underlines the importance of enteral feeding in maintaining the integrity of the gut in convalescing patients.

Complementary DNA (cDNA) expression cloning experiments suggest that some epithelial amino acid transport activities may be regulated by biosynthesis and insertion of polypeptide subunits or structural subunits in the membrane. The cloned polypeptide denoted rBAT (related to $b^{0,+}$-like amino acid transporter) is the most extensively studied

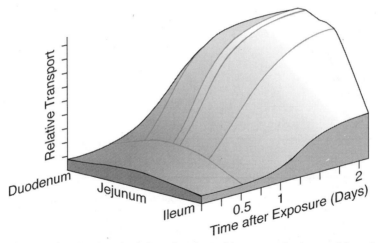

Figure 6–5. *The concept of regional upregulation of amino acid transport in the small intestine. Generally, the constitutive uptake capacity and the magnitude of transport upregulation is greater in the jejunum, compared to the ileum or duodenum. Transport is upregulated over the course of hours and days as new copies of specific transporter molecules are synthesized and inserted into the enterocytes during villus maturation and hyperplasia. From Stevens, B. R. (1992) Amino Acid Transport in Intestine. In:* Mammalian Amino Acid Transport: Mechanisms and Control *(Kilberg, M. S. and Haussinger, D., eds.), pp. 149–164, Plenum, New York. Redrawn with permission of Plenum Publishing Corporation.*

membrane protein associated with amino acid transport regulation (Palacin, 1994).

The *rBAT* gene encodes an integral membrane glycoprotein with a single transmembrane-spanning domain in the brush border membrane. The predicted protein sequence of human rBAT is 685 amino acids long. The molecular mass is about 72 kDa, with an in vitro translation product glycosylated mass of about 94 kDa. The predicted structure of rBAT is different from the structure of known transporter proteins, which normally contain about 12 to 14 transmembrane domains. The extracellular domain of rBAT possesses the carboxy-terminus, shows extensive homology with the α-amylases and α-glucosidases, and has six potential N-glycosylation sites. A cysteinyl residue is situated near the membrane surface at the extracellular face. It is thought that this cysteinyl residue forms a disulfide bridge with an adjacent transporter subunit. rBAT regulates cationic and neutral amino acid uptake via Na^+-independent system $b^{0,+}$. Figure 6–6 shows the proposed heterodimer relationship between rBAT and a $b^{0,+}$ polypeptide in the membrane. Single point mutations in the *rBAT* gene are responsible for the autosomal recessive disease cystinuria (Palacin, 1994).

Inborn Disorders of Intestinal Amino Acid Transport

The absorptive epithelium of the small intestine shares many physiological and functional traits with the reabsorptive epithelium of the kidney proximal tubule. Both tissues possess aminopeptidases on their apical membranes, and both possess the same amino acid transport systems. Several inborn disorders of amino acid transport are associated with a defective or deleted constitutive transport system in both the intestinal and kidney absorptive epithelial membranes (Mailliard et al., 1995). These are clinically observed as specific aminoacidurias, which display autosomal recessive inheritance patterns. Although specific amino acid transporters of the intestinal membrane are impaired, the aminoaciduria patient's metabolic requirements for nutrient amino nitrogen are met by other amino acid transporters with overlapping specificities or dipeptide/tripeptide transporters. No genetic defects of peptide transporter proteins are known. Peptide transporters are discussed later in this chapter.

Cystinuria is the best documented case of a specific genetic defect of amino acid transport manifested in the kidney and intestine. The clinical signature of cystinuria is the

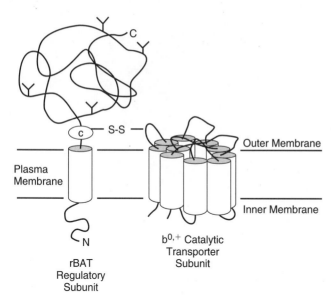

Figure 6–6. Model of rBAT regulatory subunit bound to the catalytic subunit of the system $b^{0,+}$ transporter. rBAT is a cloned polypeptide that has a single membrane-spanning domain, with most of the polypeptide chain facing extracellular fluid. Near the membrane surface, a cysteinyl residue of rBAT presumably forms a disulfide bridge with the $b^{0,+}$ transporter protein. A conserved cysteinyl residue (c) is present in the extracellular domain of rBAT. System $b^{0,+}$ has not been cloned, although its presence has been identified by kinetic experiments. Therefore its structure here is only speculative. From Palacin, M. (1994) A new family of proteins (rBAT and 4F2hc) involved in cationic and zwitterionic amino acid transport: A tale of two proteins in search of a transport function. J Exp Biol 196:123–137. Redrawn with permission of The Company of Biologists LTD.

simultaneously elevated levels of lysine, ornithine, arginine, and cystine in the urine. One variant of cystinuria has been specifically identified with a defect in the gene that encodes the rBAT protein. The *rBAT* cystinuria gene is localized to human chromosome 2, with specific mutations localized to region 2pter-12p. The most frequent *rBAT* mutation, a single threonine substitution for methionine at residue 467, abolishes amino acid transport by system $b^{0,+}$.

Other clinically observed transport defects have not been as rigorously identified and localized to specific genes by molecular biology techniques. However, most aminoacidurias have been at least associated with specific alleles. For example, it is thought that lysinuric protein intolerance—with symptoms of diarrhea and vomiting following a protein meal—likely involves a defect in one of the *CAT* genes that encode the system y^+ transporter isoforms. Hartnup disease likely involves Na^+-dependent transport system B serving the neutral amino acids. In Hartnup disease, the poor absorption of the amino acid tryptophan leads to inadequate synthesis of NAD(P)/nicotinamide; this gives rise to pellegra-like clinical symptoms of rashes and cerebellar ataxia. (See Chapter 20 for more discussion of tryptophan and the niacin requirement.) In infants, the so-called "blue diaper syndrome" is the result of excessive, unabsorbed tryptophan reaching the large intestine, where it is converted by bacteria to blue-colored indole derivatives. Other transport diseases include hyperdibasic aminoaciduria that affects lysine, ornithine, and arginine absorption with clinical signs of hyperammonemia, failure to thrive, and mental retardation; methionine malabsorptive syndrome, which leads to growth failure due to insufficient delivery and retention of the essential amino acid methionine; and dicarboxylic aminoaciduria, which is due to an impediment in the transport of glutamate and aspartate.

Brush Border Membrane Transport of Peptides

Up to this point, we have considered amino acid absorption only in terms of free amino acids. However, dipeptide and tripeptide products of protein digestion are also independently transported across the brush border membrane of absorptive enterocytes by substrate-selective carriers (Adibi, 1996). Tetra- and larger peptides are not absorbed to any appreciable extent and must be further hydrolyzed to the smaller peptides for assimilation. The ability to absorb amino acids both as peptides and as free amino acids as well as by multiple transport systems offers the advantage of a backup system that ensures

CLINICAL CORRELATION

Cystinuria

Cystinuria is a disorder of amino acid transport that affects the epithelial cells of the renal tubules and the gastrointestinal tract. It is inherited as an autosomal recessive trait and is expressed clinically as urinary tract calculus disease. The disorder results in aminoaciduria of cystine and dibasic amino acids due to their defective renal reabsorption. A urinary cystine excretion exceeding 1.2 mmol/day (compared with a normal excretion of 0.05 to 0.25 mmol/day) is usually diagnostic of homozygous cystinuria. Because cystine is very insoluble in aqueous solution, cystine stones are formed and hexagonal cystine crystals appear in the urine. Stones generally form at cystine excretion rates of greater than 300 mg cystine per gram of creatinine in acidic urine. Treatment is directed at reducing the concentration of cystine in urine by increasing urine volume, increasing cystine solubility by alkalinizing the urine, and reducing cystine excretion by use of D-penicillamine or other sulfhydryl-containing compounds to reduce the disulfide or form more soluble mixed disulfides.

Cystinuria has been classified into three subtypes on the basis of patterns of urinary excretion and intestinal transport of cystine and dibasic amino acids. The gene whose mutation is responsible for cystinuria type I has recently been identified as *SLC3A1,* which codes for the rBAT protein. The normal human rBAT protein elicited Na^+-independent, high-affinity obligatory exchange of cystine, dibasic amino acids, and some neutral amino acids ($b^{0,+}$-like) when experimentally expressed in membranes of *Xenopus* oocytes. The nature of the coupling or type of exchanger has not been defined, but it was somewhat surprising to realize that this specialized absorptive system may function as a hetero-exchanger preferring to transport basic amino acids inward and neutral amino acids outward (Palacin, 1994).

Thinking Critically

1. Adequate amino acid nutrition is not a particular problem in individuals with cystinuria. Why? Discuss several factors related to diet, intestinal absorption, or renal reabsorption that could result in this defect having minimal effect on nutrition.

2. The amount of neutral amino acids excreted in the urine is not elevated in individuals with cystinuria. What are some possible reasons for this?

3. At pH values below 7.5, about 1 mmol (250 mg) of cystine per liter is the aqueous solubility limit of cystine. Cystinuric patients may excrete more than 1 g of cystine per day. What recommendations would you give a cystinuric patient with regard to water intake?

---

efficient absorption of essential and nonessential amino acids.

Unlike amino acid transport, which is energized by the electrochemical potential of Na^+ ions, peptide transport is driven by proton (H^+) electrochemical potentials (Leibach and Ganapathy, 1996). In the lumen of the intestine, the acidic microenvironment (pH 5 to 6) near the apical surface establishes a pH gradient across the brush border membrane and supplies H^+ for cotransport with the peptides.

Dipeptides and tripeptides are absorbed more rapidly across the apical surface than the equivalent free amino acid mixture of an elemental diet composed of free amino acids. This phenomenon has been used to rationalize the clinical feeding of partially hydrolyzed casein or lactalbumin in patients with pancreatic disease. Once dipeptides are removed from the lumen, they are largely hydrolyzed to constituent free amino acids by aminopeptidases within the enterocyte cytoplasm. The free amino acids pooled in the enterocyte cytoplasm are finally transported across the basolateral membranes to the portal blood. Some data suggest that the absorption of tripeptides occurs in a manner similar to that of dipeptides. A small portion of the intact peptides originating from the diet or from digestion of dietary protein in the intestinal lumen are resistant to hydrolysis and appear intact in the circulation. Peptides such as glycylproline, which may result from the limited ability of proteolytic enzymes to cleave peptide bonds involving certain amino acids, and L-carnosine (β-alanylhistidine), a dipeptide found in food, are examples.

Although several different peptide transport systems have been predicted by uptake experiments, only one carrier protein responsible for human intestinal peptide transport has been cloned. The gene encoding this transporter *(PepT1)* has been localized to human chromosome 13q24-q33, and the 708-amino acid sequence predicts a membrane protein with 12 membrane-spanning domains (Liang et al., 1995). The molecular mass of the carrier is about 71 kDa in glycosylated

form. Figure 6–7 shows the predicted sequence of the H^+/peptide cotransporter. The large extracellular loop possesses potential N-glycosylation sites, and one of the intracellular domains possesses two potential protein kinase C-dependent regulation sites. Although the peptide transporter is similar to many membrane proteins, it shows no homology with any cloned amino acid transporter. The H^+-activated carrier protein serves a variety of dipeptides and tripeptides, as well as many of the peptide-type β-lactam antibiotic drugs.

METABOLISM OF AMINO ACIDS IN INTESTINAL EPITHELIAL CELLS

Although most dietary amino acids that are taken up by enterocytes subsequently are

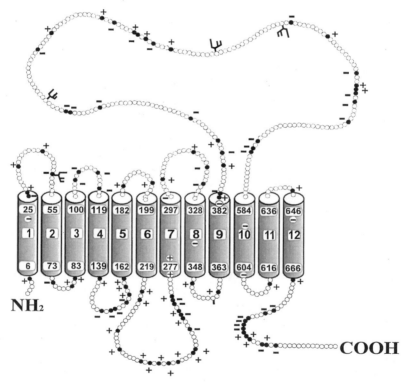

Figure 6–7. The amino acid sequence of the cloned intestinal H^+/peptide cotransporter PepT1. Shown is the predicted structure from rabbit; the human H^+/peptide cotransporter has also been cloned (81% identity and 92% similarity with rabbit). For the 708-amino acid polypeptide, there are 12 membrane-spanning regions and a large extracellular loop with several glycosylation sites. The intracellular portion contains protein kinase C-dependent phosphorylation sites. Adapted from Liang et al. (1995) and Fei et al. (1994) with permission of the authors. (Liang, R., Fei, Y-J., Prasad, P. D., Ramamoorthy, S., Han, H., Yang-Feng, T., Hediger, M. A., Ganapathy, V. and Leibach, F. H. (1995) Human intestinal H^+/peptide cotransporter cloning, functional expression, and chromosomal localization. J Biol Chem 270:6456–6463; Fei, Y-J., Kanai, Y., Nusserger, S., Ganapathy, V., Liebach, F. H., Romero, M. F., Singh, S. K., Boron, W. F. and Hediger, M. A. (1994) Expression cloning of a mammalian proton-coupled oligopeptide transporter. Nature 368:563–566.)

transported across the basolateral membrane and enter the portal blood unchanged, several of the amino acids undergo considerable metabolic conversion to other compounds before exit to the portal circulation. In particular, the enterocytes metabolize glutamate, glutamine, and aspartate taken up from the luminal contents (digesta). Glutamine is extensively metabolized by enterocytes as a major energy source. The intestine partially oxidizes glutamine as a fuel to provide ATP, and thus spares dietary glucose and fatty acids for use by other tissues. Indeed, the intestinal requirement for glutamine is so great that, in the postabsorptive state, circulating glutamine released by muscle and the lungs is avidly taken up by enterocytes via the basolateral membranes. Glutamine metabolism results in the release of ammonia, lactate, alanine, proline, and citrulline into the portal circulation. (See Chapter 11 for further discussion of amino acid metabolism.)

USE OF FREE AMINO ACIDS AND PEPTIDES FOR THERAPEUTIC ORAL REHYDRATION

Intestinal absorption normally occurs across villous epithelial cells (enterocytes), whereas secretion of fluid and electrolytes occurs via mucosal crypt cells. When the intestine becomes infected with microorganisms that release enterotoxin (e.g., *Escherichia coli*, *Vibrio cholerae*), excessive quantities of water and electrolytes are lost by intestinal crypt cells in the form of a secretory diarrhea. The fluid and electrolyte losses can be overcome by the use of oral rehydrating therapy (ORT) solutions. ORT exploits the coupled uptake of Na^+ ions, amino acids, glucose, and water that occurs in the absorptive villous cells. It has been experimentally demonstrated that intestinal amino acid absorption via systems B and y^+ remains largely intact and functional in patients with cholera infection.

Amino acid–based ORT solutions are essentially iso-osmotic or hypo-osmotic fluids containing Na^+, Cl^-, citrate, and K^+ with free amino acids such as glutamine or alanine. Alternatively, easily digested proteins/peptides may be included to serve as free amino acid

precursors. The mechanism by which enterocytes couple the absorption of Na^+ ions and amino acids was discussed earlier (see Fig. 6–4). Water absorption is subsequently osmotically coupled to the uptake of amino acids and Na^+. Enteral administration of amino acids or proteins is also beneficial in promoting the morphologic, digestive, and absorptive integrity of the mucosa. This is in contrast to long-term degradation of the intestinal mucosa's absorptive capacity that occurs with long-term TPN administration. Therefore, the use of amino acid/Na^+ rehydration has been increasingly promoted as a therapeutic aid during infection, surgery, or other trauma of the gut.

UPTAKE OF PROTEIN MACROMOLECULES AND IMMUNE RESPONSE

Virtually all proteins are completely digested and absorbed by the processes described above. Nonetheless, a small portion ($< 1\%$) of protein resists digestion, and is absorbed intact or as polypeptide fragments. Rather than serving as a simple food source of amino acids, these luminal polypeptides can potentially act as antigens, growth factors, or toxins. The intestine has specific mechanisms to control the uptake of such biologically active macromolecules (Sanderson and Walker, 1993). The uptake of certain intact peptide growth factors from the lumen, such as epidermal growth factor (EGF) or transforming growth factor alpha (TGFα), are especially important during development and maturation of the gastrointestinal mucosa.

Defects in the normal protein digestion and absorption mechanisms may compound gastrointestinal or systemic diseases. For example, chronic immune enteropathies such as inflammatory bowel disease arise from intestinal exposure to incompletely digested cereal grain gluten (celiac sprue disease) or cow's milk (bovine milk-sensitive enteropathy). Disease states associated with chronic or extensive abdominal radiation treatment, malnutrition, or invasive microorganisms (e.g., *Salmonella* or *Shigella*) can damage the epithelial cells and tight junctions of the intestinal mucosal barrier and, thereby, increase the nonspecific permeability to all macromolecules.

In the presence of a healthy mucosa with intact tight junctions, the uptake of intact polypeptides occurs by a mechanism that is quite different from the mechanisms for the membrane transport of dipeptides and amino acids described above. The process by which intact polypeptides are taken up in normal enterocytes is described in Figure 6–8 for an antigenic polypeptide resistant to hydrolysis in the lumen. In this model, the luminal polypeptide first binds to specific receptors within clathrin-

coated pits on enterocyte brush border membranes. The brush border membrane then invaginates to form an intracellular vesicle by the process of endocytosis. During invagination, additional molecules, other than receptor-bound polypeptide, can be simultaneously, nonspecifically trapped within the vesicle fluid. The vesicle then fuses with lysosomes, which are organelles that contain acid proteases such as cathepsin B and cathepsin D.

Vesicle membrane-bound macromolecules escape digestion within the lysosome, whereas the unbound molecules trapped within the vesicle are destroyed. The unbound proteins are digested to form free amino acids and small peptide fragments, both of which are transported out of the endosome to the cytosol. The peptide fragments eventually are hydrolyzed to free amino acids by the enterocyte cytosolic aminopeptidases. Polypeptide bound to the vesicle membrane subsequently traverses the cytosol, and the vesicle fuses with the basolateral membrane. The polypeptide exits the cell by exocytosis into the interstitial space, where it eventually enters the capillaries and hence the portal venous blood.

In some epithelial cells, the endocytosed peptide antigen binds to class II major histocompatibility complex molecules (MHC-II) within the Golgi apparatus (Sanderson and Walker, 1993). Subsequent fusion of the endosome to the basolateral membrane releases the antigen and MHC-II molecules for presentation to mucosal lymphocytes.

In addition to the mechanism described in Figure 6–8 for normal enterocytes, macromolecules are also transported through M cells of the intestine (Sanderson and Walker, 1993). M cells are specialized microfolded epithelial cells that overlay lymphoid follicles within the mucosa, and these M cells are involved in nonspecific uptake of peptides. The mechanism by which M cells present antigens to lymphocytes presently is not known.

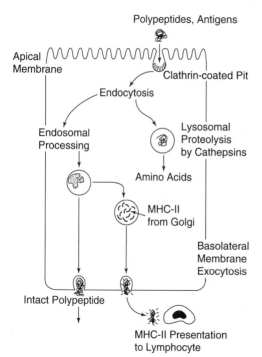

Figure 6–8. Uptake and transport of large polypeptides by intestinal enterocytes. Polypeptides and peptide antigens can bind the brush border (apical) membrane within clathrin-coated pits. The pits invaginate to form endocytic vesicles. Peptides trapped within the vesicles are shuttled to lysosomes where they are digested by cathepsin enzymes. Endosome inner membrane-bound polypeptides can be exported to the basolateral membrane, where they exit to the interstitial fluid via exocytosis. Alternatively, Golgi apparatus supplies the endosome with class II MHC molecules that bind to the polypeptide. The MHC-bound proteins are presented on the basolateral membrane surface to lymphocytes of the gastrointestinal immune system. Portions adapted from Sanderson, I. R. and Walker, W. A. (1993) Uptake and transport of macromolecules by the intestine: Possible role in clinical disorders (an update). Gastroenterology 104:622–639. Used with permission of W. B. Saunders Co.

REFERENCES

Adibi, S. A. (1996) Intestinal oligopeptide transporter: From hypothesis to cloning. News Physiol Sci 11:133–137.

Ferraris, R. P. and Diamond, J. M. (1989) Specific regulation of intestinal nutrient transporters by their dietary substrates. Annu Rev Physiol 51:125–141.

Gerencser, G. A. and Stevens, B. R. (1994) Thermodynamics of symport and antiport catalyzed by cloned or native transporters. J Exp Biol 196:59–75.

Kekuda, R., Prasad, P. D., Fei, Y.-J., Torres-Zamorano, V., Sinha, S., Yang-Feng, T. L., Leibach, F. H. and Ganapathy, V. (1996) Cloning of the sodium-dependent, broad-scope, neutral amino acid transporter B⁰ from a human placenta choriocarcinoma cell line. J Biol Chem 271:18657–18661.

Kitamoto, Y., Veile, R. A., Donin-Keller, H. and Sadler, J. E. (1995) cDNA sequence and chromosomal localization of human enterokinase, the proteolytic activator of trypsinogen. Biochemistry 34:4562–4568.

Leibach, F. H. and Ganapathy, V. (1996) Peptide transporters in the intestine and the kidney. Annu Rev Nutr 16:99–119.

Liang, R., Fei, Y.-J., Prasad, P. D., Ramamoorthy, S., Han, H., Yang-Feng, T., Hediger, M. A., Ganapathy, V. and Leibach, F. H. (1995) Human intestinal H⁺/peptide cotransporter cloning, functional expression, and chromosomal localization. J Biol Chem 270:6456–6463.

Mailliard, M. E., Stevens, B. R. and Mann, G. E. (1995) Amino acid transport by small intestinal, hepatic, and pancreatic epithelia. Gastroenterology 108:888–910.

Palacin, M. (1994) A new family of proteins (rBAT and 4F2hc) involved in cationic and zwitterionic amino acid transport: A tale of two proteins in search of a transport function. J Exp Biol 196:123–137.

Pan, M. and Stevens, B. R. (1995a) Protein kinase C-dependent regulation of L-arginine transport activity in Caco-2 intestinal cells. Biochem Biophys Acta 1239:27–32.

Pan, M. and Stevens, B. R. (1995b) Differentiation- and protein kinase C-dependent regulation of alanine transport via system B. J Biol Chem 270:3582–3587.

Sanderson, I. R. and Walker, W. A. (1993) Uptake and transport of macromolecules by the intestine: Possible role in clinical disorders (an update). Gastroenterology 104:622–639.

Stevens, B. R. (1992) Amino Acid Transport in Intestine. In: *Mammalian Amino Acid Transport: Mechanisms and Control* (Kilberg, M. S. and Haussinger, D. eds.), pp. 149–164. Plenum, New York.

Stevens, B. R., Fernandez, A., Hirayama, B., Wright, E. M. and Kempner, E. S. (1990) Intestinal brush border membrane Na⁺/glucose cotransporter functions *in situ* as a homotetramer. Proc Natl Acad Sci USA 87:1456–1460.

RECOMMENDED READING

Johnson, L. R. (ed.) 1997. Gastrointestinal Physiology. 5th ed. Mosby, St. Louis.

CHAPTER **7**

◆ ◆

Digestion and Absorption of Lipids

Patrick Tso, Ph.D., and Karen Crissinger, M.D., Ph.D.

O U T L I N E

C O M M O N   A B B R E V I A T I O N S

ACAT (acyl CoA:cholesterol acyltransferase)
FABP (fatty acid–binding protein)
SCP (sterol carrier protein)

DIETARY LIPIDS

Dietary lipids have been described as that part of the diet that can be extracted by organic solvents (Borgstrom, 1986). According to this definition, a variety of compounds qualify, including both nonpolar lipids such as triacylglycerols and polar lipids such as phospholipids. Although a variety of types of lipids are consumed in the diet, by far the greatest quantity of dietary lipids is in the form of triacylglycerols (triglycerides). Furthermore, most of these dietary triacylglycerols contain predominantly long-chain fatty acids (chain lengths of 14 to 20 carbons) esterified to the glycerol backbone. The average Western diet contains 100 to 150 g of dietary fat (triacylglycerol), which provides 900 to 1350 kcal, or about 40% of the calories consumed daily. (As discussed in Chapters 41 and 42, the American Heart Association and the Dietary Guidelines for Americans recommend that the intake of fat be reduced to 30% of calories to reduce the risk of atherosclerosis). Dietary triacylglycerol is a major source of energy, with a higher caloric density than the other macronutrients, and also it is a source of essential fatty acids in the ω3 and ω6 classes, mainly as linoleate (n-6, 18:2) and linolenate (n-3, 18:3). (See Chapter 15 for a discussion of essential fatty acids.)

Other dietary lipids include the fat-soluble vitamins A, D, E, and K (micronutrients discussed in Chapters 24 through 27), cholesterol and cholesteryl esters, and phospholipids. The amount of cholesterol/cholesteryl ester and phospholipid in the diet is considerably less than the amount of triacylglycerol; daily intake of cholesterol is generally less than 1 g and that of phospholipid is equal to 1 to 2 g. However, endogenous biliary lipids present additional cholesterol (1 g) and phospholipid (10 to 20 g) to the intestine; in the case of phospholipid, the biliary supply is much greater than that obtained from the diet (Northfield and Hofmann, 1975; Borgstrom, 1976).

LUMINAL DIGESTION OF LIPIDS

Digestion and absorption of lipids by the intestinal tract is a complex process that requires a number of steps to take place successfully in the lumen of the gastrointestinal tract, plus further processing of absorbed lipids by the enterocytes of the small intestinal mucosa.

Digestion of Triacylglycerols

The digestion of triacylglycerols begins in the stomach, with the action of gastric lipase secreted by the gastric mucosa. Gastric lipase is called an acid lipase because its activity is highest in an acidic medium. Acid lipases hydrolyze triacylglycerols that contain medium-chain fatty acids faster than they hydrolyze those containing long-chain fatty acids. Milk fat, rich in short- and medium-chain fatty acids, is hydrolyzed efficiently by acid lipases; this probably contributes to the efficient milk fat digestion observed in infants. Acid lipases do not hydrolyze cholesteryl esters or phospholipids such as phosphatidylcholine. Although the optimal pH of gastric lipase is around 4, the enzyme is still quite active at pH 6 to 6.5. Although the enzyme works well in the stomach, it probably continues to digest triacylglycerol in the upper duodenum where the pH is between 6 and 7. Acid lipase preferentially cleaves the fatty acid at the sn-3 position of the triacylglycerol molecule, regardless of the fatty acid esterified to this position. The 1,2-diacylglycerols (diglycerides) and fatty acids produced as a result of the action of acid lipases may promote the emulsification of dietary fat in the stomach. Grinding and mixing of the gastric contents also contribute to dispersion of the lipid droplets.

The lipid emulsion enters the small intestine as fine lipid droplets less than 0.5 mm in diameter. The combined action of bile and pancreatic juice brings about a marked change in the chemical and physical form of the ingested lipid emulsion. Most of the digestion of triacylglycerol is brought about by pancreatic lipase in the lumen of the upper part of the intestinal tract. Pancreatic lipase works at the interface between the oil and aqueous phases. Pancreatic lipase acts mainly on the sn-1 and sn-3 positions of the triacylglycerol molecule to release 2-monoacylglycerol and free fatty acids.

Pure pancreatic lipase works inefficiently in a bile salt–lipid mixture, and yet lipase present in pancreatic juice hydrolyzes triacylglycerols extremely efficiently. This observation led to the discovery of the cofactor called colipase. Colipase is a heat-stable protein required for lipase activity when bile salt is present; it is synthesized and secreted by the pancreas as procolipase and is activated to colipase in the small intestine by proteolytic cleavage by trypsin. As shown in Figure 7–1, the triacylglycerol lipid droplets covered with bile salts (BS in the diagram) are not accessible to pancreatic lipase. However, the binding of colipase to the triacylglycerol/aqueous in-terface allows the binding of lipase to the lipid/aqueous interface. Lipase binds with colipase in a 1:1 molar ratio.

Digestion of Phospholipids

Digestion of phospholipids occurs in the small intestine. In bile, phospholipid (predominantly phosphatidylcholine) is found in mixed micelles along with cholesterol and bile salts. Once in the intestinal lumen, the luminal phosphatidylcholine will distribute between the mixed micelles and the triacylglycerol droplets, but phosphatidylcholine tends to favor the micellar phase over the oily phase. It is phospholipid in micelles that serves as substrate for hydrolysis. Hydrolysis of phospholipids is largely brought about by phospholipase A_2, which is secreted by the pancreas as prophospholipase A_2 and then activated by trypsin within the lumen of the small intestine. Phospholipase A_2 releases the fatty acid from the *sn*-2 position of phosphatidylcholine to yield a fatty acid and lysophosphatidylcholine. Although the bulk of luminal intestinal phospholipase A_2 activity is derived from pancreatic juice, there is probably some minor contribution from the intestinal mucosa, which has an intrinsic membrane enzyme that has phospholipase and retinyl ester hydrolase activity and is known as retinyl ester hydrolase, or phospholipase B.

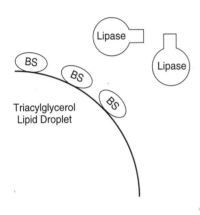

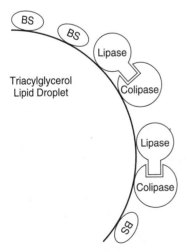

Figure 7–1. *Interaction between lipase, colipase, and triacylglycerol droplets. Lipase normally binds poorly to the triacylglycerol lipid droplets. In the presence of co-lipase, lipase molecules bind to the lipid droplets and hydrolyze the triacylglycerol to form 2-monoacylglycerol and fatty acids. BS, bile salt.*

Digestion of Cholesteryl Esters

Only free cholesterol is absorbed by the small intestine. Most dietary cholesterol is present as the free sterol, but 10% to 15% is present as the sterol ester. Biliary cholesterol is also mainly free cholesterol. Cholesteryl ester is hydrolyzed to free cholesterol in the presence of cholesterol esterase (also called carboxyl ester hydrolase), which is secreted by the pancreas as an active enzyme. The human cholesterol esterase has a broad specificity, and it can hydrolyze triacylglycerols, cholesteryl esters, phosphoglycerides, esters of vitamins A and D, and monoacylglycerols. Because it will hydrolyze all three ester linkages of triacylglycerols, it is sometimes called nonspecific esterase.

As for phospholipase A_2, cholesterol esterase is active against substrates that have been incorporated into bile salt micelles. Cholesterol esterase activity is stimulated by bile salts, particularly trihydroxy bile salts such as sodium taurocholate. The activation of cholesterol esterase by bile salts is mediated by changing the conformation of this protein. A unique property of cholesterol esterase is its self-association; the presence of trihydroxy bile salts (taurocholate or glycocholate) promotes the self-aggregation of the enzyme into polymeric forms. The self-association of cholesterol esterase protects the enzyme from proteolytic inactivation. The cholesterol esterase isolated from the pancreas exists mainly as tetramers and dimers.

UPTAKE OF LIPID DIGESTION PRODUCTS BY THE ENTEROCYTES

The digestion products of triacylglycerols, phospholipids, and cholesteryl esters are predominantly monoacylglycerols, fatty acids, lysophosphatidylcholine, and cholesterol. Although these lipid digestion products are somewhat polar, they have very limited capac-ity to dissolve in water. The epithelial surface of the small intestine is surrounded by a layer of water called the unstirred water layer, and the thickness of the unstirred water layer depends on how vigorously the small intestinal contents are mixed. Increased mixing reduces the thickness of the unstirred water layer. As illustrated in Figure 7–2, this unstirred water layer represents a barrier that lipids must cross before they can be absorbed by the enterocytes (small intestinal epithelial cells).

Importance of Micellar Solubilization

As shown in Figure 7–2, the limited solubility of lipid digestion products results in only a few individual molecules crossing the unstirred water layer and being absorbed by the enterocytes (arrow 1). To overcome this barrier, lipid digestion products are first solubilized in mixed bile salt micelles. Bile salts are biological detergents, and they will form micelles (aggregates of bile salts) when the concentration of bile salts in the lumen is at or above the critical micellar concentration. Pure micelles contain only bile salts, whereas mixed micelles contain bile salts as well as

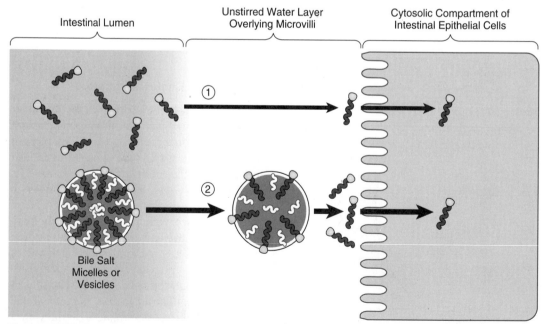

Intestinal Lumen

Unstirred Water Layer
Overlying Microvilli

Cytosolic Compartment of
Intestinal Epithelial Cells

Bile Salt
Micelles or
Vesicles

Figure 7–2. *The role of bile salt micelles in overcoming the diffusion barrier associated with the unstirred water layer. In the absence of bile salts (1), only a limited number of lipid molecules diffuse through the unstirred water layer to be taken up across the brush border membrane of the enterocytes. In the presence of bile salts (2), more lipid molecules can be delivered to the brush border membrane by bile salt micelles.*

other lipid moieties. The concentration of bile salts in the lumen is almost always above the critical micellar concentration. Free cholesterol and other lipid digestion products can be incorporated into the mixed micelles, thereby rendering these lipid molecules soluble in the bulk water phase. The mixed micelles containing polar lipids and cholesterol readily cross the unstirred water layer (arrow 2) and thereby increase the aqueous concentrations of fatty acids, monoacylglycerols, cholesterol, and lysophosphatidylcholine near the epithelial absorptive surface by a factor of 100 to 1000. This provides an efficient mechanism for transport across the unstirred water layer and the subsequent uptake of these lipid molecules by the enterocytes.

Importance of Unilamellar Vesicles

When the jejunal contents of humans are sampled during digestion of a lipid meal and subjected to ultracentrifugation, one can observe a solid particulate layer on the bottom of the tube. Next, there is a mostly clear micellar phase followed by an oily phase on the top. The oily phase is composed mainly of triacylglycerols, mono- and diacylglycerols, and fatty acids. The micellar phase contains bile salts, monoacylglycerols, and fatty acids. When Porter and Saunders (1971) performed a careful analysis of the aqueous phase after ultracentrifugation and also after the intestinal contents had been passed through a series of filters with progressively smaller pores, they observed that both the ultracentrifugation and the filtering procedure yielded a micellar phase that was slightly turbid. Furthermore, they found that there was a concentration gradient of lipids in the micellar phase, an important point that was missed previously. This observation is important because it hinted to the investigators that the micellar phase is not homogeneous.

The explanation for this intriguing observation came much later when Carey et al. (1983) proposed that the lipid in the intestinal lumen will be incorporated into mixed micelles when the bile salt concentration in the lumen exceeds the critical micellar concentration. These micelles are probably in the form of large, mixed disc-like micelles more or less saturated with lipids, with a hydrodynamic radius of about 200 Å. When the amount of lipid in the aqueous phase increases further (as occurs in some disease states), formation of lipid crystalline vesicles (liposomes) with hydrodynamic radii of 400 to 600 Å also occurs (Carey et al., 1983).

The discovery of the existence of vesicles has important pathophysiological implications. Patients with low intraluminal bile salt concentrations (Mansbach et al., 1980) and patients with bile fistulae (Porter et al., 1971) have reasonably good fat absorption, and Carey et al. (1983) proposed that liquid crystalline vesicles may play an important role in the uptake of lipid digestion products in these patients.

Permeation of Digested Fat into Enterocytes

At least two different mechanisms have been proposed for the uptake of lipid digestion products by the small intestine: passive uptake versus carrier-mediated uptake. Once digested lipid is presented to the surface of the brush border membrane of the enterocytes, the products of lipid digestion can dissolve in the lipid of the brush border membrane. The concentration gradient between the lipids in the brush border and those in the intracellular compartment of the enterocytes favors initial diffusion of these products into the cell. The rapid reesterification of the intracellular lipids to form triacylglycerols, phospholipids, and cholesteryl esters by enzymes of the endoplasmic reticulum helps maintain low intracellular concentrations of these lipids, thus favoring the continued uptake or diffusion of these lipids into the intracellular compartment of the enterocytes. The more water-soluble products of lipid digestion, such as glycerol and short-chain fatty acids, if present, are efficiently taken up by diffusion.

Specific binding proteins have been identified that may participate in the uptake processes for some lipids, including fatty acids and cholesterol. These binding proteins have been purified, and antibodies against them have been raised. Antisera raised against these binding proteins was used to demonstrate that these binding proteins are located at the apical membrane of the small intestinal epithelial cells. However, most of the studies involving these binding proteins were conducted in vitro, and data demonstrating their importance in vivo are lacking. The role of specific binding proteins in the uptake of lipid molecules across the brush border membrane remains uncertain.

The intestinal absorption of lipid-soluble vitamins is discussed in Chapters 24 through 27. Fat-soluble vitamins generally behave like the lipid digestion products and are solubilized in mixed bile salt micelles to ensure their efficient passage through the unstirred water layer. Whether they are taken up by the enterocytes by simple diffusion or by specific transporters located at the brush border membrane is unclear.

INTRACELLULAR METABOLISM OF ABSORBED LIPIDS

Once in the cytosol of the enterocyte, lipid compounds are again in an aqueous environment. Thus, various lipids must be transported intracellularly from the apical region, where they are absorbed, to the endoplasmic reticulum, where the enzymes involved in their metabolism are located. These lipid digestion products are largely reesterified in the enterocyte in preparation for export in chylomicrons.

Intracellular Transport of Absorbed Lipids

As yet, it is not fully understood how the various absorbed lipids migrate from the site of absorption to the endoplasmic reticulum where biosynthesis of complex lipids takes place. A fatty acid–binding protein (FABP) present in the small intestine has been isolated and characterized by Ockner and Manning (1974), who proposed that this FABP plays an important role in the intracellular transport of fatty acids. This hypothesis is partly supported by the finding that the concentration of FABP is greater in villi than in crypt cells, greater in jejunum than in ileum, and greater in intestinal mucosa of animals fed a high-fat diet than of those fed a low-fat diet (Ockner and Manning, 1974).

Recent studies revealed that there are at least two cytosolic FABPs in enterocytes. These are the I-FABP (intestinal FABP) and L-FABP (liver FABP). These two FABP's differ in their binding specificity (Besnard et al., 1996). I-FABP strongly binds only with fatty acids, but L-FABP will bind not only long-chain fatty acids but also lysophosphatidylcholine, retinoids, bilirubin, carcinogens, and even selenium (Glatz and Veerkamp, 1985; Bass, 1988; Bansal et al., 1989). Based on nuclear magnetic resonance (NMR) binding studies, Cistola et al. (1990) speculated that the I-FABP facilitates the intracellular transport of fatty acids, whereas L-FABP probably facilitates the intracellular transport of monoacylglycerol and lysophosphatidylcholine. Future studies in mice with various FABP genes "knocked out" may shed some light on the function of these proteins in the intracellular transport of lipids.

Two cytosolic carrier proteins for sterols have been isolated and characterized: sterol carrier protein-1 (SCP-1) and sterol carrier protein-2 (SCP-2). Experimental evidence thus far seems to indicate that SCP-2 may play a role in the intracellular transport of cholesterol.

Reesterification of Lipid Digestion Products

2-Monoacylglycerols and fatty acids are reconstituted to form triacylglycerol, mainly via the monoacylglycerol pathway. As shown in Figure 7–3, 2-monoacylglycerol is reacylated into triacylglycerol by the consecutive action of monoacylglycerol acyltransferase and diacylglycerol acyltransferase. The enzymes involved in this monoacylglycerol pathway are present in a complex called "triacylglycerol synthetase," and this has recently been purified (Lehner and Kuksis, 1995). The enzymes involved in the monoacylglycerol pathway are located on the cytosolic surface of the endoplasmic reticulum (ER). This finding has important bearing on our understanding of the intracellular formation of chylomicrons. It appears that triacylglycerols are formed at the cytosolic surface of the ER, and they then gain access to the inside of the ER.

Wetterau and Zilversmit (1984) demonstrated that there is a protein in the liver, the

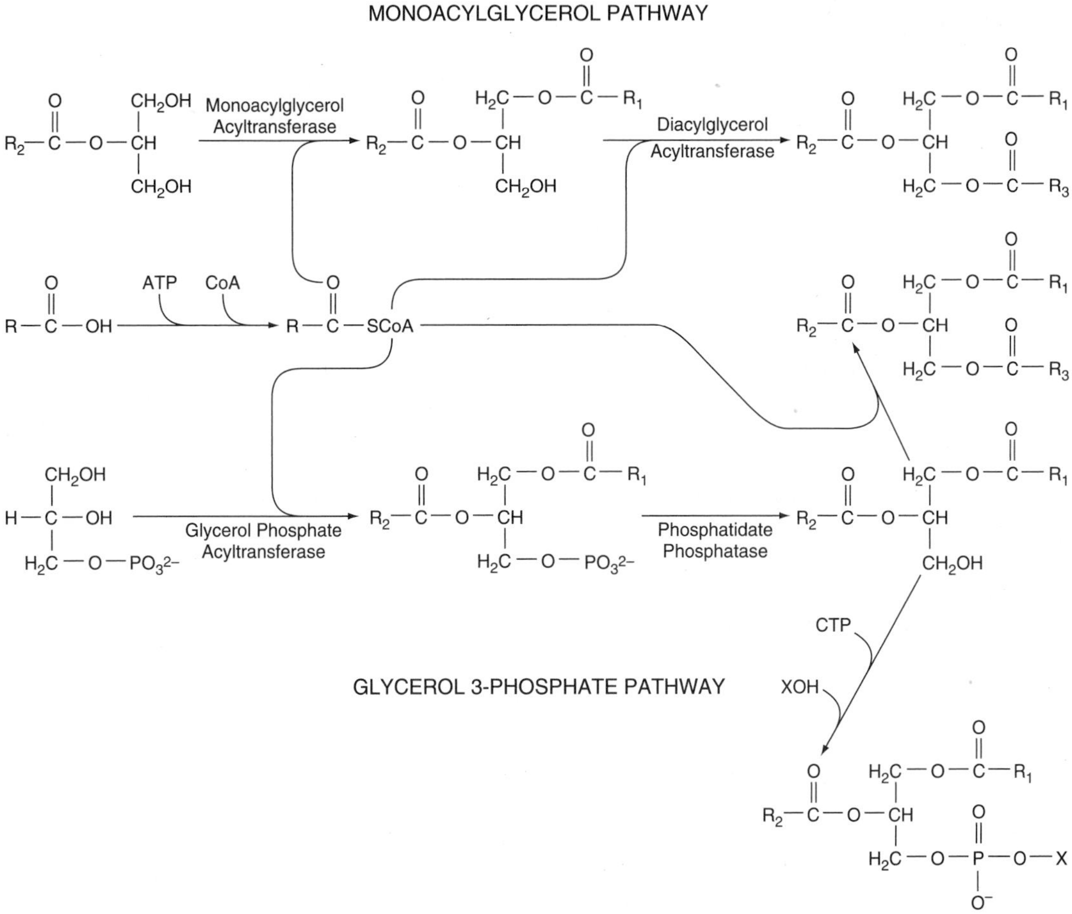

MONOACYLGLYCEROL PATHWAY

Figure 7–3. *Pathways of triacylglycerol biosynthesis in the intestinal mucosal cells (enterocytes). RCOOH, fatty acid; XOH, alcohol (e.g., choline or serine).*

small intestine, and a number of other organs that promotes the transfer of triacylglycerol and cholesteryl ester between membranes; they proposed that this transfer activity may play a role in the movement of lipids into the ER. Wetterau and his colleagues have recently provided convincing evidence that this may indeed be the case (1992). In studies of patients with abetalipoproteinemia, who lack the ability to make chylomicrons, they found that apolipoprotein B (apo B) was synthesized, but the triacylglycerol and apo B failed to associate with each other because of a lack of the microsomal (ER) triacylglycerol transfer protein.

The other pathway present in intestinal mucosa for the formation of triacylglycerol is called the glycerol 3-phosphate pathway. As shown in Figure 7–3, this pathway involves the stepwise acylation of glycerol 3-phosphate to form phosphatidic acid. In the presence of phosphatidate phosphatase, phosphatidic acid is hydrolyzed to release inorganic phosphate and to form diacylglycerol, which is then further esterified to form triacylglycerol.

The relative importance of the monoacylglycerol pathway and the glycerol phosphate pathway depends on the supply of 2-monoacylglycerol and fatty acid. During normal lipid absorption, the monoacylglycerol pathway is much more important than the glycerol phosphate pathway in enterocytes because of the abundant supply of 2-monoacylglycerol and fatty acid and their efficient conversion to triacylglycerol, and also because 2-monoacylglycerol inhibits the glycerol phosphate pathway. However, when the supply of 2-monoacylglycerol is lacking or insufficient, the glycerol phosphate pathway becomes the major pathway for the formation of triacylglycerol.

Phospholipids

Lysophosphatidylcholine and other lysophospholipids inside the enterocytes can be reacylated to form phosphatidylcholine and other phospholipids, or these lysophospholipids can be hydrolyzed to form glycerol 3-phosphorylcholine. The liberated fatty acids can be used for triacylglycerol synthesis, whereas the glycerol 3-phosphorylcholine can be readily transported via the portal blood for use in the liver. Another reaction that occurs in intestinal mucosal cells is the combination of two molecules of lysophosphatidylcholine to yield one molecule of phosphatidylcholine and one molecule of glycerol 3-phosphorylcholine.

Cholesterol

Dietary or exogenous cholesterol absorbed by the enterocytes enters a free cholesterol pool. This free cholesterol pool in the enterocyte also derives cholesterol from endogenous sources, including nondietary cholesterol (biliary cholesterol and cholesterol from cells shed from the intestinal mucosa) absorbed from the lumen of the small intestine, cholesterol derived from circulating plasma lipoproteins, and cholesterol synthesized de novo. However, enterocytes handle cholesterol from various sources quite differently. For instance, the cholesterol derived from the intestinal lumen does not mix freely with the free cholesterol pool in the enterocytes and is preferentially esterified in the enterocytes for incorporation into chylomicrons and export into the lymph. Stange and Dietschy (1985) found that very little newly synthesized cholesterol is transported into lymph during fasting; however, during active lipid absorption and chylomicron synthesis, some of the newly synthesized cholesterol can be incorporated into chylomicrons and transported in lymph.

Cholesterol is transported almost exclusively by the lymphatic system, mainly as esterified cholesterol. Therefore, the rate of es-

NUTRITION INSIGHT

Use of Structured Triacylglycerols to Enhance Absorption of Fatty Acids into the Lymphatics

Structured triacylglycerols are mixtures of long- and medium-chain fatty acids incorporated on the same glycerol backbone by hydrolysis and random reesterification of the constituent oils. Structured triacylglycerols may have different actions than do identical physical mixtures of oils that have not been reesterified. Because triacylglycerols are hydrolyzed to 2-monoacylglycerols and fatty acids in the gastrointestinal tract and because the 2-monoacylglycerols may be taken up and converted to triacylglycerol without further hydrolysis, fatty acids esterified to the 2-position of glycerol may be more likely to be absorbed into the lymphatics. For example, fatty acids with less than 12 carbons are generally transported via the portal route as free fatty acids bound to plasma albumin, but medium-chain fatty acids esterified to the 2-position may be readily absorbed as 2-monoacylglycerols, which are further acylated with long-chain fatty acids in the 1- and 3-positions for lymphatic transport.

Jensen et al. (1994) studied the lymphatic absorption of a structured triacylglycerol versus an equivalent physical mixture of the constituent medium-chain triacylglycerol and fish oils. Enhanced lymphatic absorption of medium-chain fatty acids in rats was observed when they were delivered as a structured triacylglycerol containing medium-chain fatty acid in the 2-position and long-chain fatty acids in the 1- and 3-positions, compared with the physical mixture. Fish-oil fatty acids (long- and very-long-chain polyunsaturated fatty acids) are generally not well absorbed unless they are in the 2-position of the dietary triacylglycerol. However, because most of the long-chain polyunsaturated fatty acids in fish oils are in the 2-position naturally, there was little difference in lymphatic absorption of fish oil fatty acids when structured triacylglycerols and physical mixes were compared.

terification of cholesterol probably regulates the rate of its lymphatic transport. Two enzymes have been proposed to play a role in cholesterol esterification; these are cholesterol esterase and acyl CoA:cholesterol acyltransferase (ACAT). The distribution and regulation of ACAT in the small intestinal epithelium has been studied in considerable detail. Both the jejunum and ileum have high activities of this enzyme, with the jejunum having significantly higher levels than the ileum. The activity of this enzyme can be increased by feeding a high cholesterol diet. Using immunocytochemistry, Gallo et al. (1980) demonstrated that intracellular cholesterol esterase is derived from the uptake of pancreatic cholesterol esterase. It is hypothesized that this cholesterol esterase could catalyze esterification instead of hydrolysis with the relatively high intracellular concentrations of free cholesterol and fatty acids. As yet, we do not understand the process of how pancreatic cholesterol esterase is taken up by the enterocyte, but elucidation of this process may enhance our general understanding of how intact proteins are taken up by the enterocytes. (See Chapter 6 for a description of the uptake of intact proteins from the intestine.)

There is still lack of a general agreement about whether cholesterol esterase or ACAT plays a more important role in the esterification of cholesterol by the enterocytes. However, prevailing evidence supports a more important role of ACAT in mucosal cholesterol esterification. For instance, the higher activity of ACAT is found in the segment of the small intestine most actively involved in cholesterol absorption. Furthermore, the activity present in the intestinal epithelium can adequately account for all the cholesteryl ester transported by the small intestine. Lastly, in studies employing a number of specific ACAT inhibitors, it has been demonstrated that these inhibitors significantly reduce the transport of cholesterol by the small intestine.

Plant Sterols

It has been well documented that plant sterols are handled differently from cholesterol by the mammalian gut, but the precise mechanisms responsible for this difference are not well understood. Although structurally quite similar to cholesterol, only a small percentage ($\sim$ 5%) of ingested β-sitosterol is absorbed in humans (Gould, 1955; Salen, et al., 1970). This tremendous ability of the small intestine to discriminate against the plant sterols seems to be lost in patients with β-sitosterolemia (Bhattacharyya and Connor, 1974; Salen et al., 1997). Two sisters with β-sitosterolemia had plasma cholesterol concentrations of 200 to 210 mg/100 mL and plasma plant sterol concentrations of 26 to 37 mg/100 mL (two thirds as β-sitosterol and the rest as campesterol). In most humans, the level of total plant sterols present in plasma is less than 0.9 mg/100 mL. Both sisters apparently had increased absorption of plant sterols and developed xanthomatosis (a condition characterized by the presence of xanthomas, which are nodules composed of lipid-laden foam cells). High levels of plant sterols were found in plasma, erythrocytes, adipose tissue, and skin.

β-Sitosterolemia appears to be caused by an inherited recessive trait. Field and Mathur (1983) showed that the coenzyme A–dependent esterification of cholesterol is at least 50 times more efficient than that of β-sitosterol. They proposed that inadequate esterification of this plant sterol in the enterocytes is probably responsible for the poor absorption of β-sitosterol by the small intestine. The presence of plant sterols in the intestinal lumen also inhibits the intestinal absorption of cholesterol. The mechanisms for this inhibition are the displacement of cholesterol from the bile salt–mixed micelles by plant sterols. The consumption of a sitostanol (another plant sterol) ester margarine was recently observed to lower serum cholesterol in a Finnish population with mildly elevated plasma cholesterol levels (Miettinen et al., 1995).

ASSEMBLY OF INTESTINAL LIPOPROTEINS

Lipoproteins are lipid-protein complexes formed by the small intestine and the liver for the export of lipids from these organs. The cannulation of the lymphatic vessel of rats and a number of other animal species has been used extensively for the study of chylo-

TABLE 7–1

Composition and Characteristics of Nascent Intestinal Chylomicrons and Intestinal Very Low Density Lipoproteins (Intestinal VLDL)*

	Chylomicron	Intestinal VLDL
Density	<0.95 g/mL	0.95–1.006 g/mL
Size	80–500 nm	30–80 nm
Total lipid	>90% of particle mass	>90% of particle mass
Triacylglycerol	>93%	>60%
Cholesterol (mostly as cholesteryl ester)	>1%	>15%
Phospholipids	>4%	>15%
Total protein	2% of particle weight	10% of particle mass
Major	B-48, A-I, A-IV, and A-II	Probably similar to chylomicron
Minor	C and E (both acquired through interaction with other plasma lipoproteins)	Same as chylomicron

*Nascent intestinal chylomicrons and VLDLs harvested from intestinal lymph.

micron secretion by the small intestine. This method allows the direct sampling and analysis of lipoproteins secreted by the small intestine before they enter the general circulation.

Lipoproteins Secreted by the Small Intestine

The small intestine secretes the following lipoproteins: (1) chylomicrons; (2) intestinal very low density lipoproteins (VLDLs, small chylomicrons); and (3) high density lipoproteins (HDLs). Both chylomicrons and intestinal VLDLs are triacylglycerol-rich lipoproteins. In this chapter, only chylomicrons and intestinal VLDLs are discussed because the small intestine secretes only a small amount of HDLs. High density lipoproteins are discussed in Chapter 14. During fasting, the major lipoproteins secreted by the small intestine are the intestinal (apo B-48–containing) VLDLs. Chylomicrons are the major lipoproteins secreted by the small intestine following a lipid-rich meal.

Assembly and Secretion of Chylomicrons

Only the small intestine secretes chylomicrons. The composition of the chylomicron is described in Table 7–1. The major apolipoproteins associated with chylomicrons are apo A-I, apo A-IV, and apo B-48. Traces of apo E and apo C are also added to the chylomicrons

after their entry into the circulation. Data from both animals and humans indicate that the fatty acid composition of the triacylglycerol of chylomicrons closely resembles that of the dietary lipid consumed. Kayden et al. (1963) studied the changes in human lymph triacylglycerol composition after a subject ingested 100 g of corn oil (Table 7–2). The fatty acid composition of chylomicron triacylglycerol collected 8 hours after the lipid dose was virtually identical to that of the corn oil ingested.

The fatty acid composition of the phospholipids of lymph chylomicrons is less influenced by the dietary fatty acids because phos-

TABLE 7–2

Alteration of Fatty Acid Composition (% by Weight) of Human Lymph Chylomicron Triacylglycerol After Feeding Corn Oil (100 g)

Fatty Acid	Corn Oil (%)	Fasting (%)	8–10 h* (%)
C 12:0		4	0
C 14:0		13	0
C 16:0	11	28	10
C 18:0		10	2
C 18:1	27	32	22
C 18:2	61	10	64

*Time after corn-oil feeding.
Based on data of Kayden, H. J., Karmen, A., and Dumont, A. (1963) Alterations in the fatty acid composition of human lymph and serum lipoproteins by single feeding. J Clin Invest 42:1373–1381.

NUTRITION INSIGHT

Absorption of Lipophilic Drugs and Toxins

Many lipophilic compounds, including drugs, fat-soluble vitamins, and other compounds, present in food or present on food as contaminants are incorporated into chylomicrons in the intestinal mucosal cells and transported via the lymph. Hence, absorption of these compounds depends upon normal fat digestion and absorption and upon chylomicron formation and secretion. The role of dietary fat in the absorption of fat-soluble vitamins is well known. Uptake of lipophilic drugs and toxins also may be promoted when ingested along with dietary fat. Factors that limit lipid digestion, such as blockage of biliary flow or chylomicron formation, may interfere with or protect from absorption of these compounds.

Patients are often advised to take lipophilic medications together with their meals to enhance the absorption of the drug by the gastrointestinal tract. Delivery of lipophilic drugs in forms that enhance their absorption and thus require smaller doses is of interest to pharmaceutical manufacturers. Enhancement of absorption of lipophilic compounds by the presence of dietary fat also may affect absorption of environmental contaminants or toxins. For example, absorption of DDT (1,1-*bis*(*p*-chlorophenyl)-2,2,2-trichloroethane), a toxic chlorinated hydrocarbon pesticide now banned in the United States, is enhanced by concomitant fat feeding. Enhancement of absorption of lipophilic compounds by dietary fat also may account for the observation that tetrachloroethylene, a drug used for treating hookworm infections that is not ordinarily absorbed from the gastrointestinal tract, causes toxic effects when fed with a high-fat meal.

phatidylcholine from bile is preferentially used for the coating of chylomicrons. The fatty acid composition of biliary phosphatidylcholine is rather unique.

The intestinal triacylglycerol-rich lipoproteins are transported from the endoplasmic reticulum to the Golgi apparatus. The Golgi apparatus serves as the final site of assembly for many proteins and also lipoproteins. Consequently, a block in the trafficking between endoplasmic reticulum and the Golgi apparatus results in impairment in the formation of chylomicrons. Apo B is involved in this process. Terminal glycosylation of proteins occurs at the Golgi apparatus. Golgi-derived vesicles containing the pre-chylomicrons have been clearly demonstrated by Sabesin and Frase (1977) in enterocytes actively absorbing lipid. This is illustrated in Figure 7–4. The Golgi vesicles containing the pre-chylomicrons migrate toward the basolateral membrane of the enterocytes, and pre-chylomicrons are discharged into the intercellular space through exocytosis.

Assembly and Secretion of Very Low Density Lipoproteins

As shown in Table 7–1, intestinal VLDLs are smaller than chylomicrons, and they have a

different lipid composition compared with chylomicrons. In contrast, the apolipoprotein composition is not different between lymph chylomicrons and intestinal VLDLs. The intestine secretes both chylomicrons and intestinal VLDLs. During fasting, intestinal VLDLs are the only lipoproteins produced by the small intestine. Chylomicrons are the major lipoproteins produced by the small intestine following a lipid-rich meal.

FACTORS AFFECTING FORMATION AND SECRETION OF CHYLOMICRONS

The formation and secretion of chylomicrons are tightly regulated by the synthesis of apolipoproteins and lipids in the enterocytes. Although considerable information regarding these factors has been gathered, the mechanisms of how these factors regulate the formation and secretion of chylomicrons largely remain unknown. A major reason for our limited knowledge of this is the lack of good cell models for studying these processes: it is extremely difficult to maintain intestinal epithelial cells in culture.

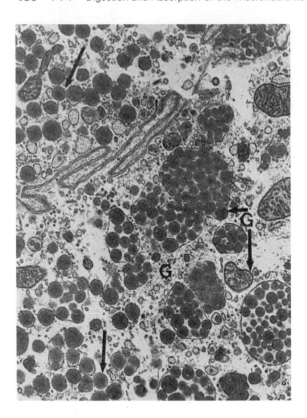

Figure 7–4. *After fat digestion, the cell is filled with numerous fat droplets located within vesiculated channels of the smooth endoplasmic reticulum (long arrows). A Golgi zone (arrows denoted by G) contains many vesicles filled with prechylomicrons measuring 600 to 3500 Å (× 11,420). (From Sabesin, S. M. and Frase, S. [1977] Electron microscopic studies of the assembly, intracellular transport, and secretion of chylomicrons by rat intestine. J Lipid Res 18:496–511.)*

Synthesis of Apolipoprotein B

Two major forms of apolipoprotein B are made by humans, apo B-100 and apo B-48. Apo B-100 and apo B-48 refer to the relative apparent molecular masses obtained by sodium dodecyl sulfate (SDS) gel electrophoresis. According to this nomenclature, the large apo B-100 was assigned an arbitrary value of 100 while apo B-48 was assigned the number 48 because it has an apparent molecular mass that is 48% that of apo B-100. In humans, the liver secretes only apo B-100, and the small intestine secretes only apo B-48. Both apo B-100 and apo B-48 are encoded by the same gene. The biogenesis of apo B-48 involves a unique mechanism by which a CAA (cytosine-adenine-adenine) codon encoding glutamine [codon 2153 of the apo B-100 messenger RNA (mRNA)] is changed to a UAA (uracil-adenine-adenine) stop codon, and thus translation is terminated earlier to form apo B-48 (Powell et al., 1987; Chen et al., 1987). Although we know that apo B is required for the formation of chylomicrons, the supply of apo B is probably not the rate-limiting step for lipid output in chylomicrons. Hayashi et al. (1990) demonstrated that apo B output by the small intestine did not change after intraduodenal infusion of lipid, despite the fact that lymphatic triacylglycerol output increased severalfold. It appears that the number of chylomicron particles made by the small intestine remains relatively constant during fasting and active lipid absorption. Instead of making more chylomicrons during active lipid absorption, the enterocyte simply fills each chylomicron particle with more triacylglycerol molecules, making them larger and lighter.

Synthesis of Apolipoproteins A-I and A-IV

The human small intestine synthesizes both apo A-I and A-IV. These apoproteins are secreted associated with chylomicrons. Despite the marked increase in chylomicron secretion by the small intestine following the ingestion of a lipid-rich meal, the synthesis and secretion of apo A-I is only marginally stimulated (20% to 30% compared with the fasting condition). In contrast, the synthesis and secretion of apo A-IV is markedly stimulated by the ingestion of fat. The roles of apo A-I and apo A-IV in the formation and secretion of chylomicrons are not clear.

When chylomicrons are metabolized in the body by lipoprotein lipase, apo A-IV detaches from these particles and circulates in the plasma either bound to HDLs or as a free protein. Although the amino acid sequence and the gene locus of apo A-IV have been known since 1984, the physiological role of apo A-IV remained unclear until recently. A number of recent reports indicate a unique physiological role for apo A-IV: apo A-IV appears to be a circulating signal released in response to fat feeding that may mediate the anorectic (inhibition of food intake) effect of a lipid meal. This function of apo A-IV is discussed later in this chapter.

Role of Luminal Phosphatidylcholine

An adequate supply of luminal phosphatidylcholine is important for the formation and secretion of intestinal chylomicrons and intestinal VLDLs. It may be important because it provides the phosphatidylcholine for the surface coat of chylomicrons. The observation that bile phosphatidylcholine has a unique fatty acid composition that closely resembles the fatty acid composition of the phosphatidylcholine in the surface coat of chylomicrons suggests that bile phosphatidylcholine is preferentially used for the coating of chylomicrons. In a model system, the lipolysis of triacylglycerol emulsions and the rates of clearance of particles from the plasma by hepatocytes versus reticuloendothelial cells depended on the cholesterol content and the phosphatidylcholine species of the lipid emulsion particles (Clark, et al., 1991). Consequently, the specific fatty acid composition of the phosphatidylcholine in the chylomicron surface coat may play an important role in the metabolism of chylomicrons by the body.

Luminal phosphatidylcholine also may be important in maintaining the normal composition, turnover, and integrity of the membranes of the subcellular organelles of the enterocytes. Normal membrane composition and integrity are important not only for membrane function but also for the function of the enzymes associated with it.

Hormones

Relatively little is known of how intestinal lipid absorption is regulated by hormones. It has been reported that neurotensin enhances lymphatic lipid transport in the rat by enhancing the processing of absorbed dietary fat. However, neurotensin also induces hemodynamic changes in the gastrointestinal tract (e.g., increased lymph flow). Further experiments are needed to ascertain whether this effect of neurotensin on intestinal lipid transport is an intracellular effect or simply a hemodynamic effect. The role of gastrointestinal hormones on intestinal lipid transport is largely unknown.

DISORDERS OF INTESTINAL LIPID ABSORPTION

The determination of the amount of fat in the stool is a common test for assessment of intestinal malabsorption. Normal humans excrete in their stool less than 6 g of fat per 24-h period, which is less than 5% of their fat intake. Thus, they absorb more than 95% of the fat consumed in their diet. The efficiency of fat absorption can be calculated as fat intake (in g per day) minus fecal fat (g per day) divided by fat intake in g per day, with the dividend multiplied by 100 to express the fraction as a percentage. Intestinal lipid malabsorption can be caused by a number of clinical conditions.

Disorders of the Small Intestine

A common disorder of the small intestine that results in malabsorption of nutrients, including lipids, is celiac sprue. Celiac sprue is characterized by lesions of the small intestinal mucosa. It is caused by gluten (a protein rich in proline and glutamine that is found in wheat, barley, oats, and some other cereals). This malabsorptive state can be corrected by feeding a gluten-free diet. The mechanism of gluten toxicity is still unclear.

Defective Digestion Caused by Pancreatic Deficiency

A major feature of pancreatic deficiency is severe abdominal pain and steatorrhea (the passage of large, pale, frothy stools), caused by the presence of a large amount of undigested fat owing to a disease of the pancreas or pancreatectomy (removal of the pancreas), which results in lack of pancreatic digestive enzymes. Pancreatic deficiency is treated by prescribing a low-fat diet or by supplementation of pancreatic enzymes with meals; severe deficiency may require diets containing partial hydrolysates of protein and starch as well.

Defective Uptake of Lipids Caused by Bile Salt Deficiency

Bile salt deficiency results in poor micellar solubilization of lipid digestion products. Unlike pancreatic deficiency, bile salt deficiency does not affect the digestion of triacylglycerol, and therefore the fats present in the stool are mainly lipid digestion products. As described earlier, the solubilization of lipid digestion products in micelles formed by the bile salts is an important method for delivery of lipid molecules to the small intestinal epithelial cells. However, because vesicles may also play a role in the delivery of lipid digestion products to the small intestine, patients with bile salt deficiency caused by liver disease or gallstone disease often can absorb a significant amount of lipids.

Abetalipoproteinemia

Apo B is required for the formation and secretion of intestinal and hepatic triacylglycerol-rich lipoproteins, as evidenced by the lack of apo B–containing lipoproteins in the circulation in patients suffering from abetalipoproteinemia. For a long time, it was generally believed that these patients lacked the ability to synthesize apo B. However, recent studies have clearly shown that apo B is being synthesized by the enterocytes of abetalipoproteinemic patients. Furthermore, Talmud et al. (1988) have performed linkage studies in kindreds of patients with abetalipoproteinemia and have shown that the apo B gene is normal. Thus, the problem in these patients may be a defect in the association of intracellular lipid with apo B, a prerequisite for the normal packaging of apo B–containing lipoproteins. Consequently, triacylglycerol droplets accumulate in the intestinal mucosa of these subjects as lipid absorption progresses (Dobbins, 1970; Fig. 7–5).

Chylomicron Retention Disorder

The chylomicron retention disorder involves failure of the discharge of pre-chylomicrons from the Golgi-derived vesicles into the intercellular space through exocytosis. Pre-chylomicrons refer to the chylomicrons that are still inside the intestinal epithelial cells. Consequently, despite the presence of numerous Golgi-derived vesicles in the cytoplasm, there is an absence of chylomicrons in the intercellular space (Roy et al., 1987). Compared with abetalipoproteinemia, chylomicron retention disorder involves a defect that is further along the chylomicron packaging pathway, probably in the trafficking of Golgi vesicles containing pre-chylomicrons to the plasma membrane.

INTESTINAL LIPID ABSORPTION AND MUCOSAL INJURY

A number of investigators have shown that long-chain fatty acids can be injurious to the intestine, especially the developing intestine. Velasquez et al. (1994) reported that the magnitude of injury caused by the presence of fatty acids in the intestinal lumen was significantly higher in piglets less than 2 weeks of age than in 1-month-old animals, suggesting that a developmental process that renders the intestinal mucosa more resistant to lipid-induced injury occurred in the piglets. The lipid-induced injury was reversible. This interesting observation is of potential clinical relevance. Immaturity or disruption of the intestinal mucosal barrier by fatty acids may result in clinical disease states to which the newborn infant is susceptible, such as necrotizing enterocolitis or toxigenic diarrhea. Velasquez et al. (1994) also showed that esterification of the injurious long-chain fatty acids with ethanol abolished their cytotoxic effects on the intesti-

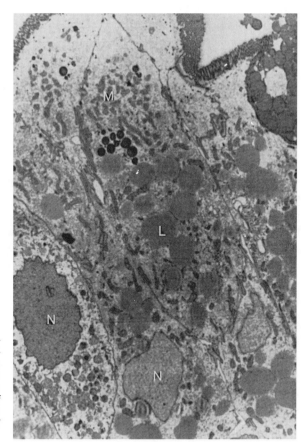

Figure 7–5. *Electron micrograph of intestinal absorptive cells from a biopsy specimen of an abetalipoproteinemic patient. The enterocytes contain massive amounts of lipid (L). Otherwise, the cells appear normal. The cell nucleus is labeled N. (From Dobbins, W. O. [1970] An ultrastructural study of the intestinal mucosa in congenital β-lipoprotein deficiency, with particular emphasis on intestinal absorptive cells. Gastroenterology 50:195–210.)*

nal mucosa. Furthermore, they showed that the ethyl esters of the long-chain fatty acids are absorbed and utilized by the developing intestine.

REGIONAL DIFFERENCES IN INTESTINAL LIPID ABSORPTION

A difference in the abilities of the proximal and distal small intestine to absorb fat has been described in rats (Wu et al., 1980; Sabesin et al., 1975). Not only was the distal intestine much less efficient than the proximal intestine in chylomicron production (Sabesin et al., 1975), but also the chylomicrons produced by the distal intestine were larger (Wu et al., 1980). The investigators suggested that this difference between intestinal segments could be due to the availability of phospholipids for the coating of pre-chylomicrons or to altered intracellular membrane lipid composition. Most phospholipids are absorbed before

the chyme reaches the distal small intestine. Although the proximal intestine is supplied with biliary phospholipids, the distal small intestine has to meet most of its phospholipid requirements by either de novo synthesis or uptake of lipoproteins from the plasma.

PORTAL TRANSPORT OF LONG-CHAIN FATTY ACIDS

The majority of absorbed fatty acids are transported by intestinal lymph as chylomicrons and intestinal VLDLs. However, there is evidence for portal transport of long-chain fatty acids, and this transport is increased when there is a defect in the intracellular esterification of fatty acids to form triacylglycerol or an impairment in chylomicron formation. In patients with abetalipoproteinemia, some dietary fat (fatty acids) may be absorbed in the virtual absence of chylomicron formation (Ways et al., 1967).

McDonald et al. (1980) demonstrated that a substantial amount of the absorbed fatty acid (58% for linoleic acid, ω6, 18:2) was transported in the portal blood of normal rats when the rates of lipid absorption were low. Recently, Mansbach et al. (1991) reported that a considerable amount of endogenous and exogenous fatty acids is transported by the portal blood. The amount of exogenous fatty acid transported via the portal route can be as much as 39% of the fatty acid infused into the small intestinal lumen. The portal transport of absorbed fatty acids by the small intestine therefore may be more important than previously recognized.

SATIETY EFFECTS OF FAT FEEDING

There is compelling evidence in the literature showing that the ingestion of fat results in satiation and the inhibition of food intake. A number of characteristics of this lipid-induced satiety provide important clues about the mechanism involved. First, long-chain fatty acids are significantly more potent in inducing satiety than are short- or medium-chain fatty acids. Because long-chain fatty acids are transported by the small intestine mainly as chylomicrons whereas medium-chain fatty acids are transported mainly in the portal blood, this observation would imply that chylomicrons are somehow involved in this lipid-induced satiety. Second, fatty acids introduced into the small intestinal lumen are more potent in inducing satiety than are fatty acids delivered by direct peripheral venous, portal, or caval routes. Again, this would imply that the gastrointestinal tract, and probably the production of chylomicrons, is somehow involved in this lipid-induced satiety. Third, the lipid-induced satiety is abolished by the presence of orlistat (an inhibitor of pancreatic lipase) in the intestinal lumen, indicating that it is the digestion products and not triacylglycerols per se that elicit the satiety response. Thus, most of the observations concerning lipid-induced satiety seem to imply that intestinal lipid absorption, in particular the formation and secretion of chylomicrons, is involved in this physiological response to the ingestion of lipid.

Fujimoto et al. (1992) reported an exciting finding that apo A-IV, an apolipoprotein made and secreted as part of the chylomicrons by the small intestinal epithelial cells, may be involved in this lipid-induced satiety. The synthesis and secretion of apolipoprotein A-IV is markedly stimulated by the ingestion of fat. It apparently acts on the central nervous system to elicit the satiety response, but the mechanism by which apo A-IV inhibits food intake is not understood. A number of recent reports (Okumura et al., 1994, 1996) suggested that apo A-IV may act as a modulator of upper gastrointestinal tract function by inhibiting gastric emptying as well as gastric acid secretion. Thus, apo A-IV appears to play an important role in the integrated control of digestive function and ingestive behavior.

REFERENCES

Bansal, M. P., Cook, R. G., Danielson, K. G. and Medina, D. (1989) A 14-kilodalton selenium-binding protein in mouse liver is fatty acid–binding protein. J Biol Chem 264:13780–13784.

Bass, N. M. (1988) The cellular fatty acid–binding proteins: Aspects of structure, regulation, and function. Int Rev Cytol 111:143–184.

Besnaed, P., Niot, I., Bernard, A. and Carlier, H. (1996) Cellular and molecular aspects of fat metabolism in the small intestine. Proc Nutr Soc 55:19–37.

Bhattacharyya, A. K., and Connor, W. E. (1974) β-Sitosterolemia and xanthomatosis. A newly described lipid storage disease in two sisters. J Clin Invest 53:1033–1043.

Borgstrom, B. (1976) Phospholipid absorption. In: Lipid Absorption: Biochemical and Clinical Aspects (Rommel, K. and Boohmer, R., eds.), pp. 65–72. MTP Press Ltd, London.

Borgstrom, B. (1986) Luminal digestion of fats. In: The Exocrine Pancreas (Go, V. L., ed.), pp. 361–373. Raven Press, New York.

Carey, M. C., Small, D. M. and Bliss, C. M. (1983) Lipid digestion and absorption. Annu Rev Physiol 45:651–677.

Chen, S. H., Habib, G., Yang, C. Y., Gu, Z. W., Lee, B. R., Weng, S. A., Silberman, S. R., Cai, S. J., Deslypere, J. P., Rosseneu, M., Gotto, A. M., Jr., Li, W. H. and Chan, L. (1987) Apolipoprotein B-48 is the product of a messenger RNA with an organ-specific in-frame stop codon. Science 238:363–366.

Cistola, D. P., Sacchettini, J. C. and Gordon, J. I. (1990) ^{13}C NMR studies of fatty acid–protein interactions: Comparison of homologous fatty acid–binding proteins produced in the intestinal epithelium. Mol Cell Biochem 98:101–110.

Clark, S. B., Derksen, A. and Small, D. M. (1991) Plasma clearance of emulsified triolein in conscious rats: Effects of phosphatidylcholine species, cholesterol content and emulsion surface physical state. Exp Physiol 76:39–52.

Dobbins, W. O. (1970) An ultrastructural study of the

intestinal mucosa in congenital β-lipoprotein deficiency with particular emphasis on intestinal absorptive cells. Gastroenterology 50:195–210.

Field, F. J. and Mathur, S. (1983) β-Sitosterol: Esterification by intestinal acyl coenzyme A: Cholesterol acyltransferase (ACAT) and its effect on cholesterol esterification. J Lipid Res 24:409–417.

Fujimoto, K., Cardelli, J. A. and Tso, P. (1992) Increased apolipoprotein A-IV in rat mesenteric lymph after lipid meal as a physiological signal for satiation. Am J Physiol 262:G1002–G1006.

Gallo, L. L., Chiang, Y., Vahouny, G. V. and Treadwell, C. R. (1980) Localization and origin at rat intestinal cholesterol esterase determined by immunocytochemistry. J Lipid Res 21:537–545.

Glatz, J. F. C. and Veerkamp, J. H. (1985) Intracellular fatty acid–binding proteins. Int J Biochem 17:13–22.

Gould, R. G. (1955) Symposium on sitosterols: IV. Absorbability of β-sitosterol. Trans NY Acad Sci 18:129–134.

Hayashi, H., Fujimoto, K., Cardelli, J. A., Nutting, D. F., Bergstedt, S. and Tso, P. (1990) Fat feeding increases size, but not number, of chylomicrons produced by small intestine. Am J Physiol 259:G709–G719.

Jensen, G. L., McGarvey, N., Taraszewski, R., Wixson, S. K., Seidner, D. L., Pai, T., Yeh, Y. Y., Lee, T. W. and DeMichele, S. J. (1994) Lymphatic absorption of enterally fed structured triacylglycerol vs physical mix in a canine model. Am J Clin Nutr 60:518–524.

Kayden, H. J., Karmen, A. and Dumont, A. (1963) Alterations in the fatty acid composition of human lymph and serum lipoproteins by single feeding. J Clin Invest 42:1373–1381.

Lehner, R. and Kuksis, A. (1995) Triacylglycerol synthesis by purified triacylglycerol synthetase of rat intestinal mucosa: Role of acyl-CoA acyltransferase. J Biol Chem 270:13630–13636.

Mansbach, C. M. II, Dowell, R. F. and Pritchett, D. (1991) Portal transport of absorbed lipids in rats. Am J Physiol 261:G530–538.

Mansbach, C. M. II, Newton, D. and Stevens, R. D. (1980) Fat digestion in patients with bile acid malabsorption but minimal steatorrhea. Dig Dis Sci 25:353–362.

McDonald, G. B., Saunders, D. R., Weidman, M. and Fisher, L. (1980) Portal venous transport of long-chain fatty acids absorbed from rat intestine. Am J Physiol 239:G141–G150.

Miettinen, T. A., Puska, P., Gylling, H., Vanhanen, H. and Vartiainen, E. (1995). Reduction of serum cholesterol with sitostanol-ester margarine in a mildly hypercholesterolemic population. N Engl J Med 333:1308–1312.

Northfield, T. C. and Hofmann, A. F. (1975) Biliary lipid output during three meals and an overnight fast. 1. Relationship to bile acid pool size and cholesterol saturation of bile in gallstone and control subjects. Gut 16:1–11.

Ockner, R. K. and Manning, J. A. (1974) Fatty acid–binding protein in small intestine. Identification, isolation and evidence for its role in cellular fatty acid transport. J Clin Invest 54:326–338.

Okumura, T., Fukagawa, K., Tso, P., Taylor, I. L. and Pappas, T. N. (1994) Intracisternal injection of apolipoprotein A-IV inhibits gastric secretion in pylorus-ligated conscious rats. Gastroenterology 107:1861–1864.

Okumura, T., Fukagawa, K., Tso, P., Taylor, I. L. and Pappas, T. N. (1996) Apolipoprotein A-IV acts in the brain to inhibit gastric emptying in the rat. Am J Physiol 270:G49–G53.

Porter, H. P. and Saunders, D. R. (1971) Isolation of the aqueous phase of human intestinal contents during the digestion of a fatty meal. Gastroenterology 60:997–1007.

Porter, H. P., Saunders, D. R., Tytgat, G., Brunster, O. and Rubin, C. E. (1971) Fat absorption in bile fistula man. A morphological and biochemical study. Gastroenterology 60:1008–1019.

Powell, L. M., Wallis, S. C., Pease, R. J., Edwards, Y. H., Knott, T. J. and Scott, J. (1987) A novel form of tissue-specific RNA processing produces apolipoprotein B-48 in intestine. Cell 50:831–840.

Roy, C. C., Levy, E., Green, P. H. R., Sniderman, A., Letarte, J., Buts, J. P., Orquin, J., Brochu, P., Weber, A. M., Morin, C. L., Marcel, Y. and Deckelbaum, R. J. (1987) Malabsorption, hypocholesterolemia, and fat-filled enterocytes with increased intestinal apoprotein B. Gastroenterology 92:390–399.

Sabesin, S. M., Bennett-Clark, S. and Holt, P. R. (1975) Intestinal lipid absorption: Evidence for an intrinsic defect in chylomicron secretion in normal rat distal intestine. Lipids 10:840–846.

Sabesin, S. M. and Frase, S. (1977) Electron microscopic studies of the assembly, intracellular transport, and secretion of chylomicrons by rat intestine. J Lipid Res 18:496–511.

Salen, G., Ahrens, E. H. Jr. and Grundy, S. M. (1970) Metabolism of beta-sitosterol in man. J Clin Invest 49:952–967.

Salen, G., Shefer, S., Nguyen, L., Ness, G. C., Tint, G. S. and Batta, A. K. (1997) Sitosterolemia. Subcell Biochem 28:453–476.

Stange, E. F. and Dietschy, J. M. (1985) The origin of cholesterol in the mesenteric lymph of the rat. J Lipid Res 26:175–184.

Talmud, P. J., Lloyd, J. K., Muller, D. P. R., Collins, D. R., Scott, J. and Humphries, S. (1988) Genetic evidence that the apolipoprotein B gene is not involved in abetalipoproteinemia. J Clin Invest 82:1803–1806.

Velasquez, O. R., Place, A. R., Tso, P. and Crissinger, K. D. (1994) Developing intestine is injured during absorption of oleic acid but not its ethyl ester. J Clin Invest 93:479–485.

Ways, P. O., Paramentier, C. M., Kayden, H. D., Jones, J. W., Saunders, D. R. and Rubin, C. E. (1967) Studies on the absorptive defect for triglyceride in abetalipoproteinemia. J Clin Invest 46:35–46.

Wetterau, J. R., Aggerbeck, L. P., Bouma, M. E., Eisenberg, C., Munck, A., Hermier, M., Schmitz, J., Gay, G., Rader, D. J. and Gregg, R. E. (1992) Absence of microsomal triglyceride transfer protein in individuals with abetalipoproteinemia. Science 258:999–1001.

Wetterau, J. R. and Zilversmit, D. B. (1984) A triglyceride and cholesteryl ester transfer protein associated with liver microsomes. J Biol Chem 259:10863–10866.

Wu, A. L., Bennett-Clark, S. and Holt, P. R. (1980) Composition of lymph chylomicrons from proximal or distal rat small intestine. Am J Clin Nutr 33:582–589.

RECOMMENDED READINGS

Thomson, A. B. R., Keelan, M., Garg, M. L. and Clandinin, M. T. (1989) Intestinal aspects of lipid absorption: In review. Can J Physiol Pharmacol 67:179–191.

Tso, P. (1994) Intestinal lipid absorption. In: Physiology of the Gastrointestinal Tract (Johnson, L. R., ed.), 3rd ed, pp. 1867–1907, Raven Press, New York.

CHAPTER **8**

◆ ◆

Dietary Fiber

Joanne R. Lupton, Ph.D., and Nancy D. Turner, Ph.D., C.N.S.

OUTLINE

DEFINITION OF FIBER

Although fiber is recognized as an important dietary component, it is not a truly essential nutrient, as evidenced by the survival of Eskimos in Arctic regions and the Masai tribes of East Africa, both of whom consume no foods of vegetable origin in their traditional diets. In fact, the benefits of fiber stem not from its assimilation by the body, but from its almost completely indigestible nature. This results in fiber being retained within the gastrointestinal tract. The presence of fiber in the gastrointestinal tract as well as the fermentation of fiber by gut microflora results in effects on gastrointestinal function that are important in health and in the prevention and management of a variety of disease states.

It would seem that the simplest thing about fiber would be its definition; unfortunately, this is not the case. Researchers in the field have long argued over what constitutes fiber, and the debate continues. Most would accept the definition of *plant material not digested by mammalian enzymes,* which is the definition we will use for this chapter. But some would disagree. Limiting fiber to "plant material" is too restrictive for those who would include chitin, which forms the exoskeleton of crustaceans, or certain heat-treated animal proteins. Others include "resistant starch" in their definition of fiber, which is not truly undigested by mammalian enzymes but may have characteristics similar to those of fiber under certain circumstances. Finally, many carbohydrate chemists prefer to have a chemical, rather than a physiological, definition of fiber. They argue that there needs to be a simple, universally accepted assay for dietary fiber in order to simplify compliance with and enforcement of labeling laws. One should be able to subject the substance to the assay and decide whether or not it is fiber and how much fiber is there. This issue will not be resolved in this chapter, but the discussion should give an appreciation for the reasons behind the disagreement over definition. Let's briefly take a look at three different ways (chemical, botanical, and physiological) to approach a definition of fiber, and what each has to offer.

Chemical Definition

With the single exception of lignin (a polyphenol), all fibers are complex carbohydrates. They differ from each other in the sugar residues making up the polysaccharide and in the arrangement of these residues. These differences in structure are discussed in Chapter 1; see Table 1–2 and Figure 1–13. Additionally, some fibers have different degrees of methylation and sulfation. Each of these differences is important. The principal residues in fibers are glucose, galactose, mannose, and certain pentoses. However, a fiber is not simply the sum of its parts. In fact, the arrangement of the parts is often more important to the physiological effect of the fiber than are the parts themselves. Branching and substitutions on the primary chains of carbohydrates can have major consequences with respect to physical properties. For example, pectin is a polymer of galacturonic acid residues, which may be methylated. If galacturonic acid is methylated, there is no ionic group to bind to calcium or trap water. This will not affect the gel-forming properties of pectin as long as there are sufficient nonmethylated portions of the molecule to form the gels. However, if methylation is randomly distributed throughout the molecule, a significant impact on gel-forming ability can occur.

One of the main reasons behind the inability of mammalian enzymes to hydrolyze certain carbohydrates, even though they may consist of primarily glucose residues, is their primary chemical structure, which is determined by the conformation of the bonds between the residues. Secondary structure also can affect digestibility. For example, the glucose linkages in starch can be attacked by enzymes. However, the same starch molecule with a different three-dimensional organization may be resistant to human digestive enzymes. In other words, the packing or arrangement of the molecule can restrict access of enzymes to the bonds they normally hydrolyze. This is why starch can become "resistant" to enzymatic hydrolysis and act like dietary fiber. Raw starches, such as potato and banana, are almost completely resistant to pancreatic amylase and thus reach the colon relatively intact.

Botanical Definition

The location of fibers within the plant and classification of their function in the plant may also be useful. The major botanical categories of fibers are cellulose, hemicellulose, pectic substances, gums, mucilage, algal polysaccharides, and lignin. Cellulose is the most widely distributed fiber of the plant kingdom. It is part of the plant cell wall and is a polymer of glucose with a β-1,4 linkage between glucose molecules. It is the only truly "fibrous" fiber. Hemicelluloses are a wide variety of polysaccharides, which contain both pentoses and hexoses. They are unrelated to cellulose; thus, their name is misleading. Pectic substances are water-soluble polysaccharides rich in galacturonic acid. Gums are not truly part of the cell wall; they are secreted by plants in response to injury, but they are classified as dietary fiber because of the way in which mammalian systems use them. Mucilages are similar to gums in that they are polysaccharides that form viscous solutions. Because of their ability to retain water, they protect seeds against desiccation. Algal polysaccharides are extracted from algae and represent a diverse group of fibers. Lignin, a polyphenolic compound, is found in woody plants.

The location of the fiber component within the plant, and whether or not fiber is extracted from the plant or eaten intact, may have significant physiological consequences. If the fiber is contained within an intact plant cell, the cell wall must first be disrupted for the physiological effects of the particular fibers to be exerted (Fig. 8–1). This in turn depends on the structure of the cell wall and its degree of lignification. The number of plant cells per particle ingested (particle size) may determine the accessibility of the cell wall to digestive enzymes, as may cooking, processing, and even chewing of the food (Bjorck et al., 1994).

Physiological Definition

Fibers are often categorized by their physiological effects. The primary physiological categories are soluble versus insoluble or, more recently, viscous versus nonviscous fibers and fermentable versus nonfermentable fibers. In

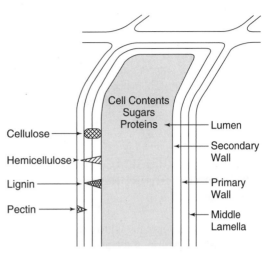

Figure 8–1. *A diagram of a plant cell, showing the location of fibrous components. The more digestible cell contents are contained within the lumen of the cell. Various fiber components are found primarily within the cell wall. The cell wall must be broken up by chewing, processing, or cooking in order for the cell contents to be made available for digestion and absorption. This also increases the surface area of the particle, increasing the ability of microbes to attach and begin fermentation of the fibrous components (cellulose, hemicellulose, lignin, and pectin). The location of greatest concentration for the various fibrous components is indicated by the hashed structures. (Modified from Maynard, L. A., Loosli, J. K., Hintz, H. F. and Warner, R. G. (1979) Animal Nutrition, 7th ed., p 88. McGraw-Hill, New York.)*

general, the structural fibers (cellulose, lignin, and some hemicelluloses) are insoluble, nonviscous, and nonfermentable. In contrast, the gel-forming fibers (pectins, gums, mucilages, and the remaining hemicelluloses) are soluble, viscous, and fermentable. However, there are exceptions: gum arabic, for example, is soluble but does not form a viscous solution. The most important characteristic of fibers with respect to upper gastrointestinal physiology is viscosity. With respect to the effect of fibers on the colon, the most important characteristic is the fiber's fermentability. Fiber fermentation depends both on the type of fiber and the colonic microflora. Fibers may be fermented to short-chain fatty acids (predominantly acetate, propionate, and butyrate) and to the gases hydrogen (H_2), carbon dioxide (CO_2), and methane (CH_4).

This chapter groups fibers in different ways to explain their effects in the body. Sometimes, in discussing food chemistry and food sources of fibers, it is most important to consider their chemical structures. In other instances, such as in describing the cholesterol-lowering effect of viscous fibers or the production of short-chain fatty acids in the colon by fermentable fibers, it is more important to classify the fiber by its physiological properties.

MAJOR PHYSIOLOGICAL EFFECTS OF FIBERS AND STRUCTURE/FUNCTION RELATIONSHIPS

The roles that fibers play within the upper and lower gastrointestinal tract are quite different, but these rely on some of the same physical and chemical attributes of the fiber. The specific physiological effects of a fiber depend on its chemical nature. Therefore, the following sections describe the various effects fibers may have within each of these segments of the gastrointestinal tract, as well as how the chemical nature of the fiber causes these results.

Effects on the Upper Gastrointestinal Tract

Satiety. One of the neurological pathways involved in the feeling of satiety is that of distention or physical fullness. Because fibers are resistant to digestion in the stomach, the bulk they add to the diet produces a feeling of fullness. Therefore, even though caloric intake may be similar, distention resulting from fiber intake and its effect on gastric emptying leads to a feeling of satiety that lasts for a longer period of time (French and Read, 1994).

Gastric Emptying and Presentation of Digesta to the Small Intestine. Viscosity of the polysaccharides and their ability to form gels in the stomach appear to slow gastric emptying. This, in turn, results in a more uniform presentation of the meal to the small intestine for absorption. Poorly soluble fibers that do not form gels (such as wheat bran and cellulose) have little effect on the rate at which the meal exits from the stomach.

Effects on Absorption from the Small Intestine. Soluble viscous polysaccharides can delay and even interfere with the absorption of nutrients such as carbohydrates, lipids, and proteins from the small intestine. The reasons for this effect on absorption include delayed gastric emptying (mentioned earlier), entrapment of nutrients in the gel-like structure, interference with micelle formation, and decreased access of enzymes to the nutrients. Fiber-rich foods may also contain lipase inhibitors. In addition, the mixing of intestinal contents appears to be impeded by the presence of viscous polysaccharides. This delay/interference with absorption has both positive and negative health benefits.

Positive Effects of Delayed Nutrient Absorption. Positive benefits of delayed nutrient absorption include an improvement of glucose tolerance and a lowering of serum cholesterol levels. Delayed absorption of carbohydrate results in a lower postprandial glucose level. In general, the more viscous the fiber, the greater the effect on blood glucose. This is similar to the effect seen with eating several small meals rather than one large meal (nibbling versus gorging). When glucose is absorbed in small amounts over an extended period, such as seen with viscous fibers, the insulin response is attenuated (Pick et al., 1996). Because high amounts of glucose appear to trigger sustained insulin secretion and insulin secretion stimulates 3-hydroxy-3-methylglutaryl coenzyme A (HMG CoA) reductase activity, high blood glucose concentrations promote cholesterol biosynthesis. Thus, fiber may also reduce plasma cholesterol levels via its effect on glucose tolerance. By lowering serum glucose and lipids, viscous fibers may produce multiple benefits in the treatment of this disease. Because of a flattened glucose curve seen with ingestion of viscous fibers, these fibers are often recommended for diabetics, who typically have lipid profiles that indicate an elevated risk of cardiovascular disease.

Effects on Properties of Lipoproteins and Serum Cholesterol. Not much is known about the effect of different fibers on the formation of lipoproteins. However, it now appears that some fibers may affect very low density lipoproteins formed in the liver, whereas others exert their primary effect on chylomicrons formed in the intestine. This

CLINICAL CORRELATION

Short-Bowel Patients

Some diseases require the removal of segments of the small intestine, leaving patients with only a short segment of the bowel remaining, with or without a preserved colon. In many of these patients, only half the calories consumed are absorbed, making dietary manipulation critical if they are to consume enough food so as not to require parenteral nutritional support. In those patients with a functional colon, energy recovery through microbial fermentation can contribute significantly to total energy availability. Mortensen and Clausen (1996) noted that an increase in carbohydrate consumption from 20% to 60% of total caloric intake provided patients with an additional 465 kcal/day, which was about 30% of the total energy absorbed. Unfortunately, there was no additional energy availability with similar diet modifications when the colon was not preserved.

Thinking Critically

1. Which type of fiber would you suggest that short-bowel patients with a functional colon include in their diet? Why?

2. How would the particle size of the fiber affect its ability to serve as a source of available energy in these patients?

means that fiber may have a different effect on lipoproteins (and thus cholesterol and triacylglycerols) depending on whether the person has eaten or is fasting. It is also clear that the effect of fiber depends on the amount of fat in the diet and the energy status of the host. Certain viscous fibers have been shown to lower serum cholesterol both in laboratory animals (Fernandez et al., 1997) and in humans (Jensen et al., 1997). These fibers include guar gum, pectin, psyllium, and oat bran. Bean products also produce this effect. In contrast, wheat bran and cellulose do not have this effect.

Possible Mechanisms by Which Fibers Lower Serum Cholesterol. The mechanism by which fibers lower serum cholesterol is still a subject of debate and may be multifactorial. Alternatively, different fibers may work by different mechanisms. The major hypotheses are summarized in Table 8–1. These hypotheses include binding of bile acids or interference with their enterohepatic recirculation. By this hypothesis, more bile acids are excreted in the feces, requiring additional synthesis of bile acids from cholesterol, thus lowering the cholesterol pool. An additional consequence of binding bile acids is that they would be less

TABLE 8–1
Possible Mechanisms by Which Fibers Lower Serum Cholesterol

Mechanism	Effect
Delayed gastric emptying	Affects the entrance of chyme into the small intestine; this in turn may affect the rate of carbohydrate and lipid absorption, which influences insulin secretion and lipoprotein formation.
Interference with digestive enzymes	Viscous fibers may sequester lipids, proteins, and carbohydrates from digestive enzymes, impairing their absorption.
Interference with micelle formation	Fibers may bind to the bile acids or interfere with micelle formation, impairing the absorption of cholesterol, bile acids, and lipids.
Interference with mixing of intestinal contents	Fibers may interfere with micelle formation and with the ability of digestive enzymes to hydrolyze lipids, proteins, and starch.
Inhibition of cholesterol biosynthesis	Fermentation of fiber in the colon results in the production of propionate, a short-chain fatty acid. Once absorbed through the portal vein, this short-chain fatty acid is thought to inhibit HMG CoA reductase activity, the rate-limiting enzyme for cholesterol biosynthesis.

NUTRITION INSIGHT

Cholesterol Manipulation

Elevated serum cholesterol can be the result of both genetic and dietary problems. Inclusion of some soluble fibers in the diet can reduce serum cholesterol as well as alter the lipoprotein profile.

Thinking Critically

1. What is the expected effect on serum cholesterol of including cellulose-containing foods in the diet?

2. What are some potential mechanisms by which a water-soluble, viscous, gel-forming fiber could reduce serum cholesterol?

available for micelle formation, which in turn could interfere with the absorption of cholesterol and triacylglycerols. A different mechanism, which remains controversial, is the production of the short-chain fatty acid propionate from fermentation of fiber in the colon. Propionate is absorbed from the colon, through the portal vein, and has been shown by some investigators to inhibit HMG CoA reductase, the rate-limiting enzyme for cholesterol biosynthesis.

Potential Interference with Mineral Absorption. Large amounts of dietary fiber also have the potential to interfere with the bioavailability of minerals. Because the charged groups on polysaccharides are usually negatively charged, the tendency of dietary fiber is to bind to cations such as calcium, magnesium, sodium, and potassium. This may limit the absorption of these minerals from the small intestine. This is not generally considered a public health concern, but it may be pertinent in certain cases when individuals have very high-fiber diets and low intake of minerals such as calcium and magnesium.

Effects on the Lower Gastrointestinal Tract

The primary way in which fiber affects the colonic luminal environment is through the fermentation of fiber, as illustrated in Figure 8–2. Fiber may be fermented to different amounts and types of short-chain fatty acids, each of which has specific properties.

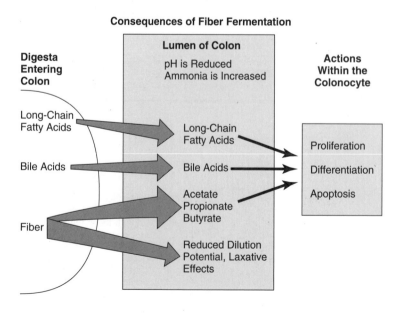

Consequences of Fiber Fermentation

Figure 8–2. Intestinal contents entering the colon are fermented by bacteria, resulting in an increase in short-chain fatty acids and a reduction in pH. As fiber is fermented, its mass is reduced as the fecal stream passes through the colon. Therefore, because the mass of fiber decreases while the mass of short-chain fatty acids increases, and the mass of bile acids and long-chain fatty acids remains the same, the concentrations of short-chain fatty acids, long-chain fatty acids, and bile acids increase in the fecal stream. Luminal pH and these molecules affect colonocyte proliferation, differentiation, and apoptosis. Absorption of these molecules can be concentration-dependent, making their concentration within the fecal milieu a key determinant of cell cycle activity.

CLINICAL CORRELATION

Ulcerative Colitis

Ulcerative colitis occurs predominantly in the distal colon (Chapman et al., 1994), a segment of the colon that is more dependent on butyrate oxidation as its metabolic fuel supply than is the proximal colon. In fact, Mortensen and Clausen (1996) have proposed that ulcerative colitis is an energy-deficiency disease. The results of Scheppach et al. (1992) indicate that supplying butyrate by enemas of short-chain fatty acids induces remission of colitis.

Thinking Critically

Patients on parenteral feeding for extended periods of time often develop ulcerative colitis. What would you recommend in order to alleviate this condition?

Roles of Acetate, Propionate, and Butyrate. Acetate is rapidly absorbed from the colonic lumen into the portal blood and then goes to the liver before entering the general circulation. Acetate is used as an energy source by most nonhepatic tissues in the body. Propionate, like acetate, is also rapidly absorbed and enters the portal vein, by which it is transported to the liver. In contrast to acetate, however, propionate is used by the liver. Some studies show that propionate inhibits HMG CoA reductase activity. Butyrate is unique in that it is the preferred energy source for colonocytes (epithelial cells lining the colon). Colonocytes metabolize butyrate to CO_2, which in part spares the use of glucose. Butyrate may also be incorporated into membrane lipids.

Dilution Potential of Fiber and Its Consequences. Different fibers have different bulking properties, depending on their degree of fermentation. Naturally, as a fiber is fermented, it is no longer available to contribute to fecal bulk; thus the poorly fermentable fibers are the best in vivo dilutors (Fig. 8–3).

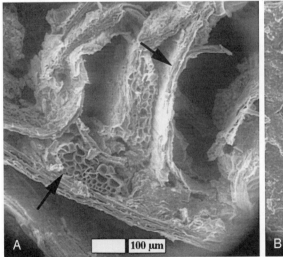 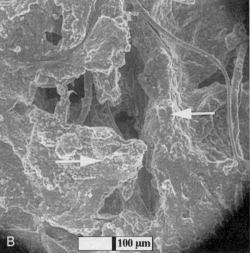

Figure 8–3. Environmental scanning electron micrographs of fecal pellets from rats consuming diets containing either wheat bran (A) or oat bran (B). More fiber (black arrows) remained in the feces of rats consuming wheat bran than consuming oat bran. The extensive amount of wheat bran fiber remaining increases the porosity (empty spaces in picture) of the feces and is able to sequester undesirable constituents in the fecal stream, thereby reducing their absorption by colonocytes. In contrast, oat bran was extensively fermented, leaving a less porous fecal pellet that was composed primarily of undigested food, endogenous secretions, and bacteria (white arrows). This increases availability of the more undesirable components and thus the potential for their absorption by colonocytes. (Assistance in image acquisition was provided by C. M. McDonough, Texas A&M University.)

This is significant because colon cancer develops and progresses in response to certain factors in the fecal stream. For example, ingested carcinogens (cancer-causing agents) have less access to the cells lining the colon if they are dispersed in a larger, rather than smaller, volume. Other factors that affect the colonocytes and are subject to dilution by dietary fibers include bile acids, diacylglycerols, long-chain fatty acids, and ammonia. There are important health consequences to keeping these factors diluted in the feces, which are explained later.

Fermentability and Its Relationship to Colonic Luminal pH. As a fiber is fermented to short-chain fatty acids, the pH of luminal contents decreases. This is significant because many bacterial reactions are pH sensitive. For example, the bacterial enzyme responsible for forming secondary bile acids from primary bile acids (7α-dehydroxylase) is inactivated

below a pH of 6.5. The colon contents, unlike the blood, often can reach this pH when fiber is fermented. The significance of luminal pH in the colon and its relation to colon cancer is discussed in detail elsewhere (Newmark and Lupton, 1990).

Colonic Epithelial Cell Proliferation, Differentiation, and Apoptosis. The cells lining the colon are only one epithelial cell deep. Unlike the case with the small intestine, no villi are found in the large intestine. Instead, the colon consists of crypts that are depressions in an otherwise smooth surface epithelia. On histological examination of a slice of colon tissue, a crypt appears as a U with the opening at the surface of the colonic lumen (Fig. 8–4). Cells are born toward the base of the crypt and migrate upward, making several divisions in transit. A cell differentiates as it reaches the upper part of the crypt and eventually is exfoliated and excreted by way of the

Lumen of the Colon

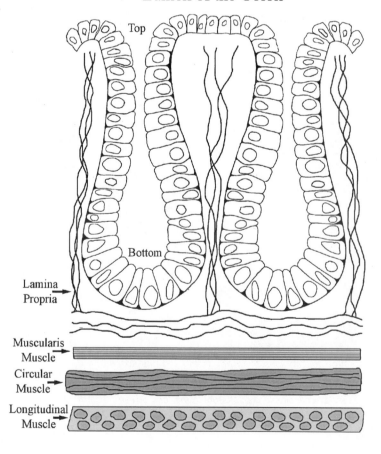

Figure 8–4. An illustration of a histological section of colon crypts, showing the arrangement of epithelial cells. The colon lumen is at the top of the picture, whereas the muscle layers surrounding the colon are represented at the bottom. Cells at the top of the crypt form the surface lining of the colon lumen. Crypts are invaginations within the colon, as opposed to the villi of the small intestine that protrude out into the lumen.

feces. This process takes from 3 to 30 days, depending on the location within the colon. During the progression of normal healthy cells to colon tumors, controls on cell division are lost. Through a series of genetic changes, cells continue to divide higher up the crypt, instead of differentiating. They may accumulate at the top of the crypt and form polyps, which then may become tumors. Tumors may invade down through the crypt and underlying muscle area. Because changes in colonic crypt cell proliferation have been shown both to precede and to accompany neoplasia, the effect of diet on cell proliferation in the colon is considered an important marker for colon tumorigenesis. Later research has found that either differentiation (transformation into the mature phenotype) or apoptosis (programmed cell death) may serve as a better prognostic indicator of colon cancer development (Chang et al., 1997). Agents or diet ingredients that stimulate cells to divide are considered to promote cancer, because dividing cells are much more vulnerable to attack by carcinogens. In contrast, dietary factors that result in a more quiescent proliferative pattern or enhance differentiation or apoptosis are considered to protect against colon cancer.

How Fiber Affects Turnover of Colonic Epithelial Cells. Fiber affects cell division by either increasing or decreasing the luminal concentration of certain mitogenic factors. As a fiber ferments, short-chain fatty acids are formed. These short-chain fatty acids increase cell proliferation in the colon. Under normal circumstances, this may be a healthy role for dietary fiber. However, in the presence of a carcinogen, this may actually enhance the tumorigenic process. Also, as a fiber is fermented, it no longer is present to dilute constituents in the fecal stream. Such fecal constituents as bile acids, long-chain fatty acids, diacyglycerols, and ammonia may also be mitogenic to colonocytes. With respect to the colon, then, the poorly fermented fibers appear to be the most protective against colon cancer. These fibers, including wheat bran and cellulose, are excellent in vivo dilutors.

Transit Time and Constipation. Colonic motility is the largest determinant of overall gastrointestinal transit times, because gastric

and small intestinal emptying averages between 2 to 5 and 3 to 6 hours, respectively (Hillemeier, 1995). Adding fiber to the diet has effects on all three transit times. Within the stomach, food is processed to reduce particle size before it is released into the intestine. Extending the amount of time required for chewing and processing in the stomach through the addition of fiber slows the passage of nutrients into the small intestine. This has benefits for individuals who need to reduce the glycemic response to certain foods (Pick et al., 1996). The presence of fiber in the diet also delays absorption of some nutrients in the small intestine because of the dilution potential that fibers have, which reduces exposure to and absorption of nutrients by epithelial cells. Within the colon, the ability of fiber to reduce transit time depends on whether or not it is soluble. Soluble fibers are more readily fermented by colonic bacteria than are insoluble fibers. Therefore, more of the insoluble fiber remains in the fecal stream, creating much more bulk than do the soluble fibers. The increase in bulk also increases the amount of water-holding capacity within the feces (Hillemeier, 1995). The combination of greater mass and greater moisture content contributes to a decrease in transit time within the colon. Hillemeier (1995) reported that including bran in the diets of control and constipated patients reduced transit time for both groups. Including bran in the diets of constipated individuals successfully decreased the time that food was present in the intestinal tract by almost half.

Constipation refers to a persistent condition in which defecation is difficult or infrequent (Camilleri et al., 1994). Whether the prevalence of constipation is related to age is currently being debated, with levels of reported constipation ranging from 3% to 20%, depending on the definitions used by the study investigators. Yet Camilleri and colleagues (1994) noted that, regardless of the study evaluated, as individual age increased above 65 years, those individuals reporting constipation increased to 10% to 30% of the population studied. Most cases of constipation are attributed to unknown causes, and most of these individuals can be treated by increasing hydration, exercise, and fiber intake (Camilleri et al., 1994). Approximately 1% of individuals may have intractable constipation, meaning it is not easily managed or cured. Further study to determine the cause of this condition is warranted, because many physiological conditions could predispose a patient to intractable constipation. Even in patients with intractable constipation, the treatment regimen may include fiber as a means of decreasing constipation (Camilleri et al., 1994).

Effects of Fiber on Whole-Body Energy Status

Because fibers may be fermented to short-chain fatty acids, which can be absorbed from the colon, the characterization of dietary fiber as contributing no energy to the host is clearly inaccurate. However, an attempt to assign a caloric value to dietary fiber is very difficult. First, one has to measure the amount of fiber in the diet (which we have already seen is a complex problem). Second, one has to know how that particular fiber is processed by an individual, which depends on several issues including other components of the diet, fermentability of the fibers, the colonic microflora, and the presence or absence of antibiotics. Last, not all the fermentation products are absorbed and metabolized. Some energy is used to support bacterial growth, and bacte-

ria, fiber, short-chain fatty acids, and other organic acids may be eliminated in the feces. A leading researcher in the area of energy contribution from dietary fiber has assigned a value of 6 kJ/g (1.44 kcal/g) for nonstarch polysaccharides and 8.4 kJ/g (2.01 kcal/g) for resistant starch (Livesey, 1995), compared with 16.7 kJ/g (4.00 kcal/g) for starch.

RECOMMENDATIONS FOR FIBER INTAKE

Currently, there is no established recommended dietary allowance (RDA) for fiber. The American Dietetic Association suggests that 10 to 13 g of fiber be eaten for every 1000 kcal of energy consumed by adults. This equates to 24 g/day for a 2000-kcal diet, or 30 g/day for a 2500-kcal diet in adults (values that are used on food labels). Similar levels of intake are suggested for elderly people. However, the concentration of fiber in the diet should be increased with age, because energy requirements decline in older folks. In addition, suggested fiber intakes for children have also been recently described by the American Dietetic Association. Fiber consumption for children over 2 years of age should be equivalent to the sum of the age plus 5 g/day. Intakes should continue to increase until 25 to 35 g/

 Food Sources of Dietary Fiber

- Whole grain products (e.g., wheat, oats)
- Legumes
- Leafy vegetables
- Fruits

Recommended Intakes Across the Life Cycle

Currently, there is no established RDA for fiber.	
Children, greater than 2 yrs	(age in yrs + 5) g per day up to an intake of 25 to 35 g per day
Adults	24 to 30 g per day or 10 to 13 g per 1000 kcal consumed; older individuals should alter their diets to maintain a total fiber intake of 24 to 30 g per day, because total energy consumption declines with age.

From American Dietetic Association. (1997) Position of the American Dietetic Association: Health implications of dietary fiber. J Am Diet Assoc 97:1157–1159.

TABLE 8–2
Food Sources of Fiber

Item	Serving	Soluble (g)	Insoluble (g)	Total (g)
Corn bread	1 piece	0.9	1.8	2.7
Pumpernickel bread	1 slice	0.6	3.7	4.3
White bread	1 slice	0.3	0.2	0.5
Whole wheat bread	1 slice	0.3	1.1	1.4
Rice, brown	1/8 cup	0.2	1.5	1.7
Rice, white	1/2 cup	0.0	0.1	0.1
All Bran cereal	1/3 cup	1.7	6.9	8.6
100% Bran cereal	1/3 cup	1.8	7.3	9.1
Product 19 cereal	3/4 cup	0.3	0.9	1.2
Raisin bran cereal	2/3 cup	0.7	2.9	3.6
Oatmeal	3/4 cup	1.4	1.4	2.8
Wheat Chex	2/3 cup	0.4	2.1	2.5
Apple, with skin	each	0.8	1.6	2.4
Figs, dried	1 medium	0.8	2.9	3.7
Orange	1 small	0.3	0.9	1.2
Prunes, dried	3	1.1	2.6	3.7
Raspberries	3/4 cup	0.3	6.5	6.8
Cauliflower, raw	1/2 cup	1.3	0.4	1.7
Corn	1/2 cup	1.7	2.2	3.9
Lettuce, raw	1/2 cup	0.1	0.2	0.3
Kidney beans	1/2 cup	2.5	3.3	5.8
Peas, blackeye	1/2 cup	5.6	6.8	12.4
Peas, green, young	1/2 cup	4.0	3.9	7.9
Pinto beans	1/2 cup	2.0	3.3	5.3
Potato, white, baked	1/2 medium	1.0	0.9	1.9
Squash, yellow, cooked	1/2 cup	0.3	0.4	0.7

Data from Anderson, J. W. (1986) Plant Fiber in Foods. HCF Diabetes Research Foundation, Lexington, KY.

day is consumed after 20 years of age. Unfortunately, Americans consume, on average, only about 11 g of fiber per day, which is far short of the suggested levels.

Food sources of fiber include whole grain products, legumes, leafy vegetables, and some fruits. As shown in Table 8–2, the levels of insoluble, soluble, and total fiber contained within a food, even within a class of foods, are quite variable. For example, green peas have similar amounts of soluble and insoluble fiber, whereas blackeye peas have considerably more total fiber, primarily because of the much greater level of insoluble fiber they contain. Similar variations in the relative quantities of soluble, insoluble, and total fiber are observed for fruits and cereals.

The incidences of heart disease, colon cancer, and obesity in populations consuming a Western diet are typically much higher, because of the lower intakes of fiber-rich foods, than is observed in most third-world communities. As described previously, the presence of fiber in the diet can have a considerable

impact on many diseases and appears to promote a healthier gastrointestinal tract. Therefore, all people should strive to include more fiber-rich foods in their diet to prevent disease onset and at least to minimize the severity of disease once it has developed.

Many difficulties are associated with the study of fiber intake and health, some of which have been addressed in this chapter. The major problem is that of defining what type of fiber is being consumed and then adequately describing how much is being consumed and utilized within the intestinal tract. In addition, diets must be designed to contain the same amount of all nutrients other than the fiber sources chosen for comparison. However, purified fiber sources do not have the same effect as intact food sources, because the intact foods contain many other biologically active chemicals, such as phytochemicals. In addition, a comparison of a high-fiber versus low-fiber diet usually indicates an alteration in the caloric density of the diet because of reductions in fat, protein, and starch consumed. Therefore, much more research must be performed under tightly controlled protocols before the real value of dietary fiber can be fully realized.

REFERENCES

American Dietetic Association. (1997) Position of the American Dietetic Association: Health implications of dietary fiber. J Am Diet Assoc 97:1157–1159.

Bjorck, I., Granfeldt, Y., Liljeberg, H., Tovar, J. and Asp, N. G. (1994) Food properties affecting the digestion and absorption of carbohydrates. Am J Clin Nutr 59(Suppl 3):699S–705S.

Camilleri, M., Thompson, W. G., Fleshman, J. W. and Pemberton, J. H. (1994) Clinical management of intractable constipation. Ann Intern Med 121:520–528.

Chang, W. -C. L., Chapkin, R. S. and Lupton, J. R. (1997) Predictive value of proliferation, differentiation and apoptosis as intermediate markers for colon tumorigenesis. Carcinogenesis 18:721–730.

Chapman, M. A., Grahn, M. F., Boyle, M. A., Hutton, M., Rogers, J. and Williams, N. S. (1994) Butyrate oxidation is impaired in the colonic mucosa of sufferers of quiescent ulcerative colitis. Gut 35:73–76.

Fernandez, M. L., Vergara-Jimenez, M., Conde, K., Behr, T. and Abdel-Fattah, G. (1997) Regulation of apolipoprotein B-containing lipoproteins by dietary soluble fiber in guinea pigs. Am J Clin Nutr 65:814–822.

French, S. J. and Read, N. W. (1994) Effect of guar gum on hunger and satiety after meals of differing fat content: Relationship with gastric emptying. Am J Clin Nutr 59:87–91.

Hillemeier, C. (1995) An overview of the effects of dietary fiber on gastrointestinal transit. Pediatrics 96:997–999.

Hove, H., Tvede, M. and Mortensen, P. B. (1996) Antibiotic-associated diarrhea, *Clostridium difficile,* and short-chain fatty acids. Scand J Gastroenterol 31:688–693.

Jensen, C. D., Haskell, W. and Whittam, J. H. (1997) Long-term effects of water-soluble dietary fiber in the management of hypercholesterolemia in healthy men and women. Am J Cardiol 79:34–37.

Livesey, G. (1995) The impact of complex carbohydrates on energy balance. Eur J Clin Nutr 49(Suppl 3):S89–S96.

Mortensen, P. B. and Clausen, M. R. (1996) Short-chain fatty acids in the human colon: Relation to gastrointestinal health and disease. Scand J Gastroenterol 31(Suppl 216):132–148.

Newmark, H. L. and Lupton, J. R. (1990) Determinants and consequences of colonic luminal pH: Implications for colon cancer. Nutr Cancer 14:161–173.

Pick, M. E., Hawrysh, Z. J., Gee, M. I., Toth, E., Garg, M. L. and Hardin, R. T. (1996) Oat bran concentrate bread products improve long-term control of diabetes: A pilot study. J Am Diet Assoc 96:1254–1261.

Scheppach, W., Sommer, H., Kirchner, T., Paganelli, G. M., Bartram, P., Christl, S., Richter, F., Dusel, G. and Kasper, H. (1992) Effect of butyrate enemas on the colonic mucosa in distal ulcerative colitis. Gastroenterology 70:211–215.

RECOMMENDED READINGS

Kritchevsky, D., and Bonfield, C. (eds.) (1995) Dietary Fiber in Health and Disease. Eagan Press, St. Paul, MN.

McNeil, N. I. (1984) The contribution of the large intestine to energy supplies in man. Am J Clin Nutr 39:338–342.

Pilch, S. M. (ed.) (1987) Physiological Effects and Health Consequences of Dietary Fiber. Federation of American Societies for Experimental Biology, Bethesda, MD.

Ripsin, C. M., Keenan, J. M., Jacobs, D. R., Elmer, P. J., Welch, R. R., Van Horn, L., Liu, K., Turnbull, W. H., Thye, F. W., Kestin, M., Hegsted, M., Davidson, D. M., Davidson, M. H., Dugan, L. D., Demark-Wahnefried, W. and Beling, S. (1992) Oat products and lipid lowering: A meta-analysis. JAMA 267:3317–3325.

Metabolism of the Macronutrients

◆ ◆

After the products of digestion are absorbed across the intestinal epithelium and enter the circulation, they are delivered to various tissues for use. The metabolism of the macronutrients by various tissues of the body is the subject of this unit. Metabolism is a term used to describe the sum of the processes by which a particular substance is handled by the living body; this includes the chemical changes occurring in cells by which energy is provided for vital processes and activities and the processes by which the body assimilates new tissue. The metabolic processes involved in the synthesis of macromolecules such

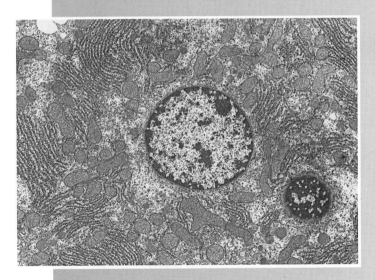

as proteins, glycogen, various lipids, and nucleic acids are called anabolic pathways or anabolism. The metabolic processes involved in the breakdown of organic compounds to CO_2 and H_2O with release of energy (which may be captured as reducing equivalents or as nucleotide triphosphate bonds) are described as catabolic pathways or catabolism. Other pathways that connect anabolism and catabolism are described as amphibolic pathways; these include pathways that serve both catabolic and anabolic purposes, such as the citric acid cycle and oxidative phosphorylation.

Nutrients are needed for the formation of the structural and functional components of tissues. Proteins, phospholipids, cholesterol, glycosaminoglycans, and nucleic acids are important structural components of cell membranes, cellular organelles, and connective tissues. In addition to these obviously structural components of the body, numerous proteins and small, nonprotein organic molecules are distributed in the body fluids, including the intracellular fluid, extracellular fluid, and plasma; these tissue components play important functions and also are essen-

Electron micrograph of liver cell; courtesy of Cornell Integrated Microscopy Center, Cornell University, Ithaca, NY.

tial. All these body components must increase during growth, reproduction, and repair of injured tissues. In addition, the body must have nutrients for maintenance—for replacement of constituents lost during the normal processes of metabolism. The chemical components of the human body are not static but are all in a state of constant turnover (breakdown or catabolism followed by resynthesis or anabolism). For example, as proteins are broken down and resynthesized, some of the amino acids are oxidized and must be replaced via the dietary supply. Small amounts of nutrients, as well as degradation products from nutrient utilization in the body, are lost from the body via the urine or via secretion in the bile and excretion in the feces. Thus, the body requires nutrients for the formation of new tissues and for the replacement or maintenance of existing ones. The processes involved in the synthesis of glycogen, glycosaminoglycans, lipids, proteins, and nonprotein, nitrogen-containing compounds such as nucleotides are discussed in this unit.

The body, of course, must have a source of energy, and dietary macronutrients serve this purpose. Cells within the body are able to use glucose, fatty acids, ketone bodies (derived from fatty acids, especially during starvation), amino acids, and other gluconeogenic (and ketogenic) precursors, such as glycerol, lactate, and propionate, as cellular fuels. Energy substrates that are taken in beyond the amount the body is able to consume immediately are converted to glycogen or fat for storage. The body's capacity for storage of glycogen is very limited. Triacylglycerol storage in adipose tissue is the major way in which animals and humans store energy, and the body's capacity for this is very large, perhaps unlimited. Thus, the body uses macronutrients in the diet as fuels and converts excess substrates to stored fuels, mainly triacylglycerol, which can be broken down when exogenous fuels are not available. These stored fuels serve an important function in providing fuels between meals and during strenuous exercise, in protecting lean body mass from immediate catabolism in the absence of food, and in extending the length of time an individual can survive with an inadequate caloric intake. The processes involved in the storage and utilization of fuels are described in this unit.

The intake of energy from carbohydrates, proteins, and fats from the diet should balance the overall needs of the body for energy and growth. Although carbohydrates, proteins, and lipids are all important components of the diet, specific compounds within these classes may be classified as essential or nonessential components, depending upon whether the body is able to synthesize them in sufficient amounts. This classification relates to metabolism; the body tissues have the enzymatic capacity to synthesize certain compounds but not others. For example, although carbohydrates make up a large proportion of healthy diets, carbohydrate per se is not an essential component of the diet. Certain cells or tissues of the body do have an absolute requirement for glucose as a fuel, but the liver is able to synthesize glucose from other sugars and from gluconeogenic substrates such as the carbon chains of amino acids or the glycerol backbone of triacylglycerols. Likewise, the body is able to synthesize the other various sugar units required for glycoprotein, glycosaminoglycan, and nucleic acid synthesis. We could say that the diet must provide either a source of glucose or a source of gluconeogenic substrate.

Protein is required in ample amounts because it serves as the source of essential amino acids and as a source of available nitrogen for synthesis of proteins and numerous other essential compounds, including purine and pyrimidine bases of nucleic acids, neurotransmitters, hormones such as thyroxin and epinephrine, creatine phosphate, carnitine, porphyrins, 1-carbon fragments of the folate coenzyme system, and small peptides such as glutathione and carnosine. Eleven of the twenty amino acids commonly found in proteins are considered essential or semi-essential for humans. Although the 9 so-called nonessential or dispensable amino acids are not strictly essential, because the body can synthesize their carbon chains from intermediates in glucose metabolism or from other amino acids, the diet still must contain a sufficient total amount of amino acids to supply amino groups for synthesis of all the nonessential amino acids.

Dietary fat is not essential as a fuel because the body can convert carbon chains of amino acids or sugars into fatty acids and glycerol phosphate and, hence, triacyglycerol and other lipids. However, certain fatty acids cannot be synthesized completely in the body. The body requires an exogenous source of the so-called essential fatty acids; a fatty acid in both the ω6 (e.g., linoleate) and the ω3 (e.g., linolenate) classes must be provided by the diet. Essential fatty acids play important structural roles in membrane phospholipids and skin ceramides and serve as precursors for synthesis of eicosanoids.

◆ ◆

Martha H. Stipanuk

CHAPTER 9

◆ ◆

Carbohydrate Metabolism—Synthesis and Oxidation

Mary M. McGrane, Ph.D.

OUTLINE

OVERVIEW OF CARBOHYDRATE METABOLISM

Carbohydrates present in food provide from 40% to 60% of the energy in the American diet. Carbohydrates, consumed as disaccharides, oligosaccharides, and polysaccharides, are digested, absorbed, and transported through the body primarily as glucose, although fructose and galactose are present as well. Glucose is the primary metabolic fuel in humans. All tissues in the human body are able to utilize glucose for energy production, and some specialized cell types such as red blood cells are completely dependent on glucose for their energy needs. Glucose is derived from either dietary carbohydrate, body glycogen stores, or endogenous biosynthesis from nonhexose precursors; these sources provide for the constant availability of glucose in the blood, which is maintained within a strictly regulated concentration range. The balance among glucose oxidation, glucose biosynthesis, and glucose storage is dependent upon the hormonal and nutritional status of the cell, the tissue, and the whole organism.

The predominant pathways of glucose metabolism vary in different cell types, depending upon physiological demand (Fig. 9–1). The liver, for example, plays the central role in glucose homeostasis in the body. In liver parenchymal cells (hepatocytes), glucose can be completely oxidized for energy, can be stored as glycogen, or can provide carbons for the biosynthesis of fatty acids or amino acids. It is important to note that the liver also can release glucose from glycogen degradation or synthesize glucose de novo under conditions of low blood glucose. The hepatocyte, like other cell types, also has the ability to utilize glucose for NADPH and ribose 5-phosphate production via the pentose phosphate pathway. Other tissues, such as adipose tissue, skeletal and cardiac muscle, and brain, respond to blood glucose changes by altering their internal usage, but they do not contribute to whole-body glucose homeostasis by releasing glucose to the blood.

In skeletal muscle and heart, glucose can be completely oxidized or it can be stored in the form of glycogen. Although glycogen is degraded in muscle and cardiac cells, the glucose 6-phosphate so produced is oxidized endogenously. Glucose is not released to the circulating blood from either skeletal or cardiac muscle. The metabolic needs of cardiac tissue, however, differ from those of skeletal tissue; the heart has a continuous need for energy to conduct regular contractions, whereas skeletal muscle has periods of high and low energy demand. In the heart, metabolism is aerobic at all times. This is in contrast to skeletal muscle, which can function metabolically with insufficient oxygen for limited time periods.

Adipose tissue presents another metabolic paradigm. In adipose cells, glucose can be partially degraded by glycolysis to provide glycerol for triacylglycerol synthesis, glucose can be completely oxidized or, under conditions of high carbohydrate intake, glucose can be metabolized to acetyl CoA and the acetyl moiety channeled to de novo fatty acid synthesis for storage. Under conditions of energy need, adipose cells release metabolic fuel in the form of fatty acids to the circulating blood supply.

The brain, which is completely dependent upon glucose for its energy needs (under normal dietary conditions), is capable of the complete oxidation of glucose to CO_2 and H_2O via glycolysis and the citric acid cycle. The brain requires a continuous supply of glucose from the blood, as there is little storage of glucose in the form of glycogen in the brain. Red blood cells, on the other hand, have a limited ability to metabolize glucose because they lack mitochondria. In red blood cells, glucose is metabolized to lactate, and lactate is released to the circulation. Other specialized cells are also primarily glycolytic because of a relative lack of mitochondria or limited blood or oxygen supply relative to their rates of metabolism; these include some cells of the cornea, lens, and retina, as well as leukocytes, white muscle fibers, cells of the testis, and the renal medulla. Intestinal cells have the capacity to oxidize glucose, but they also utilize the amino acid glutamine for their energy needs.

Overall, there are significant tissue-specific differences in the pathways of glucose oxidation, glucose storage, glucose biosynthesis, and the utilization of glucose for the syn-

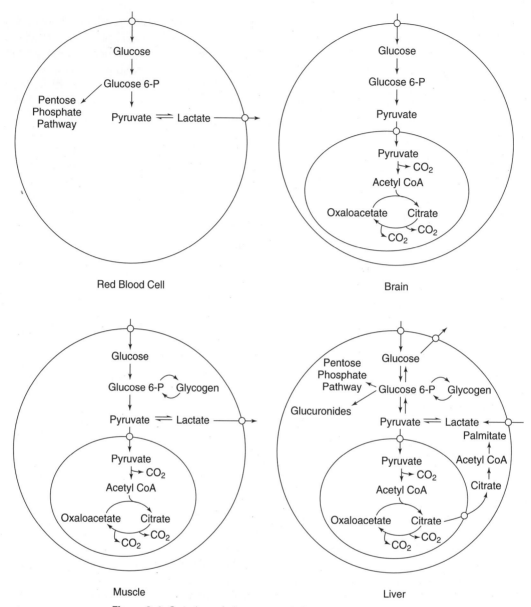

Figure 9–1. Overview of glucose metabolism in selected cell types.

thesis of other biomolecules. It is important to keep in mind the physiological context of the metabolic pathways as they occur in specific tissues.

TRANSPORT OF GLUCOSE ACROSS CELL MEMBRANES

The liver is the metabolic center of the human body and is anatomically located so that it is the first tissue exposed to elevated glucose after a carbohydrate-containing meal. After digestion, glucose and other monosaccharides are absorbed by the small intestine and transported via the portal vein to the liver. The liver has two sources of glucose: that derived from the portal vein and that derived from the hepatic artery. Dietary glucose presented via the portal route significantly increases the net uptake of glucose by the liver. A high glucose concentration in the portal vein creates a negative arterial–portal venous difference and activates hepatic glucose uptake. The portal signal relieves the sympathetic inhibition of hepatic glucose uptake and also increases hepatic glucose uptake directly by stimulating the parasympathetic innervation to the liver (Moore and Cherrington, 1996). Overall, the liver disposes of approximately 30% to 35% of the ingested glucose.

Glucose is taken up by cells in an insulin-independent manner in liver and certain nonhepatic tissues such as brain and red blood cells and in an insulin-dependent manner by cells in muscle and adipose tissue. Cellular uptake of blood glucose occurs by a facilitated transport process. Facilitated glucose uptake is mediated by a family of structurally related glucose transport proteins that have a specific tissue distribution. Five different isoforms of the glucose transporter have been identified: GLUT1 in red blood cells, GLUT2 in liver and pancreas, GLUT3 in brain, GLUT4 in skeletal muscle and adipose tissue, and GLUT5 in the small intestine. Although different glucose transporters predominate in specific tissues, a given tissue may contain more than one isoform.

Exceptions to facilitated glucose uptake occur in the brush border membrane of the small intestinal mucosal cells and the renal proximal tubules where glucose is taken up into the epithelial cells by an active symport process mediated by the sodium ion (Na^+)-dependent glucose transporter. In active symport, glucose is moved into the cell by a transport protein, which first binds Na^+. The energy for this process is provided by a Na^+,K^+-ATPase, which maintains the low intracellular Na^+ concentration. Glucose, after entry into the epithelial cell, dissociates from the transport protein and exits from the distal side by facilitated transport. (See Chapters 4 and 5 for more discussion of glucose transport in the intestine.)

The demands of glucose uptake vary depending on the tissue involved and the physiological environment of the cell. The glucose transporter isoforms serve different functions to meet these variable demands. GLUT1 is found at high levels in the brain, placenta, and fetal tissues; these are tissues in which GLUT1 mediates glucose uptake across a blood-tissue barrier (e.g., the blood-brain barrier). GLUT1, however, is also found at low

levels in all tissues and may be involved in the underlying constitutive glucose uptake of the whole organism. GLUT2 is restricted primarily to the liver and the β cells of the pancreas, but it is also found in the small intestine and kidney. In liver, GLUT2 is involved in the uptake or release of glucose by the hepatocyte, depending on the blood glucose concentration and the metabolic state of the tissue. In the pancreatic β cell, glucose uptake via GLUT2 results in glucose catabolism, which serves as a sensor of blood glucose levels and results in stimulation of insulin secretion by the β cell. In the small intestine and kidney tubules, GLUT2 is involved in glucose absorption and reabsorption, respectively, across the basolateral membranes of the epithelial cell barriers of these two tissues.

GLUT3 is present at high levels in brain and is also present in kidney and placenta. Like GLUT1, GLUT3 is also found at low levels in most adult tissues and may share with GLUT1 the task of constitutive glucose transport in the body. GLUT4, present primarily in skeletal and cardiac muscle and in white and brown adipose tissue, differs from the other isoforms in that it is stimulated by the hormone insulin. GLUT4 is responsible for insulin-stimulated glucose uptake in the aforementioned tissues in the postprandial (absorptive) state. Lastly, GLUT5 is found primarily in the jejunum of the small intestine, but also in adipocytes, skeletal muscle, and sperm. GLUT5 has the capacity to transport fructose, but it has not been determined if this is in addition to, or in place of, glucose transport.

Both GLUT1 and GLUT3 have a low K_m for glucose and transport glucose even when circulating levels are low. GLUT1 and GLUT3 appear to be responsible for basal glucose transport in most tissues of the body. This can be contrasted with glucose transport by GLUT2; GLUT2 has a high K_m for glucose and is a key transport protein involved in responding to elevated blood glucose in humans. In liver, because of the expression of GLUT2, maximal glucose uptake occurs when blood glucose levels are high, such as after a carbohydrate-containing meal. In the pancreatic β cell, glucose uptake via GLUT2 signals the cell that blood glucose concentrations have increased and begins the process by which the β cell responds to elevated blood glucose with secretion of insulin into the blood stream.

The insulin-responsive glucose transporter, GLUT4, has a unique physiological role in whole-body glucose homeostasis. In effect, GLUT4 mediates the second-tier response to elevated blood glucose. In skeletal and cardiac muscle, as well as adipose tissue, insulin stimulates the translocation of preformed GLUT4 from intracellular vesicles in the cytosol to the surface of the plasma membrane of the cell (Fig. 9–2). This translocation increases the concentration of glucose transporters at the cell surface and, hence, the capacity for glucose uptake. GLUT1 is also present in these tissues at a lower level. However, GLUT1 is present on the plasma membrane at a relative abundance that is higher than GLUT4 under basal conditions, and GLUT1 cell surface abundance is not affected by insulin-stimulated intracellular movement. Insulin, on the other hand, causes the rapid redistribution of GLUT4 to the plasma membrane from intracellular vesicles (Czech, 1995). There is, therefore, a specific insulin-responsive mechanism for the stimulation of GLUT4-mediated glucose uptake as it occurs in muscle and adipose tissue. Additionally, fasting and refeeding, as well as insulin, can affect the expression of the GLUT4 gene itself (as is discussed later in this chapter). Overall, the different glucose transporter isoforms, with variability in their kinetics and mechanisms of action, respond to the physiological demands of the body and maintain blood glucose levels within the range of 4 to 5 mmol/L.

GLYCOLYSIS

At the cellular level, the breakdown of glucose for energy can be divided into two major pathways based on the intracellular location of the enzymatic machinery involved, and on the ability of different cell types to perform the enzymatic reactions. The first of these pathways is glycolysis, the anaerobic breakdown of glucose to pyruvate. The enzymes involved in glycolysis are present in the cytosol of all cell types. The second pathway is the citric acid cycle, in which acetyl CoA is completely oxidized to CO_2 and H_2O. The citric acid cycle occurs in mitochondria and is dependent on the presence of molecular oxygen. This pathway is restricted to cells that possess mitochondria. Glycolysis and the citric acid cycle are linked by the pyruvate dehydrogenase reaction, which also takes place in the mitochondria of the cell. As a result of glycolysis, the pyruvate dehydrogenase reaction, and the citric acid cycle, energy is conserved in the chemical form of ATP, with ATP synthesis occurring both by substrate-level phosphorylation and by electron transport linked to oxidative phosphorylation.

The series of enzymatic reactions that together constitute the glycolytic pathway convert 1 molecule of glucose to 2 molecules of pyruvate. All cells of the human body contain the full complement of glycolytic enzymes and can break down glucose to this extent. The metabolic fate of pyruvate, however, is variable and depends on the cell type and the availability of oxygen. Under anaerobic conditions, when tissues such as skeletal mus-

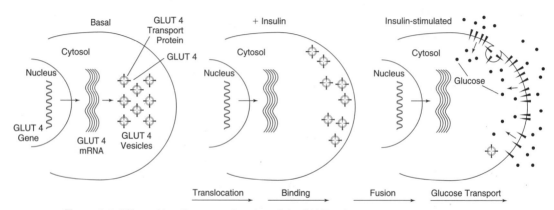

Figure 9–2. Effect of insulin on translocation of the GLUT4 glucose transporter in adipocytes.

cle are not supplied with enough oxygen to meet the metabolic need, pyruvate is reduced to lactate in the cytosol of the cells. Other tissues, such as red blood cells, produce lactate from glucose under aerobic conditions because of their lack or low abundance of mitochondria. Most tissues, under aerobic conditions, can oxidize pyruvate to acetyl CoA and CO_2 via the pyruvate dehydrogenase reaction in the mitochondria, followed by either complete oxidation of acetyl CoA to CO_2 and H_2O via the citric acid cycle or the synthesis of fatty acids from the acetyl moiety of acetyl CoA. The overall energy transfer of the glycolytic series of enzymatic reactions is exergonic, and a portion of this energy is stored as the high-energy phosphate bond of ATP. Glycolysis, however, provides a minor percentage of the ATP produced when compared with the complete oxidation of glucose to CO_2 and H_2O.

The series of enzymatic reactions that make up the glycolytic pathway are subdivided into two stages, as shown in Figure 9–3: (1) the priming of glucose, which requires ATP expenditure to generate phosphorylated intermediates, and (2) the production of reducing equivalents and the synthesis of ATP for energy provision. The enzymes that catalyze the reactions of glycolysis are present in the cytosol of the cell, organized into multienzyme complexes that function together to channel the intermediates from one enzyme to another so that they do not become diluted in the cytosol. The glycolytic enzymes are associated with cellular structures such as actin filaments, microtubules, or the outer membranes of mitochondria (Lehninger et al., 1993).

The Glycolytic Pathway

The series of enzymatic reactions that make up glycolysis utilize glucose, which enters the cell by carrier-mediated transport or glucose 6-phosphate, which is generated from glycogen degradation. Glucose, once transported inside the cell, is rapidly phosphorylated to glucose 6-phosphate in the following reaction:

$$\text{Glucose} + \text{ATP} \xrightarrow{\text{Mg}^{2+}}$$
$$\text{Glucose 6-Phosphate} + \text{ADP}$$

The mechanism of glucose phosphorylation involves the transfer of the γ phosphate from ATP to the C-6 of glucose. This essentially irreversible reaction sequesters glucose within the cell, because the phosphorylated form of glucose does not readily cross the plasma membrane. This phosphorylation reaction is catalyzed by hexokinase in most cell types and by glucokinase (hexokinase IV) in liver cells and pancreatic β cells. In all cells, the product of this reaction, glucose 6-phosphate, can be broken down in the subsequent enzymatic steps of the glycolytic pathway. However, under anabolic conditions the production of glucose 6-phosphate is also the first step in the addition of glucose to the glucose polymer, glycogen, which is synthesized and stored mainly in liver and muscle tissue. In addition to glycolysis and glycogen synthesis, glucose 6-phosphate is also metabolized by the pentose phosphate pathway. This pathway serves to provide cells with reducing equivalents in the form of NADPH and with ribose 5-phosphate for nucleotide synthesis.

The second enzymatic reaction in glycolysis is the isomerization of glucose 6-phosphate to fructose 6-phosphate, catalyzed by phosphoglucose isomerase.

$$\text{Glucose 6-Phosphate} \xoverset{\text{Mg}^{2+}}{\leftrightarrow} \text{Fructose 6-Phosphate}$$

The reaction is reversible under intracellular conditions.

6-Phosphofructo-1-kinase catalyzes the next irreversible step in the glycolytic pathway, the phosphorylation of fructose 6-phosphate to fructose 1,6-bisphosphate:

$$\text{Fructose 6-Phosphate} + \text{ATP} \xrightarrow{\text{Mg}^{2+}}$$
$$\text{Fructose 1,6-Bisphosphate} + \text{ADP}$$

The 6-phosphofructo-1-kinase reaction utilizes a second molecule of ATP and is the first committed step in glycolysis. Unlike glucose 6-phosphate, fructose 1,6-bisphosphate cannot be used directly as substrate for alternative pathways. The 6-phosphofructo-1-kinase reaction is highly regulated by allosteric modifiers and is one of the major determinants of the rate of glycolytic conversion of glucose to pyruvate.

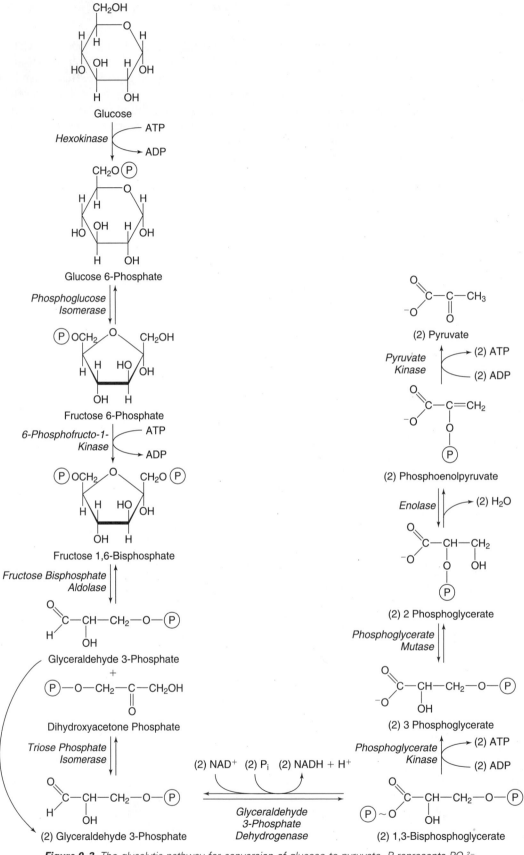

Figure 9–3. The glycolytic pathway for conversion of glucose to pyruvate. P represents PO_3^{2-}.

The next reaction involves the division of the 6-carbon sugar diphosphate, fructose 1,6-bisphosphate, to two 3-carbon phosphorylated intermediates. The enzyme aldolase catalyzes the cleavage as follows:

Fructose 1,6-Bisphosphate $\leftrightarrow$
Dihydroxyacetone Phosphate +
Glyceraldehyde 3-Phosphate

Glyceraldehyde 3-phosphate is in the direct path of glycolysis, but dihydroxyacetone phosphate is not. Dihydroxyacetone phosphate is isomerized to glyceraldehyde 3-phosphate via the action of triose phosphate isomerase. The net result of the aldolase and triose phosphate isomerase reactions is the production of 2 molecules of glyceraldehyde 3-phosphate. The series of reactions that convert 1 molecule of glucose to 2 molecules of glyceraldehyde 3-phosphate constitute the first phase of glycolysis in which the chemical energy of ATP is utilized in the generation of phosphorylated intermediates. The dihydroxyacetone phosphate generated by the aldolase reaction may also be reduced to glycerol 3-phosphate and used for synthesis of glycerolipids such as triacylglycerols; this is a particularly important source of glycerol 3-phosphate in small intestine and adipose tissue.

The second stage of glycolysis results in the generation of reducing equivalents and the synthesis of ATP. Reducing equivalents in the form NADH are produced by the reaction catalyzed by glyceraldehyde 3-phosphate dehydrogenase:

Glyceraldehyde 3-Phosphate + NAD^+ +
P_i $\leftrightarrow$ 1,3-Bisphosphoglycerate +
NADH + H^+

This reaction incorporates inorganic phosphate (P_i) to produce a high-energy phosphate bond in 1,3-bisphosphoglycerate. The second product of the reaction, NADH, provides reducing equivalents for the energy conversion of electron transport and production of ATP by oxidative phosphorylation. This is the only glycolytic reaction that generates reducing equivalents for electron transport. It is important to note that the coenzyme NAD^+ is present in limited amounts in the cytosol of the cell. For this reason, the NAD^+ utilized in the glyceraldehyde 3-phosphate reaction needs to be replaced in the cytosolic compartment so that NAD^+ availability does not limit glycolysis.

The acyl-phosphate bond of 1,3-bisphosphoglycerate has a high-energy phosphoryl transfer potential that is used to generate ATP in the next reaction of glycolysis. This is the conversion of 1,3-bisphosphoglycerate to 3-phosphoglycerate:

1,3-Bisphosphoglycerate + ADP $\leftrightarrow$
3-Phosphoglycerate + ATP

The enzyme that catalyzes this reaction is phosphoglycerate kinase. This is the first reaction in glycolysis that generates ATP. The formation of ATP by transfer of the phosphate group from 1,3-bisphosphoglycerate to ADP is a substrate-level phosphorylation.

The next step in the glycolytic pathway is the conversion of 3-phosphoglycerate to 2-phosphoglycerate, catalyzed by phosphoglycerate mutase. The mechanism of this enzymatic reaction is complex and involves a phospho-enzyme intermediate. The end products of this reaction are 2-phosphoglycerate and the regenerated phospho-enzyme. The overall series of reactions can be summarized as follows:

Enzyme-Phosphate + 3-Phosphoglycerate $\leftrightarrow$
Enzyme + 2,3-Bisphosphoglycerate

Enzyme + 2,3-Bisphosphoglycerate $\leftrightarrow$
Enzyme-Phosphate + 2-Phosphoglycerate

A second glycolytic intermediate with a high-energy phosphate bond is generated when 2-phosphoglycerate is converted to phosphoenolpyruvate via a dehydration reaction catalyzed by enolase.

2-Phosphoglycerate $\leftrightarrow$
Phosphoenolpyruvate + H_2O

The phosphoenolpyruvate generated by the enolase reaction is substrate for the last reaction of glycolysis, the conversion of phosphoenolpyruvate to pyruvate with the generation of ATP.

$$\text{Phosphoenolpyruvate} + \text{ADP} \xrightarrow{\text{Mg}^{2+}, \text{K}^+} \text{Pyruvate} + \text{ATP}$$

This reaction is catalyzed by pyruvate kinase and is the second substrate-level phosphorylation that occurs in glycolysis. The pyruvate kinase reaction is essentially irreversible under intracellular conditions. This enzyme is highly regulated by allosteric and covalent modification, much like 6-phosphofructose-1-kinase, as is discussed later in this chapter.

The total ATP produced from the reactions of glycolysis can be calculated. In this pathway, 1 molecule of glucose is converted to 2 molecules of pyruvate. Two molecules of ATP are utilized in the priming of glucose; however, 4 molecules of ATP are produced by substrate-level phosphorylation in the second phase, yielding a net increase of 2 molecules of ATP. In addition, 2 molecules of NADH are produced in the glyceraldehyde 3-phosphate dehydrogenase reaction in the cytosol of the cell. The energy gain can be summarized as follows:

$$\text{Glucose} + 2\text{ ATP} + 2\text{ NAD}^+ + 4\text{ ADP} + 2\text{ P}_i \rightarrow$$
$$2\text{ Pyruvate} + 2\text{ ADP} + 2\text{ NADH} + 2\text{ H}^+ + 4\text{ ATP} + 2\text{ H}_2\text{O}$$

or a net of

$$\text{Glucose} + 2\text{ NAD}^+ + 2\text{ ADP} + 2\text{ P}_i \rightarrow$$
$$2\text{ Pyruvate} + 2\text{ NADH} + 2\text{ H}^+ + 2\text{ ATP} + 2\text{ H}_2\text{O}$$

In electron transport, NADH transfers electrons to carrier molecules in the mitochondria of the cell, and these reactions release sufficient energy for the production of 2 to 3 molecules of ATP per pair of electrons by oxidative phosphorylation. The total amount of ATP generated from NADH depends upon the mechanism by which the reducing equivalents from NADH enter the mitochondria. The net production of ATP from glycolysis is 6 to 8 molecules of ATP from the oxidation of 1 molecule of glucose to 2 molecules of pyruvate.

Pyruvate produced by glycolysis can be metabolized in different ways, depending upon the availability of oxygen and the metabolic state of the cell. Pyruvate may enter the mitochondrion where it is converted to acetyl CoA in a complex series of reactions catalyzed by the multienzyme complex pyruvate dehydrogenase. Acetyl CoA so produced can enter the citric acid cycle for complete oxidation to CO_2 and H_2O, or it can be utilized for de novo fatty acid synthesis in certain cell types. In the absence of sufficient oxygen or in cells lacking mitochondria, pyruvate has a different fate; it is reduced to lactate by the cytosolic enzyme lactate dehydrogenase.

$$\text{Pyruvate} + \text{NADH} + \text{H}^+ \leftrightarrow \text{Lactate} + \text{NAD}^+$$

Metabolism of glucose by this anaerobic pathway may occur in active skeletal muscle, and lactate can build up when molecular oxygen becomes insufficient to meet the metabolic need. Pyruvate is also reduced to lactate in red blood cells, which do not have mitochondria. The reduction of 2 molecules of pyruvate to lactate generates 2 molecules of NAD^+ from 2 molecules of NADH. This replaces the 2 NAD^+ molecules that were reduced in the glyceraldehyde 3-phosphate dehydrogenase reaction of glycolysis. Therefore, these two reactions balance the utilization and regeneration of NAD^+ so that glycolysis can continue with no net loss of NAD^+. The lactate formed in this process can be recycled to the liver to regenerate glucose via gluconeogenesis. Heart muscle, on the other hand, is able to take up lactate and use it as a fuel for ATP production. Under conditions of heavy exercise, the heart may take up lactate released by exercising skeletal muscle and use it as a fuel.

In the presence of sufficient molecular oxygen and in cells with mitochondria, reducing equivalents ($NADH + H^+$) produced by the glyceraldehyde 3-phosphate dehydrogenase reaction can be shuttled to the mitochondria by the reduction of metabolic intermediates in the cytosol, regenerating NAD^+ in this compartment. The reduced intermediate is shuttled across the inner mitochondrial membrane with subsequent oxidation, thereby regenerating $NADH + H^+$ from NAD^+

in the mitochondria. NADH in the mitochondria is an electron donor, transferring reducing equivalents to Complex I (NADH dehydrogenase complex) in the series of oxidation/reduction reactions of electron transport (see Chapter 17, Fig. 17–2). Under these conditions, the reduction of pyruvate to lactate is not required for the regeneration of NAD^+ in the cytosol.

Metabolism of Monosaccharides Other Than Glucose

Common dietary monosaccharides other than glucose include fructose, galactose, and, in lesser amounts, mannose. Each of these is converted to intermediates in glycolysis, as shown in Figure 9–4. This occurs mainly in the liver, so these sugars are not normally present in the arterial circulation and are not available to other tissues. Although the catabolic end products of the metabolism of dietary monosaccharides are similar, these monosaccharides do not elicit the same glucose-induced hormonal response after absorption. For example, dietary fructose does not elicit a large increase in insulin secretion from the pancreas. Fructose is metabolized mainly by the liver, whereas glucose is metabolized by all tissues of the body, with only 30% to 40% of glucose intake being metabolized by the liver. A brief description of the entry of each of these monosaccharides into the glycolytic sequence of enzymatic reactions is presented here.

Fructose is a major sweetening agent in the human diet. It is present in the monosaccharide form in honey, fruit, and many vegetables and in the disaccharide sucrose (common table sugar), which is a disaccharide of fructose and glucose. Sorbitol, present in many fruits and vegetables, is also converted to fructose in the liver via the sorbitol dehydrogenase reaction. The process of fructose degradation is referred to as fructolysis. In the liver, fructose is converted to fructose 1-phosphate by the action of fructokinase, as follows:

$$\text{Fructose} + \text{ATP} \xrightarrow{\text{Mg}^{2+}}$$
$$\text{Fructose 1-Phosphate} + \text{ADP}$$

Fructose 1-phosphate is then hydrolyzed to glyceraldehyde and dihydroxyacetone phosphate by fructose 1-phosphate aldolase (aldolase B):

$$\text{Fructose 1-Phosphate} \leftrightarrow$$
$$\text{Dihydroxyacetone Phosphate} +$$
$$\text{Glyceraldehyde}$$

The majority of the triose phosphates generated from fructose are further catabolized to pyruvate, which is then converted to lactate or further degraded via the pyruvate dehydrogenase complex and the citric acid cycle. This is due, in part, to the fact that fructolysis bypasses the phosphofructo-1-kinase step, which is highly regulated and plays a major role in regulating glycolytic flux. Alternatively, to a small extent, the triose phosphates from fructose can be metabolized to glucose or glycogen. Because fructolysis provides the liver with an abundance of pyruvate and lactate, metabolites of the citric acid cycle, such as citrate and malate, also build up. Citrate can be transported out of the mitochondria and converted to acetyl CoA via the action of citrate lyase in the cytosol; acetyl CoA then serves as a precursor for fatty acid synthesis or cholesterol synthesis (as discussed in Chapter 13). Overall, a long-term increase in fructose or sucrose consumption can lead to increased hepatic lipogenesis (Shafrir, 1991). These lipids are then secreted from the liver as components of lipoprotein particles, causing hyperlipidemia, or retained in the liver if lipogenesis is in excess of lipoprotein export.

The glyceraldehyde produced by the hydrolysis of fructose 1-phosphate in the aldolase B reaction is phosphorylated by the enzyme triose kinase:

$$\text{Glyceraldehyde} + \text{ATP} \xrightarrow{\text{Mg}^{2+}}$$
$$\text{Glyceraldehyde 3-Phosphate} + \text{ADP}$$

Dihydroxyacetone phosphate produced from the hydrolysis of fructose 1-phosphate is converted to glyceraldehyde 3-phosphate by triose phosphate isomerase, the enzyme that catalyzes the same conversion of triose phosphates in the glycolytic breakdown of glucose. Overall, 1 molecule of fructose is converted

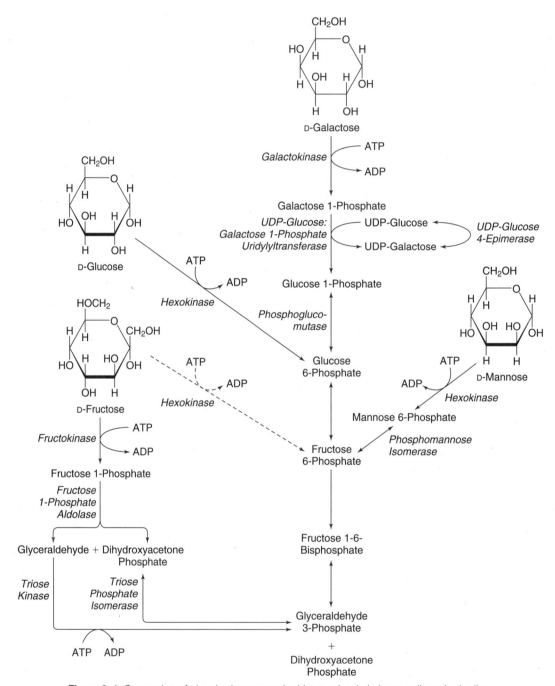

Figure 9–4. Conversion of absorbed monosaccharides to glycolytic intermediates in the liver.

Fructose Intolerance and Essential Fructosuria

Two genetic defects in fructose metabolism are known: fructose intolerance and essential fructosuria (Van den Berghe, 1995). Fructose intolerance is caused by an autosomal recessive defect in the liver fructose 1-phosphate aldolase (aldolase B) gene. The symptoms of hereditary fructose intolerance are absent in infancy if the infant is breast-fed. However, the introduction of sweetened milk formulas or the later introduction of fruits and vegetables provokes the symptoms of this disorder due to exposure to fructose. The deficiency in aldolase B leads to the buildup of fructose 1-phosphate and the depletion of P_i for ATP production in liver. The accumulation of fructose 1-phosphate blocks both glycogenolysis, owing to inhibition of phosphorylase by fructose 1-phosphate, and gluconeogenesis, owing to inhibition of the aldolase and glucose 6-phosphate isomerase reactions in the reversal of glycolysis (Van den Berghe, 1995). Furthermore, the depletion of P_i and ATP leads to a series of imbalances, including the inhibition of protein synthesis, that cause liver cell damage and a decline in liver function.

In contrast to fructose intolerance, the symptoms of essential fructosuria are essentially those of a "nondisease" (Van den Berghe, 1995). Essential fructosuria is due to a defect in fructokinase, which is normally found in liver, kidney, and intestinal mucosa. This relatively harmless disorder results in the excretion of fructose in the urine, as well as some metabolism of fructose to fructose 6-phosphate by hexokinase in adipose and muscle tissue.

Thinking Critically

In normal individuals, the capacity of the liver to phosphorylate fructose (fructokinase activity) greatly exceeds the liver's capacity to split fructose 1-phosphate (aldolase B activity). Why is deficiency of fructokinase a less serious genetic defect than a deficiency of fructose 1-phosphate aldolase? Consider what happens to fructose in each case and what effect this has on hepatic metabolism.

---

to 2 molecules of glyceraldehyde 3-phosphate. Glyceraldehyde 3-phosphate is then substrate for further glycolytic conversion.

In muscle and kidney cells, which do not have fructokinase, fructose can enter glycolysis at a different enzymatic step. In these cells, hexokinase catalyzes the phosphorylation of fructose at the C-6 position, generating fructose 6-phosphate. In this metabolic conversion, fructose enters glycolysis as fructose 6-phosphate, prior to the regulated phosphofructo-1-kinase step, rather than at the triose phosphate level. Normally, however, the liver removes fructose before it gets to these tissues.

In humans, fructose is the major fuel utilized by a specialized cell type, spermatozoa. Cells in the seminal vesicles have the ability to synthesize fructose from glucose. Fructose synthesis involves an NADPH-dependent reduction of glucose to sorbitol, followed by an NAD^+-dependent oxidation of sorbitol to fructose. Fructose is taken up by sperm cells and oxidized completely to CO_2 and H_2O by fructolysis and the citric acid cycle.

Another dietary monosaccharide, galactose, is derived from the digestion of lactose, a disaccharide of galactose and glucose. Lactose is the major carbohydrate in milk. In liver, galactose is phosphorylated by galactokinase as follows:

$$\text{Galactose} + \text{ATP} \xrightarrow{\text{Mg}^{2+}} \text{Galactose 1-Phosphate} + \text{ADP}$$

Galactose 1-phosphate then undergoes a conversion to its epimer glucose 1-phosphate through the action of UDP-glucose 4-epimerase. In this reaction, uridine diphosphate (UDP) serves as a hexose carrier, and the enzyme UDP-glucose:galactose 1-phosphate uridylyltransferase is involved in a complex exchange in which a molecule of galac-

CLINICAL CORRELATION

Hereditary Defects in Galactose Metabolism

Three inborn errors in galactose metabolism have been characterized. These are due to rare autosomal recessive defects in either galactokinase, UDP-glucose:galactose 1-phosphate uridylyltransferase, or UDP-glucose-4-epimerase. Because galactose consumption is high during infancy, the clinical symptoms of these metabolic defects are exhibited early.

Galactokinase deficiency leads to the excretion of most of the ingested galactose or its conversion to the reduced metabolite galactitol, because galactose is not phosphorylated to galactose 1-phosphate due to the defect. In newborn infants, galactitol concentrates in the lens, and the accumulation of galactitol results in the development of cataracts (Gitzelmann, 1995).

With UDP-glucose:galactose 1-phosphate uridylyltransferase deficiency, galactose 1-phosphate and galactose build up and galactitol is produced. This deficiency occurs in two forms: near-complete lack of the enzyme (classic galactosemia) and partial lack of the enzyme. Classic galactosemia affects the liver, kidney, and brain, as well as the eye, and can be life threatening.

The third metabolic deficiency syndrome, due to UDP-glucose 4-epimerase deficiency, also occurs in a mild and a severe form. Severe epimerase deficiency is very rare, and the symptoms are similar to those of classical galactosemia.

tose 1-phosphate binds to UDP with release of a molecule of free glucose 1-phosphate as the end product. Glucose 1-phosphate is a metabolic intermediate that can be channeled to glycogen synthesis under conditions that favor glucose storage. Under conditions that favor glucose utilization for energy, however, glucose 1-phosphate is converted to glucose 6-phosphate in the reversible phosphoglucomutase reaction:

Glucose 1-Phosphate $\leftrightarrow$ Glucose 6-Phosphate

Glucose 6-phosphate can then be utilized by the liver cell for glycolysis or dephosphorylated to glucose by the enzyme glucose 6-phosphatase for release to the circulating blood.

Mannose is the end product of the digestion of various polysaccharides and glycoproteins present in the diet. In the liver, mannose is phosphorylated by hexokinase at the C-6 position, generating mannose 6-phosphate:

$$\text{Mannose} + \text{ATP} \xrightarrow{\text{Mg}^{2+}} \text{Mannose 6-Phosphate} + \text{ADP}$$

The mannose 6-phosphate so produced is converted to fructose 6-phosphate by the ac-

tion of phosphomannose isomerase. Therefore, mannose can be converted to the glycolytic intermediate fructose 6-phosphate.

GLUCONEOGENESIS

The series of enzymatic reactions that make up the gluconeogenic pathway produce glucose from pyruvate, lactate, and other nonhexose precursors. The biosynthesis of glucose involves an essential reversal of glycolysis; however, the enzymatic reactions are not all a direct reversal of those of glycolysis (Fig. 9–5). Enzyme reactions specific to gluconeogenesis bypass the irreversible steps of glycolysis. Furthermore, unlike glycolysis, gluconeogenesis does not occur in all cell types—it occurs primarily in liver and to a lesser extent in kidney. In addition to having the enzymes that catalyze the reversible steps of glycolysis, liver and kidney have glycerol kinase activity, which allows glycerol to serve as a gluconeogenic substrate, entering the gluconeogenic pathway at the level of dihydroxyacetone phosphate.

The de novo synthesis of glucose by the body is critical for the maintenance of blood glucose for those tissues that are dependent upon glucose for their energy needs. In hu-

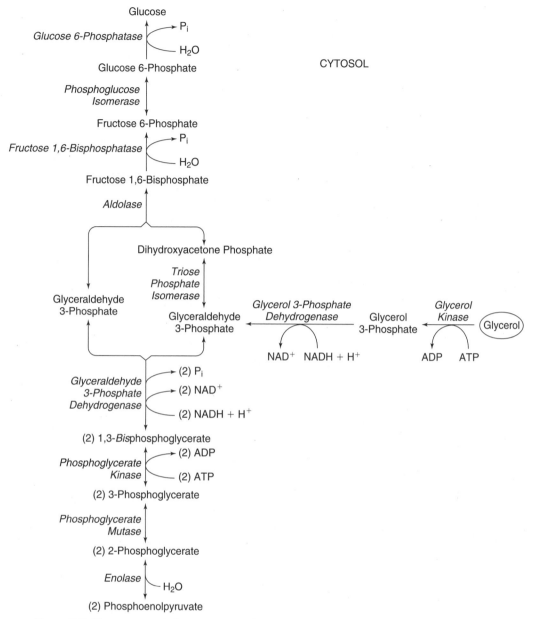

Figure 9–5. *Gluconeogenesis from pyruvate, other precursors of phosphoenolpyruvate, and glycerol.*

Illustration continued on following page

mans, in the absence of dietary carbohydrate intake, liver glycogen is depleted within 18 hours. After this time, the liver must synthesize glucose from nonhexose precursors to maintain blood glucose levels. The liver is the central gluconeogenic tissue of the human body and responds to low blood glucose by secreting newly synthesized glucose into the blood for transport to other tissues.

Although gluconeogenesis also occurs in the kidney, the kidney is a smaller organ than the liver and is less productive in de novo glucose synthesis. Overall, liver contributes approximately 90% of gluconeogenically derived glucose, whereas the kidney contributes approximately 10%. The contribution of glucose synthesis by the kidney becomes more important, however, during prolonged starvation.

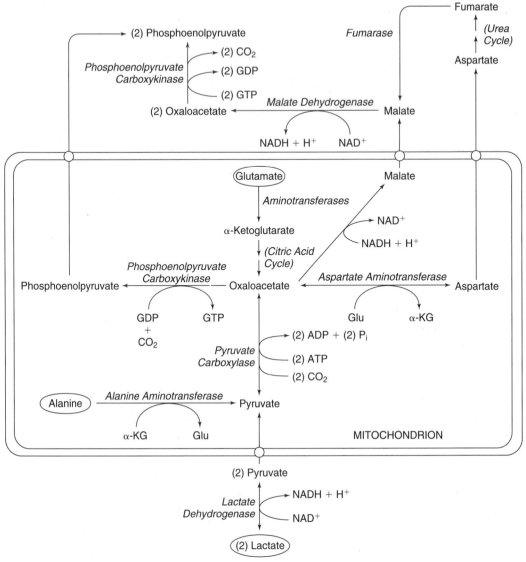

Figure 9–5 *Continued.*

The Gluconeogenic Pathway

The first step in gluconeogenesis that bypasses an irreversible glycolytic reaction is the conversion of pyruvate to phosphoenolpyruvate. This involves the activity of two enzymes, pyruvate carboxylase and phosphoenolpyruvate carboxykinase. Pyruvate is transferred from the cytosol to the mitochondrial compartment where it is substrate for mitochondrial pyruvate carboxylase. (Pyruvate also can be generated by transamination of alanine in the mitochondrion itself.) In the mitochondrion, pyruvate is carboxylated to produce oxaloace-

tate. One molecule of ATP is hydrolyzed to ADP + P_i in this reaction. Pyruvate carboxylase is a biotin-dependent enzyme in which the covalently bound coenzyme functions as the carboxyl group carrier. The reaction can be described in two stages as follows:

Enzyme-Biotin + ATP + HCO_3^- ↔
      Enzyme-Biotin-CO_2 + ADP + P_i

Enzyme-Biotin-CO_2 + Pyruvate ↔
      Enzyme-Biotin + Oxaloacetate

In addition to the requirement for biotin as a

coenzyme, this reaction also requires acetyl CoA as a positive allosteric activator. When acetyl CoA is in excess, it becomes available for activation of pyruvate carboxylase. This promotes the anabolic utilization of pyruvate, stimulating the conversion of pyruvate to oxaloacetate for gluconeogenesis. However, during metabolic conditions when there is inadequate oxaloacetate for condensation with acetyl CoA in the citric acid cycle, oxaloacetate produced by the pyruvate carboxylase reaction is used for the continuation of the citric acid cycle rather than for gluconeogenic conversion to phosphoenolpyruvate. This is referred to as an anapleurotic reaction because citric acid cycle intermediates are replenished.

In the second enzymatic step in glucose biosynthesis from pyruvate, oxaloacetate is converted to phosphoenolpyruvate. This reaction is catalyzed by phosphoenolpyruvate carboxykinase. One molecule of the high energy compound, guanosine triphosphate (GTP), is hydrolyzed in this reaction, as follows:

$$\text{Oxaloacetate} + \text{GTP} \overset{Mg^{2+}}{\longleftrightarrow}$$
$$\text{Phosphoenolpyruvate} + CO_2 + \text{GDP}$$

Although this is a reversible reaction, it is essentially irreversible in the cell because phosphoenolpyruvate is rapidly utilized.

In human liver, phosphoenolpyruvate carboxykinase is present in approximately equal concentrations in the mitochondria and the cytosol of the hepatocyte. Oxaloacetate is metabolized differently depending upon whether it is the substrate for the mitochondrial or cytosolic enzyme and whether it is derived from pyruvate or lactate. When the gluconeogenic precursor is lactate, lactate must first be converted to pyruvate by lactate dehydrogenase, a reaction that generates NADH in the cytosol. Pyruvate then enters the mitochondrion and is converted to oxaloacetate by pyruvate carboxylase. Oxaloacetate is converted to phosphoenolpyruvate by mitochondrial phosphoenolpyruvate carboxykinase, and phosphoenolpyruvate can be transported across the mitochondrial membrane to the cytosol where the remaining enzymes for gluconeogenesis are located. The lactate dehydrogenase reaction provides the required cytosolic NADH for a distal gluconeogenic step, the reversal of the glyceraldehyde 3-phosphate dehydrogenase reaction. Without this provision of cytosolic NADH, gluconeogenesis cannot continue.

A more complex process occurs when pyruvate is the gluconeogenic precursor because mitochondrial reducing equivalents must be shuttled to the cytosol to support gluconeogenesis. Pyruvate enters the mitochondrion and is converted to oxaloacetate by pyruvate carboxylase, but oxaloacetate leaves the mitochondrion as malate or aspartate. In the cytosol, malate, either directly from the mitochondria or generated by cytosolic fumarase from the fumarate released from aspartate during ureagenesis (see Fig. 11–10 in Chapter 11), is converted back to oxaloacetate by cytosolic malate dehydrogenase, with the concomitant reduction of NAD^+ to NADH. Oxaloacetate is then available as substrate for cytosolic phosphoenolpyruvate carboxykinase.

In effect, these shuttles move potential NADH from the mitochondrion to the cytosol, providing the required reduced coenzyme for the glyceraldehyde 3-phosphate dehydrogenase reaction as well as carbon substrate for gluconeogenesis. The successive actions of pyruvate carboxylase and phosphoenolpyruvate carboxykinase effectively bypass the pyruvate kinase reaction. Overall, these two reactions result in the net hydrolysis of 1 molecule each of ATP and GTP as the energy cost.

The second bypass reaction that is unique to gluconeogenesis is that catalyzed by fructose 1,6-bisphosphatase, as follows:

$$\text{Fructose 1,6-Bisphosphate} + H_2O \rightarrow$$
$$\text{Fructose 6-Phosphate} + P_i$$

This reaction reverses the 6-phosphofructo-1-kinase reaction and is essentially irreversible under intracellular conditions. It should be noted that inorganic phosphate, not ATP, is generated from the bisphosphatase reaction.

The terminal catalytic step in gluconeogenesis is the conversion of glucose 6-phosphate to glucose. This reaction provides free glucose for transport from the liver. The reaction is catalyzed by glucose 6-phosphatase and is essentially irreversible, as follows:

$$\text{Glucose 6-Phosphate} + H_2O \rightarrow$$
$$\text{Glucose} + P_i$$

The glucose 6-phosphatase reaction bypasses the glucokinase or hexokinase reaction. Glucose 6-phosphatase is important in both gluconeogenesis and glycogenolysis (glycogen breakdown) because glucose 6-phosphate is produced in both these pathways. Tissues that do not synthesize this enzyme do not have the ability to release glucose to the circulation, with the exception of some free glucose that can be released from glycogen by the debranching enzyme as discussed later in this chapter.

Glucose 6-phosphatase has a unique intracellular location. It is a membrane-bound enzyme in the endoplasmic reticulum (ER). Glucose 6-phosphatase activity is the result of the combined action of a glucose 6-phosphate translocase that moves glucose 6-phosphate into the lumen of the ER, the catalytic subunit that is responsible for the phosphohydrolase activity, and lastly, the glucose and P_i transporters that move the end products of the reaction back to the cytosol (Nordlie et al., 1993).

It should be noted that the gluconeogenic pathway is not active until after birth because the levels of phosphoenolpyruvate carboxykinase are very low until the neonatal period. Within a few hours after birth, phosphoenolpyruvate carboxykinase activity increases several-fold, and the gluconeogenic pathway becomes viable. In the human neonate, the brain is dependent on glucose for its energy needs and, therefore, is dependent on gluconeogenically derived glucose during times of carbohydrate deprivation. The premature infant is prone to hypoglycemia due to small glycogen stores and the delay in induction of phosphoenolpyruvate carboxykinase activity after birth.

Overall, the de novo synthesis of glucose requires energy in the form of ATP. Six molecules of ATP are utilized for the synthesis of one molecule of glucose from two molecules of pyruvate. In the liver, ATP is usually generated by the oxidation of fatty acids or by the partial oxidation of amino acid carbon chains, depending on fuel availability.

The Cori and Alanine Cycles

There is a metabolic connection between the liver and other tissues that depend upon glucose for their energy needs. Both lactate and alanine generated in peripheral tissues can be carried in the circulation to the liver, where they serve as substrates for hepatic gluconeogenesis. The glucose produced from these precursors can be transported from the liver and carried back to peripheral tissues for glycolytic catabolism and energy generation. This occurs in two well-defined cycles: the Cori cycle (Fig. 9–6) and the alanine cycle.

In the Cori cycle, lactate generated from pyruvate, the end product of glycolysis, is released from tissues such as muscle or red blood cells and is transported to the liver. In the liver, lactate is converted back to pyruvate by lactate dehydrogenase, and pyruvate can be used to synthesize glucose by gluconeogenesis. Gluconeogenically derived glucose is then transported from liver cells and recirculated to muscle or red blood cells for glycolysis.

A second cycle, the alanine cycle (see Fig. 11–12 in Chapter 11), involves the circulation of alanine from skeletal muscle to the

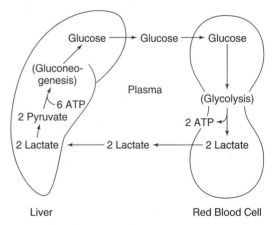

Figure 9–6. *The Cori cycle, or lactate–glucose cycle. Tissues that either lack mitochondria or have a limited blood supply depend upon glycolysis to lactate as a source of ATP. Obligate glycolytic tissues include mature red blood cells; regions of the eye including the cornea, lens, and parts of the retina; and the renal medulla.*

CLINICAL CORRELATION

Inherited Deficiencies in Gluconeogenic Enzymes

In humans, defects in both the cytosolic and mitochondrial forms of phosphoenolpyruvate carboxykinase (PEPCK) occur as rare, inherited autosomal recessive disorders. Defects in mitochondrial PEPCK are more common. A deficiency in either isoenzyme leads to hypoglycemia and lactic acidosis because sufficient glucose is not produced from pyruvate, lactate, or amino acid precursors. Therefore, individuals with this disorder are dependent upon glycogenolysis for glucose during a fast and become hypoglycemic when glycogen is depleted. The symptoms of this disorder usually present early in life. The hypoglycemia can cause seizures, coma, or lethargy. Typically, this disorder is associated with progressive neurological damage (Buist, 1995). Other symptoms include hepatomegaly, kidney dysfunction, and cardiomyopathy. This disorder can be fatal.

Inherited fructose 1,6-bisphosphatase deficiency results in impaired gluconeogenesis from any gluconeogenic precursor, including glycerol, lactate, and alanine. This disorder usually presents within the first few days of life, although in milder cases, presentation can be in early childhood. Symptoms of this disorder are similar to those described for PEPCK deficiency, i.e., hypoglycemia and lactic acidosis. Fructose 1,6-bisphosphatase deficiency, however, doesn't result in neurodegenerative disorders as does PEPCK deficiency.

One of the most common genetic diseases to affect carbohydrate metabolism in humans is Von Gierke's disease, which is caused by an autosomal recessive genetic defect in glucose 6-phosphatase. Individuals with this disease have impaired gluconeogenesis because glucose 6-phosphate cannot be converted to glucose. Because this defect results in a block in release of glucose 6-phosphate from liver as glucose, this defect also affects hepatic glucose export from the breakdown of glycogen. Because the glucose 6-phosphate is "trapped" in the liver, excessive accumulation of glycogen is observed.

---

liver. In muscle, alanine is generated from the transamination of glycolytically derived pyruvate and released. Liver cells take up the alanine and deaminate it to pyruvate, which serves as substrate for hepatic gluconeogenesis. Gluconeogenically derived glucose is then recycled from the liver back to muscle tissue. In the alanine cycle, unlike the Cori cycle, the NADH generated in skeletal muscle during glycolysis is not used for the reduction of pyruvate to lactate in the lactate dehydrogenase reaction; therefore, it is available for mitochondrial electron transport and ATP production when oxygen is sufficient.

REGULATION OF GLYCOLYSIS AND GLUCONEOGENESIS

In liver, the interconnected series of enzymatic reactions that constitute the glycolytic and gluconeogenic pathways are regulated in concert to ensure that cellular energy needs are met and that blood glucose levels are maintained. The mechanisms by which these pathways are regulated are complex and involve short-term regulation by allosteric or covalent modification of enzymes and long-term regulation by changes in expression of the genes that encode these enzymes.

The Substrate Cycle

The fine-tuned regulation of glycolysis and gluconeogenesis in liver can be understood by examining the functional concept of the substrate cycle. A substrate cycle consists of two opposing enzymatic reactions, with the potential to continuously cycle substrate and product (Fig. 9–7). If this occurs, energy is lost, with no net movement of product in either the glycolytic or gluconeogenic direction. In liver, the three substrate cycles involve the essentially irreversible reactions of glycolysis (catalyzed by glucokinase, 6-phosphofructo-1-kinase, and pyruvate kinase) and gluconeogenesis (catalyzed by pyruvate carboxylase and phosphoenolpyruvate carboxy-

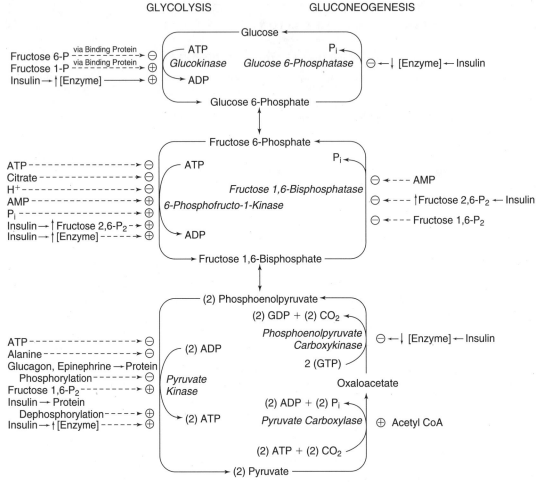

Figure 9–7. *Substrate cycles and regulation of glycolysis and gluconeogenesis in liver.*

kinase, fructose 1,6-bisphosphatase, and glucose 6-phosphatase). The paired enzymes of each specific substrate cycle are regulated in a coordinated fashion so that the stimulation of one is accompanied by the inhibition of the other. This allows for a magnification of the regulatory effect and decreases the potential for futile cycling of substrate and product (Pilkis and Claus, 1991). The rate of these enzyme reactions can be affected by allosteric modification, covalent modification, or changes in enzyme concentration. The former two mechanisms are rapid, occurring within seconds, whereas the latter mechanism is described as long-term and may require minutes to hours.

Hormonal Regulation of Glycolysis and Gluconeogenesis

In response to nutrient and physiological stimuli, hormones mediate both short- and long-term regulation of substrate cycle enzymes. Insulin, glucagon, epinephrine, and glucocorticoids are the predominant hormones that regulate enzymatic activity in carbohydrate metabolism. When blood glucose levels are elevated, such as occurs after a carbohydrate-containing meal, the anabolic hormone insulin is secreted from the β cells of the pancreas. Insulin stimulates glucose uptake via GLUT4 in skeletal muscle and adipose tissue. In liver, although insulin does not stimulate glucose uptake, insulin signals increased glycogen storage and glycolysis at the same time that it decreases glycogenolysis and gluconeogenesis. The net result is that glucose secretion from the liver is decreased. In the long term, insulin regulates the expression of genes that encode regulatory enzymes in carbohydrate metabolism; insulin activates expression of the glucokinase gene and inhibits expression of the phosphoenolpyruvate carboxykinase gene. Overall, insulin acts to decrease blood glucose levels by increasing the uptake of glucose from the blood by peripheral tissues and by decreasing glucose secretion by the liver.

When blood glucose levels are low, as in fasting or starvation, the α cells of the pancreas respond by releasing the polypeptide hormone glucagon to the blood stream. In humans, liver is the target tissue for glucagon action. Glucagon promotes increased blood glucose levels by increasing hepatic glucose production via enhanced glycogenolysis and gluconeogenesis. Glucagon, acting via 3′,5′-cyclic AMP (cAMP), regulates the expression of numerous genes encoding rate-determining enzymes, such as phosphoenolpyruvate carboxykinase. In general, glucagon stimulates increased hepatic glucose output and is a counterregulatory hormone to insulin, as are the glucocorticoids and epinephrine.

Glucocorticoids and epinephrine, from the adrenal cortex and medulla, respectively, are also released in response to decreased blood glucose. Glucocorticoids are steroid hormones that are permissive for the action of other hormones such as glucagon. Epinephrine is an adrenergic hormone that acts on many different tissues in the human body; the response of a given tissue to epinephrine depends on the predominance of specific adrenergic receptor types on the cell surface. The adrenergic receptors are grouped into α (α_1, α_2) and β (β_1, β_2, β_3) subtypes. Epinephrine stimulation of β-receptors increases glycogenolysis and gluconeogenesis, as well as lipolysis. Epinephrine stimulation of α_1-receptors results in increased glycogenolysis, whereas stimulation of α_2-receptors results in decreased lipolysis. Therefore, epinephrine in-

creases hepatic glucose output as well as lipolysis in response to fasting or starvation.

Signal Transduction. The insulin signal transduction pathway has been difficult to elucidate, but recently significant progress has been made in our understanding of the insulin receptor and the mechanism of insulin action, as described further in Chapter 16 (Fig. 16–11). The insulin receptor is made up of two α and two β subunits. The α subunits are on the extracellular face of the plasma membrane and contain the hormone-binding domains of the receptor. The two β subunits are transmembrane proteins with the carboxyl termini on the cytosolic side of the plasma membrane. The β subunits have tyrosine kinase activity, i.e., they catalyze the phosphorylation of substrate at tyrosyl residues. Insulin binding to the α subunit initiates a conformational change in the β subunit, which stimulates the tyrosine kinase domain. The initiation of tyrosine kinase activity results in autophosphorylation of tyrosyl residues in the β subunits of the receptor itself. Autophosphorylation activates the tyrosine kinase domain to phosphorylate other target proteins in the cytosol and the membrane.

Recently, a 185-kDa protein has been identified that is a substrate for the tyrosine kinase activity of the insulin receptor in most cell types. This protein is referred to as insulin receptor substrate 1 (IRS-1). A second substrate, IRS-2, has also been identified. The phosphorylation of these target proteins is one of the first postreceptor events in the pathway of insulin action within the cell. Amplification of the insulin response can occur at the level of IRS-1 and IRS-2 action independent of insulin binding to the insulin receptor or of receptor tyrosine kinase activity (White, 1998).

One outcome of the phosphorylation of IRS-1 is the association of IRS-1 with phosphatidylinositol 3-kinase (PI 3-kinase), which becomes activated. PI 3-kinase activity is involved in many of the metabolic effects of insulin (Cohen et al., 1997). Certain of these insulin effects occur in the nucleus of the cell where gene expression is activated or inhibited. Other intracellular events initiated by insulin binding to the insulin receptor are the stimulation of cyclic nucleotide phosphodiesterase, the enzyme that degrades cAMP to AMP, and the stimulation of a phosphoprotein phosphatase that dephosphorylates the bifunctional enzyme 6-phosphofructo-2-kinase/fructose 2,6-bisphosphatase. Insulin, therefore, decreases intracellular cAMP concentrations and promotes dephosphorylation of the bifunctional enzyme. The impact of these changes in cAMP levels and the phosphorylation state of the bifunctional enzyme are discussed later.

The signal transduction mechanisms for glucagon and epinephrine are similar, albeit predominant in different tissues. Glucagon and epinephrine bind to glucagon receptors and adrenergic receptors, respectively, on the plasma membrane of target cells, as described further in Chapter 16 (Fig. 16–10). These receptors are integral membrane proteins that span the lipid bilayer of the plasma membrane. The signal initiated by both glucagon binding to its receptor and epinephrine binding to β-adrenergic receptors involves the stimulatory GTP-binding protein (G_s). Binding of hormone to the cognate receptor causes a conformational change in the receptor that alters the cytoplasmic face of the receptor. This conformational change brings the hormone-receptor complex in contact with the multisubunit cytosolic protein G_s. This association causes a molecule of GDP to be exchanged for a molecule of GTP at an allosteric site of G_s. The binding of GTP stimulates G_s, causing the G_s α subunit to disassociate from the β and γ subunits; the released G_s α subunit then activates the adjoining adenylate cyclase enzyme. Adenylate cyclase, in turn, catalyzes the formation of cAMP, the intracellular second messenger of glucagon and epinephrine.

The production of cAMP stimulates the cAMP-dependent protein kinase, referred to as protein kinase A. cAMP activates protein kinase A by binding to the two regulatory subunits of the tetrameric enzyme and releasing the two catalytic subunits. The catalytic subunit of protein kinase A has numerous intracellular substrates. Relevant to the regulation of glycolysis and gluconeogenesis, protein kinase A phosphorylates both pyruvate kinase and the bifunctional enzyme, 6-phosphofructo-2-kinase/fructose 2,6-bisphosphatase (described later), both of which stimulate glycolysis. Protein kinase A also enters the nucleus of the cell and phosphorylates nuclear proteins, which can activate or inhibit the transcription of genes that encode certain glycolytic and gluconeogenic enzymes.

It should be pointed out that epinephrine also binds to α_2-adrenergic receptors. The activated α_2-receptor stimulates a series of intracellular events similar to those initiated by the β-adrenergic receptors, except that an inhibitory GTP-binding protein (G_i) is released and becomes associated with adenylate cyclase. G_i binding inhibits adenylate cyclase and leads to an overall decrease in intracellular cAMP levels. Another regulatory mechanism is contributed by epinephrine binding to α_1-adrenergic receptors. Activation of the α_1-adrenergic receptor stimulates phospholipase C on the cytoplasmic face of the plasma membrane by a GTP-binding protein mechanism similar to that for activation of adenylate cyclase. Phospholipase C hydrolyzes phosphatidylinositol 4,5-bisphosphate (PIP_2), present in the plasma membrane, to inositol 1,4,5-triphosphate (IP_3) and diacylglycerol. Diacylglycerol, in turn, stimulates protein kinase C. Protein kinase C has numerous substrates in the cell, some of which are key enzymes in hepatic glycogen metabolism, as described later in this chapter. IP_3 stimulates the release of Ca^{2+} from the ER, and calcium efflux activates the calcium/calmodulin-dependent protein kinase, as well as other enzymes. The calcium/calmodulin-dependent protein kinase catalyzes the phosphorylation and inactivation of pyruvate kinase, contributing to the diminution of the glycolytic rate (Pilkis and Claus, 1991).

Glucocorticoids differ from the polypeptide hormones such as insulin and glucagon in that the steroid hormones do not bind to plasma membrane receptors and initiate a series of intracellular events. Glucocorticoids, because they are lipid soluble, can traverse the lipid bilayer of the plasma membrane and enter the cell. Within the cytoplasm of the cell, glucocorticoids bind to their cognate receptors and subsequently enter the nucleus as an activated ligand-receptor complex. In the nucleus, the activated receptors take on the role of transcription factors and bind to regulatory regions of target genes, thereby increasing or decreasing expression of these responsive genes.

In liver, the rate of an enzymatic reaction in one substrate cycle is usually coordinated with the rates of other substrate cycle enzymes in the same pathway. For example, when blood glucose levels are low, glucagon levels increase and insulin levels decrease, resulting in an overall decrease in the insulin/glucagon ratio in the blood. This activates (by different mechanisms) phosphoenolpyruvate carboxykinase, fructose 1,6-bisphosphatase, and glucose 6-phosphatase and also inhibits pyruvate kinase, 6-phosphofructo-1-kinase, and glucokinase. These changes favor gluconeogenesis, which contributes to reestablishing normal blood glucose levels. Conversely, a high-carbohydrate diet, particularly following a fast, stimulates the release of insulin and decreases the release of glucagon from the pancreas. The rise in the insulin/glucagon ratio causes an increase in the activity of the glycolytic enzymes of the respective substrate cycles, with a concomitant decrease in the specific enzymes of gluconeogenesis. This response favors glucose utilization for energy or the synthesis of biomolecules. Clearly, this coordinated regulation allows the liver to respond to changes in the diet by determining the predominant enzymatic reaction at each substrate cycle, which in turn, determines the overall glycolytic or gluconeogenic rate of the tissue.

Regulation of the Activity of Hexokinase/Glucokinase and Glucose 6-Phosphatase

Hexokinase, which catalyzes the initial phosphorylation of glucose when it enters the cell, has different tissue-specific isoenzyme forms. Isoenzymes are different molecular forms of an enzyme that catalyze the same reaction but differ in kinetics, regulatory mechanisms, and/or tissue localization. In humans, hexokinase I predominates in skeletal muscle and other peripheral tissues. Hexokinase I has a low K_m for glucose (less than 0.1 mmol/L) relative to blood glucose concentrations (4 to 5 mmol/L). The activity of hexokinase I is

coordinated with that of the low K_m glucose carrier GLUT4, which specifically transports glucose in response to insulin stimulation. The combined action of hexokinase I and GLUT4 maintains a balance between glucose uptake and glucose phosphorylation. Hexokinase I is allosterically inhibited by its product, glucose 6-phosphate. This negative feedback assures that glucose 6-phosphate does not build up in the cell.

In liver, the predominant hexokinase is glucokinase (hexokinase IV). This isoenzyme has a high K_m for glucose (10 mmol/L) and is not inhibited by glucose 6-phosphate. The activity of glucokinase is linked to that of the high K_m glucose transporter GLUT2, which is the major glucose carrier in liver parenchymal cells. The glucokinase/GLUT2 system is very active when blood glucose levels are high. Under these conditions, the rates of glucose uptake and phosphorylation are determined by the blood glucose concentration itself. A similar coupling of GLUT2 and the high K_m glucokinase occurs in the β cells of the pancreas. In the pancreatic β cell, GLUT2 and glucokinase allow the intracellular glucose 6-phosphate concentration to equalize with the blood glucose concentration, thereby allowing the β cells to detect and respond to elevated blood glucose.

Although glucokinase in liver is not modified by its end-product, glucose 6-phosphate, it is subject to allosteric control by other intermediary metabolites. Glucokinase is indirectly inhibited by fructose 6-phosphate and activated by fructose 1-phosphate. This regulatory mechanism involves an inhibitory protein that binds to glucokinase. The affinity of this inhibitory protein for glucokinase is increased by fructose 6-phosphate; conversely, fructose 1-phosphate decreases the affinity of this inhibitory protein for glucokinase. Fructose 6-phosphate is present in the cell in equilibrium with glucose 6-phosphate because of the reversibility of the phosphoglucose isomerase reaction; therefore, fructose 6-phosphate is a negative feedback metabolite that signals the cell that glucokinase activity should decrease to prevent the buildup of this intermediate. Fructose 1-phosphate, on the other hand, is present in the liver parenchymal cell only when fructose is being metabolized; therefore, when fructose is available, the negative feedback inhibition of glucokinase is released.

In liver, reversal of the glucokinase reaction is catalyzed by glucose 6-phosphatase. Glucose 6-phosphatase is responsible for the last step in the production of glucose by either gluconeogenesis or glycogen breakdown and is required for the terminal transport of glucose from the liver cell. As indicated earlier, glucose 6-phosphatase activity is the result of the combined action of a glucose 6-phosphate translocase, the catalytic subunit that is responsible for the phosphohydrolase activity, and the glucose and P_i transporters that move the end products of the reaction back to the cytosol. Without glucose 6-phosphatase activity, glucose cannot be released to the circulation in response to low blood glucose. Glucose 6-phosphatase has a high K_m for its substrate, glucose 6-phosphate (3 mmol/L). Because the intracellular glucose 6-phosphate concentration is 0.2 mmol/L, the rate of this enzymatic reaction primarily depends upon the substrate concentration.

In liver, a substrate cycle is established between the actions of glucokinase and glucose 6-phosphatase. In the long term, the glucokinase concentration is increased in response to insulin-induced changes in expression of the glucokinase gene itself. For example, the increased insulin/glucagon ratio that occurs in response to a high carbohydrate diet stimulates expression of the glucokinase gene. Expression of the gene for the glucose 6-phosphatase catalytic subunit, on the other hand, is inhibited by insulin. Therefore, the ingestion of dietary carbohydrate results in an increase in glucokinase activity and a decrease in glucose 6-phosphatase activity, thereby favoring the net production of glucose 6-phosphate.

Regulation of 6-Phosphofructo-1-Kinase and Fructose 1,6-Bisphosphatase

In liver, the central regulatory site in glycolysis and gluconeogenesis is the substrate cycle established by the 6-phosphofructo-1-kinase and fructose 1,6-bisphosphatase reactions. Short-term regulation of this substrate cycle is critically important. Unlike the product of the glucokinase reaction, glucose 6-phosphate, which can enter glycolysis, glycogen synthesis, or the pentose phosphate pathway, the product of the 6-phosphofructo-1-kinase reaction provides a glycolytic intermediate or a substrate cycle intermediate. This reaction is the first committed step in glycolysis and, therefore, is subject to allosteric regulation by numerous metabolites that signal the energy level, pH and hormonal status of the cell. Positive regulators of 6-phosphofructo-1-kinase include AMP, P_i, and fructose 2,6-bisphosphate (described later); negative regulators include ATP, hydrogen ions, and citrate. ATP, AMP, and P_i signal the energy state of the cell; hydrogen ions signal the pH of the cell; citrate, the first metabolite of the citric acid cycle, signals the availability of sources of fuel; and fructose 2,6-bisphosphate signals the insulin/glucagon ratio.

The gluconeogenic enzyme fructose 1,6-bisphosphatase is also allosterically regulated. AMP is a strong allosteric inhibitor of this enzyme, as are fructose 2,6-bisphosphate and fructose 1,6-bisphosphate. There is a synergistic inhibition of fructose 1,6-bisphosphatase by the combined action of fructose 2,6-bisphosphate and AMP (Pilkis and Claus, 1991). When fuel for the citric acid cycle and oxygen are sufficient for oxidative phosphorylation, ATP levels in the cell are high, 6-phosphofructo-1-kinase is inhibited, and the rate of glycolysis is slow. Under the same conditions, AMP and P_i levels are low. The low concentrations of AMP and P_i contribute to the overall low 6-phosphofructo-1-kinase activity and high fructose 1-6-bisphosphatase activity.

Conversely, when oxygen pressure is low (e.g., hypoxia) or when ATP expenditure exceeds the mitochondrial capacity for oxidative metabolism and oxidative phosphorylation (e.g., when work is near or above VO_{2max}, when there are defects in mitochondrial metabolism, or in tissues with a relative or complete lack of mitochondria), lactate and hydrogen ions are increased as the end products of limited glucose catabolism. The cell releases lactate and hydrogen ions into the blood which, when in excess, can cause lactic acidosis. However, because hydrogen ions inhibit 6-phosphofructo-1-kinase activity, the glycolytic rate can be controlled to protect against lactate buildup.

A third inhibitory metabolite, citrate, signals the cell that fuel for the citric acid cycle, both oxaloacetate and acetyl CoA, is plentiful. Under these conditions, citrate is transported from the mitochondria to the cytosol, where it allosterically inhibits 6-phosphofructo-1-kinase, thereby decreasing the rate of glycolysis and sparing glucose.

The allosteric regulator fructose 2,6-bisphosphate is a potent activator of 6-phosphofructo-1-kinase and an inhibitor of fructose 1,6-bisphosphatase. The level of hepatic fructose 2,6-bisphosphate is increased by carbohydrate feeding or insulin administration. Overall, when insulin levels increase, fructose 2,6-bisphosphate levels rise and the rate of the 6-phosphofructo-1-kinase reaction is increased, thereby stimulating glycolysis. In contrast, when glucagon or epinephrine levels are elevated, fructose 2,6-bisphosphate levels are low and fructose 1,6-bisphosphatase activity is increased, resulting in an increase in gluconeogenesis. Regulation of this substrate cycle by fructose 2,6-bisphosphate is central in determining the overall flux of carbon to either glycolysis or gluconeogenesis in the liver. The end products, fructose 1,6-bisphosphate or fructose 6-phosphate, have positive feedforward effects on subsequent substrate cycles.

Regulation of 6-Phosphofructo-2-Kinase/Fructose 2,6-Bisphosphatase

Discovery of fructose 2,6-bisphosphate as an allosteric molecule in 1980 significantly advanced our understanding of the regulation of key enzymes involved in glucose metabolism. In liver, fructose 2,6-bisphosphate is a major regulatory molecule, controlling the overall direction of carbon flux toward either glycolysis or gluconeogenesis (Pilkis et al., 1990). When 6-phosphofructo-1-kinase activity is increased by fructose 2,6-bisphosphate, the increase in product, fructose 1,6-bisphosphate, allosterically activates pyruvate kinase by a feedforward mechanism. Conversely, when fructose 1,6-bisphosphatase activity is increased by a decrease in fructose 2,6-bisphosphate, more fructose 6-phosphate is produced. Fructose 6-phosphate is rapidly converted to glucose 6-phosphate, thereby providing increased substrate for glucose 6-phosphatase.

The carbohydrate content of the diet controls insulin and glucagon concentrations in the blood, which in turn regulate the production of fructose 2,6-bisphosphate. The levels of fructose 2,6-bisphosphate are controlled by a bifunctional enzyme that has both 6-phosphofructo-2-kinase and fructose 2,6-bisphosphatase activity. Regulation of the bifunctional enzyme by glucagon and insulin occurs by changes in the phosphorylation state of the enzyme. After a carbohydrate-containing meal, circulating blood glucose levels increase and stimulate insulin secretion from the β cells of the pancreas. Insulin activates phosphoprotein phosphatase 2A, which dephosphorylates the bifunctional enzyme, thereby stimulating 6-phosphofructo-2-kinase activity and favoring fructose 2,6-bisphosphate synthesis from fructose 6-phosphate and ATP. Overall, when insulin levels increase, fructose 2,6-bisphosphate levels rise and the rate of the 6-phosphofructo-1-kinase reaction is increased, thereby stimulating glycolysis (Fig. 9–8*A*).

Conversely, as an individual begins to fast, circulating insulin levels decrease and the α cells of the pancreas respond to low blood glucose by secreting glucagon. Glucagon initiates an increase in intracellular cAMP and, therefore, activates protein kinase A. Protein kinase A phosphorylates the bifunctional enzyme at a specific seryl residue. This alters the conformation of the bifunctional enzyme, decreasing the 6-phosphofructo-2-kinase activity and increasing the fructose 2,6-bisphosphatase activity. This rapidly decreases fructose 2,6-bisphosphate levels in liver, which releases the inhibition of fructose 1,6-bisphosphatase and favors gluconeogenesis (Fig. 9–8*B*). Both the 6-phosphofructo-2-kinase and the fructose 2,6-bisphosphatase reactions are also inhibited by the end products of their respective reactions, fructose 2,6-bisphosphate and fructose 6-phosphate. Overall, the predominant factors that determine fructose 2,6-bisphosphate levels in liver are the concentration of fructose 6-phosphate and the phosphorylation state of the bifunctional enzyme.

Studies done in rat liver indicate that in the fed state, fructose 6-phosphate levels are

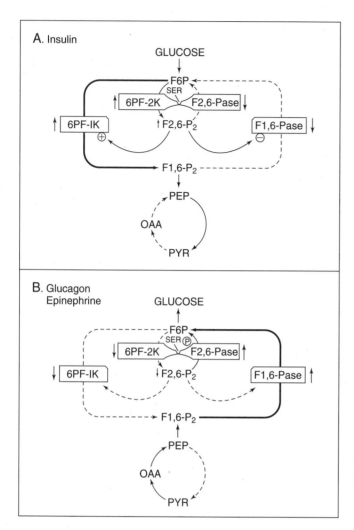

Figure 9–8. Regulation of the bifunctional enzyme 6-phosphofructo-2-kinase (6PF-2K)/fructose 2,6-bisphosphatase (F2,6-Pase) by phosphorylation (B, glucagon, or catecholamines) and dephosphorylation (A, insulin), and the allosteric regulation of 6-phosphofructo-1-kinase (6PF-1K) and fructose 1,6-bisphosphatase (F1,6-Pase) by fructose 2,6-bisphosphate (F2,6-P_2). F6P, fructose 6-phosphate; SER, seryl residue; PEP, phosphoenolpyruvate; OAA, oxaloacetate; PYR, pyruvate; P, $-PO_3^{2-}$.

in the 0.1 to 0.2 μmol/g range, and the bifunctional enzyme is in the dephosphorylated state. In this conformation, the 6-phosphofructo-2-kinase reaction is favored by a decrease in the K_m for substrate, fructose 6-phosphate. Therefore, the intracellular substrate concentration is significantly above the K_m, maximizing the rate of fructose 2,6-bisphosphate production. During fasting (or diabetes) the bifunctional enzyme becomes phosphorylated at an amino-terminal seryl residue, which activates the fructose 2,6-bisphosphatase and inhibits the 6-phosphofructo-2-kinase. The conformational change induced at the active site of 6-phosphofructo-2-kinase increases the K_m for substrate, fructose 6-phosphate. At the same time, during fasting, intracellular levels of fructose 6-phosphate decrease to below the K_m, and the rate of

fructose 2,6-bisphosphate production is concomitantly slowed (Pilkis et al., 1995). Fructose 6-phosphate is also a substrate for 6-phosphofructo-1-kinase; however, the rate of this reaction is two to three orders of magnitude greater than that of the 6-phosphofructo-2-kinase reaction. Therefore, the shunting of fructose 6-phosphate to fructose 2,6-bisphosphate production occurs at a much slower rate; the amount of glycolytic fuel used for the synthesis of this regulatory molecule is thus small.

Regulation of Pyruvate Kinase and Phosphoenolpyruvate Carboxykinase

The final substrate cycle in liver involves pyruvate kinase activity in the glycolytic direction and the combined action of pyruvate carboxylase and phosphoenolpyruvate carboxykinase in the gluconeogenic direction. The pyruvate kinase reaction is an important site of hormonal and nutritional regulation in glycolysis. In liver, the momentum of glycolysis is maintained by pyruvate kinase under conditions that increase 6-phosphofructo-1-kinase activity. This is because the end product of the 6-phosphofructo-1-kinase reaction, fructose 1,6-bisphosphate, is a positive allosteric regulator of pyruvate kinase. Pyruvate kinase is also allosterically inhibited by ATP and alanine. At physiological concentrations of substrate (phosphoenolpyruvate) and inhibitors (ATP and alanine), pyruvate kinase would be completely inhibited without the stimulatory effect of fructose 1,6-bisphosphate.

In liver, pyruvate kinase is also regulated by phosphorylation. It is a substrate for both protein kinase A, induced by interaction of glucagon with glucagon receptors or of epinephrine with β-adrenergic receptors, and the calcium/calmodulin-dependent protein kinase, induced by epinephrine interaction with α_1-adrenergic receptors. Phosphorylation of pyruvate kinase decreases the activity of the enzyme by increasing the K_m for its substrate, thereby slowing the rate of glycolysis. The reversal of this response is initiated by an increase in the insulin/glucagon ratio, which decreases cAMP and thus decreases protein kinase A activity, resulting in the dephosphorylation of pyruvate kinase and activation of the enzyme. It should be noted that the phosphorylated form of pyruvate kinase is less readily stimulated by fructose 1,6-bisphosphate and more readily inhibited by ATP and alanine. Conversely, in the dephosphorylated state, pyruvate kinase is more sensitive to allosteric activators and less sensitive to allosteric inhibitors. In the presence of fructose 1,6-bisphosphate, the protein kinase A–dependent phosphorylation of the enzyme is inhibited.

The gluconeogenic enzymes that oppose pyruvate kinase are pyruvate carboxylase and phosphoenolpyruvate carboxykinase. Pyruvate carboxylase is positively regulated by a buildup of acetyl CoA in the mitochondria, which signals the need for more oxaloacetate. However, it is the phosphoenolpyruvate carboxykinase reaction that is rate determining for gluconeogenesis. Changes in the rate of the phosphoenolpyruvate carboxykinase reac-

tion are not in response to allosteric or covalent modifiers; instead, enzyme concentration is highly regulated. The enzyme concentration is determined by regulation of the gene that encodes phosphoenolpyruvate carboxykinase.

REGULATION OF THE EXPRESSION OF GLYCOLYTIC AND GLUCONEOGENIC GENES

The pathways of glycolysis and gluconeogenesis function differently in the various tissues of the body. In liver, the rate of glycolysis is slow; the liver is more dependent on amino acids for metabolic fuel in the fed state and on fatty acids for metabolic fuel during food deprivation. Red blood cells, on the other hand, are completely dependent on glycolysis for their energy needs. Gluconeogenesis has a more restricted tissue distribution than does glycolysis; it is limited primarily to the liver and kidney. During starvation, gluconeogenesis in liver and kidney provides glucose for the body. It is clear, therefore, that different regulatory mechanisms are involved in the metabolic roles these pathways play in different tissues. Long-term regulation of the expression of specific genes dictates the concentrations of certain glycolytic and gluconeogenic enzymes as well as of transport proteins in the different cell types. Selective expression of specific genes plays a major role in determining the tissue distribution of these metabolic pathways.

A new era of metabolic investigation has been made possible by the isolation and characterization of genes encoding glycolytic and gluconeogenic enzymes. Our knowledge of long-term regulation of glycolysis and gluconeogenesis is based upon studies of individual genes that have been cloned. Genes for the key regulatory enzymes of glycolysis and gluconeogenesis: glucokinase, glucose 6-phosphatase, 6-phosphofructo-1-kinase, fructose 1,6-bisphosphatase, pyruvate kinase, phosphoenolpyruvate carboxykinase, and 6-phosphofructo-2-kinase/fructose 2,6-bisphosphatase have been isolated and sequenced. DNA elements that are responsive to hormonal and nutrient stimuli have been characterized in several of the promoter/regulatory domains of these genes. Collectively, there are a number of similarities in hormonal regulation of genes encoding the key glycolytic and gluconeogenic enzymes. Insulin increases messenger RNA (mRNA) levels and transcription rates of the glycolytic genes and decreases mRNA levels and transcription rates of the gluconeogenic genes; glucagon, acting via cAMP, has the opposite effect (Pilkis and Granner, 1992). The genes encoding the different glucose transporters and other glycolytic enzymes also have been characterized.

Expression of Glucose Transporters

The various tissue-specific glucose transporter proteins are encoded by separate genes. Expression of some of these genes is regulated by fluctuations in diet and hormones. In adipose tissue, for example, the gene for GLUT4 is regulated by fasting and carbohydrate refeeding (Charron et al., 1999). Fasting or insulin deprivation leads to a significant decrease in GLUT4 mRNA and GLUT4 protein in adipocytes. This decrease can be reversed by carbohydrate refeeding or insulin treatment. A depletion in GLUT4 mRNA and protein results

in a decrease in the vesicular GLUT4 pool that is available for translocation to the plasma membrane. The decrease in GLUT4 gene expression and the decrease in insulin-stimulated GLUT4 translocation both contribute to the decrease in glucose uptake in adipocytes with insulin deprivation (Fig. 9–9). Although the GLUT1 gene is also expressed in adipose tissue, GLUT1 mRNA levels are not significantly changed by dietary carbohydrate or insulin status.

Expression of the GLUT4 gene has also been investigated in skeletal muscle. Because the red and white muscle fiber types have different insulin sensitivities and GLUT4 concentrations, it has been difficult to determine the hormonal responsiveness of the GLUT4 gene in this tissue. Most studies indicate that insulin deficiency results in a decrease in GLUT4 mRNA in both red and white muscle, but GLUT4 mRNA levels and GLUT4 protein levels in skeletal muscle are not always correlated.

The major glucose transporter isoform in liver is GLUT2. The hepatic GLUT2 gene does not appear to be regulated by dietary carbohydrate or insulin in different experimental models. Overall, GLUT2 mRNA and protein levels

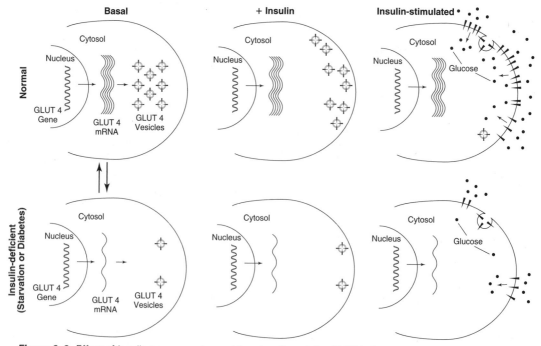

Figure 9–9. *Effect of insulin on expression and translocation of the GLUT4 glucose transporter in adipocytes.*

in liver have not been found to change consistently in response to altered metabolic states. However, it has been shown that GLUT2 gene expression in pancreatic β cells is decreased when blood glucose levels are low. Conversely, a rise in blood glucose levels results in an increase in GLUT2 mRNA and protein levels. The differential responsiveness of the GLUT2 gene in liver and pancreas provides a good example of tissue specificity in the regulation of gene expression.

Expression of Glucokinase

Glucokinase (hexokinase IV), which converts glucose to glucose 6-phosphate, is the predominant hexokinase isoform in both the liver and pancreatic β cell. However, glucokinase plays a different metabolic role in these two tissues. In liver, glucose uptake is responsible for removal of approximately 35% to 40% of portal vein glucose after a carbohydrate-containing meal. The high K_m glucokinase maintains a glucose concentration deficit across the liver cell membrane, as glucose that enters the cell is rapidly converted to glucose 6-phosphate. In pancreatic β cells, glucokinase is part of the cells' machinery for detecting the levels of glucose in the blood. The high K_m for glucose allows β cell glucose utilization to vary with alterations in the blood glucose concentration. Because glucokinase activity is optimal at elevated blood glucose concentrations, the rate of glycolytic flux increases with elevated blood glucose, thereby increasing the ATP/ADP concentration ratio. It is postulated that this ratio is involved in the complex signal that controls the rate of insulin secretion from the pancreatic β cell. Both the hepatic and pancreatic glucokinase catalyze the same reaction, but the metabolic function that is served is different in liver and pancreas. Underlying this functional difference is a divergence in expression and regulation of the glucokinase gene.

In humans, the glucokinase gene has two transcription start sites and two alternative splicing patterns that are used differentially in liver and the pancreatic β cells (Magnuson and Jetton, 1993). Transcription of the glucokinase gene and processing of the primary transcript proceed differently in these two tissues.

These are common regulatory mechanisms that increase the flexibility of gene expression in eukaryotic cells. In this case, two different promoter/regulatory domains are used to determine the transcription rate of the glucokinase gene from the different transcription start sites; these promoters are located at different positions in the 5′ noncoding region of the gene, upstream of their respective transcription start sites. Based on liver- and pancreas-specific usage of each promoter, there can be two different start sites for transcription initiation and two different first exons (or expressed sequences) in the primary transcript for glucokinase. Each first exon is linked by alternative splicing to a common second exon during processing in the nucleus of the cell. The remaining exons (2 through 10) are the same for both the liver and pancreatic form of glucokinase mRNAs. Therefore, different glucokinase mRNAs are produced in the liver and the pancreatic β cell. The translation of these mRNAs results in two glucokinase isoforms that differ in the first 15 amino acids of the protein structure. Altogether, the liver- and pancreas-specific differences in expression of the glucokinase gene involve two different promoter domains, two different start sites of transcription, alternative splicing of the primary transcript, and ultimately two different protein products.

What is the functional significance of this type of tissue-specific variation in expression of the glucokinase gene? This divergence allows for specific tissue responses to hormones and/or nutrients. In liver, but not in the pancreatic β cell, insulin stimulates transcription of the glucokinase gene and glucagon inhibits it. In the pancreatic β cell, but not in liver, expression of the glucokinase gene is responsive to glucose. Therefore, there are distinct differences in the regulation of expression of the glucokinase gene in these two tissues. It is the insulin/glucagon ratio that regulates liver glucokinase expression, whereas it is the blood glucose concentration that regulates pancreatic β-cell glucokinase expression. Differences between the glucokinase isoforms themselves (e.g., kinetic parameters) remain to be determined (Magnuson and Jetton, 1993).

Expression of 6-Phosphofructo-1-Kinase

6-Phosphofructo-1-kinase catalyzes the first committed step of glycolysis and is involved in the fructose 6-phosphate/fructose 1,6-bis-phosphate substrate cycle. In humans, there are three isoenzymes of 6-phosphofructo-1-kinase, each of which is encoded by a separate gene. The expression of the liver form has been examined under conditions of fasting and carbohydrate refeeding. Hepatic 6-phosphofructo-l-kinase mRNA levels are increased in response to carbohydrate refeeding after a fast, and this response can be partially blocked by the administration of cAMP. Hepatic 6-phosphofructo-1-kinase mRNA levels are also increased in response to insulin treatment of diabetic animals. Therefore, 6-phosphofructo-1-kinase mRNA levels in liver appear to be determined by the counterregulatory signals of insulin and glucagon (Granner and Pilkis, 1990). 6-Phosphofructo-1-kinase also is subject to short-term regulation by insulin and glucagon, as discussed earlier.

Expression of Aldolase

Aldolase converts fructose 1,6-bisphosphate to glyceraldehyde 3-phosphate in glycolysis. Under intracellular conditions, the aldolase reaction is reversible; therefore, it is active in both glycolysis and gluconeogenesis. Notably, aldolase is also active in fructose catabolism. The aldolase enzyme is made up of four subunits, consisting of different combinations of three subunit types (A, B, and C). Each of the subunits is encoded by a separate gene. The aldolase A subunit is found in most tissues but is most abundant in muscle. The aldolase B subunit is more restricted; it is found in liver, kidney proximal tubules, and enterocytes of the small intestine. Aldolase C is present in brain, fetal tissues, and cancer cells.

Of the genes for the three subunits, the aldolase B gene has been the best-characterized (Lemaigre and Rousseau, 1994). The structure of the aldolase B gene has been determined for humans and other species. This gene has a single promoter directing aldolase expression in liver, kidney, and the small intestine. The effects of dietary changes, as tested in experimental rats, show that dur-ing starvation there is a significant decrease in aldolase B mRNA abundance in liver and small intestine, but not in kidney. Refeeding a high-carbohydrate diet returns aldolase B mRNA levels to normal. The effect of refeeding on aldolase B mRNA can be blocked in liver by glucagon or cAMP. Neither glucagon nor cAMP, however, has this effect in the small intestine. It is interesting that refeeding rats a high-fructose diet increases aldolase B mRNA in kidney as well as in liver in diabetic rats.

Expression of Glyceraldehyde 3-Phosphate Dehydrogenase

Glyceraldehyde 3-phosphate dehydrogenase catalyzes the conversion of glyceraldehyde 3-phosphate to 1,3-bisphosphoglycerate, with the generation of NADH. The enzyme is a tetramer of four identical subunits encoded by one gene. The tissue distribution of glyceraldehyde 3-phosphate dehydrogenase is ubiquitous; however, the glyceraldehyde 3-phosphate dehydrogenase gene is regulated by nutrients and hormones in a tissue-specific way (Sirover, 1997). Glyceraldehyde 3-phosphate dehydrogenase mRNA levels increase in liver when fasting is followed by carbohydrate refeeding, and in adipose tissue in response to insulin treatment. Regulation of the glyceraldehyde 3-phosphate dehydrogenase gene is localized to these lipogenic tissues where glyceraldehyde 3-phosphate dehydrogenase mRNA levels increase in response to elevated blood glucose and insulin.

Expression of Pyruvate Kinase

Pyruvate kinase catalyzes the conversion of phosphoenolpyruvate to pyruvate in the last enzymatic step of glycolysis. Four pyruvate kinase isoenzymes have been characterized: the M_1 form is the predominant form in muscle, heart, and brain; the M_2 form is found in fetal tissue and in most adult tissues; the L' (or R) form is the major form in red blood cells; and the L form is the major liver form but also is present in kidney and the small intestine. Two pyruvate kinase genes have been isolated that code for the four isoenzymes identified. The pyruvate kinase L and pyruvate kinase M genes encode the L and L' isoenzymes and the M_1 and M_2 isoenzymes, respectively. The pyruvate kinase L gene has two promoters, which regulate two distinct transcription start sites, generating two unique first exons in the pyruvate kinase transcript. The pyruvate kinase M gene, on the other hand, is alternatively spliced so that the mRNAs contain either the 9th (M_1) or the 10th (M_2) exon, each expressed in the aforementioned tissue-specific manner (Noguchi and Tanaka, 1993).

In liver, regulation of the pyruvate kinase L gene involves both direct nutrient and indirect hormonal effects. Refeeding fasted rats a high-carbohydrate diet increases pyruvate kinase L mRNA levels in liver, and this stimulation is dependent on the presence of insulin. Dietary fructose also increases pyruvate kinase L mRNA levels, more rapidly than does glucose and without the insulin requirement. Glucose stimulation of pyruvate kinase L mRNA abundance appears to require the catabolism of glucose to glucose 6-phosphate or another downstream metabolite. Therefore, in liver, insulin may be required for glucose stimulation of the expression of the pyruvate kinase L gene because it stimulates glucose 6-phosphate production by increasing transcription of the glucokinase gene. Dietary glycerol is also a potent stimulant of the pyruvate kinase L gene in liver. It is possible that a downstream metabolite, common to glucose, fructose, and glycerol, is the regulatory intermediate involved in regulating pyruvate kinase L gene expression.

The first glucose response element to be identified in the promoter region of a gene was in the pyruvate kinase L gene. Two repeated DNA sequences of 6 nucleotides in length, referred to as the L4 box region, are required for glucose responsiveness of the pyruvate kinase L gene when tested in cell culture or whole animal experimental models (Vaulont and Kahn, 1993). Hypothetically, this region of the DNA within the promoter/regulatory domain of the pyruvate kinase L gene binds the metabolic intermediate generated from glucose that regulates transcription of this gene in liver.

Pyruvate kinase L is the predominant mRNA isoform in liver; however, it is also found in kidney and small intestine. All three of these tissues are major sites of fructose metabolism, and liver and kidney are major sites of glycerol metabolism. It stands to reason that pyruvate kinase L mRNA levels would be regulated by dietary fructose and glycerol in those tissues involved in their metabolism. Consistent with this assumption, refeeding a high-fructose diet to fasted rats increased pyruvate kinase L mRNA in kidney and in the small intestine, whereas refeeding a high-glycerol diet increased pyruvate kinase L mRNA in kidney alone. A high-glucose diet did not increase pyruvate kinase L mRNA in kidney or the small intestine (Noguchi and Tanaka, 1993).

Expression of Phosphoenolpyruvate Carboxykinase

Countering the activity of pyruvate kinase in liver cytosol is the activity of phosphoenolpyruvate carboxykinase, which determines gluconeogenic flux by catalyzing the conversion of oxaloacetate to phosphoenolpyruvate. A single gene encodes the cytosolic enzyme, with one promoter/regulatory domain directing transcription of the gene. This single promoter, however, is composed of a complex network of interrelated DNA response elements that are affected by nutrients, hormones, and tissue-specific transcription factors (Gurney et al., 1994). These direct the expression of the phosphoenolpyruvate carboxykinase gene at high levels in liver, kidney, and adipose tissue and at lower levels in the intestinal epithelium and mammary gland. In addition to this tissue specificity, there is a cell-specific pattern of phosphoenolpyruvate carboxykinase mRNA localization in liver. In liver, phosphoenolpyruvate carboxykinase mRNA is present in highest concentration in the hepatocytes surrounding the portal vein. Phosphoenolpyruvate carboxykinase mRNA is localized to the same periportal cells as phosphoenolpyruvate carboxykinase enzyme activity; therefore, this zonation of enzyme activity appears to be determined at the mRNA level. Other gluconeogenic enzymes and urea cycle enzymes share this periportal distribution.

Expression of the phosphoenolpyruvate carboxykinase gene is highly regulated by diet and hormones. It is well known that fasting increases phosphoenolpyruvate carboxykinase mRNA levels, and that refeeding a high-carbohydrate diet decreases phosphoenolpyruvate carboxykinase mRNA abundance (Hanson and Reshef, 1997). In the fasted state, both the transcription rate of the phosphoenolpyruvate carboxykinase gene and the stability of the phosphoenolpyruvate carboxykinase mRNA are increased by cAMP. Carbohydrate refeeding, which increases the insulin level in the blood, decreases the transcription rate of the phosphoenolpyruvate carboxykinase gene, probably mediated by active PI 3-kinase (Sutherland et al., 1996). Insulin is the dominant negative regulator of phosphoenolpyruvate carboxykinase gene expression and will inhibit cAMP- or glucocorticoid-stimulated increases in the rate of transcription of this gene. However, glucose alone decreases phosphoenolpyruvate carboxykinase mRNA levels by decreasing the transcription rate and the stability of the mRNA in hepatocytes cultured in the absence of insulin (Kahn et al., 1989). Therefore, the inhibition of phosphoenolpyruvate carboxykinase gene expression imposed by refeeding a high-carbohydrate diet may be due, in part, to a direct effect of glucose or a metabolite of glucose on the phosphoenolpyruvate carboxykinase promoter.

Expression of Glucose 6-Phosphatase

Glucose 6-phosphatase catalyzes the terminal reaction in both the gluconeogenic and glycogenolytic pathways, the conversion of glucose 6-phosphate to free glucose. As indicated previously, the enzyme activity is conferred by the action of three separate enzymes. The gene for the catalytic subunit has been isolated and partially characterized. The rate of transcription of the gene for the catalytic subunit of glucose 6-phosphatase is increased by glucocorticoids, and both basal and glucocorticoid-stimulated transcription are inhibited by insulin. The promoter for the glucose 6-phosphatase gene contains an insulin response element, similar to the phosphoenolpyruvate carboxykinase promoter. It is likely that the two genes are coordinately regulated either to increase or decrease hepatic glucose output (Streeper et al., 1997).

Expression of 6-Phosphofructo-2-Kinase/Fructose 2,6-Bisphosphatase

The bifunctional enzyme 6-phosphofructo-2-kinase/fructose 2,6-bisphosphatase catalyzes both the synthesis and breakdown of the allosteric regulator fructose 2,6-bisphosphate. There are different 6-phosphofructo-2-kinase/fructose 2,6-bisphosphatase isoenzymes, which have specific catalytic properties, tissue distributions, and responses to regulatory molecules. The 6-phosphofructo-2-kinase/fructose 2,6-bisphosphatase gene contains three promoters (L, M, and F) in its 5′ regulatory sequence. The L promoter is active in liver, adipose tissue, and skeletal muscle; the M promoter is active in a number of tissues and is predominant in muscle; and the F-type promoter is active primarily in fetal liver, muscle, lung, and thymus, as well as preterm placenta. In the fasted state, glucagon inhibits transcription from the L promoter of the 6-phosphofructo-2-kinase/fructose 2,6-bisphosphatase gene and decreases the stability of the L-type mRNA. Refeeding (or insulin treatment of a diabetic) increases 6-phosphofructo-2-kinase/fructose 2,6-bisphosphatase mRNA levels in liver within 24 to 48 hours (Lemaigre and Rousseau, 1994). Nutrient and hormonal conditions that increase the amount of 6-phosphofructo-2-kinase/fructose 2,6-bisphosphatase mRNA, also increase the amount of enzyme and increase the hepatic levels of fructose 2,6-bisphosphate, whereas those conditions that decrease 6-phosphofructo-2-kinase/fructose 2,6-bisphosphatase mRNA and protein levels decrease hepatic fructose 2,6-bisphosphate levels.

Liver Compartmentalization of Gluconeogenic Enzymes

In liver, the catabolism of glucose via glycolysis occurs at a low rate under aerobic conditions when glucose levels in the blood are not high. Gluconeogenesis, on the other hand, is carried out at a higher rate. It is interesting that there is a gradient of gluconeogenic enzyme activity, compartmentalized to different zones in the liver. These zones arise in functional subdivisions of the liver that are defined by the microcirculation of the tissue. The functional liver acinus is a subdivision that follows the symmetry of the liver cell plates. The acinus is circumscribed by terminal hepatic veins at the periphery and a terminal portal vein and terminal hepatic artery at the center (Fig. 9–10). The portal vein supplies approximately 70% of the blood that comes to the liver, and the hepatic artery supplies the rest.

The hepatocytes that surround the incoming portal venule are referred to as periportal cells, and those that surround the outgoing central venule are referred to as perivenous cells. Distinct metabolic zones occur between these regions of afferent and efferent blood flow (Jungermann, 1992). At the proximal side of the circulatory supply to the liver acinus, the cells are receiving oxygen and nutrient-rich blood from the portal vein and hepatic artery. As the blood traverses the cell population, it becomes relatively depleted of oxygen and dietary nutrients as it moves toward the hepatic central vein. It is generally accepted that the activity of gluconeogenic and urea cycle enzymes is higher in hepatocytes at the periportal side of the liver acinus. There is some debate as to whether the limited glycolysis that occurs in liver is more predominant in perivenous cells or is less compartmentalized overall than is gluconeogenesis. Because perivenous cells receive blood with a somewhat lower oxygen tension than do periportal hepatocytes, perivenous cells are thought to be more dependent upon glycolysis. It is documented that the low K_m glucose transporter GLUT1 is localized to a layer of cells surrounding the hepatic venule. The high affinity of GLUT1 for glucose assures that perivenous cells take up glucose to provide for increased glycolysis. GLUT2, on the other hand, is distributed evenly across the liver acinus.

The compartmentalization of specific enzymes and transporters of glucose metabolism appears to be due to localized gene expression. The pattern of gene expression and compartmentalization changes with alterations in dietary state. For example, the periportal to

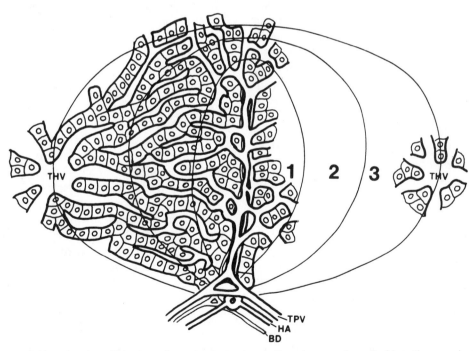

Figure 9–10. Hepatic acinus. This three-dimensional structure is the microvascular unit of hepatic parenchyma. The acinar axis is formed by the terminal portal venule (TPV), the hepatic arteriole (HA), and the bile ductule (BD). The perfusion of this unit is unidirectional from the acinar axis to the acinar periphery where two or more terminal hepatic venules (THV) empty the acinus. The arbitrary division of the acinus into functional zones is represented by 1 (periportal), 2, and 3 (perivenous). (Reprinted with permission from Gumucio, J. J. and Chianale, J. [1988] Liver cell heterogeneity and liver function. In: The Liver: Biology and Pathobiology [Arias, I. M., Jakoby, W. B., Popper, H., Schachter, D. and Shafritz, D. A., eds.], 2nd ed., pp. 931–947. Raven Press, New York.)

perivenous ratios of the activities of phospho-enolpyruvate carboxykinase, fructose 1,6-bis-phosphatase, and glucose 6-phosphatase decrease with fasting. These decreases in the periportal to perivenous ratios are due to increases in gluconeogenic enzyme activity in the perivenous cells during a fast, when total hepatic glucose output increases. Under these conditions, gluconeogenesis is activated in the larger hepatocyte population, and compartmentalization is decreased.

GLYCOGEN METABOLISM

Glucose is stored in liver and muscle tissue as glycogen, a branched-chain polymer of glucose. In humans, liver has the capacity to store glycogen up to approximately 10% of its weight. Skeletal muscle, on the other hand, has a more limited capacity to store glycogen, to approximately 1% of its weight. In humans, the overall mass of skeletal muscle is greater than that of liver, so total muscle glycogen is approximately double the amount of liver glycogen. Glycogen is stored in the postprandial state for future use when glucose levels decrease in the blood. When blood glucose levels decline, the body's first line of defense is to degrade hepatic glycogen to its individual glucose units via glycogenolysis. Glucose 6-phosphate derived from glycogenolysis has different fates in liver and skeletal muscle. The liver secretes glucose to the blood to maintain circulating blood levels for those tissues that are dependent upon glucose for energy. Skeletal muscle, on the other hand, utilizes glucose 6-phosphate produced by glycogenolysis for glycolysis and ATP production within the same cell.

Glycogen Synthesis

The glycogen polymer is a linear array of glucosyl residues linked by $\alpha1\rightarrow4$-glycosidic bonds, with branch points in $\alpha1\rightarrow6$-glycosidic linkage. The branching structure of the molecule is not random; branch points occur approximately every fourth glucosyl residue along the linear chains of the polymer. The series of enzymes that catalyze the steps of glycogen synthesis are responsible for the specificity of this structure.

The first enzymatic reaction in glycogen synthesis from glucose is the same as that in glycolysis, the glucokinase reaction in liver, and hexokinase reaction in skeletal muscle. The product of these reactions, glucose 6-phosphate, is further metabolized to glucose 1-phosphate by the action of phosphogluco-mutase.

$$\text{Glucose 6-Phosphate} \leftrightarrow \text{Glucose 1-Phosphate}$$

The third reaction in this series prepares glucose for storage as glycogen. This reaction is catalyzed by glucose 1-phosphate uridylyl-transferase.

$$\text{Glucose 1-Phosphate} + \text{UTP} \rightarrow$$
$$\text{UDP-Glucose} + \text{PP}_i$$

This is an energy-requiring step, but it is made essentially irreversible by the hydrolysis of one of the end products, pyrophosphate (PP_i), to 2 molecules of inorganic phosphate. This reaction is catalyzed by pyrophosphatase:

$$\text{PP}_i + \text{H}_2\text{O} \rightarrow 2\,\text{P}_i$$

Glycogen synthase catalyzes the addition of single glucosyl residues to a growing polymer of glycogen. The substrates for this reaction are glycogen and UDP-glucose (Fig. 9–11). The glucose moiety is added to the glycogen polymer in an $\alpha1\rightarrow4$-glycosidic linkage between C-1 of the "activated" glucose and C-4 of the terminal glucose of a linear chain of the glycogen polymer. For each new glycogen molecule, a primer is required for the attachment of the first molecule of glucose. The protein glycogenin serves this function; the first glucose moiety in a nascent chain is attached to a specific tyrosyl residue in glycogenin. Glycogen synthase then forms a complex with glucose-bound glycogenin, and extension of the polysaccharide chain is autocatalyzed by the glucosyltransferase activity of glycogenin until the linear glycogen chain reaches 8 units in length (Smythe and Cohen, 1991). The nascent glycogen chain then becomes the substrate for glycogen syn-

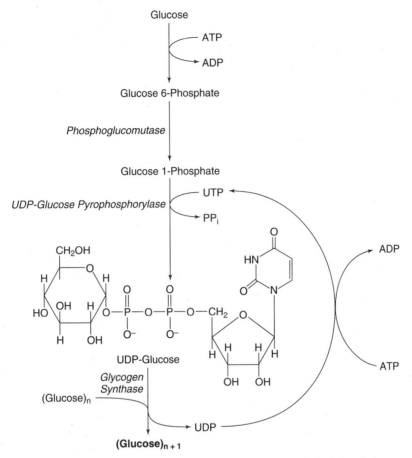

Figure 9–11. *Addition of glucosyl residues to the linear α1→4-linked chains of glycogen.*

thase. The glycogen synthase reaction can be represented as follows:

$$(\text{Glucose})_n + \text{UDP-Glucose} \rightarrow$$
$$(\text{Glucose})_{n+1} + \text{UDP}$$

Because of the UTP requirement for glycogen synthesis, an "ATP" equivalent is required for the glycogen synthase reaction. When added to the ATP used in the glucokinase reaction, this generates an overall energy expenditure of 2 molecules of ATP for the addition of 1 glucose unit to the glycogen polymer.

Glycogen synthase specifically catalyzes the addition of the glucose moiety in the α1→4 orientation; it is not involved in branching, which is the formation of an α1→6-glycosidic bond. A second enzyme, 1,4-α-glucan branching enzyme, is involved in the formation of branch points in the growing glycogen polymer. This branching enzyme cat-

alyzes the transfer of an oligosaccharide chain of approximately 7 glucosyl residues from the nonreducing end (the outer terminal glucosyl residue) of a linear glycogen segment to an interior C-6 of a glucosyl residue at least 4 units away from the last branch site, thus creating a new branch (Fig. 9–12).

Role of Gluconeogenesis in Glycogen Formation

There is an interesting paradox in the synthesis of glycogen in liver. A significant amount of glycogen synthesis in liver is dependent on gluconeogenically derived substrate rather than on glucose entering the hepatocyte directly by facilitated transport. Gluconeogenically derived glucose 6-phosphate in liver is utilized for glycogen synthesis even in the fed state when blood glucose is elevated. In

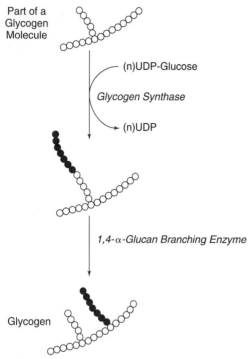

Part of a
Glycogen
Molecule

(n)UDP-Glucose

Glycogen Synthase

(n)UDP

1,4-α-Glucan Branching Enzyme

Glycogen

Figure 9–12. *Pictorial illustration of the growth of glycogen chains and the role of the branching enzyme in the translocation of linear segments of growing chains to create α1→6-linkages and, hence, new branch points.*

contrast, muscle cells directly utilize glucose for synthesis of glycogen.

In humans, approximately one third of the glucose 6-phosphate utilized for glycogen synthesis in liver is gluconeogenically derived. It is postulated that the indirect route of glycogen synthesis in liver utilizes lactate from extrahepatic tissues such as skeletal muscle and red blood cells. In the absorptive phase, it appears that a certain amount of dietary glucose may be metabolized to lactate in peripheral tissues, with the lactate being recirculated to the liver where it becomes a substrate for gluconeogenesis. In the absorptive state, other substrates present in the portal blood, such as amino acids and glycerol, are also potential sources of gluconeogenic carbon for glycogen synthesis.

Glycogenolysis

The glycogen polymer may contain as many as 100,000 glucose units in its branched-chain structure. In humans, the liver is completely depleted of glycogen by 24 hours of fasting. The degradation of this complex molecule begins at the nonreducing ends of the multiple branches and involves the phosphorolysis of single glucose units by glycogen phosphorylase. In the glycogen phosphorylase reaction, an α1→4-glycosidic bond is attacked by inorganic phosphate (P_i), generating glucose 1-phosphate and a shortened glycogen polymer (Fig. 9–13).

$$(Glucose)_n + P_i \rightarrow (Glucose)_{n-1} + \text{Glucose 1-Phosphate}$$

The phosphorylase reaction is repeated successively until the fourth glucose unit from a branch point is reached. Then the bifunctional debranching enzyme (4-α-D-glucanotransferase/amylo-α(1→6)glucosidase) comes into play. It catalyzes the transfer of 3 of the 4 glucose units to the closest nonreducing end to which they are attached in a new α1→4-glycosidic linkage. The debranching enzyme also has α1→6-glucosidase activity and removes the remaining glucose by hydrolysis of the α1→6 linkage at the branch point; this glucosyl residue is released as free glucose (Fig. 9–13). The remaining linear array is now the substrate for continued glycogen phosphorylase activity.

The product of the glycogen phosphorylase reaction, glucose 1-phosphate, is converted to glucose 6-phosphate by phosphoglucomutase. In muscle tissue, the glucose 6-phosphate produced in this reaction is broken down via the glycolytic pathway. In liver, where there is significant glucose 6-phosphatase activity and glycolysis is inhibited under the hormonal conditions that favor hepatic glycogenolysis, most glucose 6-phosphate is converted to free glucose, which is transported from the cell.

REGULATION OF GLYCOGENESIS AND GLYCOGENOLYSIS

The regulatory mechanisms affecting glycogen synthesis and degradation have been well characterized. Glycogen synthase and glycogen phosphorylase are the hormonally regulated enzymes in glycogen synthesis and deg-

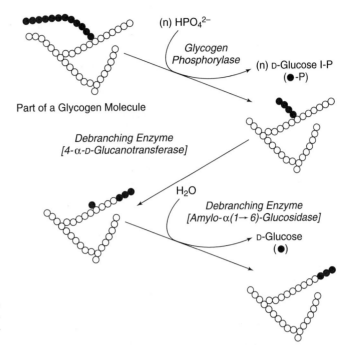

$$(n)\ HPO_4^{2-}$$

Glycogen Phosphorylase

$$(n)\ \text{D-Glucose I-P}$$
$$(\bullet\text{-P})$$

Part of a Glycogen Molecule

*Debranching Enzyme
[4-α-D-Glucanotransferase]*

$$H_2O$$

*Debranching Enzyme
[Amylo-α(1→6)-Glucosidase]*

D-Glucose
$(\bullet)$

Figure 9–13. *Pictorial illustration of the breakdown of glycogen by glycogen phosphorylase and the activities of the debranching enzyme.*

radation, respectively. The anabolic hormone insulin stimulates glycogen synthesis in liver and muscle in the absorptive state. Glucagon, on the other hand, stimulates glycogen degradation in liver when blood glucose levels decline. Epinephrine promotes glycogen degradation in both the liver and skeletal muscle. In the liver, both β-adrenergic and α-adrenergic receptors mediate the response to epinephrine via different signal transduction mechanisms. In skeletal muscle there are no glucagon receptors, but β-adrenergic receptors are stimulated by epinephrine, inducing the cAMP cascade of signaling events. Neural control of glycogen degradation is also important in skeletal muscle.

Regulation of Glycogen Synthase

Glycogen synthase is present in the cell in two different forms; the active form (*a*) is active in the absence of the allosteric modifier, glucose 6-phosphate, and the inactive form (*b*) is dependent on glucose 6-phosphate for activity. Covalent modification of glycogen synthase by phosphorylation converts the enzyme from the *a* to the *b* form. Glycogen synthase is a substrate for numerous protein kinases, including the cAMP-dependent protein kinase

A. The various protein kinases are activated as the result of different intracellular signal transduction pathways, responding to different hormonal and nutrient signals. In addition to protein kinase A, the following protein kinases phosphorylate glycogen synthase: phosphorylase kinase, which itself is phosphorylated by protein kinase A; the calmodulin-dependent protein kinase, which is regulated by calcium binding to calmodulin (see later in this section); protein kinase C, which is activated by diacylglycerol; and glycogen synthase kinase-3 and casein kinases I and II, which are signal transduction enzymes with unidentified stimuli as related to glycogen synthase inhibition.

Each of these protein kinases can convert glycogen synthase *a* to glycogen synthase *b* (Fig 9–14). The reciprocal regulation of both glycogen synthase and glycogen phosphorylase, however, is modulated primarily in response to changes in the intracellular concentration of cAMP and the activation of protein kinase A. In liver, both glucagon receptors and β-adrenergic receptors activate adenylate cyclase and induce the cAMP response; in skeletal muscle, β-adrenergic receptors are responsible for adenylate cyclase activation and increased cAMP production.

CLINICAL CORRELATION

Glycogen Storage Diseases

A lack of glucose 6-phosphatase in liver, kidney, and intestinal mucosa causes Von Gierke's disease (Type I glycogen storage disease). This is caused by a genetic defect in the glucose 6-phosphatase gene that occurs as an autosomal recessive trait in 1 of 200,000 people. This deficiency usually presents in early infancy, and the symptoms include fasting hypoglycemia, hepatomegaly, and recurrent acidosis (Dunger and Holton, 1994). A genetic defect in either the glucose 6-phosphatase enzyme (Type Ia), the glucose 6-phosphatase translocase (Type Ib), or the pyrophosphate transporter (Type Ic) can occur. Individuals with this disease lack the ability to respond to low blood glucose by releasing glucose from either glycogenolysis or gluconeogenesis. This particularly affects the liver's ability to maintain glucose balance in the body by releasing glucose from either of the latter two metabolic sources. The symptoms of this disease can be modified by providing dietary carbohydrate throughout the day so that low blood glucose does not occur.

Tissue-specific mutations in both the liver and muscle glycogen phosphorylase genes occur as rare autosomal recessive disorders. In liver, the metabolic disorder is called Hers' disease (Type VI) and presents in childhood. In this condition, liver glycogen accumulates because the first step in the degradation of glycogen is impaired. Clinical symptoms of this disorder include hypoglycemia, hepatomegaly (which develops slowly), and some growth delay (Fernandes and Chen, 1995). In muscle, the metabolic disorder is referred to as McArdle's disease (Type V), which usually presents in adult life. In early adult life, progressive muscle weakness occurs; however, hepatomegaly and fasting hypoglycemia do not. Individuals with this disease accumulate glycogen in muscle tissue and are exercise intolerant because glucose cannot be released from glycogen to meet the energy demand. There are also genetic disorders in the phosphorylase kinase gene that lead to phosphorylase kinase deficiency in liver and muscle. Phosphorylase kinase deficiency is more common than phosphorylase deficiency and is inherited as an X chromosome-linked recessive trait. Symptoms associated with this disorder are similar to those for phosphorylase deficiency.

A mutation in the gene that encodes "debranching enzyme" can occur in the liver or as a mixed liver-muscle defect. The disorder is referred to as Cori's disease (Type III). Cori's disease leads to the accumulation of glycogen in liver and muscle in the form of branched short chains. Cori's disease usually presents in infancy with symptoms of fasting hypoglycemic convulsions, hepatomegaly, and myopathy (Dunger and Holton, 1994). However, the hypoglycemia and hepatomegaly usually abate by puberty.

Thinking Critically

1. Explain the underlying metabolic basis for development of (a) hypoglycemia, (b) lactic acidosis, and (c) hypertriglyceridemia in patients with glycogen storage disease Type I.

2. What effect does treatment of patients with glycogen storage disease Type I by providing carbohydrate throughout the day (and during the night via infusion of carbohydrate into the gut through a nasogastric tube) have on the overproduction of lactate and triacylglycerol? Explain.

Glycogen synthase is dephosphorylated and converted back to the *a* form by the enzyme phosphoprotein phosphatase. This enzyme, in turn, is regulated by inhibitor-1, present in certain tissues and well-characterized in skeletal muscle. The inhibitor decreases phosphoprotein phosphatase activity, thereby maintaining glycogen synthase in the inactive phosphorylated state. Inhibitor-1, itself, is also a substrate for protein kinase A and phosphoprotein phosphatase; it is active in the phosphorylated state and inactive in the dephosphorylated state (Fig. 9–14). Therefore, cAMP is involved in another activation-inhibition cycle in muscle tissue. When glucagon levels rise, cAMP levels increase, protein kinase A is

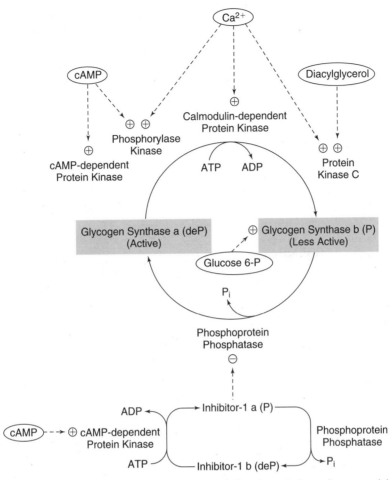

Figure 9–14. *Regulation of glycogen synthase by hormone-induced second messenger and intracellular Ca²⁺ concentrations. Phosphorylated and dephosphorylated proteins are indicated by (P) and (deP), respectively.*

activated, and glycogen synthase is phosphorylated and converted to the inactive *b* form. At the same time, inhibitor-1 is activated by phosphorylation and inhibits phosphoprotein phosphatase. The inhibition of phosphoprotein phosphatase activity maintains glycogen synthase in the *b* form. Therefore, both phosphorylation of glycogen synthase and of inhibitor-1 contribute to the "turning off" of glycogen synthase.

Regulation of Glycogen Phosphorylase

Glycogen phosphorylase is subject to covalent modification by phosphorylation and allosteric activation by AMP and inhibition by ATP (Fig. 9–15). In skeletal muscle, glycogen phosphorylase has an active form, phosphorylase *a*, and an inactive form, phosphorylase *b*.

Phosphorylation at a single seryl residue causes a conformational change to the phosphorylase *a* form. AMP can stimulate glycogen phosphorylase *b*, but not the active glycogen phosphorylase *a*. Overall, in skeletal muscle, the rate of glycogen breakdown depends on the ratio of phosphorylase *a* to phosphorylase *b*. In this tissue, the glucose 1-phosphate produced by the action of glycogen phosphorylase is converted to glucose 6-phosphate and metabolized by the glycolytic pathway to produce ATP for muscle contraction.

The phosphorylation of glycogen phosphorylase is catalyzed by phosphorylase kinase. This protein kinase, itself, is phosphorylated by protein kinase A in response to increased intracellular cAMP. The intracellular cAMP level is increased in skeletal muscle cells in response to epinephrine. The overall

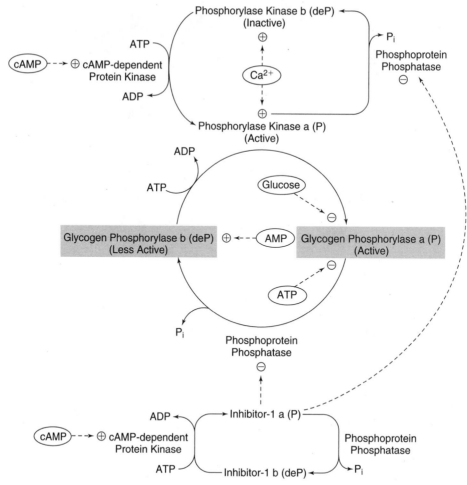

Figure 9–15. *Regulation of glycogen phosphorylase in muscle in response to cAMP and intracellular Ca^{2+} concentrations. Phosphorylated and dephosphorylated proteins are indicated by (P) and (deP), respectively.*

effect is that of a protein kinase cascade that leads to the activation of glycogen phosphorylase. In the presence of cAMP, inhibitor-1 is phosphorylated and active; it inhibits phosphoprotein phosphatase, thereby preventing dephosphorylation of glycogen phosphorylase to its less active form.

Phosphorylase kinase is also regulated by a Ca^{2+}-calmodulin regulatory mechanism. Phosphorylase kinase has a complex molecular structure and consists of 4 subunits. The γ subunit is catalytic, and the α, β, and δ subunits are regulatory. The α and β subunits are phosphorylated by protein kinase A in the activation process. The δ subunit is a Ca^{2+}-binding protein, calmodulin. Calmodulin is an intracellular Ca^{2+} receptor, and it is found in different locations in the cell, either un-

bound or in association with different enzymes. The calmodulin subunit of phosphorylase kinase binds Ca^{2+} when there is Ca^{2+} influx into the cytosol of the cell. This induces a conformational change that activates phosphorylase kinase. Phosphorylation of the α and β subunits by protein kinase A makes phosphorylase kinase more sensitive to further stimulation by calcium. Maximal activation of phosphorylase kinase is achieved by phosphorylation of the α and β subunits, plus calcium binding to the calmodulin subunit.

The importance of this regulation can be seen in skeletal muscle cells, where nerve impulses in muscle contraction depolarize the cell membrane and stimulate calcium efflux from the sarcoplasmic reticulum to the cytosol. The efflux of calcium stimulates phosphorylase kinase by calcium binding to the calmodulin subunit. At the same time, epinephrine released from the adrenal medulla stimulates the intracellular cAMP cascade, which leads to phosphorylation of the α and β subunits of phosphorylase kinase. The synergistic effects of Ca^{2+} and cAMP maximally stimulate phosphorylase kinase. Phosphorylase kinase, in turn, activates glycogen phosphorylase and thereby increases the rate of glycogen breakdown. This assures that glucose is available to meet the increased fuel demands of muscle contraction. Concurrently, Ca^{2+} stimulates the calmodulin-dependent protein kinase, which phosphorylates and inhibits the anabolic enzyme glycogen synthase.

Allosteric modification of glycogen phosphorylase by ATP and AMP is a faster mechanism (milliseconds) of regulation than is hormone-induced covalent modification (seconds to minutes). In general, these two mechanisms function in an ordered sequence. For example, in muscle contraction, glycogen phosphorylase *b*, but not glycogen phosphorylase *a*, is allosterically stimulated by AMP. When resting muscle begins to contract and AMP levels increase, this rapidly stimulates phosphorylase *b*. As muscle contraction continues, however, epinephrine stimulation of the cAMP-induced protein kinase cascade increases the concentration of phosphorylase *a*, thereby continuing the breakdown of glycogen regardless of the AMP concentration. Conversely, in the resting state, the phosphorylase *b* form predominates and ATP levels are high. Under these conditions, ATP inhibits any AMP stimulation of phosphorylase *b*, and there is no stimulation of phosphorylase *a* formation by epinephrine. Therefore, when muscle is at rest, glycogenolysis is inactive.

In the liver, glycogen breakdown serves a different metabolic function than it does in muscle tissue. Glycogenolysis provides glucose for release into the circulation to maintain normal blood glucose levels (4 to 5 mmol/L). Glycogenolysis, therefore, is regulated somewhat differently in liver than in muscle tissue. Although there is an *a* and a *b* form of glycogen phosphorylase in liver, as in muscle, the hormonal stimulus for this conversion is primarily glucagon. Furthermore, in liver, glycogen phosphorylase is allosterically regulated by glucose and not by the AMP/ATP ratio. In hepatocytes, glucose can bind to an allosteric site on phosphorylase *a* and change the conformation of the enzyme so that it becomes a good substrate for phosphoprotein phosphatase. Glucose, therefore, stimulates the dephosphorylation of phosphorylase *a* to phosphorylase *b* in liver. This regulatory mechanism ensures that glycogenolysis will be slowed under conditions of elevated blood glucose.

Although glucagon is the major hormonal stimuli for hepatic glycogenolysis, epinephrine can also stimulate the mobilization of glycogen in liver. In humans, this response involves either epinephrine stimulation of the pancreatic α cell to secrete glucagon, or the binding of epinephrine to the β-adrenergic receptor on the liver cell to stimulate adenylate cyclase and increase intracellular cAMP. A third mechanism of epinephrine action involves epinephrine binding to the $α_1$-adrenergic receptor on the liver cell. Activation of the $α_1$-adrenergic receptor stimulates phospholipase C on the cytoplasmic face of the plasma membrane by a GTP-binding protein mechanism. Phospholipase C cleaves phosphatidylinositol bisphosphate (PIP_2), present in the membrane, to inositol triphosphate (IP_3) and diacylglycerol. Diacylglycerol, in turn, stimulates protein kinase C. Protein kinase C has numerous substrates in the cell; among these is glycogen synthase *a*, which is inactivated by phosphorylation. At the same time, IP_3 stimulates the release of Ca^{2+} from the ER, and calcium efflux activates phosphorylase kinase, which activates glycogen phosphorylase. The combined effect of the second messengers derived from PIP_2 is the enhancement of glycogenolysis in response to epinephrine in liver. It is not known, however, which of the preceding mechanisms of epinephrine stimulation of hepatic glycogenolysis is physiologically predominant in humans.

Regulation of Gene Expression

There is less information on the genes that encode the enzymes of glycogen synthesis and degradation than there is on certain of the glycolytic and gluconeogenic genes. The genes for glycogen synthase, glycogen phosphorylase, and the phosphorylase kinase catalytic subunit have been isolated. Regulation of the glycogen synthase and glycogen phosphorylase genes has been studied to a limited extent. Starvation significantly decreases hepatic glycogen synthase concentration in an experimental rat model, whereas refeeding returns the glycogen synthase concentration to control values. This is thought to be due to changes in glycogen synthase mRNA translation, as glycogen synthase mRNA levels do not change significantly with starvation and refeeding. The glycogen phosphorylase gene

has been shown to be regulated by chronic diabetes and insulin treatment. The stability of glycogen phosphorylase mRNA is increased by the diabetic state and can be normalized by insulin treatment.

PYRUVATE DEHYDROGENASE COMPLEX AND CITRIC ACID CYCLE

The aerobic phase of macronutrient catabolism is referred to as cellular respiration. The metabolic stages involved in cellular respiration are the production of acetyl CoA from

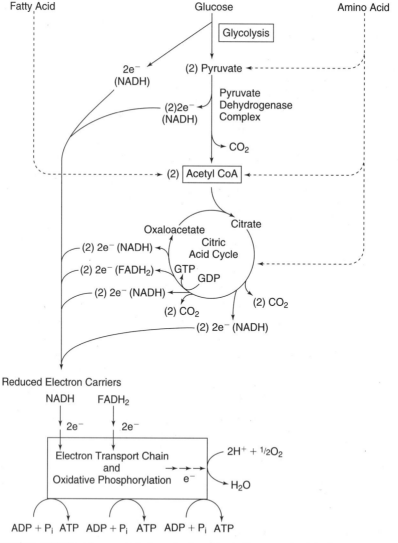

Figure 9–16. *Complete oxidation of pyruvate in the mitochondria via the pyruvate dehydrogenase complex (oxidative decarboxylation), the citric acid cycle, and the electron (e^-) transport chain.*

pyruvate (or fatty acids or specific amino acids), the complete oxidation of the acetyl moiety of acetyl CoA via the citric acid cycle, the utilization of reducing equivalents from the citric acid cycle for electron transport, and the production of ATP by oxidative phosphorylation (Fig. 9–16).

Together with the pyruvate dehydrogenase complex, the enzymes of the citric acid cycle are present in the mitochondrial compartment of the cell. The reactions of glycolysis take place in the cytosol of the cell; therefore, pyruvate produced as the end product of glycolysis needs to be translocated to the mitochondria. Pyruvate is transported across the inner mitochondrial membrane by a monocarboxylate carrier and is then converted to acetyl CoA by the pyruvate dehydrogenase complex. The acetyl CoA so produced then enters the citric acid cycle. The citric acid cycle is usually referred to as a cycle because one of the "substrates" (oxaloacetate) is regenerated in the process of oxidation of the other substrate, acetyl CoA. Although the complete citric acid cycle functions only in the mitochondria, it should be noted that some enzymes of the citric acid cycle also have cytosolic forms (i.e., cytosolic aconitase, isocitrate dehydrogenase, fumarase, and ma-

late dehydrogenase) and that particular citric acid cycle enzymes in the mitochondria also may play other roles in metabolism.

The Pyruvate Dehydrogenase Complex

The pyruvate dehydrogenase complex, associated with the mitochondrial inner membrane of mammalian cells, catalyzes the conversion of pyruvate to acetyl CoA. The overall reaction involves the activity of three individual enzymes, the activities of which are coordinated by association in a multienzyme complex. There are multiple copies of the three enzymes in this complex; the complex includes pyruvate dehydrogenase (E_1), dihydrolipoyl transacetylase (E_2), and dihydrolipoyl dehydrogenase (E_3) (Fig. 9–17). The overall reaction is essentially irreversible and converts the 3-carbon intermediate, pyruvate, to acetyl CoA. Acetyl CoA, in turn, can be either oxidized via the citric acid cycle or utilized for fatty acid synthesis, isoprenoid/cholesterol/steroid synthesis, or ketone body synthesis, as discussed in Chapter 13.

The pyruvate dehydrogenase complex in mammals contains numerous coenzymes derived primarily from the B vitamin family. These coenzymes include thiamin pyrophos-

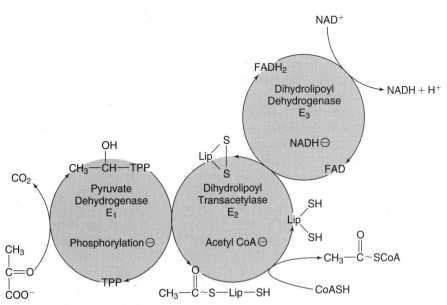

Figure 9–17. Oxidative decarboxylation of pyruvate by the pyruvate dehydrogenase complex. FAD, flavin adenine dinucleotide; Lip, enzyme-bound lipoate; NAD, nicotinamide adenine dinucleotide; TPP, thiamin pyrophosphate. Negative effectors of E_1, E_2, and E_3 enzymes are shown.

phate (TPP), derived from thiamin; flavin adenine dinucleotide (FAD), derived from riboflavin; coenzyme A (CoA), derived from pantothenic acid; nicotinamide adenine dinucleotide (NAD), derived from niacin; and lipoate. These coenzymes perform specific functions in the activity of the three individual enzymes of the pyruvate dehydrogenase complex. These coenzymes are discussed in Chapters 20 and 22.

The first reaction of the multienzyme series is the decarboxylation of pyruvate, catalyzed by pyruvate dehydrogenase (E_1), requiring the coenzyme TPP (Fig. 9–17). The two electrons removed in this reaction and the acetyl group are transferred by E_1 to lipoate, which is attached to the second enzyme, dihydrolipoyl transacetylase (E_2). In the next reaction, the acetyl group is transferred by a transesterification reaction to CoA, generating acetyl CoA; concomitantly, lipoate is fully reduced. The third enzyme, dihydrolipoyl dehydrogenase (E_3) transfers 2 hydrogen atoms from reduced lipoate to the coenzyme FAD bound to E_3, generating $FADH_2$ and regenerating the oxidized form of lipoate on E_2. A subsequent oxidation/reduction reaction transfers the hydrogen atoms of $FADH_2$ to NAD^+, forming $NADH + H^+$. The completion of these reactions produces CO_2, acetyl CoA, reducing equivalents in the form of NADH, and the regenerated enzyme complex prepared for another catalytic cycle.

Because the pyruvate dehydrogenase reaction commits carbon intermediates from glucose and amino acid catabolism to either the citric acid cycle or lipid synthesis, the enzymes of the complex are tightly regulated. The pyruvate dehydrogenase complex is regulated primarily by end product inhibition and covalent modification (Behal et al., 1993). The products of the individual enzyme reactions, acetyl CoA and NADH, act as negative feedback inhibitors of their respective reactions; acetyl CoA inhibits dihydrolipoyl transacetylase and NADH inhibits dihydrolipoyl dehydrogenase. The multienzyme complex is also inactivated by phosphorylation of pyruvate dehydrogenase (E_1) by a specific protein kinase that is bound to the enzyme.

The end product inhibitors acetyl CoA and NADH also stimulate phosphorylation of E_1, whereas pyruvate, free CoA, and NAD^+ inhibit this phosphorylation. Therefore, when the mitochondrial [NADH]/[NAD] or [acetyl CoA]/[CoA] ratio is maintained relatively high by the oxidation of fatty acids for energy, the production of acetyl CoA from pyruvate is restrained via inhibition of the activity of the pyruvate dehydrogenase complex. This allows tissues, such as the heart, to "spare" glucose and utilize fatty acids or ketone bodies for energy needs.

Fasting decreases pyruvate dehydrogenase activity significantly in tissues such as heart, kidney, and skeletal muscle, and this can be reversed by refeeding. In the brain, on the other hand, the pyruvate dehydrogenase complex is necessary for ATP production, and pyruvate dehydrogenase activity is not reduced with fasting or starvation.

The Citric Acid Cycle

The metabolic fate of acetyl CoA varies, depending upon dietary carbohydrate intake, the energy level of the cell, and the cell type. To meet the energy needs of the cell, acetyl CoA can be completely oxidized by the enzymes of the citric acid cycle (Fig. 9–18). If the energy needs of the cell have been met, an alternative route for acetyl CoA utilization is for the biosynthesis of fatty acids in liver and other lipogenic tissues. Only the oxidation of acetyl CoA via the citric acid cycle is considered in this chapter; other fates of acetyl CoA are discussed in Chapter 13. This cycle is also referred to as the tricarboxylic acid (TCA) cycle or as the Krebs cycle, after Sir Hans Krebs who proposed this pathway in 1937.

The condensation of acetyl CoA and oxaloacetate to form citrate marks the beginning of one round of the citric acid cycle, and the regeneration of oxaloacetate marks the completion of one round of the citric acid cycle. The energy transferred in the catabolism of acetyl CoA via the citric acid cycle is carried in the reduced coenzymes and in GTP produced by substrate level phosphorylation (Fig. 9–18). For each molecule of acetyl CoA that enters the cycle, 2 molecules of CO_2 are formed from the acetate moiety, and reducing equivalents are produced in the form of 3

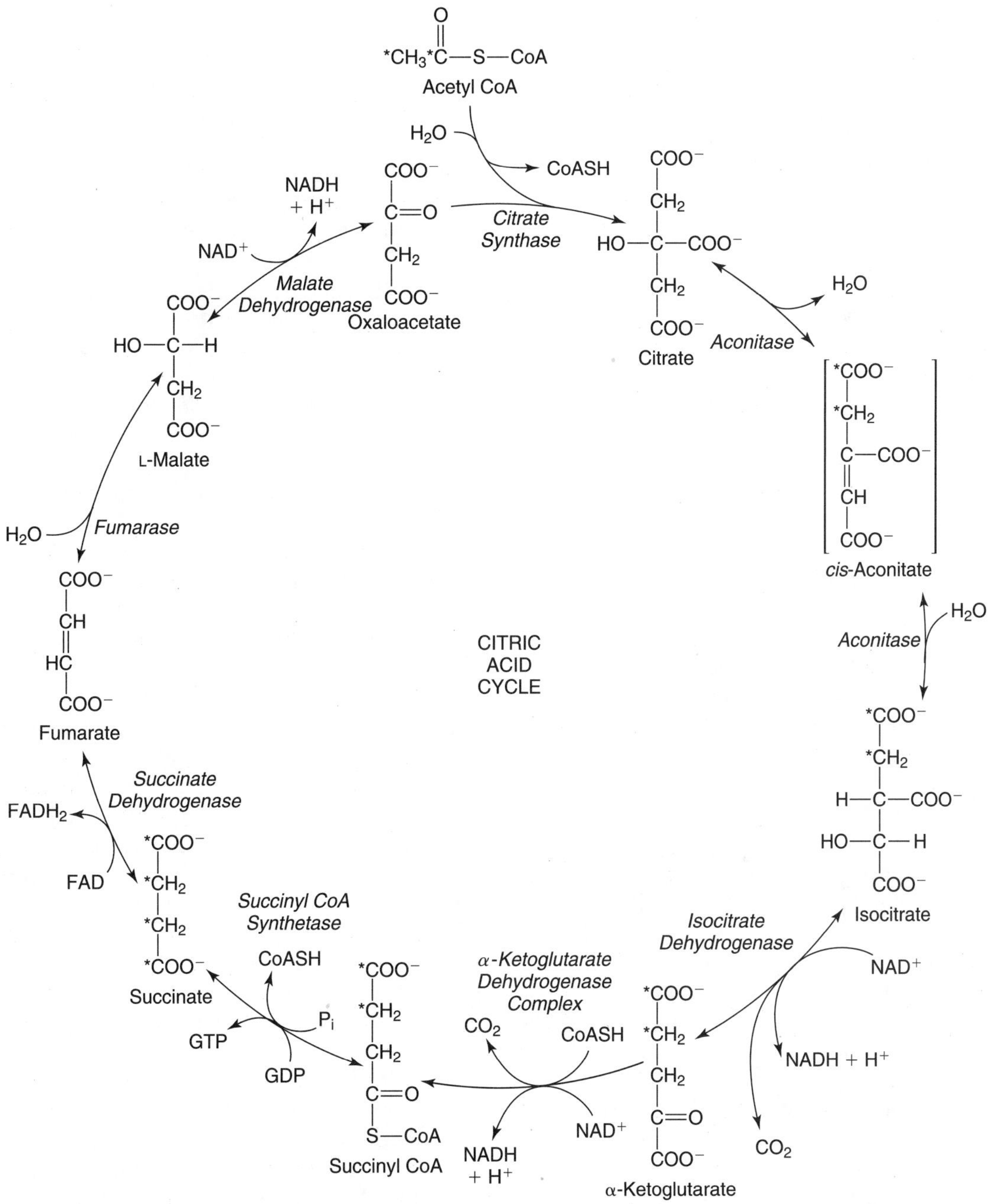

Figure 9–18. *The oxidation of acetyl CoA and generation of reducing equivalents and ATP equivalents by the citric acid cycle. Although these reactions result in the net oxidation of the acetyl group to 2 CO_2, the actual carbons lost as CO_2 in a single round of the cycle are derived from oxaloacetate. The carbons denoted by the asterisks are those from the acetate moiety of acetyl CoA. Because succinate and fumarate are symmetrical molecules, C-1 and C-2 cannot be distinguished from C-3 and C-4 once these intermediates are formed.*

molecules of NADH and 1 molecule of $FADH_2$. From 1 molecule of NADH entering the electron transport chain, a maximum of 3 molecules of ATP are produced by oxidative phosphorylation. $FADH_2$ generates a maximum of 2 molecules of ATP by oxidative phosphorylation. Therefore, the reducing equivalents produced in one round of the citric acid cycle generate a maximum of 11 molecules of ATP. To this can be added the molecule of ATP (from GTP) produced by substrate-level phosphorylation at the succinyl CoA synthetase step. Taken together, a maximum of 12 molecules of ATP are produced as a result of the complete oxidation of acetate from acetyl CoA through the citric acid cycle.

The total amount of ATP produced from the complete oxidation of glucose to CO_2 and H_2O can be summarized at this point. In glycolysis, the conversion of 1 molecule of glucose to 2 molecules of pyruvate produces a net gain of 2 molecules of ATP from substrate-level phosphorylation. Reducing equivalents (2 molecules of NADH) are also generated in the glyceraldehyde 3-phosphate dehydrogenase reaction. These reducing equivalents generate a maximum of 4 to 6 molecules of ATP after translocation of electrons to the mitochondrion (depending on the mode of transport across the inner membrane of the mitochondrion). Therefore, under aerobic conditions in those cells with mitochondria, 6 to 8 molecules of ATP are produced as a result of the breakdown of 1 molecule of glucose to 2 molecules of pyruvate. The pyruvate dehydrogenase reaction in the mitochondrion generates reducing equivalents as well; 2 molecules of NADH are produced from the conversion of 2 molecules of pyruvate to 2 molecules of acetyl CoA. Therefore, this step generates up to 6 molecules of ATP from electron transport and oxidative phosphorylation.

As detailed, 24 molecules of ATP are generated in the mitochondria from oxidation of 2 acetate moieties by the citric acid cycle coupled with the electron transport chain and oxidative phosphorylation. These ATPs are derived from 1 substrate-level ATP, 3 NADH, and 1 $FADH_2$ formed per acetyl CoA that is completely oxidized by the citric acid cycle. Overall, the total energy generated from the complete oxidation of 1 molecule of glucose to 6 molecules of CO_2 and H_2O is as much as 36 to 38 molecules of ATP.

ELECTRON TRANSPORT AND OXIDATIVE PHOSPHORYLATION

The ability of a cell to generate energy from macronutrients under aerobic conditions is dependent on the number of mitochondria it contains. Cardiac muscle cells are very dependent on aerobic metabolism; these cells contain a high concentration of mitochondria, more so than skeletal muscle cells. The mitochondrial space takes up approximately 50% of the total cytoplasmic volume in cardiac muscle cells. Liver cells contain a similarly high concentration of mitochondria. The amount of oxygen consumed by various tissues in the human adult varies, depending upon the mitochondrial respiratory capacity of the tissue and physiological activity. Skeletal muscle utilizes approximately 30% of consumed oxygen at rest, but with heavy exercise, skeletal muscle may use over 86% of consumed oxygen. The brain and abdominal tissue also consume large percentages of oxygen at rest.

In order to understand the enzymatic reactions that occur during electron transport with subsequent oxidative phosphorylation and ATP production, it is important to understand the cellular physiology that makes it possible. This requires a description of the structure of the mitochondrion as it occupies space within the cytoplasm of the cell. The mitochondrion is a very membranous organelle. The membrane structures effectively divide the mitochondrion into functional subcompartments. There is an outer membrane and an inner membrane, with numerous invaginations referred to as cristae; between these two membranes is the intermembrane space. The space inside the inner membrane is the matrix. Associated with the inner membrane are most of the enzymes involved in electron transport and oxidative phosphorylation, as well as carrier proteins for metabolic intermediates that are transported between the cytosol and the mitochondrial matrix. The inner membrane is much less permeable than the outer membrane to the metabolic intermediates and nucleotides that are important in energy metabolism. The outer membrane is permeable because it contains large, channel-forming proteins called porins. In effect, the intermembrane space is similar in composition to the cytosolic space because the outer membrane is so permeable. Consequently, it is the inner membrane that effectively separates the mitochondrial and cytosolic domains of the cell. This inner membrane is not permeable to oxaloacetate, NADH, or NAD^+, but it does have transporters for malate/α-ketoglutarate, aspartate/glutamate, and phosphoenolpyruvate, as well as pyruvate, citrate/malate, ATP, ADP, and phosphate.

Shuttle of Reducing Equivalents Across the Inner Mitochondrial Membrane

The oxidation-reduction pairs that are involved in electron transport (e.g., NAD^+/NADH, $NADP^+$/NADPH, and FAD/$FADH_2$) cannot diffuse across the inner mitochondrial membrane. Specific transport mechanisms compensate for the impermeability of this membrane to these cofactors. The transport of reducing equivalents (protons and electrons) from the cytosol to the mitochondrial matrix is carried out by substrate shuttles. The most active of these shuttle systems is the malate-aspartate shuttle. Malate carries reducing equivalents, which were generated as NADH and then used to reduce oxaloacetate to malate in the cytosol, to the mitochondrial matrix. In the mitochondria, NADH is regenerated by conversion of malate back to oxaloacetate, which can then be transaminated to aspartate and exit from the mitochondria. Cytosolic and mitochondrial isozymes of malate dehydrogenase catalyze the interconversion of malate and oxaloacetate. The malate-aspartate shuttle functions primarily in liver, heart muscle, and kidney. NADH, whether regenerated in the mitochondrial matrix from cytosolic reducing equivalents or generated within the mitochondrial matrix by the citric acid cycle and other reactions, can be oxidized by the mitochondrial respiratory chain.

In skeletal muscle and brain, another NADH shuttle mechanism occurs. This is the glycerol 3-phosphate shuttle, which does not involve transport of organic compounds but of electrons by the inner membrane flavoprotein, α-glycerol-phosphate dehydrogenase. Dihydroxyacetone phosphate, substrate for the cytosolic glycerol 3-phosphate dehydrogenase, accepts two reducing equivalents from NADH, producing glycerol 3-phosphate and NAD^+ in the cytosol. Another isozyme of glycerol 3-phosphate dehydrogenase, located on the outer face of the inner mitochondrial membrane, transfers two reducing equivalents

from glycerol 3-phosphate in the intermembrane space, via an FAD coenzyme, to ubiquinone within the inner mitochondrial membrane. The glycerol 3-phosphate shuttle is different from the malate-aspartate shuttle in that the reducing equivalents are transferred from ubiquinone to complex III (the cytochrome bc_1 complex), thus bypassing the NADH dehydrogenase complex of the electron transport chain and leading to the synthesis of a maximum of only 2 molecules of ATP rather than the 3 molecules of ATP possible when electrons enter the chain at the level of NADH. (See Figs. 17–2 and 20–7 in Chapters 17 and 20.)

Another critical transport step that occurs at the inner mitochondrial membrane is the transfer of adenine nucleotides by the adenine nucleotide translocator. In this case, cytosolic ADP produced in the hydrolysis of ATP is exchanged across the inner membrane for ATP produced by oxidative phosphorylation. This exchanger provides ADP as substrate for oxidative phosphorylation at the same time as it removes the product from the mitochondrial compartment.

Although the focus of the preceding discussion has been on the flow of reducing equivalents into the mitochondria, shuttles also exist that carry potential reducing equivalents from the mitochondrial compartment into the cytosol for use in reductive synthetic processes. The transfer of substrate as well as reducing equivalents from the mitochondria to the cytosol is discussed in Chapter 11 for gluconeogenesis from amino acids and in Chapter 13 for lipogenesis from acetyl CoA.

Electron Transport

The electron transport chain is another example of a pathway channeling metabolic intermediates in a series of linked enzymatic reactions. These are oxidation-reduction reactions, and the oxidized and reduced forms of the molecules are referred to as redox pairs. The electron carrier molecules involved in electron transport are integral membrane proteins, with cofactors or fat-soluble molecules that can freely diffuse into and out of the inner membrane. At three distinct steps in electron transport, the oxidation-reduction potential decreases and energy release is coupled to formation of a proton gradient across the inner mitochondrial membrane; the amount of energy trapped in the proton gradient at each step is sufficient to drive the synthesis of ATP. The three electron transfer steps where this occurs are the reduction of FMN by NADH in complex I, the reduction of cytochrome c_i by cytochrome b in complex III, and the reduction of molecular oxygen by cytochrome a_3 in complex IV (cytochrome c oxidase). These oxidation-reduction reactions produce sufficient energy to effectively pump protons out of the mitochondrial matrix to the intermembrane space. A proton concentration gradient is established, which changes the pH (rendering the matrix more alkaline) and electrical charge (rendering the matrix more negative) across the inner mitochondrial membrane. The electrochemical energy built up across the inner membrane is utilized, in part, for the synthesis of ATP. (See Fig. 17–2.)

The movement of electrons via a series of oxidation-reduction reactions that make up the electron transport chain in the inner membrane of the mitochondrion is a specific example of energy transfer in linked, exergonic reactions. The large free energy generated from this process is capable of producing ATP. The question remains: What is the mechanism by which energy generated by electron transport is coupled to the production of ATP? The accepted theory is the chemiosmotic theory, which postulates that the proton-motive force generated from the proton concentration difference across the inner mitochondrial membrane conserves energy for ATP production. ATP is produced when this energy is released by the movement of protons according to their downhill gradient, returning to the matrix via specific proton pores in the membrane (the inner membrane itself is impermeable to protons). The pore or channel through which protons move is provided by a subunit structure of the mitochondrial ATP synthase that spans the inner membrane. The mitochondrial ATP synthase is an F-type ATPase, which is characterized as an ATP-dependent proton pump.

Generally, F-type ATPases utilize the energy of ATP hydrolysis to move protons against a concentration gradient. The reverse occurs in oxidative phosphorylation. The spontaneous flow of protons through the channel, provided by the ATP synthase subunit (F_0) in the membrane, releases energy for the synthesis of ATP from enzyme-bound ADP and P_i. The latter enzymatic reaction is catalyzed by the second ATP synthase subunit (F_1) on the interior side of the inner mitochondrial membrane.

Thus, the three sites in electron transport that pump protons to the intermembrane space generate the electrochemical energy for ATP synthesis. The electrochemical energy difference generated across the inner mitochondrial membrane is referred to as the proton-motive force. This force is the amount of free energy available to do work when protons flow passively back into the mitochondrial

---

CLINICAL CORRELATION

Mutations in Mitochondrial DNA

Autosomal recessive defects occur in the proteins of the respiratory chain. Two genomes are involved in the coding of respiratory chain proteins: the nuclear genome and the mitochondrial genome. Mitochondrial DNA (mtDNA) is circular and encodes 13 proteins, which are synthesized in this compartment of the cell. These proteins include 7 subunits of complex I, one subunit of complex III, three subunits of cytochrome C oxidase, and two subunits of the ATP synthase (Bindoff and Turnbull, 1994).

Current evidence shows that mutations in the mtDNA are responsible for numerous degenerative disorders of skeletal muscle, heart, central nervous system, and the eye (Shoffner and Wallace, 1994). Biochemical analyses indicate that many of the clinical syndromes caused by mtDNA mutations involve multiple respiratory chain defects, although single deficiencies have also been reported.

matrix. The electrochemical energy generated by complexes I, III, and IV is each sufficient for, and coupled to, ATP synthesis. Therefore, 3 molecules of ATP are generated from the oxidation-reduction reactions initiated by NADH entry into the electron transport chain. Only 2 molecules of ATP are generated from $FADH_2$, which donates electrons to oxidized ubiquinone, bypassing the oxidation-reduction reactions of complex I and the free energy derived therefrom. Approximately 40% of the free energy generated in electron transport is conserved in the form of ATP; the remaining energy is dissipated as heat. (See Chapter 17 for more about electron transport and oxidative phosphorylation.)

OTHER PATHWAYS OF CARBOHYDRATE METABOLISM

Pentose Phosphate Pathway

The pentose phosphate pathway serves as a secondary pathway of glucose oxidation, a source of reducing equivalents in the form of NADPH, and as a means of generation of 5-carbon sugar phosphates, particularly ribose 5-phosphate. The pentose phosphate pathway is also called the hexose monophosphate shunt or the phosphogluconate pathway. The first three steps of the pathway shown in Figure 9–19 are involved in the oxidation of glucose 6-phosphate to ribulose 5-phosphate,

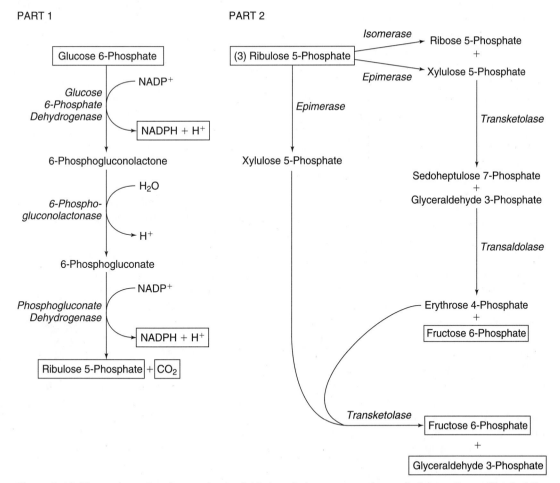

Figure 9–19. The pentose phosphate pathway. Oxidation of glucose occurs in part I of the pathway. Part II of the pathway shows the rearrangement of 3 molecules of ribulose 5-P to re-form glycolytic intermediates, fructose 6-phosphate and glyceraldehyde 3-phosphate.

which can be transformed to ribose 5-phosphate or xylulose 5-phosphate.

NADPH is formed in the first and third steps, which are catalyzed by glucose 6-phosphate dehydrogenase and phosphogluconate dehydrogenase, respectively. Glucose 6-phosphate dehydrogenase is regulated by the $NADP^+$ concentration (substrate availability), and the need for NADPH regeneration determines flux through this pathway. Glucose 6-phosphate dehydrogenase is considered a lipogenic enzyme because the NADPH generated by the pentose phosphate pathway is required for synthesis of fatty acids, cholesterol, and other sterols. The tissues most heavily involved in fatty acid and cholesterol biosynthesis (mammary gland, adipose tissue, liver, adrenal cortex, and testis) are rich in pentose phosphate pathway enzymes. The gene that encodes glucose 6-phosphate dehydrogenase has been isolated and shown to be regulated by fasting and refeeding and by dietary fatty acids in the liver, consistent with the important role of the encoded enzyme in lipogenesis in liver (Stabile et al., 1996). The pentose phosphate pathway is also active in red blood cells, which require NADPH for reduction of glutathione. Reduced glutathione is required by red blood cells for maintenance of their redox state and thus of the integrity of the red blood cell membrane. Without adequate NADPH, the red blood cell membrane lyses and hemolytic anemia results. Oxidation of glucose by the pentose phosphate pathway occurs in the cytosol and is not dependent upon the presence of mitochondria.

The ribulose 5-phosphate produced from glucose 6-phosphate by the first three steps of the pentose phosphate pathway serves as a source of ribose 5-phosphate, which can be formed by isomerization of ribulose 5-phosphate. Ribose 5-phosphate is essential for the biosynthesis of nucleotides and nucleic acids, including ATP, CoA, NAD, NADP, FAD, RNA, and DNA. If the cell needs the pentose phosphates produced from glucose 6-phosphate, the pathway may stop at the level of the pentose phosphates. Alternatively, a series of reversible reactions can convert excess ribose 5-phosphate and xylulose 5-phosphate to the glycolytic intermediates fructose 6-phosphate and glyceraldehyde 3-phosphate, as shown in part II of Figure 9–19. Fructose 6-phosphate and glyceraldehyde 3-phosphate can reenter glycolysis or be converted to glucose 6-phosphate and enter other pathways of glucose metabolism. These sugar rearrangements also allow for degradation of ribose 5-phosphate from nucleotide degradation. Because the reactions involved in these sugar rearrangements are freely reversible, cells that need pentose phosphates also can form them by conversion of glycolytic intermediates to pentoses without net oxidation of glucose to CO_2 and without NADPH production.

Although only the 1-carbon of glucose 6-phosphate is lost as CO_2 in the pentose phosphate pathway, net oxidation of glucose can occur if both parts I and II of the pathway, as shown in Figure 9–19, are operative. This occurs when the need for NADPH is greater than the need for ribose 5-phosphate. If 6 molecules of glucose 6-phosphate are oxidized to 6 molecules of pentose 5-phosphate, and these pentoses are further rearranged to form 4 molecules of fructose 6-phosphate and 2 molecules of glyceraldehyde 3-phosphate (the equivalent of 5 molecules of hexose), net conversion of 1 molecule of glucose to 6 CO_2 will have occurred with net production of 12 NADPH.

Formation of Sugar Derivatives for Synthesis of Glucuronides, Lactose, and Other Carbohydrates

Various sugars and sugar derivatives are formed from glucose phosphate. These have a variety of functions in the body, including serving as substrate for glucuronidation pathways; for synthesis of glycosaminoglycans, glycoproteins, and glycolipids; and as substrate for lactose synthesis by the mammary gland. The amount of glucose that is consumed by these pathways is generally small relative to the amount that is catabolized via glycolysis and the citric acid cycle.

Glururonide formation is an important pathway of glucose consumption in the liver. UDP-glucose, formed by reaction of glucose 1-phosphate with UTP, is oxidized to UDP-glucuronate. UDP-glucuronate serves as the glucuronosyl donor in various detoxification and elimination reactions in which conjugates of glucuronate and nonpolar acceptor molecules are formed.

$$\text{UDP-Glucuronate} + \text{R-OH} \rightarrow$$
$$\text{R-O-Glucuronate} + \text{UDP}$$

Many drugs, such as the anti-AIDS drug 3'-azido-2'-3'-dideoxythymidine (AZT) or the over-the-counter drug acetaminophen, and endogenous compounds, such as bilirubin, are conjugated with glucuronate to form more polar compounds that are more readily excreted in the urine and bile. (See Chapter 40 for further discussion of the role of glucuronidation in detoxification processes.) UDP-glucuronate can be converted to glucuronate, which can be converted to xylulose 5-phosphate, a pentose phosphate pathway intermediate. In most species other than primates, glucuronate serves as a substrate for ascorbic acid synthesis (see Chapter 23; Fig. 23–1). Because humans and other primates lack one of the enzymes in this pathway, gulonolactone oxidase, ascorbic acid must be supplied in the diet.

Pathways for interconversion of galactose, glucose, fructose, and mannose were shown in Figure 9–4. Additional pathways exist to form a number of other sugar derivatives, many in the form of nucleotide diphosphate sugars. These include GDP-L-fucose from GDP-mannose; UDP-*N*-acetylglucosamine, UDP-*N*-acetylgalactosamine, and CMP-*N*-acetylneuraminic acid (one of the sialic acids) from glucose phosphate or fructose phosphate; dTDP-rhamnose from glucose phosphate; and UDP-galactose from galactose phosphate or UDP-glucose.

The disaccharide lactose is synthesized by the lactating mammary gland. The mammary enzyme lactose synthase is induced in response to release of the hormone prolactin. UDP-galactose and glucose are substrates; a glycosidic bond is formed between galactose and glucose to form β-galactosyl(1→4)glucose, commonly known as lactose.

Synthesis of Glycosaminoglycans and Proteoglycans

Glycosaminoglycan chains are long, unbranched, heteropolysaccharide chains made up largely of disaccharide repeating units, with a hexosamine and a uronic acid commonly found in the repeating structure. In many glycosaminoglycans, these sugars are sulfated. Both the carboxylate groups of the uronic acid units and sulfate groups, linked either to hydroxyl groups of the sugar residues or to amino groups of the hexosamine residues, are responsible for the large number of negative charges associated with these compounds. Six classes of glycosaminoglycans are recognized: hyaluronate, chondroitin sulfate, dermatan sulfate, heparin, heparan sulfate, and keratan sulfate. Most of these are found covalently attached to protein in proteoglycan and are present mainly in the extracellular matrix of tissues. Exceptions include hyaluronate, which is not known to exist covalently attached to protein, and heparin, which is found as an intracellular component of mast cells.

The oligosaccharide chains of glycosaminoglycans contain sugars linked to other sugars by glycosidic bonds. Chrondroitin sulfate, dermatan sulfate, heparin, heparan sulfate, and keratan sulfate chains are synthesized in the lumen of the ER by transfer of glycosyl units from nucleotide diphosphate (NDP) derivatives to the nonreducing end of an acceptor sugar or oligosaccharide chain.

$$\text{NDP-Sugar (Donor)} +$$
$$\text{Sugar or Oligosaccharide (Acceptor)} \rightarrow$$
$$\text{Glycosyl-O-Glycose (Glycoside)} + \text{NDP}$$

Hyaluronic acid, on the other hand, is synthesized in association with the plasma membrane using UDP-glucuronate and UDP-*N*-acetylglucosamine as precursors; sugar units are added to the reducing end of the chain by hyaluronan synthase.

Proteoglycans are high molecular weight polyanionic substances that consist of many different glycosaminoglycan chains linked covalently to a protein core. Because proteoglycans may contain as much as 95% carbohydrate, their properties tend to resemble those of polysaccharides more than those of proteins. The polysaccharide chains (glycosaminoglycan chains) of proteoglycans are assembled by the sequential action of a series of glycosyltransferases in the lumen of the ER.

These glycosyltransferases catalyze the transfer of a monosaccharide from an NDP-sugar to the appropriate acceptor, either the nonreducing end of another sugar or an amino acid side chain on a polypeptide. In chrondroitin sulfate proteoglycan formation, for example, sugar units are added to the core protein to form a tetrasaccharide linkage region followed by alternate addition of the characteristic repeating N-acetylgalactosamine and glucuronate units of chrondroitin sulfate and by sulfation of the N-acetylgalactosamine residues in either the 4 or 6 position.

Proteoglycans are found in tissues such as cartilage, tendons, ligaments, aorta, skin, blood vessels, and heart valves. Proteoglycans are usually found together with fibrous proteins, such as collagen and elastin, in the extracellular matrix. The network of proteoglycans and the cross-linked fibers of collagen or elastin provide the extracellular matrix with tensile strength, as is found in tendons, or elasticity, as is found in ligaments. Additionally, an intricate attachment is formed between cells and the proteoglycans of extracellular matrix. Integrins, integral membrane proteins of the cell, have an extracellular domain that binds members of a family of adhesion proteins, and these adhesion proteins also bind to proteoglycans. Thus, integrins and the extracellular adhesion proteins form an attachment between cells and the surrounding proteoglycans of the extracellular matrix. Common adhesion proteins are fibrin and laminin.

Chondroitin sulfates are the most abundant glycosaminoglycan in the body. Most chains consist of between 60 and 100 sugar residues made up mainly of alternating N-acetylgalactosamine and glucuronate units. A typical chondroitin sulfate proteoglycan has about 100 chondroitin sulfate chains attached to the protein core. These chondroitin sulfate proteoglycans are abundant in cartilage, tendons, ligaments, and aorta.

Although hyaluronate chains are not covalently attached to proteins, hyaluronate can serve as a central strand around which proteoglycan molecules are organized. Hyaluronate chains can be very long (approximately 10^6 sugar residues). Because of its large molecular weight and anionic character, hyaluronate holds large volumes of water and serves as an effective lubricant and shock absorbent. It is found predominantly in synovial fluid of the joints and the vitreous humor of the eye.

Synthesis of Glycoproteins

Glycoproteins are defined as proteins that contain one or more saccharide chains (usually less than 12 to 15 sugar residues per chain) that lack serial repeat units and that are bound covalently to the polypeptide chain. This definition distinguishes them from the carbohydrate-rich proteoglycans. Glycoproteins are found in cell membranes with the oligosaccharide portion of the glycoprotein on the external face of the plasma membrane. The carbohydrate portion of glycoproteins can range from 1% to 70% of the glycoprotein by weight. The carbohydrate chains are covalently linked to glycoproteins by N- or O-glycosyl bonds. A variety of monosaccharide units linked by either α- or β-glycosidic bonds result in the diversity of oligosaccharide moieties that are found in glycoproteins.

Glycosylation of proteins occurs in the ER and Golgi apparatus. Glycosylation serves to alter the properties of proteins, and the oligosaccharide structures also act as recognition signals for various aspects of protein targeting and for cellular recognition of proteins and of other cells. The O-linked oligosaccharides are synthesized in the Golgi apparatus by serial addition of monosaccharide units to a completed polypeptide chain. The sugar residues are added by the sequential action of a series of glycosyltransferases. This process begins with transfer of a sugar such as N-acetylgalactosamine from UDP-N-acetylgalactosamine to a seryl or threonyl residue on the polypeptide. This is then followed by stepwise addition of other sugars.

The N-linked oligosaccharides are synthesized somewhat differently and usually contain a core structure made up of mannose and N-acetylglucosamine residues. This common core is preassembled as a dolichol-linked oligosaccharide prior to incorporation into the polypeptide. First N-acetylglucosamine from UDP-N-acetylglucosamine is attached to dolichol phosphate to form N-acetylglucosaminylpyrophosphoryldolichol, with release of UMP from the nucleotide sugar. Addition of other core sugars occurs and, in the final step, the core oligosaccharide is transferred from the dolichol pyrophosphate to an asparaginyl residue in the polypeptide chain. After synthesis and transfer of the specific core region, extensive processing of the oligosaccharide chain occurs in the Golgi apparatus. Processing involves removal of some of the precursor core's sugar units and addition of other sugar residues to the remaining core oligosaccharide; these reactions are catalyzed by glycosyltransferases and do not require the participation of dolichol intermediates.

Glycoproteins are important components of cell membranes where the oligosaccharide portion of the glycoprotein is on the external face of the plasma membrane. Glycoproteins make up a major part of the mucus secreted by epithelial cells. Many secreted proteins such as follicle-stimulating hormone, chorionic gonadotropin, and luteinizing hormone are glycoproteins, and many plasma proteins such as immunoglobulins, prothrombin, plasminogen, and ceruloplasmin are also glycoproteins. A well-characterized erythrocyte glycoprotein called glycophorin is widely studied as a model of plasma membrane glycoproteins. The glycophorin C complex in human erythrocyte membranes regulates the stability and mechanical properties of the plasma membrane. Components of the glycophorin C complex are implicated in ion channel clustering, cytoskeletal organization, cell signaling, and cell proliferation (Chishti, 1998). The oligosaccharide component of glycoproteins also marks soluble glycoproteins in the plasma for continued circulation or degradation by the liver. A specific unit of the oligosaccharide, a sialic acid residue at the terminus of the oligosaccharide chain, marks glycoproteins for continued circulation; the loss of this sialic acid residue results in the uptake of the asialoglycoprotein and its degradation by the liver. Liver contains asialoglycoprotein receptors that recognize, bind, and internalize glycoproteins that lack terminal sialic acid residues.

Synthesis of Glycolipids

Sphingoglycolipids are glycosyl derivatives of sphingolipids. Structure and synthesis of the glycosphingolipids, including glucocerebrosides, galactocerebrosides, globosides, and gangliosides, are discussed in Chapters 1, 3, and 13. The more complex globosides and gangliosides contain glucose and/or galactose as well as additional sugars such as L-fucose, N-acetylgalactosamine, and sialic acids (e.g., N-acetylneuraminic acid).

Another important glycolipid is glycosyl phosphatidylinositol (GPI), which functions to anchor a variety of proteins to the exterior surface of the plasma membrane. The core GPI is synthesized on the luminal side of the ER from phosphatidylinositol, UDP-N-acetylglucosamine, dolicholphosphomannose, and phosphatidylethanolamine. The core GPI structure is modified by addition of a variety of additional sugar residues, which vary with the protein to which the GPI attaches. Target proteins in the ER become attached to preformed GPI when the amino group of the GPI phosphoethanolamine moiety nucleophilically attacks a specific residue of the protein near its C-terminus, resulting in a transamidation reaction that releases a 20- to 30-amino acid residue C-terminal peptide and attaches GPI to the new C-terminal amino acid residue of the target protein. These GPI-anchored proteins are found on the exterior surface of the plasma membrane of cells; the fatty acids of GPI are inserted into the lipid membrane to provide the anchor.

REFERENCES

Behal, R. H., Buxton, D. B., Robertson, J. G. and Olson, M. S. (1993) Regulation of the pyruvate dehydrogenase multienzyme complex. Annu Rev Nutr 13:497–520.

Bindoff, L. A. and Turnbull, D. M. (1994) Defects of the mitochondrial respiratory chain. In: The Inherited Metabolic Diseases (Holton, J. B., ed.), 2nd ed., pp. 265–295. Churchill Livingstone, London.

Buist, N. R. M. (1995) Disorders of gluconeogenesis. In: Inborn Metabolic Diseases: Diagnosis and Treatment (Fernandes, J., Saudubray, J.-M. and van den Berghe, G., eds.), pp. 101–106. Springer-Verlag, Berlin.

Charron, M. J., Katz, E. B. and Olson, A. L. (1999) GLUT4 gene regulation and manipulation. J Biol Chem 274:3253–3256.

Chishti, A. H. (1998) Function of p55 and its nonerythroid homologues. Curr Opin Hematol 5:116–121.

Cohen, P. T., Alessi, D. R. and Cross, D. A. (1997) PDK1, one of the missing links in insulin signal transduction? FEBS Lett 410:3–10.

Czech, M. P. (1995) Molecular actions of insulin on glucose transport. Annu Rev Nutr 15:441–471.

Dunger, D. B. and Holton, J. B. (1994) Disorders of carbohydrate metabolism. In: The Inherited Metabolic Diseases (Holton, J. B., ed.), 2nd ed., pp. 21–65. Churchill Livingstone, London.

Fernandes, J. and Chen, Y.-T. (1995) Carbohydrate metabolism: Glycogen storage diseases. In: Inborn Metabolic Diseases: Diagnosis and Treatment (Fernandes, J., Saudubray, J.-M. and van den Berghe, G., eds.), pp. 71–131. Springer-Verlag, Berlin.

Gitzelmann, R. (1995) Disorders of galactose metabolism. In: Inborn Metabolic Diseases: Diagnosis and Treatment (Fernandes, J., Saudubray, J.-M. and van den Berghe, G., eds.), pp. 87–92. Springer-Verlag, Berlin.

Granner, D. K. and Pilkis, S. J. (1990) The genes of hepatic glucose metabolism. J Biol Chem 265:10173–10176.

Gurney, A. L., Park, E. A., Liu, J., Giralt, M., McGrane, M. M., Patel, Y. M., Crawford, D. R., Nizielski, S. E., Savon, S. and Hanson, R. W. (1994) Metabolic regulation of gene transcription. J Nutr 124:1533S–1539S.

Hanson, R. W. and Reshef, L. (1997) Regulation of phosphoenolpyruvate carboxykinase (GTP) gene expression. Annu Rev Biochem 66:581–611.

Jungermann, K. (1992) Zonal liver cell heterogeneity. Enzyme 46:5–7.

Kahn, C. R., Lauris, W., Koch, S., Crettaz, M. and Granner, D. K. (1989) Acute and chronic regulation of phosphoenolpyruvate carboxykinase mRNA by insulin and glucose. Molec Endocrinol 3:840–845.

Lehninger, A. L., Nelson, D. L. and Cox, M. M. (1993) Glycolysis and the catabolism of hexoses. In: Principles of Biochemistry, 2nd ed., pp. 400–439. Worth Publishers, New York.

Lemaigre, F. P. and Rousseau G. G. (1994) Transcriptional control of genes that regulate glycolysis and gluconeogenesis in adult liver. Biochem J 303:1–14.

Magnuson, M. A. and Jetton, T. L. (1993) Tissue-specific regulation of glucokinase. In: Nutrition and Gene Expression (Berdanier, C. D. and Hargrove, J. L., eds.), pp. 143–167. CRC Press, Boca Raton, Florida.

Moore, M. C. and Cherrington, A. D. (1996) Regulation of net hepatic glucose uptake: Interaction of neural and pancreatic mechanisms. Reprod Nutr Dev 36(4):399–406.

Noguchi, T. and Tanaka, T. (1993) Dietary and hormonal regulation of L-type pyruvate kinase gene expression. In: Nutrition and Gene Expression (Berdanier, C. D. and Hargrove, J. L., eds.), pp. 143–167. CRC Press, Boca Raton, Florida.

Nordlie, R. C., Bode, A. M. and Foster, J. D. (1993) Recent advances in hepatic glucose 6-phosphatase regulation and function. Proc Soc Exp Biol Med 203:274–285.

Pilkis, S. J., El-Maghrabi, M. R. and Claus, T. H. (1990) Fructose-2,6-bisphosphate in control of hepatic gluconeogenesis. From metabolites to molecular genetics. Diabetes Care 13(6):582–599.

Pilkis, S. J. and Claus, T. H. (1991) Hepatic gluconeogenesis/glycolysis: Regulation and structure/function relationships of substrate cycles. Annu Rev Nutr 11:465–515.

Pilkis, S. J., Claus, T. H., Kurland I. J. and Lange, A. J. (1995) 6-Phosphofructo-2-kinase/fructose-2,6-bisphos-

phatase: A metabolic signaling enzyme. Annu Rev Biochem 64:799–835.

Pilkis, S. J. and Granner, D. K. (1992) Molecular physiology of the regulation of hepatic gluconeogenesis and glycolysis. Annu Rev Physiol 54:885–909.

Shafrir, E. (1991) Metabolism of disaccharides and monosaccharides with emphasis on sucrose and fructose and their lipogenic potential. In: Sugars in Nutrition. Nestle Nutrition Workshop Series (Gracey, M., Kretchmer, N. and Rossi, E., eds.), Vol. 25, pp. 131–152. Raven Press, New York.

Shoffner, J. M. and Wallace, D. C. (1994) Oxidative phosphorylation diseases and mitochondrial DNA mutations: Diagnosis and treatment. Annu Rev Nutr 14:535–568.

Sirover, M. A. (1997) Role of the glycolytic protein, glyceraldehyde-3-phosphate dehydrogenase, in normal cell function and in cell pathology. J Cell Biochem 66:133–140.

Smythe, C. and Cohen, P. (1991) The discovery of glycogenin and the priming mechanism for glycogen biogenesis. Eur J Biochem 200:625–631.

Stabile, L. P., Hodge, D. L., Klautky, S. A. and Salati, L. M. (1996) Posttranscriptional regulation of glucose-6-phosphate dehydrogenase by dietary polyunsaturated fat. Arch Biochem Biophys 332:269–279.

Streeper, R. S., Svitek, C. A., Chapman, S., Greenbaum, L. E., Taub, R. and O'Brien, R. M. (1997) A multicomponent insulin response sequence mediates a strong repression of mouse glucose-6-phosphatase gene transcription by insulin. J Biol Chem 272:11698–11701.

Sutherland, C., O'Brien, R. M. and Granner, D. K. (1996) New connections in the regulation of PEPCK gene expression by insulin. Philos Trans R Soc Lond B Biol Sci 351:191–199.

Van den Berghe, G. (1995) Disorders of fructose metabolism. In: Inborn Metabolic Diseases: Diagnosis and Treatment (Fernandes, J., Saudubray, J.-M. and van den Berghe, G., eds.), pp. 95–99. Springer-Verlag, Berlin.

Vaulont, S. and Kahn, A. (1993) Transcriptional control of metabolic regulation genes by carbohydrates. FASEB J 8:28–36.

White, M. (1998) The IRS-signalling system: A network of docking proteins that mediate insulin action. Mol Cell Biochem 182:3–11.

RECOMMENDED READINGS

Berdanier, C. D. (1995) Advanced Nutrition: Macronutrients, pp. 160–207. CRC Press, Boca Raton, Florida.

Devlin, T. M., ed. (1992) Textbook of Biochemistry with Clinical Correlations, pp. 291–386. Wiley-Liss, New York.

Guyton, A. C. (1991) Textbook of Medical Physiology, 8th ed., pp. 771–774. W. B. Saunders, Philadelphia.

Lehninger, A. L., Nelson, D. L. and Cox, M. M. (1993) Principles of Biochemistry, 2nd ed., pp. 400–475. Worth Publishers, New York.

◆ ◆

CHAPTER 10

Protein Synthesis and Degradation

Margaret A. McNurlan, Ph.D. and Peter J. Garlick, Ph.D.

OUTLINE

COMMON ABBREVIATIONS

DNA (deoxyribonucleic acid)
EF (elongation factor)
eIF (eukaryotic initiation factor)
ER (endoplasmic reticulum)
hnRNA (heterogeneous nuclear RNA)
IGF (insulin-like growth factor)
IL (interleukin)
mRNA (messenger ribonucleic acid)
TNF (tumor necrosis factor)
tRNA (transfer ribonucleic acid)

ESSENTIALITY OF PROTEIN

The importance of dietary protein to life was demonstrated in the early 1800s by the nutritional experiments of François Magendie. He found that adult dogs fed on diets containing only flour (carbohydrate) or oil (fat) died, whereas dogs lived indefinitely on diets of eggs or cheese; that is, on diets containing protein (Munro, 1964).

In the young, the provision of dietary protein is not only necessary for maintaining body protein but also contributes to the increase in protein mass associated with growth. If either dietary protein or energy is limited, therefore, growth is retarded. In the adult, an adequate intake of protein maintains the body protein mass and the capacity to adapt to changing conditions. Loss of body protein is not compatible with health and accompanies many disease states. Renal, gastrointestinal, and liver disease, as well as cancer and infections such as human immunodeficiency virus (HIV), are associated with the loss of body protein, which in turn is associated with increased mortality. In HIV-infected individuals, for example, the loss of less than 30% of body protein mass is associated with about 80% survival. When the loss of body protein exceeds 30%, the survival rate drops to about 20% (Süttman et al., 1995). It becomes imperative, therefore, to understand what functions proteins serve, why body protein is lost, and how these losses can be prevented.

Functions and Distribution of Body Protein

Proteins consist of linear polymers of amino acids and make up approximately 17% of the body mass. Protein molecules function to maintain body structure (e.g., collagen), to facilitate mobility (e.g., actin and myosin for muscle contraction), in transport (e.g., oxygen transport by hemoglobin, membrane transport systems), in metabolism (e.g., enzymes), in regulation (e.g., growth factors), and in immune fuction (e.g., immunoglobulins). Although the diversity in function of body proteins is reflected in the large number of different protein species, almost half of body protein is contained in just four: the structural proteins collagen, actin, and myosin and the oxygen-transporting protein hemoglobin.

Body protein is distributed throughout the various organs, with the majority (about 40%) in muscle tissue. In addition to providing for locomotion and work, muscle protein also provides amino acids that can be mobilized in times of stress. However, muscle protein is not a storage form, like glycogen or fat, and loss of muscle protein represents a loss of functional protein. The functions of muscle tissue are given a lower priority than the functions of the visceral tissues such as liver and intestine, which contain about 10% of body protein. The protein of these tissues is not mobilized rapidly in times of stress, thereby preserving their more vital functions (Kinney, 1978). Another 30% of body protein is contained in skin and blood, and both skin lesions and anemia accompany deficit of dietary protein. Some proteins such as collagen are preserved during malnutrition, not because of their essential function but because their structure is such that they are not readily degraded.

Nitrogen Balance

Protein and amino acids are unique among the compounds of the body in the amount of nitrogen they contain. Although other compounds such as amino sugars and nucleic acids contain nitrogen, they do not contain the substantial amounts that are contained in body protein. On average, protein contains 16% nitrogen, leading to the familiar factor of 6.25 (i.e., 100/16) for converting measured values of nitrogen into corresponding amounts of protein. Because nitrogen is relatively easy to measure, changes in the protein mass of the body can be assessed by the difference between nitrogen intake and nitrogen excretion. Historically and clinically, one of the most common ways of assessing changes in body protein mass is through the assessment of the difference between the intake of nitrogen and the loss of nitrogen from the body, the nitrogen balance:

Nitrogen Balance =
        Nitrogen Intake − Nitrogen Excretion

Using 6.25 as the average conversion factor

for converting grams of nitrogen to grams of protein, protein balance can then be derived from nitrogen balance:

$$\text{Protein (gained or lost)} = \text{N (gained or lost)} \times 6.25$$

When the body is in nitrogen equilibrium, nitrogen excretion is equal to nitrogen intake. Thus, for the average American consuming about 100 g of protein per day, both nitrogen intake and nitrogen excretion will be about 16 g per day. Whenever nitrogen intake exceeds excretion, protein is being retained by the body, resulting in growth. When nitrogen excretion exceeds nitrogen intake, body protein is being lost, such as during starvation and disease.

Although the concept of nitrogen balance is useful in that it can provide information on the overall balance of body protein, this concept is a static one. For example, it cannot answer questions about whether negative balance arises from depressed protein synthesis or accelerated protein degradation. The nitrogen balance technique is neither able to determine which organs within the body are retaining protein and which are losing it nor to assess details of the adaptive changes that occur in body protein metabolism in order to preserve balance. Questions such as these require a more dynamic assessment of protein metabolism.

DYNAMIC PROTEIN METABOLISM

During any day an adult human makes, and degrades, about 300 g of protein. In contrast, the normal intake of protein from the diet for an affluent, well-fed individual is about one third of that amount, or 100 g. This means that the body not only processes the protein that is taken in but also degrades about three times as much body protein. Thus, about 400 g of protein is broken down to amino acids by digestion and protein degradation. Amino acids are used to resynthesize about 300 g of body protein; most of the remaining amino acids are catabolized.

Interchange of Protein and Amino Acids

The interchange between body protein and the pool of free amino acids is depicted schematically in Figure 10–1. The process by which body protein is continually degraded and resynthesized is called protein turnover, a term that has been used colletively to include both protein synthesis and degradation. In addition to the exchange of amino acids into and out of protein, amino acids also are irreversibly lost through degradative pathways. For most adults who are in protein balance, the amount of amino acids degraded is equivalent to the amount in the diet. The degradative pathways are also shown schematically in Figure 10–1. Degradation involves the removal of nitrogen, primarily as urea and ammonia, and the degradation of the carbon skeleton. The end result of the degradation of the carbon skeleton of amino acids is the provision of energy either directly or through the formation of compounds such as glucose and fatty acids, which can then be stored or metabolized to provide energy. The pathways for the oxidative metabolism and nitrogen excretion of amino acids are discussed in detail in Chapter 11, but it is important to understand the integrated nature of protein metabolism that is represented by Figure 10–1. The needs of the body regulate which of the possible pathways predominates; that is, when amino acids are used for the synthesis of protein, when they are oxidized for energy, and when they are used to form glucose.

Also, within the body, there are pathways for conversion of amino acids to end products other than protein. These reactions are depicted in Figure 10–1 as nonprotein derivatives. Nonprotein derivatives include compounds such as purine and pyrimidine bases, neurotransmitters (serotonin, tyramine), and nonpeptide hormones (catecholamines, thyroid hormones). The quantities of amino acids involved in these nonprotein pathways are, in general, much smaller than the amounts of amino acids involved in protein synthesis and degradation. Because the amounts of amino acids irreversibly consumed in the synthesis of nonprotein compounds are normally much smaller than those

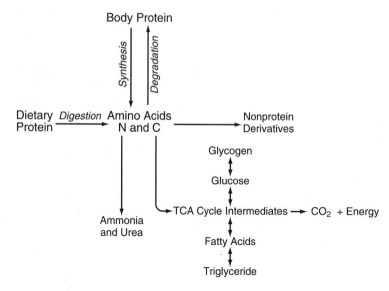

Figure 10–1. Overview of protein and amino acid metabolism. Amino acids are primarily incorporated into protein or degraded to provide energy. The synthesis of nonprotein compounds does not consume quantitatively important amounts of amino acids. Degradation of amino acids involves removal of the nitrogen and catabolism of the carbon skeleton.

consumed by either protein synthesis or amino acid oxidation, these pathways often are ignored in the assessment of protein turnover and nitrogen balance. However, the amounts of some of these compounds that are synthesized can be substantial (e.g., creatine, heme, and nucleic acids) and, for some amino acids, these pathways can become quantitatively significant during periods of protein deprivation.

Protein Turnover

The pathways shown in Figure 10–1 can be simplified to focus specifically on the interactions of amino acids with body protein (Fig. 10–2) through protein synthesis and protein degradation. In this simplified scheme, all the tissue and circulating proteins are considered together and, likewise, the free amino acid pool is simplified to a single, homogeneous pool, rather than the complex arrangements of pools in blood, individual tissues, and subcellular compartments that are known to exist. This simplification has proved helpful in conceptualizing and developing methods for measuring the exchange of amino acids between the free amino acid pool and the protein pool.

This simple model in Figure 10–2 highlights the exchange of free amino acids with body protein through the processes of protein synthesis and protein degradation and also

the entry and exit of amino acids by dietary intake and oxidation. Amino acids enter the body free pool from the digestion of dietary protein (I) and from the degradation of body protein (D). Removal of amino acids from the free pool occurs either by the synthesis of protein (S) or through excretion (E) via oxidation to CO_2 with the concurrent excretion of nitrogen, mainly as ammonia and urea.

If the amount of free amino acid in the

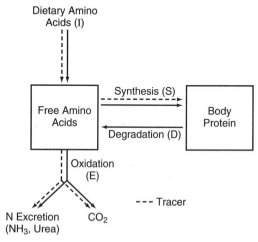

Figure 10–2. Protein turnover. The complexity of body protein and free amino acid pools is simplified in this two-compartment model, which can be used to assess kinetic data from labeled tracers (shown as dashed lines). In this model, amino acids enter a free amino acid pool via the diet (I) or from the degradation of body protein (D). Amino acids leave the free amino acid pool through protein synthesis (S) and oxidation (E).

pool is constant, then the sum of the processes that remove amino acids (protein synthesis + oxidation) is equal to the sum of the processes by which amino acids enter the free pool (protein degradation + dietary amino acid intake).

$$S + E = D + I = Q$$

Q, the sum of the rates of either entry or exit from the free amino acid pool, has been termed the flux rate, appearance rate (R_a), or disappearance rate (R_d). In an adult in nitrogen equilibrium or protein balance, nitrogen intake (I) is equal to nitrogen excretion (E), and protein synthesis (S) is equal to protein degradation (D). For an individual to be in positive nitrogen balance, there must be net protein synthesis or accretion (S>D), whereas there must be net protein degradation or loss for an individual to be in negative nitrogen balance (S<D).

Protein Balance = Protein Synthesis − Protein Degradation

From the aforementioned relationships, it is clear that protein is retained in the body when synthesis exceeds degradation and that protein is lost from the body when degradation exceeds synthesis. Unlike the technique of nitrogen balance, which measures only net changes in body protein, estimates of protein synthesis and degradation indicate that changes in balance arise in a number of different ways.

For example, as shown in Figure 10–3, loss of body protein can occur from a decrease in the synthesis of protein with no change in protein degradation (Fig. 10–3A), an increase in the degradation with no change in protein synthesis (Fig. 10–3B), or from either an increase (Fig. 10–3C) or a decrease (Fig. 10–3D) in both synthesis and degradation, with protein degradation exceeding protein synthesis. In a number of pathological conditions, body protein degradation exceeds synthesis with both protein synthesis and degradation rates elevated over the rates in healthy individuals (Fig. 10–3C). In the case of infection in malnourished children, body

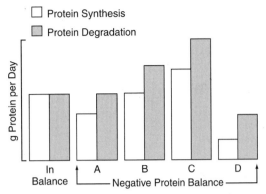

Figure 10–3. *Four ways of achieving negative nitrogen balance. Negative nitrogen balance (degradation > synthesis) arises from changes in either protein synthesis (A) or protein degradation (B), or from changes in both (C, D). Similarly, positive balance (synthesis > degradation) arises whenever synthesis exceeds degradation. This can occur with changes in the rates of synthesis or degradation or with changes in both.*

protein is lost, but both synthesis and degradation rates are depressed (Fig. 10–3D).

Likewise, positive protein balance can be achieved by increases in protein synthesis, by decreases in protein degradation, or with changes in both protein synthesis and degradation, such that synthesis exceeds degradation. For example, in children recovering from malnutrition (see Fig. 10–8), both the rates of protein synthesis and degradation were increased, but the increase in synthesis was larger than the increase in protein degradation. Unlike the information from nitrogen balance studies, measurements of protein synthesis and degradation provide information about how the changes in balance are brought about.

Although the illustration of protein turnover in Figure 10–2 is presented in terms of whole-body protein, the balance between the processes of synthesis and degradation also determines the net protein balance at the level of individual tissues or organs and for individual proteins. Examples of this type of regulation are discussed later in this chapter.

MEASUREMENT OF PROTEIN SYNTHESIS AND DEGRADATION

The methods used for measuring protein synthesis, protein degradation, and amino acid

TABLE 10–1
Stable Isotopes of Elements Commonly Used in Metabolic Research

Element	Normal*	Radioactive	Stable*
Hydrogen	^1H	^3H	^2H (0.015%)
Carbon	^{12}C	^{14}C	^{13}C (1.1%)
Nitrogen	^{14}N	—	^{15}N (0.37%)
Oxygen	^{16}O	—	^{17}O (0.037%)
			^{18}O (0.2%)

*The "normal" isotope is the most abundant naturally occurring form. The "stable" isotopes also occur naturally, and the average natural abundance is shown in parentheses.

oxidation, in general, incorporate isotopic tracer techniques. Amino acids labeled with either radioactive (^{14}C, ^3H) or stable (^{15}N, ^{13}C, ^2H) isotopes have been used, although the trend is toward the exclusive use of stable isotopes for humans (Table 10–1). Like their radioactive counterparts, stable isotopes differ in atomic mass from the abundant natural form of the element, but they are not radioactive and occur as a small proportion of all naturally occurring materials. Because of this, they are totally harmless and can be used for multiple repeat studies in the same subject. No radioactive isotope of nitrogen is suitable for use in laboratory studies, so the stable isotope ^{15}N is the only commonly available tracer for this element. Measurement of stable isotopes is by mass spectrometry, which requires more expensive and elaborate equipment than radioactivity counting but has the advantage of greater selectivity and sensitivity.

The earliest work on protein turnover, by Schoenheimer and colleagues in the 1930s used ^{15}N-labeled amino acids. They first demonstrated the concept of turnover of protein by observing that a labeled amino acid was incorporated into body protein even when the animals were not growing. They reasoned that the body protein pool was turning over, so that some of the label was incorporated into protein, replacing some of the unlabeled body protein that was degraded and excreted (Waterlow et al., 1978).

Methods Based on the Disappearance of Label from the Free Pool

Protein Turnover in the Whole Body.
Since the time of Schoenheimer, a variety of techniques for assessing protein turnover have

been developed. The isotopic labeling procedure usually is performed by giving the tracer amino acid as an intravenous injection or infusion, although sometimes the less invasive intragastric route is used. Two alternative methods of measurement have been developed. One method measures the disappearance of the label from the free amino acid pool, and the other method assesses the rate of appearance of label in protein. The former approach has been used extensively to measure rates of protein turnover in the whole body, because the free pool is easier to sample than the body protein pool. When a ^{13}C-labeled amino acid is given (e.g., L-[1-^{13}C]leucine), rates of whole-body protein synthesis and degradation, as well as amino acid oxidation, can be determined by monitoring the labeling of the amino acid in the blood and the labeling of expired CO_2 in the breath. The rates of whole-body synthesis in humans of different ages shown in Figure 10–4 were measured with this technique.

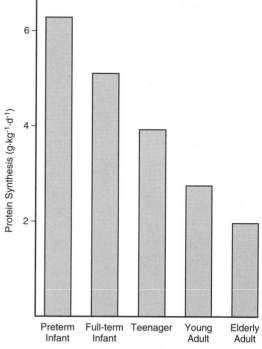

Figure 10–4. *The decline in whole-body protein synthesis with advancing age. Rates of whole-body protein synthesis were measured with L-[1-^{13}C]leucine infusion in subjects of various ages. [Based on the data of Mitton et al. (1991), Denne and Kalhan (1987), Mauras et al. (1994), Mauras (1995), and Welle et al. (1994).]*

If the tracer is an amino acid labeled with ^{15}N (e.g., [^{15}N]glycine), the excretion of the label in urinary end products (urea or ammonia) can be used to calculate whole-body protein synthesis and degradation. This approach also assumes a single pool of free amino acid, which is sampled via urinary urea or ammonia. The rates of protein synthesis and degradation in malnourished and recovering children shown in Figure 10–8 were measured with [^{15}N]glycine.

Measurements of Protein Turnover from Arterial–Venous Differences. Measurement of the disappearance of label from the free amino acid pool has also been used to determine rates of protein synthesis in individual organs or limbs by monitoring the extraction of the label as the blood passes through the tissue. Sampling of both arterial and venous blood allows for the estimation of extraction of label by the organ or limb. This measurement is referred to as the arterial–venous or A–V difference. Using a similar approach, the dilution of label in the free amino acid pool by release of unlabeled amino acids from tissue proteins as the blood passes through the organ or limb has been used to determine rates of protein degradation.

Methods Based on the Incorporation of a Labeled Amino Acid into Protein

Measurement of Protein Synthesis in Tissues. The determination of rates of protein synthesis in individual organs or tissues is based on the amount of a labeled amino acid that is incorporated into protein in a given amount of time. A range of tissue protein synthetic rates measured from the incorporation of a labeled amino acid is shown in Figure 10–5. The technique does not yield estimates of protein degradation, but it has the advantage that individual tissue responses can be monitored, which is valuable in conditions in which there are different responses in different tissues. In cancer, for example, the responses in the tumor can be differentiated from the responses in the host tissues. The disadvantage of the technique based on the incorporation of label is that tissue samples must be obtained and, therefore, the technique is more invasive than the methods based on the disappearance of label from the free pool.

Turnover Rates of Individual Proteins. These are measured by basically the same technique as that used for individual tissues. The range of turnover rates for individual pro-

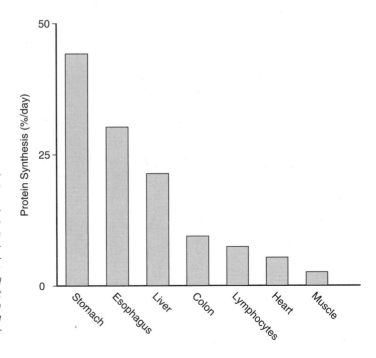

Figure 10–5. Fractional rates of protein synthesis in a range of human tissues. Rates of protein synthesis, assessed from the incorporation of L-[1-^{13}C]leucine or L-[^{2}H$_5$]phenylalanine into tissue protein, are expressed as a fractional rate; that is, as the fraction of the protein pool that is synthesized each day. (Data from Garlick, P. J., McNurlan, M. A., Essén, P. and Wernerman, J. [1994] Measurement of tissue protein synthesis rates in vivo: A critical analysis of contrasting methods. Am J Physiol 266:E287–E297.)

teins is extremely wide and is listed in Table 10–2. Some proteins, such as hemoglobin, do not turn over unless their environment changes. Within the red blood cell, hemoglobin is stable and is degraded only when the cell is broken down. Other proteins turn over extremely rapidly. Rapid turnover facilitates a rapid change in the amount of protein present and is commonly found for regulatory proteins.

Isotopic Measurement of Protein Degradation in Tissues. Rates of protein degradation in tissues are more difficult to determine than are synthesis rates. The direct method involves isotopic labeling of protein and the determination of the rate at which label is lost. This technique, however, is complicated by the fact that label from degraded protein can be reincorporated into protein and, consequently, not included in the measurement of the rate of degradation. A more indirect method, which is not affected by recycling, involves the measurement of synthesis together with the rate of change of protein mass. Protein degradation is determined from the difference between the rate of growth (or loss) of tissue and the rate of protein synthesis (i.e., growth = synthesis − degradation). Neither of these techniques is entirely satisfactory, however, because they cannot be used in humans and require measurements of large numbers of animals over extended periods of time. Because many factors that regulate protein turnover do so over short time periods, the long time period for degradation measurements is a serious disadvantage.

Myofibrillar Degradation from 3-Methylhistidine

For muscle, a nonisotopic method can be used to measure protein degradation. The amino acid 3-methylhistidine (N^3-methylhistidine) is produced by posttranslational methylation of histidyl residues of actin and myosin. After release by protein degradation, the 3-methylhistidine cannot be reincorporated into protein, is not metabolized further in most species such as rats and humans, and so is excreted quantitatively in the urine. The rate of 3-methylhistidine excretion, therefore, is used as a measure of the rate of muscle or, more specifically, myofibrillar protein degradation. Although there are myofibrillar proteins in tissues other than muscle (e.g., the smooth muscle of the intestinal tract), studies on the release of 3-methylhistidine by arterial–venous difference across the leg have shown good agreement with urinary 3-methylhistidine excretion (Sjölin et al., 1989), and this method is used widely to estimate human muscle protein degradation. The excretion of 3-methylhistidine also depends on the total muscle mass, so that data are most often expressed as the ratio of 3-methylhistidine to creatinine, because urinary creatinine is an indicator of total muscle mass. The ratio of 3-methylhistidine to creatinine is, therefore, an indication of how actively protein is being degraded. However, because dietary protein from meat contains 3-methylhistidine, which would complicate the interpretation of 3-methylhistidine excretion, the measurement of excretion must be made when subjects

TABLE 10–2
Turnover Rates of Enzymes in Rat Liver

Enzyme	Cellular Compartment	$t_{1/2}$	k_d
Ornithine decarboxylase	Cytosol	11 min	91
5-Aminolevulinate synthetase	Cytosol	20 min	50
5-Aminolevulinate synthetase	Mitochondria	72 min	14
Hydroxymethylglutaryl CoA reductase	Endoplasmic reticulum	4.0 h	4.2
Phosphoenolpyruvate carboxykinase	Cytosol	5.0 h	3.3
Alanine-glyoxylate aminotransferase	Cytosol	3.5 days	0.20
Arginase	Cytosol	4.0 days	0.17
NAD^+ nucleosidase	Endoplasmic reticulum	16 days	0.04

Turnover rates are expressed as half-lives ($t_{1/2}$, the time to replace half the molecules originally present) and fractional turnover rates (k_d, fraction turned over per day). Data from Waterlow, J. C., Garlick, P. J., and Millward, D. J. (1978) Protein Turnover in Mammalian Tissues and in the Whole Body, pp. 490–492. North-Holland Publishing, Amsterdam.

are on a meat-free diet. An example of the assessment of muscle protein degradation from 3-methylhistidine excretion is shown in Figure 10–9, which illustrates increased muscle degradation in acquired immunodeficiency syndrome (AIDS) patients with wasting.

PROTEIN TURNOVER AND ADAPTATION

What are the advantages and disadvantages of this highly inefficient protein turnover system that uses energy to cycle proteins and amino acids? Obviously, the system is inefficient with respect to energy, because energy is needed both for the degradation of protein and for the synthesis of new protein. Estimates of the energy cost of protein turnover suggest that 15% of basal energy expenditure is associated with the turnover of protein (Reeds and Garlick, 1984). However, substantial advantages also are conferred by the dynamism. One example of the value of this capacity to adapt is seen in the response of malnourished children to infection with measles. Whereas well-nourished children with measles increase both protein synthesis and degradation with a net loss of body protein, malnourished children respond to the infection with both a blunted increase in protein turnover and a blunted loss of body protein. Although the loss of body protein is smaller in the malnourished children, the impact of the disease is greater, and these children often die from measles infection (Tomkins et al., 1983). Protein turnover provides benefit in the capacity to adapt to infection, at the expense of the loss of some body protein and the expenditure of energy.

Individual proteins vary in their rate of turnover (see Table 10–2), and the higher rates of turnover are found in regulatory proteins. The higher rates of turnover in these proteins allow for more rapid adaptation in the levels of regulatory proteins in response to changing conditions than is seen in proteins with much longer turnover times.

At the level of individual tissues, higher turnover rates are found in tissues that respond rapidly to changes in the environment. The turnover rates for a selection of human tissues are shown in Figure 10–5. The high rates of protein synthesis in tissues like stomach and esophagus reflect both the secretory function and the rapid replacement of cells of the gastric and esophageal mucosa. The liver also has a relatively high rate of turnover, which facilitates adaptation to changes such as alterations in nutrient intake. By contrast, the rate of protein synthesis is relatively slower in muscle tissue, and the response of this tissue to altered conditions (e.g., work-induced hypertrophy) occurs more slowly.

In response to altered demands or alterations in the environment, tissues can respond both by altering the overall rates of protein synthesis and degradation and by changing the spectrum of individual proteins being made. This adaptation allows the body to meet continually changing demands such as those associated with growth and development, health and illness, and pregnancy and lactation. Protein turnover is, therefore, a "substrate cycle" (or futile cycle; see Chapters 9 and 18 for related discussions relative to energy metabolism); that is, there is continual synthesis and degradation, which requires energy but accomplishes no net change in amount of protein. The benefit is that protein turnover provides the capacity for rapid adaptation when needed.

REGULATION OF PROTEIN SYNTHESIS AND DEGRADATION AT THE MOLECULAR LEVEL

The regulation of the amount of a specific protein or of the total protein of a cell or organ involves molecular changes at a number of different sites. Figure 10–6 represents these regulatory areas in a schematic form: the shaded areas represent points of regulation of protein synthesis, involving transcription of DNA to messenger RNA (mRNA), stability of mRNA, translation of mRNA into protein, and the synthesis and degradation of ribosomes. From an understanding of the molecular basis of protein synthesis, it is possible to see where regulation can occur, and this understanding sets the framework for investigating the mechanisms by which changes in protein metabolism are brought about.

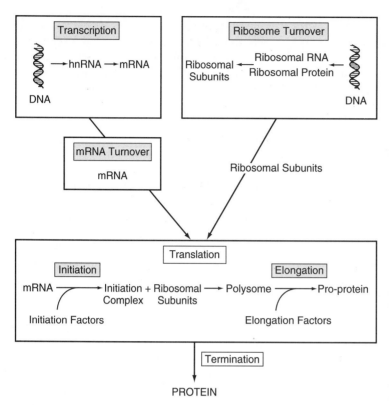

Figure 10–6. *Protein synthesis. The scheme shows the processes involved in the synthesis of protein. The boxes all denote points of regulation. Transcription of DNA produces heterogeneous nuclear RNA (hnRNA), which is processed into messenger RNA (mRNA). mRNA undergoes continuous synthesis and degradation, shown as mRNA turnover. Ribosomal subunits cycle between subunits and polyribosomes. Ribosomes also undergo synthesis and degradation of both ribosomal RNA and ribosomal protein. Translation of mRNA into protein involves the processes of initiation and elongation, which are also regulated by initiation and elongation factors. The final step in protein formation is termination, the separation of the protein from the polyribosome, which also releases mRNA and ribosomal subunits.*

Transcription of DNA and Translation of mRNA

The overall sequence of events begins with the transcription of a particular gene to produce an mRNA template. This heterogeneous nuclear RNA (hnRNA) is then processed to provide a final mRNA template to which ribosomes attach to translate the nucleic acid code into a particular sequence of amino acids, forming a specific protein molecule.

Transcription. Transcription of a particular region of DNA into the corresponding mRNA (Fig. 10–6) involves the binding of RNA polymerase to the genome. The site of binding and the frequency of transcription are regulated by parts of the genome that are not themselves transcribed. These noncoding regions are located both near the site of transcription (promoter regions) and at sites that are distant from the coding regions (regulatory regions). The regulatory regions can either enhance or repress the transcription of the coding region.

Coordinate transcription of a number of genes simultaneously influences the amount of message available for each of the corres-

ponding proteins and, therefore, the amount of each protein that accumulates. An example of this type of coordinate regulation can be seen in the enzymes of metabolic pathways, such as the urea cycle (see Chapter 11), that are inducible under the appropriate stimulus. Enzymes of this pathway, which removes nitrogen from the body by the formation of urea, are induced by an increase in the amount of protein in the diet.

Translation. The process of translating the code on the mRNA into a protein with a specific sequence of amino acids is divided into three phases: initiation, elongation, and termination. Initiation involves the formation of an active complex with the 40S subunit of the ribosome, a specific methionyl–tRNA complex, and at least four regulatory proteins, eukaryotic initiation factors (eIF 1, 2, 3, and 4). With the binding of the initiation complex to the mRNA, a second (60S) ribosomal subunit is bound to form an active 80S ribosome.

The process of elongation involves the movement of the ribosome along the message in sequences of three bases, called codons, which each encode for a specific transfer RNA (tRNA) complexed to a specific amino acid. Translation begins at the 5' end traversing the mRNA to the 3' end. There is a noncoding region of the mRNA, rich in adenosine residues (referred to as a poly A tail), which has been exploited in the isolation of mRNA. More than one ribosome can be bound to a given mRNA so that a polyribosome (or polysome) is formed, which includes a single mRNA and several attached ribosomes. Because polysomes are formed during the active translation of mRNA, the degree to which ribosomes are aggregated into polysomes in a cell is a function of the activity of protein synthesis. The ratio of active to inactive ribosomes is, therefore, a measure of the activity of protein synthesis. Elongation involves the formation of a peptide bond between successive amino acids and the translocation of the growing polypeptide chain from one adjacent site to another, so that the next aminoacyl-tRNA can be bound, ready for the formation of the next peptide bond. Elongation is also under the control of regulatory proteins, including elongation factors 1 and 2 (EF-1, EF-2).

When the ribosomes reach a nonsense or terminating codon for which there is no corresponding tRNA, releasing factors promote the hydrolysis of the bond between the protein and the tRNA binding it to the message. As the protein is released, the 80S ribosome dissociates into 40S and 60S subunits. These subunits are then available to begin the synthesis of a new protein.

Regulation of the Amount of Specific mRNAs. For individual proteins within the cell, the amount of protein is determined by a balance between synthesis and degradation. In general, synthesis of a particular protein is increased by increasing the amount of mRNA for that protein, rather than enhancing the rate of translation of its mRNA. Such a system of regulation can be readily seen in the alterations that occur in the amount of particular enzyme proteins. For example, when a nutrient is chronically consumed in amounts in excess of requirement, the enzymes for its degradation may be induced. Thus, enzymes for the degradation (oxidation) of some amino acids are induced by dietary consump-

tion that exceeds the body's need for that amino acid.

Increased levels of particular mRNA species occur as a result of increased formation by transcription or of increased stability (decreased degradation) of the mRNA. When the degradation of a particular mRNA is reduced, that mRNA accumulates and hence the total amount of protein translated from that mRNA is increased. An example of this type of regulation is seen in the stabilization of the mRNA for the enzyme phosphoenolpyruvate carboxykinase (PEPCK) by cyclic AMP (cAMP). In fact, this enzyme, which is the key regulatory enzyme in gluconeogenesis, is regulated in multiple ways. Hormones, including glucagon, glucocorticoids, and insulin, alter the transcription rate of the gene for PEPCK, thereby affecting the amount of PEPCK mRNA. By contrast, cAMP increases the amount of mRNA by stabilizing the message and reducing the rate at which it is degraded (Nachaliel et al., 1993).

It should be noted that an increase in enzyme activity due to an increase in the amount of enzyme present in the cell is in contrast to forms of acute regulation of amino acid oxidation that do not depend on changes in protein synthesis or turnover. After a meal, the oxidation of amino acids rises acutely, not because of increased synthesis of the enzymes that catabolize the amino acid, but because of activation of existing enzymes (e.g., via dephosphorylation). In addition, because the K_m values for the amino acid oxidative enzymes are generally high relative to normal tissue concentrations, when the concentrations of amino acid substrates increase, the rate of oxidation also increases due to increased saturation of enzymes. This is how the body regulates oxidation with the diurnal pattern of food intake, with increased oxidation during feeding and a reduction in oxidation in the postabsorptive state. But there is also adaptation to the chronic level of intake, which is brought about by changes in the amount of enzyme (due to changes in turnover of the protein as described above). Individuals who habitually eat higher levels of protein have increased amounts of amino acid degradative enzymes relative to individuals who habitually consume lower amounts of protein.

Regulation of Protein Synthesis by the Quantity of Ribosomes

In addition to regulation that alters the synthesis of individual proteins by altering the amount of mRNA for that protein, regulation of protein synthesis and degradation also occurs at the level of the tissue by changes that affect all the proteins of that tissue or organ. Protein synthesis at the tissue level is regulated by the number of ribosomes in the cell and also by the amount of work done by each ribosome.

An example of the regulation of protein synthesis at the tissue level is seen in the responses to starvation, when there is a substantial loss of protein from skeletal muscle. Within hours of food withdrawal, there is a fall in the rate of synthesis per ribosome, followed by a slower decline in the total number of ribosomes, which becomes the dominant factor as starvation progresses. There are also changes in protein degradation with starvation that are discussed later in this chapter.

The exact way in which protein metabolism is controlled in response to any particular stimulus depends on the particular tissue or cell type. Each tissue responds in a way determined by the needs of the body as a whole. For example, diseases can alter the pattern of regulation of protein metabolism and impose priorities. This is observed in tumor-bearing mice, in which protein synthesis in muscle declines while the synthesis of liver proteins is enhanced, presumably because liver function is more important to survival than preservation of function in skeletal muscle. In rats with malaria, there is also evidence of priority among tissues. In response to the anemia that accompanies infection with malaria, heart and spleen protein synthesis are maintained, whereas that in tissues such as skeletal muscle decline.

Molecular Aspects of Protein Degradation

Once a protein is made, it is immediately a target for degradation. Some proteins, such as collagen and hemoglobin, are relatively resistant to degradation and so turn over slowly. Other proteins, especially those that have an important regulatory function, or those that are damaged in some way or with errors in amino acid sequence due to errors in transcription, are readily degraded. The details of the molecular basis of protein degradation have not been as fully described as the system for protein synthesis. However, like synthesis, the regulation of protein degradation includes both a component that targets specific proteins and a component that regulates the overall rate of protein degradation in a tissue and facilitates overall changes in protein content. Increased proteolysis of muscle tissue protein occurs, for example, in response to a number of stresses, including fasting, acidosis, denervation, cancer, and thermal injury (Mitch and Goldberg, 1996).

The degradation of protein involves two different systems: lysosomal and nonlysosomal. The regulation of these two systems is somewhat different, as is their specificity for individual proteins and their distribution within tissues. In general, lysosomal proteolysis begins with the formation of vesicles (Fig. 10–7A). Vesicles are formed when portions of the cell membrane enclose a portion of extracellular matrix (this process is called endocytosis) or a portion of intracellular matrix (this process is called autophagy). These vesicles, or autophagic vacuoles, then fuse with organelles (primary lysosomes) within the cell that contain the degradative enzymes (e.g., cathepsins B, D, H, and L). Membrane-bound insulin receptors, for example, are degraded by the lysosomal system, and the process is enhanced when insulin is bound to the receptor. In general, this system is thought to be less selective than the nonlysosomal system, because portions of cellular membrane or cell matrix are engulfed rather nonselectively into lysosomes. Much of the information about the lysosomal system comes from studies in rat liver. In the liver, the activity of the lysosomal system is the major system that responds to variations in nutrient supply. The system is activated by starvation and suppressed by the presence of amino acids (Lee and Marzella, 1994).

In addition to lysosomal degradation, there are also a number of cytosolic proteases. In general, the cytosolic enzymes degrade rapidly, turning over proteins and abnormal pro-

A   Lysosomal Degradation

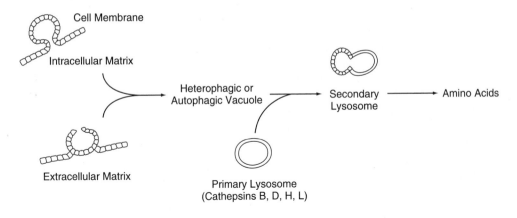

B   ATP-Dependent Ubiquitin–Proteasome Degradation

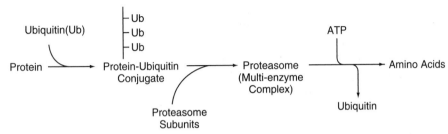

Figure 10–7. *Protein degradation. The two primary pathways of protein degradation are (A) lysosomal degradation, and (B) ATP-dependent ubiquitin–proteasome degradation. Lysosomal degradation proceeds when a portion of either intracellular or extracellular matrix is enclosed by a portion of cell membrane, forming an autophagic or heterophagic vacuole. Vacuoles fuse with primary lysosomes containing proteases such as cathepsins B, D, H, and L. The resulting secondary lysosome degrades the engulfed protein. ATP-dependent ubiquitin–proteasome degradation proceeds when ubiquitin molecules bind to a protein. The protein–ubiquitin conjugate binds with proteasome subunits to form a large, multi-enzyme complex called a proteasome. Within the complex, the degradation of protein proceeds by an ATP-dependent process, and ubiquitin and amino acids are released.*

teins. The majority of degradation of this type is thought to proceed through a multi-enzyme complex, the ATP-dependent ubiquitin–proteasome system. This complex includes activity of both an ATP-requiring system and a system involving ubiquitin. Ubiquitin is a highly basic, 76-amino acid peptide, which is bound, under the regulation of several enzymes, to lysyl residues on the targeted protein. This pathway of protein degradation is shown in Figure 10–7B. Multiple molecules of ubiquitin are bound to proteins for degradation, and then the complex is degraded by lysosomes or by a large (26S), multicatalytic protease complex known as a proteasome. In this ubiquitin-dependent system, there is much more specificity than in the lysosomal

system. Specific proteins are targeted for degradation by the addition of ubiquitin molecules. Many abnormal and regulatory proteins are degraded by this system, including proteins that must turn over very rapidly, such as those that control DNA repair and cell cycle progression. Animal studies have shown that the acceleration of muscle degradation seen in fasting, sepsis, and cancer cachexia is due to an activation of the ubiquitin–proteasome system (Mitch and Goldberg, 1996). This system also may play an important part in increased muscle catabolism in some pathological states in humans. Studies in head trauma patients have confirmed an increase in ubiquitin–proteasome activity in these individuals (Mansoor et al., 1996), suggesting that this system may be important in the accelerated protein degradation that accompanies many catabolic states.

There are also a number of proteases with special functions, such as the calcium-dependent calpains. These proteases are responsible for processing proteins within the cell before the proteins are secreted. Although functionally very important, these proteases do not contribute substantially to the total amount of body protein that is degraded.

In addition to general degradation of cellular proteins, the proteolytic systems can also select individual proteins, either through specific inactivating factors or because enzymes are more susceptible to degradation in the absence of their substrate or coenzyme. For example, animal studies have shown that feeding a diet with excess amounts of tryptophan results in an increase in the activity of the tryptophan dioxygenase, an enzyme involved in the degradation of tryptophan. The enzyme is stabilized by its substrate, so that the increased levels of tryptophan decrease the degradation of the enzyme (Cihak et al., 1973).

REGULATION OF PROTEIN METABOLISM

The steps in the synthesis and degradation of protein delineated in the preceding section are the potential sites of regulation. Some of these processes are controlled through the action of mediators such as hormones. Although hormones do not act in isolation, an understanding of the individual actions of hormones is necessary for understanding the coordinated regulation involved in the responses of protein turnover to feeding, growth, and injury. These aspects of regulation are under study, but some examples of the ways in which protein metabolism is controlled are given in the following section.

Hormones and Cytokines

Anabolic Hormones. Growth hormone and insulin are both considered to be anabolic, in that reduced circulating levels of these hormones are associated with loss of body protein or decreased growth. Normally, the blood

insulin concentration increases with feeding and decreases with fasting, which is associated with cyclic responses of carbohydrate, fat, and protein metabolism between anabolism and catabolism. An inability to mount an anabolic response to the influx of nutrients is accompanied by a loss of body protein, and individuals who lack insulin because of diabetes lose body protein. Measurements in animal models show that insulin stimulates the synthesis of protein, although some human studies suggest that this requires that amino acids are also provided. The most consistent finding in human studies is that protein degradation is inhibited by insulin in both the whole body and in skeletal muscle (Long and Lowry, 1990).

The mechanism for the acute action of insulin to stimulate protein synthesis occurs at the level of initiation of translation of mRNA with phosphorylation of initiation factors (e.g., eIF-2) already present in the cell. The precise way in which insulin inhibits protein degradation is not known, but some depression in protein degradation, particularly in the liver, may be brought about through increased amino acid concentrations that inhibit lysosomal degradation (Lee and Marzella, 1994).

Growth hormone is associated with longer-term regulation of growth. Growth hormone levels are higher in children, especially during growth spurts, and children are dwarfed when growth hormone is absent. The effect of growth hormone is, in part, mediated by insulin-like growth factors IGF-I and IGF-II, which are peptides produced by the liver in response to circulating growth hormone. Local production of these hormones at their site of action in tissues might also be important in regulating protein metabolism. Muscle protein synthesis in adults is stimulated by provision of growth hormone or IGFs, whereas there is no observable stimulation of whole-body protein synthesis. Muscle degradation is also enhanced by growth hormone, as evidenced by an increase in the excretion of 3-methylhistidine. This response may be a necessary consequence of the remodeling necessary for the growth of muscle, but the precise details of how these hormones regulate protein metabolism are not yet fully understood. However, growth hormone has been used in clinical experiments to stimulate an anabolic response in protein metabolism in patients with severe illness (Garlick and Wernerman, 1997).

In addition to growth hormone and insulin, the male sex hormone testosterone also promotes protein synthesis, particularly in muscle. Synthetic testosterone-like compounds, classed as anabolic steroids, are also capable of promoting the retention of body protein. These have been used in animal production but are not routinely used clinically.

Catabolic Hormones. The three hormones cortisol, glucagon, and epinephrine are often collectively termed the stress hormones, because their plasma concentrations are elevated after injury or during infection. Infusion of these hormones together mimics stress, causing loss of body protein and an inhibition of muscle protein synthesis. Glucagon promotes gluconeogenesis from amino acids and from lactate. The ratio of glucagon to insulin levels is an important factor in both acute regulation (such as after a meal) and with prolonged deprivation. At physiological levels, glucagon is not known to have a direct effect on tissue or whole-body protein synthesis, but elevated glucagon does interfere with the ability of insulin to inhibit protein degradation (Long and Lowry, 1990).

Cortisol, from the adrenal cortex, has a catabolic effect similar to that of glucagon. In addition, cortisol decreases protein synthesis and increases protein degradation in muscle. The synthesis of several liver proteins is increased, including the synthesis of enzymes involved in amino acid oxidation, which facilitates the conversion of amino acids into energy-yielding compounds or gluconeogenic precursors.

Few studies have been performed with epinephrine, but it appears that at moderate levels of the hormone, protein metabolism is not affected, whereas at higher levels of epinephrine, protein degradation in the whole body and in muscle may be reduced (Matthews et al., 1990). This anabolic action of epinephrine may limit the loss of body protein brought about by elevated cortisol and glucagon.

Cytokines. Cytokines are peptides produced by cells of the immune system (macrophages) in response to injury or inflammation. High circulating levels of cytokines, particularly interleukin-1β (IL-1β), interleukin-6 (IL-6), and tumor necrosis factor-α (TNF-α), are associated with catabolism of body protein. Direct action of these cytokines on muscle in vitro has not been demonstrated. However, when given in vivo to growing rats, both IL-1β and TNF-α stimulate protein synthesis in liver and depress protein synthesis in muscle. Protein degradation is inhibited in liver and stimulated in muscle by TNF-α, and these effects are potentiated by treatment with IL-1β. These effects on muscle protein synthesis and degradation mimic those observed in injury or inflammation. Further evidence for cytokine involvement in the catabolic response to infection is provided by studies that show a diminished catabolic state in septic animals treated with TNF-α antibody and IL-1β receptor antagonist (Garlick and Wernerman, 1997).

Responses of Protein Metabolism to Nutrient Supply

Anabolic Responses to Eating. One of the most fundamental anabolic responses is that observed after the ingestion of a meal. Substrates in the form of amino acids and energy-yielding substances are provided by the influx of nutrients. The hormonal responses include an increase in the circulating levels of insulin and a decrease in the levels of catabolic hormones such as glucagon. Rates of protein degradation are decreased in the whole body, and rates of synthesis might, in addition, be stimulated. Although the oxidation of amino acids is increased in the immediate postprandial period, there is a net positive balance of protein.

Studies in animals suggest that, at the tissue level, protein synthesis in the liver is stimulated and protein degradation is inhibited by the ingestion of a meal. The liver protein mass is increased, and the synthesis of hepatic proteins is increased. Increased synthesis is also observed for proteins such as albumin that are made in the liver and then exported into the circulation. Muscle protein synthesis in growing animals can be stimulated acutely by the intake of food, and this effect depends on the increase in circulating insulin. However, not only are there problems when extrapolating from animal experiments to humans, but there is often an additional complication in that the animal studies are often carried out in young, growing animals, whereas the studies in humans are most often carried out in adults. Sensitivities to the effects of feeding on muscle protein synthesis vary in rats of different ages, with decreased responses in protein synthesis in adult rats, suggesting that differences in maturity and growth rate are important determinants of the response to feeding (Garlick et al., 1992).

In addition to the role of insulin in the feeding response, studies in vitro suggest that amino acid concentrations, which rise after feeding, regulate protein synthesis through an enhancement in initiation factor activation. Stimulation of protein synthesis by amino acids in humans in vivo has also been demonstrated. Amino acids may also alter the sensitivity of tissues to hormones, such as insulin. However, the precise roles of insulin and amino acid concentrations in mediating the observed effects on protein metabolism are still somewhat uncertain.

Catabolism Associated with Brief Fasting. As the body moves from the absorptive period following a meal (also known as postprandial) to the postabsorptive period before the consumption of the next meal, protein balance changes from net accumulation to net loss. At the level of the whole body, the change is predominantly an increase in protein degradation. Amino acids are mobilized from tissues such as muscle and redirected to maintain synthesis in tissues such as the liver, as well as to provide the substrates for gluconeogenesis, which maintain the level of blood glucose. The hormonal changes associated with fasting include a reduction in the circulating levels of insulin along with increased levels of glucagon.

Starvation. If fasting is prolonged and the body's stores of liver glycogen are exhausted, the body adapts to use muscle protein to meet most of the needs for glucose. Although body fat is mobilized to meet most of the energy needs as fasting proceeds, this mobilization results in only limited usable energy for the brain and obligate glycolytic tissues such as

red blood cells and the renal medulla. The brain requires glucose, because fatty acids that are mobilized during starvation are not an energy source for the brain. Only the small glycerol component of fat, which is converted to glucose, can be used by the brain. During starvation, the major portion of the brain's glucose requirement is met by mobilization of amino acids from protein, with subsequent gluconeogenesis by the liver. The mobilization of body protein for glucose production is evidenced by the relatively high excretion of urinary nitrogen.

However, if gluconeogenesis were to continue at an accelerated rate, skeletal muscle would soon be exhausted. An adaptation in lipid metabolism occurs in longer-term starvation, so that ketone bodies (acetoacetate, β-hydroxybutyrate) are formed. Ketone bodies can cross the blood-brain barrier to provide energy for the brain and thus spare body protein. These changes involve further adaptations, with reductions in protein synthesis and degradation and in oxidation of amino acids. These adaptations help conserve both energy and amino acids and are reflected in the output of nitrogen, which is decreased to about 3 g nitrogen per day by several weeks of starvation (Cahill, 1976). When body fat stores are exhausted, body protein is again mobilized for energy by means of an increase in muscle protein degradation. This final increase in the degradation of body protein cannot be sustained for long, and, if feeding does not occur, death ensues.

The hormonal changes that bring about alterations in protein metabolism in starvation are, for the most part, an amplification of the response to an overnight fast, with a further reduction in insulin and a further elevation in glucagon. In addition, the level of thyroid hormone decreases, thereby reducing both basal energy expenditure and the energy expenditure due to the turnover of protein. Reduced levels of thyroid hormones result in a reduction in proteolysis by both lysosomal and ubiquitin–proteasome pathways (Mitch and Goldberg, 1996).

Malnutrition. Prolonged undernutrition of energy and protein (see Chapter 19) shares many of the same characteristics as starvation, but these develop over a longer time frame. There are reductions in the circulating levels of insulin and increases in the levels of glucagon. Growth hormone levels are elevated, but the levels of IGF-I are depressed. Thyroid hormone levels are reduced, with a similar conservation of energy and amino acids as is seen in starvation. The oxidation of amino acids is reduced, as is protein turnover (both synthesis and degradation).

In children, a reduction in food intake is accompanied by a cessation of growth. Chronic malnutrition results in both stunting (reduction in height for age) and wasting (reduction in weight for height). Nutrient deprivation also results in reductions of particular proteins. Albumin concentration often is reduced, as scarce amino acids are directed to more essential proteins. This selective reduction in albumin is mediated through a reduction in the amount of mRNA for albumin in the liver. Because circulating levels of albumin respond to nutritional intake, albumin concentration has been used to assess nutritional status, but the relation of albumin levels to nutritional status often is confused by the fall in albumin associated with injury or disease. Immunity and the resistance to infection are also impaired by chronic undernutrition. Infections are both more frequent than normal and accompanied by increases in mortality and morbidity.

The data in Figure 10–8 demonstrate the reduction in protein synthesis and degradation in malnourished children in Jamaica. These children were studied sequentially with [^{15}N]-glycine as they recovered from their malnutrition. During recovery from malnutrition, both synthesis and degradation were accelerated compared with measurements made either when the children were malnourished or after they had recovered from malnutrition. This increased synthesis and degradation is associated with catch-up growth (i.e., growth rates that are more rapid than normal). When the children reach more appropriate weight and height for age, the rate of growth slows to more age-appropriate rates.

Protein Metabolism in Growth and Development

Normal Growth. Growth is an anabolic process that occurs over a much longer time

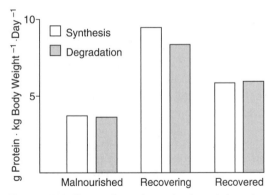

Figure 10–8. Rates of protein synthesis and degradation in children suffering from malnutrition, during the recovery process (recovering), and when recovery was complete (recovered). The rates of protein synthesis and degradation, expressed in g of protein per kg body weight per day, were assessed with [^{15}N]glycine. (Based on the data of Golden, M. H. N., Waterlow, J. C., and Picou, D. [1977] Protein turnover, synthesis and breakdown before and after recovery from protein-energy malnutrition. Clin Sci Mol Med 53:473–477.)

period than do the acute responses to the intake of nutrients. Although the overall process of growth includes a net increase in the amount of body protein, this is often accompanied by significant remodeling so that protein degradation is also elevated. The capacity for growth can be seen in the difference in turnover rates between growing children and adults. In newborn infants, rates of protein synthesis are about twice the rates in adults, and this decline in protein synthesis is progressive throughout life, from preterm infants to old age (see Fig. 10–4).

Growth rates for children recovering from malnutrition are greater than those observed in healthy children, and the rate of growth is positively correlated with the rate of protein synthesis, even though protein degradation also is increased to some extent. A similar phenomenon with increases in both synthesis and degradation associated with protein accumulation can occur in specific tissues in conditions such as hypertrophy of muscle in response to increased work. In this latter case, net protein is retained within the tissue, and this is accomplished by an increase in protein synthesis that exceeds the increase in degradation.

Increased protein synthesis sustained during growth is accomplished with increased levels of RNA in the tissue, including both messenger and ribosomal RNA, so that the capacity of the body to make protein is increased. Growth is under hormonal regulation, primarily by growth hormone and IGF-I. The capacity for growth may also include responses to other anabolic agents that do not occur in the adult. For example, insulin has the capacity to stimulate protein synthesis in the young, growing rat, but this anabolic response to insulin is diminished in the nongrowing adult rat.

In addition to an acceleration of the overall process of turnover and the positive balance between protein synthesis and degradation, growth and development also involve the selective accumulation of specific proteins at the appropriate period of development. At puberty and during pregnancy and lactation, for example, appropriate hormone concentrations are increased by the selective transcription of the appropriate genes. These hormones, in turn, provide for further alterations in protein metabolism. Androgens, for example, are anabolic, providing for an increase in protein mass. This increase may be mediated, in part, through a potentiation of the effect of growth hormone or by a reduction in the catabolic action of corticosteroids.

Hypertrophy and Atrophy. Certain organs are capable of growth even in the adult; most notably, increased muscle tissue brought about by increased use of the muscle. This phenomenon, known as work-induced hypertrophy, is associated with increased levels of protein synthesis with smaller increases in protein degradation.

Protein also can be lost from individual tissues during disuse. In humans, the loss of muscle tissue is apparent during immobilization, such as that which accompanies bone fracture. This disuse atrophy is associated with decreased synthesis of muscle protein with little change in protein degradation (Gibson et al., 1987).

Protein Loss in Injury and Disease

Loss of body protein accompanies many disease states, such as trauma, cancer, and infection. These disease states contrast to malnutrition and overt starvation in that adaptation to preserve lean body mass does not occur. In response to starvation, energy is conserved with a lowering of metabolic rate, whereas disease states are hypermetabolic; that is, the basal metabolic rate is higher than in healthy individuals. In addition to the increased demands for energy, there is an accompanying metabolic abnormality that prevents the adaptation to the use of ketone bodies for energy. The lack of this adaptive response means that body protein is not preserved but rather continues to be the supply of substrates for energy through the formation of glucose. The mobilization of amino acids from muscle involves an acceleration in the rate of protein degradation. Although some amino acids, such as leucine, valine, and isoleucine, are oxidized in muscle tissue, other amino acids pass into the blood stream for transport to the liver. Within the liver, the amino acids are available for gluconeogenesis and for the synthesis of liver proteins, especially acute-phase proteins, including C-reactive protein and fibrinogen, which rise in concentration after injury or during illness.

Burns, Surgery, and Sepsis. Conditions such as burn injury, surgery, and systemic infection or sepsis are all accompanied by the loss of body protein. The metabolic responses to these conditions often are considered together as stress responses. Stress responses include increased energy expenditure, loss of body protein, and the synthesis of acute-phase proteins. The magnitude of the responses varies with the condition and the severity of the injury. In patients with burn injury, for example, there is loss of body heat to the environment, and energy expenditure is increased to compensate for this loss. Raising the ambient temperature and humidity can reduce the loss of body heat. With major surgery, the degree of surgical trauma has an impact on the magnitude of the response. At the level of the whole body, there is an observable increase in protein synthesis and degradation following surgery, with degradation increased more than synthesis so that there is net loss of body protein. However, this whole-body response is a composite of different responses in different tissues. For example, the rate of protein synthesis in skeletal muscle is depressed after surgery, whereas a variety of inflammatory conditions cause an increase in liver protein synthesis.

The complete response to stress involves the mobilization of muscle amino acids through decreased protein synthesis and accelerated degradation and the production of acute-phase proteins by the liver. These effects are mediated by the concerted actions of stress hormones—glucagon, cortisol, and epinephrine. In addition to catabolic responses such as an inhibition of muscle protein synthesis and increased muscle degradation, higher levels of stress hormones are also associated with a failure of normal anabolic responses, such as the ability of insulin to reduce the rate of protein degradation. The catabolic responses in trauma are also associated with increased levels of cytokines. Of the more than 30 of these peptides produced by leukocytes in response to stress, those particularly associated with protein catabolism include TNF-α, IL-1, and IL-6. In burn injury, the strongest correlations of increased whole-body protein degradation are observed with IL-6 (Long and Lowry, 1990). Neither the actions of the stress hormones nor those of the catabolic cytokines are sufficient to mimic the entire stress hormone response, and an interaction between the two systems has been postulated.

For some types of surgery, an attenuation of the increase in plasma cortisol can be achieved by epidural anesthesia, with a reduction in the negative nitrogen balance that normally accompanies the surgical stress. This suggests that neural regulation also is an important factor in the catabolic response to trauma. Immobilization also might be a contributing factor in muscle loss, because unused muscles are known to atrophy.

Muscle wasting is part of the response to stress and may be viewed as beneficial in that amino acids are mobilized from expendable to essential tissues, to provide more vital functions such as the synthesis of acute-phase proteins. As with starvation, such short-term adaptation may be beneficial to the organism; however, in stress, the longer this state continues, the more detrimental it becomes. Nutritional support therefore becomes obligatory in long-term critical illness, and there is much active research on strategies for optimizing nutrition by altering the composition of nutrients given in particular illnesses and also by combining nutrition with anabolic agents such as growth hormone.

Cancer. In catabolic conditions such as cancer, the loss of body protein can be due in part to the anorexia that accompanies the disease. However, some forms of cancer, such as small cell cancer of the lung, are associated with the loss of body protein, which occurs even when nutrients are supplied. This wasting condition is called cachexia. The mechanism by which this loss is mediated is not fully delineated, but reduction in dietary intake or diversion of nutrients to the tumor is not sufficient to account for the loss of lean body mass. Researchers have hypothesized that there may be an unidentified factor that induces the loss of protein. Recently, a glycoprotein, which may be such a factor, has been isolated from tumor-bearing mice. This protein induces the loss of body protein when it is given to healthy mice (Todorov et al., 1996).

It has been suggested that energy expenditure might be elevated in cancer, thus contributing to body weight loss, but this has not been a consistent finding. Studies on whole-body protein metabolism in cancer have, in general, demonstrated an elevation in both synthesis and degradation. In animal studies in which it is possible to study the responses at the tissue level, differential responses among different tissues have been reported. For example, in tumor-bearing mice, protein synthesis rates in muscle were depressed, whereas the synthesis of liver protein was enhanced. This is similar to the response seen with other forms of stress.

Attempts to retard the loss of body protein by nutritional means in cancer patients must be considered in terms of the effects on both body tissue and the tumor. Because feeding can stimulate protein synthesis in some tumors, researchers are attempting to devise a feeding regimen that preserves host tissue at the expense of tumor growth.

Human Immunodeficiency Virus. Infection with HIV results in substantial loss of body weight, known as AIDS wasting. This condition is somewhat different from starvation and other wasting conditions in that body fat is preserved, but lean tissue is lost. Poor nutrient intake may contribute to AIDS wasting through anorexia, diarrhea, and malabsorption. However, the wasting associated with AIDS is not simply due to poor nutrient intake but has many features of catabolic states such as burns, surgery, and sepsis. The loss of body protein arises from the use of amino acids for the formation of glucose, similar to the mobilization of amino acids during the early stages of starvation. Unlike starvation, however, the adaptive responses to spare body protein are blunted. HIV disease also is associated with increased rates of whole-body protein synthesis and degradation.

The catabolic condition of AIDS wasting at the level of muscle tissue can be seen in the measurements of protein synthesis and protein degradation shown in Figure 10–9. The rates of protein synthesis are similar in healthy controls and AIDS patients, but the rates of protein degradation, based on the excretion of 3-methylhistidine, are higher. Moreover, the increased rates of protein degradation in muscle are apparent in patients with AIDS even without weight loss, indicating that these changes in muscle metabolism precede the onset of significant loss of body weight.

Resting energy expenditure is also increased in AIDS patients, particularly during the periods of secondary infection that frequently accompany the disease. This increase may be due in part to the increased energy requirement imposed by increased protein turnover. Adaptive mechanisms to reduce voluntary energy expenditure, i.e., by reduced physical activity, may balance some of the increase in resting energy expenditure, so that total energy expenditure is not elevated.

Circulating levels of several anabolic hormones are reduced in AIDS patients, including growth hormone, IGF-I, and insulin. Levels of thyroid hormone (T_3) are also reduced, as are gonadal hormones such as testosterone. Glucagon and cortisol levels are elevated, as they are in other conditions of stress/trauma. The hormonal changes are, in general, similar to the changes seen in starvation (Sellmeyer and Grunfeld, 1996), but the failure of the adaptive responses suggests resistance to hor-

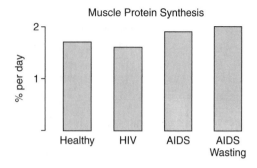

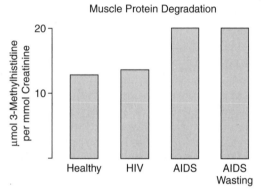

Figure 10–9. *Muscle protein metabolism in healthy subjects and patients with HIV, patients with AIDS but no weight loss, and patients with AIDS wasting. The rate of synthesis of vastus lateralis muscle was determined from the incorporation of L-[²H₅]phenylalanine. Muscle protein degradation was measured from the ratio of urinary 3-methylhistidine to urinary creatinine. HIV subjects were asymptomatic. AIDS patients previously had an AIDS-defining illness but no significant weight loss. Patients with AIDS wasting had lost >10% of their pre-illness weight. (Based on the data of McNurlan, M. A., Garlick, P. J., Steigbigel, R. T., et al. [1997] Responsiveness of muscle protein synthesis to growth hormone administration in HIV-infected individuals declines with severity of disease. J Clin Invest 100:2125–2132.)*

monal effects at the level of the tissue. Furthermore, the levels of catabolic cytokines, TNF-α, interferon α and γ, and IL-1 and IL-6, are increased in the later stages of HIV disease, particularly during episodes of secondary infections (Grunfeld and Feingold, 1992). These cytokines may contribute directly to wasting and may also mediate hormonal resistance, exacerbating the loss of body protein that is characteristic of this disease.

Current Challenges in Protein Metabolism

The preservation of body protein in diseases such as HIV and other long-term illnesses is

CLINICAL CORRELATION

Is AIDS Wasting Simply Starvation?

Infection with HIV is associated with a profound and selective loss of body protein that gives rise to the condition known as AIDS wasting. Although AIDS wasting superficially appears to be like simple starvation in that there is a loss of body protein, there are a number of differences between this state of stress and uncomplicated starvation.

Thinking Critically

1. What are the similarities/differences between starvation and AIDS wasting?

2. Which hormones might potentially be involved in AIDS wasting? What other possible mediators might be different in the adaptation to starvation compared with adaptation to the stress of HIV infection?

one of the current challenges in the field of protein metabolism. The approach to solving this problem has been both to understand the underlying mechanisms and to reverse the loss of body protein, either by nutritional means or by combining specific nutritional regimens with anabolic agents. For example, investigations into stress responses have delineated both hormonal mechanisms and those involving cytokines such as TNF. The link to cytokines has led to treatment modalities that include antibodies to either the cytokine or its receptor. Although early parenteral nutrition does not completely prevent the loss of body protein associated with stress such as surgery, certainly the loss of body protein is attenuated over that observed without provision of nutrition. The amino acids that are supplied help preserve body tissue and also may facilitate responses by the body such as the synthesis of acute-phase proteins, activation of the immune system, or synthesis of specific proteins involved in wound healing. Provision of anabolic agents such as insulin and growth hormone in conjunction with adequate nutrition has been demonstrated to be more effective than nutrition alone in preventing the loss of body protein.

Increasingly, the focus in catabolic illness is not only on the provision of adequate nutrition but also on altering nutrition to reflect the particular problems associated with particular diseases. For example, patients with severe liver disease may benefit from the provision of nutrition enriched with branched-chain amino acids. As the capacity of the liver to degrade amino acids such as methionine, phenylalanine, and tyrosine is diminished, plasma levels of these amino acids rise, while concentrations of amino acids degraded in the periphery, such as the branched-chain amino acids, fall. Enhancing the supply of branched-chain amino acids may help correct the amino acid imbalance caused by the disease.

In addition to illnesses that result in specific amino acid imbalances, provision of extra amounts of single amino acids sometimes has been demonstrated to have therapeutic benefit. For example, glutamine-enriched nutrition has been used clinically in patients after surgery. Glutamine is released from muscle tissue in response to stress such as surgery, and provision of glutamine-containing nutritional regimens to surgical patients reduces negative nitrogen balance. Both glutamine and arginine have been used in conjunction with adequate nutrition to stimulate the immune system and to promote healing. Ongoing research seeks to understand how protein metabolism is altered by disease states and how nutrition may be employed for benefit.

REFERENCES

Cahill, G. F. Jr. (1976) Starvation in man. Clin Endocrinol Metab 5:397–415.

Cihak, A., Lamar, C. Jr. and Pitot, H. C. (1973) L-Tryptophan inhibition of tyrosine aminotransferase degradation in rat liver in vivo. Arch Biochem Biophys 156:188–194.

Denne, S. C. and Kalhan, S. C. (1987) Leucine metabolism in human newborns. Am J Physiol 253:E608–E615.

Garlick, P. J., Baillie, A. G. S., Grant, I. and McNurlan, M. A. (1992) In vivo action of insulin on protein metabolism in experimental animals. In: Protein Metabolism in Diabetes Mellitus (Nair, K. S., ed.), pp. 163–171. Smith Gordon and Co., London.

Garlick, P. J., McNurlan, M. A., Essén, P. and Wernerman, J. (1994) Measurement of tissue protein synthesis rates in vivo: A critical analysis of contrasting methods. Am J Physiol 266:E287–E297.

Garlick, P. J. and Wernerman, J. (1997) Protein metabolism in injury. In: Scientific Foundations of Trauma (Cooper, G. J., Dudley, H. A. F., Gann, D. S., Little, R. A. and Maynard, R. L., eds.), pp. 690–728. Butterworth-Heinemann Reed, Oxford, England.

Gibson, J. N. A., Halliday, D., Morrison, W. L., Stoward, P. J., Hornsby, G. A., Watt, P. W., Murdoch, G. and Rennie, A. J. (1987) Decrease in human quadriceps muscle protein turnover consequent upon leg immobilization. Clin Sci 72:503–509.

Golden, M. H. N., Waterlow, J. C. and Picou, D. (1977) Protein turnover, synthesis and breakdown before and after recovery from protein-energy malnutrition. Clin Sci Mol Med 53:473–477.

Grunfeld, C. and Feingold, K. R. (1992) Seminars in Medicine of the Beth Israel Hospital, Boston. Metabolic disturbances and wasting in the acquired immunodeficiency syndrome. N Engl J Med 327:329–337.

Kinney, J. M. (1978) The tissue composition of surgical weight loss. In: Advances in Parenteral Nutrition (Johnson, J. A., ed.), pp. 511–520. Medical and Technical Press, Lancaster, England.

Lee, H. K. and Marzella, L. (1994) Regulation of intracellular protein degradation with special reference to lysosomes: Role in cell physiology and pathology. Int Rev Exp Pathol 35:39–147.

Long, C. L. and Lowry, S. F. (1990) Hormonal regulation of protein metabolism. J Parenter Enteral Nutr 14:555–562.

Mansoor, O., Beaufrere, B., Boirie, Y., Ralliere, C., Taillandier, D., Aurousseau, E., Schoeffler, P., Arnal, M. and Attaix D. (1996) Increased mRNA levels for components of the lysosomal, Ca^{2+}-activated, and ATP-ubiquitin-dependent proteolytic pathways in skeletal muscle from head trauma patients. Proc Natl Acad Sci USA 93:2714–2718.

Matthews, D. E., Pesola, G. and Campbell, R. G. (1990) Effect of epinephrine on amino acid and energy metabolism in humans. Am J Physiol 258:E948–E956.

Mauras, N. (1995) Estrogens do not affect whole-body protein metabolism in the prepubertal female. J Clin Endocrinol Metab 80:2842–2845.

Mauras, N., Haymond, M. W., Darmaun, D., Vieira, N. E., Abrams, S. A. and Yergey, A. L. (1994) Calcium and protein kinetics in prepubertal boys: Positive effects of testosterone. J Clin Invest 93:1014–1019.

McNurlan, M. A., Garlick, P. J., Steigbigel, R. T., DeCristofaro, K. A., Frost, R. A., Lang, C. H., Johnson, R. W., Santasier, A. M., Cabahug, C. J., Fuhrer, J. and Gelato, M. C. (1997) Responsiveness of muscle protein synthesis to growth hormone administration in HIV-infected individuals declines with severity of disease. J Clin Invest 100:2125–2132.

Mitch, W. E. and Goldberg, A. L. (1996) Mechanisms of muscle wasting: The role of the ubiquitin-proteasome pathway. N Engl J Med 335:1897–1905.

Mitton, S. G., Calder, A. G. and Garlick, P. J. (1991). Protein turnover rates in sick, premature neonates during the first few days of life. Pediatr Res 30:418–422.

Munro, H. N. (1964) Historical introduction: The origin and growth of our present concepts of protein metabolism. In: Mammalian Protein Metabolism (Munro, H. N. and Allison, J. B., eds.), vol. 1, pp. 1–29. Academic Press, New York.

Nachaliel, N., Jain, D. and Hod, Y. (1993) A cAMP-regulated RNA-binding protein that interacts with phosphoenolpyruvate carboxykinase (GTP) mRNA. J Biol Chem 268:24203–24209.

Reeds, P. J. and Garlick, P. J. (1984) Nutrition and protein turnover in man. In: Advances in Nutritional Research (Draper, H. H., ed.), vol. 6, pp. 93–138. Plenum Press, New York.

Sellmeyer, D. E. and Grunfeld, C. (1996) Endocrine and metabolic disturbances in human immunodeficiency virus infection and the acquired immune deficiency syndrome. Endocr Rev 17:518–532.

Sjölin, J., Stjernström, H., Henneberg, S., Andersson, E., Mårtensson, J., Friman, G., and Larsson, J. (1989) Splanchnic and peripheral release of 3-methylhistidine in relation to its urinary excretion in human infection. Metabolism 38:23–29.

Süttman, U., Ockenga, J., Selberg, O., Hoogestraat, L., Deicher, H. and Muller, M. J. (1995) Incidence and prognostic value of malnutrition and wasting in human immunodeficiency virus-infected outpatients. J Acquir Immune Defic Syndr Hum Retrovirol 8:239–246.

Todorov, P., Cariuk, P., McDevitt, T., Coles, B., Fearon, K. and Tisdale, M. (1996) Characterization of a cancer cachectic factor. Nature 379:739–742.

Tomkins, A. M., Garlick, P. J., Schofield, W. N. and Waterlow, J. C. (1983) The combined effects of infection and malnutrition on protein metabolism in children. Clin Sci 65:313–324.

Waterlow, J. C., Garlick, P. J. and Millward, D. J. (1978) Protein Turnover in Mammalian Tissues and in the Whole Body. North-Holland Publishing, Amsterdam.

Welle, S., Thornton, C., Statt, M. and McHenry, B. (1994) Postprandial myofibrillar and whole body protein synthesis in young and old human subjects. Am J Physiol 267:E599–E604.

RECOMMENDED READINGS

Frayn, K. N. (1996) Metabolic Regulation and Human Perspective. Portland Press, London.

Garlick, P. J. and Wernerman, J. (1997) Protein metabolism in injury. In: Scientific Foundations of Trauma (Cooper, G. J., Dudley, H. A. F., Gann, D. S., Little, R. A. and Maynard, R. L., eds.), pp. 690–728. Butterworth-Heinemann Reed, Oxford, England.

CHAPTER **11**

◆ ◆

Amino Acid Metabolism

Martha H. Stipanuk, Ph.D., and Malcolm Watford, D.Phil.

OUTLINE

OVERVIEW OF AMINO ACID METABOLISM

This discussion of amino acid metabolism focuses on the 20 α-amino, α-carboxylic acids that are the precursors for protein synthesis. Many other compounds in the body, perhaps as many as 300, also could be considered amino acids, because this term can be used more broadly to describe any compound with an amine group and an acidic group. For example, other amino acids are formed when some of the 20 amino acids used for protein synthesis undergo limited posttranslational modification to form derivatized residues that are released as free amino acids on proteolysis; these include N-methylhistidine, γ-carboxyglutamate, hydroxyproline, and hydroxylysine. Additionally, some serine is specifically converted to selenocysteine cotranslationally. A number of other amino acids (including citrulline, ornithine, γ-aminobutyrate, homocysteine, and taurine) are formed during metabolism of specific amino acids. In addition, these and other amino acid derivatives, including some that are not synthesized by mammalian tissues, are consumed in the diet.

The 20 amino acids required for protein synthesis include some whose carbon chains cannot be synthesized in the body (essential or indispensable amino acids) and others whose carbon skeletons can be made from common intermediates in metabolism (nonessential or dispensable amino acids). The nutritional requirement for protein is actually a requirement for the indispensable (essential) amino acids and a source of nitrogen for synthesis of dispensable (nonessential) amino acids, as is discussed in more detail in Chapter 12. Most of the nitrogen for synthesis of dispensable amino acids must be provided by α-amino groups of amino acids because the body has a limited ability to incorporate inorganic nitrogen (ammonia; NH_3 and NH_4^+) into amino acids. The indispensable amino acids for humans include leucine, isoleucine, valine, lysine, threonine, tryptophan, phenylalanine, methionine, and histidine. Tyrosine and cysteine are termed semi-essential because they can be synthesized only if their indispensable amino acid precursors (phenylal-

anine and methionine, respectively) are provided. Many, but not all, of these indispensable amino acids actually can be made from their keto- or hydroxy-acid analogs if these are fed instead of the amino acids because of widespread transamination reactions in mammalian tissues. In practice, food proteins provide all 20 amino acids, but the body can adjust the proportions by transferring nitrogen to nonessential carbon skeletons and by catabolizing the excess amino acids.

An overview of amino acid metabolism is shown in Figure 11–1. The free amino acid pool is shown in the center of this figure; free amino acid pool is the term used to describe the amino acids that exist in the body in free form at any moment and to distinguish these free amino acids from those that exist in peptide or polypeptide/protein form. The size of this free amino acid pool in humans is approximately 150 g, and the flux of amino acids through this pool typically amounts to 400 to 500 g per day (Bergstrom et al., 1974; Jungas et al., 1992).

As can be seen from arrows leading toward the free amino acid pool, the major sources of amino acids are (1) digestion of endogenous proteins and peptides secreted or sloughed off into the gastrointestinal tract and absorption of the resulting amino acids into the circulation (about 70 g per day), (2) dietary protein after digestion and absorption of the resulting amino acids into the circulation (about 100 g per day depending on diet), and (3) intracellular protein turnover or degradation (about 230 g per day). These processes are discussed in Chapters 6 and 10. As shown by the arrows leading away from the free amino acid pool, the major metabolic fates of amino acids include (1) their use for protein synthesis, (2) their use as precursors for the synthesis of numerous nonprotein nitrogenous molecules, and (3) their catabolism with excretion of the nitrogen and use of the carbon chains as energy substrates. Note that the amino acids incorporated into proteins may eventually reenter the amino acid pool as a result of protein degradation and become available for reutilization, but those amino acids that were irreversibly modified, used for synthesis of nonpeptide metabolites, or under-

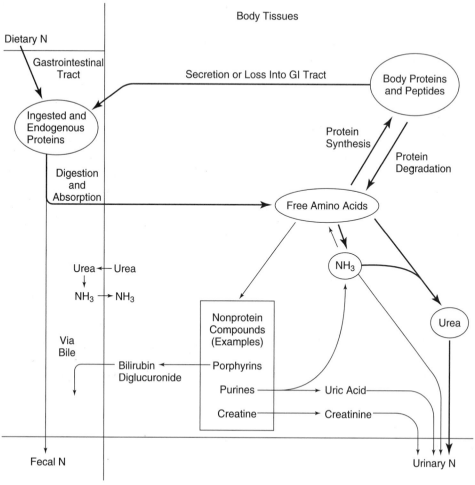

Figure 11–1. Schematic outline of the flow of nitrogen through the body. Major routes of nitrogen movement are indicated by the heavy lines.

went oxidative catabolism will, for the most part, no longer exist as amino acids.

The utilization of amino acids for protein synthesis was discussed in the preceding chapter. Catabolism of amino acids with the utilization of their carbon chains as fuels is described in the present chapter. These two fates of amino acids account for most of the amino acids that move through the amino acid pool. Although quantitatively not as large, the very important role of amino acids in synthesis of a large range of nonprotein compounds with specialized functions also is described in this chapter under the sections for metabolism of individual amino acids. Synthesis of dispensable amino acids, which often is simply the reverse of their catabolism

and which involves catabolism of another amino acid to provide the α-amino group, also is discussed.

In discussing the metabolism of amino acids in the body, it is important to recognize that amino groups can be transferred from one carbon skeleton to another by a number of reactions. Hence, the fate of amino groups and carbon skeletons must be considered somewhat separately, and the amino acid via which nitrogen enters a particular cell or tissue may be the same as or different from the amino acid that carries the nitrogen out of the cell or tissue. For example, glutamine or glutamate catabolism by the small intestine can result in release of the carbon chain as CO_2 and pyruvate, lactate, or alanine, and release of the nitrogens as alanine, ammonia, or both. The small intestine also converts glutamine to citrulline and proline, which contain both carbon and the α-amino nitrogen from glutamine or glutamate.

TRANSPORT OF AMINO ACIDS

As discussed in Chapter 6, amino acids taken up from the gastrointestinal tract are released by intestinal mucosal cells into the portal circulation. Specific transport proteins with overlapping specificities are responsible for the uptake and release of amino acids from cells. A number of transport systems for amino acids have been categorized in mammalian

cells (Christensen, 1990; McGivan and Pastor-Anglada, 1994) as summarized in Table 11–1. Major systems for the transport of small aliphatic amino acids include Na$^+$-dependent systems A and ASC and the Na$^+$-independent system L. Other, more restricted systems probably are responsible for the transport of glutamine, acidic amino acids, basic amino acids, and imino acids. In general, the amino acid transport systems serve to carry several amino acids across the cell membrane, and the transport of a particular amino acid is subject to competitive inhibition by the presence of other amino acids that share the same transport system.

Amino acid transport is subject to short- and long-term regulation. Most of the amino

TABLE 11–1
Some Major Amino Acid Transport Systems in Mammalian Cells

System	Specificity	Distribution	Comments
I. Na$^+$-dependent transport systems			
A	Small aliphatic amino acids; methyl-AIB	Widespread	Inducible by starvation, hormones, growth factors
ASC	Small aliphatic amino acids; nonmethyl-AIB	Widespread	Not usually inducible
N	Glutamine, histidine, asparagine	Liver	Variant system N^m in skeletal muscle
X$_{AG}^-$	Glutamate, aspartate	Widespread	Electrogenic; more than one Na$^+$ per amino acid; high affinity
β	β-Alanine, taurine, α-aminobutyrate	Widespread	Also Cl$^-$-dependent
Gly	Glycine, sarcosine	Liver, erythrocytes, central nervous system	Also Cl$^-$-dependent
B	Broad specificity; most neutral amino acids	Brush border membrane of epithelial cells of intestinal mucosa and renal tubules	Transports branched-chain and aromatic amino acids, unlike ASC
B$^{0,+}$	Broad specificity; most neutral and basic amino acids	Brush border membrane of epithelial cells of intestinal mucosa and renal tubules; vascular smooth muscle cells; microvillous membrane of placenta	Restricted distribution; also Cl$^-$-dependent; variant of B?
IMINO	Proline	Brush border membrane of epithelial cells of intestinal mucosa	Also Cl$^-$-dependent?
II. Na$^+$-independent systems			
L	Mainly branched-chain and aromatic amino acids	Widespread	Not usually inducible
y$^+$	Lysine, histidine, arginine	Widespread	Electrogenic
b$^{0,+}$	Neutral and basic amino acids and cystine	Brush border membrane of epithelial cells of intestinal mucosa and renal tubules	Exchanger? Electrogenic?
x$_c^-$	Glutamate, cystine	Macrophages, fetal and cultured cells	Electroneutral; exchanger

Me-AIB = methyl-aminoisobutyrate is a marker substrate for system A and is excluded by ASC.
Modified from McGivan, J. D. and Pastor-Anglada, M. (1994) Regulatory and molecular aspects of mammalian amino acid transport. Biochem J 299:321–334; and from Christensen, H. (1990) Role of amino acid transport and countertransport in nutrition and metabolism. Physiol Rev 70:43–77.

acid transporters have not been fully characterized, and relatively little is known about their regulation. System A has been studied most extensively, particularly in hepatocytes and hepatoma cells, in which it is subject to a variety of regulatory signals. System A activity is rapidly increased in response to glucagon or epidermal growth factor (EGF) by mechanisms that involve hyperpolarization of the cell membrane by changes in Na^+/H^+ exchange. In addition, system A is sensitive to pH changes. In response to acidosis, there is evidence that amino acid transport in the liver may be decreased, with a resultant decrease in urea synthesis.

System A is also subject to long-term regulation brought about by changes in the amount of transporter protein. System A can be induced by insulin in most cell types and by either insulin or glucagon in liver cells. This apparent paradox of induction of system A in liver by two opposing hormones probably is explained by the increased hepatic uptake of amino acids required in response to food intake (when protein synthesis and catabolism of excess exogenous amino acids predominate in the liver) and in response to starvation or diabetes (when amino acids from muscle protein degradation are taken up and catabolized by the liver as gluconeogenic precursors).

REACTIONS INVOLVED IN THE TRANSFER, RELEASE, AND INCORPORATION OF NITROGEN

Because each amino acid has one or more individual pathways for metabolism, it is difficult to present a simplified scheme for amino acid metabolism. Some general types of reactions that are involved in the movement of amino groups and fixation of inorganic nitrogen (NH_3 or NH_4^+) are described first, followed by a summary of the fate of the carbon skeletons released by amino acid catabolism. This is followed by a summary of specific metabolic pathways for each amino acid or related group of amino acids. Finally, the pathways for excretion of nitrogen from the body are summarized. The reader should also refer to Chapter 21 for a discussion of the roles vitamin B_6, vitamin B_{12}, and folate coenzymes play in many of the reactions of amino acid metabolism.

Transamination

The α-amino group may be moved from one carbon chain to another by transamination reactions to form the respective amino and keto acids. Transamination is the most general route for removing nitrogen from an amino acid and transferring it to another carbon skeleton. The transfer of the amino group from an amino acid to a keto acid to form another amino acid is catalyzed by aminotransferases, which are pyridoxal 5′-phosphate-dependent enzymes. The general reaction catalyzed by an aminotransferase is shown in Figure 11–2. Most physiologically important aminotransferases have a preferred amino acid/keto acid substrate and utilize α-ketoglutarate/glutamate as the counter keto acid/amino acid; an example is aspartate aminotransferase, which accepts aspartate or oxaloacetate as substrate and uses glutamate or α-ketoglutarate as co-substrate. Alanine, aspartate, glutamate, tyrosine, serine, valine, isoleucine, and leucine are actively transaminated in human tissues. Histidine, phenylalanine, methionine, cysteine, glutamine, asparagine, and glycine also may undergo transamination in human tissues, but these amino acids primarily are metabolized by other types of reactions under normal physiological conditions. In contrast, threonine, lysine, proline, tryptophan, and arginine do not directly participate in transami-

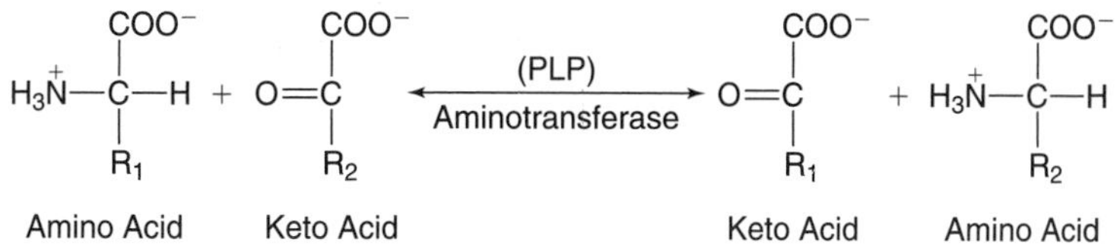

Figure 11–2. Example of a transamination reaction. The amino acid substrate is converted to a keto acid product, whereas the keto acid cosubstrate is converted to an amino acid product.

nation reactions in mammalian tissues; intermediates in the degradation pathways of lysine, proline, tryptophan, and arginine may, however, undergo transamination for transfer of the amino group. Because α-ketoglutarate is used so widely as the acceptor of amino groups in transamination reactions, the α-amino groups of numerous amino acids are funneled through glutamate in the process of amino acid catabolism.

Deamination

A limited number of reactions in the body are capable of direct deamination of amino acids to release ammonia and form a keto acid. The major reaction in the body in which α-amino groups are released as ammonia is catalyzed by glutamate dehydrogenase. As shown in Figure 11–3, glutamate dehydrogenase brings about the interconversion of glutamate with α-ketoglutarate and ammonia. Glutamate dehydrogenase is mitochondrial and is present at high activity in liver, kidney cortex, and brain. The fate of the ammonia released by glutamate dehydrogenase is tissue specific. In liver, the ammonia is mainly incorporated into urea; in the kidney, it can be excreted as urinary ammonium; in the brain, it is incorporated predominantly into glutamine.

Specific reactions in the metabolism of individual amino acids also give rise to free ammonia from the α-amino nitrogen. In particular, ammonia is released from histidine by histidine ammonia lyase (commonly called histidase), from methionine in the process of transsulfuration (in the reaction catalyzed by cystathionine γ-lyase, commonly called cystathionase), from glycine by the glycine cleavage system, and from serine or threonine by serine-threonine dehydratase. In some tissues that lack significant glutamate dehydrogenase activity, such as skeletal muscle, the purine nucleotide cycle can function to release ammonia from adenosine via adenosine deaminase, with the subsequent resynthesis of adenosine using nitrogen obtained from aspartate (Lowenstein, 1972). The net effect of this purine nucleotide cycle is the release of amino groups from aspartate (or from glutamate via transamination of glutamate with oxaloacetate to form aspartate) as ammonia and with salvage of the aspartate (or glutamate) carbon chains.

L-Amino acid oxidase activity is very low in mammals and is probably of little importance in amino acid catabolism in humans. However, some foodstuffs contain small amounts of D-amino acids, and these appear to be degraded mainly by D-amino acid oxidase, which is expressed at high levels in the kidney (D'Aniello et al., 1993). The overall reaction catalyzed by amino acid oxidase is shown in Figure 11–4. Once a keto acid is formed from a D-amino acid, the keto acid can be transaminated by an L-amino acid aminotransferase to form an L-amino acid, allowing some utilization of D-amino acid carbon chains.

Deamidation/Transamidation

Glutamine and asparagine contain carboxamide groups, from which the amide nitrogen can be released by glutaminase or asparaginase. The reaction catalyzed by glutaminase is shown in Figure 11–5. The hydrolysis of glutamine to glutamate and ammonia occurs in many tissues and is catalyzed by phosphate-dependent glutaminase, which is located in the mitochondria. In most cells, the ammonia

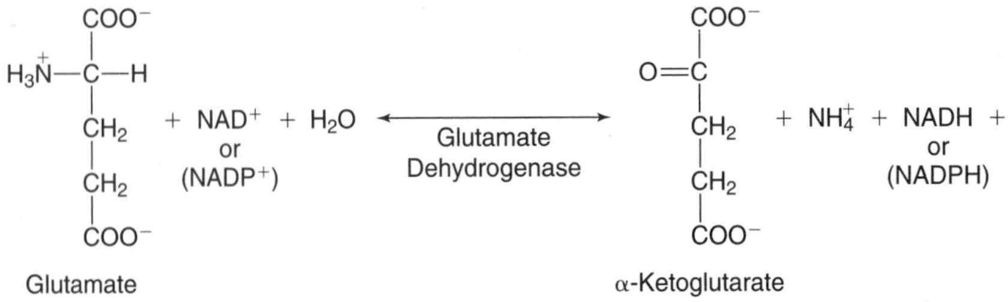

Figure 11–3. Interconversion of glutamate and α-ketoglutarate plus ammonia by glutamate dehydrogenase.

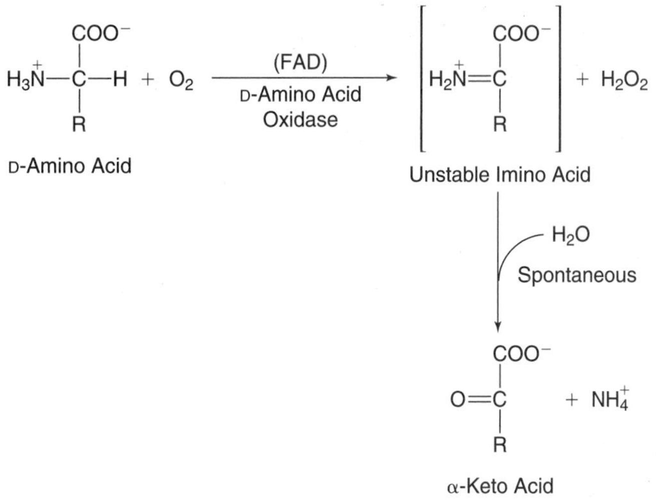

Figure 11–4. *Oxidative deamination of a D-amino acid by D-amino acid oxidase.*

liberated is released from the cell without further modification. The glutaminase of liver is a different isozyme from that found in other tissues; in the liver, the ammonia generated by this reaction is channeled efficiently to the carbamoyl phosphate synthetase I reaction and incorporated into urea. A similar reaction, catalyzed by asparaginase, deamidates asparagine to yield aspartate plus ammonia. Transfer of the amide group from glutamine also plays an important role in synthetic reactions, including the synthesis of purine and pyrimidine nucleotides, NAD^+, and amino sugars, as is discussed further in a subsequent section of this chapter.

Incorporation of Ammonia into the α-Amino Pool

Although most of the interconversions and metabolism of amino acids and other nitrogenous compounds within the body occur with fixed nitrogen, primarily amino and amide groups, some reactions can utilize ammonia. Glutamate dehydrogenase (see Fig. 11–3), which was discussed as the mitochondrial enzyme responsible for release of α-amino nitrogen as ammonia, can also function in the reverse direction to allow incorporation of ammonia into glutamate and, hence, into the α-amino nitrogen pool. This enzyme catalyzes a near-equilibrium reaction in tissues with high activity (liver, kidney, and brain) and can operate to either incorporate ammonia into or release ammonia from the α-amino acid pool. The direction of flux depends on the provision and removal of reactants. Because glutamate and α-ketoglutarate are key intermediates in many transamination reactions, the glutamate dehydrogenase reaction plays a central role in the movement of nitrogen between the inorganic and organic pools, as

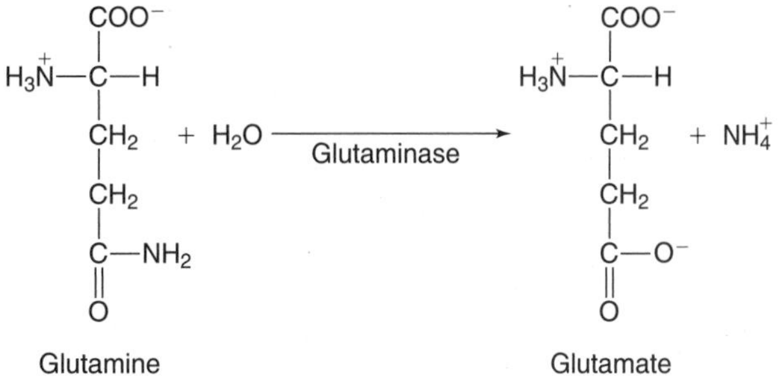

Figure 11–5. *Hydrolysis of amide nitrogen from glutamine by glutaminase.*

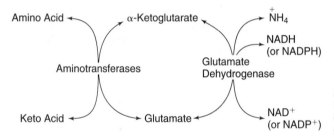

Figure 11–6. *The equilibrium nature of aminotransferases and glutamate dehydrogenase activities in brain, liver, and kidney maintain ammonia, amino acid, and keto acid levels.*

illustrated in Figure 11–6. The equilibrium nature of the glutamate dehydrogenase and transamination reactions in these tissues also acts to maintain intracellular ammonia levels in a narrow range.

Incorporation of Ammonia into Glutamine as an Amide Group

A second major ammonia-fixing reaction in the body is the synthesis of glutamine from glutamate and ammonia; this reaction is catalyzed by glutamine synthetase and involves the addition of ammonia to form a carboxamide group from the γ-carboxyl group of glutamate (Fig. 11–7). Glutamine, which has two nitrogenous groups, plays an important role in the transfer of nitrogen between cells and tissues, and glutamine synthetase activity is particularly high in muscle, adipose tissue, lung, brain, and the perivenous parenchymal cells of the liver (the cells located closest to the terminal hepatic venule or central veins by which blood exits the liver; see Fig. 9–10).

Asparagine synthetase catalyzes a similar reaction by which asparagine is synthesized from aspartate, but this enzyme can use either ammonia or glutamine as the substrate for the amidation reaction. This reaction plays a small role in overall nitrogen transfer in the body compared with that of glutamine synthetase.

Incorporation of Ammonia into Carbamoyl Phosphate for Formation of Urea Cycle Intermediates and Urea

Although it does not incorporate inorganic nitrogen into the amino acid pool (except into the guanidinium group of arginine), carbamoyl phosphate synthetase I, which is found in the mitochondria of liver and small intestinal cells, produces carbamoyl phosphate for citrulline production (Fig. 11–8). Within the liver, this citrulline is an integral part of the urea cycle, but in the intestine the citrulline may be released into the circulation as citrulline for further metabolism to arginine in the kidney.

METABOLISM OF THE CARBON CHAINS OF AMINO ACIDS

The use of amino acids as a fuel requires the removal of the amino group and the conversion of the carbon chain to an intermediate that can enter the central pathways of fuel metabolism. The processes of amino acid catabolism, ureagenesis or ammoniagenesis, the

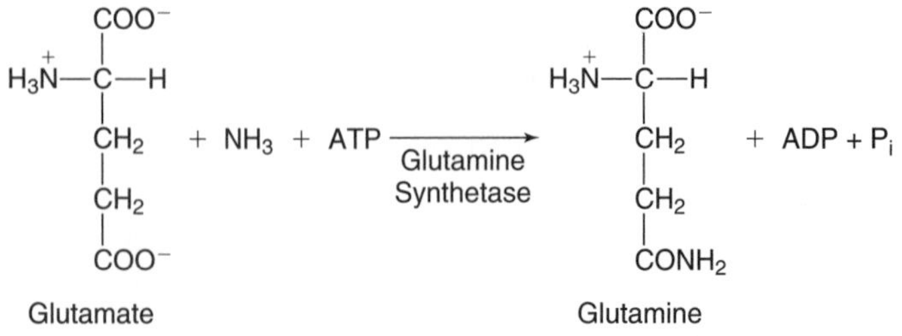

$$
\begin{array}{l}
\text{COO}^- \\
| \\
\overset{+}{\text{H}_3\text{N}}-\text{C}-\text{H} \\
| \\
\text{CH}_2 \quad + \text{NH}_3 + \text{ATP} \xrightarrow[\text{Synthetase}]{\text{Glutamine}} \\
| \\
\text{CH}_2 \\
| \\
\text{COO}^-
\end{array}
\qquad
\begin{array}{l}
\text{COO}^- \\
| \\
\overset{+}{\text{H}_3\text{N}}-\text{C}-\text{H} \\
| \\
\text{CH}_2 \quad + \text{ADP} + \text{P}_i \\
| \\
\text{CH}_2 \\
| \\
\text{CONH}_2
\end{array}
$$

Glutamate　　　　　　　　　　　　　Glutamine

Figure 11–7. *Synthesis of glutamine from glutamate and NH₃ by glutamine synthetase.*

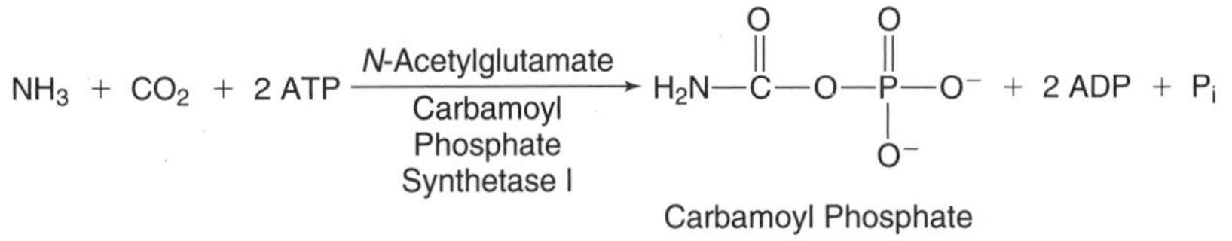

$$NH_3 + CO_2 + 2\,ATP \xrightarrow[\substack{\text{Carbamoyl} \\ \text{Phosphate} \\ \text{Synthetase I}}]{\text{\textit{N}-Acetylglutamate}} H_2N\text{—}\overset{\displaystyle O}{\overset{\|}{C}}\text{—}O\text{—}\overset{\displaystyle O}{\overset{\|}{\underset{\underset{\displaystyle O^-}{|}}{P}}}\text{—}O^- + 2\,ADP + P_i$$

Carbamoyl Phosphate

Figure 11–8. Synthesis of carbamoyl phosphate from NH_3 and CO_2 in mitochondria of hepatocytes and enterocytes.

conversion of amino acid carbon chains to glucose or other fuels, and the eventual complete oxidation of the amino acid carbon skeleton are all metabolically interrelated.

Catabolism of Amino Acid Carbon Chains

The rate of amino acid catabolism varies with amino acid supply. When amino acids are abundant, after a meal or during conditions of net proteolysis (e.g., uncontrolled diabetes, hypercatabolic states, or starvation), the extent of amino acid catabolism increases markedly. Conversely, when the diet is adequate in energy but deficient in amino acids, the catabolism of amino acids is reduced significantly.

The points at which the carbon skeletons of various amino acids enter central pathways of metabolism during their catabolism are shown in Figure 11–9. The carbon skeletons of most amino acids are metabolized to glycolytic or citric acid cycle intermediates and hence have the potential to be used for gluconeogenesis. Isoleucine, phenylalanine, tryptophan, and tyrosine also give rise to acetyl CoA in addition to a potentially glucogenic intermediate, whereas catabolism of leucine and lysine results only in the formation of acetyl units (as acetyl CoA or as acetoacetate). Amino acids often are classified as glu-

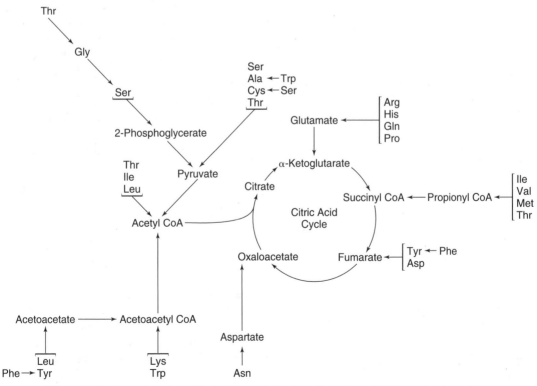

Figure 11–9. Formation of amphibolic intermediates from the carbon skeletons of amino acids.

cogenic, ketogenic, or both glucogenic and ketogenic based on their metabolic fates, but any amino acid that is potentially glucogenic is also potentially ketogenic. Once the carbon skeleton of an amino acid enters central pathways of fuel metabolism, it may be further oxidized for energy or used for synthesis of other compounds such as dispensable amino acids, glucose and glycogen, cholesterol, or triacylglycerols.

It is often stated that amino acids are oxidized in the liver, which is the major site of amino acid catabolism and urea production. Similar statements also are made about amino acid catabolism in other tissues, such as glutamine oxidation in the small intestine or branched-chain amino acid oxidation in the muscle. Such statements seem to imply that the amino acids are completely oxidized to CO_2 and H_2O. However, apart from some evidence for leucine oxidation in skeletal muscle, the complete oxidation of amino acids does not occur in any single tissue. Jungas et al. (1992) calculated that the amount of energy that would be produced by complete catabolism of amino acids at a rate equivalent to their net uptake by the liver would exceed the total energy used by the liver. Thus, amino acids are only partially oxidized within the liver (and other tissues), and the carbon skeletons are converted to glucose, glycogen, carbon chains of dispensable amino acids, lipids, and small amounts of ketone bodies for utilization or storage by various tissues.

Amino acids are quantitatively important as a fuel for the liver, small intestine, and other specialized cells such as reticulocytes and cells of the immune system. It has been estimated that liver derives at least half of its ATP need from the partial oxidation of amino acids, and that the small intestinal jejunum may derive up to 80% of its fuel needs from amino acids. The intestinal jejunum uses glutamine, glutamate, and aspartate taken up from the luminal contents (digesta), as well as arterial glutamine (Matthews et al., 1993). Although branched-chain amino acid oxidation at least partially occurs in muscle, other fuels are quantitatively much more important for muscle; muscle releases nitrogen primarily as glutamine and alanine (Elia and Livesey, 1983; Darmaun and Dechelotte, 1991). The

kidneys consume large amounts of glutamine and significant, but lesser, amounts of glycine (Tizianello et al., 1982). The kidneys also release serine. The net uptake of amino acids by the liver (from the arterial and portal circulation) differs substantially from the dietary input. In particular, the uptake of alanine and serine are high, whereas net uptake of aspartate, glutamate, and the branched-chain amino acids is very low, and the liver may actually exhibit net glutamate release. Although the gastrointestinal tract extracts large amounts of glutamine from the circulation and also metabolizes dietary glutamine (and glutamate), there is evidence that human liver also takes up considerable amounts of glutamine (Felig et al., 1973; Elia, 1993).

Gluconeogenesis

In the liver, amino acid catabolism is accompanied by both ureagenesis and gluconeogenesis, which is the synthesis of glucose from nonglucose precursors. Amino acids are an important source of carbon skeletons for gluconeogenesis, and gluconeogenesis plays an important role in the process of amino acid catabolism in the liver. Although gluconeogenesis in the liver traditionally has been considered to operate predominantly during fasting or starvation in response to hypoglycemia and breakdown of muscle protein, it is now apparent that gluconeogenesis also functions postprandially while amino acids are being absorbed and processed. Estimates of glucose synthesis from amino acid carbon in the fed human are 50 to 60 g of glucose per 100 g of protein partially oxidized (Jungas et al., 1992). Thus, ureagenesis can be viewed as operating together to produce glucose (or glycogen), urea, and CO_2 from amino acids whenever the liver is processing amino acids.

A general overview of the processes by which the liver converts amino acid carbon chains to the "universal fuel" glucose and at the same time incorporates the nitrogen groups into urea for excretion is shown in Figure 11–10. This scheme demonstrates that, when a balanced mixture of amino acids is being oxidized, most of the glucogenic carbon will be carried out of the mitochondria as aspartate, which also serves as the immediate

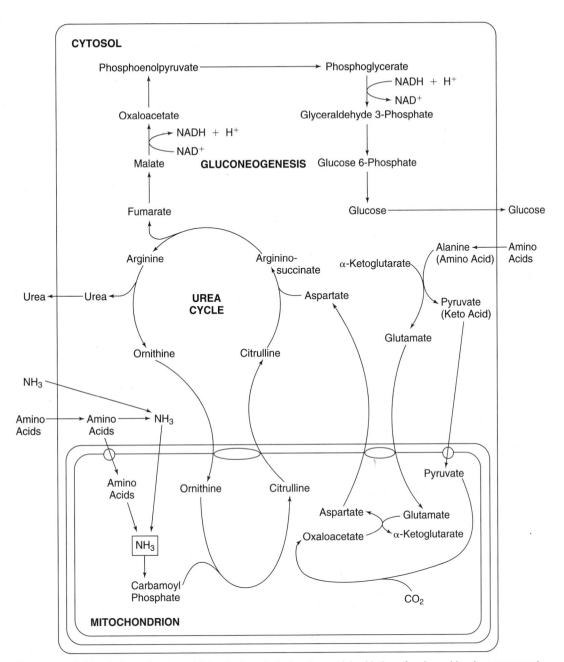

Figure 11–10. *Metabolism of amino acids by the liver, including the partial oxidation of amino acids, gluconeogenesis, and ureagenesis. Although not shown in the figure, α-ketoglutarate generated in the mitochondria can be transported out of the mitochondria to replenish the cytosolic α-ketoglutarate pool.*

donor of one of the two nitrogens for urea synthesis. Within the mitochondria, pyruvate is carboxylated to oxaloacetate by pyruvate carboxylase, whereas α-ketoglutarate and other glucogenic carbon chains of amino acids are converted to oxaloacetate by citric acid cycle enzymes. Gluconeogenesis and

ureagenesis can be considered as sharing the common steps (catalyzed by argininosuccinate synthetase and lyase) by which aspartate is converted to fumarate and citrulline is converted to arginine (Jungas et al., 1992). Because metabolism of aspartate by argininosuccinate synthetase and lyase releases the carbon as fumarate (a precursor of malate, which in turn is oxidized to oxaloacetate in a reaction that generates cytosolic NADH + H$^+$), aspartate also carries reducing equivalents out of the mitochondria to the cytosol, where they are needed for gluconeogenesis. Gluconeogenesis is discussed in detail in Chapter 9. Urea synthesis is discussed in more detail in the last section of this chapter.

Energetics of Amino Acid Oxidation

Jungas et al. (1992) detailed the processes involved in amino acid oxidation in liver and calculated that the partial oxidation of dietary amino acids provides sufficient energy to support the ATP requirements for synthesis of both glucose and urea; hence, the liver is not dependent on oxidation of another fuel besides amino acids to provide ATP to support these processes. Based on the detailed calculations of Jungas et al. (1992), complete oxidation of 1 g of meat protein by the body yields a net gain of approximately 195 mmol of ATP (an average of 21.5 mol ATP per mole of amino acids). They also estimated that, on a whole-body basis, about 35% of this net ATP production results from amino acid oxidation in muscle and small intestine, 60% from oxidation of the glucose generated by hepatic gluconeogenesis, and 5% from oxidation of acetoacetate.

Regulation of Amino Acid Oxidation and Gluconeogenesis

Clearly, amino acid oxidation, gluconeogenesis, and ureagenesis are processes that are metabolically interrelated in the liver. These metabolic pathways are predominantly expressed in the periportal parenchymal cells (cells that surround the terminal portal venule and hepatic arteriole by which blood enters the liver) rather than in the perivenous cells. These processes are active in both the fed (protein-containing meal) and in the starved states. Glucagon, glucocorticoids, and thyroid hormones play a role in increasing the rates of amino acid catabolism as well as ureagenesis and gluconeogenesis in the liver, whereas insulin may decrease these metabolic processes. Many amino acid catabolic enzyme ac-

tivities are increased under conditions that result in higher rates of amino acid catabolism, and some of these changes involve responses to hormonal signals, whereas others seem to be specific responses to high concentrations of amino acid subtrates. Glucocorticoids, catecholamines, and cytokines, which are elevated during stress, infection, and trauma, play a role in increasing net muscle protein breakdown and thus the availability of amino acids to the liver for gluconeogenesis.

In the fed state, dietary glutamine, glutamate, and aspartate (~20% of dietary protein) essentially are metabolized within the enterocyte with the resultant production of alanine. Thus, the portal blood contains higher amounts of alanine but lower amounts of glutamine, glutamate, and aspartate when compared with the amino acid pattern of dietary protein. In addition, the portal-drained viscera also extract glutamine from the arterial circulation even during protein feeding. Because the intestine catabolizes glutamine, glutamate, and aspartate to alanine, which is subsequently released and taken up by the liver, the gluconeogenic potential of amino acid carbon chains largely is conserved in spite of the intestine's use of these amino acids as fuels (Watford, 1994). Uptake of alanine by the liver exceeds gut release (with additional alanine originating from the peripheral tissues), whereas hepatic uptake of branched-chain amino acids is substantially below gut output such that the systemic blood levels of valine, leucine, and isoleucine rise in response to protein ingestion. There is a net uptake of these branched-chain amino acids by peripheral tissues (muscle, brain) in the absorptive period.

In the starved state, large amounts of glutamine as well as large amounts of alanine are released from muscle, and these can be utilized as fuels or substrate for gluconeogenesis. The increase in hepatic removal of alanine and in hepatic gluconeogenesis in early starvation or uncontrolled diabetes probably is related to the rise in glucagon and the fall in insulin. A rise in the concentration of plasma branched-chain amino acids is noted in early starvation and probably is due to hypoinsulinemia of starvation and decreased net uptake of amino acids by the muscle. Although the initial response to starvation is directed at maintenance of hepatic glucose output by increasing gluconeogenesis, the later response is directed at maintenance of body protein reserves by minimizing protein catabolism. The replacement of glucose by ketone bodies as the major oxidative fuel utilized by the brain is accompanied by a decrease in hepatic gluconeogenesis and urinary nitrogen excretion (particularly as urea, such that the ratio of ammonia to urea in the urine markedly increases). A general decline in plasma amino acid levels is observed, but the fall in plasma alanine is most obvious. Decreased output of alanine from muscle contributes to the decreased alanine uptake and decreased gluconeogenesis by liver. Ketone bodies seem to contribute to protein conservation by limiting amino acid (alanine) availability for gluconeogenesis.

Acid-Base Considerations of Amino Acid Oxidation

Amino acid oxidation generates nonvolatile or fixed acids, primarily SO_4^{2-} ($+ 2 H^+$) from catabolism of the sulfur-containing amino acids methionine and cysteine. The body can compensate for some of this excess fixed anion by increasing its excretion of dietary HPO_4^{2-} as $H_2PO_4^-$ (titratable acidity) or by consumption of HCO_3^- (bicarbonate) generated from the metabolism of dietary carboxylate anions (malate, citrate, etc.). The kidney excretes additional acid by generating NH_3 from glutamine (and to a lesser extent glycine) catabolism and by excreting NH_4^+ (net acid) while simultaneously producing and retaining HCO_3^- (net base) from the glutamine carbon skeleton. Note that ureagenesis in the liver is not capable of adjusting acid-base balance because both HCO_3^- and NH_4^+ are consumed in ureagenesis.

Metabolic acidosis results in an increased release of glutamine from skeletal muscle, which raises circulating glutamine levels. Within the kidney, a stimulation of α-ketoglutarate dehydrogenase by the lower pH results in increased glutamine utilization and ammonia production. The glutamine carbon skeleton is then further metabolized to bicarbonate and, in some species, glucose. Long-term regulation during metabolic acidosis involves increased synthesis of the key kidney enzymes glutaminase and phosphoenolpyruvate carboxykinase (Curthoys and Watford, 1995).

SYNTHESIS OF DISPENSABLE AMINO ACIDS

For the synthesis of the carbon chains of dispensable amino acids, glucose or glucogenic substrates (such as the carbon skeletons of many amino acids) are required. Pyruvate or other 3-carbon glycolytic intermediates serve as substrates for synthesis of alanine, serine, and glycine. Oxaloacetate, a 4-carbon keto acid, is the carbon skeleton of aspartate and asparagine. The 5-carbon keto acid α-ketoglutarate, or its metabolites, provides the carbon skeleton for glutamate, glutamine, proline, and arginine (Fig. 11–11). Nitrogenous groups are added to these carbon chains by direct transamination of other amino acids with pyruvate, 3-phosphohydroxypyruvate, oxaloacetate, and α-ketoglutarate; by amidation of glutamate and aspartate; and by the formation of metabolites of pyrroline 5-carboxylate as is discussed in more detail in the section on proline and arginine.

METABOLISM OF SPECIFIC AMINO ACIDS

For the reader who is interested in metabolism of individual amino acids, the pathways by which amino acid carbon chains are used as fuels, by which amino acids are used for synthesis of numerous nonprotein compounds, and by which dispensable amino acids are synthesized are discussed in this section. To the extent possible, an effort has been made to describe the pathways and interorgan fluxes that are most significant in humans. The dispensable amino acids are discussed first, followed by discussion of the indispensable amino acids.

Alanine

The only reactions that use alanine in mammalian tissues are its incorporation into pro-

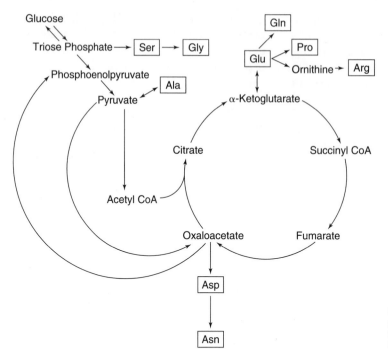

Figure 11–11. *Synthesis of dispensable amino acids from the carbon skeletons of amphibolic intermediates.*

teins and its participation in transamination. In skeletal muscle, liver, and small intestine, alanine aminotransferase catalyzes a reaction close to equilibrium, and alanine flux increases when a high carbohydrate diet is ingested and tissues are using glucose as a major fuel (Yang et al., 1986). (A minor source of alanine is its formation from the aliphatic portion of tryptophan during tryptophan catabolism.)

As already mentioned, alanine is a major amino acid that is released from muscle and small intestine. The muscle normally releases large quantities of alanine in the basal postabsorptive state, and this release is increased during early starvation and reduced when branched-chain amino acids from a protein-containing meal are abundantly available as a fuel for muscle (in which case glutamine is the major amino acid released by muscle). The carbon skeleton of alanine is derived primarily from glucose in muscle; the nitrogen (as well as a small amount of the carbon of alanine) is derived from catabolism of branched-chain and other amino acids in muscle. The catabolism of dietary glutamate, aspartate, and glutamine, together with arterial glutamine, in the enterocytes of the small

intestine results in the synthesis and release of lactate, pyruvate and alanine. Hence, these cells only partially oxidize these amino acids, and the gluconeogenic potential is conserved within the body (Watford, 1994).

Alanine is removed from the circulation primarily by the liver, which uses the alanine for ureagenesis and gluconeogenesis (Felig, 1975; Jungas et al., 1992). Alanine alone accounts for more than 25% of the total amino acids removed from the blood by the liver. It should be noted that most production of alanine in muscle, especially during exercise when glycolytic activity is high, does not represent a net contribution of alanine to body glucose because most of the pyruvate for alanine synthesis in muscle is derived from glycolysis of glucose. The role of the glucose-alanine cycle in transporting nitrogen to the liver for ureagenesis is shown in Figure 11–12. This cycle serves to transport nitrogen out of the muscle but does not generate any new glucogenic substrates. In contrast, the synthesis and release of glutamine by skeletal muscle does represent provision of new gluconeogenic substrate (Nurjhan et al., 1995). Although not definitively known, because of problems in sampling the portal vein in humans, there is evidence that approximately 30% to 40% of the glutamine used by the splanchnic bed (portal-drained viscera) is taken up directly by the liver (Felig et al., 1973; Elia, 1993). In addition, as indicated earlier, intestinal glutamine catabolism also results in the synthesis of alanine, which is then taken up by the liver for gluconeogenesis.

Glutamate, Glutamine, Aspartate, and Asparagine

Roles of Glutamate, Glutamine, and Aspartate in the Movement of Amino Acid Nitrogen and Carbon in the Body.

Glutamate, glutamine, and aspartate play central roles in nitrogen metabolism within the body. Glutamate and aspartate are involved in numerous reactions, such as the transfer of α-amino acid nitrogen in the synthesis of dispensable amino acids, purines, and pyrimidines. However, most glutamate and aspartate metabolism is intracellular, and the turnover of the plasma pools is relatively low (Battezzati et al., 1995). Glutamine, in contrast, not only plays a major role in intracellular metabolism (e.g., pyrimidine and purine synthesis), but also is the major transport form of nitrogen among tissues in the circulation.

Glutamate and aspartate are interconvertible with two citric acid cycle intermediates, α-ketoglutarate and oxaloacetate, respectively. Hence, like alanine, they have carbon skeletons that play central roles as amphibolic intermediates (serving both anabolic and catabolic purposes) in metabolism. Aspartate aminotransferase catalyzes the interconversion of aspartate and oxaloacetate, and two isozymes, cytosolic and mitochondrial, play important roles in the movement of carbon and reducing equivalents across mitochondrial membranes by the malate-aspartate shuttle. Additionally, during ureagenesis and gluconeogenesis in the liver, as shown in Figure 11–10, aspartate carries carbon and reducing equivalents for hepatic gluconeogenesis as well as nitrogen for ureagenesis from the mito-

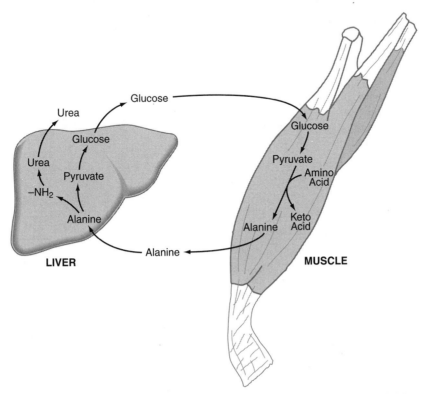

Figure 11–12. The glucose-alanine cycle for amino group transport. The carbon chain is cycled between glucose and pyruvate.

chondria to the cytosol. Glutamate and α-ketoglutarate are interconverted by a number of other aminotransferases, especially alanine aminotransferase and branched-chain aminotransferase, in addition to aspartate aminotransferase. In some tissues glutamate is also interconverted with its keto acid via the mitochondrial glutamate dehydrogenase reaction (Fig. 11–6).

In addition to the α-carboxylic acid group, aspartate and glutamate (or aspartic acid and glutamic acid) possess a second carboxylic acid group. The β-carboxylic acid group of aspartate and the γ-carboxylic acid group of glutamate can be amidated to form amino acids with carboxamide groups; these amino acids are asparagine and glutamine, respectively. Their synthesis was described earlier in the discussion of fixation of inorganic nitrogen (Fig. 11–7).

Glutamine catabolism occurs predominantly by the hydrolysis of the amide group from the carboxamide, a process called deamidation. A mitochondrial enzyme, glutaminase, catalyzes the reaction, resulting in the production of glutamate and ammonia (see Fig. 11–5). Asparagine catabolism occurs in the same manner in a reaction catalyzed by asparaginase; aspartate and ammonia are released. Glutamine also serves as a donor of its carboxamide nitrogen via transamidation reactions. Although of minor physiological importance, both asparagine and glutamine can also undergo transamination with keto acids, especially in the mitochondria of some cells, to produce α-ketosuccinamate or α-ketoglutaramate. These keto acids can be deamidated to form ammonia plus oxaloacetate or α-ketoglutarate.

Tissue-Specific Metabolism of Glutamine.
Glutamine is the most abundant free α-amino acid in the body; the body contains about 80 g of free glutamine, with more than 95% of this located intracellularly. The branched-chain amino acids are a major source of carbon and nitrogen for glutamine synthesis (as well as of the nitrogen for alanine synthesis) by muscle. In addition to branched-chain amino acids, there is evidence that muscle also takes up some glutamate from the circulation. During the fed state, large amounts of

dietary branched-chain amino acids are taken up and catabolized in the muscle. During times of net proteolysis, the branched-chain amino acids from muscle proteins are catabolized within the muscle. In both cases, the release of glutamine serves to transport carbon and nitrogen that originated from the branched-chain amino acids to other tissues such as small intestine, immune cells, kidney, and liver.

The source of the carbon skeleton for net glutamine synthesis in muscle is not firmly established, but the propionyl CoA derived from valine and isoleucine metabolism may be carboxylated to succinyl CoA, which is then converted to oxaloacetate, which in turn may condense with acetyl CoA to form citrate and hence α-ketoglutarate as shown in Figure 11–13. This can be transaminated to glutamate (probably in concert with the transamination of a branched-chain amino acid to form a branched-chain keto acid) and amidated to glutamine by glutamine synthetase (using ammonia released from glutamate or other amino acids). Thus, glutamine seems to transport branched-chain amino acid carbon skeletons as well as nitrogen out of the muscle. Net

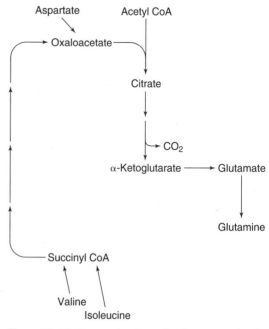

Figure 11–13. *Proposed pathway for de novo synthesis of glutamine in skeletal muscle. The precursors are aspartate and branched-chain amino acids.*

synthesis of glutamine also occurs in the lungs, adipose tissue, brain, and, under certain conditions, liver.

In the healthy individual, the major site of glutamine catabolism is the small intestine, where glutamine is the principal respiratory fuel of the enterocytes. The catabolism of glutamine in the intestine results in the production of CO_2, alanine, pyruvate, and lactate from the carbon skeleton and of ammonia and alanine from the amide and amino groups. Proline and citrulline are additional products of intestinal glutamine/glutamate catabolism. Thymocytes, lymphocytes, and macrophages all use glutamine as the principal respiratory fuel, and these cells show increased rates of glutamine utilization when they are activated. In these immune system cells, the major carbon end product is aspartate, with little or no production of alanine, proline, or citrulline. Glutamine plays an important role in acid-base balance and is taken up by the kidney during metabolic acidosis. The kidney uses the glutamine to produce ammonia, bicarbonate, and glucose, which allows the excretion of acid and conservation of important cations. In the liver, glutamine is taken up and catabolized in periportal cells with the resultant production of urea and glucose, whereas perivenous cells synthesize glutamine for release into the circulation.

Role of Aspartate and *N*-Acetylglutamate in Urea Synthesis. In the urea cycle (Fig. 11–10), aspartate serves as the donor of an α-amino group to citrulline to form argininosuccinate. This nitrogen, along with the nitrogen (from ammonia) and the carbon (from CO_2) contributed via carbamoyl phosphate, ultimately is released as urea. Hence, aspartate serves as a direct donor of α-amino nitrogen to the urea cycle, with release of the aspartate carbon chain as fumarate, whereas carbamoyl phosphate serves as a direct donor of inorganic nitrogen to the urea cycle. Both nitrogen donors serve to funnel nitrogen that originated in various dietary and endogenous amino acids into the urea cycle for ultimate excretion from the body. As discussed earlier (Fig. 11–10), the fumarate derived from aspartate metabolism in the urea cycle serves as a carrier of both carbon and reducing equivalents that can be used for the process of gluconeogenesis from amino acid carbon skeletons.

N-Acetylglutamate, an allosteric activator of carbamoyl phosphate synthetase I, is synthesized from acetyl CoA and glutamate in liver and in the small intestine (the two tissues that have carbamoyl phosphate synthetase I activity). *N*-Acetylglutamate can be hydrolyzed by a specific deacylase.

Roles of Aspartate and Glutamine in Purine and Pyrimidine Nucleotide Synthesis. Purine nucleotides (adenine and guanine nucleotides) are synthesized by a sequence of reactions that involve glutamine and aspartate, as well as glycine, as direct participants (Fig. 11–14). Both of the carbons and the nitrogen of glycine are incorporated into purines; the amide groups of two or three glutamine molecules and the amine group of one aspartate molecule (with the aspartate carbons being released as fumarate) are contributed to each purine molecule that is synthesized. Two one-carbon units from the folate coenzyme system are also required; these likely originate from serine or other amino acids. This process results in the formation of inosine monophosphate, from which the other purine nucleotides can be formed. Formation of adenosine monophosphate (AMP) requires transfer of one more amine group from aspartate, with subsequent release of the aspartate carbon chain as fumarate. Formation of guanosine monophosphate (GMP) requires transfer on one more amide nitrogen from glutamine.

Pyrimidine nucleotides (uridine, thymidine, and cytosine nucleotides) are synthesized by a sequence of reactions that involve glutamine and aspartate (Fig. 11–15). Glutamine donates only a nitrogen, whereas aspartate donates carbons and nitrogen. The synthetic sequence begins with formation of carbamoyl phosphate by the carbamoyl phosphate synthetase II cytosolic reaction, which uses glutamine (amide group) as the nitrogen donor. Carbamoyl phosphate is condensed with aspartate to form *N*-carbamoyl aspartate. Three of the four carbons of aspartate become part of the newly synthesized pyrimidine, whereas the α-carboxyl carbon of aspartate is

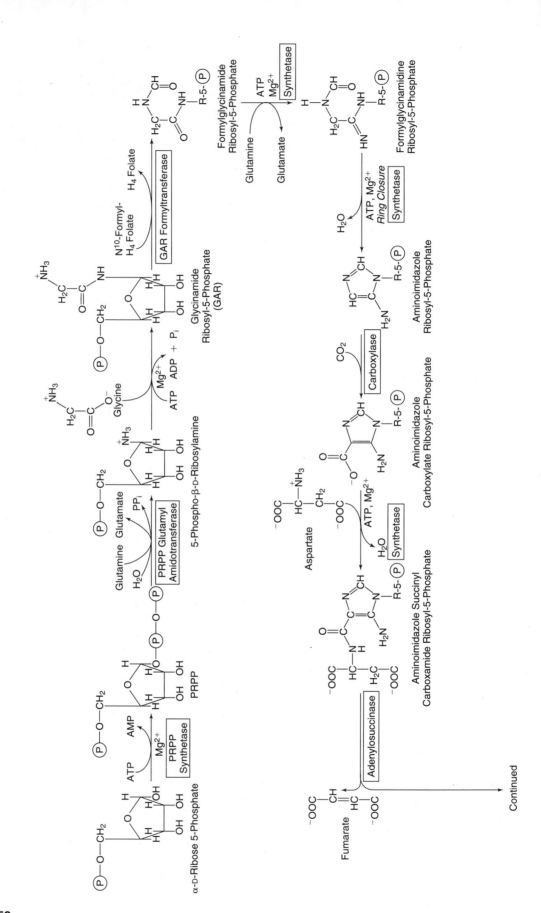

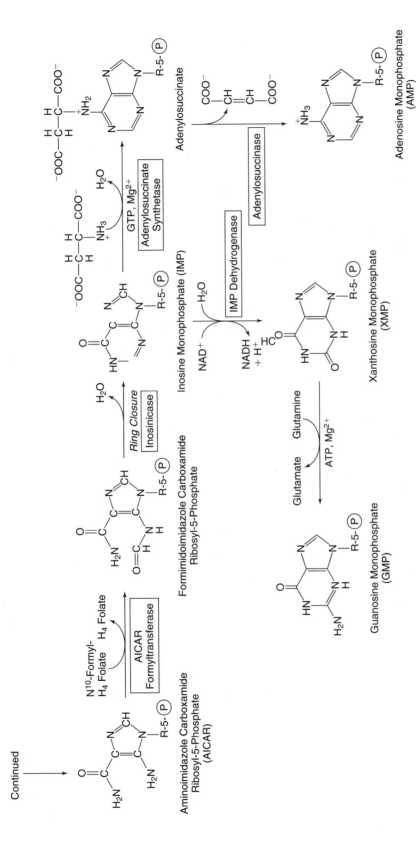

Figure 11–14. Pathway of de novo purine nucleotide biosynthesis from ribose 5-phosphate, ATP, glycine, glutamine amide groups, aspartate amino group, and 1-carbon units from the folate coenzyme system. R5P, ribosyl-5-phosphate; PRPP, 5-phosphoribosyl-1-pyrophosphate; P_i, inorganic phosphate; PP_i, inorganic pyrophosphate.

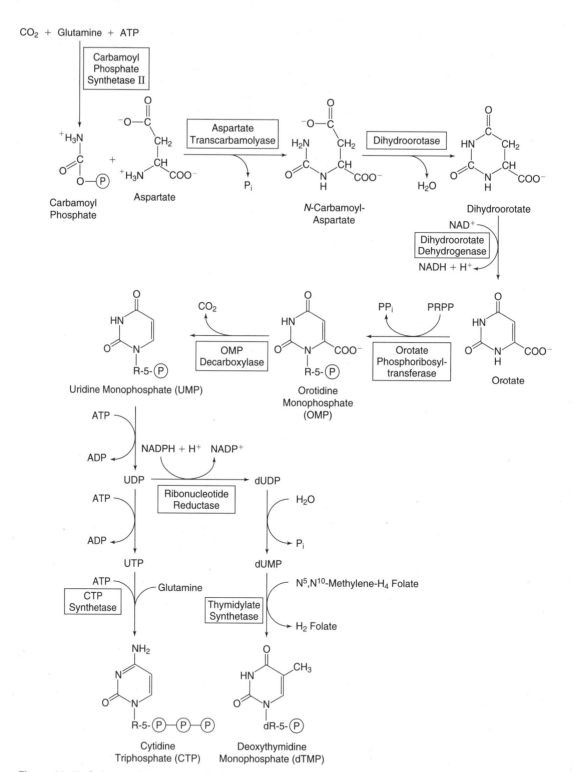

Figure 11–15. *Pathway of de novo synthesis of pyrimidine nucleotides from CO₂, ATP, glutamine amide groups, aspartate, ribose phosphate, and 1-carbon units from the folate coenzyme system. R5P, ribosyl-5-phosphate; dRP, deoxyribosyl-5-phosphate; PRPP, 5-phosphoribosyl-1-pyrophosphate; Pᵢ, inorganic phosphate; PPᵢ, inorganic pyrophosphate.*

lost as CO_2 in the conversion of orotidine 5'-phosphate to uridine 5'-phosphate. Conversion of uridine triphosphate (UTP) to cytidine triphosphate (CTP) requires donation of an additional amide nitrogen from glutamine. Conversion of deoxyuridine monophosphate (dUMP) to deoxythymidine monophosphate (dTMP) requires donation of a methyl group from the folate coenzyme system; again, this one-carbon fragment likely originates from serine or another amino acid.

Other Processes That Require Glutamate or Glutamine. In the central nervous system, glutamate is an important excitatory neurotransmitter, and it also serves as the precursor for γ-aminobutyric acid (GABA), an important inhibitory neurotransmitter. The conversion of glutamate to γ-aminobutyrate is catalyzed by glutamate decarboxylase, which releases the α-carboxyl group as CO_2, as shown in Figure 11–16. GABA is removed by transamination with α-ketoglutarate to yield glutamate and succinate semialdehyde, which is then oxidized to succinate, which can be used to regenerate α-ketoglutarate via citric acid cycle enzymes. The cycling of α-ketoglutarate to glutamate to GABA to succinate and back to α-ketoglutarate is called the GABA shunt. Nerve terminals and neurons also may use glutamine for synthesis of glutamate (and hence GABA) because neurons have high glutaminase activity. Some of the glutamate and GABA released by neurons is taken up by glial cells, which have high glutamine synthetase activity, and is used in the resynthesis of glutamine.

Glutamate is part of the tripeptide glutathione, in which its γ-carboxyl group is in peptide linkage to the α-amino group of cysteine. Glutathione synthesis is covered in the discussion of sulfur amino acids in this chapter. Glutamate forms a similar linkage with other glutamate residues to form the polyglutamate chain that is added to folate coenzymes in cells; see Chapter 21.

Glutamine is the donor of nitrogen for synthesis of amino sugars such as glucosamine 6-phosphate (formed from fructose 6-phosphate and glutamine). Glucosamine is further metabolized to synthesize N-acetylglucosamine and sialic acids. Other amino sug-

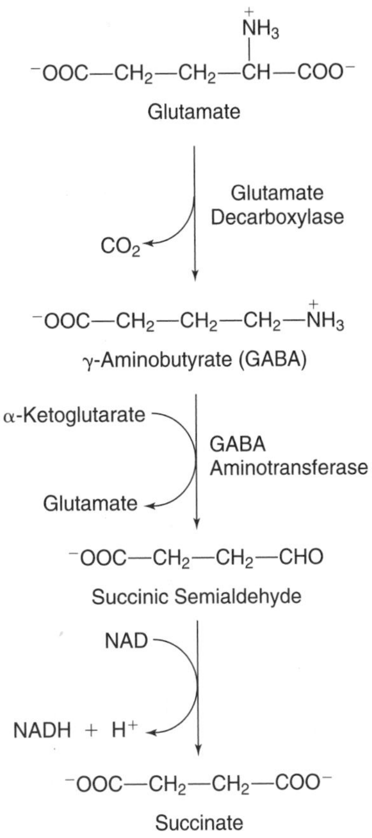

Figure 11–16. Synthesis and degradation of γ-aminobutyric acid (GABA).

ars include galactosamine and N-acetylgalactosamine. Amino sugars are found in both glycoproteins and proteoglycans. The transfer of glutamine amido nitrogen is catalyzed by a family of eight amidotransferases that possesses a conserved active site sequence.

In contrast to the major role played by glutamine, asparagine is not known to have any function in mammals other than incorporation into protein. In some glycoproteins, the oligosaccharide unit is attached to the side chain of an asparaginyl residue in the protein by an N-glycosidic linkage with the carboxamide group. This linkage is formed by transfer of the oligosaccharide chain from dolichol pyrophosphate. (See Chapters 1 and 9 for a discussion of glycoproteins.)

Proline and Arginine

Proline and Arginine Synthesis and Degradation: Interconversion of Proline and

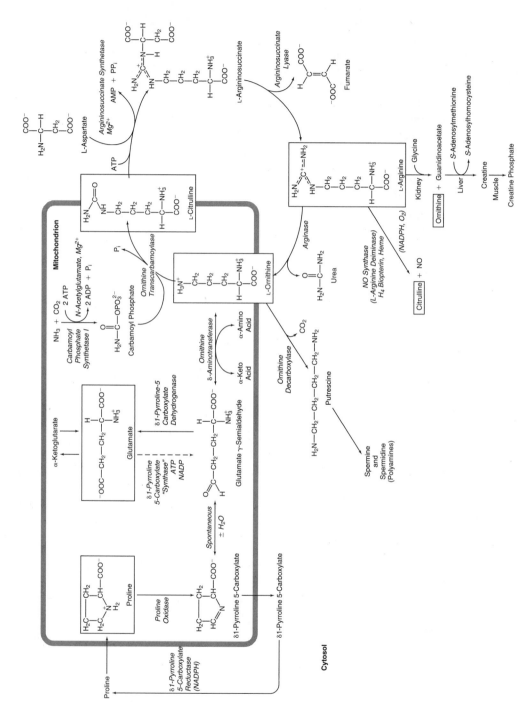

Figure 11–17. Reactions involved in the metabolism of arginine and proline, illustrating the interconversion of the 5-carbon skeletons and α-amino group of glutamate, ornithine, citrulline, arginine, and proline.

Arginine with Glutamate, Ornithine, and Citrulline. Glutamate and ornithine are key intermediates in the metabolism of proline and arginine, because all these amino acids share the same 5-carbon skeleton. The dispensability of proline and arginine (Carey et al., 1987) is related to the body's ability to synthesize these two amino acids from glutamate or α-ketoglutarate and amino groups (Cynober et al., 1995; Rabier & Kamoun, 1995). These interrelationships are illustrated in Figure 11–17. The reactions shown are intended to illustrate whole body metabolism of these amino acids and not metabolism within any single tissue. Of particular importance for arginine and proline synthesis, ornithine carbamoyltransferase, carbamoyl phosphate synthetase I, and N-acetylglutamate synthetase are expressed in both liver and small intestine, and pyrroline 5-carboxylate synthase is abundant only in small intestine. The synthesis of both arginine or proline from glutamate depends on the presence of an adequate level of pyrroline 5-carboxylate synthase (the enzyme that catalyzes the step that allows the glutamate carbon and nitrogen to enter the proline/ornithine/citrulline/arginine pool) in the small intestine. Hence, the small intestine plays a critical role in the synthesis of both arginine and proline (or their precursors, citrulline and ornithine) from glutamate or glutamine.

In adults, metabolism of glutamate and glutamine within small intestinal cells (enterocytes) results in the formation and release of proline and citrulline and lesser amounts of arginine and ornithine. These amino acids are released into the portal circulation and provide arginine and proline or their precursors to various tissues. Ornithine is readily used for proline synthesis through ornithine aminotransferase and pyrroline 5-carboxylate reductase activities; the liver and intestine probably are important sites of proline synthesis. Plasma citrulline is not actively taken up from the circulation by the liver, but rather passes through to be removed by other tissues, especially by the kidney. The kidney has relatively high levels of argininosuccinate synthetase and arginosuccinate lyase, which allows the kidney to convert citrulline to arginine for use by peripheral tissues. Although the liver has an active urea cycle, it cannot use glutamate

to produce ornithine/citrulline/arginine or proline. Extensive hydrolysis of arginine to ornithine occurs in liver, but the ornithine is recycled back to citrulline and arginine via the urea cycle.

The rate of arginine synthesis in the adult has been estimated to be about 25 mmol/day (Castillo et al., 1994), and arginine synthesis in adults seemed adequate to meet arginine requirements of subjects who consumed an arginine-devoid diet for several days (Carey et al., 1987). In adult subjects, the rate of de novo synthesis of arginine did not change in response to changes in arginine intake or need, but the rate of arginine catabolism (formation and oxidation of ornithine) was diminished in subjects with low arginine intakes; arginine catabolism rather than arginine synthesis seems to be regulated to conserve arginine when arginine availability is low (Beaumier et al., 1995).

The pre-weanling pig, which is often used as a model for human infants, has a low rate of intestinal proline and arginine synthesis due to low intestinal pyrroline 5-carboxylate synthase activity, which limits the formation of citrulline/arginine/ornithine or proline from glutamate carbons in enterocytes (Wu et al., 1994). An arginine requirement (despite an adequate supply of dietary proline) can be demonstrated when intestinal synthesis of citrulline is limited or blocked, but it has been difficult in practice to demonstrate a requirement for proline (when arginine supply is adequate) even in pigs with massive resection of the small intestine. Apparently, the rate of arginine catabolism in the body is high enough to allow ornithine to be used for proline synthesis, whereas the reverse does not occur at an adequate rate.

Conditions that result in a decreased capacity for synthesis (premature birth of an infant or intravenous feeding) or increased demand (tissue injury and repair) for arginine and proline may result in a need for dietary arginine. Because of the role of urea cycle enzymes in arginine synthesis, individuals with inborn errors of the urea cycle (other than a lack of arginase) require arginine in the diet.

Use of the Guanidinium Group of Arginine in the Synthesis of Creatine, Nitric

CLINICAL CORRELATION

Role of Extrahepatic Tissues in Arginine Synthesis

The urea cycle enzymes are required to prevent the accumulation of toxic nitrogenous compounds and for the de novo synthesis of arginine. Genetic defects that result in abnormal synthesis of carbamoyl phosphate synthetase I, ornithine transcarbamoylase, argininosuccinate synthetase, and argininosuccinate lyase are characterized by the accumulation of ammonia and glutamine.

Rabier et al. (1991) reported their experience with two patients with urea cycle defects. One patient was a girl who presented at 18 months of age with hyperammonemic coma; she had high urinary orotate levels, and a diagnosis of ornithine transcarbamoylase deficiency was made following liver biopsy. The second patient was a boy who developed hyperammonemia on the third day after birth. He had a high plasma concentration of citrulline, and a diagnosis of argininosuccinate synthetase deficiency was confirmed by enzyme assay on liver biopsy. Both patients were placed on a protein-restricted diet supplemented with arginine and sodium benzoate.

Both patients subsequently underwent orthotopic liver transplantation because of recurrent ammonia intoxication; liver transplantation was done at 6 years of age for the girl and 3 years of age for the boy. Following liver transplantation, both patients were placed on diets with 50 g of protein per day through normal meals. Liver transplantation was effective in normalizing plasma ammonia concentration, and it reduced the urinary excretion of orotate in the female patient. However, plasma citrulline and arginine concentrations did not return to normal values. In the patient with ornithine transcarbamoylase deficiency, citrulline remained significantly lower than control values. In the patient with argininosuccinate synthetase deficiency, plasma citrulline was decreased compared with values observed before transplantation but was still higher than control values. Both patients had low plasma arginine concentrations before the liver transplant despite arginine supplementation, and their plasma arginine concentrations remained low compared with control levels after transplantation.

Thinking Critically

1. Why did citrulline and arginine remain low after liver transplantation? What is the role of extrahepatic tissues in arginine synthesis?

2. What is the purpose of the conventional diet/supplement therapies used prior to liver transplantation? Would you make any specific dietary recommendations for these patients who had undergone successful liver transplantation?

3. In total parenteral (intravenous) nutrition, the gut is bypassed in supplying nutrients. What effect might this have on the synthesis of arginine and proline from precursor glutamate?

Oxide, and Urea. The guanidinium group of arginine is crucial for synthesis of urea, nitric oxide, and creatine (Cynober et al., 1995; Rabier and Kamoun, 1995). In the liver, which has a complete urea cycle, arginine is formed from ornithine, carbamoyl phosphate, and the amino group of aspartate. The terminal guanidinium group of arginine is cleaved in the final step of the urea cycle to release the amidino portion of the guanidinium group as urea and to replenish the ornithine used as the starting substrate. This cyclic process consumes nitrogen and CO_2 but does not result in any net synthesis of arginine. In the urea cycle, urea essentially is synthesized by forming and cleaving the amidino portion of the guanidinium group of arginine.

Some of the arginine made in the kidney is used for synthesis of guanidinoacetate, which then goes to the liver to be used for creatine synthesis. The amidino group of arginine is transferred to glycine to form guanidinoacetate, and the 5-carbon skeleton of arginine is released as ornithine; this reaction is catalyzed by a transamidinase. Arginine is also the substrate for nitric oxide synthase, which forms nitric oxide (NO) and citrulline. Two general types of NO synthase have been identified: a calcium-dependent form found in endothelial cells and neurons, and a calcium-independent inducible form found in cells of the immune system. Nitric oxide is an effector molecule that is produced by a number of cell types, including macrophages, which use it for cytotoxicity, and endothelial cells, which produce it as a vasodilator of smooth muscle in blood vessels. Analogs of arginine such as N-monomethyl arginine are effective inhibitors of nitric acid synthase and can be used to lower NO production. As for urea synthesis, creatine synthesis and NO synthesis do not consume the 5-carbon skeleton of arginine. The citrulline or ornithine released by arginine guanidinum group metabolism can be recycled back to arginine or, alternatively, can be used for proline synthesis or catabolized to α-ketoglutarate.

Other Requirements for Arginine and Proline.

In mammalian brain, arginine decarboxylase brings about decarboxylation of arginine to agmatine, which may, like other bioactive amines, serve a neurotransmitter or neuromodulator function.

The 5-carbon skeleton of arginine or proline (as ornithine) is substrate for polyamine synthesis (Cynober et al., 1995; Pegg et al., 1995). Arginase is present in many extrahepatic tissues, where it can function to produce the ornithine needed for polyamine synthesis. The major polyamines include putrescine and derivatives of putrescine, spermine and spermidine, that are formed by transfer of one or two aminopropyl groups from decarboxylated S-adenosylmethionine to the 5-carbon skeleton of putrescine. These compounds are found in all tissues and appear to play important roles in cell growth and division.

Additional dietary arginine may be beneficial in times of tissue injury and repair, because arginine is required for synthesis of NO (effector molecule produced in response to cytokines; inflammation), polyamines (as mediators of cell growth; tissue repair), and proline (needed for collagen synthesis; fibrogenesis). In this context, dietary arginine might be considered as a conditionally indispensable amino acid in states of tissue injury and repair.

Catabolism of Proline and Arginine via Conversion to α-Ketoglutarate.

As shown in Figure 11–17, the 5-carbon skeleton of proline and ornithine and the 5-carbon portion of arginine and citrulline are degraded mainly via glutamate and α-ketoglutarate. The ultimate fate of the α-amino nitrogen of these amino acids largely depends on the fate of glutamate. The 5-carbon portion of arginine is released as citrulline or ornithine in the synthesis of urea, NO, and creatine, allowing salvage of the carbon skeleton and some of the nitrogen atoms. Some loss of 5-carbon skeleton and α-amino nitrogen occurs via the conversion of ornithine to putrescine and other polyamines.

Glycine and Serine

Glycine Degradation by the Glycine Cleavage System.

Glycine and serine play very important roles in nitrogen homeostasis and in 1-carbon metabolism, as illustrated in Figure 11–18. Glycine is degraded by a complex enzyme system, the glycine cleavage system. In mammals, the expression of this enzyme system is restricted to liver, kidney, and brain astrocytes; it is located on the inner mitochondrial membrane of these cells. Primarily it operates to degrade glycine and not to synthesize it. The overall reaction mechanism consists of a pyridoxal 5′-phosphate-dependent glycine decarboxylation, followed by transfer of the aminomethyl group to a lipoylaminomethyltransferase and finally to an N^5,N^{10}-methylenetetrahydrofolate synthesizing protein. The overall products are CO_2, ammonia, and N^5,N^{10}-methylenetetrahydrofolate. (NAD$^+$ is reduced to NADH + H$^+$ in order to oxidize the dihydrolipoyl-dehydrogenase component of the system; this enzyme is the same as the lipoyl-dehydrogenase that is present in the α-keto acid dehydrogenase complexes discussed in Chapter 20.) The importance of the glycine cleavage system in humans is well established due to inborn errors of metabolism that result in absent or very low glycine cleavage system activity in the tissues that normally express this activity. These defects give rise to nonketotic hyperglycinemia, a condition in which glycine accumulates in body fluids. In rats, the activity of the glycine cleav-

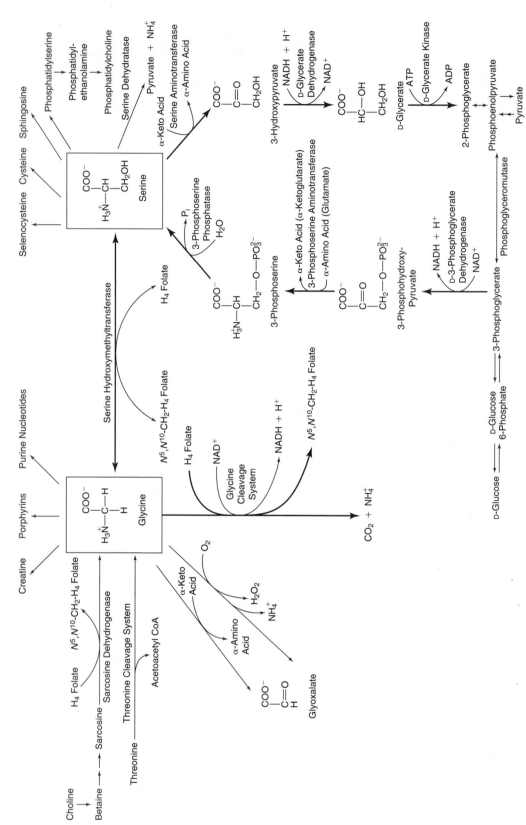

Figure 11–18. Reactions of glycine and serine metabolism. Major pathways of glycine and serine metabolism are indicated by the heavy lines.

age system in liver is stimulated rapidly by high protein intakes, by glucagon administration, or by Ca^{2+} (dependent on presence of inorganic phosphate); the activity of the system is increased in kidney of rats with metabolic acidosis, which is associated with net ammonia production from glycine (Ewart et al., 1992; Lowry et al., 1985).

Other minor pathways of glycine catabolism have been described, including the deamination and transamination pathways that lead to glyoxalate production. These enzymes seem to be of little physiological importance in glycine catabolism in mammals. In vitamin B_6-deficient animals, increased excretion of oxalate in the urine is thought to be due to decreased serine hydroxymethyltransferase (see next section) or glycine cleavage system activity that results in increased metabolism of glycine by deamination to oxalate.

Interconversion of Glycine and Serine via Serine Hydroxymethyltransferase. Serine and glycine are freely interconvertible via the enzyme serine hydroxymethyltransferase. Serine hydroxymethyltransferase is a pyridoxal 5′-phosphate-dependent enzyme; it uses tetrahydrofolate as a substrate and transfers the C-3 of serine, which is at the oxidation level of formaldehyde, to the tetrahydrofolate acceptor, where it bridges the nitrogen atoms at positions 5 and 10. By this reaction, serine serves as the major donor of 1-carbon units to the folate coenzyme system. The product, N^5,N^{10}-methylenetetrahydrofolate, can transfer the 1-carbon element back to glycine. Hence, this enzyme allows synthesis of either serine or glycine, provided that the other amino acid is available, or this reaction can permit serine catabolism via conversion to glycine with further catabolism of glycine. Although glycine contains only two carbon atoms, it can be considered glucogenic because of its ability to be converted to serine and hence to glucose.

Both mitochondrial and cytosolic forms of serine hydroxymethyltransferase are found in tissues. The mitochondrial serine hydroxymethyltransferase is distributed widely in tissues and seems to be involved mainly in serine catabolism to glycine plus formate (via N^5,N^{10}-methylenetetrahydrofolate). Serine degradation is the major route of glycine synthesis. A cytosolic form of serine hydroxymethyltransferase is abundant only in liver and kidney of humans, with some activity also being found in skeletal muscle (Girgis et al., 1998). The cytosolic serine hydroxymethyltransferase seems to be involved in net synthesis of serine from glycine in these tissues.

The combined action of the glycine cleavage system and serine hydroxymethyltransferase allows conversion of two molecules of glycine to one molecule each of serine, ammonia, and CO_2 (Cowan et al., 1996). This allows the kidney to use glycine as a contributor to net ammoniagenesis (by taking up glycine, releasing serine, and excreting ammonium). Glycine contributes about 5% of the urinary ammonium, much less than is contributed by glutamine. Also, the combined action of glycine cleavage and serine hydroxymethyltransferase allows glycine to supply all three carbons (via serine and hydroxypyruvate) for gluconeogenesis in liver. Glycine seems to play an important role in nitrogen-carbon transfer among organs and in renal ammoniagenesis. Glycine, in addition to alanine and glutamine, is released by muscle during starvation, and the renal uptake of glycine is increased in prolonged starvation.

Serine Synthesis from Glycolytic Intermediates. In addition to being synthesized from glycine via serine hydroxymethyltransferase, serine can be synthesized from the glycolytic intermediate 3-phosphoglycerate via an NAD^+-linked dehydrogenase that converts this intermediate to 3-phosphohydroxypyruvate. The latter then undergoes transamination with glutamate to 3-phosphoserine, followed by the irreversible removal of the phosphate by a phosphatase. This cytosolic pathway from 3-phosphoglycerate is distributed widely and is considered the major pathway of serine synthesis de novo in mammals. Once serine is formed from glycolytic intermediates, it can be converted to glycine via serine hydroxymethyltransferase, permitting de novo synthesis of glycine as well.

Other Routes of Glycine Synthesis. A limited amount of glycine can be synthesized from catabolism of threonine by the threonine cleavage complex (Darling et al., 1997). Glycine also can be produced from metabolism of betaine (or its precursor, choline) by successive removal of the methyl groups from the amine group of betaine. This leads to formation of dimethylglycine and monomethylglycine (sarcosine) and, ultimately, glycine, with transfer of the first methyl group to homocysteine to form methionine and donation of the second and third methyl groups to the folate coenzyme system as N^5,N^{10}-methylenetetrahydrofolate. Direct methylation of glycine also occurs; this is catalyzed by glycine methyltransferase, which transfers the methyl group from *S*-adenosylmethionine to glycine to form sarcosine. Sarcosine formation by methylation of glycine seems to be an important route for removal of excess methyl groups via the folate system and, ultimately, for their release as CO_2 (see Chapter 21). The significance of the betaine/sarcosine pathway in glycine production/turnover depends on the dietary intake of choline or betaine and on the turnover of choline-containing phospholipids. Nevertheless, the major route of glycine synthesis is clearly the serine hydroxymethyltransferase reaction.

Other Pathways of Serine Degradation. As discussed previously, serine degradation can be accomplished by conversion of serine to glycine by serine hydroxymethyltransferase, followed by catabolism of glycine by the glycine cleavage system. Serine also can be degraded by other routes. Transamination of serine to yield 3-hydroxypyruvate occurs in liver mitochondria and may be an important pathway of serine degradation in human liver, which contains a substantial level of serine aminotransferase. The 3-hydroxypyruvate can be further converted to glycerate and phosphorylated to 2-phosphoglycerate, an intermediate in glycolysis and gluconeogenesis. In some species, serine (as well as threonine) is degraded by a cytosolic enzyme called serine (threonine) dehydratase, which increases markedly in liver of animals fed high-protein diets. Serine dehydratase catalyzes the deamination of serine to pyruvate plus ammonia. The activity of serine dehydratase is reported to be low in human liver (Ogawa et al., 1989), and serine deamination to pyruvate seems unlikely to be quantitatively significant in human liver. The relative roles of various pathways of serine synthesis and degradation, however, remain to be clarified for human tissues.

Essential Roles of Glycine in the Synthesis of Nonprotein Compounds. Glycine is a substrate for synthesis of purine nucleotides, porphyrins, creatine, 1-carbon fragments for the folate coenzyme system, glutathione, and glycine-conjugated bile acids. The glycine cleavage system is involved in the donation of 1-carbon units to the folate coenzyme system, as shown in Figure 11–17. Glycine is incorporated (as an intact molecule) into purine nucleotides, as shown in Figure 11–13. δ-Aminolevulinate, a precursor of porphyrins, is synthesized from glycine and succinyl CoA with the α-carbon and the α-amino group of glycine retained in the porphobilinogen, but with the carboxyl carbon lost as CO_2. Some of the glycine nitrogen is lost when porphobilinogen is converted to porphyrinogen in the process of porphyrin/heme synthesis. Glycine is used by the kidney in the synthesis of guanidinoacetate, a precursor of creatine phosphate. Both the glycine carbons and the nitrogen remain in creatine phosphate or its elimination product, creatinine.

Glycine is a major inhibitory neurotransmitter in the central nervous system. Glycine, along with glutamate and cysteine, is a component of the tripeptide glutathione, and glycine can be released from glutathione during its hydrolysis. Glycine is used to conjugate bile acids in the liver, and glycine-conjugated bile acids are secreted in the bile. Other compounds also can form glycine conjugates; the best-known example is the conjugation of glycine with benzoic acid to form hippuric acid, which is excreted in the urine. The conjugation of benzoic acid with glycine facilitates the excretion of nitrogen from the body (as glycine), and this is presumed to be the basis of its therapeutic effect in patients with hyperammonemia.

Essential Roles of Serine in the Synthesis of Nonprotein Compounds. Serine is a precursor for synthesis of 1-carbon fragments for the folate coenzyme system, for synthesis of phospholipids and sphingosine, and for synthesis of cysteine and selenocysteine. The 3-carbon of serine is the major source of

NUTRITION INSIGHT

Neurotransmitters

The nervous system uses many biogenic amines and neuropeptides as neurotransmitters. The biogenic amines include the amino acids glutamate and glycine, as well as many decarboxylation products or derivatives of amino acids such as GABA (γ-aminobutyric acid), serotonin, catecholamines, and histamine.

Glycine and GABA are the major neuroinhibitory peptides in the central nervous system. Glycine acts predominately in the spinal cord and brain stem, and GABA acts predominately in all other parts of the brain. The receptors for glycine and GABA are ligand-gated channels that are selectively permeable to Cl⁻. When these channels are open, the membrane potential becomes more negative (hyperpolarized) rather than depolarized (as occurs when excitatory cation channels are opened). A neuron inhibited by hyperpolarization requires a more intense depolarization than is otherwise required to trigger an action potential. In the brain cortex, glycine acts as an excitatory agonist of the N-methyl-D-aspartate (NMDA)-type of glutamate receptor-channel complex.

Nonketotic hyperglycinemia is an inborn error caused by a biochemical defect in one of the components of the glycine cleavage system complex that results in the accumulation of large quantities of glycine in all body tissues. Most individuals born with nonketotic hyperglycinemia show severe neurologic abnormalities, including lethargy, hypotonia and myoclonic jerks, and apnea, often progressing to coma and death. Those who regain spontaneous respiration develop intractable seizures and profound mental retardation. It is thought that the apnea and hiccuping seen early in the course of the disease is the result of the neuroinhibitory effects of glycine in the spinal cord and brain stem. The intractable seizures and brain damage observed in individuals with nonketotic hyperglycinemia may be related to excessive stimulation of excitatory NMDA-glutamate receptors.

1-carbon fragments for the folate coenzyme system via the reaction catalyzed by serine hydroxymethyltransferase (see Fig. 11–18 and Chapter 21). This same reaction allows serine to be converted to glycine.

Serine is used in production of phosphatidylserine, phosphatidylethanolamine and phosphatidylcholine. Thus, serine serves as the precursor of choline. The details of the conversion are not well established, but phosphatidylserine undergoes decarboxylation to phosphatidylethanolamine, followed by transfer of three methyl groups from S-adenosylmethionine to form phosphatidylcholine. Because choline can be degraded to betaine, sarcosine, and glycine, this synthetic route provides another possible route of glycine synthesis from serine or from dietary choline or betaine. Serine, along with palmitoyl CoA, is used for the synthesis of the amino alcohol sphingosine, which is a component of ceramide and other sphingolipids.

Serine is the precursor of the carbon chain of both cysteine and selenocysteine.

The incorporation of the 3-carbon chain of serine into cysteine is accomplished enzymatically in the methionine transsulfuration pathway, by which the sulfur of methionine is transferred to serine to form cysteine. The utilization of the carbon chain of serine for synthesis of selenocysteine is accomplished in a very different manner. A limited number of proteins contain the modified amino acid selenocysteine in specific location(s). This amino acid is named selenocysteine because it has the structure of cysteine, except that the sulfur is replaced by selenium. Unlike other modified amino acid residues found in proteins, selenocysteine is formed by cotranslational, rather than by posttranslational, modification of an amino acid residue in the protein. Serine esterified to a specific transfer RNA (tRNA) that contains an anticodon complementary to the stop codon UGA (uracil-guanine-adenine) is the substrate for selenocysteine synthesis. In certain messenger RNAs (mRNAs), this codon acts as a codon for selenocysteine rather than as a termination sequence. Proteins may contain selenomethionyl residues at random locations owing to incorporation of selenomethionine in place of methionine; this incorporation reflects dietary intake of selenomethionine and not its specific synthesis and incorporation. See Chapter 34 for details of selenocysteine synthesis.

Threonine

Threonine Catabolism. Threonine is an indispensable amino acid for humans; its carbon skeleton cannot be synthesized in the body. The major pathway of threonine degradation in humans is uncertain. Threonine is catabolized in mammals by cytosolic threonine (serine) dehydratase or by a mitochon-

drial threonine cleavage complex, as shown in Figure 11–19.

Although threonine (serine) dehydratase does not seem to play a major role in serine catabolism in human liver, this cytosolic enzyme may play a significant role in threonine catabolism. Recently, Darling et al. (1997) reported results of kinetic studies in humans that suggested that threonine was metabolized predominantly to CO_2. They attributed threonine oxidation to the conversion of threonine to α-ketobutyrate plus ammonia (catalyzed by threonine dehydratase), with only a small proportion of threonine being converted to glycine (via the mitochondrial threonine cleavage complex). The α-ketobutyrate, which is formed from both threonine and methionine

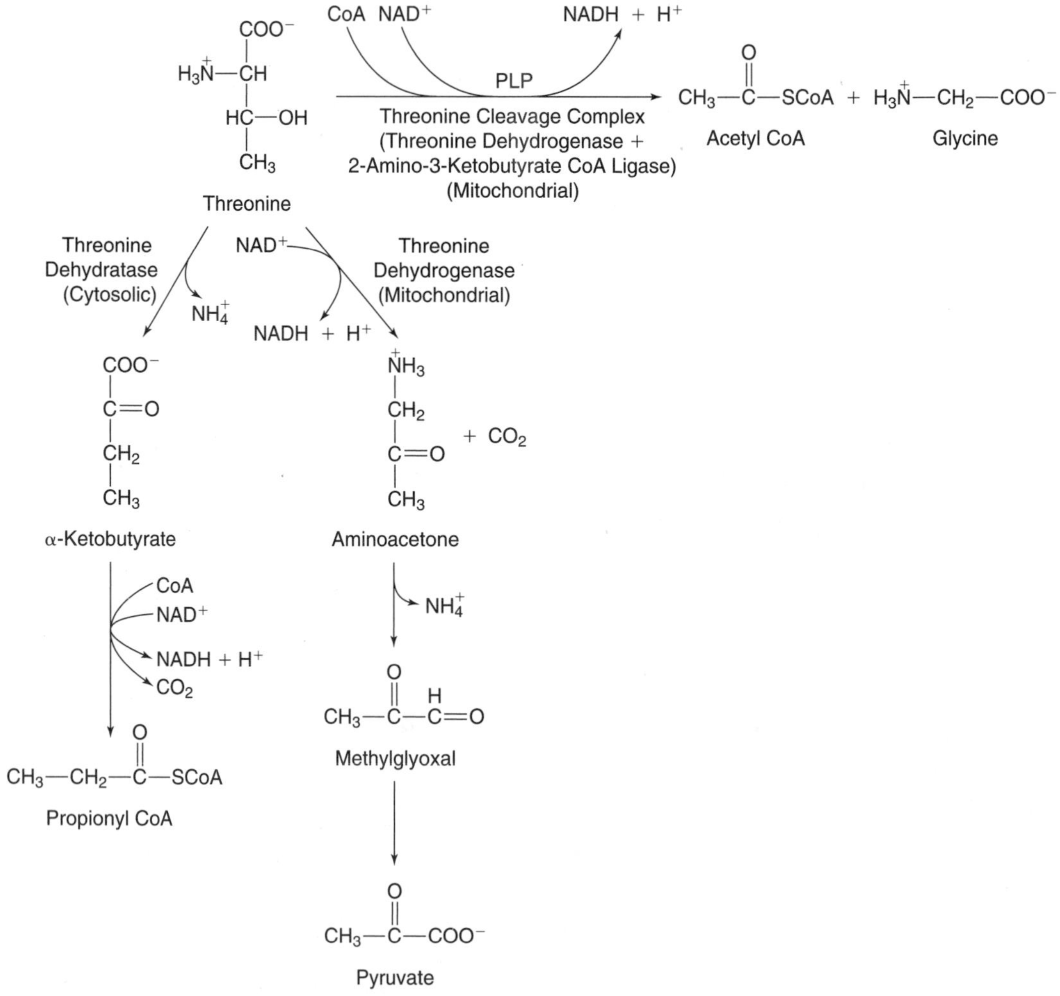

Figure 11–19. Catabolism of threonine in mammalian cells.

catabolism, is oxidatively decarboxylated to propionyl CoA by action of the branched-chain keto acid dehydrogenase or pyruvate dehydrogenase complex (Paxton et al., 1986). Propionyl CoA can be converted to succinyl CoA, a glucogenic precursor, and further metabolized.

Studies in pigs have suggested that this species, which has low serine (threonine) dehydratase activity, converts threonine to glycine through the threonine cleavage complex in both liver and extrahepatic tissues (Ballevre et al., 1991). Studies with liver mitochondria suggest that the coupled activities of threonine dehydrogenase and 2-amino-3-ketobutyrate CoA ligase act as a threonine cleavage complex, which converts threonine to glycine plus acetyl CoA in the presence of coenzyme A and NAD^+. However, when coenzyme A is limiting, threonine carbon may be released from the enzyme complex as aminoacetone + CO_2 as a result of the threonine dehydrogenase activity. Bird et al. (1984) calculated that at physiological concentrations of threonine and coenzyme A, at least 65% of threonine in intact rat liver mitochondria was metabolized to glycine and acetyl CoA. At higher threonine concentrations, more aminoacetone was formed (and excretion of aminoacetone in the urine increased); at lower threonine levels, more glycine was formed. Hence, mitochondrial threonine catabolism can give rise to either a glucogenic metabolite (aminoacetone) or to both a glucogenic (glycine) and a ketogenic metabolite (acetyl CoA) upon its degradation. Aminoacetone can be converted to pyruvate by the reactions shown in Figure 11–19, and glycine can be converted to pyruvate via serine, as shown in Figure 11–18.

Histidine

Essentiality of Histidine. Histidine is essential in infants, but it has been difficult to establish adult requirements. In long-term studies, histidine is essential for maintenance of nitrogen balance of adults (Cho et al., 1984). There is very little evidence of de novo histidine synthesis in humans, and no pathway for histidine synthesis in mammalian tissues has been described. The presence of histidine in dipeptides (carnosine, anserine), which are found in very high concentrations in human skeletal muscle and which can be degraded to release histidine, and the ability of the body to selectively degrade hemoglobin, a histidine-rich protein, may allow the body to maintain a supply of histidine in the face of a deficiency.

Histidine Catabolism. The first step in histidine degradation involves the conversion of histidine to urocanate with release of the α-amino group as ammonia; this step is catalyzed by histidine ammonia lyase, more commonly called histidase. Histidase activity is located only in the liver and in the surface layer (stratum corneum) of the skin. In the skin, the breakdown of histidine stops with the production of urocanic acid, which is an ultraviolet-absorbing compound that plays an important protective role. Urocanate is found in the sweat. The inborn error of metabolism called histidinemia, which is relatively benign, is due to a lack of histidase activity.

In the liver, the urocanate formed from histidine is further metabolized to ammonia (2 mol ammonia per mole of histidine), glutamate, and a 1-C fragment for the folate coenzyme system (Fig. 11–20). Additional steps convert the urocanate to N-formiminoglutamate (Figlu), which participates in the transfer of the formimino group, a 1-carbon fragment bearing a nitrogen atom, to the N^5 of tetrahydrofolate, with release of glutamate. Hence, the α-amino group of histidine is lost as ammonia, the 2-carbon of the imidazole ring is donated to the folate coenzyme system, and the adjacent imidazole nitrogen is lost as ammonia in conversion of N^5-formiminotetrahydrofolate to N^{10}-formyltetrahydrofolate; the other carbons and the second ring nitrogen are converted to glutamate. The histidine catabolic pathway in liver is regulated at the level of histidase, which is subject to induction by glucagon, glucocorticoids, and estrogens. Hepatic histidase activity also increases in liver of animals fed high levels of protein (Torres et al., 1998).

Although the liver possesses very high histidine aminotransferase activity, this does not appear to be of much physiological importance under normal conditions. However, individuals with a histidase deficiency, who have decreased or blocked urocanate

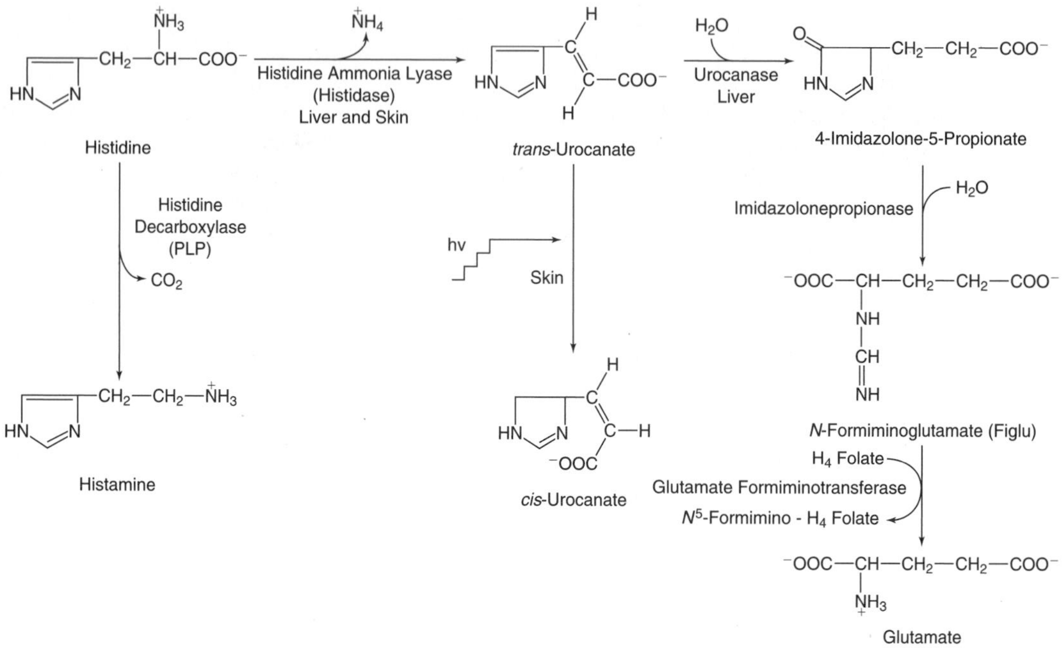

Figure 11–20. Histidine metabolism in mammalian cells.

formation, do transaminate histidine to imidazolepyruvate, and this keto acid and its metabolites (imidazoleacetate and imidazolelactate) are excreted in their urine (Lam et al., 1996).

Synthesis of Nonprotein Compounds from Histidine. The decarboxylation of histidine to the corresponding amine, histamine, occurs in various organs. Histamine synthesis is catalyzed by a specific histidine decarboxylase, as shown in Figure 11–20. In most tissues, histamine is located predominantly in mast cells. Most tissues contain type H_1-histamine receptors, and histamine acts as a paracrine agent in the physiological control of various functions. In the stomach, histamine acts on type H_2-receptors to stimulate the secretion of gastric acid by the parietal cells. H_2-receptor antagonists are used to treat gastric and duodenal ulcers. Histamine-containing neurons are present in the hypothalamus, and histamine acts as a neurotransmitter in histaminergic pathways. Additionally, histamine release is part of immune cell function. Binding of antigen to IgE molecules bound to mast cells stimulates the release of granules that contain histamine. Excess reaction to histamine

causes the symptoms of asthma and various allergic reactions. Antihistamine medications are H_1-receptor blockers; they minimize the symptoms caused by histamine release. Histamine is inactivated by deamination to imidazoleacetate or by methylation followed by oxidation by monoamine oxidase.

Two unusual peptides that contain histidine, carnosine and homocarnosine, are synthesized in human tissues and may be present at concentrations near 1 mmol/g in skeletal and cardiac muscle and in central nervous tissues (MacFarlane et al., 1991). Carnosine (β-alanyl-L-histidine) is synthesized in muscle from histidine and β-alanine (a catabolite of cytosine as well as of β-alanylpeptides); homocarnosine (γ-aminobutyryl-L-histidine) is synthesized in brain from histidine and γ-aminobutyric acid (GABA) or putrescine (an ornithine catabolite that serves as the donor of the GABA moiety). Both are synthesized by carnosine synthetase and degraded by plasma or brain carnosinase. The roles of these peptides are not well established; carnosine may play a functional role in the muscle, and homocarnosine could be an alternate route of GABA synthesis in brain. Two other histidine-containing peptides are present in foods and are concentrated by some tissues; these are ergothioneine (2′-thiolhistidine betaine), which accumulates in red blood cells, and anserine (β-alanyl-L-l-methylhistidine), which accumulates in skeletal muscle.

Methionine and Cysteine

Methionine Metabolism—Transmethylation and Transsulfuration. Methionine is metabolized almost entirely via the transmethylation/transsulfuration pathway, as shown in Figure 11–21 (Stipanuk, 1986). Liver is the most active site of methionine metabolism. Methionine is activated by synthesis of S-adenosylmethionine, which converts the sulfur of methionine (a thioether) to a positively charged sulfonium atom. S-Adenosylmethionine serves as the methyl donor for numerous methyltransferases, which transfer the methyl group from S-adenosylmethionine to acceptor substrates. S-Adenosylmethionine is the direct donor of methyl groups for almost all transmethylation reactions in the body. The S-adenosylhomocysteine that is generated by transfer of the methyl group subsequently is hydrolyzed to release homocysteine and adenosine. These reactions are collectively referred to as the methionine transmethylation pathway.

Homocysteine may be remethylated to methionine by a widespread N^5-methyltetrahydrofolate:homocysteine methyltransferase (methionine synthase) or by a liver-specific betaine:homocysteine methyltransferase. The remethylation of homocysteine allows the body to use methyl groups from choline (betaine) or from de novo synthesis from 1-carbon fragments via the folate coenzyme system for the numerous methylation reactions for which S-adenosylmethionine serves as the methyl donor. In male subjects fed methionine-adequate diets, approximately 40% of the homocysteine formed per transmethylation cycle underwent remethylation to methionine (Storch et al., 1990). The extent of remethylation increased in subjects fed methionine-deficient diets.

Homocysteine that is not remethylated condenses with serine to form the thioether cystathionine, as shown in Figure 11–21. This step commits the methionine molecule to degradation via the transsulfuration pathway. Cystathionine is cleaved on the other side of the sulfur atom to release α-ketobutyrate and ammonia as products of the homocysteine moiety, and cysteine, which contains the sulfur from homocysteine and the carbon chain and nitrogen donated by serine. Thus, transsulfuration allows cysteine to be synthesized from serine and the methionine sulfur atom and also accomplishes the process of methionine degradation. The carbon skeleton of methionine, α-ketobutyrate, is oxidatively decarboxylated to propionyl CoA, which enters the citric acid cycle at the level of succinyl CoA. Because transsulfuration permits methionine to serve as the precursor of cysteine sulfur, the sulfur amino acid requirement can be met either by methionine alone or by a mixture of methionine and cysteine. Studies in young men have indicated that about 50% of the total sulfur amino acid requirement can be supplied as cysteine (Storch et al., 1990).

A number of inborn errors of sulfur amino acid metabolism have served to verify the steps in the methionine metabolic pathway in humans. Inborn errors or vitamin deficiencies that limit the removal of homocysteine, either by remethylation to methionine or by transsulfuration, result in elevated levels of homocysteine in the blood and urine. A mildly elevated level of plasma homocysteine is considered a risk factor for cardiovascular disease and neural tube defects (Guba et al., 1996; Robinson et al., 1994). In patients with inborn errors associated with homocystinuria, numerous abnormalities, including premature thromboembolic and atherosclerotic disease and mental deficiencies, are observed. Treatment by restriction of methionine intake and supplementation with betaine have been found to lower the homocysteine level in these homocystinuric patients.

Methionine also can be degraded by transamination to its keto acid and further catabolism of that keto acid, but this does not appear to be a substantial route of methionine degradation in humans under normal conditions. Hence, methionine degradation depends almost entirely on the transmethylation

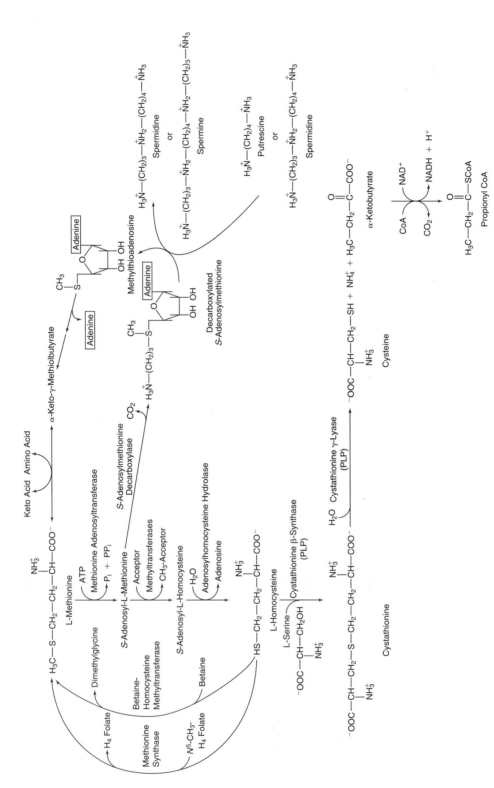

Figure 11–21. Pathways of methionine transmethylation, transsulfuration, and polyamine synthesis. Note that the remethylation allows the body to use methyl groups from de novo synthesis in the folate coenzyme system or from choline/betaine for S-adenosylmethionine-dependent transmethylation reactions. The transsulfuration pathway is required for cysteine synthesis and for methionine catabolism. Polyamine synthesis transfers aminopropyl groups from decarboxylated S-adenosylmethionine to putrescine (formed from ornithine) with salvage of the methylthioribose moiety of S-adenosylmethionine for resynthesis of methionine.

and transsulfuration pathways, with transfer of the methionine sulfur to cysteine.

Role of Methionine as the Donor of Aminopropyl Groups for Polyamine Synthesis. An alternative route of S-adenosylmethionine metabolism is polyamine synthesis (Pegg et al., 1995). This pathway involves the decarboxylation of S-adenosylmethionine and the transfer of the aminopropyl group from the decarboxylated S-adenosylmethionine (S-adenosylmethylthiopropylamine) to putrescine to form spermidine or to spermidine to form spermine (Fig. 11–21). Polyamines are essential molecules that seem to be involved in cell division and cell growth. The byproduct of polyamine synthesis, methylthioadenosine, is efficiently salvaged with little loss of sulfur. The sulfur atom, methyl carbon, and ribose chain of methylthioadenosine all are reincorporated into methionine by a series of reactions in which α-keto-γ-methiolbutyrate (methionine keto acid) is formed and then transaminated to methionine in the final step.

Cysteine Catabolism to Pyruvate and Inorganic Sulfur or to Taurine. Cysteine catabolism results in production of several essential compounds, including taurine, reduced inorganic sulfur, and sulfate or 3′-phosphoadenosine-5′-phosphosulfate. Formation of these metabolites is accomplished by the cysteine catabolic pathways, as shown in Figure 11–22. Cysteine catabolism may occur by desulfuration of cysteine to yield pyruvate and reduced sulfur (often in the form of a persulfide such as thiocysteine or thiosulfate). Cysteine desulfuration can be catalyzed by the β-cleavage of cysteine (or cystine) by cystathionine γ-lyase or by transamination of cysteine to β-mercaptopyruvate followed by de- or transsulfuration by mercaptopyruvate sulfurtransferase. Individuals with a rare inborn error of metabolism in which β-mercaptopyruvate sulfurtransferase is deficient excrete the mixed disulfide of cysteine and β-mercaptolactate, suggesting that transamination of cysteine to mercaptopyruvate occurs to some extent in humans. These patients excrete normal levels of urinary sulfate, indicating that overall cysteine catabolism is not impaired. The reduced sulfur may be used for synthesis of iron-sulfur proteins or other molecules that require a source of reduced sulfur or sulfide, or the reduced inorganic sulfur is further oxidized to thiosulfate (inner sulfur), sulfite and, finally, sulfate.

In the liver of animals fed high-protein or high-sulfur amino acid–containing diets, the major pathway of cysteine catabolism involves the oxidation of cysteine to cysteinesulfinate by cysteine dioxygenase, an inducible enzyme. Cysteinesulfinate may be decarboxylated to hypotaurine, which is subsequently oxidized to taurine, or cysteinesulfinate may be transaminated (with α-ketoglutarate) to the putative intermediate β-sulfinylpyruvate, which spontaneously decomposes to pyruvate and sulfite. Sulfite is further oxidized to sulfate by sulfite oxidase. In all pathways except that which results in taurine formation, the carbon chain of cysteine is released as pyruvate, the sulfur is released as inorganic sulfur (reduced or oxidized), and the amino group is released as ammonia or transferred to a keto acid acceptor. When taurine is the end product, only the carboxyl carbon of the cysteine is released, and the other three carbons as well as the nitrogen and sulfur atoms remain in the end product. Both sulfate and taurine are excreted in the urine, but sulfate normally accounts for more than 80% of the total sulfur excreted. The inorganic sulfate produced from methionine and cysteine sulfur largely accounts for the acidogenic potential of protein-containing diets (Bella and Stipanuk, 1995).

Inorganic sulfur and taurine are not necessarily essential dietary nutrients because they are provided via sulfur amino acid degradation. Nevertheless, both taurine and inorganic sulfur are essential nutrients for many nonhepatic cells that cannot synthesize them at adequate rates. Reduced sulfur is required for synthesis of iron-sulfur proteins and other compounds. The activated form of sulfate, 3′-phosphoadenosine-5′-phosphosulfate (PAPS), serves as the substrate for sulfation of a number of molecules. Many structural compounds are sulfated. In particular, proteoglycans contain oligosaccharide chains that contain many sulfated sugar residues. In addition, many compounds of both endogenous and exogenous origin are excreted as sulfo-esters; sulfo-

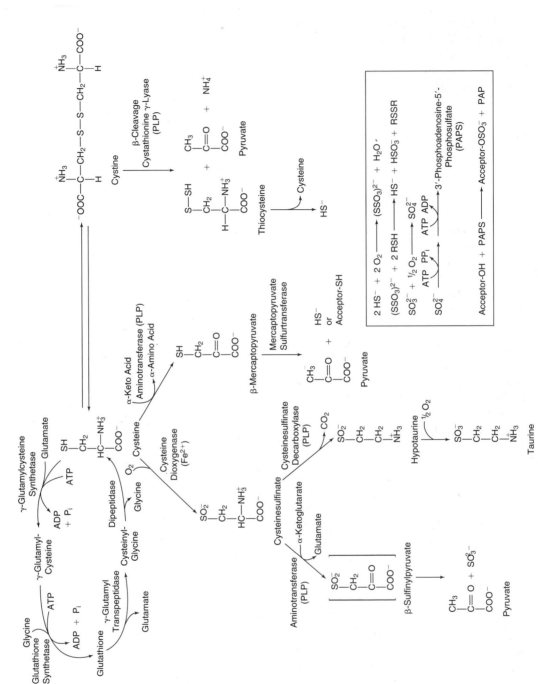

Figure 11–22. Pathways of cysteine and inorganic sulfur metabolism, including glutathione synthesis and degradation.

esters of steroid hormones and of the drug acetaminophen are examples.

Taurine, like glycine, is used for conjugation of bile acids in the liver. (See Chapters 4 and 7 for the role of bile acids in digestion and absorption.) In addition, taurine seems to be essential for other physiological functions; studies with animal models, including primates, indicate that abnormalities in retinal and neurological development and function may occur when taurine is deficient (Huxtable, 1992). Taurine is present in high concentrations in human milk and is added to infant formulas in the United States.

Role of Cysteine in the Synthesis of Glutathione and Coenzyme A. A large amount of available cysteine is used for synthesis of the tripeptide γ-glutamylcysteinylglycine, as illustrated in Figure 11–22; this tripeptide is better known as glutathione. At sulfur amino acid intakes near the requirement, a large proportion of available cysteine is used for synthesis of glutathione; the normal turnover of glutathione in adults has been estimated to be 40 mmol per day, which is slightly greater than the estimated normal turnover of cysteine in protein (Fukagawa et al., 1996). A large part of the normal glutathione turnover is related to glutathione's role as a reservoir of cysteine and as a means for transporting cysteine. The enzyme γ-glutamyl transpeptidase is located on the outer surface of the plasma membrane of cells in extrahepatic tissues such as kidney and lung, and it can hydrolyze the γ-glutamyl linkage of glutathione to yield cysteinylglycine (with or without transpeptidation of glutamate to another amino acid). The cysteinylglycine dipeptide can be hydrolyzed to cysteine and glycine either extracellularly or intracellularly by dipeptidases. Thus, cysteine may be released into the plasma or provided to peripheral tissues by hepatic glutathione synthesis and extrahepatic glutathione hydrolysis. (If a γ-glutamyl amino acid is formed, this dipeptide is transported into cells and then hydrolyzed; the glutamate spontaneously undergoes cyclization to form 5-oxoproline, which can be used to regenerate glutamate.)

Glutathione (GSH) has a reactive sulfhydryl group and can readily form disulfides with itself (oxidized glutathione or GSSG) or with other thiol compounds (GSSR). The ratio of GSH to GSSG in most cells is greater than 500, so GSH serves as a supply of reducing equivalents or electrons. Glutathione is involved in protection of cells from oxidative damage because of its role in the reduction of hydrogen peroxide and organic peroxides via glutathione peroxidases and because of its ability to inactivate free radicals by donating hydrogen to the radical; these processes result in oxidation of GSH to GSSG (DeLeve and Kaplowitz, 1991; White et al., 1994). Oxidized glutathione and GSH can be interconverted via the glutathione reductase reaction, which uses $NADP^+/NADPH$ as the oxidant/reductant; hence, glutathione plays a role in maintenance of the cellular redox state.

Glutathione also serves as cosubstrate for several reactions, including certain steps in leukotriene synthesis and melanin polymer synthesis. Glutathione is the substrate for a group of enzymes, glutathione *S*-transferases, that form glutathione conjugates from a variety of acceptor compounds, including various xenobiotics (foreign compounds such as drugs and carcinogens). These conjugates are normally degraded by γ-glutamyl transpeptidase and cysteinylglycine dipeptidase to yield the cysteinyl derivatives, which may be acetylated using acetyl CoA to become mercapturic acids, which are excreted in the urine. This process usually is a detoxification and excretion process.

Cysteine is necessary for the synthesis of the cysteamine (decarboxylated cysteine) portion of the coenzyme A molecule (see Chapter 22). It contributes the reactive sulfhydryl group that forms thioesters with fatty acids and related metabolites.

Formation of Cystine from Cysteine. Cysteine readily reacts with itself or other thiols to form disulfides. The disulfide formed from two molecules of cysteine is cystine. Most of the cyst(e)ine present in the plasma is present as cystine. Also, some cysteinyl residues in proteins react to form disulfide bridges; when the protein is hydrolyzed, these residues are released as cystine. Hence, there is a need to reduce cystine and other disulfides in order to release cysteine for use in metabolic reactions that require cysteine as substrate. Glutathione is an important source of reducing equivalents for this reduction, which can occur by thiol-disulfide exchange or enzymatically by thioltransferase, with glutathione providing the reducing equivalents.

High concentrations of cystine are found in the urine of patients with cystinuria, an inborn error of cystine and dibasic amino acid transport by the brush border membranes of the small intestinal mucosa and the renal tubules. Because cystine is very insoluble, it causes cystine stones to form in the renal tubules if it is present above its aqueous solubility limit (250 mg/L or 1 mmol/L). In another genetic disease, cystinosis, there is a defect in the transport of cystine out of lysosomes, and high concentrations of cystine accumulate in lysosomes of various tissues.

Phenylalanine and Tyrosine

Conversion of Phenylalanine to Tyrosine.
The major catabolism of phenylalanine and tyrosine occurs in the liver, but tyrosine is an important precursor for synthesis of several essential compounds in other tissues. As shown in Figure 11–23, phenylalanine is converted to tyrosine by phenylalanine hydroxylase, which is a tetrahydrobiopterin-dependent, mixed-function oxidase that hydroxylates phenylalanine at the 4-carbon of the aromatic ring. This reaction is the first step in phenylalanine degradation and also is the step that allows phenylalanine to serve as a dietary precursor of tyrosine (Clarke and Bier, 1982). The reverse reaction does not occur, so tyrosine cannot totally replace phenylalanine

---

CLINICAL CORRELATION

Cystinosis

Cystinosis is a rare, autosomal recessively inherited disorder caused by a defect in the lysosomal transport system for the amino acid cystine. In cystinosis, free cystine accumulates to 15 to 1000 times normal concentrations in the lysosomes. The cystine forms crystals within the lysosomes of most tissues, which are damaged at different rates.

Children born with cystinosis are normal at birth, but signs of the renal tubular Fanconi syndrome (failure of the kidney to reabsorb small molecules properly) develop, usually when the child is between 6 and 12 months of age. Symptoms of renal tubular Fanconi syndrome include dehydration, acidosis, vomiting, electrolyte imbalances, hypophosphatemic rickets, and failure to grow. The renal glomerular damage progresses, and children typically require dialysis or transplantation by 6 to 12 years of age. In individuals who receive a kidney transplant, cystine accumulation does not occur in the transplanted kidney but continues in other tissues, resulting in retinal blindness, corneal erosions, diabetes mellitus, distal myopathy, swallowing difficulties, pancreatic insufficiency, and primary hypogonadism in patients between 13 and 35 years of age. Plasma cystine concentrations and the intestinal absorption of cystine are normal in individuals with cystinosis, unlike in the disorder known as cystinuria (described in Chapter 6). Urinary cystine levels are slightly elevated due to renal damage, but the cystine levels are no more elevated than those of other amino acids.

The reasons for the variable rates of cystine accumulation among different tissues are unknown, but they may be related to different rates of protein turnover and lysosomal protein degradation. Lysosomes are involved in protein degradation, and cysteinyl residues in protein that have formed disulfide linkages give rise to free cystine upon hydrolysis of the peptide linkages. Oral cysteamine (β-mercaptoethylamine) has been used successfully to lower the cystine content of cystinotic fibroblasts. The cysteine-cysteamine mixed disulfide resembles lysine structurally and is transported across cystinotic lysosomal membranes in a carrier-mediated fashion by the intact lysine transporter, whereas cystine remains trapped inside the lysosomes. Long-term oral cysteamine therapy lowers the cystine content of tissues, preserves renal function, and improves growth. Cysteamine also is used in eyedrops to dissolve corneal crystals in children and to remove the haziness from the corneas of older patients.

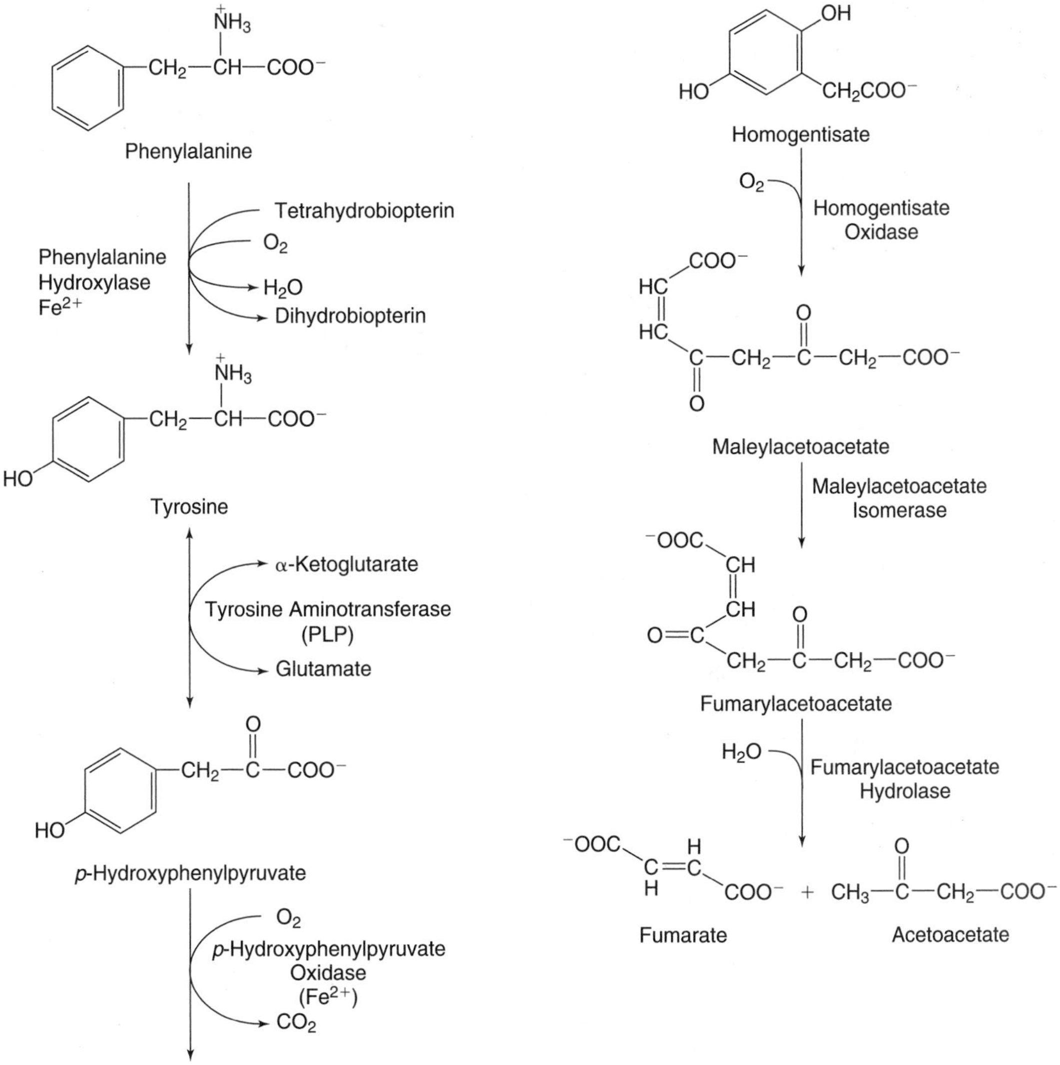

Figure 11–23. *Metabolism of phenylalanine and tyrosine.*

in the diet; only approximately 50% of the total phenylalanine + tyrosine requirement can be provided as tyrosine.

Conversion of phenylalanine to tyrosine and, hence, phenylalanine catabolism are regulated by changes in the activity of phenylalanine hydroxylase, which is regulated by its phosphorylation state (Doskeland et al., 1996; Kaufman, 1993). Phosphorylation of a seryl residue in a regulatory domain of the enzyme activates phenylalanine hydroxylase by increasing its specific activity. Phenylalanine also activates the enzyme, and the potency of phenylalanine as an activator of phenylalanine hydroxylase is greater for the phosphor-

ylated form of the enzyme. Thus, either an increase in phenylalanine concentration (high-protein diet) or an increase in the circulating glucagon level acts to increase phenylalanine hydroxylase activity. In the rat, phosphorylation of the enzyme is catalyzed by both cAMP-dependent protein kinase and calcium/calmodulin-dependent protein kinase. (See Chapter 16 for a discussion of these signal transduction pathways.)

The absence of phenylalanine hydroxylase activity is the basis of the inborn error of metabolism, phenylketonuria (PKU); PKU is the most common disease caused by a deficiency of an enzyme of amino acid metabolism, and infants routinely are screened at birth for this defect. Children with an absence of phenylalanine hydroxylase accumulate high levels of phenylalanine in their tissues and also metabolize some phenylalanine via abnormal routes such as transamination. The keto acid of phenylalanine, phenylpyruvate, along with its products phenyllactate and phenylacetate, accumulates in body fluids and is excreted in the urine of individuals with phenylketonuria who are not treated with a low-phenylalanine (adequate tyrosine) diet. In normal individuals, transamination of phenylalanine plays a very small role because the K_m for phenylalanine transamination is much higher than normal hepatic phenylalanine concentrations.

Tyrosine Catabolism. Tyrosine is primarily catabolized via transamination to *p*-hydroxyphenylpyruvate (Fig. 11–23); tyrosine aminotransferase is expressed only in the liver, has a short half-life, and is subject to regulation by a number of hormones, including insulin, glucagon, and glucocorticoids. The keto acid *p*-hydroxyphenylpyruvate is further metabolized to homogentisate and ultimately to fumarate plus acetoacetate.

The role of the tyrosine transamination pathway in phenylalanine and tyrosine catabolism is demonstrated by the inborn error of metabolism called alcaptonuria. Alcaptonuria results from a deficiency of homogentisate oxidase. Individuals with alcaptonuria excrete almost all ingested tyrosine (and phenylalanine) as homogentisate in their urine. If urine that contains homogentisate is allowed to stand or if alkali is added, it gradually turns dark as the homogentisate is oxidized to a melanin-like product. This darkening of the urine led to early recognition of this disease, and alcaptonuria was the first condition to be identified as an inborn error of metabolism. Alcaptonuria and other inborn errors of metabolism have provided much information about metabolism of amino acids in humans.

Role of Tyrosine in the Synthesis of Neuroactive Amines, Hormones, and Pigments. Tyrosine also is hydroxylated to 3,4-dihydroxyphenylalanine (DOPA) by tyrosine hydroxylase, which is a tetrahydrobiopterin-dependent enzyme similar to phenylalanine

hydroxylase (Dix et al., 1987). DOPA is further metabolized to various products, depending on the tissue (Fig. 11–24). In specific regions of the brain, DOPA is decarboxylated to dopamine, which functions as a neurotransmitter. Decreased production of dopamine is the cause of Parkinson's disease. In noradrenergic neurons, DOPA is converted to dopamine and further hydroxylated to norepinephrine. Norepinephrine is the chemical transmitter at most sympathetic postganglionic nerve endings. Norepinephrine is synthesized by the noradrenergic neurons and stored in vesicles in the termini of the axons; these cells also have an active mechanism for reuptake of norepinephrine. In chromaffin granules in the adrenal medulla, dopamine and norepinephrine also are produced, but most of the norepinephrine is methylated (by a transmethylase that uses *S*-adenosylmethionine) to epinephrine, the major hormone secreted by the adrenal medulla of humans. Epinephrine, norepinephrine, and dopamine, collectively called catecholamines, are stored in these chromaffin granules and subsequently released from these granules into the blood. Inactivation of catecholamines is accomplished by the reactions catalyzed by monoamine oxidase and catechol-*O*-methyltransferase and by conjugation of catecholamines with sulfate or glucuronate.

In melanin-producing cells (melanocytes), DOPA is oxidized by tyrosinase to form dopaquinone and various derivatives of dopaquinone. These compounds condense to form melanins or dark pigments, which are contained in cellular organelles called melanosomes. Melanins are a family of high molecular weight polymers that contain various metabolites of dopaquinone and, in the case of reddish pigments, cysteine. Melanins are concentrated in the skin, hair, and parts of the eye and brain. Genetic defects in melanin synthesis are responsible for albinism.

Tyrosyl residues in the protein thyroglobulin serve as precursors of thyroid hormones. Thyroglobulin in the thyroid gland contains iodinated aromatic amino acids derived from tyrosine. Posttranslational iodination and coupling of tyrosyl residues in thyroglobulin is followed by release of triiodothyronine (T_3)

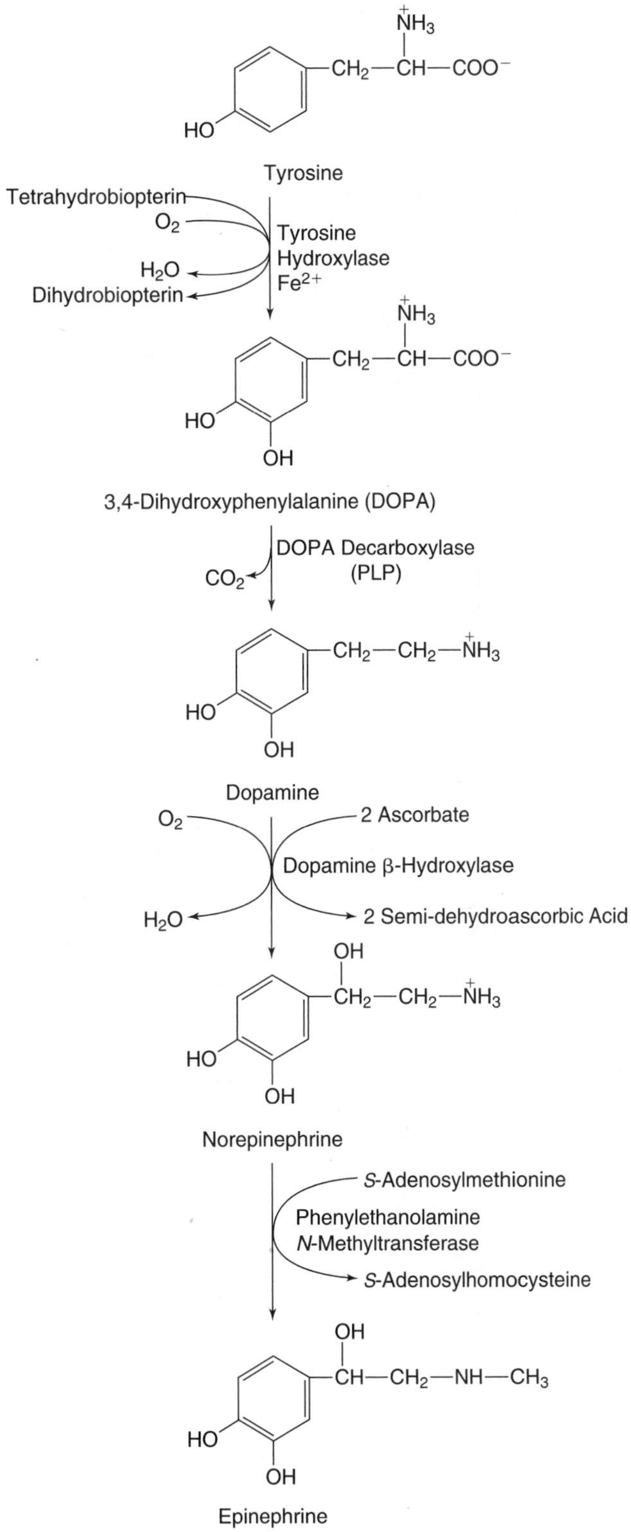

Figure 11–24. Synthesis of catecholamines from tyrosine.

and thyroxin (T_4) from the thyroid gland after proteolysis of thyroglobulin (see Chapter 33).

Tryptophan

Tryptophan Catabolism and NAD Synthesis. Tryptophan is degraded primarily in the liver. The first step in the catabolic pathway is an oxygenation that opens the 5-membered ring of the indole nucleus of tryptophan to yield *N*-formylkynurenine; this reaction is catalyzed by tryptophan dioxygenase (also called tryptophan pyrrolase) in the liver but can also be catalyzed by indoleamine 2,3-dioxygenase in other tissues (Fig. 11–25). Tryptophan dioxygenase has a short half-life and is highly regulated. Glucagon and other hormones such as glucocorticoids increase the amount of the enzyme; high levels of nicotinamide nucleotide coenzymes can inhibit the enzyme; and tryptophan can stabilize the enzyme against proteolysis, resulting in higher steady-state levels of enzyme.

The hydrolytic removal of formate (which can be used by the folate coenzyme system) from *N*-formylkynurenine yields kynurenine, a compound that lies at the first branch point of the catabolic pathway (Peters, 1991). As shown in Figure 11–25, kynurenine can be converted to kynurenate, anthranilate, or 3-hydroxykynurenine. Another branch point occurs at 3-hydroxykynurenine; 3-hydroxykynurenine can be metabolized to 2-amino-3-carboxymuconate semialdehyde or to xanthurenate. The major metabolite produced as a result of the second branch of normal tryptophan catabolism, 2-amino-3-carboxymuconate semialdehyde, lies at a third important branch point in tryptophan metabolism, leading to production of NAD⁺ (nicotinamide adenine dinucleotide) by one route and aminomuconate by the other route. Hence, tryptophan catabolism by the various branches of the catabolic pathway results in formation of kynurenate, anthranilate, xanthurenate, NAD⁺, or aminomuconate semialdehyde from the ring structure of tryptophan.

Both kynurenine and 3-hydroxykynurenine are converted to anthranilate or 3-hydroxyanthranilate by kynureninase, which is a pyridoxal 5′-phosphate-dependent enzyme. The kynureninase-catalyzed steps result in pro-duction of anthranilate or 3-hydroxyanthranilate from the benzene ring of tryptophan and of alanine from the 3-carbon aliphatic portion of the amino acid, including its α-amino and carboxyl groups. In contrast, in the branches of the pathway that lead to formation of kynurenate and xanthurenate, kynurenine or 3-hydroxykynurenine undergoes transamination with α-ketoglutarate, such that the amino group of tryptophan is incorporated into glutamate, and the remainder of the aliphatic side chain condenses to form a second 6-membered ring.

Loss of kynurenine, kynurenate, 3-hydroxykynurenine, or xanthurenate in the urine represents a loss of both gluconeogenic and ketogenic precursors; the basal excretion of these tryptophan catabolites normally accounts for about 3% to 6% of the ingested tryptophan (Leklem, 1971). A deficiency of vitamin B_6 results in decreased catabolism of tryptophan by kynureninase to kynurenine derivatives and in increased excretion of kynurenine, 3-hydroxykynurenine, kynurenate, and xanthurenate in the urine. During pregnancy, increased urinary excretion of these same tryptophan metabolites is observed; this seems to result from a pregnancy-specific decrease in kynureninase activity that is not related to a vitamin B_6 deficiency (Van De Kamp and Smolen, 1995).

At the 2-amino-3-carboxymuconate semialdehyde branch point, the 2-amino-3-carboxymuconate semialdehyde can undergo nonenzymatic cyclization to quinolinate, which can be converted to NAD⁺ or NADP⁺ by a pathway similar to that used for conversion of nicotinic acid to NAD⁺ or NADP⁺, or it can be decarboxylated by picolinate carboxylase to form 2-aminomuconate semialdehyde (Ikeda et al., 1965). (The 2-aminomuconate semialdehyde also can spontaneously undergo cyclization to form picolinate, which is the basis for the name of the enzyme that forms 2-aminomuconate semialdehyde.) Hence, the synthesis of quinolinate and subsequently NAD(P)⁺ depends on a nonenzymatic step that competes with an enzymatic route of tryptophan catabolism via 2-aminomuconate semialdehyde. Species with high picolinate carboxylase activity rapidly metabolize 2-amino-3-carboxymuconate semialdehyde by

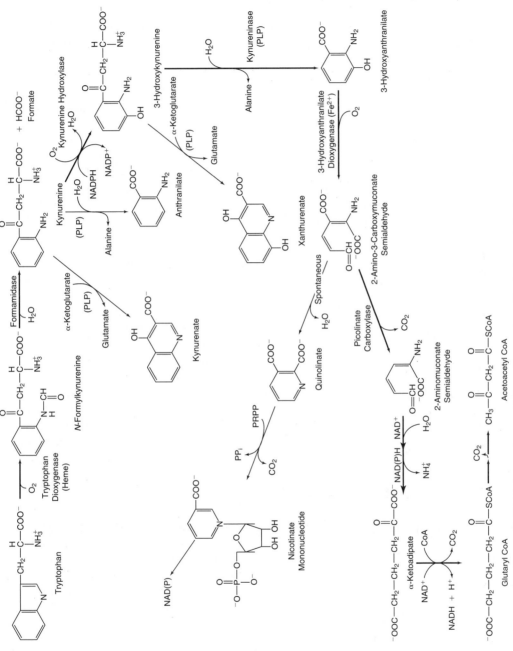

Figure 11-25. *Pathways for metabolism of tryptophan. The major route is shown by the heavy arrows.*

the enzymatic reaction and, hence, convert little tryptophan to NAD$^+$. Humans have moderate levels of picolinate carboxylase, and the synthesis of NAD$^+$ and NADP$^+$ (the niacin-containing coenzymes) from tryptophan is sufficient to provide a major portion of the body's need for the vitamin niacin, provided dietary tryptophan intake is sufficient, even though this pathway is a minor route of tryptophan catabolism. See Chapter 20 for more discussion of NAD(P)$^+$ synthesis from tryptophan.

In humans, most of the 2-aminomuconate semialdehyde formed in the picolinate carboxylase-catalyzed reaction at the last major branch point is dehydrogenated, deaminated, and further oxidized. The pathway for further oxidation of 2-aminomuconate semialdehyde involves its conversion via poorly understood reactions to α-ketoadipate, which is oxidatively decarboxylated to glutaryl CoA. Glutaryl CoA ultimately is converted to acetoacetyl CoA by a sequence of reactions that are similar to those involved in the metabolism of the α-aminoadipate that is formed in lysine catabolism (see Fig. 11–27). Glutaric aciduria type I results from a deficiency of glutaryl CoA dehydrogenase; when patients with this inborn error of metabolism are treated with dietary restrictions of both tryptophan and lysine, the urinary excretion of glutarate is decreased (Yannicelli et al., 1994). (Compare with glutaric aciduria type II discussed in Chapter 20.) This, along with the observed patterns of metabolite excretion, suggests that metabolism of tryptophan via kynurenine, 3-hydroxykynurenine, 2-amino-3-carboxymuconate semialdehyde, 2-aminomuconate semialdehyde, and glutaryl CoA is the major route of tryptophan catabolism under normal conditions.

Although some loss of tryptophan carbon and nitrogen does occur via the formation and excretion of kynurenine, kynurenate, 3-hydroxykynurenine, and xanthurenate in the urine, most of the tryptophan carbon skeleton is funneled into central pathways of energy metabolism. The formation of alanine in the two reactions catalyzed by kynureninase (conversion of kynurenine to anthranilate or conversion of 3-hydroxykynurenine to 3-hydroxyanthranilate) would be considered glu-

cogenic, and the formation of acetoacetyl CoA from 2-aminomuconate semialdehyde in the major branch of the catabolic pathway would be considered ketogenic.

Conversion of Tryptophan to Serotonin and Melatonin. Tryptophan is also converted to serotonin, an important neurotransmitter that also may have functions outside the central nervous system (Peters, 1991). Serotonin synthesis involves the hydroxylation of tryptophan at the 5-carbon by a mixed-function oxygenase that uses tetrahydrobiopterin as a co-substrate, followed by decarboxylation of the resulting 5-hydroxytryptophan by a pyridoxal 5′-phosphate-dependent enzyme to give 5-hydroxytryptamine (serotonin), as shown in Figure 11–26. Tryptophan hydroxylase normally is not saturated with substrate, and increased uptake of tryptophan by a tissue can result in increased serotonin synthesis. Serotonergic neurons have an active reuptake mechanism, and they can inactivate the serotonin by oxidation to 5-hydroxyindoleacetic acid and by methylation. The inactive metabolites and their conjugates are excreted in the urine. Serotonin is methylated and acetylated to form melatonin (N-acetyl-5-methoxytryptamine) in the pineal gland and, perhaps, other tissues. Melatonin production in the pineal gland is elevated during the dark phase of the daily cycle and may play a role in maintenance of daily and seasonal rhythms.

Lysine

Lysine Catabolism. Most degradation of lysine occurs by the saccharopine pathway, shown in Figure 11–27, which is present in liver mitochondria of mammals (Vianey-Liaud et al., 1991). This pathway involves the reaction of the ε-amino group of lysine with the carbonyl group of α-ketoglutarate to form saccharopine, which is further metabolized to α-aminoadipic semialdehyde plus glutamate. These two reactions result in transfer of the ε-amino group of lysine to the α-ketoglutarate that was used to form saccharopine; the net effect of these two reactions is to incorporate the ε-amino group of lysine into the α-amino nitrogen pool via glutamate. The α-aminoadipate semialdehyde is oxidized to α-amino-

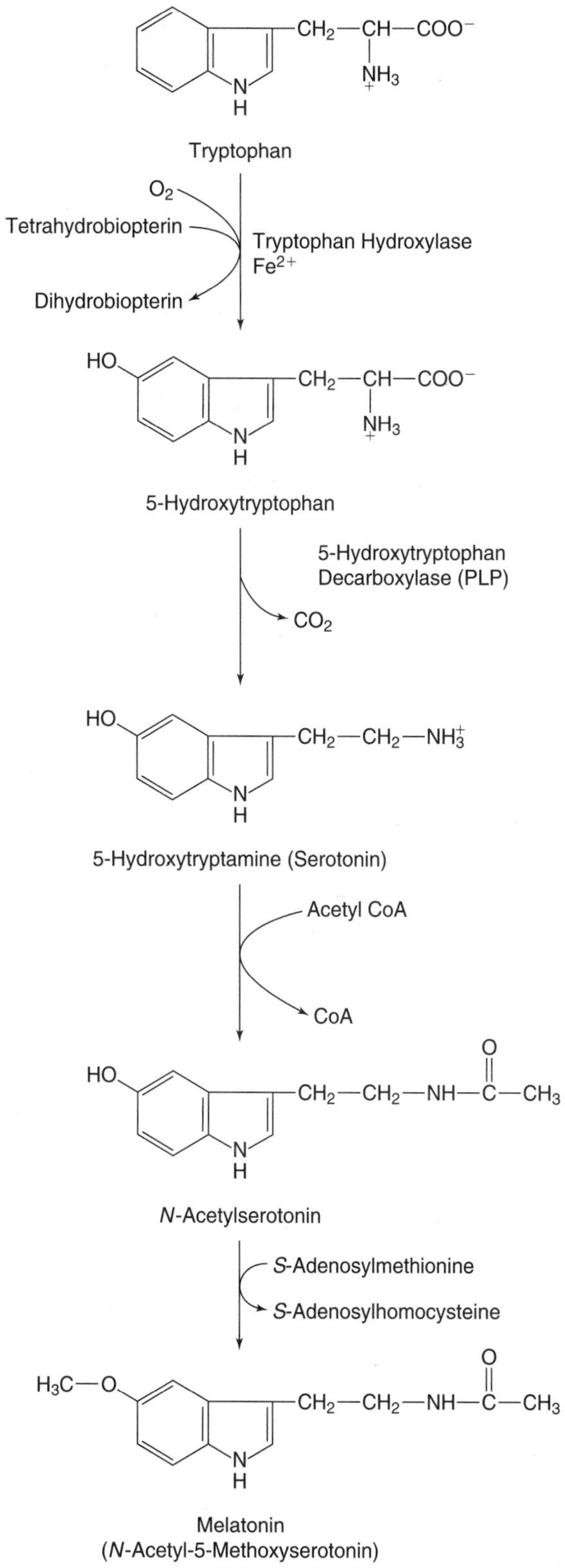

Figure 11–26. *Synthesis of serotonin and melatonin from tryptophan.*

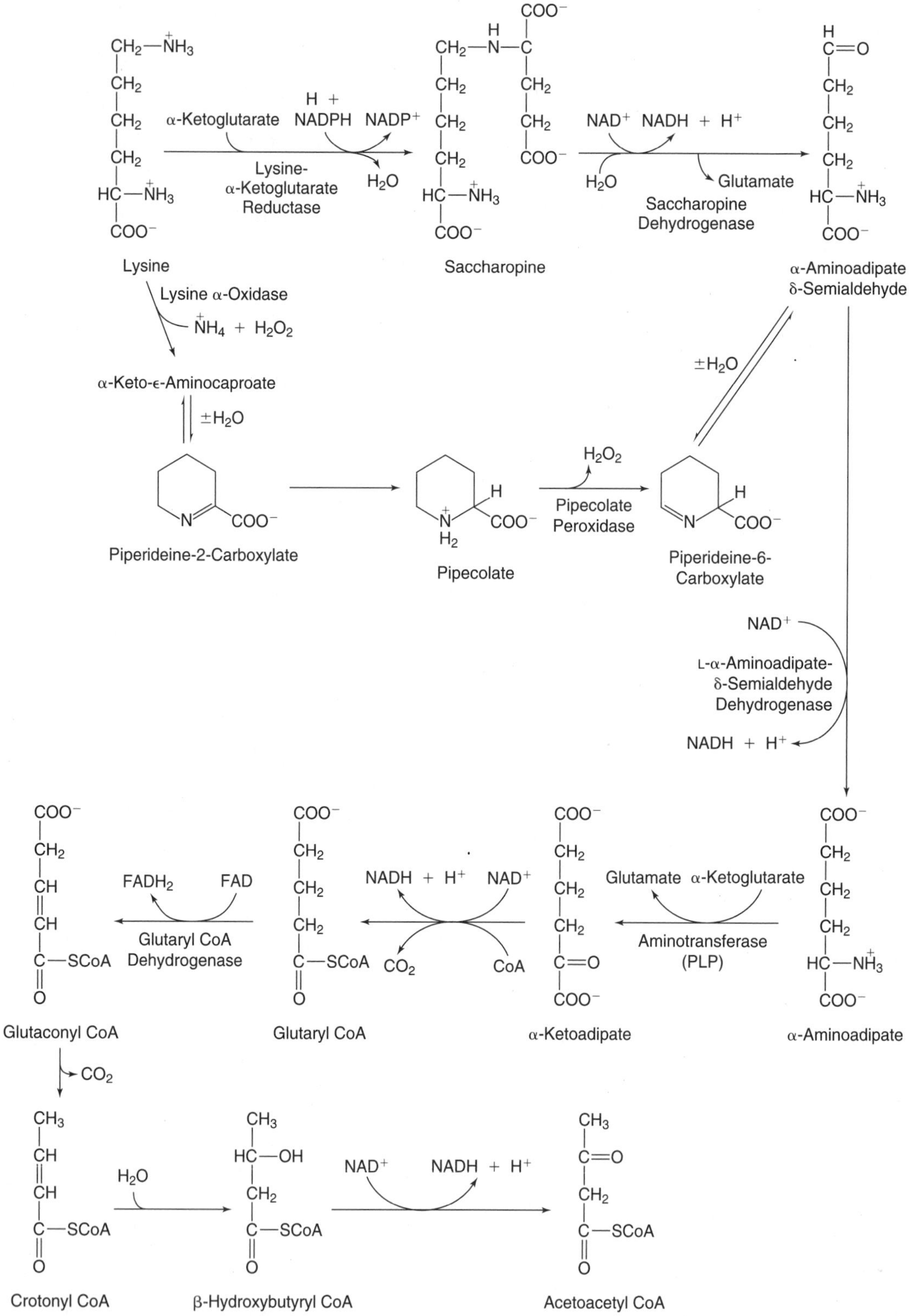

Figure 11–27. *The saccharopine and the pipecolate pathways of lysine catabolism. The two pathways merge at the intermediate, α-aminoadipate semialdehyde.*

adipate, which undergoes a conventional transamination with α-ketoglutarate to transfer the α-amino group of lysine to glutamate with formation of α-ketoadipate from the lysine carbon chain. The α-ketoadipate, which is a higher homologue of α-ketoglutarate, is oxidized to glutaryl CoA and ultimately to acetoacetyl CoA (Yannicelli et al., 1994); these final steps of lysine catabolism are analogous to those involved in the final steps of tryptophan catabolism (see Fig. 11–25).

The formation and dehydrogenation of saccharopine are catalyzed by the same protein, and a rare inborn error of metabolism in which both lysine-α-ketoglutarate reductase and saccharopine dehydrogenase activities are deficient results in hyperlysinemia and excretion of lysine and smaller amounts of saccharopine in the urine (Divry et al., 1991). The saccharopine pathway is regulated by changes in the activity of lysine-α-ketoglutarate reductase/saccharopine dehydrogenase, which is increased in animals fed diets high in lysine or protein (increased enzyme protein) and in rats treated with glucagon (increased specific activity) (Scislowski et al., 1994).

Although not sufficient to compensate for deficiency in the saccharopine pathway, other pathways of lysine degradation may play a role, especially in nonhepatic tissues (Broquist, 1990). The α-amino group of lysine can be released as ammonia by a lysine α-oxidase reaction with formation of a cyclic derivative, piperideine-2-carboxylate, which is reduced to form pipecolate, a cyclic imino acid. The pipecolate is oxidized by pipecolate peroxidase, which is found in peroxisomes in human liver, brain, and kidney (and perhaps in brain mitochondria). Pipecolate accumulates in individuals with peroxisomal disorders. The oxidation of pipecolate by pipecolate peroxidase yields hydrogen peroxide and piperideine-6-carboxylate, which is hydrolyzed spontaneously to α-aminoadipate δ-semialdehyde, an early intermediate in the saccharopine pathway of lysine catabolism. Hence, the two pathways converge, and the process of lysine catabolism is completed by the same series of reactions.

Carnitine Formation from Lysine. The residues of the ε-amino groups of lysyl residues in many proteins are methylated to mono-, di-, or trimethyllysyl residues by an N-methyltransferase that uses S-adenosylmethionine as the methyl donor. Trimethyllysine is released when these proteins undergo proteolysis, and this trimethyllysine serves as the precursor of carnitine (Rebouche, 1988). Carnitine synthesis is discussed in Chapter 23 (Fig. 23–8). The role of carnitine in the transport of long-chain fatty acids into the mitochondria is discussed in Chapters 13 and 22.

Leucine, Isoleucine, and Valine

Branched-Chain Amino Acid Catabolism. The branched-chain amino acids (leucine, isoleucine, and valine) make up a considerable part of the diet (20% to 30% of all amino acids). In contrast to other amino acids, these amino acids are not metabolized substantially by the human intestine or by liver, both of which have low levels of branched-chain amino acid transaminase activity and very low levels of the branched-chain keto acid dehydrogenase complex (Taniguchi et al., 1996). Although some transamination of branched-chain amino acids may occur in the splanchnic organs, the transamination is probably reversible due to the slow removal of branched-chain keto acids. Hence, the concentration of branched-chain amino acids in peripheral plasma rises considerably after a meal. Branched-chain amino acids in excess of amounts needed for protein synthesis are catabolized in peripheral tissues such as skeletal muscle, heart, adipose tissue, and kidney. Catabolism begins by transamination of the amino acids with α-ketoglutarate to form the corresponding branched-chain α-keto acids, as shown in Figure 11–28. Both mitochondrial and cytosolic forms of branched-chain aminotransferase exist, and the mitochondrial form is widespread in human tissues (Suryawan et al., 1996). Both isoenzymes are capable of using all three branched-chain amino or keto acids as substrate.

The branched-chain keto acids formed as a result of transamination are oxidized via a mitochondrial branched-chain keto acid dehydrogenase complex, similar to the pyruvate and α-ketoglutarate dehydrogenase complexes, to CO_2, NADH, and the branched-chain acyl CoAs. (See Chapters 20 and 22 for

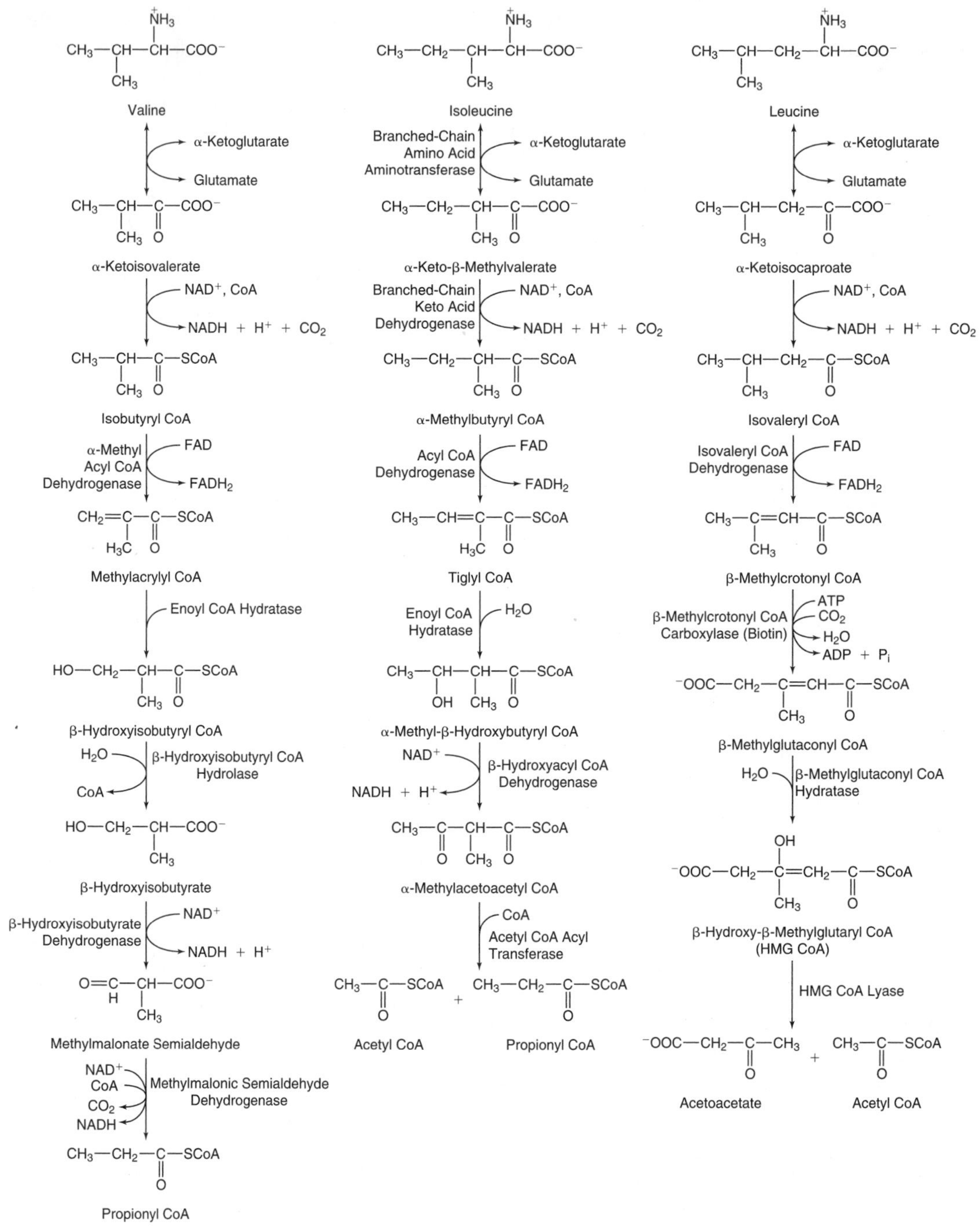

Valine

CH₃—CH—CH—COO⁻ (NH₃⁺, CH₃)

Branched-Chain Amino Acid Aminotransferase → α-Ketoglutarate → Glutamate

α-Ketoisovalerate
CH₃—CH—C—COO⁻ (CH₃, O)

Branched-Chain Keto Acid Dehydrogenase — NAD⁺, CoA → NADH + H⁺ + CO₂

Isobutyryl CoA
CH₃—CH—C—SCoA (CH₃, O)

α-Methyl Acyl CoA Dehydrogenase — FAD → FADH₂

Methylacrylyl CoA
CH₂=C—C—SCoA (H₃C, O)

Enoyl CoA Hydratase

β-Hydroxyisobutyryl CoA
HO—CH₂—CH—C—SCoA (CH₃, O)

β-Hydroxyisobutyryl CoA Hydrolase — H₂O, CoA

β-Hydroxyisobutyrate
HO—CH₂—CH—COO⁻ (CH₃)

β-Hydroxyisobutyrate Dehydrogenase — NAD⁺ → NADH + H⁺

Methylmalonate Semialdehyde
O=C—CH—COO⁻ (H, CH₃)

Methylmalonic Semialdehyde Dehydrogenase — NAD⁺, CoA, CO₂, NADH

Propionyl CoA
CH₃—CH₂—C—SCoA (O)

Isoleucine
CH₃—CH₂—CH—CH—COO⁻ (NH₃⁺, CH₃)

→ α-Ketoglutarate → Glutamate

α-Keto-β-Methylvalerate
CH₃—CH₂—CH—C—COO⁻ (CH₃, O)

— NAD⁺, CoA → NADH + H⁺ + CO₂

α-Methylbutyryl CoA
CH₃—CH₂—CH—C—SCoA (CH₃, O)

Acyl CoA Dehydrogenase — FAD → FADH₂

Tiglyl CoA
CH₃—CH=C—C—SCoA (H₃C, O)

Enoyl CoA Hydratase — H₂O

α-Methyl-β-Hydroxybutyryl CoA
CH₃—CH—CH—C—SCoA (OH, CH₃, O)

β-Hydroxyacyl CoA Dehydrogenase — NAD⁺ → NADH + H⁺

α-Methylacetoacetyl CoA
CH₃—C—CH—C—SCoA (O, CH₃, O)

Acetyl CoA Acyl Transferase — CoA

Acetyl CoA
CH₃—C—SCoA (O)

Propionyl CoA
CH₃—CH₂—C—SCoA (O)

Leucine
CH₃—CH—CH₂—CH—COO⁻ (CH₃, NH₃⁺)

→ α-Ketoglutarate → Glutamate

α-Ketoisocaproate
CH₃—CH—CH₂—C—COO⁻ (CH₃, O)

— NAD⁺, CoA → NADH + H⁺ + CO₂

Isovaleryl CoA
CH₃—CH—CH₂—C—SCoA (CH₃, O)

Isovaleryl CoA Dehydrogenase — FAD → FADH₂

β-Methylcrotonyl CoA
CH₃—C=CH—C—SCoA (CH₃, O)

β-Methylcrotonyl CoA Carboxylase (Biotin) — ATP, CO₂, H₂O → ADP + Pᵢ

β-Methylglutaconyl CoA
⁻OOC—CH₂—C=CH—C—SCoA (CH₃, O)

β-Methylglutaconyl CoA Hydratase — H₂O

β-Hydroxy-β-Methylglutaryl CoA (HMG CoA)
⁻OOC—CH₂—C=CH₂—C—SCoA (OH, CH₃, O)

HMG CoA Lyase

Acetoacetate
⁻OOC—CH₂—C—CH₃ (O)

+

Acetyl CoA
CH₃—C—SCoA (O)

Figure 11–28. *Catabolism of the branched-chain amino acids.*

the roles of coenzymes in the catabolism of the branched-chain keto acids.) In the rat, much of the branched-chain keto acid formed in muscle is released into the circulation to be further metabolized in the liver, but the oxidative decarboxylation of branched-chain keto acids in humans occurs largely in the peripheral tissues, rather than in liver. The branched-chain keto acid dehydrogenase complex is subject to feedback regulation by high ratios of NADH/NAD⁺ and acyl CoA/CoA and also is regulated by phosphorylation/dephosphorylation. The activity state of the branched-chain keto acid dehydrogenase complex is regulated by the phosphorylation state of specific seryl residues of the E1 component of the complex, which in turn is regulated by the relative activities of a specific kinase and phosphatase (Harris et al., 1994, 1995). The complex is inactive in its phosphorylated state. In animals, adaptation to higher protein diets results in the association of less kinase with the branched-chain keto acid dehydrogenase complex, which favors the dephosphorylated, active state. Short-term regulation of the complex is achieved by inhibition of the branched-chain keto acid dehydrogenase kinase by branched-chain keto acids (e.g., α-ketoisocaproate), which are the substrates for the branched-chain dehydrogenase complex.

An inborn error of branched-chain amino acid metabolism, called maple syrup urine disease because of the odor of the urine, results from defective synthesis of the branched-chain keto acid dehydrogenase. Plasma and urinary levels of branched-chain amino acids and their α-keto acids are elevated. Small amounts of branched-chain α-hydroxy acids (formed by reduction of α-keto acids) also are found in the urine of patients with this inborn error (Parsons et al., 1990).

The branched-chain acyl CoAs are further oxidized by specific branched-chain acyl CoA dehydrogenases to form the corresponding α,β-unsaturated compounds (Taniguchi et al., 1996). Catabolism of valine and isoleucine then continues through several steps to produce propionyl CoA from valine and both propionyl CoA and acetyl CoA from isoleucine. Release of β-hydroxyisobutyrate from muscle and heart has been observed in animals; this valine catabolite can be converted to glucose in the liver or kidney. The branched-chain acyl CoA formed from leucine, isovaleryl CoA, is catabolized to yield β-hydroxy-β-methylglutaryl CoA (HMG CoA). A biotin-dependent carboxylation step is required for conversion of β-methylcrotonyl CoA to β-methylglutaconyl CoA prior to HMG CoA formation in the leucine catabolic pathway. The HMG CoA can be further catabolized to yield acetoacetate and acetyl CoA. As discussed previously, much of the branched-

chain amino acid nitrogen is carried out of muscle as alanine and glutamine (Darmaun and Dechelotte, 1991). Defects in branched-chain amino acid metabolism that affect a number of these intermediary steps have been identified in human patients (Gibson et al., 1994).

NITROGEN EXCRETION

The major end products of amino acid catabolism in humans are CO_2, H_2O, and urea, with a small amount of ammonia. Because energy is required for urea synthesis and urea has a heat of combustion of 151.6 kcal/mol, the net physiological fuel value mammals can gain from dietary protein is less than would be predicted based on complete oxidation of protein. In adults in nitrogen balance, nitrogen excretion as urea approximates the daily intake of nitrogen from protein. Urine also contains smaller amounts of other nitrogenous end products formed from catabolism of amino acids or of nonprotein compounds formed from amino acids (Table 11–2). Although most of the body's loss of nitrogen occurs via the urine, nitrogen is also lost via the feces (including loss of remnants from digestion of dietary and endogenous proteins in the gastrointestinal tract and endogenous nitrogenous compounds excreted by the liver in the bile) and via loss of proteins and other nitrogenous compounds in the hair, nails,

TABLE 11–2
Major Nitrogen-Containing Components of Normal Human Urine

End Product	Excreted Nitrogen (g N/24 h)
Urea	10–15 g*
Creatinine	0.3–0.8 g
$NH_3 + NH_4^+$	0.4–1.0 g
Uric acid	0.1–0.2 g
Amino acids	0.1–0.2 g
Other nitrogen	0.2–0.8 g†
Total nitrogen	12–18 g

*Urea N depends heavily on the amount of dietary protein and may vary from less than 2 to more than 20 g N per day.

†Other N includes trace amounts of proteins, δ-aminolevulinic acid, porphobilinogen, 5-hydroxyindole acetic acid, catecholamine metabolites, tryptophan metabolites, etc.

sloughed-off skin, various bodily secretions, and blood losses.

Incorporation of Nitrogen into Urea by the Urea Cycle in the Liver

The urea cycle was first described by Krebs and Henseleit in 1932, based on experiments in which they found that ornithine stimulated urea synthesis by rat liver without itself being utilized in the process. In mammals, a complete urea cycle functions only in liver, the major site of urea synthesis. (Some urea cycle enzymes are expressed in the intestine, kidney, and other tissues, where they play a role in the synthesis of citrulline, arginine, and ornithine, as discussed earlier in this chapter.) The urea cycle is shown in Figures 11–10 and 11–17. The pathway begins with the fixation of ammonia and carbon dioxide into carbamoyl phosphate by the mitochondrial enzyme carbamoyl phosphate synthetase I. The carbamoyl phosphate then combines with ornithine to form citrulline, which exits from the mitochondria in exchange for ornithine (Indiveri et al., 1992). In the cytosol, argininosuccinate synthetase and argininosuccinate lyase effectively add another nitrogen, from aspartate, to the citrulline to produce arginine. The arginine is then hydrolyzed by arginase liberating urea and ornithine; ornithine reenters the mitochondria to begin the cycle again.

The urea cycle is subject to both short- and long-term regulation. The first step, catalyzed by carbamoyl phosphate synthetase I, is subject to activation by N-acetylglutamate. A relatively small change in carbamoyl phosphate synthetase I activity can result in a large change in urea cycle flux. This first step in urea synthesis also is regulated by substrate availability; high rates of amino acid uptake and catabolism in the liver result in increased levels of N-acetylglutamate and ammonia. With an increase in carbamoyl phosphate synthesis, flux through the rest of the urea cycle also increases because all the subsequent enzymes have K_m values that are below or near the physiological concentrations of their substrates.

Long-term regulation is brought about by adaptive changes in the amounts of urea cycle enzymes. Conditions that result in high rates of urea synthesis (high-protein diets, hypercatabolic states) are accompanied by increases in the activities of all the urea cycle enzymes, whereas conditions that result in low rates of urea synthesis (low-protein diets) result in decreased activities of the urea cycle enzymes. Although the enzymes of the urea cycle appear to be coordinately regulated, the mechanisms involved in regulation of different enzymes vary. Regulation occurs both by changes in the rate of protein degradation and by changes in the rate of enzyme synthesis, with changes in protein synthesis being primarily due to changes in the rate of gene transcription (Takiguchi and Mori, 1995).

In the postabsorptive state, the principal extrahepatic sources of nitrogen used for ureagenesis are glutamine and alanine released by muscle and ammonia from the portal blood. Glutamine is largely taken up by the intestine, and glutamine nitrogen is released back into the portal blood as citrulline, alanine, proline, and ammonia. The ammonia delivered by the portal blood originates predominately from this glutamine catabolism in the small intestinal cells (enterocytes) and from formation by bacterial metabolism of urea in the lumen of the large intestine; it is estimated that nearly 25% of the urea that is synthesized by the liver over the course of a day is broken down to ammonia in the large intestine and returned to the liver as ammonia for reincorporation into urea. Alanine and ammonia are readily removed by the liver. In the fed state, most amino acids that reach the liver can serve as precursors for ureagenesis. For each molecule of urea, one nitrogen is derived from ammonia via the carbamoyl phosphate synthetase I reaction; the second nitrogen is donated to the urea cycle from the α-amino nitrogen of aspartate, with the carbon chain of aspartate being released as fumarate. The immediate sources of hepatic ammonia funneling into the urea cycle have been estimated to include ammonia from the portal blood (33%), glutamine deamidation (6% to 13%), release of α-amino nitrogen from glutamate by the glutamate dehydrogenase-catalyzed reaction, with the amino groups of various amino acids being transferred to glutamate via transamination (20%), and direct catabolism of certain amino acids such as glycine to release ammonia (33% to 40%) (Meijer et al., 1990). A variety of amino acids, especially alanine, contribute amino groups to aspartate (via the coupled activities of alanine or another aminotransferase and aspartate aminotransferase), with glutamate being the direct donor of the amino group to oxaloacetate to form aspartate. These α-amino groups are funneled into the urea cycle to provide the second nitrogen atom for urea synthesis.

Excretion of Ammonium by the Kidney

Ammonia excretion usually is low, because most ammonia is incorporated into urea. However, in metabolic acidosis (resulting from diabetic ketosis, lactic acidosis, or excess protein catabolism), the urinary output of ammonium is increased. The production and excretion of strong acids (such as acetoacetic, β-hydroxybutyric, lactic, and sulfuric acids) requires the co-excretion of a cation. Excretion of ammonium (NH_4^+) as the cation allows the body to conserve cations such as Na^+, K^+, and Ca^{2+}; facilitates the excretion of excess H^+; and has the net effect of conserving bicarbonate ion, which serves as an important buffer. The ammonia that is excreted by the kidney is generated predominately in the kidney by deamidation of glutamine by glutaminase, followed by deamination of glutamate by glutamate dehydrogenase. The process of acidosis-increased ammonium excretion also is facilitated by net glutamine production by the liver and increased release of glutamine from skeletal muscle during acidosis. A small proportion of ammoniagenesis in the kidney is accomplished by the metabolism of glycine.

Nitrogenous End Products of Purine and Pyrimidine Catabolism

Purines are present in relatively large amounts in the body because they are present both in nucleic acids and in the form of free adenine and guanine nucleotides (ATP, ADP, AMP, GTP, NAD, FAD, etc.). Purine degradation results in formation of uric acid rather than urea; this uric acid also is excreted in the urine. Purine degradation involves the deamination of AMP or adenosine to release ammo-

nia and form inosine. Inosine and guanosine undergo phosphorylysis by purine nucleoside phosphorylase to yield hypoxanthine (from inosine) and guanine (from guanosine). The guanine is deaminated to yield xanthine, and the hypoxanthine is oxidized to xanthine. Finally, xanthine is converted to uric acid by xanthine oxidase. Hence, both ammonia and uric acid result from catabolism of purine bases. Uric acid is not very soluble in water, and deposition of urate in the joints causes gout. Gout usually is treated with the drug allopurinol, which inhibits oxidation of xanthine to uric acid and results in excretion of soluble purine metabolites (hypoxanthine, xanthine, and guanine).

Degradation of pyrimidines results in release of β-amino acids and ammonia. Cytidine monophosphate (CMP) loses ammonia in its degradation to uridine monophosphate (UMP) or uridine. Degradation of the pyrimidine base, uracil, results in release of ammonia and formation of β-alanine. Degradation of the base of dTMP, thymine, results in release of ammonia and formation of β-aminoisobutyrate. The β-amino acids may be excreted in the urine, although further metabolism occurs, and the nitrogen from pyrimidine degradation is thought to be excreted largely as urea. β-Aminoisobutyrate is a specific product of thymine catabolism, and the level of β-aminoisobutyrate in urine increases in cancer patients undergoing chemotherapy or radiation therapy due to the increased death of cells and degradation of DNA. β-Alanine is found in the urine, but it is not a specific product of pyrimidine metabolism because it is also formed from pantothenic acid, carnosine, and other peptides. In comparison with purine degradation, pyrimidine degradation makes a smaller contribution to urinary nitrogen because of the more limited occurrence of pyrimidines in the body (mainly in the nucleic acids).

Excretion of Creatinine

Creatine phosphate is present in muscle cells at a rather high concentration of about 25 mmol/kg. Both creatine and creatine phosphate undergo spontaneous loss of water and cyclization to creatinine, and this creatinine is excreted from the body in the urine. About 1.7% ($\sim$12 mmol) of the total body creatine is replaced each day by synthesis from glycine, arginine, and S-adenosylmethionine. The rate of creatinine formation reflects the amount of creatine/creatine phosphate present in the muscle mass and is relatively constant from day to day in adults who are not losing or gaining muscle mass. Because of this relation, creatinine excretion (of individuals on creatine-free diets) has been used to estimate the completeness of 24-hour urine collections, as a basis for normalizing urinary concentrations of various metabolites, and to estimate the lean body mass of individuals. Because the renal tubules do not reabsorb creatinine, creatinine excretion also can be used to calculate the volume of plasma filtered by the kidneys, which is used as a measure of renal clearance or renal function.

Reabsorption of Amino Acids from the Renal Filtrate

Amino acids are efficiently reabsorbed from the renal filtrate, and only small amounts are lost in the urine. A few milligrams of nitrogen per day are accounted for by excretion of derivatives of amino acids such as N^3-methylhistidine and hydroxyproline. Trace amounts of a large variety of other compounds also are normal constituents of urine. These include trace amounts of albumin and other proteins, δ-aminolevulinate, porphobilinogen, tryptophan metabolites, and catecholamine catabolites. All together, amino acids, proteins, and miscellaneous nitrogenous metabolites account for about 0.3 to 1.0 g of urinary nitrogen per day.

REFERENCES

Ballevre, O., Houlier, M.-L., Prugnaud, J., Bayle, G., Bercovici, D., Seve, B. and Arnal, M. (1991) Altered partition of threonine metabolism in pigs by protein-free feeding or starvation. Am J Physiol 261:E748–E757.

Battezzati, A., Brillon, D. J. and Matthews, D. E. (1995) Oxidation of glutamic acid by the splanchnic bed in humans. Am J Physiol 269:E269–E276.

Beaumier, L., Castillo, L., Ajamik A. M. and Young, V. R. (1995) Urea cycle intermediate kinetics and nitrate excretion at normal and "therapeutic" intakes of arginine in humans. Am J Physiol 269:E884–E896.

Bella, D. L. and Stipanuk, M. H. (1995) Effects of protein, methionine, or chloride on acid-base balance and on cysteine catabolism. Am J Physiol 269:E910–E917.

Bergstrom, J., Furst, P., Noree, L. -O. and Vinnars, E. (1974) Intracellular free amino acid concentration in human muscle tissue. J Appl Physiol 36:693–697.

Bird, M. I., Nunn, P. B. and Lord, L. A. J. (1984) Formation of glycine and aminoacetone from L-threonine by rat liver mitochondria. Biochim Biophys Acta 802:229–236.

Broquist, H. P. (1990) Lysine-pipecolic acid metabolic relationships in microbes and mammals. Annu Rev Nutr 11:435–448.

Carey, G. P., Kime, Z., Rogers, Q. R., Morris, J. G., Hargrove, D., Buffington, C. A. and Brusilow, S. W. (1987) An arginine-deficient diet in humans does not evoke hyperammonemia or orotic aciduria. J Nutr 117:1734–1739.

Castillo, L., Sanchez, M., Chapman, T. E., Ajami, A., Burke, J. F. and Young, V. R. (1994) The plasma flux and oxidation rate of ornithine adaptively decline with restricted arginine intake. Proc Natl Acad Sci USA 91:6393–6397.

Cho, E. S., Anderson, H. L., Wixom, R. L., Hanson, K. C. and Krause, G. F. (1984) Long-term effects of low histidine intake on men. J Nutr 114:369–384.

Christensen, H. (1990) Role of amino acid transport and countertransport in nutrition and metabolism. Physiol Rev 70:43–77.

Clarke, J. T. R. and Bier, D. M. (1982) The conversion of phenylalanine to tyrosine in man. Direct measurement by continuous intravenous tracer infusions of L-[ring-^{2}H$_5$]phenylalanine and L-[1-^{13}C]tyrosine in the postabsorptive state. Metabolism 31:999–1005.

Cowan, G. J., Willgoss, D. A., Bartley, J. and Endre, Z. H. (1996) Serine isotopomer analysis by ^{13}C-NMR defines glycine-serine interconversion in situ in the renal proximal tubule. Biochim Biophys Acta 1310:32–40.

Curthoys, N. P. and Watford, M. (1995) Regulation of glutaminase activity and glutamine metabolism. Annu Rev Nutr 15:133–159.

Cynober, L., Le Boucher, J. and Vasdson, M.-P. (1995) Arginine metabolism in mammals. J Nutr Biochem 6:402–413.

D'Aniello, A., Vetere, A. and Petrucelli, L. (1993) Further study on the specificity of D-amino acid oxidase and of D-aspartate oxidase and time course for complete oxidation of D-amino acids. Comp Biochem Physiol 105B:731–734.

Darling, P., Rafii, M., Grunow, J., Ball, R. O., Brookes, S. and Pencharz, P. B. (1997) Threonine dehydrogenase is not the major pathway of threonine catabolism in adult humans. FASEB J 11:A119.

Darmaun, D. and Dechelotte, P. (1991) Role of leucine as a precursor of glutamine α-amino nitrogen in vivo in humans. Am J Physiol 260:E326–E329.

DeLeve, L. D. and Kaplowitz, N. (1991) Glutathione metabolism and its role in hepatotoxicity. Pharmacol Ther 52:287–305.

Divry, P., Vianey-Liaud, C. and Mathieu, M. (1991) Inborn errors of lysine metabolism. Ann Biol Clin 49:27–35.

Dix, T. A., Kuhn, D. M. and Benkovic, S. J. (1987) Mechanism of oxygen activation by tyrosine hydroxylase. Biochemistry 26:3354–3361.

Doskeland, A. P., Martinez, A., Knappskog, P. M. and Flatmark, T. (1996) Phosphorylation of recombinant human phenylalanine hydroxylase: Effect on catalytic activity, substrate activation and protection against nonspecific cleavage of the fusion protein by restriction protease. Biochem J 313:409–414.

Elia, M. (1993) Glutamine metabolism in human adipose tissue in vivo. Clin Nutr 12:51–53.

Elia, M. and Livesey, G. (1983) Effects of ingested steak and infused leucine on forelimb metabolism in man and the fate of the carbon skeletons and amino groups of branched-chain amino acids. Sci Lond 64:517–526.

Ewart, H. S., Jois, M. and Brosnan, J. T. (1992) Rapid stimulation of the hepatic glycine-cleavage system in rats fed on a single high-protein meal. Biochem J 283:441–447.

Felig, P. (1975) Amino acid metabolism in man. Annu Rev Nutr 44:933–955.

Felig, P., Wahren, J. and Raf, L. (1973) Evidence of interorgan amino acid transport by blood cells in man. Proc Natl Acad Sci USA 70:1775–1779.

Fukagawa, N. K., Ajami, A. M. and Young, V. R. (1996) Plasma methionine and cysteine kinetics in response to an intravenous glutathione infusion in adult humans. Am J Physiol 270:E209–E214.

Gibson, K. M., Lee, C. F. and Hoffmann, G. F. (1994) Screening for defects of branched-chain amino acid metabolism. Eur J Pediatr 153:S62–S67.

Girgis, S., Nasrallah, I. M., Suh, J. R., Oppenheim, E., Zanetti, K. A., Mastri, M. G. and Stover, P. J. (1998) Molecular cloning, characterization and alternative splicing of the human cytoplasmic serine hydroxymethyltransferase gene. Gene 210:315–324.

Guba, S. C., Fink, L. M. and Fonseca, V. (1996) Hyperhomocysteinemia: An emerging and important risk factor for thromboembolic and cardiovascular disease. Am J Clin Pathol 105:709–722.

Harris, R. A., Popov, K. M., Zhao, Y. and Shimomura, Y. (1994) Regulation of branched-chain amino acid metabolism. J Nutr 124:1499S–1502S.

Harris, R. A., Popov, K. M. and Zhao, Y. (1995) Nutritional regulation of the protein kinases responsible for the phosphorylation of the α-ketoacid dehydrogenase complexes. J Nutr 125:1758S–1761S.

Huxtable, R. J. (1992) Physiological actions of taurine. Physiol Rev 72:101–163.

Ikeda, M., Tsuji, H., Nakamura, S., Ichiyama, A., Nishizuka, Y. and Hayaishi, O. (1965) Studies on the biosynthesis of nicotinamide adenine dinucleotide. J Biol Chem 240:1395–1401.

Indiveri, C., Tonazzi, A. and Palmieri, F. (1992) Identification and purification of the ornithine/citrulline carrier from rat liver mitochondria. Eur J Biochem 207:449–454.

Jungas, R. L., Halperin, M. L. and Brosnan, J. T. (1992) Quantitative analysis of amino acid oxidation and related gluconeogenesis in humans. Physiol Rev 72:419–448.

Kaufman, S. (1993) The phenylalanine hydroxylating system. Adv Enzymol Relat Areas Mol Biol 67:77–264.

Lam, W. K., Cleary, M. A., Wraith, J. E. and Walter, J. H. (1996) Histidinaemia: A benign metabolic disorder. Arch Dis Child 74:343–346.

Leklem, J. E. (1971) Quantitative aspects of tryptophan metabolism in humans and other species: A review. Am J Clin Nutr 24:659–672.

Lowenstein, J. M. (1972) Ammonia production in muscle and other tissues: The purine nucleotide cycle. Physiol Rev 52:383–414.

Lowry, M., Hall, D. E. and Brosnan, J. T. (1985) Increased activity of renal glycine-cleavage-enzyme complex in metabolic acidosis. Biochem J 231:477–480.

MacFarlane, N., McMurray, J., O'Dowd, J. J., Dargie, H. J. and Miller, D. J. (1991) Synergism of histidyl dipeptides as antioxidants. J Mol Cell Cardiol 23:1205–1208.

Matthews, D. E., Marano, M. A. and Campbell, R. G. (1993) Splanchnic bed utilization of glutamine and glutamic acid in humans. Am J Physiol 264:E848–E854.

McGivan, J. D. and Pastor-Anglada, M. (1994) Regulatory and molecular aspects of mammalian amino acid transport. Biochem J 299:321–334.

Meijer, A. J., Lamers, W. H. and Chamuleau, R. A. F. M. (1990) Nitrogen metabolism and ornithine cycle function. Physiol Rev 70:701–749.

Nurjhan, N., Bucci, A., Stumvoll, M., Bailey, G., Bier, D. M., Toft, I., Jenssen, T. G. and Gerich, J. E. (1995) Glutamine: A major gluconeogenic precursor and vehicle for interorgan carbon transport in man. J Clin Invest 95:272–277.

Ogawa, H., Gomi, T., Konishi, K., Date, T., Nakashima, H., Nose, K., Matsuda, Y., Peraino, C., Pitot, H. C. and Fujioka, M. (1989) Human liver serine dehydratase: cDNA cloning and sequence homology with hydroxyamino acid dehydratases from other sources. J Biol Chem 264:15818–15823.

Parsons, H. G., Carter, R. J., Unrath, M. and Snyder, F. F. (1990) Evaluation of branched-chain amino acid intake in children with maple syrup urine disease and methylmalonic aciduria. J Inherit Metab Dis 13:125–136.

Paxton, R., Scislowski, P. W. D., Davis, E. J. and Harris, R. A. (1986) Role of branched-chain 2-oxo acid dehydrogenase and pyruvate dehydrogenase in 2-oxobutyrate metabolism. Biochem J 234:295–303.

Pegg, A. E., Poulin, R. and Coward, J. K. (1995) Use of aminopropyltransferase inhibitors and of non-metabolizable analogs to study polyamine regulation and function. Int J Biochem Cell Biol 27:425–442.

Peters, J. C. (1991) Tryptophan nutrition and metabolism: An overview. In: Kynurenine and Serotonin Pathways (Schwarcz, R., Young, S. N. and Brown, R. R., eds.), pp. 345–358. Plenum Press, New York.

Rabier, D. and Kamoun, P. (1995) Metabolism of citrulline in man. Amino Acids 9:209–316.

Rabier, D., Narcy, C., Bardet, J., Parvy, P., Saudubray, J. M. and Kamoun, P. (1991) Arginine remains an essential amino acid after liver transplantation in urea cycle enzyme deficiencies. J Inherit Metab Dis 14:277–280.

Rebouche, C. J. (1988) Carnitine metabolism and human nutrition. J Appl Nutr 40:99–111.

Robinson, K., Mayer, E. and Jacobsen, D. W. (1994) Homocysteine and coronary artery disease. Cleve Clin J Med 61:438–450.

Scislowski, P. W. D., Foster, A. R. and Fuller, M. F. (1994) Regulation of oxidative degradation of L-lysine in rat liver mitochondria. Biochem J 300:887–891.

Stipanuk, M. H. (1986) Metabolism of sulfur-containing amino acids. Annu Rev Nutr 6:179–209.

Storch, K. J., Wagner, D. A., Burke, J. F. and Young, V. R. (1990) [1-^{13}C;$methyl$-^{2}H$_3$]methionine kinetics in humans: Methionine conservation and cystine sparing. Am J Physiol 258:E790–E798.

Suryawan, A., Bledsoe, R., Shimomura, Y. and Hutson, S. (1996) Towards a human model of branched chain amino acid metabolism. FASEB J 10:A285.

Takiguchi, M. and Mori, M. (1995) Transcriptional regulation of genes for ornithine cycle enzymes. Biochem J 312:649–659.

Taniguchi, K., Nonami, T., Nakao, A., Harada, A., Kurokawa, T., Sugiyama, S., Fujitsuka, N., Shimomura, Y., Hutson, S. M., Harris, R. A. and Takagi, H. (1996) The valine catabolic pathway in human liver: Effect of cirrhosis on enzyme activities. Hepatology 24:1395–1398.

Tizianello, A., Deferrari, G., Garibotto, G., Robaudo, C., Acquarone, N. and Ghiggeri, G. M. (1982) Renal ammoniagenesis in an early stage of metabolic acidosis in man. J Clin Invest 69:240–250.

Torres, N., Martinez, L., Aleman, G., Bourges, H. and Tovar, A. R. (1998) Histidase expression is regulated by dietary protein at the pretranslational level in rat liver. J Nutr 128:818–824.

Van De Kamp, J. L. and Smolen, A. (1995) Response of kynurenine pathway enzymes to pregnancy and dietary level of vitamin B-6. Pharmacol Biochem Behav 51:753–758.

Vianey-Liaud, C., Divry, P., Poinas, C. and Mathieu, M. (1991) Lysine metabolism in man. Ann Biol Clin 49:18–26.

Watford, M. (1994) Glutamine metabolism in rat small intestine: Synthesis of three-carbon products in isolated enterocytes. Biochim Biophys Acta 1200:73–78.

White, A. C., Thannickal, V. J. and Fanburg, B. L. (1994) Glutathione deficiency in human disease. J Nutr Biochem 5:218–226.

Wu, G., Borbolla, A. G. and Knabe, D. A. (1994) The uptake of glutamine and release of arginine, citrulline and proline by the small intestine of developing pigs. J Nutr 124:2437–2444.

Yang, R. D., Matthews, D. E., Bier, D. M., Wen, Z. M. and Young, V. R. (1986) Response of alanine metabolism in humans to manipulation of dietary protein and energy intakes. Am J Physiol 250:E39–E46.

Yannicelli, S., Rohr, F. and Warman, M. L. (1994) Nutrition support for glutaric acidemia type I. J Am Diet Assoc 94:183–191.

RECOMMENDED READINGS

Abcouwer, S. F. and Souba, W. W. (1999) Glutamine and arginine. In: Modern Nutrition in Health and Disease (Shils, M. E., Olson, J. A., Shike, M. and Ross, A. C., eds.), 9th ed., pp. 559–569. Williams & Wilkins, New York.

Jungas, R. L., Halperin, M. L. and Brosnan, J. T. (1992) Quantitative analysis of amino acid oxidation and related gluconeogenesis in humans. Physiol Rev 72:419–448.

Stipanuk, M. H. (1999) Homocysteine, cysteine, and taurine. In: Modern Nutrition in Health and Disease (Shils, M. E., Olson, J. A., Shike, M. and Ross, A. C., eds.), 9th ed., pp. 543–558. Williams & Wilkins, New York.

Wu, G. and Morris, S. M., Jr. (1998) Arginine metabolism: Nitric oxide and beyond. Biochem J 336:1–17.

CHAPTER **12**

◆ ◆

Protein and Amino Acid Requirements

Malcolm F. Fuller, M.A., Ph.D., Sc.D.

O U T L I N E

C O M M O N   A B B R E V I A T I O N S

BV (biological value)
NPU (net protein utilization)
PER (protein efficiency ratio)

THE PHYSIOLOGICAL BASIS OF PROTEIN AND AMINO ACID REQUIREMENTS

In the early part of the 19th century, it was discovered that protein (or a substance containing nitrogen) was required in the diet, but it was more than a century later (the 1930s) before all the constituent amino acids were identified and work could begin on assessing human requirements for these nutrients. Because nonreproductive adults form such a large proportion of the total human population, it is appropriate that most effort has been directed to establishing their requirements, although the special needs of mothers and children have also received attention.

Dispensable and Indispensable Amino Acids

It is normally considered that a dietary requirement for protein represents only the need for the amino acids that constitute it. As described in Chapter 11, of the 20 or so amino acids found in natural proteins, about half, the dispensable or nonessential amino acids, can be synthesized in the body from other amino acids or from still simpler substances. (The term "dispensable" is preferred by some nutritionists to "nonessential," because all the amino acids found in protein are metabolically essential, even though some are dispensable in the diet.) Of the others, nine are indispensable for humans, who do not possess the pathways for their synthesis. These nine are threonine, valine, leucine, isoleucine, phenylalanine, methionine, lysine, histidine, and tryptophan. A further two are called semidispensable or semi-essential and must be considered when evaluating indispensable amino acid intake. These are cysteine (or its disulfide form, cystine), which can be synthesized in the body from serine and the sulfur group of methionine, and tyrosine, which can be formed in the body by the hydroxylation of phenylalanine. Both of these syntheses are irreversible. This means that, whereas a lack of tyrosine in the diet can be compensated by an excess of phenylalanine, the reverse is not true: no matter how much tyrosine is provided by the diet, tyrosine cannot compensate for a deficiency of phenylalanine. The same is true of methionine and cyst(e)ine.

A fourth category of amino acids includes dispensable amino acids that may behave as indispensable amino acids if the rate at which they are provided by endogenous synthesis is below the rate of their disposal. In these cases, the amino acid is said to be "conditionally dispensable." Arginine, for instance, as one of the intermediates in the urea cycle, is synthesized in large amounts in the body, most of it in the liver. There is also high arginase activity, especially in the liver, so that most of what is synthesized is then broken down to liberate urea. However, other organs, notably the kidney, although synthesizing less arginine than the liver, also have lower arginase activity, so that there is a net production of arginine that is sufficient to meet the needs of most individuals. Nevertheless, in some circumstances, when the requirement is particularly high, such as during catch-up growth, the rate of endogenous production may be less than the rate of utilization, so that dietary arginine is needed to satisfy the requirement. There are suggestions that glycine may similarly behave as an indispensable amino acid in infants (especially premature infants), who have a limited capacity for glycine synthesis and who are usually fed milk, which is low in glycine (Jackson et al., 1981). Clearly, an amino acid cannot be classified as dispensable solely because a pathway for its synthesis exists; whether it behaves as a dispensable or an indispensable amino acid depends on the functional state of that pathway relative to the rate of metabolic utilization of the product.

Needs for Dietary Amino Acids to Replace Losses and to Allow for Growth

Amino acids are used for a great variety of functions in the body, as discussed in Chapters 10 and 11. Both dispensable and indispensable amino acids are required for the synthesis of protein; as intermediates in various pathways of metabolism, including the transport of nitrogen between organs; and for synthesis of numerous nonprotein compounds that require amino acids as precursors. The requirements for indispensable amino acids and total amino acid nitrogen are basically a requirement for net tissue accretion (during growth, pregnancy, and lactation) and for maintenance or replacement of obligatory losses. The major routes of obligatory amino acid or protein loss are by irreversible modification (such as by posttranslational modification as described in Chapters 2 and 10), loss of proteins through the epithelia, the loss of amino acids in the urine, use of amino acids for synthesis of nonprotein substances (see Chapter 11), and by oxidation of amino acids as fuels (see Chapter 11).

As discussed in Chapter 10, the rate of utilization of amino acids for protein synthesis usually accounts for several-fold the daily intake. During growth and in pregnancy, when protein synthesis is greater than protein degradation, the use of amino acids for body protein accretion is a major component of requirements. Likewise, in lactation, the needs of the mammary gland for milk protein synthesis become a large component of requirements. However, when there is no change in body protein mass, protein synthesis does not of itself result in much net disposal of amino acids, because the concomitant process of protein degradation returns amino acids almost entirely to the free pool.

Nevertheless, protein turnover in the adult does result in some irreversible losses of amino acids. Some amino acids, after they are incorporated into proteins, are irreversibly modified by processes such as methylation (methylhistidine, methyllysine) or hydroxylation (hydroxylysine, hydroxyproline); these modified amino acids cannot be reutilized for protein synthesis and are excreted in the urine.

Protein and amino acid losses also occur from the skin and gastrointestinal tract. Dermal losses of protein include the keratins of skin, hair, and nails, which together in adults amount to about 300 mg of protein per day. Because keratins are very rich in cystine, these losses may account for about 5% of the methionine + cyst(e)ine requirements for maintenance. Additional and highly variable quantities of nitrogen are lost in sweat, but this is mainly urea and represents little loss of amino acids per se. Proteins, including mucins and pancreatic digestive enzymes, also are contin-uously secreted into the gastrointestinal tract via salivary, gastric, and intestinal secretions. Furthermore, the enterocytes, which form the gastrointestinal epithelium, are themselves continuously shed from the villi. Although much of the protein passing into the gastrointestinal tract from these sources is itself digested, with the resulting amino acids and small peptides being reabsorbed, a substantial amount, especially of mucins and other proteins that are inherently resistant to proteolysis, escapes digestion.

Those incompletely digested proteins that pass into the large intestine may be utilized by the gastrointestinal microflora, and a large proportion of this nitrogen is voided in the microbial biomass of the feces. There is experimental evidence, mainly from animals, that there is little absorption of amino acids from the large intestine. There is, however, substantial absorption of nitrogen from the large intestine, most of it as ammonia and much of it originating from hydrolysis of urea secreted into the gastrointestinal tract. Measurements of amino acid losses in ileostomy fluid when subjects were given protein-free diets suggest that losses of nitrogen via the gastrointestinal tract may account for 15% to 30% of maintenance requirements for most indispensable amino acids and an even greater percentage of the requirement for threonine (Fuller et al., 1994).

Amino acids, both dispensable and indispensable, are precursors or donors of essential groups for the synthesis of many essential substances such as hormones, neurotransmitters, pyrimidines, and purines. Although the amounts of amino acids that are used over the course of a day for synthesis of nonprotein compounds are much less than the amounts used for protein synthesis, the irreversible disposal of amino acids into the various nonprotein synthetic pathways accounts for a small but significant proportion of the requirements for indispensable amino acids and amino acid nitrogen. The rates at which amino acids are consumed for these nonprotein purposes depend, to some extent, on the turnover rate of the pools of the individual compounds and on net tissue accretion.

Small amounts of amino acids and an even smaller amount of protein are lost in the urine. The highly efficient reabsorption of nutrients by the kidneys means that losses of amino acids through urine are small: for most amino acids, urinary excretion accounts for less than 5% of total requirements, although some derivatized amino acids such as N-methylhistidine and hydroxyproline are essentially quantitatively excreted.

Replacement of obligatory losses due to oxidation or catabolism of amino acids is the largest single component of maintenance requirements. The rate of amino acid oxidation is modulated so as to dispose of amino acids in excess of requirements, not only preventing their potentially toxic accumulation but converting them into energy-yielding substrates (see Chapter 11, Fig. 11–9). This control is exercised partly as a direct response to alterations in plasma or intracellular amino acid concentrations and partly by activation or induction (or both) of the relevant oxidative enzymes. When the dietary intake is less than the requirement, oxidation is suppressed to conserve the limited supply as fully as possible. However, oxidation is not shut down completely and the residual rate of oxidation, although small compared with the rate on normal diets, is nevertheless the major route of obligatory loss. Minimum rates of oxidation have not been estimated for all amino acids; values for those that have are given in Table 12–1. Although the diets used were not devoid of the amino acid under investigation, the amino acid concentrations were low and the rates of oxidation accordingly were near to their minimums. Amino acid oxidation is usually estimated by the infusion of an isotopic tracer with measurement of the production of labeled end product. In humans, this most commonly involves the use of a ^{13}C-labeled amino acid and measurement of ^{13}CO$_2$ production. It should be noted, however, that with ^{13}C-labeled amino acids, the measurement involves giving a nutritionally significant amount of amino acid, in contrast to the use of radiolabeled amino acids, which can be used as tracers without administration of a significant mass of amino acid.

Maintenance Requirements

In a nutritional context, it is not convenient to consider the amino acid requirements for each of the individual processes, even if they could be measured (and many have not), but to consider them collectively in terms of the overall status of the individual. All individuals require amino acids for maintenance, simply to replace inevitable losses. The obligatory loss of an amino acid is the sum of the losses by all routes, and the maintenance requirement is the dietary intake needed to replace this obligatory loss.

In the context of protein metabolism, maintenance is the condition where there is no change in the amino acid content of the body, which is usually considered to occur at nitrogen equilibrium. In this condition, the dietary intake of every amino acid is exactly balanced by losses in digestion, secretion, and metabolism. Because dietary intake can vary enormously, it is obvious that the body has mechanisms to adjust the rate of amino acid disposal according to the supply, the major mechanism being the modulation of amino acid oxidation. Because the body can maintain nitrogen equilibrium over a wide range of intakes, the protein or amino acid "requirement" is usually defined as the minimum intake consistent with nitrogen equilibrium.

Requirements for Body Protein Accretion and for Milk Protein Secretion

In addition to their maintenance needs, children require additional quantities of amino

TABLE 12–1
Minimum Rates of Oxidation of Indispensable Amino Acids in Normal Adults

	Rate of Amino Acid Oxidation*	Amino Acid Intake of Subjects
	mg · kg^{-1} · day^{-1}	
Lysine	15	2–6
Threonine	13	3–10
Valine	11	40
Leucine	22	4–8
Methionine	14	13
Phenylalanine	5	5–10

*Estimates not adjusted for the labeled amino acid infused.
Data from Fuller, M. F. and Garlick, P. J. (1994) Human amino acid requirements: Can the controversy be resolved? Annu Rev Nutr 14:217–241.

acids for the growth of their body protein mass. Although there have been no studies in humans to confirm the point, experiments with animals suggest that the pattern of amino acids required for growth is very close to the composition of whole-body protein (see Table 12–3 for the composition of whole-body protein), which means that all amino acids are used with much the same efficiency. However, the utilization of absorbed amino acids for body protein accretion is not completely efficient: estimates of efficiency vary, with a mean of approximately 0.7. This means that to retain 1 g of amino acid, 1/0.7 or approximately 1.4 g of the amino acid must be supplied in the diet. It should be noted, however, that the rate of body protein accretion in normally growing children is at most only of the order of 5 g/day, so the amino acid requirements to support it are correspondingly small. Thus, except for the first months of life, during which the infant's requirement for growth exceeds its requirement for maintenance, maintenance requirements account for the major proportion of the dietary protein needs of children and adolescents (Table 12–2). The same is true for the mother during gestation, for the actual rate of body accretion in the fetus and other products of conception is not high relative to the mother's total nitrogen needs, and maternal maintenance needs still predominate. An exception to the small proportionate contribution of body protein accretion (net protein synthesis) to total amino acid requirements is during catch-up growth, which occurs when children whose growth has been retarded by malnutrition are fed well. Their fractional growth rate may then reach 2% to 3% per day: the amino acid needs for this rapid rate of body protein gain may increase requirements to two or three times the normal levels.

As with growth, the additional amino acid requirements for lactation derive primarily from the quantity and composition of the protein and amino acids secreted in the milk. The amino acid composition of milk changes substantially over the course of lactation (Table 12–3). The amount of milk secreted also changes during lactation and varies greatly among individuals. Again, there are no direct estimates of the efficiency of amino acid utilization for milk protein production in women; as an approximation, a value derived from animal studies is usually taken to apply equally to humans for the purpose of estimating amino acid requirements for lactating women.

FOOD PROTEINS AND PROTEIN QUALITY

Although the physiological requirement is for a mixture of indispensable amino acids plus other amino acids to provide the total amount of required amino acid nitrogen, these re-

---

TABLE 12–2

The Factorial Assessment of the Protein Requirements of Infants (Sexes Combined), Compared with Typical Intakes from Breast Milk

Age (months)	Protein (mg N · kg⁻¹ · day⁻¹)			
	Allowance for Maintenance	*Allowance for Growth*	*Total Requirement, Allowing for Efficiency of Utilization**	*Typical Intake from Breast Milk*
1–2	120	168	360	303
2–3	120	120	291	273
3–4	120	81	236	234
4–5	120	66	214	NA
5–6	120	62	209	NA
6–9	120	56	200	NA
9–12	120	45	184	NA

*Assumed to be 0.7.
NA, not applicable.
Data from World Health Organization. (1985) Energy and Protein Requirements. Report of a Joint FAO/WHO/UNU Expert Consultation. WHO Technical Report Series 724. World Health Organization, Geneva.

TABLE 12–3

The Amino Acid Composition of Mixed Body Proteins and of Human Milk at Three Stages of Lactation

	Body Protein (mg/g protein)	Milk Protein (mg/g total amino acids)		
		Colostrum	*Intermediate*	*Mature*
Threonine	48	55	45	44
Valine	62	54	51	51
Methionine	19	13	16	16
Cystine	24	40	25	20
Isoleucine	48	36	50	53
Leucine	77	91	104	104
Phenylalanine	53	43	42	37
Tyrosine	33	44	44	46
Lysine	82	59	71	71
Histidine	24	23	25	23
Tryptophan	14	ND	ND	ND
Arginine	ND	55	42	36

ND, not determined.

Data from Smith, R. H. (1980) Comparative amino acid requirements. Proc Nutr Soc 39:71–78; and from Davis, T. A., Nguyen, H. V., Garcia-Bravo, R. et al. (1994) Amino acid composition of the milk of some mammalian species changes with stage of lactation. Br J Nutr 72:845–853.

quirements normally are met by a mixture of food proteins. Consequently, requirements and recommended dietary intakes are usually expressed in terms of dietary protein rather than amounts of individual amino acids. Different individual proteins (e.g., casein, gelatin) or different food proteins (which are actually mixtures of proteins; e.g., milk protein, soy protein) are not identical in terms of their amino acid composition and their ability to replace losses or support net protein accretion. Hence, we need a way to describe the ability of particular proteins or mixtures of proteins to meet requirements. The term *protein quality* has been developed for this purpose. Hence, we can talk about total protein in a food or diet and also about the quality of the protein or mixture of proteins in the food or diet.

Dietary protein is usually measured not as protein but as nitrogen, and then nitrogen is converted to protein by use of a factor. Factors have been developed for the conversion of weight of nitrogen to weight of protein (e.g., 6.25 g protein per g of nitrogen; nitrogen makes up 16% of the weight of protein on average). The term "crude protein" implies the use of the factor 6.25, but other factors are more appropriate for specific foods (e.g., 6.38 for milk and 5.7 for wheat). These differ-

ent factors are appropriate because the nitrogen concentration in proteins varies with differences in their amino acid composition. (This is obvious if one considers that the nitrogen concentration in tyrosine is 77 mg/g and in arginine is 322 mg/g.) It must be noted, too, that not all the nitrogen in food is in the form of amino acids. Substances such as nitrates, amides, urea, amino sugars, and nucleic acids may account for a significant proportion of the total nitrogen in some foods, and these components affect the relationship between nitrogen and protein contents. For mixed diets, it is a matter of convenience to use the factor 6.25 to calculate protein content, but it must be borne in mind that for particular foods, this average factor may be substantially in error.

Definition of Protein Quality

Protein quality, or the ability of a given amount of a particular protein or mixture of proteins to meet the body's amino acid requirements, depends on three attributes of the protein: its digestibility, the availability of the amino acids, and the pattern of amino acids.

Digestibility. It is rather obvious that only that part of the protein that is digested can contribute amino acids to meet requirements. Apparent protein digestibility (d) is conventionally described as

$$d = (I - F)/I$$

where I is the protein or nitrogen intake and F is fecal nitrogen or protein excretion, with both measured in the same units (e.g., g/day, usually as nitrogen). This is called *apparent digestibility* in recognition of the fact that the fecal nitrogen output does not consist entirely of undigested dietary matter, but includes nitrogen from endogenous sources (i.e., secretions and sloughed intestinal cells). By deducting this endogenous component, which can be estimated by measuring fecal nitrogen in individuals consuming protein-free diets, a value for the *true digestibility* of the dietary protein can be derived. True digestibility is higher than apparent digestibility because of this correction. In practice, these measurements are not routinely made in human subjects but commonly are made when protein quality is evaluated in experimental animals. The true digestibility of most animal proteins such as milk, meat, and eggs is high, between 90% and 99%. Many plant proteins, conversely, especially when eaten raw, are less digestible (70% to 90% digestibility), partly because they are contained within cell walls, which are resistant to mammalian digestive enzymes and are broken down only by the gastrointestinal microflora.

Availability. There is some confusion in the use of the terms "digestibility" and "availability," and these terms are sometimes used interchangeably. The original use of availability was to describe the chemical integrity of an amino acid, which is a quite separate attribute from its digestibility, and it seems preferable to preserve the distinction. Loss of availability is principally associated with Maillard reactions, which modify lysine through conjugation of its ε-amino group with sugars. These reactions occur readily during drying of milk, meat, fish, and other animal proteins. Severe heat damage can also reduce the availability of methionine and tryptophan and of protein as a whole.

Amino Acid Pattern. The major factor de-termining the quality of a protein is usually its amino acid composition: essentially, how closely the pattern of its amino acids conforms to the needs of the subject. It is therefore not a fixed attribute of the protein, but a measure of its suitability for a particular use. In practice, its value is determined by the amino acid that is most deficient in the protein relative to the requirements. This is the limiting amino acid. A protein that supplies indispensable amino acids in exactly the same pattern as the requirements, along with a sufficient supply of dispensable amino acids, can be considered an "ideal" or "complete" protein. In order to establish which amino acid is limiting and how closely a given protein conforms to the ideal, both a reference pattern and a method for comparing the dietary protein with the reference pattern are needed. This pattern must include a value for each of the indispensable amino acids, together with the sum of the dispensable amino acids. The pattern of the dispensable amino acids is of little consequence in terms of protein quality, although a mixture of dispensable amino acids such as occurs in proteins is preferable to one or a few of the dispensable amino acids (e.g., glutamate). This is because some may be synthesized at a limited rate when all the dispensable amino acids must be synthesized from a single nitrogen source.

Methods of Evaluating Protein Quality

Methods of assessing protein quality are basically of two kinds. Those in the first category, which can be considered integrative assays, simply describe the utilization of the dietary protein without regard for its amino acid composition. Those in the second category are based on comparing the amino acid composition of the protein with an "ideal" or reference pattern.

Integrative Bioassays. In the earliest of the integrative assays, proteins were compared in terms of their growth-promoting values, most commonly using rats or chicks as the test species. Protein efficiency ratio (PER) is defined as the weight gain per gram of protein consumed. However, weight gain reflects aspects of the diet other than the quality of the protein, and PER gives no information on the value of a protein for meeting maintenance requirements. These two factors limit the usefulness of PER as a measure of the quality of protein for use in human diets. Later methods such as biological value (BV) and net protein utilization (NPU) are based on the nitrogen gained. Biological value describes the efficiency with which truly digested nitrogen is utilized for both maintenance and body nitrogen gain. It is calculated as

$$BV = \frac{N_{int} - (N_u - N_{eu}) - (N_f - N_{mf})}{N_{int} - (N_f - N_{mf})}$$

where N_{int} is nitrogen intake, N_u is urinary nitrogen excretion, N_{eu} is endogenous urinary nitrogen excretion, N_f is fecal nitrogen excretion, and N_{mf} is metabolic fecal nitrogen. N_{eu} and N_{mf} are measured as the urinary and fecal nitrogen excretion of comparable animals given a protein-free diet or, alternatively, as their body nitrogen loss. NPU is similar to BV in being a measure of nitrogen utilization for both maintenance and body protein accretion, but is expressed in relation to nitrogen intake rather than nitrogen truly digested; it is numerically equal to BV multiplied by true digestibility and is likewise determined using two groups of animals, one fed the test protein and the other fed a protein-free diet.

The values obtained with integrative assays are meaningful when determined for whole diets, but are of limited usefulness when applied to individual foods that are components of mixed diets. Values for the protein quality of individual foods are additive only when the limiting amino acid in all the foods happens to be the same. If not, the deficiency of a particular amino acid in one of the foods can be compensated by a relative excess of that amino acid in another; this effect is called complementation. The complementation of cereals, which typically are limiting in lysine, and legumes, which typically are limiting in sulfur amino acids, is an important example.

Amino Acid Scoring. The protein quality of proteins in individual mixtures of foods may be evaluated based on their amino acid com-

position. In order to evaluate proteins on the basis of their amino acid composition, a reference pattern is needed against which to compare them. Block and Mitchell (1946) devised the system of chemical score, in which the concentration of each amino acid in the test protein is expressed as a proportion of the corresponding concentration in the reference pattern. The lowest of these proportions identifies the limiting amino acid and defines the score of the protein, which is usually expressed as a percentage.

When this method of protein evaluation was first devised, Block and Mitchell (1946) used egg protein as the standard, because in assays with rapidly growing rats, chicks, or other animals, egg protein was found to be unsurpassable in quality (i.e., a minimum amount of protein was required to support maximal weight gain). The high quality of egg protein, however, does not mean that its amino acid pattern closely matches the "ideal" pattern; it could contain excesses of many of the essential amino acids relative to the total amino acid requirement. Also, because young, rapidly growing animals utilize most of their amino acid intake for growth, whereas the amino acid requirements of humans (at least after the first 2 months of postnatal life) are dominated by their maintenance needs, egg protein is not necessarily an appropriate reference pattern for humans. Clearly, the pattern of amino acids required for maintenance is profoundly different from that required for tissue protein accretion. As a consequence of one or both of these factors, the egg protein reference pattern is not appropriate for application to human diets and undervalues some proteins used in human nutrition. However, the same scoring principle can be used with reference patterns more appropriate to the needs of the human population being considered, such as those proposed by a joint FAO/WHO/UNU committee (WHO, 1985).

As for animal bioassay values, chemical score values for various food proteins are not additive unless the limiting amino acid is the same for all proteins. However, amino acid contents of individual proteins can be added, and the overall chemical score for the diet can be calculated. This is the only system by

NUTRITION INSIGHT

Chemical Scores and Amino Acid Complementation

The indispensable and conditionally dispensable amino acid composition of two sources of dietary protein are given in the following table, expressed as g amino acid per 100 g protein (i.e., not per amount of food, but as the amino acid pattern in the food protein). Also shown are two amino acid patterns that could be used as reference patterns: the reference pattern for the preschool child (2 to 5 years) suggested by FAO/WHO/UNU (WHO, 1985) and the adult reference pattern used by the National Research Council (1989), which is based on the FAO/WHO/UNU recommendations except for histidine.

	Peanut Butter	White Bread (wheat)	Preschool Child Reference Pattern	Adult Reference Pattern
	g amino acid/100 g protein			
Histidine	3.0	1.8	1.9	1.1
Isoleucine	4.0	3.4	2.8	1.3
Leucine	7.7	6.2	6.6	1.9
Lysine	3.9	1.7	5.8	1.6
Methionine plus cyst(e)ine	2.4	3.6	2.5	1.7
Phenylalanine plus tyrosine	10.8	6.4	6.3	1.9
Threonine	3.0	2.4	3.4	0.9
Tryptophan	1.2	1.0	1.1	0.5
Valine	4.6	3.8	3.5	1.3

Thinking Critically

1. For each of the two food proteins, calculate its amino acid score and determine its limiting amino acid using the preschool reference pattern. Which amino acid is first limiting in each protein? Which of the two proteins has the higher amino acid score?

2. If a mixture of the two protein-containing foods were consumed such that the mixture provided equal amounts of each protein, what would be the amino acid score of the mixture relative to the preschool pattern?

3. What can you say about quality of these two proteins relative to the adult reference pattern?

which information about individual proteins can be used additively to evaluate a mixture.

Chemical score methods do not correct for digestibility of the protein, but digestibility can be determined separately and applied to correct the score; hence, these methods yield values that closely correlate with BV determinations. However, some amino acids in the protein may be more available than others, and this would not be detected with the chemical score method. Another assumption of the chemical score method that is not made in the animal bioassay methods is that excesses of nonlimiting amino acids do not affect the utilization of the protein. This is not entirely true: relative excesses of some amino acids can affect the utilization of others with which they interact in metabolism. In practice, significant effects are likely to be confined to situations where there are gross imbalances among the branched-chain amino acids or between lysine and arginine. Despite these limitations, amino acid pattern is the major factor determining protein quality, and chemical scores and BV have been shown to be closely correlated in animal studies. Although all indispensable amino acids are considered in determination of chemical score, only lysine, methionine + cyst(e)ine, tryptophan, or threonine are normally limiting in the mixed proteins of human diets.

Because most population groups consume a mixture of dietary proteins, the quality of individual proteins is of less concern than the quality of the mixture of proteins present in the total diet. When mixtures of proteins are consumed, complementation occurs such that the amino acid score for the mixture of proteins may be higher than that of any of the individual proteins. Protein quality is most likely to be a concern when a very limited variety of protein sources is consumed and particularly when the major dietary staples contain a small amount of total protein and that protein has a low amino acid score. In these cases, complementation of proteins or supplementation of the diet with a small amount of high-quality protein can be of significant benefit.

ASSESSMENT OF REQUIREMENTS FOR DIETARY PROTEIN OR AMINO ACIDS

There have been essentially four approaches to the assessment of protein and amino acid requirements. The first and simplest is to examine the protein and amino acid contents of diets that are found to be satisfactory in practice. An example is the derivation of infant requirements from the yield and composition of milk by the mothers of normally growing infants.

The second approach is the factorial method, in which the relevant components of the requirement (maintenance, growth, pregnancy, lactation) are estimated separately and summed. Although this approach ostensibly provides a logical system for determination of requirements, the direct estimation of the component requirements is difficult. This approach is normally applied to protein rather than amino acid requirements, because nitrogen losses (mainly as urea) cannot be directly related to the catabolism or loss of specific amino acids.

The third approach is an empirical analysis of dose responses. In experiments of this kind, the response of some important parameter such as growth rate or nitrogen balance is measured at various intakes of protein or amino acid. This approach, using the criterion of nitrogen balance, provided the basis of the

first quantitative estimates of the amino acid needs of human adults, and these remained unchallenged until recently (see Fuller and Garlick, 1994). The current Recommended Dietary Allowances (RDAs) for protein are based on results of nitrogen balance studies for protein (National Research Council, 1989).

The fourth and most recent approach to the assessment of amino acid requirements is based on studies of amino acid kinetics in which isotopically labeled amino acids are used to measure the rate of amino acid disposal. Usually, only disposal by oxidation is considered.

Content in Satisfactory Diets

Requirements for infants are based on intake data because of the difficulty in accurately determining requirements for growth and development. Infant formula or human milk will meet an infant's needs for protein up to 4 months of age if energy needs are met. Average protein intake of breast-fed infants in the United States is about 1.68 g/kg per day. The National Research Council (1989) accepted an average intake of 1.68 g/kg body weight and adjusted it upward by 25% to allow for variation in requirements in establishing the protein RDA for infants (0 to 0.5 y) at 2.2 g/kg. Although this approach results in safe allowances, such diets might include more than enough protein or indispensable amino acids and, hence, are not close estimates of minimum requirements.

Factorial Method

In the factorial approach, the protein needs for each function (maintenance, body protein accretion, and milk protein secretion) are summed. The amino acid requirements of infants shown in Table 12–2 were determined by the factorial method in that the requirements were estimated from infants' maintenance needs and their requirements for growth. These calculations involve assumptions about the efficiency with which dietary protein is utilized both to replace obligatory losses and for body protein accretion. It is important to note that, although, for want of information, a constant efficiency is assumed, variation in the efficiency with which individuals utilize protein or amino acids may be an important source of variation in requirements. To calculate the requirements of a population of children (as opposed to a single child) also requires a factor to account for the variability in mean growth rate.

The basis of adult protein requirements is the need to replace obligatory nitrogen and amino acid losses. There is a remarkable consistency in the minimum urinary nitrogen losses of adults despite a range of ethnic and nutritional backgrounds (Table 12–4). These losses, determined on protein-free diets (or diets very low in protein) typically amount to 36 mg of nitrogen per kg body weight each day. Obligatory nitrogen losses in feces add approximately $10 \text{ mg} \cdot \text{kg}^{-1} \cdot \text{day}^{-1}$ and losses by other routes such as sweat, skin, and hair add up to a further $8 \text{ mg} \cdot \text{kg}^{-1} \cdot \text{day}^{-1}$, giving a total of approximately 54 mg of nitrogen $\cdot \text{kg}^{-1} \cdot \text{day}^{-1}$. If digested protein were used with an efficiency of 100% in replacing these obligatory losses, the daily maintenance requirement of a human adult would be this same amount, equivalent to a daily supply of approximately 340 mg of digestible protein per kg body weight (54 mg N $\times$ 6.25 mg protein/mg N). In reality, much more protein than this is required to replace these losses and to prevent the loss of body protein. From a collation of data from long-term nitrogen balance studies, it appears that approximately

600 mg of digestible protein per kg body weight is required daily, implying that this protein is utilized with an efficiency of only 0.57 (340/600). This additional protein is required partly because obligatory losses are increased and partly because there is increased oxidation as protein and amino acid intakes are increased.

The factorial method can be illustrated with the approach used by the National Research Council (1980) for the ninth edition of the Recommended Dietary Allowances. The daily adult protein allowance was based on an estimate of the average daily obligatory losses of nitrogen [per kg body weight, 37 mg N in urine, 12 mg N in feces, 3 mg N in cutaneous losses, and 2 to 3 mg N losses by other routes (probably low) for a total of 54 mg N per kg body weight], which was converted to its protein equivalent (0.34 g protein/kg body weight), adjusted for variability of requirements in the population by adding 30% (0.34 + 0.11 = 0.45 g protein/kg body weight), adjusted for efficiency of utilization of protein as the maintenance requirement was approached (+30% based on nitrogen balance studies with egg protein; 0.45 + 0.14 = 0.59 g protein/kg body weight), and finally for an assumed average biological value of 75% (0.59/0.75 = 0.79) for a final RDA of 0.79 mg protein per kg body weight.

The different efficiencies with which protein is used at different protein intakes makes estimation of requirements from obligatory nitrogen losses difficult. It is clear that dietary protein is more efficiently used at intakes below the maintenance requirement and less efficiently used at intakes above the maintenance requirement. Furthermore, the efficiency of utilization of protein changes with adaptation to a change in nutritional state and differs among individuals accustomed to different protein intakes. The data in Figure 12–1, for example, show the nitrogen balances of Nigerian students who were given a range of intakes of beef protein in either an ascending or a descending sequence (Atinmo et al., 1988). Results such as these suggest that gradual adaptation to a low intake (descending series) allows more effective conservation of body protein than does gradual adaptation to a high intake (ascending series). The rea-

---

TABLE 12–4
Obligatory Urinary Nitrogen Losses in Adult Males from Various Studies

Source	Age (years)	Weight (kg)	Urinary Nitrogen Loss ($\text{mg} \cdot \text{kg}^{-1} \cdot \text{day}^{-1}$)
USA	20	71	38
USA	21	74	37
Taiwan	23	55	33
India	27	46	38
Nigeria	26	54	34
Japan	*	63	33
Mean			36
SD			2.2

*Unknown.

Data from World Health Organization. (1985) Energy and Protein Requirements. Report of a Joint FAO/WHO/UNU Expert Consultation. WHO Technical Report Series 724. World Health Organization, Geneva.

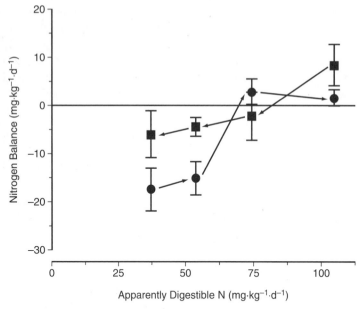

Figure 12–1. *Influence of previous level of protein intake on nitrogen balance. Each diet was given for 10 days and subjects were given the same series of four diets in either an ascending (●) or descending series (■). Mean value with standard deviation. Based on data of Atinmo, T., Mbofung, C. M. F., Egun, G. N. and Osotomehin, B. O. (1988) Nitrogen balance study in young Nigerian male adults using four levels of protein intake. Br J Nutr 60:451–458.*

sons for this are not obvious. It has long been known that protein metabolism adapts to changes in protein intake. On moving from a high to a low intake, there is a fall in urinary nitrogen excretion, reflecting a decreased rate of amino acid oxidation (Fig. 12–2). The change, whether a decrease (as in Figure 12–2) or an increase, is not immediate but takes several days to reach a new steady state. Part of the reason for this is the slow turnover of the urea pool; part is due to the time course of changes in the activities of amino acid degrading enzymes and perhaps also of amino acid transport systems.

Dose-Response Studies—Nitrogen Balance

In nitrogen balance experiments, the rate of body nitrogen retention is estimated as the difference between the dietary nitrogen intake

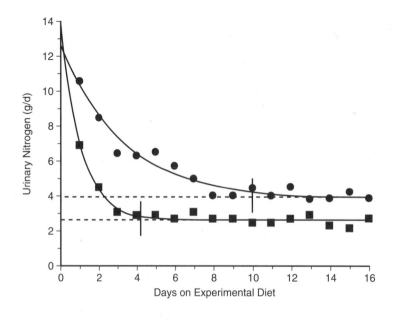

Figure 12–2. *Time course of changes in the urinary nitrogen excretion of two subjects (■; ●) on changing, at day 0, from a high to a low level of protein intake. Based on data of Rand, W. M., Young, V. R. and Scrimshaw, N. S. (1976) Change of urinary nitrogen excretion in response to low-protein diets in adults. Am J Clin Nutr 29:639–644.*

and the sum of the losses in urine and feces and by other routes.

Nitrogen Balance =
Nitrogen Intake − Nitrogen Losses

The first estimates of the amino acid requirements of human adults were made by Rose and his colleagues in a series of nitrogen balance studies in the 1940s. First, young men were given diets devoid of a single amino acid so as to establish which amino acids were dispensable and which were indispensable or dietary essentials. Eight amino acids were determined to be indispensable. (In these studies, removal of histidine from the diet did not lead to a negative nitrogen balance; this was interpreted to mean that histidine was dispensable, and this conclusion was only reversed by longer-term experiments much later.) Rose and his colleagues then conducted a series of quantitative studies in which they gave each subject a succession of diets with different concentrations of the amino acid under investigation. From the changes in nitrogen balance that ensued, they attempted to identify the intake of each amino acid that was required for nitrogen equilibrium to be achieved.

The findings of these experiments were summarized by Rose (1957) and are given in Table 12–5. These pioneering experiments provided valuable information on amino acid requirements but had several limitations. First, they were made with very few subjects, in some instances as few as three. Second, the energy intakes of subjects were excessive, which would tend to minimize amino acid oxidation and so yield lower estimates of apparent requirements than would be obtained if subjects were in both nitrogen and energy equilibrium. Third, many of the diets included D-amino acids, which introduced uncertainties about the extent to which these might have been utilized.

Similar experiments were conducted on young women, but using more subjects and with several improvements in experimental procedures, such as moderate energy intakes and only L-amino acids. The results of these experiments were summarized by Leverton et al. (1959) and they are also given in Table 12–5. The results of these early experiments in determining the amino acid requirements of men and women formed the basis of the current international estimates of adult amino acid requirements (World Health Organization, 1985), which are also shown in Table

TABLE 12–5

Estimates of the Indispensable Amino Acid Requirements for the Maintenance of Nitrogen Equilibrium in Adult Men and Women

	Amino Acid Requirements (mg per day)		
	Rose *(Men)*	*Leverton (Adjusted)* *(Women)*	*FAO/WHO/UNU* *(Adults)*
Threonine	500	305 (942)	455
Valine	800	650 (811)	650
Methionine	165	180 (287)	ND
Methionine + cyst(e)ine	1100	550 (1827)	845
Isoleucine	700	450 (1083)	650
Leucine	1100	620 (1580)	910
Phenylalanine	300	220 (414)	ND
Phenylalanine + tyrosine	1100	ND (ND)	910
Lysine	800	544 (1044)	780
Histidine	*	* *	520–780
Tryptophan	250	157 (222)	228

ND, not detected.
*Histidine was considered dispensable.
Values are from nitrogen balance experiments in men (Rose, 1957) and women (Leverton et al., 1959). Also given in parentheses are the Leverton et al. values in women adjusted to allow for unmeasured losses (Fuller and Garlick, 1994). The current international estimates established by a joint FAO/WHO/UNU committee (WHO, 1985) are also given.

12–5. The FAO/WHO/UNU (World Health Organization, 1985) estimates of amino acid requirements for various age groups were accepted by the National Research Council (1989) for calculations of amino acid requirement patterns, for amino acid scoring of diets, and for the establishment of the RDA for protein.

Nitrogen balance studies in adults were used as the basis for calculating the RDA for protein for the 10th edition of the RDAs (National Research Council, 1989). The average requirement for reference protein (highly digestible, high-quality protein such as egg, meat, milk, or fish) was determined to be 0.6 g/kg per day based on long- and short-term nitrogen balance studies. This value was increased by 25%, based on a coefficient of variation of 12.5%, so that the requirement would cover the needs of 97.5% of a normally distributed population. Based on data from studies in which men were fed habitual mixed diets of ordinary foods, the RDA subcommittee concluded that the adult requirement for absorbed protein did not differ between reference and practical diets (i.e., that the amino acid score of typical American diets is 100 and that digestibility is equal to that of the reference protein). Thus, the RDA was set at 0.75 g protein/kg, close to the 1980 RDA, which was calculated by the factorial method (National Research Council, 1980).

The main problem with estimates based on nitrogen balance experiments is the well-known tendency for the balance technique to overestimate nitrogen retention. The size of the error depends on the exact procedures used. Commonly, and this is true in both the experiments of Rose and of Leverton and associates described above, nitrogen losses other than those in urine and feces are ignored. Additionally, errors from the small amounts of unconsumed food and from small losses of urine or feces both tend to exaggerate retention. This means that a subject apparently receiving sufficient amino acid (or protein) to maintain nitrogen equilibrium is actually in negative nitrogen balance and needs more of the amino acid (or protein) to maintain true nitrogen equilibrium. The over-

Food Sources of Protein

• Meat
• Dairy products
• Cereals and legumes

RDAs Across the Life Cycle

	g per day
Infants, 0–0.5 y	13
0.5–1.0 yr	14
Children, 1–3 yr	16
4–6 yr	24
7–10 yr	28
Males, 11–14 yr	45
15–18 yr	59
19–24 yr	58
25+ yr	63
Females, 11–14 yr	46
15–18 yr	44
19–24 yr	46
25+ yr	50
Pregnant	60
Lactating	62–65

From National Research Council. (1989) Recommended Dietary Allowances, 10th ed. National Academy Press, Washington, D. C.

estimation of nitrogen retention in the experiments of Rose and coworkers and of Leverton et al. (1959) was probably around 300 mg N/day; recalculating the estimates to correct for this overestimation gives substantially higher estimates for the amino acid requirements. Recalculated values for the amino acid requirements of women are shown in Table 12–5.

A further problem with the nitrogen balance approach, especially in short-term studies, may arise through the implicit assumption that a subject in nitrogen equilibrium must also be in amino acid equilibrium. This is not necessarily so. Histidine, for example, is stored in the form of the peptide carnosine (β-alanyl-histidine). Carnosine, in experimental animals at least, is depleted during dietary histidine deficiency. This allows obligatory losses of histidine to be met, for a time, without loss of body protein, despite an inadequate histidine intake. There may also be a potential to adapt to an indispensable amino acid deficiency through modification of the amino acid composition of the body protein pool as a whole. Of course, it is not possible to modify the amino acid composition of any of the body's proteins, but it is possible to vary the relative amounts of the various proteins. Because proteins have different amino acid compositions, there is the potential to adapt, at least temporarily, to a deficiency of one amino acid by depleting the body of proteins rich in that amino acid. This also happens in histidine deficiency when hemoglobin, which is very rich in histidine, is gradually depleted. The mechanism of this adaptation is not known. This ability of the body to use endogenous sources of histidine explains why histidine was not identified as an indispensable amino acid in the early balance studies.

It is also important to note that most estimates of amino acid requirements have been made using purified diets with free amino acids. The use of diets based on natural foods may lead to higher estimates of requirements because the amino acids may be incompletely digested.

Oxidation of Isotopically Labeled Amino Acids

The availability of isotopically labeled amino acids has opened up the possibility of making direct measurements of the rate of amino acid disposal. For human studies, stable isotopes—^{13}C, ^{15}N, and ^{2}H (deuterium)—are preferred to radioactive isotopes. Particularly for the measurement of amino acid oxidation, it is important that the amino acid be labeled in such a way that, when it is catabolized, the label is completely and exclusively transferred to the measured end product. This means, for example, that uniformly labeled [^{13}C]amino acids are unsuitable because, when the amino acid is catabolized, much of the label may be sequestered via synthetic pathways (dispensable amino acids, fatty acids, glucose), rather than appearing in expired CO_2. Conversely, [1-^{13}C]leucine is a good choice because the carboxyl carbon is lost during the initial step of catabolism of the branched-chain keto acid.

Measurements of amino acid oxidation can be used in one of two ways. In the first, called the breakpoint method, amino acid oxidation is measured over a range of intakes to establish the intake above which there is a steep increase in the rate at which the amino acid is oxidized. The approach is based on the principle that, when intakes are below the requirement, amino acids are conserved and oxidation remains at a low level, whereas when amino acid intakes are greater than the requirement, the excesses are disposed of by oxidation. When the results of these measurements are plotted, a distinct break point is seen and the amino acid intake associated with the break point is an approximation of the amino acid requirement. This approach is analogous to the empirical dose-response approach, but uses amino acid oxidation rather than growth or nitrogen balance as the criterion of adequacy.

The second approach, called the amino acid balance method, is to use isotopically labeled amino acids to estimate amino acid oxidation at various rates of amino acid intake and thereby estimate the intake required to achieve amino acid equilibrium. Because oxidation is not the only route of amino acid loss, true rates of amino acid balance may be overestimated, leading to an underestimate of requirements. Estimates of minimal rates of amino acid oxidation are shown in Table 12–1. By comparison of these values with the estimates of amino acid requirements shown in Table 12–5 (after converting to similar units; assume ~70 kg body weight for an adult), it is clear that the present estimates based on oxidation studies suggest that amino acid requirements are higher than those that have been determined by nitrogen balance studies.

FACTORS THAT AFFECT AMINO ACID REQUIREMENTS

Protein and amino acid requirements of healthy individuals are affected by several important factors, some intrinsic (mainly genetic), others extrinsic, of which the most important are dietary.

Dietary Energy

Perhaps the most important dietary factor affecting protein utilization is dietary nonprotein energy; that is, carbohydrate and fat. When amino acids are oxidized as a fuel, most of their carbon enters the citric acid cycle and other central pathways of fuel metabolism via pyruvate, oxaloacetate, α-ketoglutarate, or acetyl CoA (see Chapter 11, Fig. 11–9). This ability of amino acids to substitute for other energy sources is important, for example, in starvation, when body protein is depleted to provide amino acids both as precursors for important synthetic pathways and as a source of glucose and other energy-yield-ing substrates. It follows that, when energy is available in other forms, either from body glycogen and fat or from dietary carbohydrate and fat, the need for net breakdown of body protein with oxidation of amino acids is diminished.

Dietary energy, in the form of carbohydrate or fat, has a profound effect on protein utilization in both the growing and the adult states. With generous intakes of nonprotein energy, in excess of immediate energy needs, amino acid oxidation is minimized and amino acids are utilized with maximal efficiency. This is called the protein-sparing effect of dietary carbohydrate and fat. In adults, the effect is typically to spare 2 mg of nitrogen for each kcal added to a nutritionally adequate basal diet, which is associated with an increase in lean body mass that accompanies the deposition of body fat. In growing animals, the magnitude of the effect is similar or rather greater and diminishes as the highest levels of energy intake are approached. The effect is that apparent amino acid requirements, for maintenance in adults and for normal growth in the immature, are minimized. Conversely, when carbohydrate and fat intakes are limited, amino acid oxidation rises and apparent requirements are increased. This means that amino acid requirements cannot be stated without reference to the provision of other nutrients. Deficiencies of many other nutrients, such as vitamins and minerals, limit the utilization of dietary protein. In all published

NUTRITION INSIGHT

Protein Requirement as a Percentage of Calories

Based on the RDAs for protein (e.g., 63 g per day for an adult male) and estimated energy allowances (e.g., 2900 kcal per day for an adult male), one can calculate that approximately 8% to 9% of total food calories needs to be supplied as protein in order for a diet to meet the protein needs of adult humans. Some major tropical foods such as cassava, plantain, and yam (*Dioscorea* species) have a low protein content relative to their total caloric yield (2% to 5% of calories as protein) and thus are inadequate as the only or major dietary source of protein for a population; they would be inadequate even if the protein in these vegetables had as high a biological value as typical animal proteins. In contrast, rice supplies about 8% of total calories as protein, and lean fish supplies 93% of its caloric value in the form of high-quality protein. More than 12% of the caloric intake of individuals consuming typical American diets is in the form of protein; thus, the RDA for protein is easily met or exceeded in typical American diets.

estimates of requirements, it is assumed that other nutrients are also provided at the appropriate level.

Possible Contribution of Microbial Synthesis of Amino Acids

It is normally assumed that the indispensable amino acids can only be derived from the diet. However, this may not be entirely true. From the evidence of both human and animal studies, it now seems likely that some amino acids synthesized by gastrointestinal microorganisms may be absorbed, augmenting the dietary supply. It has not been established whether this route makes a significant contribution to meeting human requirements, but the available evidence suggests that it may.

As pointed out earlier, the gut is also a route of amino acid loss through the unrecovered endogenous secretions. How this balance of gains and losses comes out in practice has yet to be established, but it is very likely to depend on factors such as the amount of fermentable carbohydrate in the diet, which affects microbial growth in the intestine. If it turns out to be true that there can be a net gain of amino acids from the gastrointestinal flora, the amount of an amino acid required in the diet may be less than the amount utilized in the body, the difference being supplied by microbial synthesis. How big this difference might be has yet to be established, but it could explain why estimates of amino acid requirements based on amino acid intake are lower than those derived from measurements of metabolic disposal.

Criterion of Adequacy

As we have seen, amino acid requirements may be derived in a number of different ways. It is perhaps not surprising that these should yield rather different estimates. However, most have been based on some measure of body protein status. In considering maintenance requirements, for example, it has been assumed that the requirement is that amount needed to preserve the total protein or amino acid content of the body. This may be too limited a definition as a basis of dietary recommendations. We need to ask if there are aspects of

health and well-being that benefit from greater amounts than are needed simply to maintain protein homeostasis. There is some evidence for this. For example, higher tryptophan intakes are associated with greater synthesis of nicotinamide-adenine dinucleotide (NAD), and higher sulfur amino acid intakes are associated with greater synthesis of glutathione and taurine. The relation of dietary supply to optimal production or tissue concentrations of these nonprotein metabolites is not considered by current methods used for establishing amino acid and protein requirements and allowances. Also, it is possible that intakes of specific dispensable amino acids affect metabolic state and health. For example, arginine supplements have been shown to enhance aspects of immune function and to have beneficial effects on wound healing, possibly due to its roles in the formation of nitric oxide and polyamines. Likewise, glutamine, another amino acid normally considered dispensable, may improve recovery from injury or disease. This may relate to the fact that glutamine is a major fuel for rapidly proliferating cells, including lymphocytes. There is, however, little reliable evidence on the long-term effects of different habitual protein intakes on mortality, morbidity, or longevity.

Benefits of Intact Dietary Proteins and Peptides

Although dietary requirements for protein are correctly viewed as requirements for the amino acids contained in the proteins, there are some examples of intact peptides or even proteins that are of nutritional significance, such as the immunoglobulins and lactoferrin passed to the infant in its mother's milk. Other bioactive proteins, such as retinol-binding protein, transforming growth factor, and epidermal growth factor, may also be derived from maternal milk. It is also possible, as discussed by Reeds and Hutchens (1994), that certain peptides resulting from the incomplete hydrolysis of dietary proteins may sufficiently resemble bioactive peptides as to mimic their function in the body. Proteins in the diet also include antigens, toxins, and other proteins with antinutritional effects such as the trypsin inhibitors in a number of legumes. Some of these have their effects in the gut lumen; others are absorbed. All these can be important in determining to what extent protein nutriture may amount to more than simply the provision of amino acids and nitrogen.

REFERENCES

Atinmo, T., Mbofung, C. M. F., Egun, G. N. and Osotomehin, B. O. (1988) Nitrogen balance study in young Nigerian male adults using four levels of protein intake. Br J Nutr 60:451–458.

Block, R. J. and Mitchell, H. H. (1946) The correlation of the amino-acid composition of proteins with their nutritive value. Nutr Abstr Rev 16:249–278.

Davis, T. A., Nguyen, H. V., Garcia-Bravo, R., Fiorotto, M. L., Jackson, E. M. and Reeds, P. J. (1994) Amino acid composition of the milk of some mammalian species changes with stage of lactation. Br J Nutr 72:845–853.

Fuller, M. F. and Garlick, P. J. (1994) Human amino acid requirements: Can the controversy be resolved? Annu Rev Nutr 14:217–241.

Fuller, M. F., Milne, A., Harris, C. I., Reid, T. M. S. and Keenan, R. (1994) Amino acid losses in ileostomy fluid on a protein-free diet. Am J Clin Nutr 59:70–73.

Leverton, R. M., Waddill, F. S. and Skellenger, M. (1959) The urinary excretion of five essential amino acids by young women. J Nutr 67:19–28.

Jackson, A. A., Shaw, J. C. L., Barber, A. and Golden, M. H. N. (1981) Nitrogen metabolism in preterm infants fed human donor breast milk: The possible essentiality of glycine. Pediatr Res 15:1454–1461.

National Research Council. (1980) Recommended Dietary Allowances, 9th ed. National Academy Press, Washington, D.C.

National Research Council. (1989) Recommended Dietary Allowances, 10th ed. National Academy Press, Washington, D.C.

Rand, W. M., Young, V. R. and Scrimshaw, N. S. (1976) Change of urinary nitrogen excretion in response to low-protein diets in adults. Am J Clin Nutr 29:639–644.

Reeds, P. J. and Hutchens, T. W. (1994) Protein requirements: From nitrogen balance to functional impact. J Nutr 124:1754S–1764S.

Rose, W. C. (1957) The amino acid requirements of adult man. Nutr Abstr Rev 27:631–647.

Smith, R. H. (1980) Comparative amino acid requirements. Proc Nutr Soc 39:71–78.

World Health Organization. (1985) Energy and Protein Requirements. Report of a Joint FAO/WHO/UNU Expert Consultation. WHO Technical Report Series 724. World Health Organization, Geneva.

RECOMMENDED READINGS

Fuller, M. F. and Garlick, P. J. (1994) Human amino acid requirements: Can the controversy be resolved? Annu Rev Nutr 14:217–241.

Millward, D. J., Jackson, A. A., Price, G. and Rivers, J. P. W. (1989) Human amino acid and protein requirements: Current dilemmas and uncertainties. Nutr Res Rev 2:109–132.

Waterlow, J. C. (1996) The requirements of adult man for indispensable amino acids. Eur J Clin Nutr 50:S151–S179.

CHAPTER 13

Lipid Metabolism—Synthesis and Oxidation

Alan G. Goodridge, Ph.D., and Hei Sook Sul, Ph.D.

OUTLINE

BIOLOGICAL ROLES FOR LIPIDS

There are four major and a multitude of minor roles for lipids in living organisms. Major roles include serving as an energy source or fuel, as structural components of membranes, as lubricants, especially of the body surfaces, and as signaling molecules. These four major functions require specific classes of lipids that differ in general structure. Each class contains numerous members with small but substantive structural differences. These lipid structures and their functions are discussed in Chapter 3.

Lipids in the form of triacylglycerol play a critical role in metabolism as the primary form of stored energy in the mammalian body. About 85% of the energy stored in the body of a 70-kg normal-weight man is in the form of triacylglycerol, primarily stored in adipose tissue. Triacylglycerol in the diet provides a concentrated source of energy. Triacylglycerol in milk is important for supplying calories to the newborn infant. When the caloric content of the diet exceeds the immediate energetic requirements of the individual, carbohydrates (and to some extent amino acids) may be converted to fatty acids and esterified to glycerol to form triacylglycerol. Triacylglycerol is a very efficient chemical form for storing energy because it contains about 9 kcal/g as opposed to about 4 kcal/g for carbohydrate and protein. In addition, triacylglycerol is advantageous because it can be stored in a relatively anhydrous form requiring about 1 g of water per gram of fat, whereas carbohydrate and protein require about 4 g of water per gram of glycogen or protein. Conversion of carbohydrate and protein to triacylglycerol is regulated by diet; it is high in the fed state, especially if the diet is rich in carbohydrate, and it is low in the fasting state. Storage of triacylglycerol also is high in the fed state and low in the fasting state, regardless of the composition of the diet.

The principal structural role of lipids is in the membranes—both the plasma membrane and subcellular membranes. A lipid bilayer constitutes the external boundary of every mammalian cell. Similarly, lipid membranes form the boundaries of numerous subcellular organelles. The principal components of the lipid bilayer are phospholipids, sphingolipids, and cholesterol, whose proportions vary with the membrane type.

Lipids also play an important role in lubrication and conditioning of body surfaces. Most sebaceous glands, which are microscopic in size, are found in skin and the mucous membranes of external orifices of the mammalian body, and they secrete a lipid product composed of triacylglycerol, squalene, and wax esters. This secretion lubricates mucous membranes and conditions skin and hair. Some larger glands are modified sebaceous glands with specific functions. The meibomian glands in the eyelids, for example, provide lubricant and protection for the surface of the eye.

Lipids are important signaling molecules, both outside and inside cells. Sex hormones, adrenocortical hormones, and vitamin D are derived from cholesterol and play important extracellular signaling roles. Eicosanoids derived from arachidonic acid, and platelet-activating factor, which is a phospholipid-like compound, are also important in extracellular signaling. Inside cells, diacylglycerol and molecules derived from phospholipids and sphingolipids are involved in the transmission of signals from the plasma membrane to enzymes in the cytosol or other subcellular compartments and to proteins that regulate the expression of specific genes in the nucleus.

SYNTHESIS OF LONG-CHAIN FATTY ACIDS FROM ACETYL CoA

The primary anatomic sites for synthesis of fatty acids are the liver and adipose tissue. In humans, the extent and the contribution of each of these tissues to de novo lipogenesis are still debated (Hellerstein et al., 1996). The lipogenic pathway may be suppressed by the high fat content of the modern diet (~40% of total energy). Thus, in most individuals consuming typical Western diets, de novo lipogenesis may not contribute significantly to triacylglycerol biosynthesis. However, low but regulated rates of lipogenesis still may be critical for overall control of fatty acid metabolism in humans. As discussed later, malonyl CoA, the product of the acetyl CoA carboxylase reaction, inhibits fatty acid oxidation. In addition, in some physiological and pathophysiological conditions, de novo lipogenesis may play a quantitatively significant role. For example, developmental needs for lipid in the fetus may be met by de novo lipogenesis, and its rate is extremely high in premature infants. De novo lipogenesis also contributes significantly to the hypertriglyceridemia of alcoholic liver diseases. Some of the metabolic abnormalities in untreated type 1 diabetes mellitus arise from the impaired fatty acid synthesis caused by low insulin levels.

Another calorically important site of fat synthesis is the lactating mammary gland in which medium-chain fatty acids are synthesized and esterified to glycerol for milk fat. Branched-chain fatty acids for conditioning body surfaces are synthesized in sebaceous and other more specialized glands.

Transfer of Acetyl CoA from Inside the Mitochondria to the Cytosol

The enzymes that catalyze the reactions for fatty acid synthesis are cytosolic. This localization is important because it separates processes of fatty acid synthesis and fatty acid oxidation (mitochondrial). Although the enzymes that catalyze the reactions in these two pathways are different, the substrate of one pathway is the product of the other and vice versa. Because the reactions are in different compartments, the strategy for regulating these competing processes is different from that used in gluconeogenesis and glycolysis in which most of the competing reactions are in the same compartment. Thus, fatty acid synthesis is regulated by both phosphorylation and allosteric control of the key regulatory enzyme of fatty acid synthesis, acetyl CoA carboxylase, whereas fatty acid oxidation is regulated primarily by the rate of uptake of substrate by the mitochondria.

The substrate for fatty acid synthesis, acetyl CoA, is formed from pyruvate in the mitochondria. The inner mitochondrial membrane is impermeable to acetyl CoA and does not contain a carrier to transport the acetyl CoA into the cytosol. When production of acetyl CoA from pyruvate is high, the rate of formation of citrate catalyzed by citrate synthase in

the citric acid cycle also is elevated, resulting in the accumulation of intramitochondrial citrate. Under these conditions, citrate can be translocated to the cytosol in exchange for a dicarboxylate anion, probably malate, by the tricarboxylate anion carrier in the inner mitochondrial membrane (Fig. 13–1). Citrate, therefore, serves as the intermediary for the transfer of acetyl CoA from mitochondria to cytosol. As described later in this chapter, citrate as a feed-forward activator of acetyl CoA carboxylase plays a key role in regulating fatty acid synthesis. In the cytosol, therefore, fatty acid synthesis actually starts by cleavage of citrate back to acetyl CoA.

Cytosolic citrate is cleaved to acetyl CoA and oxaloacetate in a reaction catalyzed by ATP-citrate lyase:

$$Citrate + CoA + ATP + H_2O \rightarrow$$
$$Acetyl\ CoA + Oxaloacetate + ADP + P_i$$

Oxaloacetate formed in the cytosol cannot be returned to the mitochondria because the mitochondrial membrane lacks the necessary transporter. Oxaloacetate can be reduced to malate by cytosolic malate dehydrogenase.

$$Oxaloacetate + NADH + H^+ \leftrightarrow Malate + NAD^+$$

Malate can be returned to mitochondria on a tricarboxylate anion carrier in exchange for another molecule of citrate. Malate can then be converted back to oxaloacetate by mitochondrial malate dehydrogenase. This cycle results in the net transport of acetyl CoA at an energetic cost of 1 mol of ATP per mole of acetyl CoA translocated. In addition, it results in transfer of NADH formed in the cytosol to the mitochondria, where it can contribute to the generation of ATP via oxidative phosphorylation.

Alternatively, or perhaps in addition, malate generated by reduction of oxaloacetate in the cytosol can, in turn, be oxidized to pyruvate and carbon dioxide (malic enzyme). The pyruvate can then be returned to the mitochondria. Oxidation of malate to pyruvate by the malic enzyme requires NADP as the hydrogen acceptor and generates NADPH. As discussed later, NADPH is the required donor

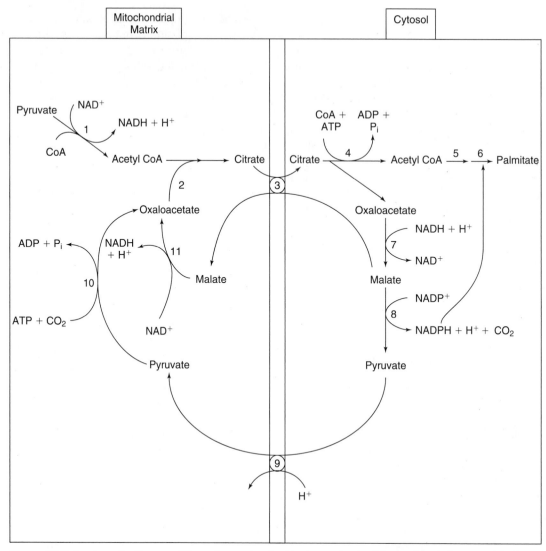

Figure 13–1. *A schematic diagram of the pathways involved in the synthesis of fatty acids. 1, Pyruvate dehydrogenase; 2, citrate synthase; 3, tricarboxylate transporter; 4, ATP-citrate lyase; 5, acetyl CoA carboxylase; 6, fatty acid synthase; 7, malate dehydrogenase; 8, malic enzyme; 9, pyruvate transporter; 10, pyruvate carboxylase; 11, malate dehydrogenase.*

for the reductive step in fatty acid biosynthesis. This longer cycle is then completed in the mitochondria by the ATP-dependent carboxylation of pyruvate to form oxaloacetate (pyruvate carboxylase). The malic enzyme cycle thus translocates 1 mol of acetyl CoA and generates 1 mol of NADPH per 2 mol of ATP expended. By this pathway, reducing equivalents from cytosolic NADH are transferred to NADP so that the resulting NADPH is used for fatty acid synthesis along with NADPH produced by the pentose phosphate pathway.

Conversion of Acetyl CoA to Malonyl CoA

The next reaction in the synthesis of fatty acids is catalyzed by acetyl CoA carboxylase and involves an ATP-dependent carboxylation of acetyl CoA to malonyl CoA (see Fig. 22–8 in Chapter 22). This is the first committed step in fatty acid synthesis and is highly regulated. Like pyruvate carboxylase, acetyl CoA carboxylase utilizes bicarbonate as a source of carbon dioxide, has a two-step reaction mechanism, and requires a covalently bound biotin.

$$HCO_3^- + ATP + \text{Biotin-Enzyme} \rightarrow$$
$$\text{Carboxybiotin-Enzyme} + ADP + P_i$$

$$\text{Carboxybiotin-Enzyme} + \text{Acetyl CoA} \rightarrow$$
$$\text{Malonyl CoA} + \text{Biotin-Enzyme}$$

$$\text{NET: Acetyl CoA} + HCO_3^- + ATP \rightarrow$$
$$\text{Malonyl CoA} + ADP + P_i$$

In the first step, the biotin, which is bound to a specific lysyl residue of the enzyme, is carboxylated with the energy furnished by the hydrolysis of ATP (biotin carboxylation). In the second step (transcarboxylation), the activated, biotin-bound carboxyl group is transferred to acetyl CoA, regenerating enzyme-bound biotin and synthesizing malonyl CoA. Both of these reactions are catalyzed by a single polypeptide chain that also contains a domain for the covalently linked biotin. In biotin deficiency, the acetyl CoA carboxylase reaction is impaired, and thus fatty acid synthesis from acetyl CoA is decreased. (See Chapter 22 for more discussion of biotin-dependent carboxylation.)

Acetyl CoA carboxylase is regulated by an array of control mechanisms, permitting the rate of fatty acid synthesis to fluctuate in response to physiological and developmental conditions (Hillgartner et al., 1995). The activity of acetyl CoA carboxylase is stimulated by the allosteric activator citrate and inhibited by an allosteric inhibitor, long-chain acyl CoA. Production of cytosolic citrate is increased under conditions favoring fatty acid synthesis. The level of long-chain acyl CoAs increases during starvation when fatty acid synthesis is inhibited, and conversely, the long-chain acyl CoA level decreases in the fed state when fatty acid synthesis is stimulated. These allosteric mechanisms thus represent examples of feed-forward and feedback regulation.

Acetyl CoA carboxylase also is regulated by covalent modification. Each molecule of enzyme contains up to seven seryl residues that can be phosphorylated. The phosphorylated enzyme is less active, less sensitive to the stimulatory effects of citrate, and more sensitive to the inhibitory action of long-chain acyl CoA. A number of different protein kinases catalyze phosphorylation of acetyl CoA carboxylase and do so at different specific seryl residues on the enzyme. As a conse-

quence, the enzyme is regulated by a number of different extracellular signals. In liver, glucagon is an important effector increasing production of cAMP, which, in turn, activates protein kinase A. Unlike the situation for other enzymes regulated by glucagon, the signaling pathway appears to be indirect. Protein kinase A phosphorylates and activates an AMP-dependent protein kinase, which in turn phosphorylates acetyl CoA carboxylase and regulates its activity (Fig. 13–2).

In addition to regulation by allosteric and phosphorylation-dephosphorylation mechanisms, acetyl CoA carboxylase also is regulated by the changes in the number of molecules present in the cell. The concentration of the enzyme is high in the liver of fed animals, especially if the diet is high in carbohydrate, and low in the liver of starved animals. Changes in acetyl CoA carboxylase protein concentration in cells are controlled primarily by changes in the rate of transcription of the acetyl CoA carboxylase gene. Changes in circulating insulin and glucagon, as well as glucose levels during the fasting and fed states, participate in regulating acetyl CoA carboxylase gene transcription: insulin and glucose increase and cAMP decreases the rate of transcription.

Synthesis of Palmitate from Malonyl CoA, Acetyl CoA, and NADPH by Fatty Acid Synthase

The second and final committed step in fatty acid synthesis is catalyzed by a multifunctional polypeptide, fatty acid synthase. The substrates for this reaction are 7 molecules of malonyl CoA, 1 of acetyl CoA, 14 of NADPH, and 14 of H^+. The products are 1 molecule of palmitate (C16), 8 of CoA, 7 of CO_2, 14 of $NADP^+$, and 6 of H_2O. The reaction is complex in two ways. First, the fatty acid is built up by the serial addition of 2-carbon fragments to a growing chain. Second, after each addition, the added carbons are reduced, dehydrated, and reduced again. The process then repeats itself—condensation, reduction, dehydration, reduction—until a 16-carbon fatty acid has been formed and is released from the enzyme (Fig. 13–3).

The first step in this complicated process

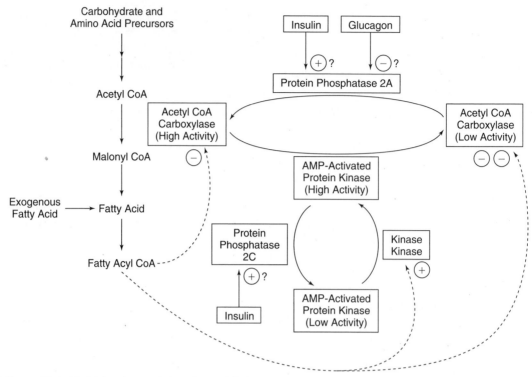

Figure 13–2. *Model for the regulation of acetyl CoA carboxylase. Acetyl CoA carboxylase is phosphorylated and converted to a less active form by AMP-activated protein kinase. The latter enzyme is phosphorylated and activated by a kinase kinase. Arrows with dotted lines indicate either positive (+) or negative (−) allosteric effects of fatty acyl CoA on the specified enzyme. Extent of allosteric inhibition is indicated by the number of (−) symbols. The phosphatases that inactivate AMP-activated protein kinase or activate glucagon inhibition of this step have not been demonstrated definitively.*

involves an acyl transferase activity that transfers the acetyl moiety of acetyl CoA to a seryl residue in the acyltransferase domain of the enzyme. The acetyl group is then transferred from the seryl residue in the acyltransferase domain to the 4′-phosphopantetheine if the sulfhydryl of the covalently linked 4′-phosphopantetheine group in the acyl carrier protein domain of the enzyme is free. The 4′-phosphopantetheine group of the acyl carrier protein domain of fatty acid synthase is described in Chapter 22. The β-ketoacyl synthase (the "condensing enzyme") activity of fatty acid synthase then catalyzes transfer of the acetyl group to a cysteinyl residue at the active site of the condensation reaction. The seryl residue in the acyl transferase domain is now free to accept a malonyl group. The malonyl group is then transferred to the sulfhydryl group of the phosphopantetheine side arm (see Fig. 13–3), which has been freed of its acetyl

group, and the enzyme is poised to carry out the first condensation reaction.

During the condensation reaction, the methylene carbon of the malonyl-phosphopantetheine form of the enzyme attacks the carbonyl group of the acetyl moiety in the active site of the β-ketoacyl transferase, forming the acetoacetyl-phosphopantetheine form of the enzyme and releasing the carboxyl group at carbon 2 of the malonyl moiety as CO_2. The energy for this reaction is provided by coupling condensation of the acetyl and malonyl groups with decarboxylation. A condensation that started with two acetyl CoAs would be energetically unfavorable. As a result, the energy for this reaction really comes from the hydrolysis of ATP during the carboxylation of acetyl CoA to form malonyl CoA; malonyl CoA is thus an activated form of acetyl CoA. The carboxyl group added by acetyl CoA carboxylase is the same one that is removed during the condensation reaction. Even though bicarbonate is a required substrate for the fatty acid synthesis pathway, net incorporation of bicarbonate into the fatty acid does not occur.

The phosphopantetheine side arm in the acyl carrier protein domain of fatty acid synthase is long and flexible, so that its attached acetoacetyl group can interact sequentially with the active sites of the β-ketoacyl reductase, β-hydroxyacyl dehydratase, and enoyl reductase domains to form a four-carbon saturated fatty acyl group. At the end of this reaction sequence, the butyryl moiety is still attached to the phosphopantetheinyl moiety, but it is then transferred to a cysteinyl residue in the active site of the β-ketoacyl synthase domain. This leaves the sulfhydryl of the phosphopantetheinyl moiety free to receive a new malonyl CoA moiety from the seryl residue in the acyltransferase domain. The next cycle of condensation, reduction, dehydration, and reduction then forms a six-carbon saturated fatty-acyl group (hexanoyl) attached to the phosphopantetheine side arm. The hexanoyl group is transferred to the active site cysteinyl residue of the β-ketoacyl synthase domain, and another malonyl group is condensed, reduced, dehydrated and reduced. After 7 cycles, the growing acyl chain reaches 16 carbons, and a thioesterase activity in the thioesterase domain of fatty acid synthase cleaves the free fatty acid from the enzyme (see Fig. 13–3).

All the reactions required for fatty acid synthesis from acetyl CoA and malonyl CoA are catalyzed by a single polypeptide that contains all the activities in separate domains. Therefore, the multifunctional fatty acid synthase can provide a greater efficiency by channeling intermediates from one active site to the next rather than relying on diffusion of intermediates between separate enzymes. In addition, the relative amounts of each enzyme can be regulated simultaneously by controlling expression of a single gene. Mammalian fatty acid synthase is synthesized as an inactive monomer of about 270 kDa. The active enzyme is a homodimer. The dimer is assembled with the head of one monomer bound to the tail of the other, resulting in the formation of two catalytic centers in each homodimer. Each catalytic center has components from each monomer (Fig. 13–4).

The activity of fatty acid synthase, similar to that of acetyl CoA carboxylase and other enzymes involved in fatty acid synthesis, such as ATP-citrate lyase, malic enzyme, and some of the enzymes in the pentose phosphate pathway, is high in the fed state (especially if the diet is high in carbohydrate) and low in the fasting state. Fat, especially polyunsaturated fatty acids in the diet, decreases fatty acid synthase activity. Neither allosteric nor phosphorylation-dephosphorylation mechanisms appear to contribute to these changes in fatty acid synthase activity. Regulation is at the level of protein concentration, and both transcriptional and posttranscriptional mechanisms are involved.

SYNTHESIS OF FATTY ACIDS OTHER THAN PALMITATE

The product of the reaction catalyzed by fatty acid synthase is exclusively palmitate, a 16-carbon saturated fatty acid. However, fatty acids with chain lengths of 18 or more carbons, in both saturated and unsaturated forms, are abundant in animal tissues. For example, more than 50% of the human adipose tissue triacylglycerol contains fatty acids of 18 carbons in length. Acyl chain length and the degree of saturation can influence membrane function, and polyunsaturated long-chain fatty acids serve as precursors for biologically active signaling molecules such as eicosanoids. Therefore, although a variety of fatty acids are provided by the diet, the capacity to modify and elongate fatty acid chains prior to esterification is required to maintain specific fatty acid composition in cells. Many specialized organs, such as mammary and sebaceous glands, synthesize fatty acids with shorter acyl chains and branched acyl chains. The de novo synthesis of these fatty acids requires separate enzymes and enzyme systems.

Elongation of Fatty Acids

Fatty acids can be elongated in 2-carbon steps. There are two systems for elongating

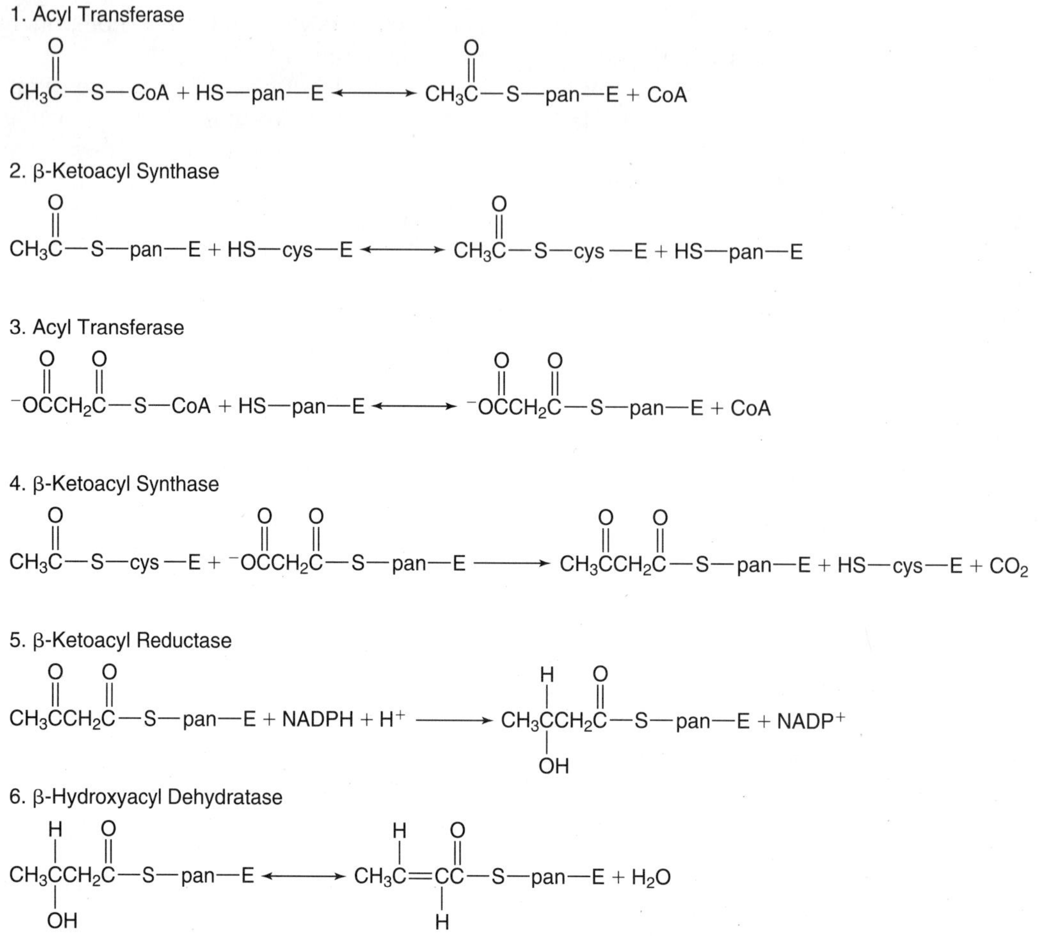

1. Acyl Transferase

$$CH_3C(=O){-}S{-}CoA + HS{-}pan{-}E \longleftrightarrow CH_3C(=O){-}S{-}pan{-}E + CoA$$

2. β-Ketoacyl Synthase

$$CH_3C(=O){-}S{-}pan{-}E + HS{-}cys{-}E \longleftrightarrow CH_3C(=O){-}S{-}cys{-}E + HS{-}pan{-}E$$

3. Acyl Transferase

$$^-OCCH_2C(=O){-}S{-}CoA + HS{-}pan{-}E \longleftrightarrow {}^-OCCH_2C(=O){-}S{-}pan{-}E + CoA$$

4. β-Ketoacyl Synthase

$$CH_3C(=O){-}S{-}cys{-}E + {}^-OCCH_2C(=O){-}S{-}pan{-}E \longrightarrow CH_3CCH_2C(=O){-}S{-}pan{-}E + HS{-}cys{-}E + CO_2$$

5. β-Ketoacyl Reductase

$$CH_3CCH_2C(=O){-}S{-}pan{-}E + NADPH + H^+ \longrightarrow CH_3C(H)(OH)CH_2C(=O){-}S{-}pan{-}E + NADP^+$$

6. β-Hydroxyacyl Dehydratase

$$CH_3C(H)(OH)CH_2C(=O){-}S{-}pan{-}E \longleftrightarrow CH_3C(H){=}C(H)C(=O){-}S{-}pan{-}E + H_2O$$

Figure 13–3. *The component reactions of fatty acid synthase. The abbreviations HS–cys–E and HS–pan–E indicate an enzyme-bound cysteinyl residue and an enzyme-bound 4′-phosphopantetheine group, respectively.*

(Continued on next page)

fatty acids, one in the endoplasmic reticulum (ER) and the other in mitochondria. Although neither system is well characterized, the ER system is more active and better understood and uses both saturated and unsaturated fatty acyl CoAs as substrates. The individual reactions are analogous to those catalyzed by fatty acid synthase, except that only long-chain acyl CoAs are used as primers, and different gene products catalyze the individual reactions. The sequence of reactions is condensation, reduction, dehydration, and reduction. Malonyl CoA is the elongating group, and NADPH is the electron donor (see Fig.13–3). The mitochondrial system appears to utilize acetyl CoA as the elongating unit and NADH or NADH plus NADPH as electron donors. The mitochondrial elongation system is not a simple reversal of fatty acid oxidation involving two-

carbon units (β-oxidation) because flavoenzymes are not involved in catalysis for either the first or second reduction in each cycle.

Desaturation of Fatty Acids

Monounsaturated fatty acids are formed by direct oxidative desaturation of preformed long-chain saturated fatty acids in reactions catalyzed by a complex of enzymes located in the ER. The first double bond introduced into a saturated acyl chain is generally in the Δ9 position. The Δ9 desaturase complex (also called stearoyl CoA desaturase) uses saturated fatty acids with 14- to 18-carbons; stearate is the most active. This complex, sometimes called a "mixed function oxidase," utilizes two electrons and two protons donated by NADH ($+H^+$) and two electrons and two protons

7. Enoyl Reductase

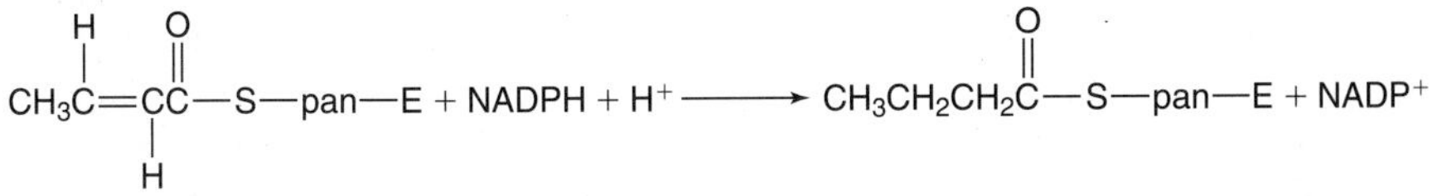

$$CH_3C=CC-S-pan-E + NADPH + H^+ \longrightarrow CH_3CH_2CH_2C-S-pan-E + NADP^+$$

8. β-Ketoacyl Synthase (#2)

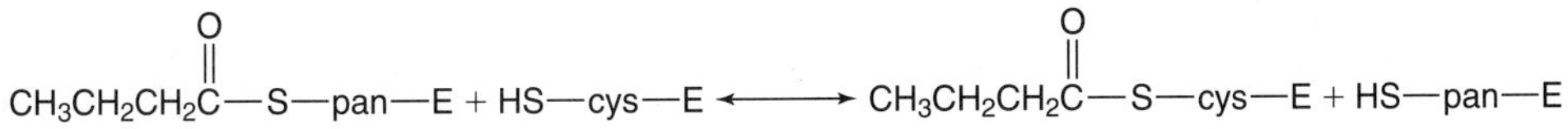

$$CH_3CH_2CH_2C-S-pan-E + HS-cys-E \longleftrightarrow CH_3CH_2CH_2C-S-cys-E + HS-pan-E$$

9. Acyl Transferase (#3)

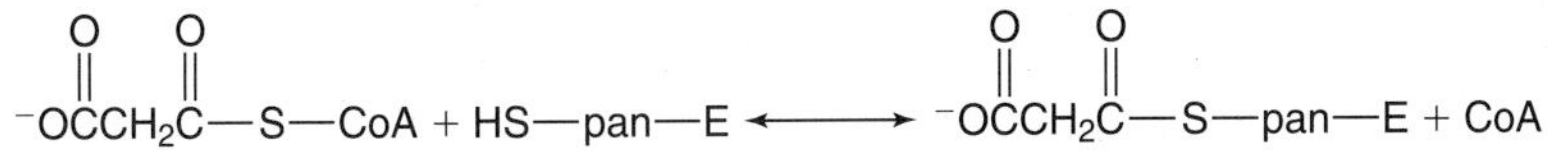

$$^-OCCH_2C-S-CoA + HS-pan-E \longleftrightarrow ^-OCCH_2C-S-pan-E + CoA$$

10. β-Ketoacyl Synthase (#4)

$$CH_3CH_2CH_2C-S-cys-E + ^-OCCH_2C-S-pan-E \longrightarrow CH_3CH_2CH_2C-CH_2C-S-pan-E$$
$$+ HS-cys-E + CO_2$$

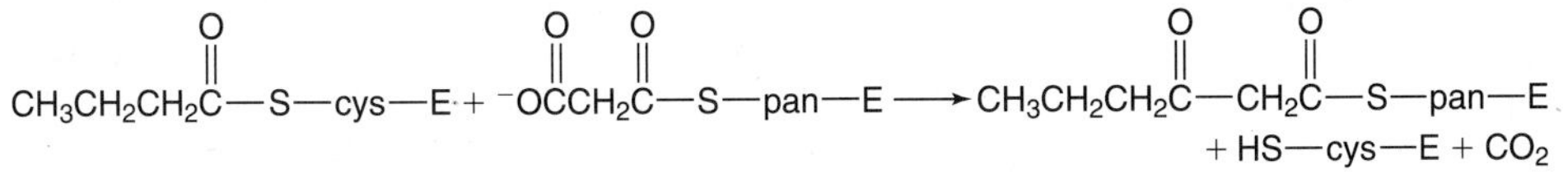

11-13. Repeat 5-7; Forming Hexanoyl—pan—E

14-38. Five Repeats of Reactions 3-7; Forming Palmitoyl—pan—E

39. Thioesterase

Palmitoyl—pan—E + H$_2$O $\longrightarrow$ Palmitate + HS—pan—E

Figure 13–3 Continued.

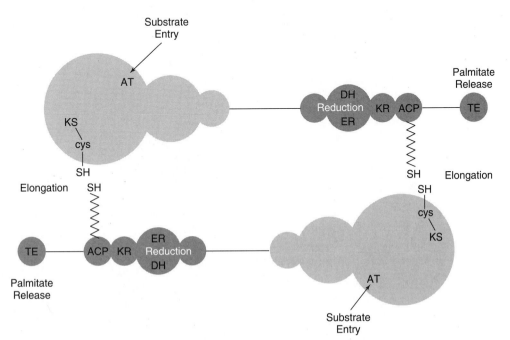

Figure 13–4. The fatty acid synthase model. Two identical subunits of fatty acid synthase are juxtaposed head-to-tail. Two centers for acyl chain assembly and release are shown. ACP, acyl carrier protein; AT, acyl transferase; DH, β-hydroxyacyl dehydratase; ER, enoyl reductase; KR, β-ketoacyl reductase; KS, β-ketoacyl synthase; SH, the free sulfhydryl group of the 4'-phosphopantetheine moiety of ACP or of a cysteinyl residue of KS; TE, thioesterase.

from the fatty acid, plus oxygen as an electron acceptor, to generate the oxidized fatty acid and two water molecules. The substrates and products are the acyl CoA derivatives of the fatty acid. Electrons donated by NADH are passed via $FADH_2$ to the heme iron of cytochrome b_5, reducing it to the ferrous form, in a reaction catalyzed by NADH:cytochrome b_5 reductase. Cytochrome b_5 then donates two electrons to the nonheme iron of the desaturase component, reducing it to the ferrous form. This form then interacts with molecular oxygen and the fatty acyl CoA to form water and the unsaturated fatty acyl CoA (Fig. 13–5). The desaturase activity regulates the overall reaction. Its activity is controlled by diet and hormones in much the same manner as are the activities of the lipogenic enzymes, mainly by regulation of enzyme concentration.

Polyunsaturated fatty acids, usually containing double bonds interrupted by methylene groups, are produced in mammalian tissues. Using the same enzymatic mechanism described earlier for the first desaturation at the Δ9 position, mammalian cells can further introduce double bonds into long-chain fatty acids at the Δ5 and Δ6 positions. However, due to the lack of Δ12 and Δ15 desaturases, double bonds cannot be introduced beyond the Δ9 position. As a consequence, linoleate (18:2, Δ9, Δ12) or linolenate (18:3, Δ9, Δ12, Δ15) cannot be synthesized in humans, and they or longer chain members of the ω3 or ω6 class must be provided in the diet. These fatty acids are essential for the synthesis of polyunsaturated fatty acids such as arachidonate (20:4, Δ5, Δ8, Δ11, Δ14) or docosahexaenoate (22:6, Δ4, Δ7, Δ10, Δ13, Δ16, Δ19). An alternating pattern of desaturation and elongation produces arachidonate from the essential

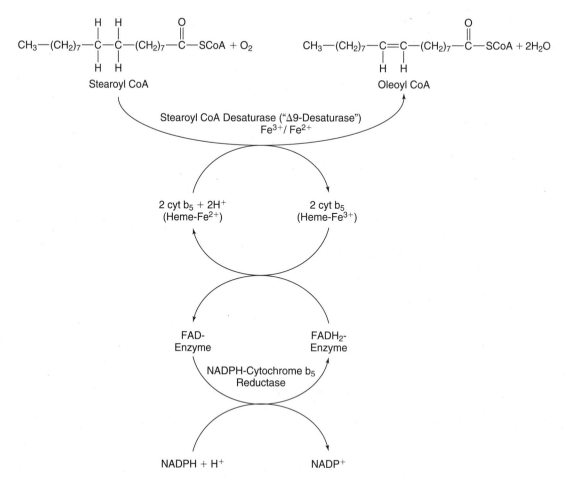

Figure 13–5. *Stearoyl CoA desaturase reaction.*

fatty acid linoleate; these reactions, plus a retroconversion step, are involved in synthesis of docosahexaenoate from α-linolenate (see Fig. 15–2; see Chapter 15 for more discussion of essential fatty acids).

Synthesis of Medium-Chain Fatty Acids

Medium-chain fatty acids are synthesized in mammary gland and are present as triacylglycerol in milk. Mammary gland has the same fatty acid synthase as does liver. Therefore, fatty acid synthase purified from either tissue can synthesize palmitate because the thioesterase activity of fatty acid synthase is specific for 16-carbon acyl groups. However, secretory cells of the mammary gland contain a second thioesterase that is specific for medium-chain fatty acids. This enzyme interacts with growing acyl chains on the fatty acid synthase and cleaves them from the enzyme when they are 8 to 12 carbons in length.

Production of Simple Branched-Chain Fatty Acids

Sebaceous glands and certain derivatives of sebaceous glands, such as the meibomian glands in the eyelids, synthesize fatty acids with 1-carbon side chains. The "normal" fatty acid synthase carries out these reactions using unusual substrates. Thus, propionyl CoA can be used as a primer for fatty acid synthase rather than acetyl CoA, and the resulting fatty acid will have a methyl branch at the 2(α) position. Methyl groups also can be inserted at other positions along the fatty acid chain. Although it has a lower affinity for the condensing enzyme than does malonyl CoA, methylmalonyl CoA is used as an elongating group if the concentration of malonyl CoA is lower than that of methylmalonyl CoA. In sebaceous glands and their derivatives, propionyl CoA is converted to methylmalonyl CoA in a reaction catalyzed by acetyl CoA carboxylase. The enzyme uses both substrates equally efficiently so that the group actually incorporated depends on the relative concentrations of acetyl CoA and propionyl CoA. In sebaceous glands, a soluble malonyl CoA carboxylase keeps malonyl CoA levels low.

The mechanism for generating high levels of propionyl CoA is not known.

SYNTHESIS AND STORAGE OF TRIACYLGLYCEROL

Esterification of Fatty Acids

Triacylglycerols are esters of glycerol and 3 molecules of fatty acids. The substrates for this pathway are glycerol 3-phosphate and fatty acyl CoA. Two reactions catalyze formation of glycerol 3-phosphate. First, dihydroxyacetone phosphate, a glycolytic (and gluconeogenic) intermediate, can be reduced to glycerol 3-phosphate. NADH is the electron donor in the reaction catalyzed by glycerol 3-phosphate dehydrogenase.

Dihydroxyacetone Phosphate + NADH +
$$H^+ \leftrightarrow \text{Glycerol 3-Phosphate} + NAD^+$$

This reaction is freely reversible, allowing glycerol 3-phosphate to enter the glycolytic or gluconeogenic pathways under certain conditions. Second, in some tissues such as liver, but not in adipose or muscle tissues, glycerol can be phosphorylated to glycerol 3-phosphate in a reaction catalyzed by glycerol kinase.

Glycerol + ATP →
$$\text{Glycerol 3-Phosphate} + ADP$$

Fatty acids synthesized de novo, taken up from the plasma, or derived from plasma or tissue triacylglycerols by the action of lipases, are unesterified and unactivated. Prior to esterification or oxidation, they must be activated to their CoA derivatives. This reaction is catalyzed by fatty acyl CoA synthetase (also called fatty acyl CoA ligase or fatty acid thiokinase). Fatty acyl CoA synthetase is present in the membranes of mitochondria, ER, and peroxisomes, where fatty acids are utilized for either esterification or oxidation.

This ATP-dependent reaction has three steps. In the first step, fatty acid reacts with ATP to form a fatty acyl-AMP intermediate plus pyrophosphate. In the second step, the acyl moiety is transferred to CoA, and AMP is generated:

(1) Fatty Acid + ATP $\leftrightarrow$ Fatty Acyl-AMP + PP$_i$
(2) Fatty Acyl-AMP + CoASH $\leftrightarrow$
$\qquad\qquad\qquad$ Fatty Acyl CoA +AMP

As written, the reactions are freely reversible: one high-energy bond is cleaved between PP$_i$ and AMP, and one is formed between the fatty acid and CoA. In the third step, the reaction is driven in the direction of formation of fatty acyl CoA by a ubiquitous pyrophosphatase that rapidly cleaves pyrophosphate to inorganic phosphate.

(3) PP$_i$ + H$_2$O $\rightarrow$ 2 P$_i$
NET: Fatty Acid + ATP + CoASH $\rightarrow$
$\qquad\qquad$ Fatty Acyl CoA + AMP + 2P$_i$

As will be shown in other pathways in this chapter, the hydrolysis of pyrophosphate is a relatively common mechanism for driving reactions to completion.

The glycerol 3-phosphate reaction pathway for the synthesis of triacylglycerols starts with fatty acyl CoA and glycerol 3-phosphate (Fig. 13–6). The acyl group of a fatty acyl CoA is transferred to the *sn*-1 position of glycerol 3-phosphate in the reaction catalyzed by glycerol 3-phosphate acyltransferase. This is the first committed step in glycerolipid biosynthesis. The 1-acylglycerol 3-phosphate (lysophosphatidic acid) is esterified by a second molecule of fatty acyl CoA to form 1,2-diacylglycerol 3-phosphate (phosphatidic acid). The enzyme that catalyzes this reaction is 1-acylglycerol 3-phosphate acyltransferase. Usually, the *sn*-1 position of the glycerol backbone is esterified with a saturated fatty acid, whereas the *sn*-2 position is esterified with an unsaturated fatty acid. However, the fatty acid composition of lipids in the diet influences the fatty acid composition of triacylglycerol in adipose tissue.

(1) Glycerol 3-Phosphate + Fatty Acyl CoA $\rightarrow$
$\qquad$ 1-Acylglycerol 3-Phosphate + CoA

(2) 1-Acylglycerol 3-Phosphate + Fatty Acyl CoA $\rightarrow$ 1,2-Diacylglycerol 3-Phosphate + CoA

In the third reaction of this pathway, 1,2-diacylglycerol 3-phosphate is dephosphorylated to 1,2-diacylglycerol and inorganic phosphate.

The enzyme that catalyzes this reaction is 1,2-diacylglycerol 3-phosphate phosphatase (also called phosphatidic acid phosphohydrolase).

(3) 1,2-Diacylglycerol 3-Phosphate $\rightarrow$
$\qquad\qquad\qquad$ 1,2-Diacylglycerol + P$_i$

Up to this point the reactions of triacylglycerol synthesis are the same as those leading to synthesis of phospholipids, some of which utilize 1,2-diacylglycerol 3-phosphate as substrate and some of which utilize diacylglycerol. The final reaction for triacylglycerol synthesis involves acylation of diacylglycerol to form triacylglycerol. This reaction is catalyzed by 1,2-diacylglycerol acyltransferase, which is particularly active in liver and adipose tissue.

(4) 1,2-Diacylglycerol + Fatty Acyl CoA $\rightarrow$
$\qquad\qquad\qquad$ Triacylglycerol + CoA

Dihydroxyacetone phosphate also can be used in the first acylation of fatty acyl CoA. The first reaction is catalyzed by a dihydroxyacetone acyltransferase that is present in ER and also in peroxisomes, which forms 1-acyl dihydroxyacetone as the product. This compound is then reduced by 1-acyl dihydroxyacetone reductase with NADPH as the electron donor and 1-acylglycerol 3-phosphate and NADP$^+$ as products. The remaining steps are the same as outlined for the glycerol 3-phosphate pathway. The role of this second pathway in phosphatidic acid biosynthesis is not clear. It is generally accepted that 1-acyldihydroxyacetone phosphate is an intermediate in the synthesis of alkyl and alkenyl lipids, a process that occurs exclusively in peroxisomes.

Glycerolipid biosynthesis occurs mostly in ER; and the enzymes reside on the ER membrane, but the catalytic activities must face the cytosol where substrates reside. Because these enzymes are membrane-bound, their characterization has been difficult, and their regulation is largely unknown. It is presumed that 1,2-diacylglycerol 3-phosphate phosphatase may be a rate-controlling step in triacylglycerol synthesis, and that the enzyme activity is regulated via translocation of the enzyme from cytosol to ER, where it becomes active. However, 1,2-diacylglycerol acyltrans-

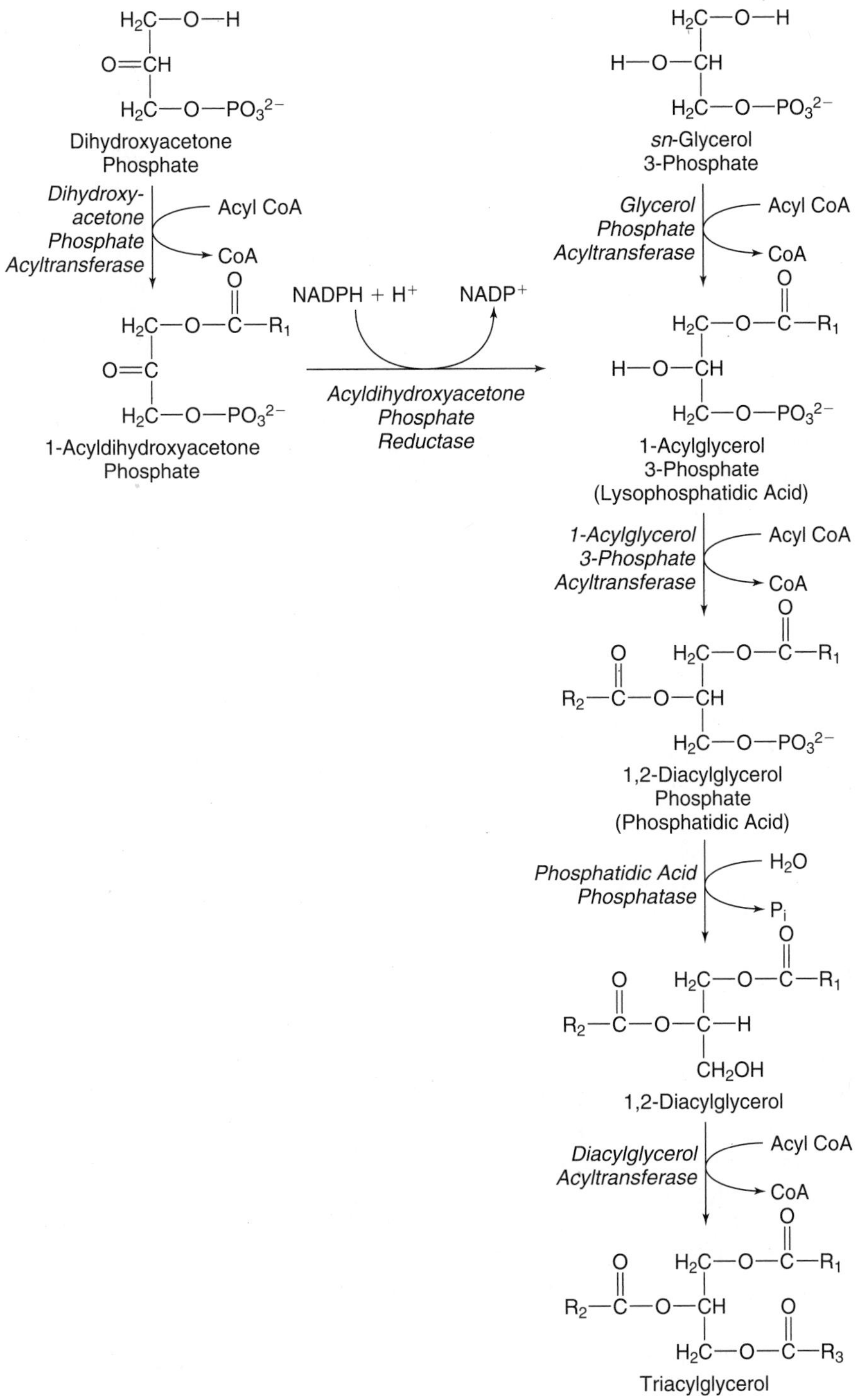

H₂C—O—H → H_2C-O-H

$$H_2C-O-H$$
$$O=CH$$
$$H_2C-O-PO_3^{2-}$$

Dihydroxyacetone Phosphate

Dihydroxyacetone Phosphate Acyltransferase — Acyl CoA → CoA

$$H_2C-O-\overset{O}{\overset{\|}{C}}-R_1$$
$$O=C$$
$$H_2C-O-PO_3^{2-}$$

1-Acyldihydroxyacetone Phosphate

NADPH + H⁺ → NADP⁺

Acyldihydroxyacetone Phosphate Reductase

$$H_2C-O-H$$
$$H-O-CH$$
$$H_2C-O-PO_3^{2-}$$

sn-Glycerol 3-Phosphate

Glycerol Phosphate Acyltransferase — Acyl CoA → CoA

$$H_2C-O-\overset{O}{\overset{\|}{C}}-R_1$$
$$H-O-CH$$
$$H_2C-O-PO_3^{2-}$$

1-Acylglycerol 3-Phosphate (Lysophosphatidic Acid)

1-Acylglycerol 3-Phosphate Acyltransferase — Acyl CoA → CoA

$$R_2-\overset{O}{\overset{\|}{C}}-O-CH$$
$$H_2C-O-\overset{O}{\overset{\|}{C}}-R_1$$
$$H_2C-O-PO_3^{2-}$$

1,2-Diacylglycerol Phosphate (Phosphatidic Acid)

Phosphatidic Acid Phosphatase — H₂O → Pᵢ

$$R_2-\overset{O}{\overset{\|}{C}}-O-CH$$
$$H_2C-O-\overset{O}{\overset{\|}{C}}-R_1$$
$$CH_2OH$$

1,2-Diacylglycerol

Diacylglycerol Acyltransferase — Acyl CoA → CoA

$$R_2-\overset{O}{\overset{\|}{C}}-O-CH$$
$$H_2C-O-\overset{O}{\overset{\|}{C}}-R_1$$
$$H_2C-O-\overset{O}{\overset{\|}{C}}-R_3$$

Triacylglycerol

Figure 13–6. *Triacylglycerol biosynthesis.*

ferase also may be a target for regulating triacylglycerol synthesis, because this is the only unique step not involved in phospholipid synthesis. Glycerol 3-phosphate acyltransferase also may be a regulatory step. An isoform of glycerol 3-phosphate acyltransferase, with characteristics different from those of the form present in ER, is found in mitochondrial membrane. The mitochondrial enzyme is expressed mostly in lipogenic tissues (the liver and adipose tissue) and is regulated by nutritional changes as described earlier for the enzymes involved in fatty acid synthesis. During the fasting state, enzyme activity is very low; in the fed state, especially on a high carbohydrate diet, enzyme activity is increased. Regulation is at the transcriptional level.

Much of the triacylglycerol synthesized in the liver is destined for export to peripheral tissues, especially to adipose tissue where it is stored. Triacylglycerol is not soluble in water, so special arrangements must be made to permit its transport in the blood. Lipoproteins perform this function, as described in detail in Chapter 14. Triacylglycerol synthesized in liver from fatty acids derived from dietary fat or from de novo synthesis is packaged into lipoproteins in liver and secreted into the blood as VLDL.

Synthesis of triacylglycerol in enterocytes (intestinal cells) follows a somewhat different pathway than that just described for liver and adipose tissue and is described in Chapter 7. The products of the hydrolysis of triacylglycerol in the lumen of the intestine are unesterified fatty acids and 2-monoacylglycerol. These compounds are taken up by enterocytes and recombined to form triacylglycerol. The triacylglycerol then is packaged into lipoproteins and secreted into the lymph; ultimately it passes into the blood stream as chylomicrons. In the first reaction of triacylglycerol resynthesis in enterocytes, 2-monoacylglycerol reacts with fatty acyl CoA to form diacylglycerol (2-monoacylglycerol acyltransferase). The next step is the same as that in other tissues and is catalyzed by the same enzyme, diacylglycerol acyltransferase. The 2-monoacylglycerol pathway is dominant in enterocytes, but because some triacylglycerol is hydrolyzed to glycerol and fatty acids in the intestinal lumen, the glycerol 3-phosphate pathway also is essential.

Uptake and Storage of Triacylglycerol in Lipoproteins

Triacylglycerol in lipoproteins is taken up by extrahepatic tissues such as muscle, where it provides a source of oxidizable fatty acids, and adipose tissue, where it is reconverted

to triacylglycerol and stored in the "signet ring–like" adipocytes until needed. Lipoprotein lipase facilitates uptake of fatty acids by extrahepatic tissues from blood by hydrolyzing plasma triacylglycerol in the circulating lipoproteins (Goldberg, 1996). Lipoprotein lipase is localized on the luminal face of the endothelial cells that form the "walls" of capillaries (Fig. 13–7). The enzyme is synthesized by myocytes (muscle cells) or adipocytes (adipose cells) and secreted into the interstitial space. It then is taken up at the interstitial (basal) side of the endothelial cells, transported across those cells, secreted, and bound to the plasma side of the luminal surface. As discussed in more detail in Chapter 14, triacylglycerol in lipoproteins is hydrolyzed by lipoprotein lipase, producing unesterified fatty acids. The unesterified fatty acids cross the endothelial cells by an unknown mechanism and are probably taken up by transporter-mediated processes by adipocytes or myocytes. Synthesis and secretion of lipoprotein lipase in muscle and adipose tissue are regulated differentially. In the fed state, synthesis and secretion of adipose tissue lipoprotein lipase are increased. During a shortage of energy (such as overnight fasting or exercise), muscle lipoprotein lipase is increased. Inside adipocytes, the fatty acids are activated to their CoA derivatives, esterified to triacylglycerol via the glycerol 3-phosphate pathway, and stored as a lipid droplet in those cells. Inside myocytes the fatty acids are used primarily for oxidation.

MOBILIZATION OF STORED TRIACYLGLYCEROL

Another lipase, hormone-sensitive lipase, catalyzes release of fatty acids from the lipid droplet stored in the adipocytes. It acts at the surface of the triacylglycerol droplet and hydrolyzes fatty acids at the sn-1 and sn-3 positions. Subsequently, monoacylglycerol lipase present at high activity hydrolyzes the fatty acids at the sn-2 position. Hormone-sensitive lipase is regulated by a phosphorylation-dephosphorylation mechanism. In the fed state, the insulin level in the blood rises and brings about dephosphorylation and inactivation of

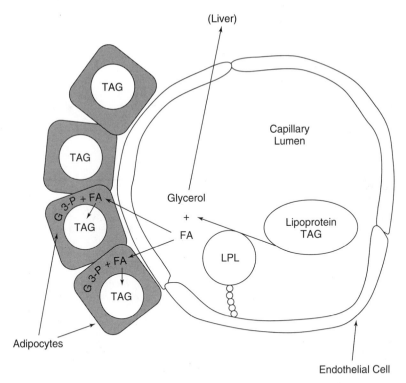

Figure 13–7. Model for hydrolysis of lipoprotein-bound triacylglycerol (TAG) and uptake of fatty acids (FA) into adipocytes resulting in assimilation of TAG for storage. Hydrolysis of FA from TAG-rich lipoproteins by lipoprotein lipase (LPL) bound to the capillary endothelial surface via sulfated proteoglycans is shown. Released FA are then taken up by adipocytes and reesterified to TAG for storage.

hormone-sensitive lipase (Fig. 13–8). Fat mobilization from adipose tissue is therefore decreased. In addition, insulin promotes uptake of glucose into the adipocyte. Because the rate of glycolysis is limited by the rate of uptake of glucose, there is a steady production of triose phosphate and glycerol 3-phosphate under these conditions. As a consequence, in fed animals, any fatty acid produced by the adipose tissue hormone-sensitive lipase is reesterified.

On the other hand, in the fasting state, stored triacylglycerol in adipose tissue is the major source of energy. Hormone-sensitive lipase is phosphorylated by protein kinase A, which is activated by increased intracellular cAMP. In isolated rat adipocytes, glucagon, which rises during starvation, is a potent stimulator of fat mobilization. In humans, however, epinephrine and norepinephrine probably play the major role in increasing intracellular cAMP levels and thus phosphorylation and activation of hormone-sensitive lipase. This leads to the accelerated hydrolysis of triacyl-

glycerol (Fig. 13–8). At the same time, the decrease in insulin levels during starvation inhibits glucose uptake and, therefore, production of triose phosphate. Because adipose tissue lacks the enzyme glycerol kinase, the glycerol 3-phosphate required for esterification of fatty acids must be derived from glycolysis. As a consequence, during starvation, there is little reesterification to restrain the increased production of fatty acids by the activated hormone-sensitive lipase, and release of fatty acids to the blood proceeds at a high rate. Once in the blood, unesterified fatty acids are bound noncovalently to albumin and transported in that form to other tissues, primarily destined for oxidation. Glycerol produced in adipose tissue during triacylglycerol hydrolysis also is released to the blood and is transported to the liver for reutilization.

OXIDATION OF FATTY ACIDS

The rate of oxidation of fatty acids is proportional to their concentration in the plasma.

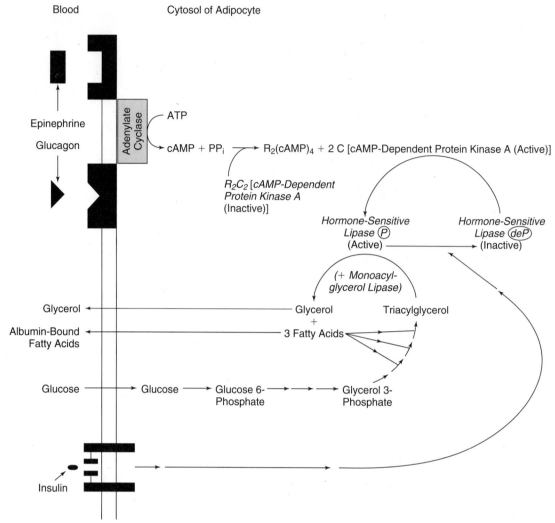

Figure 13–8. *Hydrolysis of stored triacylglcerol in adipose tissue by hormone-sensitive lipase. R and C represent the regulatory and catalytic subunits of cAMP-dependent protein kinase A.*

Fatty acid oxidation is high in muscle and liver during starvation because rapid mobilization of fatty acids in adipose tissue causes an increase in the level of plasma unesterified fatty acids. The converse is true in the fed state. The positive correlation between plasma fatty acid concentration and the rate of fatty acid oxidation is due to the fact that uptake of fatty acids from the plasma and the rate of activation of intracellular fatty acid to the acyl CoA derivative are proportional to the concentration of unesterified fatty acids in the plasma. During exercise, fatty acid oxidation in muscle also increases, although the plasma fatty acid level may remain the same. This is due to the increase in delivery of fatty acids that accompanies higher blood flow during exercise.

Role of Carnitine in Transport of Acyl Groups from Cytosol to Mitochondria

Synthesis of fatty acyl CoA is catalyzed by fatty acyl CoA synthetase, as outlined earlier in this chapter. Oxidation of fatty acids is localized in the mitochondrial compartment. Neither unesterified long-chain fatty acids nor their fatty acyl CoA derivatives can diffuse across the inner mitochondrial membrane. Entry of the acyl groups is catalyzed by a "carnitine" cycle (Fig. 13–9) (McGarry and Brown, 1997). On the outer mitochondrial membrane, an

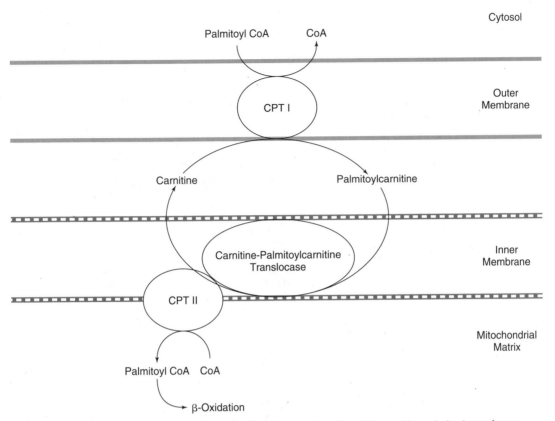

Figure 13–9. *Transport of long-chain fatty acyl CoA into mitochondria. CPT, carnitine palmitoyl transferase.*

enzyme called carnitine palmitoyltransferase-I (CPT I) catalyzes the transfer of long-chain acyl groups from CoA to carnitine.

Fatty Acyl CoA + Carnitine ↔
               Fatty Acylcarnitine + CoA

Carnitine-palmitoylcarnitine translocase catalyzes transport of the acylcarnitine across the impermeable inner mitochondrial membrane in exchange for free carnitine. On the inner surface of the inner mitochondrial membrane, carnitine palmitoyltransferase-II (CPT II) catalyzes the reesterification of acylcarnitines to form acyl CoA esters.

Fatty Acylcarnitine + CoA ↔
               Fatty Acyl CoA + Carnitine

The free carnitine is exchanged for acylcarnitine, allowing the process to continue. Rapid oxidation of the fatty acyl CoA in the β-oxidation pathway likely provides the driving force to keep everything moving in the same direction through these largely freely reversible reactions. Both saturated and unsaturated long-chain fatty acids are metabolized via this pathway.

In the fed state, the rate of lipolysis in adipose tissue is slow, and the concentration of plasma free fatty acids and hence their availability for β-oxidation in other tissues are decreased. In liver, the rate of production of malonyl CoA and its intracellular concentration are elevated in the fed state, because acetyl CoA carboxylase, the key regulatory enzyme in de novo lipogenesis, is activated by insulin. Malonyl CoA, is a potent allosteric inhibitor of carnitine palmitoyltransferase-I. Malonyl CoA limits entry of fatty acyl CoA into the mitochondrial compartment and consequently depresses hepatic β-oxidation. This reciprocal regulatory mechanism minimizes futile cycling by ensuring that the opposing processes of β-oxidation and fatty acid biosynthesis are not activated simultaneously.

CLINICAL CORRELATION

Defects in Fatty Acid Transport into Mitochondria for Oxidation

Genetic disorders in any of the enzymes in the carnitine cycle, including carnitine palmitoyltransferases-I and -II (CPT I and CPT II) and carnitine-acylcarnitine translocase (see Fig. 13–9), block oxidation of long-chain fatty acids due to impaired transport of long-chain fatty acids into the mitochondrial matrix (Scriver et al., 1995). There are two tissue-specific isoforms of CPT I encoded by separate genes: the liver form is expressed mainly in liver and kidney, and the muscle form is expressed in muscle and heart. On the other hand, there appears to be only one form of CPT II. Reported cases of CPT I deficiency have primarily involved defects of liver metabolism: enlarged fatty livers, hypoketotic hypoglycemia, and possibly coma during fasting. Neither muscle weakness nor cardiomyopathy was associated with CPT I deficiency. Although the molecular basis of CPT I deficiency has not been elucidated, the finding that patients diagnosed with this genetic defect mainly have liver defects suggests that the liver isoform of CPT I is defective.

CPT II deficiency can take two distinct clinical forms. Classical CPT II deficiency in adults affects primarily fatty acid metabolism in skeletal and/or cardiac muscle. In these patients, long-chain acylcarnitine translocated across the inner mitochondrial membrane is not reconverted to acyl CoAs. The accumulated long-chain acylcarnitine species are then transported out of the mitochondria and into plasma. Under normal conditions, fuel metabolism is still adequate. During sustained exercise or starvation, however, fatty acid oxidation is important quantitatively, and patients experience cramps and fatigue. Although the CPT II deficiency primarily affects muscle, defects in CPT II also occur in other tissues. The manifestation of a severe infantile form of CPT II deficiency is hypoketotic hypoglycemia with cardiomyopathy; it is usually fatal. In the adult-onset form, there is a partial deficiency of CPT II activity. In the more severe infantile form, CPT II activity is less than 10% of normal. CPT II in a patient with an infantile form of the disease was shown to have an arginine to cysteine substitution at amino acid residue 631; this variant CPT II has decreased CPT II activity.

Carnitine deficiency causes a similar impairment of fatty acid oxidation, but fatty acid oxidation in this case can be restored by administering carnitine. Carnitine in the diet is absorbed in the intestine. Also, human tissues can synthesize carnitine de novo, mostly in liver and kidney. Endogenous synthesis normally meets the metabolic need, provided that the diet contains sufficient lysine and methionine (precursors) and ascorbic acid, vitamin B_6, niacin, and iron (cofactors) for the biosynthesis. (Synthesis of carnitine is outlined in Figure 23–8 and is discussed in Chapters 11 and 23.) Carnitine deficiency is rare in adults. However, patients undergoing kidney dialysis or those with organic aciduria may lose large amounts of carnitine; they and patients on long-term parenteral nutrition may exhibit carnitine deficiency. Carnitine deficiency also may occur in neonates, particularly in premature infants.

Thinking Critically

1. Why does hypoketotic hypoglycemia occur in CPT I deficiency?

2. What dietary recommendations would you make for patients with CPT I or CPT II deficiency?

3. Why are the symptoms of CPT I and CPT II deficiencies in patients more severe during starvation?

4. What changes in plasma carnitine and acylcarnitine levels could be used to distinguish between CPT I and CPT II deficiencies?

Mitochondrial β-Oxidation

Fatty acids are oxidized by a series of reactions that overall are the reverse of those catalyzed by fatty acid synthase. The two processes, however, are catalyzed by different enzymes, have different subcellular localizations, and have a number of chemical differences (Eaton et al., 1996). Instead of condensation, reduction, dehydration, and reduction, the β-oxidation cycle involves oxidation, hydration, oxidation, and cleavage, catalyzed by four enzymes (Fig. 13–10). The intermediates, however, have not been detected. It is probable that the product of one reaction is transferred directly to the next enzyme. In fact, some of the steps in β-oxidation are catalyzed by a multifunctional enzyme. β-Oxidation occurs in 2-carbon steps, as with fatty acid synthesis.

The first step in β-oxidation is catalyzed by acyl CoA dehydrogenase. In contrast to fatty acid synthesis in which NADPH is the electron donor, a tightly but noncovalently linked flavin adenine dinucleotide (FAD) is the electron acceptor in the first reaction of β-oxidation.

Acyl CoA + Enzyme-FAD →
2-*trans*-Enoyl CoA + Enzyme-FADH$_2$

FAD is used as the electron acceptor because the ΔG of this reaction is not sufficient to drive production of NADH. The FADH$_2$ generated in this first reaction of β-oxidation donates its electrons to the FAD prosthetic group of electron-transferring flavoprotein, which, in turn, transfers its electrons to ubiquinone in the electron transfer chain (see Fig. 20–7 in Chapter 20). Oxidation of each mole of FADH$_2$ generates a maximum of 2 mol of ATP. Separate enzymes encoded by different genes catalyze the oxidation of long-, medium-, and short-chain fatty acids.

The second step in β-oxidation is catalyzed by enoyl CoA hydratase and involves hydration of the *trans* double bond created by the first oxidation.

2-*trans*-Enoyl CoA + H$_2$O ↔
L-3-Hydroxyacyl CoA

Hydration of the double bond is stereospecific; L-3-hydroxyacyl CoA is the product when a *trans* double bond is hydrated. Enoyl CoA hydratase also hydrates *cis* double bonds; this produces the D-isomer of 3-hydroxyacyl CoA. Two enzymes, one specific for long-chain fatty acids and the other for short- and medium-chain fatty acids, are present in the mitochondria and cooperate in the hydration of fatty acyl chains of different lengths.

In the third step, a dehydrogenase that is specific for the L isomer of hydroxyacyl CoA catalyzes a second oxidation step. NAD$^+$ is the electron acceptor. (See Fig. 20–7 in Chapter 20 for reactions involved in transfer of electrons through the electron transport chain.)

L-3-Hydroxyacyl CoA + NAD$^+$ ↔
3-Ketoacyl CoA + NADH + H$^+$

Two enzymes, one specific for long-chain fatty acids and the other for short- and medium-chain fatty acids, also cooperate in the oxidation of 3-hydroxyacyl CoA chains of different lengths.

In the final step of each 2-carbon cycle of β-oxidation, 3-ketothiolase catalyzes the thiolytic cleavage of the 3-ketoacyl CoA to acetyl CoA plus an acyl CoA that is 2 carbons shorter.

3-Ketoacyl CoA + CoASH →
Acetyl CoA + Acyl CoA (n-2)

Several types of thiolases have been described. Mitochondria contain two: acetoacetyl CoA thiolase, which cleaves acetoacetyl CoA and functions during ketone metabolism, and 3-ketothiolase, which catalyzes the thiolytic cleavages that occur during β-oxidation of fatty acids. A single 3-ketothiolase appears to catalyze the cleavages of acyl groups of all chain lengths.

Deficiencies in each of the enzymes in the β-oxidation pathway, including specific short-, medium-, and long-chain fatty acyl CoA dehydrogenase deficiencies, cause disorders in metabolic adaptation during starvation owing to an impairment of fatty acid oxidation. The most common deficiency is that of medium-chain fatty acyl CoA dehydrogenase, an inherited disease with an incidence similar to that of phenylketonuria (Scriver et al., 1995). Intermediates of fatty acid oxidation accumu-

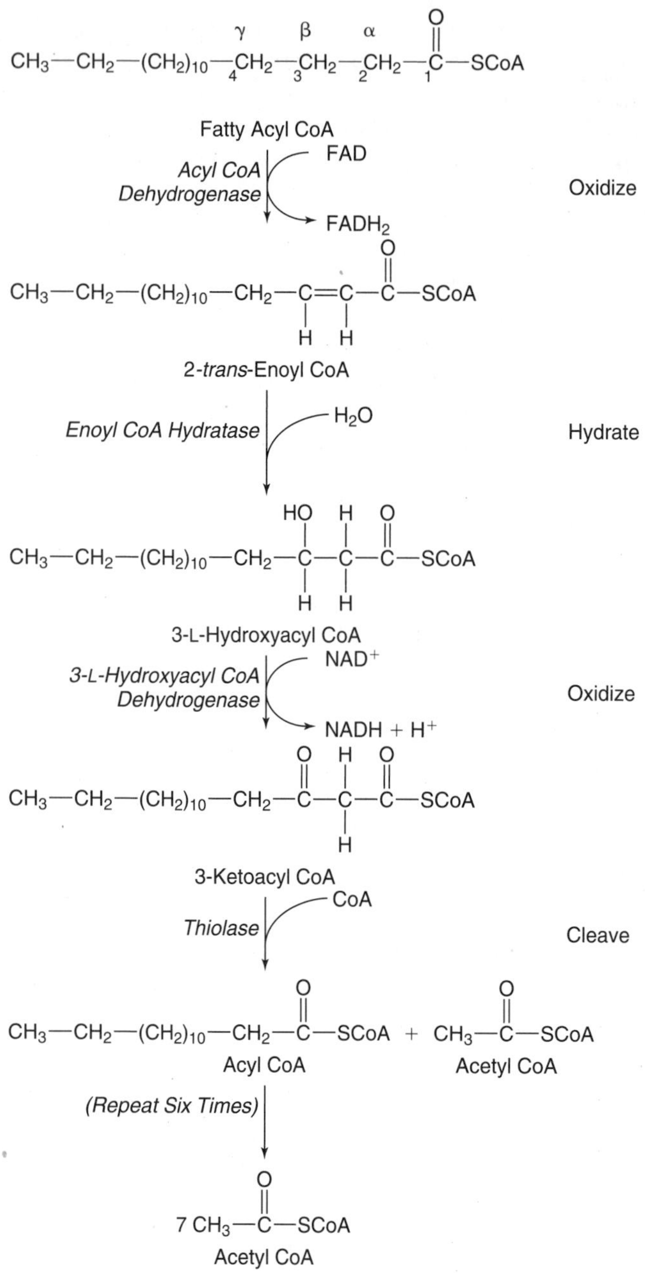

Figure 13–10. *β-Oxidation of fatty acids. Example is for oxidation of palmitoyl CoA.*

late and result in increases in levels of related plasma and urinary metabolites, especially during conditions such as fasting and infection when the rate of lipolysis is increased. Accumulation of some intermediates, such as dicarboxylic acids, is due to the metabolic block of fatty acid oxidation in general. Accumulation of some others, such as *cis*-4-decenoic acid, phenylpropionylglycine, and octanoyl- and *cis*-4-decenoylcarnitine, is unique to

the deficiency of medium-chain fatty acyl CoA dehydrogenase. Carnitine supplementation has been used to treat patients with medium-chain acyl CoA dehydrogenase deficiency. Although the supplementation does not correct the underlying defect, it may help remove these potentially toxic intermediates as acylcarnitines. In patients with this deficiency, nonketotic hypoglycemia can be provoked by fasting during the first 2 years of life. Avoidance of fasting and administration of glucose in acute episodes of hypoglycemia are recommended. Deficiencies in long-chain fatty acyl CoA dehydrogenase, long-chain 3-hydroxyacyl CoA dehydrogenase, and short-chain acyl CoA dehydrogenase cause muscle weakness similar to that caused by a deficiency of carnitine palmitoyltransferase-II. A deficiency in mitochondrial acetoacetyl CoA thiolase does not impair fatty acid oxidation but affects isoleucine and ketone body metabolism.

The function of mitochondrial fatty acid oxidation is primarily to supply energy. Peroxisomes also carry out β-oxidation, and some fatty acids, including very-long-chain fatty acids, are preferentially oxidized in peroxisomes. One function of peroxisomal β-oxidation may be to supply acetyl CoA for anabolic reactions. As discussed later in this chapter, diagnosis of peroxisome defects such as Zellweger syndrome can be based on measurement of the concentrations of very long-chain fatty acids.

Energy Yield from β-Oxidation of Palmitate

For each cycle—oxidation, hydration, oxidation, and cleavage—an acyl CoA is shortened by 2 carbons, and 1 molecule each of $FADH_2$, NADH, hydrogen ion, and acetyl CoA are produced. For the oxidation of palmitate, therefore, the balanced equation is:

$$\text{Palmitoyl CoA} + 7 \text{ CoASH} + 7 \text{ FAD} \\ + 7 \text{ NAD}^+ + 7 \text{ H}_2\text{O} \rightarrow 8 \text{ Acetyl CoA} \\ + 7 \text{ FADH}_2 + 7 \text{ NADH} + 7 \text{ H}^+$$

Each $FADH_2$ yields a maximum of 2 ATPs as it passes its electrons down the electron transport chain; each NADH yields a maximum of 3 ATPs. Thus, oxidation of palmitoyl CoA as shown in the preceding equation yields a maximum of 35 ATPs. As noted in Chapter 9, the complete oxidation of acetyl CoA to CO_2, H_2O, and CoASH yields a maximum of 12 ATPs. In sum, therefore, the complete oxidation of palmitoyl CoA yields 131 ATPs. Two high-energy bonds are used up in the activation of palmitate to palmitoyl CoA because ATP is split into AMP and PP_i. The complete oxidation of palmitate to CO_2 and

H_2O thus yields a net of 129 mol of ATP per mole of palmitate.

The standard free energy for the complete oxidation of palmitate is about 9800 kJ/mol (2344 kcal/mol). The standard free energy for the hydrolysis of ATP is 30.5 kJ/mol (7.3 kcal/mol). Thus, palmitate oxidation in the living cell, if it were under standard conditions, would conserve a maximum of 131×30.5, or 3995 kJ/mol (956 kcal/mol) in ATP. This represents a very respectable efficiency of about 34%. If, however, the free energy changes were calculated under the conditions that exist in vivo, the energy conservation is closer to 80%. Living cells are remarkably efficient at capturing the energy available in lipid foodstuffs.

Additional Reactions Required for β-Oxidation of Unsaturated Fatty Acids

Unsaturated fatty acids are abundant in nature and are also degraded via β-oxidation. Most of the double bonds in natural mono- and polyunsaturated fatty acids are in the *cis* configuration and can be put into two classes: ones that extend from odd- (e.g., Δ9 of oleic acid or Δ9 of linoleic acid) or from even- (e.g., Δ12 of linoleic acid) numbered carbons in the fatty acid chain. Neither of these double bonds is a natural intermediate in β-oxidation, so auxiliary enzymes must rearrange the double bonds to permit complete oxidation. The simplest of these rearrangements involves double bonds extending from odd-numbered carbons (Fig. 13–11). Oleoyl CoA (9-*cis*-octadecenoyl CoA) undergoes three rounds of β-oxidation to form 3-*cis*-dodecenoyl CoA. This intermediate is not a substrate for either of the dehydrogenases or enoyl CoA hydratase. This problem is circumvented by isomerization of the double bond to yield 2-*trans*-dodecenoyl CoA. The auxiliary enzyme that catalyzes this reaction is 3-*cis*-2-*trans*-enoyl CoA isomerase (enoyl CoA isomerase). This enzyme also isomerizes 3-*trans*-enoyl CoA to its 2-*trans*-enoyl CoA isomer. The product of the enoyl CoA isomerase-catalyzed reaction is 2-*trans*-dodecenoyl CoA, a substrate for enoyl CoA reductase. This reaction allows β-oxidation to continue, but, in the fourth cycle of β-oxidation, the first dehydrogenase step cata-

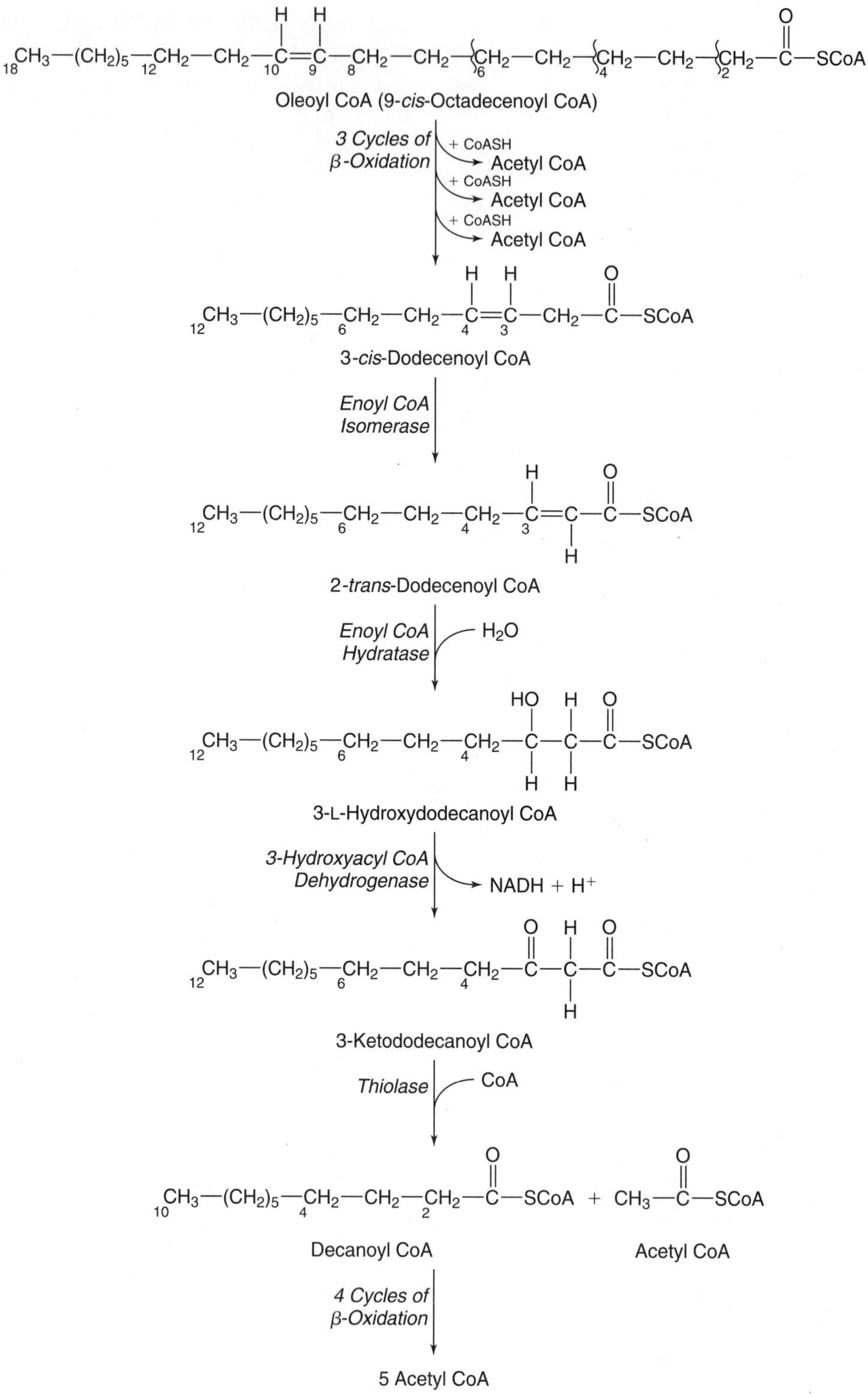

Figure 13–11. Oxidation of oleoyl CoA.

lyzed by acyl CoA dehydrogenase is omitted. Thus, complete oxidation of oleate (18:1) yields one less FADH$_2$—or 2 less ATPs—than complete oxidation of stearate (18:0).

The oxidation of linoleate (Fig. 13–12) proceeds like that of oleate, including the isomerase step just described, for four cycles plus the first dehydrogenase reaction of the fifth cycle. At this point the product is 2-*trans*, 4-*cis* decadienoyl CoA, an intermediate that is not a substrate for the enoyl CoA hydratase or the β-hydroxyacyl CoA dehydrogenase. This potential block to β-oxidation is circumvented by two reactions catalyzed by auxiliary enzymes. First, 2-*trans*, 4-*cis*-decadienoyl CoA is reduced to 3-*trans*-decenoyl CoA. This reaction utilizes NADPH as the electron donor and is catalyzed by 2,4-dienoyl CoA reductase. The product of this reaction, 3-*trans*-decenoyl CoA, is not a substrate for the enzymes of β-oxidation and must be isomerized to 2-*trans*-decenoyl CoA, a substrate for the enoyl CoA hydratase. β-oxidation then continues to complete the fifth cycle, and three more complete cycles as shown in Figure 13–12. In the oxidation of linoleate, one FADH$_2$ (2 ATPs) is lost in the third cycle, as with oleate. The fifth cycle utilizes both dehydrogenases, generating both FADH$_2$ and NADH. However, the utilization of 1 NADPH balances the production of 1 NADH, meaning that 3 ATPs are lost. Overall then, the complete oxidation of linoleate (18:2) generates 5 less ATPs than that of stearate (18:0).

Although most naturally occurring unsaturated fatty acids contain *cis* double bonds, small amounts of *trans* fatty acids are found in cow's milk fat. During hydrogenation of polyunsaturated fatty acids by rumen microorganisms, the double bonds are isomerized from the *cis* to the *trans* configuration. A similar process occurs during hydrogenation in manufacturing margarine, and large amounts of *trans* fatty acids are found in margarine products. Although they have a lower affinity for isomerases, *trans* fatty acids are oxidized by the isomerases. Dietary *trans* fatty acids seem to have effects similar to or potentially worse than saturated fatty acids in the development of atherosclerosis. (See Chapter 41 for a discussion of dietary fat and cardiovascular disease.)

β-Oxidation of Fatty Acids with an Odd Number of Carbons or with Methyl Side Chains to Generate Propionyl CoA

Fatty acids of odd-chain length are not synthesized in animals and, therefore, are not commonly found in meat. However, small amounts of odd-chain fatty acids are found in vegetables. The β-oxidation of straight-chain fatty acids containing an odd number of carbons requires three auxiliary enzymes (Fig. 13–13). Oxidation proceeds as described above for other saturated fatty acids until the last step of the last cycle, producing FADH$_2$, NADH, and acetyl CoA in each cycle. However, the product of the final cleavage reaction is 1 acetyl CoA and 1 propionyl CoA. Propionyl CoA is more abundantly generated by metabolism of certain amino acids (valine, isoleucine, threonine, and methionine), as described in Chapter 11. Propionyl CoA is carboxylated to D-methylmalonyl CoA in an ATP-dependent reaction catalyzed by propionyl CoA carboxylase. The reaction mechanism is similar to that for acetyl CoA carboxylase. The enzyme methylmalonyl CoA racemase catalyzes the isomerization of the D-isomer to the L-isomer, and L-methylmalonyl CoA is isomerized to succinyl CoA in a reaction catalyzed by methylmalonyl CoA mutase. Succinyl CoA is an intermediate in the citric acid cycle. Unlike acetyl CoA, which is the final product of β-oxidation of fatty acids containing an even number of carbons, succinyl CoA can be converted to phosphoenolpyruvate and hence to glucose. Therefore, fatty acids with an odd number of carbons, especially propionic acid, can be considered gluconeogenic. Methylmalonyl CoA mutase requires as a cofactor deoxyadenosylcobalamin, a derivative of vitamin B$_{12}$. Individuals develop pernicious anemia when they lack intrinsic factor, a specific vitamin B$_{12}$-binding glycoprotein required for vitamin B$_{12}$ absorption. These patients have impaired conversion of methylmalonyl CoA to succinyl CoA and excrete methylmalonate in their urine.

Odd- or even-numbered fatty acids that contain methyl side chains are oxidized by the usual β-oxidation scheme. A methyl side chain on the carbon does not interfere with β-oxidation. The products of the thiolytic

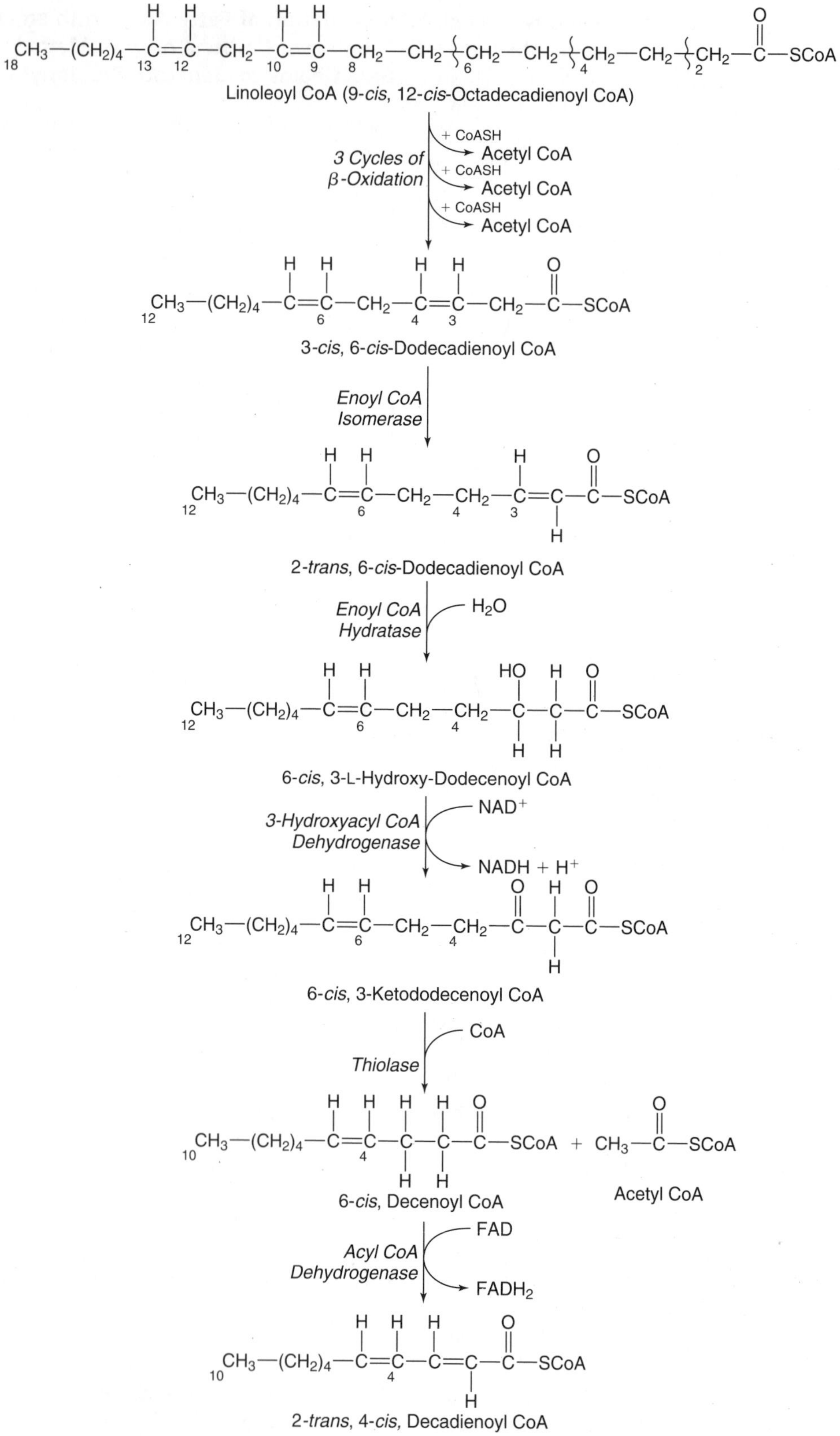

Figure 13–12. Oxidation of linoleoyl CoA.

(Continued on next page)

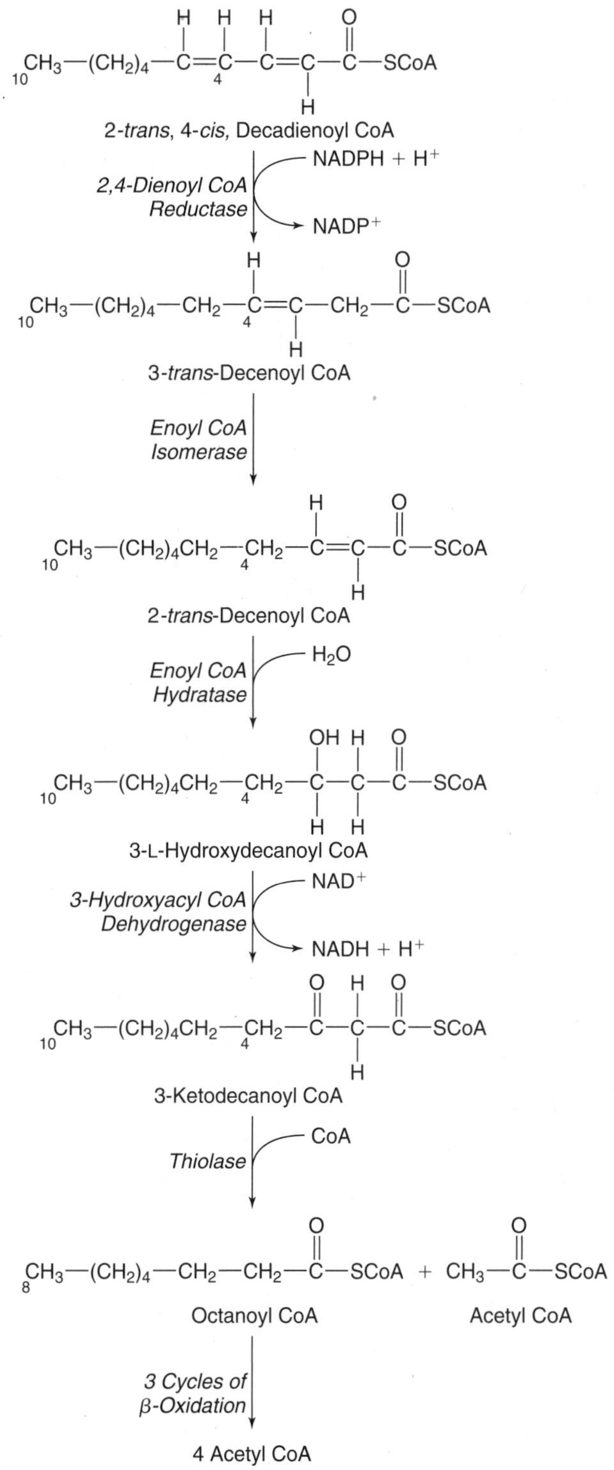

Figure 13–12 Continued.

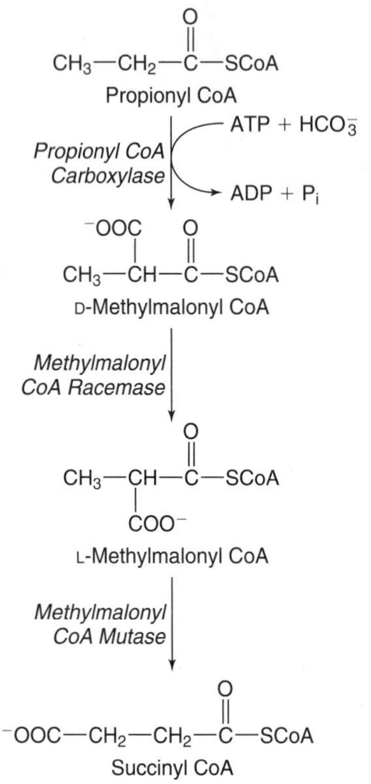

$$CH_3-CH_2-\overset{\overset{\displaystyle O}{\|}}{C}-SCoA$$

Propionyl CoA

Propionyl CoA Carboxylase

ATP + HCO_3^-

ADP + P_i

$$\underset{\underset{\displaystyle}{|}}{\overset{\overset{\displaystyle^-OOC}{|}}{CH_3}}-CH-\overset{\overset{\displaystyle O}{\|}}{C}-SCoA$$

D-Methylmalonyl CoA

Methylmalonyl CoA Racemase

$$CH_3-\underset{\underset{\displaystyle COO^-}{|}}{CH}-\overset{\overset{\displaystyle O}{\|}}{C}-SCoA$$

L-Methylmalonyl CoA

Methylmalonyl CoA Mutase

$$^-OOC-CH_2-CH_2-\overset{\overset{\displaystyle O}{\|}}{C}-SCoA$$

Succinyl CoA

Figure 13–13. *Propionate metabolism.*

cleavage are propionyl CoA and chain-shortened acyl CoA. The latter continues through additional cycles of β-oxidation. Propionyl CoA is metabolized to succinyl CoA as described earlier.

FORMATION OF KETONE BODIES FROM ACETYL CoA IN THE LIVER AS A FUEL FOR EXTRAHEPATIC TISSUES

In muscle and other nonhepatic tissues in any nutritional state, and in the liver in the well-fed state, acetyl CoA formed during the β-oxidation of fatty acid is oxidized to CO_2 and H_2O in the citric acid cycle. When the rate of mobilization of fatty acids from adipose depots is accelerated, as, for example, during starvation, the liver converts acetyl CoA generated from fatty acid oxidation into ketone bodies—acetoacetate and 3-hydroxybutyrate. The rate of formation of ketone bodies is directly proportional to the rate of fatty acid oxidation. Thus, when the rate of mobilization of fatty acids from adipose tissue is high, he-

patic fatty acid oxidation and production of acetoacetate and 3-hydroxybutyrate are high. Ketone bodies are "water-soluble" metabolites of fatty acids that are readily transported to other organs for oxidation to CO_2 and water.

Synthesis of Acetoacetate and 3-Hydroxybutyrate in Liver Mitochondria

Ketone bodies are synthesized in mitochondria. This is important because production of acetyl CoA, the substrate for synthesis of ketone bodies, occurs in the mitochondria via β-oxidation of fatty acids. Furthermore, initial steps for the de novo synthesis of cholesterol utilize some of the same reactions, but the enzymes for synthesis of cholesterol precursors are present in the cytosol of the liver. Differential localization permits independent regulation of ketone body and cholesterol synthesis.

The first step in ketone body synthesis is condensation of two molecules of acetyl CoA to form acetoacetyl CoA (Fig. 13–14). This reaction is catalyzed by β-ketothiolase:

Acetyl CoA + Acetyl CoA →
Acetoacetyl CoA + CoA

The second step involves condensation of a third molecule of acetyl CoA with acetoacetyl CoA to form 3-hydroxy-3-methylglutaryl CoA (HMG CoA). This reaction is catalyzed by HMG CoA synthase:

Acetyl CoA + Acetoacetyl CoA →
3-Hydroxy-3-Methylglutaryl CoA + CoA

In the third step of ketone body synthesis, HMG CoA is cleaved to acetoacetate and acetyl CoA in a reaction catalyzed by HMG CoA lyase.

3-Hydroxy-3-Methylglutaryl CoA →
Acetoacetate + Acetyl CoA

Both acetoacetate and 3-hydroxybutyrate are considered ketone bodies because they are rapidly interconverted via a reaction catalyzed by 3-hydroxybutyrate dehydrogenase. This NAD^+-requiring enzyme catalyzes a reversible reaction in which the concentrations

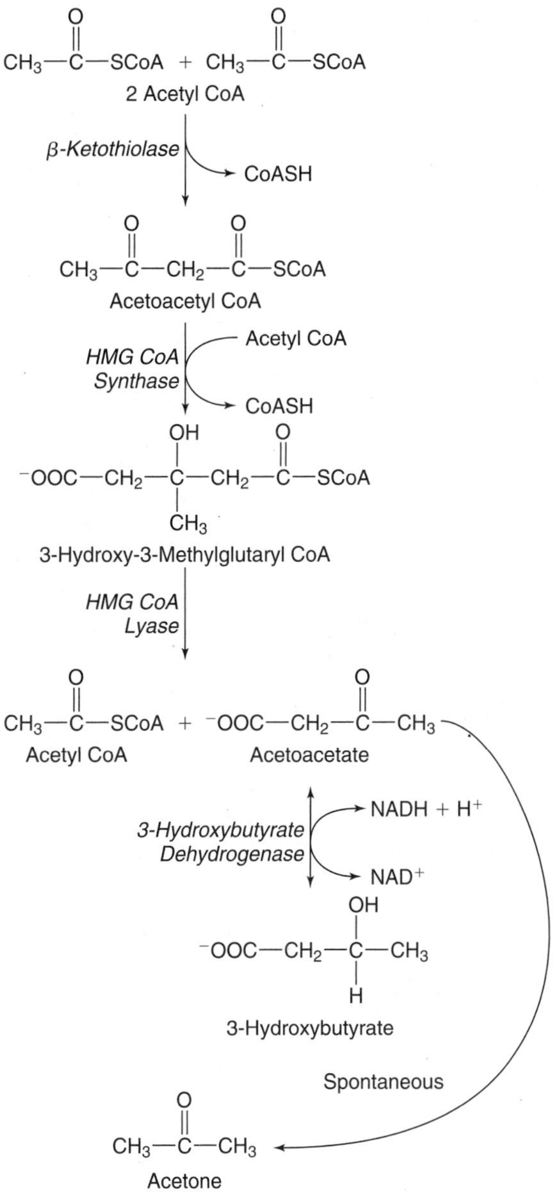

Figure 13–14. Ketone body formation.

of the products are nearly in thermodynamic equilibrium with NAD$^+$ and NADH in the mitochondria. Both acetoacetate and 3-hydroxybutyrate circulate in the blood. The ratio of their concentrations reflects the molar ratio of NAD$^+$ to NADH in liver mitochondria.

$$\text{Acetoacetate} + \text{NADH} + \text{H}^+ \leftrightarrow$$
$$\text{3-Hydroxybutyrate} + \text{NAD}^+$$

Of the two "ketone bodies," only one is a keto compound. So, how did these compounds become known as ketone bodies?

Acetoacetate decarboxylates slowly and spontaneously to acetone in the blood. When the plasma concentration of ketone bodies is very high—as in untreated diabetics—sufficient acetone accumulates in the blood to be detectable by a smell in the breath. This led early investigators to call the chemically uncharacterized material that accumlated in the blood of diabetics ketone bodies. The name has been retained even though we now know that acetone is only a minor component, and 3-hydroxybutyrate, a non-keto compound, is the major component.

Oxidation of Ketone Bodies in Peripheral Tissues

The liver produces ketone bodies, but it cannot utilize them because it lacks the mitochondrial enzyme succinyl CoA:3-ketoacid CoA transferase required for activation of acetoacetate to acetoacetyl CoA. High activity of the enzymes involved in ketone body formation and the lack of an enzyme required for its mitochondrial oxidation result in the net flow of ketone bodies from the liver to extrahepatic tissues for use as a fuel. The plasma concentration of albumin-bound fatty acids can increase from approximately 0.5 mmol/L to 2 mmol/L from the fed to fasting state. During prolonged starvation, glucose concentration can decrease from 5.5 mmol/L to 3.5 mmol/L. The concentration of ketone bodies is approximately 10 μmol/L in the fed state, and 0.1 mmol/L after an overnight fast, but can reach 2 mmol/L after 3 days of starvation or over 5 mmol/L after a week of starvation. At these increased concentrations, ketone bodies become effective fuels. In peripheral tissues such as muscle, ketone bodies are an important source of energy, especially when fatty acid mobilization has been activated. The brain also requires a large and constant source of energy. In the fed state, the brain depends exclusively on glucose for energy and cannot oxidize either fatty acids or ketone bodies. During starvation, however, ketone body metabolism is increased in the brain, and acetoacetate and 3-hydroxybutyrate become important sources of energy, sparing the limited sources of glucose. In untreated type I diabetes mellitus, ketosis (i.e., ketonemia and ketonuria) can occur. Because acetoacetic and 3-hydroxybutyric acids are moderately strong acids, ketonuria causes loss of sodium ions and metabolic acidosis, causing coma and death.

Both 3-hydroxybutyrate and acetoacetate diffuse into peripheral tissues along their concentration gradients. The rates of their metabolism are related directly to their concentration in the blood, which, in turn, are proportional to the rate of release of fatty acids from adipose tissue. The reaction pathway is shown in Figure 13–15. 3-Hydroxybutyrate must be converted to acetoacetate before

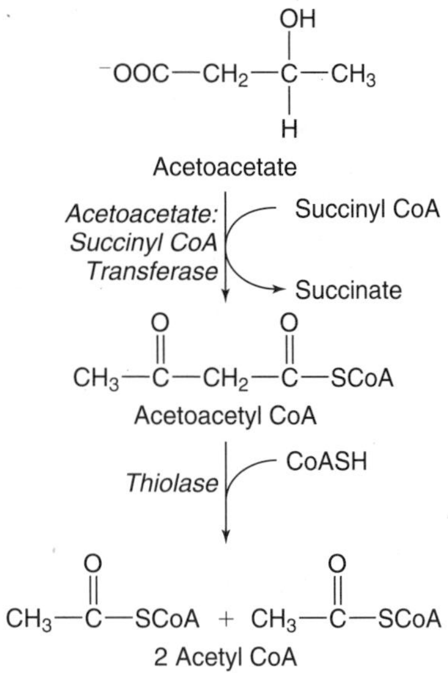

Figure 13–15. *Ketone body metabolism.*

it can be used. The same enzyme, 3-hydroxybutyrate dehydrogenase, that catalyzes interconversion of 3-hydroxybutyrate and acetoacetate in liver also does so in peripheral tissues. In peripheral tissues, acetoacetate is then activated to acetoacetyl CoA in a reaction catalyzed by acetoacetate:succinyl CoA transferase:

Acetoacetate + Succinyl CoA →
　　　　　Acetoacetyl CoA + Succinate

Acetoacetyl CoA is then cleaved to two molecules of acetyl CoA by the action of β-ketothiolase.

Acetoacetyl CoA → 2 Acetyl CoA

The reactions of ketone body metabolism are localized in mitochondria, so that the acetyl CoA that is formed enters the citric acid cycle and is oxidized to CO_2 and water.

Energy Yield from Oxidation of Palmitate via the Ketone Body Pathway

Oxidation of palmitoyl CoA to acetyl CoA in the liver will yield 8 acetyl CoA, 7 $FADH_2$, and 7 NADH and, therefore, a maximum of 35 mol of ATP per mole of palmitoyl CoA—as described earlier in this chapter. An additional

96 mol of ATP can be generated from the oxidation of the 8 mol of acetyl CoA in the mitochondria of peripheral tissues. However, ketone body utilization in extrahepatic tissues requires energy expenditure. Conversion of acetoacetate to 2 acetyl CoAs utilizes the equivalent of 1 ATP (succinate + CoA + GTP→succinyl CoA + GDP + P_i). The β-ketothiolase-catalyzed synthesis of 2 acetyl CoAs from 1 acetoacetyl CoA utilizes the energy released in the cleavage of the 4-carbon ketone body to drive synthesis of the second molecule of CoA derivative. The NADH used to reduce acetoacetate to 3-hydroxybutyrate in the liver is recovered in the peripheral organs when the 3-hydroxybutyrate is converted back to acetoacetate via the same reaction. The net result is utilization of 1 mol of ATP per mole of ketone body. Because there are 4 molecules of acetoacetyl group per molecule of palmitoyl CoA, oxidation of palmitoyl CoA via ketone body formation costs 4 mol of ATP per mole of palmitoyl CoA, resulting in a net production of a maximum of 125 mol of ATP instead of 129 mol of ATP per mole of palmitate oxidized.

Why has this apparently wasteful pathway of ketone body formation been preserved during evolution? A simple explanation is that the brain cannot metabolize fatty acids and therefore needs ketone bodies as a fuel during prolonged starvation. Moreover, by generating ketone bodies, the liver does not completely use the energy derived from fatty acids but distributes it as ketone bodies for other tissues to use during metabolic adaptation to starvation (or other dietary conditions that cause production and utilization of ketone bodies).

SYNTHESIS OF CHOLESTEROL FROM ACETYL CoA UNITS

Cholesterol is a sterol that is important as an essential structural component of cell membranes, as a precursor to the sex and adrenal steroid hormones, and as a precursor for the synthesis of bile acids. Moreover, isoprenoids, intermediates in the cholesterol biosynthetic pathway, also are used for production of small amounts of molecules that have important biological functions. These include dolichol re-quired for glycoprotein synthesis and ubiquinone (coenzyme Q) involved in electron transport in mitochondria. Isoprenoids also are used for posttranslational farnesylation or geranylgeranylation of specific proteins. Cholesterol itself also may be used for modification of specific proteins. Cholesterol is provided by foods of animal origin. In addition, de novo synthesis of cholesterol occurs in all nucleated cells, and its de novo synthesis is regulated by the availability of cholesterol in the blood. Quantitatively, the liver and intestine are the major sites of cholesterol synthesis. On average, cholesterol intake from the diet is about 0.6 g/day, whereas cholesterol from synthesis is about 1 g/day. Cholesterol homeostasis is discussed further in Chapters 14 and 41. The enzymes of cholesterol synthesis are extramitochondrial. Mevalonate and squalene are intermediates in the synthesis of cholesterol.

Conversion of Acetyl CoA to Mevalonate in the Cytosol

Synthesis of HMG CoA (Fig. 13–16) follows the same pathway described earlier for the synthesis of ketone bodies, except that it occurs in the cytosol instead of the mitochondria. Two molecules of acetyl CoA condense to form acetoacetyl CoA (acetyl CoA:acetoacetyl CoA acetyltransferase). Another molecule of acetyl CoA then condenses with a molecule of acetoacetyl CoA to form HMG CoA (HMG CoA synthase). HMG CoA is converted to mevalonate (Fig. 13–16) by HMG CoA reductase:

$$HMG\ CoA + 2\ NADPH + 2\ H^+ \rightarrow$$
$$Mevalonate + 2\ NADP^+ + CoA$$

This NADPH-requiring enzyme catalyzes the committed step in isoprenoid synthesis. It is the regulatory step in cholesterol biosynthesis and is highly regulated as described in the material that follows.

Synthesis of Squalene from Mevalonate

Mevalonate is converted to 3-phospho-5-pyrophosphomevalonate by three sequential phosphorylations (Fig. 13–17):

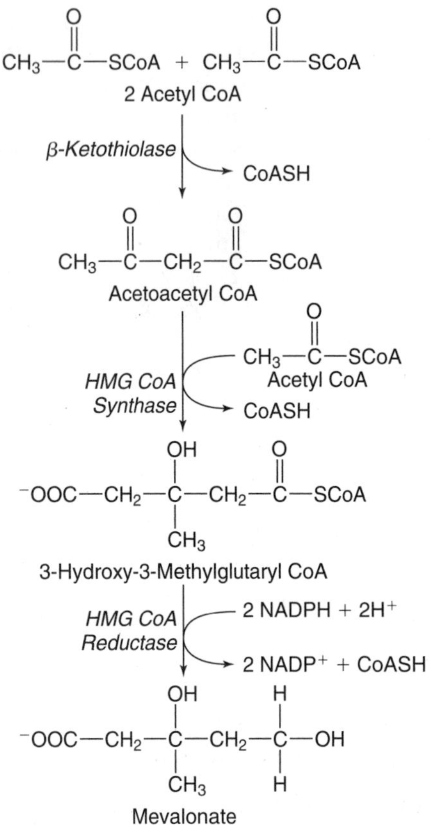

Figure 13–16. *Mevalonate biosynthesis.*

(1) Mevalonate + ATP →
$\qquad$ 5-Phosphomevalonate + ADP
(2) 5-Phosphomevalonate + ATP →
$\qquad$ 5-Pyrophosphomevalonate + ADP

Synthesis of isopentenyl pyrophosphate from 5-pyrophosphomevalonate involves the decarboxylation of 5-pyrophosphomevalonate and the hydrolysis of ATP:

(3) 5-Pyrophosphomevalonate
$\qquad$ + ATP → Isopentenyl Pyrophosphate
$\qquad\qquad$ + CO_2 + ADP + P_i

Squalene, and thus the sterol molecule, is built up from isopentenyl groups. The reaction sequence involves condensation of two 5-carbon molecules to form one of 10 carbons. A third 5-carbon molecule is added to form a 15-carbon intermediate. Two 15-carbon intermediates are linked to form the 30-carbon squalene (Fig. 13–18).

$$C5 \rightarrow C10 \rightarrow C15 \rightarrow C30$$

Formation of the 10-carbon geranyl pyrophosphate involves two enzymatic reactions. First, isopentenyl pyrophosphate isomerase catalyzes the isomerization of isopentenyl pyrophosphate to dimethylallyl pyrophosphate (Fig. 13–17). One molecule of each of these two activated isoprenes condenses. As shown in Figure 13–18, C-1 one of one isoprene bonds with C-5 of the other (head-to-tail) to form geranyl pyrophosphate:

Isopentenyl Pyrophosphate +
$\qquad$ Dimethylallyl Pyrophosphate →
$\qquad\qquad$ Geranyl Pyrophosphate + PP_i

In a mechanistically similar reaction, a third 5-carbon isopentenyl pyrophosphate condenses with geranyl pyrophosphate—in a head-to-tail manner—to form farnesyl pyrophosphate. Farnesyl pyrophosphate is a precursor of cholesterol, dolichol, ubiquinone, and the isoprenoid groups on a number of proteins and thus is located at a branch point in the synthesis of steroid and isoprenoid compounds. Squalene synthase, the next step in cholesterol biosynthesis is thus the committed step in sterol biosynthesis. This enzyme catalyzes the head-to-head condensation of two farnesyl pyrophosphates to form an intermediate, pre-squalene pyrophosphate. Presqualene pyrophosphate then undergoes NADPH-dependent reduction and pyrophosphate elimination to form squalene. Several further rearrangements, with lanosterol as one of the intermediates, convert the 30-carbon squalene to the 28-carbon cholesterol.

Earlier in this chapter, we noted that activation of fatty acids to their acyl CoA derivatives involved hydrolysis of ATP to AMP and PP_i. There are ubiquitous pyrophosphatases in cells, which then rapidly degrade PP_i to two inorganic phosphates. This biochemical mechanism is used to drive to completion several of the intermediate reactions in cholesterol biosynthesis.

Cholesterol synthesis is tightly regulated in cells. Along with the LDL receptor, the enzymes in the cholesterol biosynthetic pathway—HMG CoA synthase, HMG CoA re-

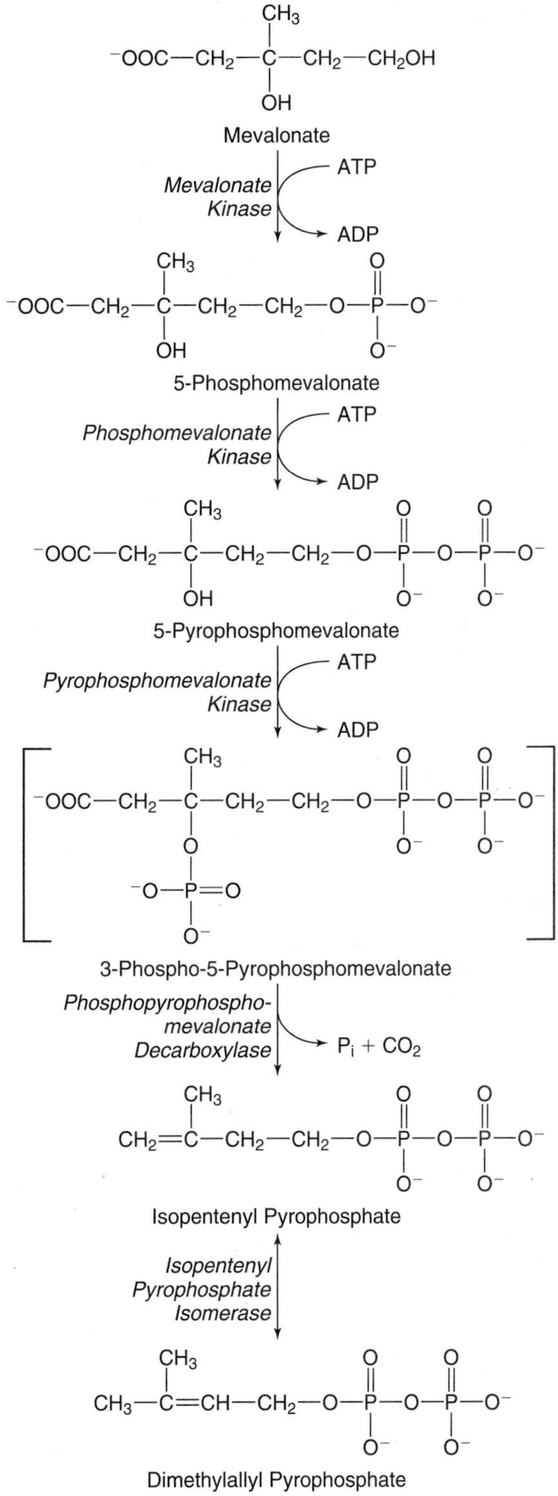

Figure 13–17. Synthesis of isoprenoid units.

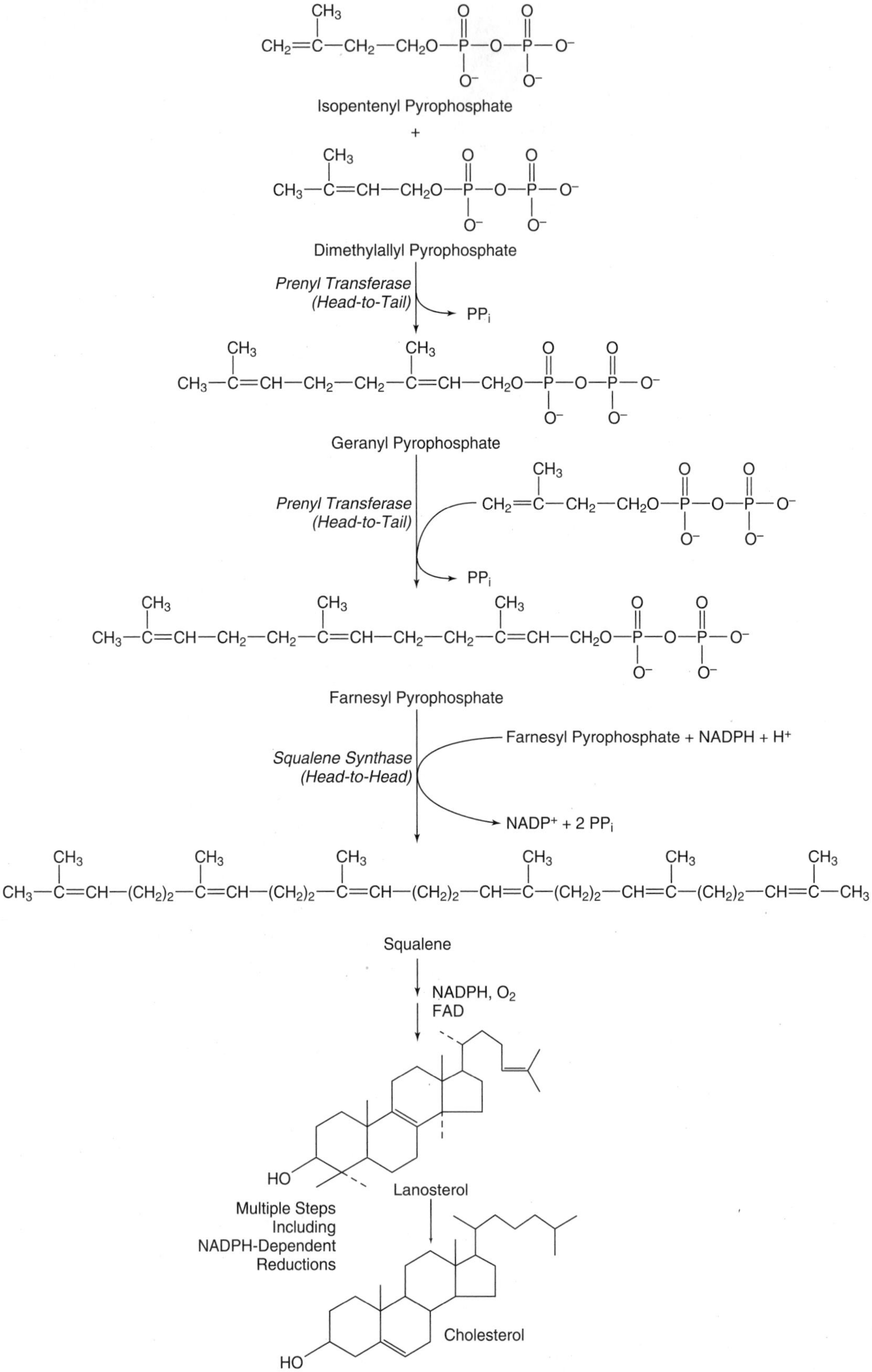

Figure 13–18. Synthesis of squalene and cholesterol.

ductase, farnesyl diphosphate synthase, and squalene synthase—are regulated coordinately at the transcriptional level. The primary target for regulation, however, is HMG CoA reductase, which catalyzes the main regulatory step in the overall cholesterol biosynthetic pathway. HMG CoA reductase is under negative feedback control by the immediate product, mevalonate, and by the eventual main product, cholesterol. The principal mechanism involves regulation of the number of enzyme molecules per cell, which, in turn, is regulated at several levels: transcription of the gene, stability of the mRNA, translation of the mRNA, and stability of protein. Moreover, the activity of HMG CoA reductase also is regulated by a phosphorylation-dephosphorylation mechanism, which explains why it responds faster than could be accounted for by changes in the concentration of HMG CoA reductase.

PHOSPHATIDATE AND DIACYLGLYCEROL AS PRECURSORS OF PHOSPHOLIPIDS

Phospholipids are amphipathic lipids that contain acyl groups esterified to the *sn*-1 and *sn*-2 positions of the glycerol moiety. The amphipathic nature of phospholipids makes them suitable for their roles as components of membranes and as surfactants. They contain

NUTRITION INSIGHT

Regulation of Gene Transcription by Cholesterol

In the 1930s, Schoenheimer and Breusch demonstrated that mice synthesize less cholesterol when fed a diet containing cholesterol. In the 1950s, it was shown that cholesterol synthesis from [^{14}C]acetate in liver in vitro was suppressed profoundly by feeding cholesterol to the donor animal. Cholesterol inhibits expression of HMG CoA reductase, the key regulatory enzyme in cholesterol biosynthesis. It also decreases expression of other enzymes in the cholesterol biosynthetic pathway: HMG CoA synthase and farnesyl pyrophosphate synthase. Expression of the LDL receptor, a protein that mediates cholesterol uptake by the cell, also is inhibited. Thus, cholesterol acts as an end-product feedback inhibitor.

How do cells monitor the cellular levels of cholesterol, a lipid present in cell membranes? Brown and Goldstein and their collaborators (1997) have elucidated the mechanism by which sterols regulate transcription. Members of a novel family of membrane-bound transcription factors called sterol regulatory element–binding proteins (SREBPs) bind to a specific sequence in the 5′-flanking region of sterol-regulated genes. SREBPs belong to the family of basic helix-loop-helix-zipper proteins. In addition to DNA binding and transcription activation domains, SREBPs contain two hydrophobic transmembrane domains. These hydrophobic domains anchor SREBPs in the plasma membrane. When the amino-terminal region containing the DNA binding and activation domains is released from the membrane, SREBPs can enter the nucleus and regulate transcription. Proteolytic cleavage is regulated by a cholesterol-sensing transmembrane protein that binds to SREBPs. High cholesterol levels inhibit this cleavage and release of SREBP and prevent activation of the transcription of sterol-responsive genes.

Cholesterol is one of the most investigated of all small molecules; investigators of cholesterol metabolism have received 13 Nobel prizes since 1928, including one awarded to Brown and Goldstein in 1985 for their work on the LDL receptor. During studies of the enzymes in the cholesterol synthetic pathway, potent inhibitors of HMG CoA reductase, including compactin and mevinolin, were isolated from fungi; some of these inhibitors are effective therapeutic agents that lower blood cholesterol levels and thus cholesterol-induced coronary heart disease. Compactin and mevinolin are structurally similar to HMG CoA and mevalonate and inhibit HMG CoA reductase competitively. Inhibition of HMG CoA reductase decreases the cellular sterol concentration, which, in turn, causes cleavage of the SREBP and activation of sterol-responsive genes. Understanding regulation of transcription by cholesterol will undoubtedly bring new therapeutic strategies in the future.

an alcohol in the sn-3 position that is linked to the diacylglycerol by a phosphodiester bond. In eukaryotic phospholipids, the most common alcohols are choline, ethanolamine, serine, glycerol, and inositol. The number of different molecular species of phospholipids is enormous because the long-chain fatty acyl groups in the sn-1 or sn-2 positions can vary in length and degree of unsaturation. Synthesis of triacylglycerols and phospholipids follows a common pathway up to the diacylglycerol stage. In this section, the reactions that occur in higher animals are described (Vance and Vance, 1996; van den Bosch and Vance, 1997). Most of the reactions occur in the ER, as do those of triacylglycerol biosynthesis.

Synthesis of Phosphatidylcholine from Activated Choline and Diacylglycerol

Phosphatidylcholine (lecithin) is the most abundant phospholipid in eukaryotic cells. Choline from the diet is phosphorylated to phosphocholine by choline kinase (Fig. 13–19). Choline kinase also uses ethanolamine as a substrate. This lack of substrate specificity suggests that it is not a regulatory step but may serve as a means of trapping choline inside the cell.

$$\text{Choline} + \text{ATP} \rightarrow \text{Phosphocholine} + \text{ADP}$$

Phosphocholine then reacts with cytidine triphosphate (CTP) to yield the activated form of

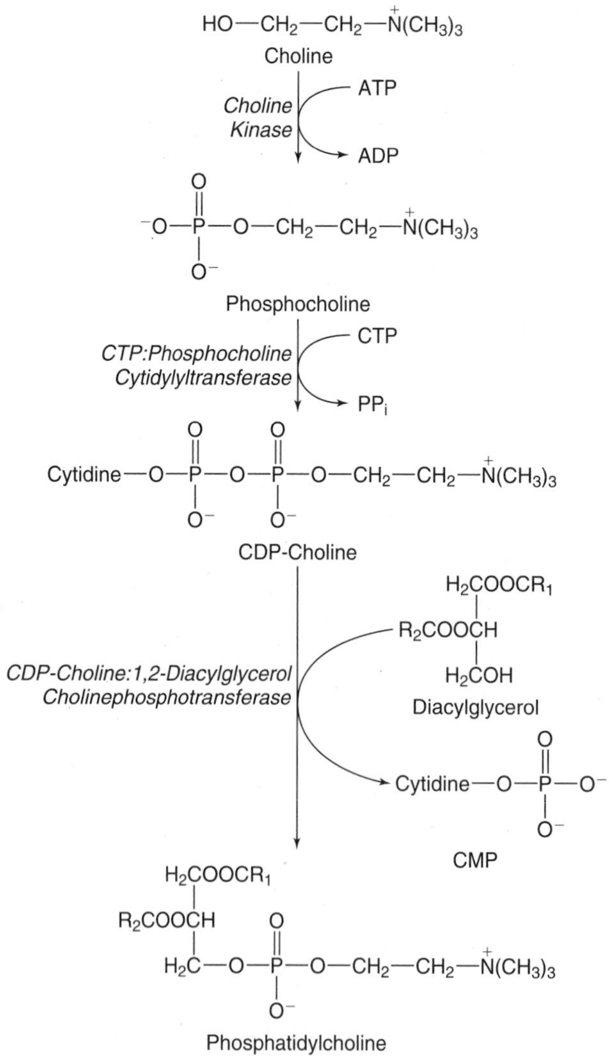

Figure 13–19. Phosphatidylcholine synthesis from choline and diacylglycerol. R_1COOH and R_2COOH represent fatty acids.

choline, cytidine diphosphate (CDP)-choline. The other product, pyrophosphate, is rapidly degraded to two inorganic phosphates by the ubiquitous pyrophosphatase. As noted before, this assures that the reaction will proceed in the direction of CDP-choline synthesis. The enzyme, CTP:phosphocholine cytidylyltransferase catalyzes this reaction:

$$\text{Phosphocholine} + \text{CTP} \rightarrow \text{CDP-Choline} \\ + \text{PP}_i$$
$$\text{PP}_i + \text{H}_2\text{O} \rightarrow 2\,\text{P}_i$$

Cytidylyltransferase catalyzes the main regulatory step in this pathway and is found in both soluble and membrane fractions. The enzyme requires phospholipid for activity so translocation between the ER membrane (with phospholipid, active enzyme) and the cytosol (no phospholipid, inactive enzyme) is a regulatory mechanism. Diacylglycerol and phosphatidylcholine are potential feedforward (positive) and feedback (negative) regulators of cytidylyltransferase activity, respectively.

In the final reaction in this pathway, CDP-choline reacts with diacylglycerol to form phosphatidylcholine (CDP-choline:1,2-diacylglycerol cholinephosphotransferase):

$$\text{CDP-choline} + \text{Diacylglycerol} \rightarrow \\ \text{Phosphatidylcholine} + \text{CMP}$$

The enzyme catalyzing this reaction is localized in the ER and does not appear to be limiting for phosphatidylcholine synthesis.

Phosphatidylcholine also is formed from phosphatidylethanolamine (Fig. 13–20). The three methyl groups are donated by S-adenosylmethionine in a series of three reactions catalyzed by phosphatidylethanolamine N-methyltransferase:

$$3\ S\text{-Adenosylmethionine} + \\ \text{Phosphatidylethanolamine} \rightarrow \\ 3\ S\text{-Adenosylhomocysteine} + \\ \text{Phosphatidylcholine}$$

Normal diets provide sufficient choline. In humans, choline cannot be synthesized directly but is produced indirectly via the foregoing phosphatidylethanolamine N-methyltransferase reaction. The metabolism of choline, methionine, and folate is closely interrelated. The three methyl groups of choline can be made available for 1-carbon metabolism upon conversion of choline to betaine. One-carbon metabolism is discussed in detail in Chapter 21. In malnutrition, when stores of choline, methionine, and folate are depleted, or in total parenteral nutrition, choline may become deficient. Carbohydrate loading, due to enhanced hepatic triacylglycerol synthesis, also increases the amount of choline required. Phosphatidylcholine is required for lipoprotein synthesis and secretion. In choline deficiency, biosynthesis of phosphatidylcholine is inhibited, causing development of fatty liver.

Pathways for the Synthesis of Phosphatidylethanolamine and Phosphatidylserine

The first and most prevalent pathway for synthesis of phosphatidylethanolamine is de novo synthesis. This pathway involves phosphorylation of ethanolamine which is catalyzed by choline kinase, the same enzyme that is involved in the synthesis of phosphatidylcholine. The remainder of the pathway is also similar to that for the de novo pathway for synthesis of phosphatidylcholine (see Fig. 13–19). Ethanolamine reacts with CTP to produce its activated form, CDP-ethanolamine (CTP:ethanolaminephosphate cytidylyltransferase). Reaction of CDP-ethanolamine with diacylglycerol forms phosphatidylethanolamine (CDP-ethanolamine:1,2-diacylglycerol ethanolaminephosphotransferase).

In addition, there are two pathways for synthesis of phosphatidylethanolamine via modification of preexisting phospholipids. First, phosphatidylserine decarboxylase catalyzes the decarboxylation of phosphatidylserine to form phosphatidylethanolamine (Fig. 13–20):

$$\text{Phosphatidylserine} + \text{H}^+ \rightarrow \\ \text{Phosphatidylethanolamine} + \text{CO}_2$$

The second route involves an exchange reaction with phosphatidylserine in which phosphatidylserine reacts with ethanolamine to form phosphatidylethanolamine and serine.

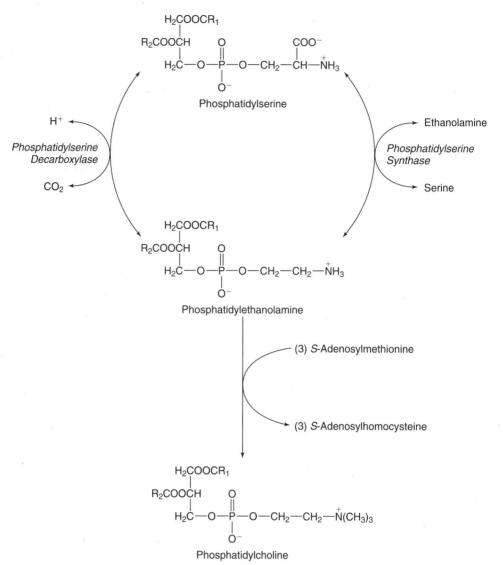

Figure 13–20. *Synthesis of phosphatidylcholine from phosphatidylethanolamine and interconversion of phosphatidyl-serine and phosphatidylethanolamine. R_1 and R_2 represent fatty acid chains.*

The reaction is catalyzed by phosphatidylserine synthase (Fig. 13–20):

$$\text{Phosphatidylserine} + \text{Ethanolamine} \leftrightarrow$$
$$\text{Phosphatidylethanolamine} + \text{Serine}$$

Phosphatidylserine constitutes only 5% to 15% of phospholipids in cells. Although the CDP-diacylglycerol pathway, similar to that described in the next section for phosphatidylglycerol, is used in de novo synthesis of phosphatidylserine in bacteria, the enzyme catalyzing the reaction of CDP-diacylglycerol

and serine does not appear to be present in mammalian tissue. Instead, phosphatidylethanolamine or phosphatidylcholine reacts with serine to undergo base exchange to form phosphatidylserine and ethanolamine (phosphatidylserine synthase) or choline.

CDP-Diacylglycerol as an Intermediate in the Synthesis of Phosphatidylglycerol and Diphosphatidylglycerol

In this pathway, CTP is used to activate diacylglycerol to CDP-diacylglycerol. Pyrophosphate is the other product in this reaction catalyzed by phosphatidate cytidylyltransferase. Cleavage of the resulting pyrophosphate drives the reaction toward completion:

Diacylglycerol + CTP → CDP-Diacylglycerol + PP_i
$$PP_i + H_2O → 2 P_i$$

In the next reaction, CDP-diacylglycerol reacts with sn-glycerol 3-phosphate to form phosphatidylglycerol phosphate and CMP. The reaction is catalyzed by glycerophosphate phosphatidyltransferase (Fig. 13–21):

CDP-Diacylglycerol + sn-Glycerol 3-Phosphate →
Phosphatidylglycerol Phosphate + CMP

In the second step, phosphatidylglycerol phosphate phosphatase catalyzes hydrolysis of phosphate from phosphatidylglycerol phosphate to form phosphatidylglycerol:

Phosphatidylglycerol Phosphate →
Phosphatidylglycerol + P_i

Finally, another molecule of CDP-diacylglycerol reacts with phosphatidylglycerol to form diphosphatidylglycerol and CMP (Fig. 13–21, reaction catalyzed by phosphatidate phosphatidyltransferase). Diphosphatidylglycerol (cardiolipin) is synthesized exclusively in the mitochondria and is found only in these organelles. Cardiolipin is rich in unsaturated 18-carbon fatty acids such as oleate and linoleate.

Phosphatidylglycerol + CDP-Diacylglycerol →
Diphosphatidylglycerol + CMP

CDP-Diacylglycerol as an Intermediate in Inositol Phospholipid Synthesis

Inositol reacts with CDP-diacylglycerol to form phosphatidylinositol in a reaction localized in the ER and catalyzed by phosphatidylinositol synthase:

Inositol + CDP-Diacylglycerol →
Phosphatidylinositol + CMP

The inositol phospholipids (Fig. 13–22) are constituents of membranes. A small portion of the phosphatidylinositols that are phosphor-

ylated serve as precursors to the important intracellular second messengers diacylglycerol and inositol polyphosphates as described later. Phosphatidylinositol phosphate and phosphatidylinositol bisphosphate are formed by the sequential addition of phosphate using ATP; the reactions are catalyzed by phosphatidylinositol kinase and phosphatidylinositol phosphate kinase, respectively. Several inositol polyphosphates with more than three phosphates can be derived from the inositol triphosphate released by the hydrolysis of phosphatidylinositol bisphosphate catalyzed by phospholipase C. The additional phosphorylations of inositol triphosphate to form polyphosphates are catalyzed by kinases that use free inositol polyphosphates as substrates.

Ether-Linked Lipids

There are two major classes of ether-linked lipids in the cells. Glycerol ethers have O-alkyl groups; plasmalogens have O-alk-1-enyl groups. In each case, the ether linkage is to the sn-1 position. Some ether-linked lipids have potent biological activity. Platelet activating factor, 1-alkyl-2-acetyl-sn-glycerol 3-phosphocholine, for example, causes aggregation of blood platelets at concentrations as low as 10^{-11} mol/L. Plasmalogens, the other class of ether-linked lipids, constitute about 5% to 20% of the phospholipids of cell membranes; that they are important is suggested by the plasmalogen deficiency described later. The exact biological function(s) of these compounds is not known. Plasmalogen is especially abundant in nervous tissue and in the membranes of the myelin sheath; for example, ethanolamine plasmalogen may represent as much as 80% of phospholipids in the myelin sheath membranes. Elevated levels of choline plasmalogens are found in heart tissue.

One of the substrates for the synthesis of ether-linked lipids is a fatty alcohol. This compound is produced from acyl CoA in a reaction that requires NADPH. This reaction involves an aldehyde intermediate and is catalyzed by a membrane-associated acyl CoA reductase:

(1) Acyl CoA + NADPH + H^+ →
Fatty Aldehyde + $NADP^+$ + CoA
(2) Fatty Aldehyde + NADPH + H^+ →
Fatty Alcohol + $NADP^+$

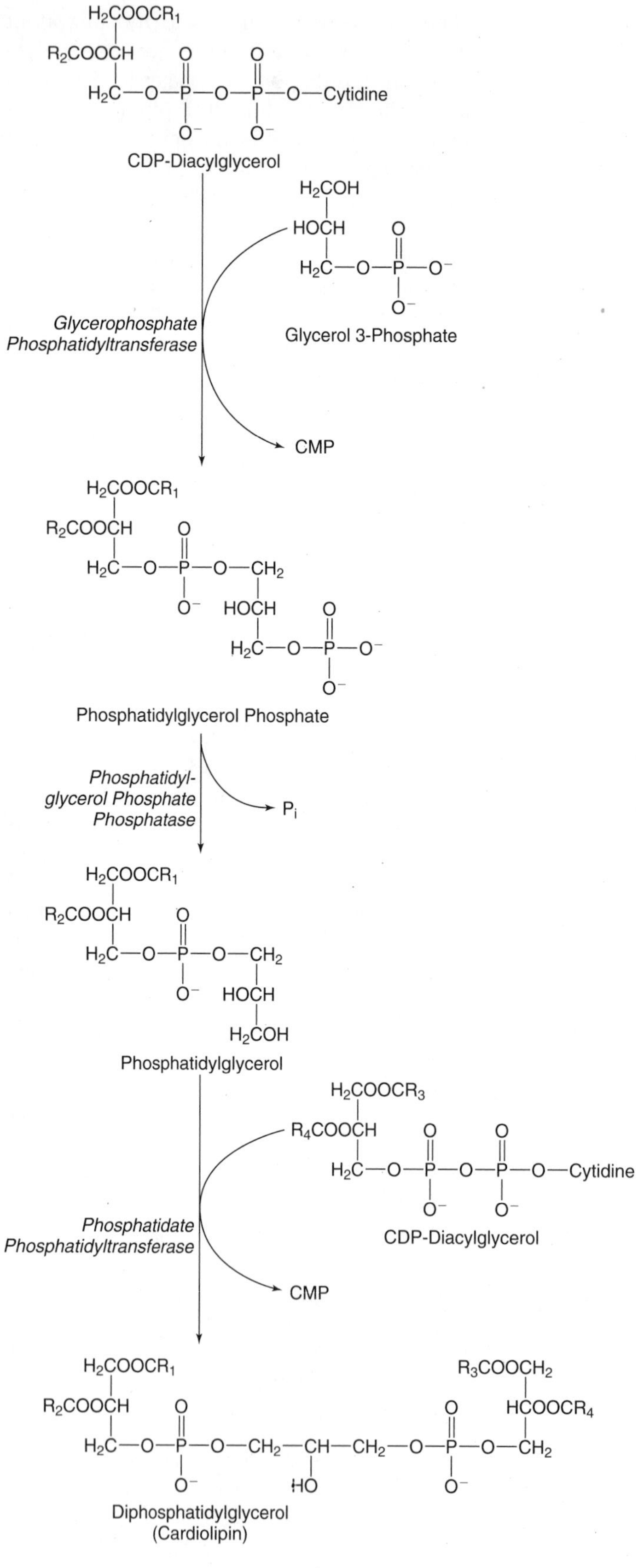

Figure 13–21. Synthesis of phosphatidylglycerol and cardiolipin. Fatty acids are represented as R_1COOH, R_2COOH, R_3COOH, and R_4COOH.

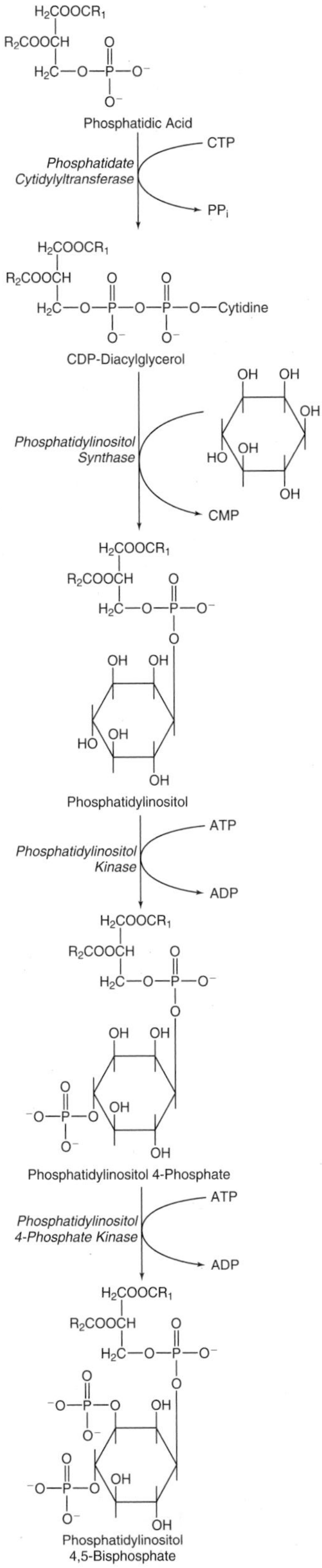

Figure 13–22. Inositol phospholipid synthesis.

The other substrate for synthesis of ether-linked lipids is 1-acyldihydroxyacetone phosphate. This is produced by the dihydroxyacetone phosphate acyltransferase that was described in the section on synthesis of triacylglycerol:

Dihydroxyacetone Phosphate +
Fatty Acyl CoA →
1-Acyldihydroxyacetone Phosphate + CoA

In triacylglycerol synthesis, the next step is reduction of the keto group to a hydroxyl group to form lysophosphatidic acid. In ether-lipid synthesis the next step is an exchange reaction with a fatty alcohol to produce 1-alkyldihydroxyacetone phosphate in a reaction catalyzed by 1-alkyldihydroxyacetone phosphate synthase (Fig. 13–23):

1-Acyldihydroxyacetone Phosphate +
Fatty Alcohol →
1-Alkyldihydroxyacetone Phosphate +
Fatty Acid

This reaction is specific for a substrate with a ketone function. Synthesis of ether lipids thus utilizes only the dihydroxyacetone phosphate pathway. The next reaction is a reduction of the keto group of alkyldihydroxyacetone phosphate to yield alkylglycerol 3-phosphate. This reaction is catalyzed by NADPH-dependent alkyldihydroxyacetone phosphate reductase. This reductase is capable of reducing both acyl and alkyl analogs of dihydroxyacetone phosphate.

1-Alkyldihydroxyacetone Phosphate +
$NADPH + H^+$ → 1-Alkylglycerol
3-Phosphate + $NADP^+$

In the next reaction, the alkyl analog of phosphatidic acid is synthesized by adding an acyl group to the *sn*-2 position. This reaction is catalyzed by 1-alkylglycerol phosphate acyltransferase:

1-Alkylglycerol 3-Phosphate + Acyl CoA →
1-Alkyl-2-Acylglycerol 3-Phosphate + CoA

The next step in this pathway creates an alkyl-acylglycerol by dephosphorylation. This com-

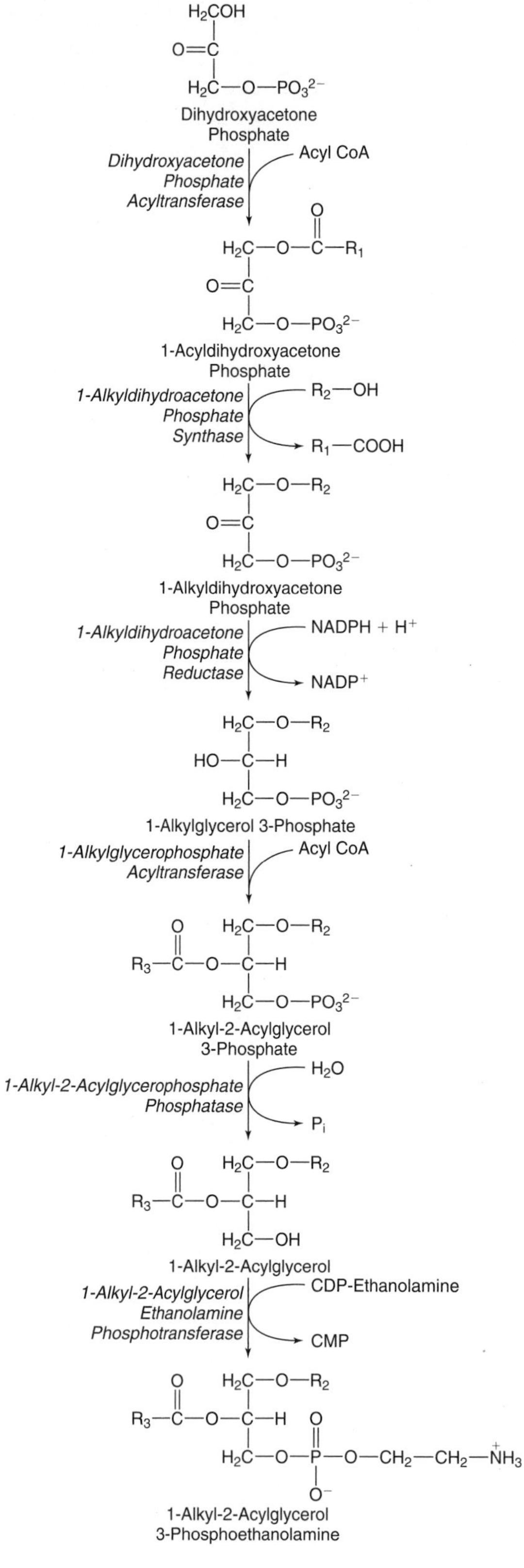

Figure 13–23. Ether-lipid synthesis. R_1COOH represents a fatty acid, and R_2OH represents a fatty alcohol.

pound represents a branch point in ether lipid synthesis in much the same way as diacylglycerol is at a branch point for synthesis of triacylglycerol and glycerophospholipids.

1-Alkyl-2-Acylglycerol 3-Phosphate +
$\quad$ H_2O → 1-Alkyl-2-Acylglycerol + P_i

Next, analogous to the reactions that form phosphatidylethanolamine or phosphatidylcholine, an alcohol base is transferred to 1-alkyl-2-acylglycerol from CDP-ethanolamine or CDP-choline:

1-Alkyl-2-Acylglycerol +
CDP-Ethanolamine → 1-Alkyl-2-Acylglycerol
$\quad\quad\quad$ 3-Phosphoethanolamine + CMP

Plasmalogens are formed by desaturation of the alkyl moiety of the ethanolamine or choline derivative to form an O-alk-1-enyl substituent. Platelet activating factor is synthesized from 1-alkyl-2-acetylglycerol and is 1-alkyl-2-acetyl-glycerol 3-phosphocholine.

The enzymatic reaction that creates the double bond in 1-alkyl-2-acylglycerol 3-phosphoethanolamine is unusual in that the intact phospholipid is the substrate for the desaturase. Fatty acyl groups are usually desaturated prior to making them part of more complex lipids. Δ1-Alkyl desaturase behaves like a typical acyl CoA desaturase; it is a mixed function oxidase that requires oxygen, NADH, cytochrome b_5 reductase, and a terminal desaturase protein (see Fig. 13–5, which illustrates a similar reaction mechanism for stearoyl CoA desaturase).

Dihydroxyacetone phosphate acyltransferase and 1-alkyldihydroxyacetone phosphate synthase catalyze the first two reactions in ether-lipid biosynthesis and are localized in peroxisomes. One of the manifestations of Zellweger's syndrome, a block in peroxisome biogenesis, is decreased tissue plasmalogen levels, and these deficiencies may contribute to pathological features of this disease, including profound neurological deficits and death within the first year of life. Some types of β-oxidation of fatty acids, including oxidation of very long-chain fatty acids, polyunsaturated fatty acids, and dicarboxylic fatty acids, occur in peroxisomes. Zellweger patients, therefore, show both accumulation of very long-chain fatty acids and decreased plasmalogen levels.

Remodeling of Phospholipids in Situ

The phospholipid composition of different cellular membranes is usually specific for each organelle. Differences involve both the fatty acyl groups in the sn-1 and sn-2 positions and the alcohol base on the sn-3 position. In general, the sn-1 position of phospholipids contains saturated fatty acids, whereas the sn-2 position contains unsaturated fatty acids. However, dietary content of fatty acids influences fatty acid composition of phospholipids. The specificity of insertion of fatty acids at the sn-1 and sn-2 positions is usually determined by the specificities of glycerol 3-phosphate acyltransferase and 1-acylglycerol 3-phosphate acyltransferase. An additional mechanism for generating and/or maintaining these specific compositions is to remove acyl groups from phospholipids through the action of phospholipases and to reesterify with a specific acyl group. The abundance of polyunsaturated fatty acids at the sn-2 position is due to phospholipid remodeling. The alcohol bases also can be rearranged when a specific phospholipase generates diacylglycerol or phosphatidic acid.

The phospholipases that cleave acyl groups or alcohol bases can be put into five groups, based on the specific phospholipid bond that they attack (Fig. 13–24). Phospholipases A and B are acyl hydrolases. Phospholipase A_1 cleaves the ester bond between the sn-1 position and its acyl group, generating 2-acylglycerol 3-phospholipid. Phospholipase A_2 attacks the ester bond between the sn-2 position and its acyl group, generating 1-acylglycerol 3-phospholipid. Phospholipase B cleaves the ester bonds at either the sn-1 or sn-2 position but is relatively rare. Phospholipases C and D are phosphodiesterases. Phospholipase C cleaves the bond between the sn-3 position and the phosphate (glycerophosphate bond) and encompasses a family of enzymes that generate diacylglycerol and the free phosphorylated alcohol as products. Phospholipase D attacks the bond between the alcohol base and the glycerol phosphate.

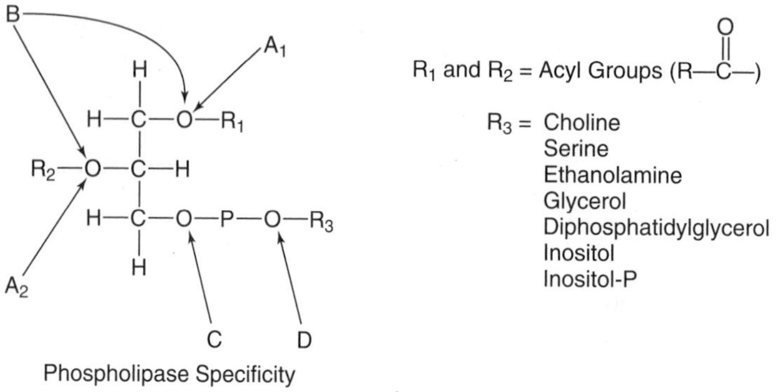

Phospholipase Specificity

R_1 and R_2 = Acyl Groups $(R—\overset{\overset{\displaystyle O}{\|}}{C}—)$

R_3 = Choline
Serine
Ethanolamine
Glycerol
Diphosphatidylglycerol
Inositol
Inositol-P

Figure 13–24. *Phospholipase specificity.*

Generation of Signaling Molecules by Regulated Phospholipases

In addition to the remodeling of molecular species of membrane lipids, some of the phospholipases play important roles in cell signaling. When certain hormones or growth factors occupy their cell surface receptors, phosphoinositide-specific plasma membrane phospholipase Cs are activated. The reaction catalyzed by phospholipase C generates the second messengers inositol 1,4,5-triphosphate and diacylglycerol, which cause Ca^{2+} release and activation of protein kinase C, respectively. This mechanism is discussed in more detail in Chapters 15 and 16. Inositol polyphosphates and diacylglycerol are recycled, and recycling accomplishes two purposes. First, it ends the action of the second messenger. Second, it regenerates the substrates upon which phospholipase can act. Thus, specific phosphatases remove the phosphates, ultimately yielding free inositol. Diacylglycerol can be converted to phosphatidic acid via the action of diacylglycerol kinase, or it can react with CDP-inositol to form phosphatidylinositol or with other compounds activated with CDP to yield other phospholipids. Lithium, a drug that is used to treat bipolar disorders, exerts its therapeutic effects by inhibiting hydrolysis of inositol monophosphate to inositol. This depletes the intracellular supply of inositol and therefore interrupts the phosphatidylinositol signaling pathway, which is presumably hyperactive in bipolar disorders.

Phospholipase A_2 also can be activated by extracellular stimuli, including local mediators, by a receptor-mediated process. Arachidonic acid released by phospholipase A_2 can

be used for synthesis of prostaglandins and thromboxanes via the cyclooxygenase pathway, and leukotrienes via the lipoxygenase pathway (see Chapter 15 for further discussion of these eicosanoids). Antiinflammatory corticosteroids induce an inhibitory protein for phospholipase A_2, lipocortin, and thereby decrease arachidonic acid release.

SPHINGOLIPIDS AS STRUCTURAL AND SIGNALING MOLECULES

More than 300 structurally distinct sphingolipids occur in nature. The hydrophobic portion of sphingolipids is ceramide; ceramide contains a fatty acid that is amide-linked to sphingosine or a related sphingoid base. Sphingolipids also contain a hydrophilic moiety, usually phosphocholine (sphingomyelin) or one or more sugar residues (cerebrosides and gangliosides). Sphingolipids play both structural and regulatory roles. Ceramide and sphingosine likely play important physiological roles in intracellular signaling (Ghosh et al., 1997; Spiegel et al., 1996). Numerous gangliosides are displayed on the external face of mammalian cells and probably play roles in recognition of other cells and basement membranes. Many bacteria have developed specific adhesion mechanisms that recognize and result in their binding to specific gangliosides. Further evidence for the importance of these compounds is the inherited mutations in the pathway for degradation of sphingolipids that result in the accumulation of specific gangliosides, cerebrosides, and ceramides. These lipid accumulations account for the pathologies of several lipid storage diseases.

Ceramide, the Precursor of Most Mammalian Sphingolipids

Enzymes involved in the synthesis of ceramide are localized in the ER. In the first reaction, palmitoyl CoA reacts with serine to form 3-ketosphinganine. This reaction requires pyridoxal phosphate (vitamin B_6 coenzyme) for decarboxylation and is catalyzed by serine palmitoyltransferase (Fig. 13–25):

Palmitoyl CoA + Serine →
$\qquad$ 3-Ketosphinganine + CoA + CO_2

The next reaction is a reductase that requires NADPH and converts the keto group at C-3 of the long-chain base to a hydroxyl, forming sphinganine (dihydrosphingosine):

3-Ketosphinganine + NADPH + H^+ →
$\qquad$ Sphinganine + $NADP^+$

Addition of a long-chain acyl group to sphinganine to produce dihydroceramide is catalyzed by ceramide synthase:

Sphinganine + Fatty Acyl CoA→
$\qquad$ Dihydroceramide + CoA

Finally, dihydroceramide is converted to ceramide by the introduction of a 4,5-*trans*-double bond. Ceramide is the precursor of all complex sphingolipids.

Sphingomyelin

Sphingomyelin is the only major sphingolipid that contains phosphate. Sphingomyelin is synthesized when ceramide reacts with phosphatidylcholine to form sphingomyelin and diacylglycerol (Fig. 13–26).

Ceramide + Phosphatidylcholine →
$\qquad$ Sphingomyelin + Diacylglycerol

Sphingomyelin is hydrolyzed by sphingomyelinase to produce ceramide and phosphocholine. Ceramide is hydrolyzed by ceramidase to produce the sphingoid base sphingosine. Activations of sphingomyelinase and ceramidase are linked to activation of cell surface receptors that initiate multiple cellular responses. Ceramide acts as a second messenger in a signaling cascade regulating cell growth and differentiation, cellular functions, and programmed cell death. Sphingosine also activates or inhibits a number of cellular events.

Gangliosides and Sulfatoglycosphingolipids

Gangliosides are built up from cerebroside by the addition of sugars. The neutral glycosphingolipids galactosylceramide and glucosylceramide are intermediates in the synthesis of more complex gangliosides and sulfatoglycosphingolipids. They are formed by the reaction of ceramide with uridine diphosphate (UDP)-galactose or UDP-glucose to form the corresponding cerebroside and UDP (Fig. 13–26):

Ceramide + UDP-Glucose →
$\qquad$ Cerebroside + UDP

Gangliosides are created by adding one or more sugars to the nonreducing end of the carbohydrate moiety of cerebroside or of the growing carbohydrate chain. The sugar donors are nucleotide diphosphate sugars. The "terminal" sugar of all gangliosides is *N*-acetyl neuraminic acid. Specific glycosyl transferases catalyze these reactions.

Galactocerebroside 3-sulfate is a major sulfolipid. It is synthesized by the reaction of galactosyl ceramide with 3'-phosphoadenosine-5'-phosphosulfate (PAPS). PAPS is a common donor of sulfate groups in the synthesis of sulfated compounds.

Degradation of Gangliosides by Specific Lysosomal Exoglycosidases

Specific acid hydrolases localized in lysosomes degrade plasma membrane–bound and extracellular gangliosides. The pathway for this sequential removal of sugars has been worked out based on the metabolic consequences of known genetic defects in humans that are often manifested in childhood. In Tay-Sachs, Fabry's, Sandhoff's, and Gaucher's diseases, specific gangliosides accumulate because degradation of a specific ganglioside is blocked while synthesis and the initial steps of

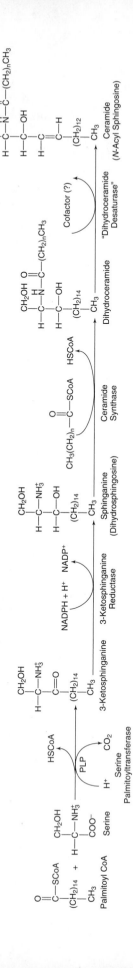

Figure 13-25. *Ceramide synthesis.*

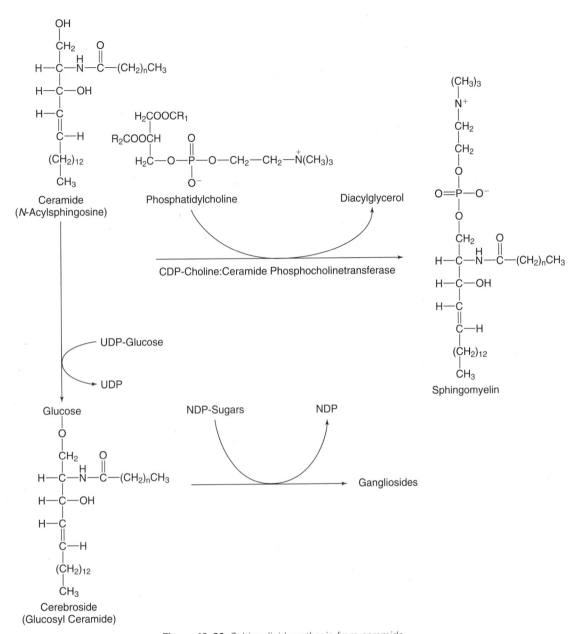

Figure 13–26. *Sphingolipid synthesis from ceramide.*

degradation occur at normal rates. Abnormal accumulations of these lipids, particularly in nervous tissues, cause the pathologies of these diseases, including mental retardation.

Lysosomal defects in acid ceramidase (Farber's lipogranulomatosis) and acid sphingomyelinase (Niemann-Pick disease) result in tissue accumulation of ceramide and sphingomyelin, respectively, and metabolic disturbances. Acid ceramidase catalyzes the hydro-

lysis of ceramide to release sphingosine and long-chain fatty acid. Acid sphingomyelinase catalyzes the degradation of sphingomyelin to form ceramide plus phosphocholine. All these defects are lysosomal disorders of sphingolipid catabolism. Nonlysosomal ceramidases and sphingomyelinases with neutral to alkaline pH optima probably are involved in turnover of ceramide and sphingomyelin, respectively, for cell signaling.

REFERENCES

Brown, M. S. and Goldstein, J. L. (1997) The SREBP pathway: Regulation of cholesterol metabolism by proteolysis of a membrane-bound transcription factor. Cell 89:331–340.

Eaton, S., Bartlett, K. and Pourfarzam, M. (1996) Mammalian mitochondrial β-oxidation. Biochem J 320:345–357.

Ghosh, S., Strum, J. C. and Bell, R. M. (1997) Lipid biochemistry: Functions of glycerolipids and sphingolipids in cellular signaling. FASEB J 11:45–50.

Goldberg, I. J. (1996) Lipoprotein lipase and lipolysis: Central roles in lipoprotein metabolism and atherogenesis. J Lipid Res 37:693–707.

Hellerstein, M. K., Schwartz, J.-M. and Neese, R. A. (1996) Regulation of hepatic de novo lipogenesis in humans. Annu Rev Nutr 16:523–557.

McGarry, J. D. and Brown, N. F. (1997) The mitochondrial carnitine palmitoyltransferase system. From concept to molecular analysis. Eur J Biochem 244:1–14.

Hillgartner, F. B., Salati, L. M. and Goodridge, A. G. (1995) Physiological and molecular mechanisms involved in nutritional regulation of fatty acid synthesis. Physiol Rev 75:47–76.

Scriver, C. R., Beaudet, A. L., Sly, W. S. and Valle, D. (eds.) (1995) The Metabolic and Molecular Bases of Inherited Disease, 7th ed. McGraw-Hill, New York.

Spiegel, S., Foster, D. and Kolesnick, R. (1996) Signal transduction through lipid second messengers. Curr Opin Cell Biol 8:159–167.

van den Bosch, H. and Vance, D. E. (eds.) (1997) Phospholipid biosynthesis: Current status of the Kennedy and related pathways. Biochim Biophys Acta 1348:1–256.

Vance, D. E. and Vance, J. (1996) Biochemistry of Lipids, Lipoproteins, and Membranes; New Comprehensive Biochemistry, Vol 31. Elsevier Science B.V., New York.

RECOMMENDED READINGS

Brown, M. S. and Goldstein, J. L. (1997) The SREBP pathway: Regulation of cholesterol metabolism by proteolysis of a membrane-bound transcription factor. Cell 89:331–340.

Hillgartner, F. B., Salati, L. M. and Goodridge, A. G. (1995) Physiological and molecular mechanisms involved in nutritional regulation of fatty acid synthesis. Physiol Rev 75:47–76.

Vance, D. E. and Vance, J. (1996) Biochemistry of Lipids, Lipoproteins, and Membranes; New Comprehensive Biochemistry, Vol 31. Elsevier Science B.V., New York.

CHAPTER 14

◆ ◆

Lipoprotein Synthesis, Transport, and Metabolism

Christopher J. Fielding, Ph.D.

OUTLINE

COMMON ABBREVIATIONS

Apo A-I (apolipoprotein A-I)
Apo B (apolipoprotein B)
Apo C-II (apolipoprotein C-II)
Apo E (apolipoprotein E)
CETP (cholesteryl ester transfer protein)
HDL (high density lipoprotein)
IDL (intermediate density lipoprotein)
LCAT (lecithin:cholesterol acyltransferase)
LDL (low density lipoprotein)
LPL (lipoprotein lipase)
PLTP (phospholipid transfer protein)
VLDL (very low density lipoprotein)

CLASSIFICATION OF PLASMA LIPOPROTEINS

As discussed in Chapters 7 and 13, the small intestine and the liver package triacylglycerol, cholesteryl ester, cholesterol, and phospholipid along with certain apolipoproteins into large lipoprotein particles, nascent chylomicrons, or nascent very low density lipoproteins (VLDL), respectively, for transport in the circulation. These lipoprotein particles contain many molecules of triacylglycerol, cholesteryl ester, cholesterol, and phospholipid and smaller numbers of various apolipoproteins. Chylomicrons secreted by the intestine following a fat-containing meal can have average molecular weights more than 100 times those of the VLDL secreted by the liver. Once the nascent lipoproteins enter the plasma, they pick up additional apolipoproteins (such as apo C and apo E lipoproteins) to become circulating or mature chylomicrons and VLDL. Products of chylomicron and VLDL metabolism in the plasma (i.e., chylomicron remnants; intermediate density lipoproteins, IDL; and low density lipoproteins, LDL) are smaller and denser, largely due to the loss of triacylglycerol from the core of the lipoprotein complexes. Nascent high density lipoproteins (HDL) are involved in chylomicron and VLDL metabolism as well as in cholesterol transport. HDL originate from the liver and intestine, which synthesize apolipoproteins A-I and A-II, but unlike VLDL and LDL, HDL are also regenerated in the plasma.

Plasma lipoproteins can be separated by ultracentrifugation or electrophoresis, giving rise to nomenclature based on their density or electrophoretic migration. Density is inversely proportional to the percentage lipid content of the lipoproteins, with HDL being denser than VLDL, for example. In electrophoresis, lipoprotein complexes are separated based on their charge to mass ratio, with alpha-migrating particles (HDL) migrating farther and beta-(LDL) or prebeta- (VLDL) particles migrating less distance.

The lipoproteins found in normal plasma are listed in Table 14–1. The most abundant of the circulating lipoproteins are HDL and LDL. As shown in Table 14–1, plasma lipoproteins generally may be grouped into two classes of particles by the presence of an essential apolipoprotein: the apolipoprotein A-I (apo A-I)-containing lipoproteins and the apolipoprotein B (apo B)-containing lipoproteins (Fielding and Fielding, 1996).

The presence of apo A-I identifies HDL particles. HDL are small particles (mainly 9 to 12 nm in diameter) with a "core" of cholesteryl esters and a small amount of triacylglycerol and a surface composed of free cholesterol, phospholipid (particularly phosphatidyl choline, commonly called lecithin), and protein. The amino acid sequence of apo A-I includes a series of amphipathic helical repeats, each containing 22 amino acids. Lipid-binding, hydrophobic amino acids are preferentially localized to one face of the helix, and charged and other hydrophilic residues are mostly confined to the other.

These amphipathic helical repeats are located on the surface of the HDL particles. Their hydrophobic face is turned toward the lipid core of the HDL lipoprotein particle, while the hydrophilic face is turned out to the aqueous medium. Individual helical repeats within the apo A-I sequence are separated by helix-breaking prolyl or glycyl residues. There are no cystine cross-links in apo A-I, and its free energy of denaturation (~2 kcal/mole) is small. This means the apo A-I polypeptide is flexible, and its association with the surface of HDL is relatively weak. As a result, the shape of apo A-I on the surface of HDL can adapt as the lipid core of the particle expands, and lipid-free or lipid-poor apo A-I easily dissociates from the surface of HDL if the diameter of the HDL particles is reduced by loss of core lipids (triacylglycerol, cholesteryl ester).

Many HDL particles contain smaller amounts of other apolipoproteins in addition to apo A-I (i.e., apo A-II, apo A-IV, apo C-I, apo C-III, and apo E). The functions of several of these proteins are clearly established, and their mechanisms of lipid binding are similar to that described for apo A-I. In addition to being an essential structural component of HDL, apo A-I promotes the desorption of free cholesterol from cell membranes, and it activates cholesterol esterification in plasma. These activities also depend on one or more of the lipid-binding helical repeats of this apolipoprotein.

TABLE 14–1
Classification of Plasma Lipoproteins

Major Lipoproteins		Other Major Apolipoproteins	Density (g/mL)
Apo B-48 lipoproteins:	chylomicrons	Apo C-II, apo C-III, apo E	<1.00
Apo B-100 lipoproteins:	VLDL	Apo C-II, apo C-III, apo E	<1.006
	IDL	Apo E	1.006–1.019
	LDL	None	1.019–1.063
Apo A-I lipoproteins:	prebeta-HDL	None	>1.21
	alpha-HDL	Apo A-II	1.063–1.21

The apo B–containing lipoproteins include chylomicrons and VLDL and their circulating lipoprotein lipolysis products (remnants). Each VLDL particle contains a single copy of the 4536 amino acid (512 kDa) form of apo B polypeptide (apo B-100). IDL and LDL are formed in the circulation as lipolysis products of VLDL. As a result, these particles also contain one copy of apo B-100. In spite of its high molecular mass, apo B makes only a single turn around the circumference (~75 nm) of an LDL particle. Other apolipoproteins adsorbed to the VLDL surface, including both lipase cofactors (apo C-II) and cellular receptor ligands (apo E), increase the stability of these large particles, regulate the catabolism of VLDL lipids, and control the removal of partially lipolyzed VLDL particles (IDL) from the circulation.

Chylomicrons contain one copy of a shortened (2152 amino acid, 241 kDa) form of apo B (apo B-48). This is a product of the same apo B gene responsibile for apo B-100, generated as the result of a posttranscriptional modification of the apo B-100 messenger RNA (mRNA) base sequence by an intestine-specific cytosine deaminase, which converts cytosine to uracil. A new stop signal is introduced half-way through the sequence. Essentially all the apo B secreted in chylomicrons by the human intestine is apo B-48, whereas essentially all the apo B secreted in VLDL by the human liver is apo B-100. This tissue specificity is less complete in other mammals. For example, liver of rats and mice secretes VLDL-sized particles containing either apo B-100 or apo B-48.

The large apo B-48 and B-100 polypeptides, like apo A-I, contain stretches of amphipathic helix, but these helical regions form a smaller proportion of the whole sequence in apo B than in apo A-I. Apo B-100 contains at least 11 cystine bridges. Most of these are present in the N-terminal half of the polypeptide. Overall, apo B is more hydrophobic than apo A-I. It does not dissociate during the metabolism of VLDL to IDL and LDL. Apo B plays an essential role in VLDL and chylomicron secretion, in the binding of triacylglycerol-rich lipoproteins to the capillary endothelium prior to lipolysis, and in the removal of apo B-100–containing lipoprotein particles from the circulation (Hussain et al., 1996). The amino acid sequence that binds to the high-affinity apo B (LDL) receptor of liver cells is in the C-terminal half of apo B-100, which is absent from apo B-48. Whereas the removal of VLDL remnants by the liver is mediated by apo B, the removal of chylomicron remnants is mediated mainly by apolipoprotein E (apo E), using the same receptor (Cooper, 1997). An earlier report of a distinct hepatic apo E receptor has not been confirmed. A small proportion of chylomicron remnants may be internalized via an LDL receptor-like protein (LRP).

Plasma normally contains a relatively large amount of apo B-100 and only a very small amount of apo B-48. Most of the apo B-100 is in LDL, with only small amounts in IDL and VLDL. About 5% to 10% of the total apo B in plasma is in the VLDL. An even smaller proportion is present in the IDL, which are normally present at low concentration. The reason for this distribution of lipids is that chylomicrons and VLDL are rapidly catabolized by lipases, and chylomicron remnants are effectively removed via hepatic receptors. Some VLDL are removed as remnants (IDL), but most are converted to LDL, which have a much longer circulation time (~2 days) than lighter apo B–containing lipoproteins. As a result, even though only one LDL particle is formed per VLDL particle, there are many more LDL than VLDL particles in normal plasma.

The contributions of the major lipoprotein fractions to the triacylglycerol and total cholesterol content of normal plasma are shown in Table 14–2.

SYNTHESIS AND SECRETION OF PLASMA LIPOPROTEINS

Long-chain free (unesterified) fatty acids, absorbed by the apical microvilli of mucosal cells in the duodenum and ileum, are reesterified within these enterocytes prior to their secretion as triacylglycerol in chylomicrons. Although mucosal cells can somewhat modify the composition of the saturated fatty acids present in secreted triacylglycerol, the fatty acid composition of chylomicron triacylglycerol closely resembles that of the dietary lipids. Dietary free cholesterol internalized from the intestinal lumen by the mucosal cell is almost completely esterified prior to its secretion in chylomicrons. Free cholesterol present in newly synthesized chylomicrons appears to represent small amounts of free cholesterol synthesized within the mucosal cell, together with some preformed free cholesterol transferred from the basolateral membrane of intestinal cells or from other lipoproteins present in the interstitial fluid.

Intestinal cells store apo B-48, the structural protein of chylomicrons, in the form of lipid-poor precursor particles. These intracellular precursor particles contain most of the cholesteryl ester of mature chylomicrons and a much smaller proportion of their triacylglycerol. The initial addition of triacylglycerol to chylomicron precursor particles requires a triacylglycerol transfer protein that is found in the endoplasmic reticulum (ER). A second step of triacylglycerol addition, which leads to the formation of mature, triacylglycerol-rich chylomicrons, is considered to be independent of this transfer protein. It is not clear whether this second step involves triacylglycerol transfer under the influence of a second, unidentified transfer protein, or whether fusion takes place between precursor particles containing apo B-48 and preformed triacylglycerol-rich lipid droplets; the first mechanism appears more likely on thermodynamic grounds. Nascent chylomicrons, assembled within the Golgi apparatus, are released from the enterocyte as mature Golgi vesicles fuse with the basolateral region of the plasma membrane. These newly secreted particles enter the lymphatic system via the lacteals of the intestinal villi and subsequently enter the venous plasma compartment via the left thoracic lymph duct.

The assembly of VLDL within the hepatocyte follows a parallel course, although with some important differences. A comparable two-step assembly process takes place, with the formation of precursor particles containing apo B-100, cholesteryl ester, and some triacylglycerol (Thompson et al., 1996). The measurement of equal contents of cholesteryl esters (relative to apo B-100) in nascent triacylglycerol-rich VLDL and in smaller VLDL produced by lipolysis in plasma suggests that most of the cholesteryl ester in human VLDL originates in the liver.

The second step of VLDL assembly involves the addition of triacylglycerol to precursor particles in the ER, probably by molecular transfer. Whereas triacylglycerol in chylomicrons originates mainly from the dietary fat, some of the fatty acids in the triacylglycerol in VLDL are synthesized de novo from dietary carbohydrate. VLDL triacylglycerol secretion and circulating concentrations both increase

---

TABLE 14–2
Distribution of Triacylglycerol and Cholesterol Among Fasting Plasma Lipoproteins

	Cholesterol	Triacylglycerol
	(mg/100 mL plasma)	
Plasma	176.4 ± 20 (100%)	84.9 ± 19.1 (100%)
VLDL	9.1 ± 3.7 (5.1%)	46.5 ± 12.8 (54.8%)
IDL	3.5 ± 4.3 (1.9%)	5.8 ± 6.2 (6.6%)
LDL	114.8 ± 28 (65.1%)	15.9 ± 8.8 (18.7%)
HDL	45.3 ± 11.8 (25.7%)	12.2 ± 1.6 (14.3%)

Recalculated from Fielding, P. E. and Fielding, C. J. (1966) Dynamics of lipoprotein transport in the circulatory system. In: Biochemistry of Lipids (Vance, D. E. and Vance, J., eds.), pp. 495–516. Elsevier Science-NL, Amsterdam: Adapted with kind permission from Elsevier Science-NL.

after a carbohydrate-rich meal. Other fatty acids in triacylglycerol of VLDL originate from long-chain free fatty acids internalized from plasma by the liver. The proportions of fatty acids in newly secreted VLDL that are contributed by new synthesis or by recycling probably vary widely among individuals and under different conditions.

CLEARANCE OF TRIACYLGLYCEROL IN CHYLOMICRONS AND VLDL BY LIPOPROTEIN LIPASE

Most cholesteryl ester and triacylglycerol are concentrated in the core of plasma lipoprotein particles, but this core is in rapid equilibrium with small amounts of the same lipids dissolved within the surface monolayer, which is made up mainly of phospholipid and free cholesterol. The hydrolysis or transfer of triacylglycerol on apo B lipoproteins by plasma lipases and transfer proteins directly depletes only the surface pool, but the surface lipids are replenished by equilibration from the core of the particle. Lipoprotein lipase (LPL) is a triacylglycerol hydrolase present on the capillary endothelium of various tissues, with highest concentrations present in muscle and adipose tissues. Molecules of LPL protein, synthesized by the parenchymal cells of these tissues, migrate to the vascular face of the endothelial cells, where they are anchored by glycosaminoglycans (Braun and Severson, 1992). Only the endothelial fraction of adipose or muscle tissue LPL is directly involved in triacylglycerol lipolysis.

Chylomicrons and VLDL are competitive substrates for lipoprotein lipase bound to the endothelial surface of adipose and muscle tissues. Much of the free fatty acid produced by lipolysis is internalized locally, though some escapes into the general circulation. In fasting plasma, the VLDL (hepatic) triacylglycerol concentration is relatively low and chylomicron (intestinal) triacylglycerol almost absent. During fasting, the expression of lipoprotein lipase in adipose tissue, which is insulin-dependent, is downregulated, while levels of LPL in heart and other muscle tissues are maintained. Lipoprotein lipase on the capillary endothelial surface of the heart has a

higher affinity (lower K_m) for lipoprotein substrate than does lipoprotein lipase in the adipose tissue. This difference in affinity of lipoprotein lipase for lipoprotein substrate may provide a mechanism for the self-regulation of the partitioning of lipoprotein triacylglycerol uptake between storage in adipose tissue and oxidation in muscle tissues.

According to this model, triacylglycerol hydrolysis by the vascular bed of the heart would be determined mainly by lipoprotein lipase levels, because its lipoprotein lipase has a low K_m and as a result is saturated at low circulating VLDL concentrations. In contrast, in adipose tissue, where the apparent K_m exceeds normal circulating triacylglycerol concentrations, triacylglycerol hydrolysis also would be influenced by VLDL and chylomicron concentrations. In this way, the energy needs of muscle cells utilizing triacylglycerol fatty acids (such as those of the heart) would receive priority, particularly during fasting, whereas adipose tissue would reesterify and store most of the excess fatty acids resulting from hydrolysis of lipoprotein triacylglycerol by adipose endothelial lipoprotein lipase after a fatty meal. These stores can be liberated, during extended periods of exercise or fasting, by activation of adipose tissue hormone-sensitive lipase, as described in Chapter 13.

The hydrolysis of triacylglycerol by lipoprotein lipase depends on the presence of its activator/co-protein (apo C-II) on the surface of chylomicron and VLDL particles. Apo C-II preferentially equilibrates from other lipoproteins (e.g., HDL) onto newly secreted VLDL and chylomicrons as these particles are released into the plasma.

The later metabolism of chylomicrons and VLDL differs in significant aspects (Goldberg, 1996). As the chylomicron triacylglycerol is hydrolyzed by lipoprotein lipase and the chylomicron remnant decreases in size, apo C-II dissociates from its surface. After ~80% of the initial triacylglycerol has been lost, insufficient apo C-II remains to support lipoprotein lipase activity. The remaining triacylglycerol, together with most of the chylomicron cholesteryl ester, is removed by the liver.

VLDL, IDL, and LDL make up a lipolysis cascade, as illustrated in Figure 14–1. All LDL in the plasma are formed from the catabolism

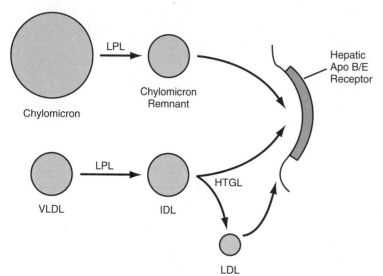

Figure 14–1. *Catabolism of apolipoprotein B–containing lipoproteins in human plasma. LPL, lipoprotein lipase; HTGL, hepatic triacylglycerol lipase.*

of VLDL and IDL, but not all VLDL become LDL. As VLDL triacylglycerol is catabolized, apo C-II dissociates, as it does from chylomicrons, leaving a VLDL remnant or IDL that still contains both apo B-100 and apo E. Part of this IDL is cleared via hepatocyte LDL receptors, but the rest of the IDL particles lose their apo E, along with additional lipid, at the hepatocyte surface. The product of this reaction is released back into the circulation as LDL. The details and regulation of the conversion of IDL to LDL are still not fully understood, but hepatic triacylglycerol lipase activity at the endothelial surface of the liver is probably involved. This enzyme, structurally related to the lipoprotein lipases found in muscle and adipose tissue, also plays an important role in hydrolyzing HDL triacylglycerol and probably HDL phospholipid.

ROLE OF HDL AND LECITHIN: CHOLESTEROL ACYLTRANSFERASE IN PLASMA CHOLESTEROL METABOLISM

About 95% of HDL consists of spherical particles with a hydrophobic lipid core; these are called α-HDL because they display α-electrophoretic migration. Most of these particles contain apo A-II, a small protein implicated in HDL turnover, as well as apo A-I. A small proportion of spherical HDL also contains other proteins (including apo C-II and apo E)

whose main functions are in the metabolism of plasma VLDL and chylomicron triacylglycerol. The rest of the HDL are very small particles (6 to 7 nm in diameter) that, unlike α-HDL, lack a significant lipid core. These HDL have preβ-electrophoretic migration and are called preβ- or lipid-poor HDL.

Preβ-HDL can be formed from spherical HDL by several reactions, all of which reduce the surface to volume ratio of the particle. Reduction of HDL core volume leads to dissociation of some of the apo A-I, probably as a complex with a small amount of phospholipid (Barrans et al., 1996). The hydrolysis of HDL triacylglycerol by hepatic triacylglycerol lipase, the activity of plasma phospholipid transfer protein (PLTP), and a hepatic cell-surface receptor SR-BI (scavenger receptor BI) that selectively internalizes HDL cholesteryl esters all probably contribute to preβ-HDL formation. As shown in Figure 14–2, preβ-HDL (molecular mass: 65 to 70 kDa) cross the endothelium freely. Preβ-HDL are enriched in the extracellular fluid of peripheral tissues, compared with the larger, spherical, α-migrating HDL, most of which have a molecular mass of 180 to 250 kDa. Preβ-HDL are exceptionally active as acceptors of free cholesterol and phospholipid from the parenchymal cells of extrahepatic tissues (Fielding and Fielding, 1995a). Many peripheral tissues are rich in caveolae. These small cell-surface indentations appear to represent a major loca-

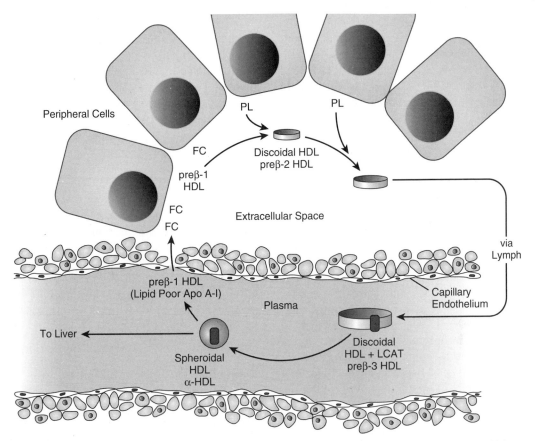

Figure 14–2. *The HDL cycle. Lipid-poor apo A-I (preβ HDL) passes through the vascular bed to the interstitial space and accumulates free cholesterol (FC) and phospholipid (PL) from the parenchymal cells of peripheral tissues. The discoidal HDL formed reenter the plasma compartment via the lymph. Free cholesterol in HDL is esterified by LCAT (lecithin:cholesterol acyltransferase) as HDL discs become spheres. After hepatic triacylglycerol lipase and/or cholesteryl ester transfer protein (CETP) activity, preβ HDL or lipid-poor apo A-I is released for recycling. (Modified from Fielding, C. J. and Fielding, P. E. [1995] Molecular physiology of reverse cholesterol transport. J Lipid Res 36:211–228.)*

tion from which free cholesterol in these tissues is transferred to preβ-HDL (Fielding and Fielding, 1995a). Other cells directly secrete complexes of apo E, cholesterol, and phospholipid. Additionally, some cholesterol may transfer by simple diffusion from the cell surface to lipoprotein acceptors, particularly HDL.

Within the extracellular space, the small preβ-HDL become enlarged into disc-shaped particles by the continuing transfer of lecithin and free cholesterol from cell membranes. Discoidal HDL formed in this way reenter the plasma via the main lymph trunks. Within the plasma compartment, discoidal HDL react with lecithin:cholesterol acyltransferase (LCAT). The LCAT reaction in plasma:

Free Cholesterol + Lecithin →
Lysolecithin + Cholesteryl Ester

generates the spherical α-migrating particles that make up the majority of plasma HDL. The transfer of phospholipid out of tissues is much slower than that of free cholesterol. As a result, much of the lecithin needed for the LCAT reaction may come from apo B-100–containing lipoproteins (VLDL, IDL, and LDL) in a reaction catalyzed by PLTP.

About one third of LCAT-derived cholesteryl ester is transferred from HDL to apo B-100–containing lipoproteins through the action of the plasma cholesteryl ester transfer protein (CETP). The optimal substrate of CETP (i.e., the recipient of the cholesteryl ester) appears to be an apo B-100–containing parti-cle with a density on the IDL-LDL boundary, but some HDL-derived cholesteryl ester is also transferred to VLDL. Triacylglycerol is moved from the apo B-100–containing particle to HDL in exchange for the cholesteryl ester. Although the CETP reaction is an integral part of the normal reaction sequences by which the composition and properties of HDL and LDL are determined, it is unlikely that CETP by itself generates preβ-HDL. The molecular volumes of cholesteryl ester and of triacylglyc-erol, which replaces it in HDL, are similar. CETP-mediated exchange would not modify the core volume of HDL appreciably, unless this was followed by hepatic lipase-mediated hydrolysis of HDL triacylglycerol.

Most of the rest of the cholesteryl ester generated by LCAT activity is selectively inter-nalized from HDL by hepatocytes, and to a lesser extent by adrenal and gonadal cells, via the scavenger receptor SR-BI (Acton et al., 1996). These cells use the HDL cholesteryl ester for bile acid or steroid hormone synthe-sis.

REMOVAL OF PLASMA LIPOPROTEINS BY RECEPTOR-MEDIATED PROCESSES

Lipoprotein synthesis and removal rates have an impact on steady-state fasting levels of the major lipoprotein classes. Available evidence strongly suggests that hepatic lipoprotein re-ceptors normally play the major role in re-moval of lipoprotein remnants and LDL and, hence, in regulation of human plasma choles-terol levels (Spady et al., 1993).

Chylomicron remnants, VLDL remnants (IDL), and LDL are all removed via the high-affinity LDL receptor, which recognizes both apo B-100 and apo E. By far the greatest num-ber of functional LDL receptors is expressed in the liver. Smaller amounts are expressed by adrenal and gonadal cells. Functional LDL receptors are essentially absent from other tis-sues. Because the circulating concentration of apo B lipoproteins exceeds that required for saturation of the high-affinity LDL receptor, the rate of internalization of LDL by the liver is determined by the amount of LDL receptors rather than by the concentration of LDL.

There is also considerable nonspecific (receptor-independent) uptake of intact LDL particles by the liver. This nonspecific pathway predominates when circulating LDL levels are high. The detailed mechanism for the nonspe-cific uptake of LDL by the liver remains to be determined.

HDL particles containing apo E, which make up only a small proportion of apo A-I–containing lipoproteins, are also recognized and internalized by the LDL receptor. There is insufficient evidence to show that this path-way is an important element of total HDL clearance in normal human plasma. Most HDL protein is removed from the circulation as lipid-poor or lipid-free apo A-I. The kidney seems to play a major role; radioactivity is found in urine following the injection of isoto-pically labeled apo A-I in HDL into human subjects.

POSTPRANDIAL LIPOPROTEIN METABOLISM

The concentration and proportions of plasma lipoproteins following an overnight (16-h) fast are often used as a baseline state from which the effects of postprandial lipemia can be determined. The proportions and types of di-etary fat and carbohydrate consumed have major effects upon postprandial plasma lipid levels. The effects of a moderate meal (one-third of daily caloric requirements) can be observed over a 9- to 12-h period postprandi-ally as changes (from the fasting baseline) in plasma lipid concentrations and in activities of lipoprotein-metabolizing enzymes. This means that humans who consume regular meals are in a nonfasting or absorptive state for most of each day or 24-h period.

Changes in Plasma Triacylglycerol and Total Cholesterol Concentrations in Response to a Meal

In humans, the size, frequency, and composi-tion of meals are often unpredictable. Lipid metabolic rates must respond rapidly to con-tinuously changing inputs of cholesterol and fatty acids. Lipid and carbohydrate in excess of immediate needs must be selectively trans-

CLINICAL CORRELATION

Familial Hypercholesterolemia

Familial hypercholesterolemia (FH) is characterized by a congenital defect in LDL receptors. A variety of mutations in the LDL receptor gene have been identified that affect synthesis, processing, binding, or clustering of the receptor on the cell surface. The homozygous phenotype may result from a compound heterozygote with two different genetic defects that affect the same gene. Homozygotes for FH have high levels of LDL in their plasma, resulting in plasma cholesterol levels that are typically six or more times normal.

Patients with FH often deposit cholesterol in their skin and tendons, forming nodules known as xanthomas. When cultured in lipoprotein-containing media, fibroblasts taken from either normal subjects or FH homozygotes do not express LDL receptors at their cell surfaces. However, when these cells are equilibrated in vitro in lipoprotein-deficient plasma to reduce their cellular free cholesterol content, normal cells express LDL receptors but cells from FH homozygotes do not. Cells from heterozygotes remove LDL at about half the normal rate. These results with fibroblasts are considered to model hepatic LDL clearance in vivo.

Coronary artery disease typically occurs during childhood in homozygotes, and it occurs early in adulthood and with a prevalence about 25 times that of the general population in heterozygotes. The prevalence of heterozygotes for FH in the population is about 1 in 500 individuals. The prevalence of homozygotes is rare and is estimated at 1 in 1 million people.

Thinking Critically

What effects [direction of change (i.e., increase or decrease?) and degree of change (i.e., little, moderate, or major?)] would you anticipate a genetic defect in the LDL receptor to have on the following features of plasma lipid concentration and metabolism in vivo? Why?

A. Plasma cholesterol in VLDL and HDL

B. Extrahepatic cholesterol synthesis

C. Nonspecific uptake of LDL by the liver

D. LCAT activity

---

ferred to appropriate storage sites and released later upon demand. Postprandial lipid metabolism represents an ordered biochemical response to these physiological realities.

Plasma triacylglycerol levels peak about 3 h following a moderate meal of whole foods. Both the magnitude of the increase in plasma triacylglycerol levels and the duration of the postprandial response depend on the fat content of the meal. After ingestion of a normal meal containing one third of daily caloric intake, plasma triacylglycerol levels typically double at 3 h, then decrease toward or even below fasting levels by 9 h, and finally rebound to fasting levels again by 12 h. This pattern varies little with the saturation of dietary fat or with the presence of higher or lower levels of dietary cholesterol.

The concentrations of circulating apo B-48 and apo B-100 in triacylglycerol-rich lipoproteins increase postprandially, but, even at peak triacylglycerol levels, apo B-48 makes up only a small part of the total apo B lipoproteins circulating within the triacylglycerol-rich lipoproteins. The greater abundance of apo B-100 than of apo B-48 in plasma is due to several factors. The triacylglycerol content of a newly secreted chylomicron is 10- to 100-fold greater than that of a nascent hepatic VLDL particle, yet both lipoprotein particles contain a single apo B polypeptide. As a result, the apo B-48/apo B-100 ratio greatly underrepresents the proportion of triacylglycerol of intestinal origin that is present in postprandial plasma. Additionally, chylomicron triacylglycerol is hydrolyzed more rapidly by lipoprotein lipase ($t_{1/2}$ 5 to 15 min) than is triacylglycerol in VLDL ($t_{1/2}$ 1 to 5 h). Chylomicron or apo B-48–containing remnants also are cleared rapidly, whereas the plasma concentration of apo B-100–containing LDL remains relatively high at all times.

Dietary free cholesterol appears as cholesteryl ester in chylomicrons. It is retained within the chylomicron remnant and rapidly cleared by the liver. Because of their relatively rapid clearance, chylomicrons contain an insignificant part of total plasma cholesterol, even after a meal rich in free cholesterol. Loss of free cholesterol from LDL, and a comparable increase within the triacylglycerol-rich lipoprotein fractions, have been observed during the postprandial response. This probably reflects mainly a passive transfer of free cholesterol, driven by the low free cholesterol content of newly secreted VLDL. There is little change postprandially in the cholesterol or triacylglycerol content of HDL.

Chylomicrons also transport fat-soluble vitamins from the small intestine to the liver. Retinol is esterified in the intestinal mucosa. Chylomicrons retain retinyl ester, as they do cholesteryl ester, during the peripheral lipolysis of triacylglycerol by lipoprotein lipase. After chylomicron remnants are taken up by the liver, the retinyl ester they contained is hydrolyzed. Free retinol is then distributed from the liver in a complex with plasma retinol–binding protein. In view of the specificity of this pathway, the level of retinyl ester in plasma lipoproteins has been used to estimate the contribution of chylomicrons to total triacylglycerol-rich lipoproteins in the postprandial state (Cohn et al., 1993). Because retinyl ester is a substrate for CETP, although less effective than cholesteryl ester, a small amount of retinyl ester is probably distributed from chylomicrons to apo B-100 lipoproteins and HDL. This redistribution would result in only a small error in calculation of chylomicron abundance in normal plasma because of the rapid removal of chylomicron remnants by the liver.

The major effect of postprandial lipemia is to increase transiently the number and triacylglycerol content of both apo B-48–and apo B-100–containing triacylglycerol-rich lipoproteins. These changes have significant consequences for plasma lipoprotein metabolism,

including the lipid composition and concentrations of the other plasma lipoproteins, all of which are modified in plasma by the chylomicron and VLDL lipids.

Postprandial Changes in Plasma Lipid Metabolism

Adipose tissue lipoprotein lipase regulates fatty acid storage after a meal. Postprandially, the level of lipoprotein lipase activity at the endothelial surface of adipose tissue is increased. The principal factor mediating this effect is a rise in the circulating level of insulin. Insulin increases the transcription of lipoprotein lipase in the adipocyte and stimulates the processing of polysaccharide chains in newly synthesized lipoprotein lipase to the trimmed state found in the secreted lipase.

Lipemia in postprandial plasma also stimulates the activity of CETP in exchanging VLDL triacylglycerol for HDL cholesteryl ester. Because the proportion of plasma triacylglycerol in acceptor lipoproteins (VLDL, IDL, LDL) has increased, there is a greater likelihood, on average, that a cholesteryl ester molecule transferred from HDL to VLDL or LDL will be replaced by a triacylglycerol molecule, rather than by a VLDL or LDL cholesteryl ester molecule. As a result, the net exchange of HDL cholesteryl ester mass for triacylglycerol mass increases. There is no increase in the plasma concentration of CETP protein postprandially. Although increased free fatty acid levels raise CETP activity in vitro, the high level of albumin (which binds free fatty acids) in plasma probably rules out this mechanism as an important regulator of CETP activity in vivo. By 9 h postprandially, the flux of cholesteryl ester through CETP has usually decreased again to baseline fasting levels (Fig. 14–3).

Postprandial lipemia also stimulates free cholesterol mass transfer from cells into plasma. Increased transfer of triacylglycerol to HDL in exchange for cholesteryl ester, followed by hydrolysis of the triacylglycerol by hepatic triacylglycerol lipase, leads to a significant decrease in the size of HDL. If sequential plasma samples obtained during the course of postprandial lipemia are incubated in vitro with monolayers of peripheral cells, an increase in the mass transfer of free choles-

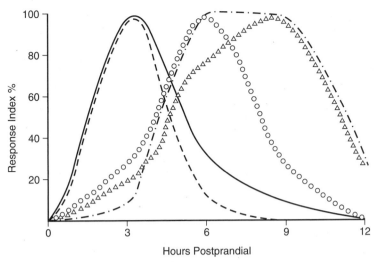

Figure 14–3. *The postprandial response of triacylglycerol and plasma metabolic activities following a moderate meal (~one third of daily calories) of whole foods. Shown on the figure are plasma triacylglycerol concentration (————); net exchange of cholesteryl ester in HDL for triacylglycerol, catalyzed by CETP (— — — —); transfer of cellular free cholesterol to plasma (ooooooooo); cholesterol esterification by LCAT (—•—•—); and phospholipid transfer catalyzed by PLTP (△△△△). Values have been scaled between 0% (fasting) and 100% (peak postprandial response) to facilitate comparison among different factors. Data are from Castro and Fielding (1985) and Fielding (unreported data).*

terol from the cells to plasma lipoproteins is seen for plasma samples obtained at 6 to 9 h postprandially. The model shown in Figure 14–2 suggests that small, lipid-poor preβ-HDL, generated from HDL, first cross the endothelium into the interstitial space of the peripheral tissues. "Discoidal" HDL, formed extravascularly from small preβ-HDL by accumulation of phospholipid and free cholesterol from peripheral cells, accumulate in the lymph and are returned to the plasma via the lymphatic ducts. Finally, LCAT activity (but not the plasma concentration of LCAT protein) is also increased postprandially, normally peaking after about 9 h and favoring esterification of the free cholesterol picked up by the preβ-HDL. Thus postprandial lipemia is associated with a stimulation in the reverse transport of cholesterol from peripheral tissues to the liver.

The extravascular phase of postprandial lipid metabolism is likely to explain the 3-h lag between the sequential rise first of net exchange of HDL cholesteryl ester for triacylglycerol (catalyzed by CETP) and second of LCAT activity (esterification of free cholesterol to form HDL cholesteryl ester) that is characteristic of postprandial lipemia. The difference in the shape of the response curves of LCAT and CETP activities means that the ratio of

LCAT to CETP activity is increased at 6 h postprandially relative to that of their fasting levels. As a result, the mean diameter of HDL, which decreases early in postprandial metabolism (3 h), increases back to its fasting value later in the postprandial period (6 h) as LCAT-derived cholesteryl ester accumulates in the spherical, α-migrating particles.

The sequential changes that characterize postprandial lipid metabolism in plasma have several effects. Fatty acids in triacylglycerols are directed for storage to adipose tissue through the properties and regulation of adipose tissue lipoprotein lipase. The accumulation of unstable, cholesterol-enriched remnant lipoproteins is prevented by the efficient removal of these particles by the liver. Fat-soluble vitamins are delivered efficiently to the liver as part of the chylomicron remnants. Finally, postprandial lipemia promotes reverse free cholesterol transport from peripheral tissues to the liver by accelerating the recycling of apo A-I through preβ-HDL.

At a time when dietary fats often have a negative connotation, it is important to consider that, in normal metabolism, the postprandial phase appears to play a beneficial role in reestablishing the whole body homeostasis of glycerides and cholesterol.

CHRONIC EFFECTS OF DIETARY LIPIDS ON PLASMA LIPOPROTEINS AND LIPID METABOLISM

The major differences among diets that affect plasma lipids are the percentage of total calories consumed as fat, the proportions of saturated and polyunsaturated fats (monounsaturated fats being considered neutral), and the mass of dietary cholesterol (Grundy and Denke, 1990). The major effects of dietary lipids are on circulating levels of triacylglycerol and of LDL cholesterol. Wide variations in individual response to a standard meal are typically seen. In lower primates, there is convincing evidence for inherited differences in response to diet. In human subjects, the response of individuals tested several times with the same diet was consistent in some individuals but not in others. Probably humans, like lower primates, have a genetic element in their response to diet, but this can easily be obscured through environmental factors.

Most studies of the effects of dietary cholesterol on LDL concentrations have identified both responders and nonresponders. The extent to which differences in intestinal absorption of cholesterol contributes to this classification remains controversial. The LDL response to dietary cholesterol is mediated mainly by the level of expression of hepatic LDL receptors, but changes in the activity of CETP, which regulates the distribution of lipoprotein cholesterol between apo A-I–containing and apo B–containing particles, may also contribute. Hyporesponders to dietary cholesterol reduce endogenous cholesterol synthesis in proportion to the amount of chylomicron cholesterol entering the liver, whereas hyperresponders do not.

Most studies of the response of plasma lipids to dietary lipid intake have been done with young, white, male subjects. There are insufficient data at present to determine the extent to which variables such as gender, age, and ethnicity contribute to the response to dietary lipids, although this information is urgently needed in the ongoing debate on public health effects of dietary lipids.

Effects of Changes in Total Dietary Fat Level on Fasting Plasma Lipids

Switching from a typical American diet to a low-fat diet, in which fat has been replaced isocalorically by carbohydrate, typically leads to an increase in circulating fasting triacylglycerol levels (mainly in VLDL) and to a decrease, probably secondary and CETP-mediated, in both fasting LDL and HDL cholesterol levels. This increase in triacylglycerol has been attributed to the influence of carbohydrate in stimulating the synthesis of long-chain fatty acids and the secretion of triacylglycerol-rich VLDL from the liver. An increase in dietary fat has been shown to be associated with modest increases (10% to 20%) in the levels of lipoprotein lipase and hepatic triacylglycerol lipase. Whether comparable reductions in lipase activities occur when individuals switch to low-fat diets is unclear, although such reductions would also be consistent with the modest hypertriglyceridemia observed.

Effects of Dietary Fat Saturation on Fasting Plasma Lipid Levels

The degree of dietary fat saturation is often expressed as a P/S (polyunsaturated/saturated) ratio. A lower P/S ratio indicates the presence of a lower proportion of polyunsaturated fatty acids and a higher proportion of saturated fatty acids in dietary triacylglycerol. Until recently it was believed that the effects of dietary cholesterol and fat saturation on fasting plasma total cholesterol levels were independent and additive. However, the study shown in Figure 14–4, among others, demonstrated that the effects of dietary fat saturation were dependent upon the dietary cholesterol level. When cholesterol intake was low (~200 mg/day), there was no significant effect of P/S ratios of 0.8 as compared with 0.2 (at constant total fat and constant monounsaturated fat) on the plasma cholesterol level. In contrast, when the cholesterol intake was ~600 mg/day, a decrease in the P/S ratio from 0.8 to 0.2 (more saturated fat and less polyunsaturated fat) resulted in a doubling of the fasting plasma cholesterol concentration (Hayes and Khosla, 1992). In contrast to effects on plasma cholesterol, an increase in saturated fat (with unchanged dietary cholesterol and total fat calories) had negligible effects on plasma triacylglycerol concentration, provided that weight was maintained constant.

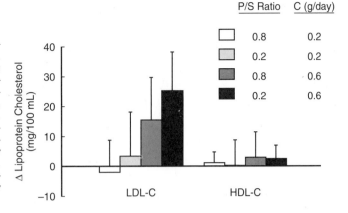

Figure 14–4. Changes in the concentration of LDL cholesterol (LDL-C) and HDL cholesterol (HDL-C) in response to diets differing in cholesterol (C) and polyunsaturated/saturated fat content (P/S ratio). (Redrawn from Fielding, C. J., Havel, R. J., Todd, K. M., Yeo, K. E., Schloetter, M. C., Weinberg, V. and Frost, P. H. [1995] Effects of dietary cholesterol and fat saturation on plasma lipoproteins in an ethnically diverse population of healthy young men. J Clin Invest 95:611–618. Used by copyright permission of The American Society for Clinical Investigation.)

Effects of Dietary Cholesterol on Fasting Plasma Lipid Levels

In responsive individuals, increased dietary cholesterol is generally associated with an increase in LDL cholesterol without a significant change in cholesterol in other fractions. This effect is mediated, at least in part, by downregulation of hepatic LDL receptor expression and receptor mRNA levels. Increases in dietary cholesterol (+400 to 600 mg/day) at different levels of total fat and fat saturation are usually associated with ~20% increases in the flux of lipids through both LCAT and CETP. Because of the long circulation time of LDL ($t_{1/2}$~2 days), even modest changes in CETP activity could of themselves lead to a significant redistribution of cholesteryl esters among plasma lipoproteins. For example, a 20% increase in CETP activity could generate an increase of 5 to 10 mg of LDL cholesterol/100 mL of plasma if LDL removal rate were unchanged. Corroborating an influence of CETP levels on circulating LDL concentrations, responders to dietary cholesterol on average had higher basal CETP activities than did nonresponders (Fielding et al., 1995). These preliminary data suggest that CETP activity could affect the circulating level of LDL cholesterol in human plasma, but more infor-

NUTRITION INSIGHT

Effect of Degree of Fat Saturation on Plasma Lipids

A typical American diet might provide a total of 15% of calories as protein and 36% of calories as fat. If this fat is made up of equal parts of saturated, monounsaturated, and polyunsaturated fats, the P/S ratio of this diet would be about 1.0. If 80% of the polyunsaturated fat is replaced isocalorically with saturated fat, the P/S ratio would be markedly reduced to 0.11.

Thinking Critically

Assuming that no other changes are made in the diet and that no changes in body weight result from this dietary change, what effect would you predict on the following parameters? Give the direction of change (increase/decrease) and the magnitude of the change (little/moderate/major).

A. Plasma fasting triacylglycerol concentration

B. Plasma HDL cholesterol concentration

C. Plasma postprandial triacylglycerol concentration

D. Plasma LDL cholesterol concentration

mation is needed to determine the importance of this parameter relative to that of hepatic LDL receptor levels.

Effects of Diet on Postprandial Lipid Metabolism

Effects of diet on postprandial lipid metabolism are relatively small. There have been few studies in this area, in spite of its possible contribution to plasma lipid levels throughout most of the day. In human subjects fed moderate cholesterol levels (up to 600 mg/day), there was no significant effect of elevated cholesterol levels on the magnitude of the postprandial response of LCAT and CETP activities above the enhanced fasting baseline of these activities. The same was found for plasma triacylglycerol concentration and for lipase activities.

REFERENCES

Acton, S., Rigotti, A., Landschultz, K. T., Xu, S., Hobbs, H. H. & Krieger, M. (1996) Identification of scavenger receptor SR-BI as a high density lipoprotein receptor. Science 271:518–520.

Barrans, A., Jaspard, B., Barbaras, R., Chap, H., Perret, B. and Collet, X. (1996) Prebeta HDL: Structure and metabolism. Biochim Biophys Acta 1300:73–85.

Braun, J. E. A. and Severson, D. L. (1992) Regulation of the synthesis, processing, and translocation of lipoprotein lipase. Biochem J 287:337–347.

Castro, G. R. and Fielding, C. J. (1985) Effects of postprandial lipemia on plasma cholesterol metabolism. J Clin Invest 75:874–882.

Cohn, J. S., Johnson, E. J., Millar, J. S., Cohn, S. D., Milne, R. W., Marcel, Y. L., Russell, R. M. and Schaefer, E. J. (1993) Contribution of apo B-48 and apo B-100 triglyceride-rich lipoproteins (TRL) to postprandial increase in the plasma concentration of TRL triglycerides and retinyl esters. J Lipid Res 34:2033–2040.

Cooper, A. D. (1997) Hepatic uptake of chylomicron remnants. J Lipid Res 38:2173–2192.

Fielding, P. E. and Fielding, C. J. (1996) Dynamics of lipoprotein transport in the circulatory system. In: Biochemistry of Lipids, Lipoproteins, and Membranes (Vance, D. E. and Vance, J., eds.), pp. 495–516. Elsevier Press, New York.

Fielding, C. J. and Fielding, P. E. (1995a) Molecular physiology of reverse cholesterol transport. J Lipid 36:211–228.

Fielding, P. E. and Fielding, C. J. (1995b) Plasma membrane caveolae mediate the efflux of cellular free cholesterol. Biochemistry 34:14288–14292.

Fielding, C. J., Havel, R. J., Todd, K. M., Yeo, K. E., Schloetter, M. C., Weinberg, V. and Frost, P. H. (1995) Effects of dietary cholesterol and fat saturation on plasma lipoproteins in an ethnically diverse population of healthy young men. J Clin Invest 95:611–618.

Goldberg, I. J. (1996) Lipoprotein lipase and lipolysis: Central roles in lipoprotein metabolism and atherogenesis. J Lipid Res 37:693–707.

Grundy, S. M. and Denke, M. A. (1990) Dietary influences on serum lipids and lipoproteins. J Lipid Res 31:1149–1172.

Hayes, K. C. and Khosla, P. (1992) Dietary fatty acid thresholds and cholesterolemia. FASEB J 6:2600–2607.

Hussain, M. M., Kancha, R. K., Zhou, Z., Luchoomun, J., Zu, H. and Bakillah, A. (1996) Chylomicron assembly and catabolism: Role of apolipoproteins and receptors. Biochim Biophys Acta 1300:151–170.

Spady, D. K., Woollett, L. A. and Dietschy, J. M. (1993) Regulation of plasma LDL-cholesterol levels by dietary cholesterol and fatty acids. Annu Rev Nutr 13:355–381.

Thompson, G. R., Naoumova, R. P. and Watts, G. F. (1996) Role of cholesterol in regulating apolipoprotein B secretion by the liver. J Lipid Res 37:439–447.

RECOMMENDED READINGS

Fielding, C. J. and Fielding, P. E. (1995) Molecular physiology of reverse cholesterol transport. J Lipid Res 36:211–228.

Fielding, P. E. and Fielding, C. J. (1996) Dynamics of lipoprotein transport in the circulatory system. In: Biochemistry of Lipids, Lipoproteins and membranes (Vance, D. E. and Vance, J., eds.), pp. 495–516. Elsevier Press, New York.

Spady, D. K., Woollett, L. A. and Dietschy, J. M. (1993) Regulation of plasma LDL-cholesterol levels by dietary cholesterol and fatty acids. Annu Rev Nutr 13:355–381.

CHAPTER 15

◆ ◆

Lipid Metabolism: Essential Fatty Acids

Arthur A. Spector, M.D.

OUTLINE

COMMON ABBREVIATIONS

DHA (docosahexaenoic acid)
DHET (Dihydroxyeicosatrienoate)
EET (epoxyeicosatrienoate)
EPA (eicosapentaenoic acid)
G-protein (guanosine triphosphate (GTP)-binding protein)
HETE (hydroxyeicosatetraenoate)
HODE (hydroxyoctadecadienoate)
HPETE (hydroperoxyeicosatetraenoate)
LT (leukotriene)
PG (prostaglandin)
PPAR (peroxisome proliferator-activator receptor)
PPRE (peroxisome proliferator response element)
TX (thromboxane)

Essential fatty acids are polyunsaturated fatty acids that cannot be completely synthesized in the body. They must be obtained from the diet because they are necessary for certain physiological functions. Two types of polyunsaturated fatty acids are present in the body, the omega-6 ($\omega 6$) class and the omega-3 ($\omega 3$) class. Both of these classes are considered to be essential nutrients.

HISTORICAL PERSPECTIVE

Early work demonstrated that a small amount of dietary fat was necessary for laboratory rats to reproduce, grow normally, and remain healthy. Two opposing views were put forward to explain this observation. Some thought that the protective action was due entirely to the vitamin E present in the dietary fat. Others believed that in addition to vitamin E, some component of the fat itself was an essential dietary factor. This controversy was resolved in 1929 when Burr and Burr demonstrated that linoleic acid, an $\omega 6$ polyunsaturated fatty acid, was an essential nutrient for the rat. In the rat, the syndrome produced by a lack of $\omega 6$ fatty acids, called essential fatty acid deficiency, causes a cessation of growth, dermatitis, loss of water through the skin, loss of blood in the urine, fatty liver, and loss of reproductive capacity. Subsequent work showed that linoleic acid also is an essential nutrient for other mammals, including humans. The main clinical signs of a deficiency in humans are dermatitis and poor wound healing.

No distinct disease occurs if the second type of polyunsaturated fatty acid, which is normally present in human and animals, the $\omega 3$ class, becomes deficient. Therefore, it initially appeared that $\omega 3$ fatty acids were not essential nutrients. This view has changed during the last 20 years because of increasing evidence indicating that $\omega 3$ fatty acids are required for optimum vision and central nervous system development (Connor et al., 1992; Uauy et al., 1992). There is now a growing consensus that, like the $\omega 6$ class, the $\omega 3$ polyunsaturated fatty acids are essential nutrients for humans.

STRUCTURE OF POLYUNSATURATED FATTY ACIDS

Fatty acids contain a hydrocarbon chain attached to a carboxyl group. The carboxyl group is ionized at physiological pH. Therefore, we usually refer to the fatty acid as the anionic form; that is, linoleic acid commonly is called linoleate. All fatty acids that contain two or more double bonds are classified as polyunsaturated. The double bonds in a polyunsaturated fatty acid normally are three carbons apart; they are interrupted by a carbon atom that is fully saturated.

$$-CH=CH-CH_2-CH=CH-$$

The presence of the methylene carbon between each pair of double bonds reduces the tendency of the fatty acid to undergo spontaneous oxidation in air as compared with conjugated pairs of double bonds ($-CH=CH-CH=C-$).

The double bonds in all naturally occurring unsaturated fatty acids are in the *cis* configuration. This introduces a rigid, 45-degree bend at each double bond in the fatty acid chain. The bent conformation reduces the tightness with which adjacent fatty acid chains can pack, producing a more fluid physical state and thereby decreasing the melting point.

The carbon atoms of a polyunsaturated fatty acid are numbered in two different ways. In the delta (Δ) numbering system, the carboxyl carbon is designated as carbon 1. The reverse occurs in the ω numbering system, in which the carbon at the methyl end of the hydrocarbon chain is designated as carbon 1. Another notation for numbering double bonds from the methyl end is the "n minus" notation, with n equal to the total number of carbon atoms (e.g., $n-3$ to indicate $\omega 3$ and $n-6$ to indicate $\omega 6$). Note that this system actually numbers carbons and double bonds from the carboxyl end (e.g., $n-3$ places the double bond closest to the methyl end at carbon 15 in a C18 fatty acid such as linoleic acid, and $n-6$ places the double bond at carbon 12 in a C18 fatty acid such as linoleic acid).

	CH_3-	CH_2-	$\ldots\ldots\ldots$	$-CH_2-$	$COOH$
Δ system				2	1
ω system	1	2			
n minus system	n	$n-1$			

All of these numbering systems are used; the delta system to indicate the position of the double bonds numbering from the carboxyl carbon, and the ω or n system to indicate the location of the first double bond from the methyl end of the unsaturated fatty acid chain. In every member of the ω3 class, the closest double bond to the methyl end is located 3 carbons from the methyl end.

$$\omega3\ CH_3—CH_2—CH=CH—$$

The closest double bond to the methyl end is six carbons from the methyl end in ω6 fatty acids.

$$\omega6\ CH_3—CH_2—CH_2—CH_2—CH_2—CH=CH—$$

Mammals do not have the capacity to completely synthesize either of these two types of polyunsaturated fatty acids because they cannot desaturate the 16- or 18-carbon products of fatty acid synthesis any further than nine carbons from the carboxyl end.

If an essential fatty acid deficiency develops, a 20-carbon polyunsaturated fatty acid in which the first double bond is nine carbons removed from the methyl end of the hydrocarbon chain is synthesized and accumulates in the plasma and tissues. It is derived from oleate, the most abundant monounsaturated fatty acid, and can be completely synthesized from acetyl CoA in humans and animals. The accumulation of polyunsaturated ω9 derivatives is abnormal and can be a diagnostic sign of essential fatty acid deficiency.

Another class of monounsaturated fatty acids, the ω7 series, also can be synthesized by mammals. Normally, polyunsaturated ω7 forms do not accumulate even in essential fatty acid deficiency. Only very small amounts of ω9 and ω7 polyunsaturated fatty acids ordinarily are present in human tissues, and almost all of the polyunsaturated fatty acids are either ω6 or ω3. Therefore, except in abnormal situations, essentially all of the polyunsaturated fatty acids in the body are essential fatty acids.

ω6 Polyunsaturated Fatty Acids

The structures of the most abundant ω6 fatty acids are shown on the left side of Figure 15–1. Fatty acids are abbreviated as number

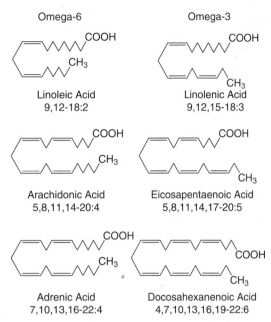

Figure 15–1. Structures of the most abundant ω6 and ω3 polyunsaturated fatty acids.

of carbons:number of double bonds. If the fatty acid is unsaturated, the location of the double bonds is given first, using the delta nomenclature. Thus, the notation for linoleate is 9,12-18:2, indicating that it contains 18 carbons and two double bonds that are 9 and 12 carbons distant, respectively, from the carboxyl carbon. The position of the double bonds often is omitted, and the commonly used designation for linoleate is 18:2. Although this shortened designation is convenient, it does not indicate where the double bonds are located. However, in cases such as 18:2, only one form is ordinarily present in biological preparations, and it is generally recognized to indicate the ω6 form unless otherwise stated. *Linoleate* is the main polyunsaturated fatty acid synthesized by terrestrial plants, and it is a major component of the triacylglycerols contained in corn oil, sunflower seed oil, and safflower oil.

The most prominent member of the ω6 family is *arachidonate* (20:4). It is the main substrate for the synthesis of eicosanoid mediators, including the prostaglandins and leukotrienes. It is also a major fatty acid component of the inositol phosphoglycerides. Although a small amount usually is present in meat and other animal products in the diet, much of the arachidonate contained in the body is synthesized from linoleate. *Adrenate* (22:4), the elongation product of arachidonate, accumulates in tissues that have a high arachidonate content. It functions as an intracellular storage form of arachidonate.

ω3 Polyunsaturated Fatty Acids

The ω3 fatty acids are present in large amounts in the retina and certain areas of the brain. Like their ω6 counterparts, ω3 fatty acids cannot by synthesized completely by mammalian tissues and are obtained from the diet. The structures of representative ω3 fatty acids are shown on the right side of Figure 15–1. α-*Linolenate* (18:3), the 18-carbon member of the family, has a structure identical to linoleate except for the presence of an additional double bond at carbon 15. It is synthesized by some terrestrial plants and is present in soybean and canola oil. Currently, it is the only ω3 fatty acid contained in com-

mercially prepared infant formulas. Although the intestinal mucosa can desaturate α-linoleate, most of the dietary intake that is absorbed remains unmodified and is incorporated into chylomicrons.

In addition to α-linolenate, more highly polyunsaturated derivatives present in fish and products containing fish oils also are consumed in the diet. These include *eicosapentaenoate* (20:5; EPA) and *docosahexaenoate* (22:6; DHA). Thus, most people who consume a balanced diet take in a mixture of 18-, 20-, and 22-carbon ω3 fatty acids. This differs from the ω6 dietary intake, which is mostly in the form of the 18-carbon constituent, linoleate.

POLYUNSATURATED FATTY ACID SYNTHESIS IN MAMMALIAN TISSUES

Although neither ω3 nor ω6 fatty acids can be synthesized completely, the essential fatty acid requirements of humans ordinarily can be sat-

---

Food Sources of Essential Fatty Acids

Food Sources of ω6 Fatty Acids

- Safflower oil (73% 18:2 ω6)
- Corn oil (57% 18:2 ω6)

Food Sources of Both ω6 and ω3 Fatty Acids

- Canola oil (8% to 11% 18:3 ω3; 22% 18:2 ω6)
- Soybean oil (7% 18:3 ω3; 51% 18:2 ω6)

Food Sources of Longer-Chain ω3 Fatty Acids (20:5 and 22:6)

- Cod liver oil (9% to 12% 20:5 ω3; 9% to 12% 22:6 ω3)
- Salmon oil (9% 20:5 ω3; 11% 22:6 ω3)

Recommended Intakes of Essential Fatty Acids

RDAs have not been established for either ω6 or ω3 fatty acids. To prevent essential fatty acid deficiency, a normal human requires about 1% of the daily energy intake in the form of ω6 polyunsaturated fatty acids, usually between 2 and 4 g per day in adults. A well-fed person consumes a much larger amount, because 5% to 10% of the daily caloric intake, about 20 to 35 g per day, normally is in the form of polyunsaturated fatty acids (mainly ω6). A deficiency of ω6 fatty acids is very rare under typical dietary conditions.

The typical Western diet contains much less ω3 fatty acid. Available evidence suggests that between 0.2 and 0.4 g of ω3 fatty acids should be consumed daily. Some experts recommend that a higher intake of ω3 fatty acids is desirable, between 2 and 4 g per day. The higher intake may provide a better balance between ω6 and ω3 fatty acid intake, with the ω3 fatty acids comprising about 10% of the total polyunsaturated fatty acid intake.

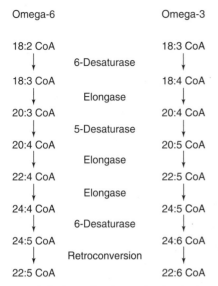

Figure 15–2. Pathway for the synthesis of ω6 and ω3 polyunsaturated fatty acids in mammalian tissues.

only can be converted to another ω3 fatty acid.

The fatty acids in all of the reactions in this pathway are in the form of acyl CoA derivatives. The complete pathway involves three elongations, three desaturations, and one retroconversion step. Similar structures occur in both the ω3 and ω6 pathways, for example, 18:3, 20:4, and 22:5. However, they are not the same fatty acids; they are positional isomers. Thus, the 18:3 in the ω3 pathway is 9, 12, 15-18:3 (α-linolenate), whereas the corresponding member in the ω6 pathway is 6,9,12-18:3 (γ-linoleate). Likewise, the 20:4 fatty acids or 22:5 fatty acids that occur in both pathways are isomeric pairs. Although the synthetic pathway produces 24-carbon fatty acids, they are intermediates that do not normally accumulate in either the plasma or tissues.

Figure 15–3 shows the fatty acid composition of normal human erythrocytes. The ω6 fatty acids detected are 18:2, 20:3, 20:4, and 22:4, with linoleate and arachidonate accounting for about 75% of these components. Much less total ω3 fatty acid is present, and the small amount is distributed roughly equally between 22:5 and DHA (22:6). This distribution is representative of many human tissues, the most notable exceptions being retina, brain, and testes.

isfied as long as the 18-carbon member of that class is available in the diet. The synthesis of the other forms from the 18-carbon precursors occurs through the pathway illustrated in Figure 15–2. It involves fatty acid chain elongation, desaturation, and retroconversion (Voss et al., 1991; Mohammed et al., 1995). However, one class cannot be interconverted to another. Thus, an ω6 fatty acid only can be converted to another ω6 fatty acid, and an ω3 fatty acid

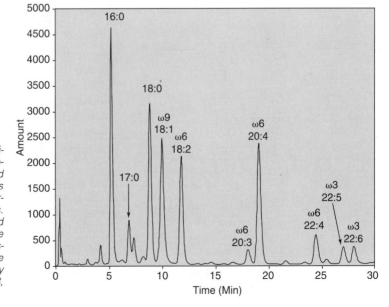

Figure 15–3. Fatty acid composition of the normal human erythrocyte as determined by gas-liquid chromatography. The fatty acids are indicated as number of carbons:number of double bonds. Margaric acid, 17:0, was added as an internal standard for the analysis and is not ordinarily present in the erythrocyte lipids. The classes of the unsaturated fatty acids are ω9, 18:1; ω6, 18:2, 20:3, 20:4, 22:4; ω3, 22:5, 22:6.

Fatty Acid Elongation

Fatty acids are elongated in the endoplasmic reticulum (ER). The available evidence indicates that mammalian tissues contain only one fatty acid elongase, and the same enzyme operates at each of the three elongation steps in the synthetic pathway shown in Figure 15–2. The mechanism by which elongation occurs is illustrated in Figure 15–4. The fatty acid must be in the form of an acyl CoA. The chain is lengthened by the addition of two carbons to the carbonyl group. Malonyl CoA, which contains three carbons, is the elongating agent, but only two of the carbons add to the fatty acid. In the condensation reaction, the free carboxyl group of the malonyl CoA is discharged as CO_2, and the CoA originally attached to the fatty acid carbonyl group is displaced. Because the CoA of the malonyl group remains attached, the resulting product is still an acyl CoA. The original carbonyl group subsequently is reduced to a methylene group in a series of reactions that require NADPH.

The double bonds do not move when a

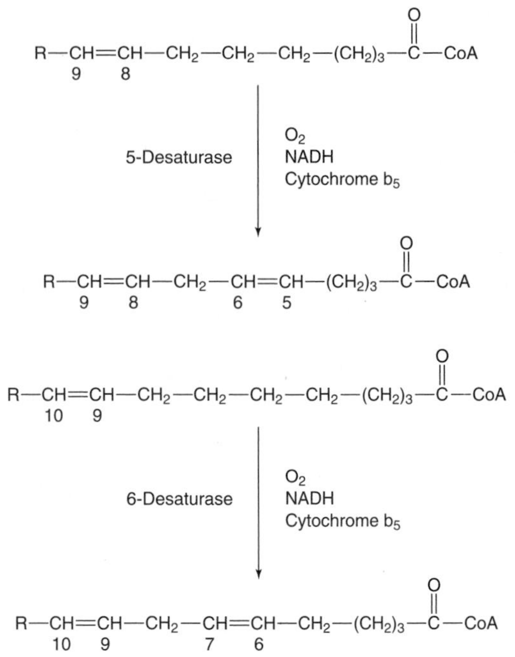

Figure 15–5. *Function of fatty acid Δ5- and Δ6-desaturases.*

polyunsaturated fatty acid is elongated. However, their numbering changes in the delta system because the two-carbon fragment that adds to the carboxyl end becomes carbons 1 and 2 of the lengthened product. Thus, when 6,9,12–18:3 undergoes one elongation, the resulting 20-carbon fatty acid is 8,11,14-20:3.

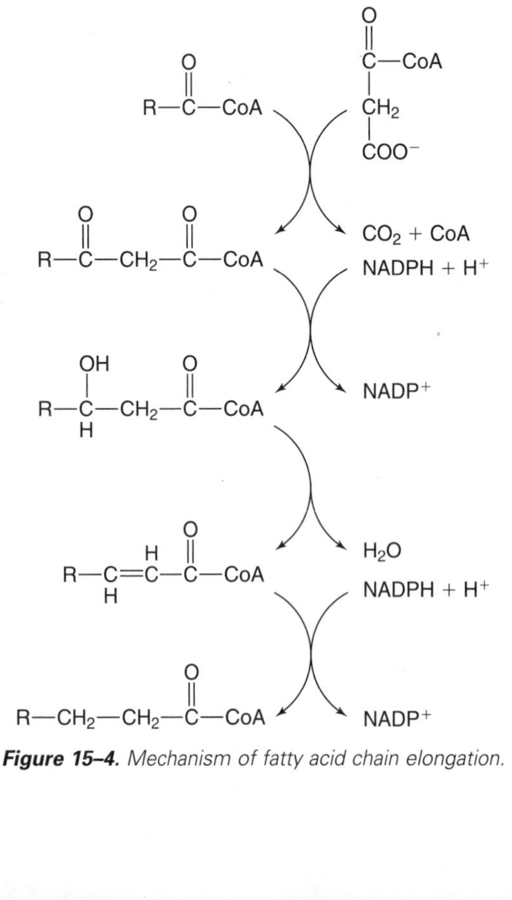

Fatty Acid Desaturation

Double bonds are inserted into a fatty acid by a process called desaturation which takes place in the ER. There are two desaturases that act on polyunsaturated fatty acyl CoA, Δ5-desaturase and Δ6-desaturase. The reactions, which require O_2, NADH, cytochrome b_5, and cytochrome b_5 reductase, are illustrated in Figure 15–5. The double bonds that they form are always in the *cis* configuration. These desaturases act on the segment of the fatty acyl chain between the carboxyl carbon and the first double bond, inserting the new double bond three carbons removed from the existing double bond. Acyl CoA Δ5-desaturase operates on a polyunsaturated acyl CoA that has a double bond at carbon 8, and the new double bond is inserted at carbon 5. It acts at only

Figure 15–4. *Mechanism of fatty acid chain elongation.*

one point in the pathway, converting 20:4 to EPA in the ω3 pathway and 20:3 to arachidonate in the ω6 pathway.

Only one acyl CoA Δ6-desaturase has been detected (Geiger et al., 1993), so this enzyme functions at two places in the synthetic pathway (Fig. 15–2). It utilizes a polyunsaturated acyl CoA that has a double bond at carbon 9, and the new double bond is inserted at carbon 6. With ω3 fatty acids, this enzyme converts α-linolenate to 18:4, and 24:5 to 24:6. With ω6 fatty acids, it converts linoleate to 18:3, and 24:4 to 24:5.

Retroconversion

The shortening of the 24-carbon intermediates to form the 22-carbon end products occurs through the process of retroconversion that takes place in the peroxisomes. Retroconversion utilizes an acyl CoA substrate, and the process removes two carbons from the carboxyl end of the fatty acid as acetyl CoA. In this way, 24:5 is retroconverted to 22:5 in the ω6 pathway, and 24:6 is retroconverted to 22:6 in the ω3 pathway. As shown in Figure 15–6, the fatty acid product formed in each case has a double bond four carbons removed from the new carboxyl group.

Studies in patients with Zellweger's syndrome and in normal skin fibroblasts indicate that this retroconversion mechanism for double bond formation at carbon 4 operates in humans (Martinez, 1996; Moore et al., 1995). Peroxisomal fatty acid oxidation (a β-oxidation system that functions to shorten very long-chain fatty acids) is deficient in Zellweger's syndrome, a severe neurological disease

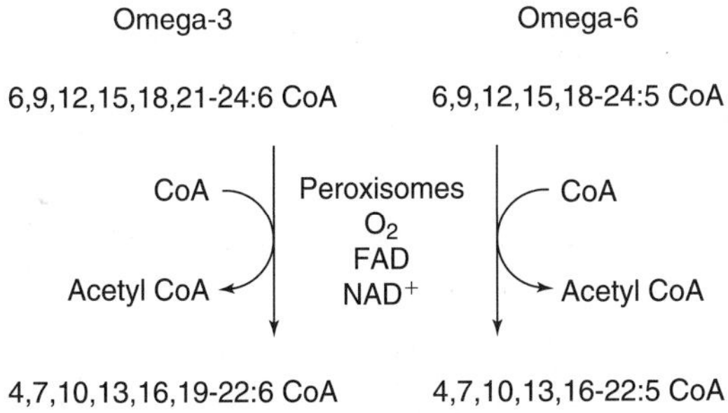

Omega-3   Omega-6

6,9,12,15,18,21-24:6 CoA   6,9,12,15,18-24:5 CoA

4,7,10,13,16,19-22:6 CoA   4,7,10,13,16-22:5 CoA

Figure 15–6. *Retroconversion reactions that occur in the ω3 and ω6 polyunsaturated fatty acid synthetic pathways.*

that results from a genetic defect in peroxisome biogenesis. Patients who inherit this disease have low levels of DHA because they cannot carry out the peroxisomal retroconversion step needed to convert 24:6 to DHA (Martinez, 1996).

There are other reactions involving ω3 and ω6 polyunsaturated fatty acids in which chain shortening through retroconversion occurs. For example, DHA can be retroconverted to 20:5, and 22:4 can be retroconverted to arachidonic acid. Therefore, just as linoleate and α-linolenate can serve as a source of longer, more highly polyunsaturated forms, the 22-carbon members can serve as a source of the shorter, 20-carbon members. This provides considerable flexibility because the body can utilize whatever forms are available in the environment to generate the members of the ω3 and ω6 classes needed for metabolic or functional purposes.

Products Formed

The ω3 and ω6 pathways function to generate different arrays of products. The main ω6 fatty acids that accumulate in plasma and most tissues are linoleate and arachidonate. By contrast, there is very little 18-carbon ω3 fatty acid in the plasma or tissues, and unless the diet is supplemented with fish oil, little EPA. Instead, the ω3 pathway is geared to produce 22-carbon products. Tissues that have a high content of ω3 fatty acid such as the retina and brain contain large amounts of DHA. Two hypotheses have been put forward to explain these differences. One is based on the specificity of the desaturases and elongase that act on the 18- and 20-carbon fatty acids. The other is that the specificity of the enzymes that incorporate fatty acids into the tissue phospholipids is selective for DHA and, therefore, is the controlling factor (Sprecher et al., 1995).

Tissue Differences

Hepatocytes have the complete polyunsaturated fatty acid synthetic pathway shown in Figure 15–2, but many other cells cannot carry out all of these reactions. When dietary α-linolenate is delivered to the liver, it is converted to DHA and then circulated to other tissues, such as the retina. This process is called "long-loop" transport (Scott and Bazan, 1989). Through a similar long-loop process, some of the dietary linoleate is converted to arachidonate in the liver and then transported to other tissues.

Studies done in tissue culture suggest that certain cells obtain arachidonate and DHA through cooperative interactions with other types of cells in the same organ. This is called short-loop transport. For example, primary cultures of neurons do not convert ω3 precursors to DHA, whereas cultured astrocytes (neuroglial cells) can convert all ω3 precursors to DHA and release much of the DHA that they produce (Moore et al., 1991). Likewise, retinal microvessel endothelial cells convert the ω3 docosapentaenoate (22:5) to DHA (Delton-Vanderbroucke et al., 1997). Taken together, these findings suggest that a short-loop mechanism exists in the brain. The microvessel endothelium and glial cells function to produce DHA from circulating ω3 precursors and then release some of the DHA to supply the neurons.

ESSENTIAL FATTY ACIDS IN PLASMA

As shown in Table 15–1, plasma contains a wide variety of polyunsaturated fatty acids.

These data were obtained from human subjects who consumed ordinary Western diets. The ω3 class comprises only 1% to 3% of the fatty acids in any of the lipid fractions. By contrast, the ω6 class accounts for 17% of the fatty acids in the plasma free fatty acid fraction, 37% in phospholipids, 22% in triacylglycerols, and 60% in cholesteryl esters. Linoleate and arachidonate comprise most of the ω6 fatty acid contained in these lipids.

After eating, the fatty acid composition of the chylomicron triacylglycerols reflects that of the dietary fat. Therefore, in the immediate postprandial state, chylomicrons supply extrahepatic tissues with essential fatty acids, and chylomicron remnants supply these fatty acids to the liver. Other plasma lipoproteins and albumin transport these fatty acids between different organs after the chylomicrons are removed from the circulation. Because they turn over rapidly, it is likely that the plasma free fatty acids and lipoprotein triacylglycerols are the primary sources of essential fatty acids for the tissues between meals. However, these plasma lipid fractions contain very little DHA or arachidonate, and there is evidence that phospholipids also are involved. For example, lysophosphatidylcholine is a source of DHA for blood cells (Brossard et al., 1997). Lysophosphatidylcholine is produced by partial hydrolysis of phosphatidylcholine,

TABLE 15–1
Essential Fatty Acid Composition of Human Serum Lipids

| | | Fraction of Total Fatty Acids (% by Weight) | | |
| | | Lipoproteins | | |
Fatty Acid	Free Fatty Acid	Phospholipids	Triglycerides	Cholesteryl Esters
ω3				
18.3	0.71	0.21	1.18	0.50
20.5	0.02	0.65	0.40	0.70
22.5	0.12	0.77	0.29	0.04
22.6	0.34	2.23	0.35	0.49
ω6				
18.2	15.60	22.94	19.50	48.82
18.3	0.04	0.13	0.48	1.07
20.3	0.14	3.11	0.36	0.91
20.4	1.25	10.95	1.64	8.08
22.4	0.02	0.42	0.22	0.01
22.5	0.03	0.41	0.17	0.05

Adapted from data compiled in Edelstein, C. (1986) General properties of plasma lipoproteins and apolipoproteins. In: Biochemistry and Biology of the Plasma Lipoproteins (Scanu, A. M. and Spector, A. A., eds.), pp. 495–505. Marcel Dekker, New York.

the main phospholipid in plasma lipoproteins, through the action of a phospholipase.

ESSENTIAL FATTY ACID DEFICIENCY

Essential fatty acid deficiency is the disease that occurs when there is an insufficient amount of ω6 fatty acid in the body to meet functional needs. The ω9 polyunsaturated fatty acids, which do not normally accumulate in plasma or tissues, are produced in abnormally high amounts when humans or animals become deficient in essential fatty acids. Figure 15–7 shows the pathway for synthesis of the ω9 polyunsaturated fatty acids.

These ω9 polyunsaturated fatty acids are produced from oleate, the main monounsaturated fatty acid in mammalian tissues. Oleate can be obtained from either the diet or by complete synthesis. The acyl CoA Δ6-desaturase utilizes oleate only if linoleate and α-linolenate are unavailable. Under these conditions, the main product that accumulates is (ω9) eicosatrienoic acid, 5,8,11-20:3. This is not the same isomer as the 20:3 that is part of the ω6 family, which is 8,11,14-20:3. The ω9 isomer cannot replace the ω6 form, and it cannot be converted to arachidonate. The prevailing opinion is that the ω9 form of 20:3 provides some compensation for essential fatty acid deficiency by partially substituting for arachidonate in membrane structure. Because the isomeric form is incorrect, however, the eicosanoid products normally synthesized from arachidonate cannot be made from this

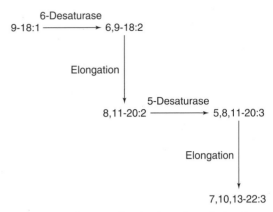

Figure 15–7. *Pathway for the formation of ω9 polyunsaturated fatty acids that occurs in essential fatty acid deficiency.*

form of 20:3, so there is no benefit in terms of lipid mediator synthesis.

POLYUNSATURATED FATTY ACID FUNCTION

The two main reasons why polyunsaturated fatty acids are essential for humans and animals are synthesis of lipid mediators and the production of membranes that have the optimum lipid bilayer structure and functional properties. Because these are very basic functions, it is surprising that a number of animal cell lines can grow in culture for many passages in the absence of any detectable polyunsaturated fatty acid. Many of these cell lines lack Δ6-desaturase and were derived from malignant tumors. A few biochemical functions

---

CLINICAL CORRELATION

Triene/Tetraene Ratio in Essential Fatty Acid Deficiency

An elevated triene/tetraene ratio in the plasma usually is a sign of essential fatty acid deficiency. Triene and tetraene refer to the number of double bonds in polyunsaturated fatty acids. A trienoic fatty acid has three double bonds; a tetraenoic fatty acid has four. Arachidonate is the main tetraenoic fatty acid in plasma, and it normally composes 8% to 10% of the plasma fatty acid. Because little trienoic fatty acid ordinarily is present in plasma, the normal triene/tetraene ratio is very low, about 0.1 to 0.2. This ratio becomes abnormally high in essential fatty acid deficiency. Due to a lack of ω6 fatty acid, the arachidonate content of the plasma decreases and is replaced by the (ω9) eicosatrienoic acid (5,8,11-20:3). This produces an increase in the triene/tetraene ratio of the plasma. An increase in the triene/tetraene ratio of plasma lipids is one of the clinical tests that is used to establish a diagnosis of essential fatty acid deficiency.

appear to be slightly compromised, but the cells are viable, grow well, and look healthy. Based on this finding, it appears that polyunsaturated fatty acids are not essential for the maintenance of basic life processes in isolated cells. The advantages that they provide apparently become important in the multicellular organism, where intercellular communication and highly differentiated membrane functions are vital.

The ω6 fatty acids play a major role in the formation of lipid mediators. These include the eicosanoids and the inositol phosphoglycerides. Arachidonate is the main ω6 component involved in these processes. Although EPA also can play a role in eicosanoid formation, the main function of the ω3 fatty acids appears to be membrane structure. DHA is the ω3 component that has the primary role in this regard.

Lipid Mediators

Eicosanoids are lipid mediators synthesized from 20-carbon polyunsaturated fatty acids. The fatty acids utilized for this purpose are 8,11,14-20:3 and arachidonate, both members of the ω6 family, and EPA, an ω3 member. These fatty acids are contained in membrane phospholipids and released by activation of a phospholipase. There still is some debate about which class of phospholipid and which type of phospholipase are involved, and this may vary in different cells or in response to different kinds of stimuli. However, in many cases, the main phospholipid class that releases the fatty acid is the choline phosphoglycerides, and the main enzyme that catalyzes the hydrolysis is phospholipase A_2. In addition, extracellular polyunsaturated fatty acid present as free fatty acid or contained in plasma lipoproteins can be taken up and utilized directly for eicosanoid synthesis. Because ordinarily there is much more arachidonate than any other 20-carbon polyunsaturated fatty acid in cell phospholipids and plasma lipids (see Fig. 15–3 and Table 15–1), the eicosanoids are formed predominantly from arachidonate. An overview of the mechanism is illustrated in Figure 15–8.

The arachidonate is channeled into one of three pathways of eicosanoid synthesis, de-

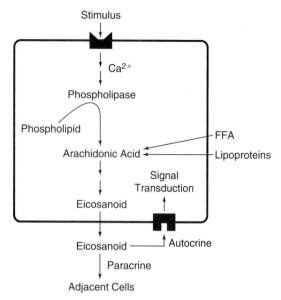

Figure 15–8. *Production and mechanism of action of eicosanoids.*

pending on which of the enzymes the cell expresses. Each of these pathways involves the addition of oxygen to one or more of the unsaturated bonds, forming oxygenated derivatives of arachidonate. Figure 15–9 lists the types of products formed by each of these pathways and illustrates the structures of some of the main arachidonate products.

The cyclooxygenase pathway produces prostaglandins (PGs) and thromboxanes (TXs). The first enzyme in the cyclooxygenase pathway is prostaglandin H synthase. Two isoforms have been detected: a constitutive form, called prostaglandin H synthase-1, and an inducible form, called prostaglandin H synthase-2 (DeWitt, 1991). Arachidonate products formed by this pathway contain two double bonds and are called dienoic cyclooxygenase products. The structures of two of these products, PGE_2 and TXA_2, are illustrated in Figure 15–9.

Lipoxygenases convert arachidonate to hydroperoxyeicosatetraenoate (HPETE). There are three lipoxygenases, 5-, 12-, and 15-lipoxygenase. They differ in their positional specificity for the double bonds in arachidonate. Other enzymes convert the HPETE to hydroxyeicosatetraenoate (HETE), leukotrienes (LTs), and lipoxins. Lipoxygenase products derived from arachidonate contain

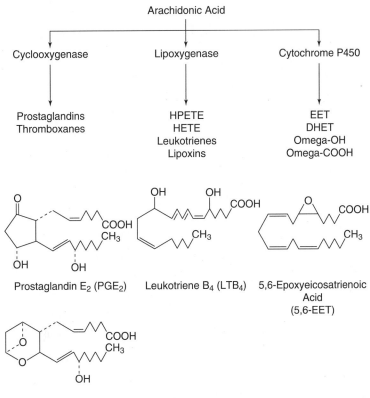

Figure 15–9. Pathways of eicosanoid synthesis and structures of some representative products.

four double bonds. The structure of one of the major LTs, LTB$_4$, is illustrated.

The cytochrome P450 monooxygenase pathway converts arachidonate to epoxyeicosatrienoate (EET) and dihydroxyeicosatrienoate (DHET). Four different EET and DHET positional isomers are formed, because the oxidation can take place at any of the four double bonds in arachidonate. The structure of 5,6-EET is illustrated in Figure 15–9. In addition to these products, ω-oxidized derivatives of arachidonate can be formed by the cytochrome P450 pathway.

Most cells express only one or two of the pathways and, therefore, make significant amounts of just one or two of the products. For example, arterial endothelial cells make PGI$_2$ as their main eicosanoid product, platelets make TXA$_2$ and 12-HETE, and neutrophil leukocytes make LTB$_4$ and 5-HETE.

Cell Biology of Eicosanoid Action

As shown in Figure 15–8, eicosanoids are released into the extracellular fluid after they are synthesized. They then bind to cell surface receptors, which initiate the response in the target cell. Table 15–2 lists the prostaglandin receptors, the main prostaglandin that each one binds, the physiological response, and the mechanism of action.

One of the main functions of prostaglandins is cell-to-cell communication. For example, PGI$_2$ released from the arterial endothelial cells acts on adjacent platelets to inhibit aggregation and thereby prevent blood clotting. PGI$_2$ also acts on the underlying arterial smooth muscle cells to induce relaxation. The process of one cell releasing a bioactive mediator that acts on a different kind of cell in the same localized environment is called a paracrine regulatory mechanism.

Prostaglandins and other eicosanoids also can act through an autocrine regulatory mechanism. In this mechanism, a released mediator acts on the same cell that secreted it; for example, an endothelial cell releases a mediator that affects it as well as other endothelial cells in the localized environ-

TABLE 15-2
Function and Mechanism of Action of Prostaglandins

Receptor	Main Prostaglandin that Binds	Response	Mechanism
IP	PGI_2	Relaxes arterial smooth muscle; inhibits platelet aggregation	Activates adenylate cyclase
TP	TXA_2	Contracts arterial smooth muscle; activates platelet aggregation	Phosphatidylinositol 4,5-bisphosphate hydrolysis, raises calcium
EP_1	PGE_2	Contracts smooth muscle	Phospholipid signaling, raises calcium
EP_2	PGE_2	Relaxes smooth muscle	Activates G_s, raises cAMP
EP_3	PGE_2	Inhibits water absorption, inhibits gastric acid secretion	Activates G_i, reduces cAMP
EP_4	(unknown)	Relaxes smooth muscle	(unknown)
FP	PGF_{2a}	Promotes uterine contraction, promotes bronchoconstriction	Phosphatidylinositol 4,5-bisphosphate hydrolysis, raises calcium
DP	PGD_2	Relaxes smooth muscle, inhibits platelet aggregation, inhibits neurotransmitter release	Activates adenylate cyclase

ment. One purpose of autocrine function is to coordinate the response of a group of similar cells, such as the endothelial lining of a blood vessel.

Most paracrine and autocrine processes occur through binding of the released mediator to specific receptors present on the target cell surface. The PGs, TXs, and LTs act in this way. Eight different prostaglandin receptors so far have been cloned. Each has a different specificity for the cyclooxygenase products, and they are designated according to the main product that they bind. For example, IP is the PGI receptor, and EP is the PGE receptor. Where more than one subtype of a receptor exists, they are designated by a subscript; that is EP_1, EP_2, etc. The tissue distribution of these receptors is different, and they are linked to different signal transduction systems. Binding of a cyclooxygenase product either activates or modulates the activation of a signal transduction process within the target cell.

This very complicated process can occur in a number of different ways, depending on the type of cyclooxygenase product and the receptor on the target cell to which it binds. One mechanism is activation of adenylate cyclase by the eicosanoid-receptor complex. PGI_2 operates in this way; it binds to the IP receptor and causes a large increase in cyclic adenosine monophosphate (cAMP) within the target cell. Another mechanism is modula-

tion of the adenylate cyclase response to another stimulus. PGE_2 acts in this way when it binds to a receptor that is coupled to a guanosine triphosphate (GTP)-binding protein (G-protein) linked to adenylate cyclase. The PGE receptor, EP_2 is linked to a stimulatory G-protein, G_s and binding to EP_2 amplifies the amount of cAMP formed. In contrast, EP_3 is linked to an inhibitory G-protein, G_i, and binding to EP_3 reduces the amount of cAMP formed. Finally, some cyclooxygenase products bind to receptors that lead to an increase in intracellular calcium by stimulating inositol phospholipid hydrolysis. The EP_1 receptor, which also binds PGE_2, functions in this way by activating phospholipase C.

Eicosapentaenoate

The mechanism of action of EPA is illustrated schematically in Figure 15–10. The cyclooxygenase pathway can convert EPA to cyclooxygenase products that contain three double bonds. Two of the main trienoic products are PGI_3 and TXA_3. However, EPA generally is a much poorer substrate for prostaglandin H synthase than arachidonate, and its usual effect is to suppress the conversion of arachidonate to dienoic prostaglandins and TXA_2. The amount of trienoic products formed in their place is either too small to compensate for the decrease in arachidonate products, or the trienoic products have less bioactivity. There-

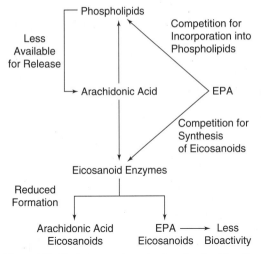

Figure 15–10. *Suggested mechanism for the bioactive effects of ω3 fatty acids on eicosanoid formation and function. These effects are produced primarily by eicosapentaenoic acid (EPA). EPA competes with arachidonate for incorporation into the phospholipids that provide the fatty acid for eicosanoid synthesis, and it also competes with arachidonate for access to the enzymes for eicosanoid synthesis.*

the arachidonate content of the phospholipids decreases and is replaced by EPA and its elongation product, 22:5. When the phospholipase subsequently is activated, there is less arachidonate available in the phospholipids for release, further contributing to a reduction in the formation of eicosanoid products derived from arachidonate. This, combined with the competition at the level of prostaglandin H synthase, makes EPA an effective inhibitor of arachidonate metabolism.

This suggests two possible reasons why ω3 fatty acids are essential for optimum health. One is that the eicosanoids produced from EPA play some vital functional role, even though the amounts formed are usually small. The other is that EPA prevents the excessive production of eicosanoid from arachidonate, thereby fine-tuning processes such as intercellular signaling and reducing eicosanoid-mediated responses such as inflammation so that they do not become uncontrolled.

Inositol phosphoglycerides

The inositol phosphoglycerides are important components of one of the main membrane signal transduction systems in the cell. Prostaglandin receptors, such as the TP, EP_1, and FP, and several mitogen receptors transmit signals across the cell membrane through hydrolysis of inositol phospholipids. These receptors are linked to a GTP-binding protein that activates phospholipase C, an enzyme that hydrolyzes phosphatidylinositol 4,5-bisphosphate. Two

fore, if substantial amounts of EPA are present, there is a reduction in the usual eicosanoid-mediated response to a stimulus. The result is that EPA reduces or prevents the effects produced by arachidonate and its products.

EPA also competes with arachidonate for incorporation into tissue lipids, including the phospholipid pools that supply substrate for eicosanoid synthesis (Yerram et al., 1989). When cells are exposed to supplemental EPA,

---

CLINICAL CORRELATION

Fish Oil for the Prevention of Coronary Thrombosis

Daily fish oil supplements are being recommended by some physicians to reduce the risk of coronary thrombosis. Patients often take between 3 and 9 g/day, usually administered in the form of fish oil capsules. The approach is based on the pioneering work of Dyerberg and Bang (1979), who observed that the very low incidence of coronary thrombosis in Greenland Eskimos was due to a high dietary intake of ω3 fatty acids, primarily EPA.

Thinking Critically

1. How do ω3 fatty acids act to reduce the risk of coronary thrombosis?

2. Would the administration of soybean or canola oil, which also contain ω3 fatty acid, be as effective as fish oil for this purpose?

products are formed, 1,2-diacylglycerol and inositol triphosphate. The diacylglycerol activates protein kinase C, which phosphorylates a number of intracellular regulatory proteins, and the inositol triphosphate releases calcium from the ER. The resulting increase in cytosolic calcium also activates protein kinase C and other processes that produce the cellular response to the signal.

Inositol phosphoglycerides contain a high percentage of arachidonate. It is attached to the middle carbon of the glycerol moiety, the *sn*-2 position. When hydrolysis is mediated by phospholipase C, arachidonate remains a part of the diacylglycerol that is formed. Why inositol phosphoglycerides contain large amounts of arachidonate is not known. The possibilities include targeting to specific intracellular locations or enzymes, imparting special properties to the diacylglycerol that is formed, or hydrolysis of the diacylglycerol by diacylglycerol lipase so that the arachidonate becomes available for eicosanoid synthesis. Although the mechanism remains to be determined, it is clear that the ω6 polyunsaturated fatty acids, through arachidonate formation, are necessary for the inositol phosphoglyceride signal transduction system.

Membrane Lipid Structure

About 25% to 35% of the fatty acyl chains in most mammalian cell membranes are polyunsaturated. Almost all of these are ω6 or ω3 fatty acids under normal conditions (see Fig. 15–3). They are contained in phospholipids that make up the membrane lipid bilayer. The phospholipid fatty acyl chains in the lipid bilayer are a major determinant of the overall physical state of the membrane, and the presence of some polyunsaturated fatty acid probably is essential for the optimum function of certain processes that take place in the membrane.

The packing and degree of motion of the fatty acyl chains in the lipid bilayer, called membrane fluidity, is a commonly used measure of the physical state. The degree of fluidity depends on the ratio of saturated to unsaturated fatty acyl chains. Cells can adjust the extent to which saturated fatty acids are converted to monounsaturated fatty acids, and

this may be all that is required to maintain the average fluidity of the membrane within acceptable limits. The increases in average fluidity produced by adding polyunsaturated acid is either small or negligible. What must be recognized, however, is that fluidity measurements indicate the average physical state of the membrane lipid bilayer. Even if there is little average change, a change in the structural properties of a localized region may have a profound effect on the function of a protein that is contained within that region.

Lipid Domains

Localized regions within the membrane lipid bilayer are called domains. Polyunsaturated fatty acids play a key role in certain domains that interact with integral membrane proteins. If the protein fits in better with the structure of its surrounding lipid, it will function more effectively. This mechanism has been suggested as an explanation of why the presence of DHA in membrane phospholipids facilitates the action of rhodopsin, the light receptor in the retina (Litman and Mitchell, 1996).

Nonbilayer Structures

Physical studies suggest that some phospholipids have a tendency not to form a bilayer structure. One of the alternate arrangements is an inverted configuration in which the polar head groups of the phospholipids cluster together on the inside and the hydrocarbon chains point outward. This is called a hexagonal configuration (see Chapter 3, Fig. 3–10). Phosphatidylethanolamine has an increased tendency to form this type of hexagonal arrangement when it contains a high percentage of DHA. Such a structure would allow the passage of a polar solute through the lipid bilayer by forming a channel in the center of the clustered phospholipid head groups. Also, the tendency to form such a structure may affect the packing of the phospholipid head groups at the surface of the lipid bilayer and thereby change the surface properties of the membrane. The functional advantages provided by these alternative structures may be another reason why highly polyunsaturated fatty acids, especially DHA, are required for specialized membrane functions.

NUTRITION INSIGHT

Dietary Effects on Membrane Fatty Acid Composition

The fatty acid composition of cell membranes can be altered substantially by modifying the dietary fat intake. Even the fatty acid composition of the heart, which one might think of as a very stable tissue, can be modified rapidly in experimental animals. The brain is the only organ that is resistant to such diet-induced change. Therefore, the fatty acid composition of most membranes adapts to some extent to the type of fat available in the diet. This flexibility is surprising, considering the vital role that membranes play in so many cellular functions. Diet-induced changes in membrane lipid composition support the old saying that "you are what you eat." However, there are limits to the extent of change that can take place in mammalian cells. Most of the variation occurs in the relative proportions of unsaturated fatty acids. For example, if the diet is enriched in sunflower seed oil, which contains 70% linoleate, the ω6 polyunsaturated fatty acid content of the membrane phospholipids increases and is counterbalanced by a decrease in oleate. This reduction in monounsaturated fatty acid content is a compensation that protects against an excessive increase in membrane fluidity.

Linoleate

The average requirement for ω6 fatty acids, about 2 to 4 g/day, greatly exceeds the amount of arachidonate needed for the synthesis of lipid mediators. This suggests that ω6 fatty acids may have other essential roles besides providing the tissues with arachidonate. Emphasis has focused on the skin, because essential fatty acid deficiency leads to a breakdown of the epidermal barrier to water loss. Linoleate is strongly preferred for the synthesis of two sphingolipids, acylceramide and acylglucosylceramide, that maintain the structure of the outer layer of the skin (the stratum corneum) (Downing, 1992). This suggests that linoleate may be required to impart a barrier property to the skin surface sphingolipids, thereby preventing excessive water loss through the skin.

Furthermore, linoleate can be oxygenated by several different types of cells to form a hydroperoxyoctadecadienoate. The addition of oxygen can occur at either carbon 9 or 13, forming the 9- or 13-isomer. These hydroperoxides subsequently are reduced, forming the corresponding hydroxyoctadecadienoate (HODE), 9- or 13-HODE. The oxygenation reaction that forms 13-HODE is catalyzed by 15-lipoxygenase. Although the functions of 9- and 13-HODE presently are unknown, the formation of these oxidized metabolites is another reason why linoleate itself may be essential.

LIPID PEROXIDATION

Polyunsaturated fatty acids are susceptible to lipid peroxidation. Figure 15–11 illustrates the mechanism. This is a nonenzymatic process that is initiated when a free radical attacks the methylene carbon present between a pair of double bonds in the fatty acid chain. The process is propagated by the presence of oxygen and transition metal ions like Fe^{2+} (Buettner, 1993). It is autocatalytic, because the polyunsaturated fatty acid initially attacked is converted to a free radical that attacks a second polyunsaturated fatty acid. This becomes a free radical and attacks a third polyunsaturated fatty acid, and so on, continually spreading the effect, and leading to membrane damage and cytotoxicity.

The initial lipid radical produced, $FA_1 \cdot$, reacts with oxygen to form a fatty acid peroxide, $FA_1OO \cdot$. Because the peroxyl group also is a free radical, it can attack a second polyunsaturated fatty acid, forming another lipid radical, $FA_2 \cdot$. This radical reacts with oxygen to start a second branch of the chain reaction. At the same time, the fatty acid hydroperoxide, FA_1OOH, formed in this reaction is converted to an alkoxyl radical, $FA_1O \cdot$. This radical can attack a third polyunsaturated fatty acid, forming $FA_3 \cdot$, which reacts with oxygen to start the third branch of the chain reaction. Alternatively, the alkoxyl radical can be converted to short-chain aldehydes or hydrocarbons. The

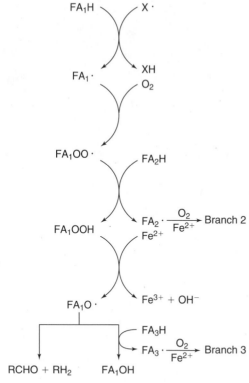

Figure 15–11. *Mechanism of lipid peroxidation. FAH, polyunsaturated fatty acid; X·, initiating free radical; FA·, fatty acid carbon-centered radical; FAOO·, fatty acid peroxyl radical; FAOOH, fatty acid hydroperoxide; FAO·, fatty acid alkoxyl radical; FAOH, hydroxy fatty acid; RCHO, short-chain aldehyde; RH_2, short-chain hydrocarbon. The numbers after FA designate the order in which different polyunsaturated fatty acids entered the peroxidation process. Two pathways are shown for FAO·; this indicates that the alkoxyl radical generated by each branch can take one of these two paths, but not both simultaneously.*

oxidation and breakdown of the polyunsaturated fatty acyl chains perturb the structural organization of the membrane lipid bilayer. In addition, some of the radicals generated can attack proteins and DNA, injuring or even killing the cell. (Lipid peroxidation is discussed further in Chapters 25 and 40; see Fig. 40–2.)

Effect of Polyunsaturated Fatty Acid Content

Tissues are protected against lipid peroxidation by antioxidants such as vitamin E (see Chapter 25) and antioxidant enzymes such as superoxide dismutase, catalase, and glutathione peroxidase. However, a substantial increase in the polyunsaturated fatty acid con-

tent can overcome the protective action and increase the susceptibility to lipid peroxidation. For example, plasma low density lipoproteins (LDL) become more susceptible to peroxidation if the diet is high in polyunsaturated fat, resulting in LDL that are enriched with linoleate (Reaven et al., 1993). Likewise, studies with cultured cells indicate that tissues also become more susceptible to free radical induced lipid peroxidation when they accumulate polyunsaturated fatty acid (North et al., 1994). Thus, either initiation or propagation of the peroxidation process is enhanced as the relative number of polyunsaturated fatty acid chains in a lipid structure increases.

EFFECTS ON PLASMA CHOLESTEROL AND LIPOPROTEINS

One of the factors that regulate the plasma cholesterol concentration is the degree of saturation of the dietary fat intake. A diet high in saturated fat content, especially when the fat contains 12-, 14-, and 16-carbon saturated fatty acids, leads to an increase in the plasma cholesterol concentration. In particular, it raises the amount of cholesterol present in LDL. When elevated, LDL cholesterol is a major risk factor for the development of atherosclerosis and its most prevalent complication, coronary thrombosis.

The plasma total cholesterol and LDL cholesterol concentrations usually decrease if some of the saturated fat in the diet is replaced by foods that are rich in linoleate. It is generally accepted that this protects against atherosclerosis and coronary heart disease by reducing the plasma LDL concentration. The current recommendation is that, in a well-balanced diet, the content of polyunsaturated fat (P) to saturated fat (S) should be equal, so that the P/S ratio of the dietary fat is 1.0. Such dietary modification can be achieved by reducing the intake of animal products that are rich in saturated fat and replacing them with fruits, vegetables, and vegetable oils that have a high polyunsaturated fatty acid content. The most likely mechanism by which this dietary modification acts is to increase LDL receptors in the tissues (Mustad et al., 1997). This increases the clearance of LDL from the

CLINICAL CORRELATION

Oxidized Low Density Lipoproteins and Atherosclerosis

Lipid peroxidation is a key event in one of the most widely held theories concerning the mechanism of atherosclerosis, the disease in which cholesterol accumulates in the intima of an artery. According to this theory, plasma low density lipoproteins (LDL) penetrate into the arterial wall. The LDL, which are rich in cholesteryl esters, undergo lipid peroxidation in the arterial intima, forming oxidized LDL. Oxidation converts LDL into a form that can be taken up by macrophages attracted into the arterial wall. The cholesterol content of the oxidized LDL cannot be degraded. As a result, the macrophages accumulate cytoplasmic lipid droplets rich in cholesteryl esters. These lipid-filled macrophages, called foam cells, form the fatty streak lesions in the arterial intima. In the process, the macrophages become activated and induce a locally damaging inflammatory reaction. This eventually progresses into an atherosclerotic plaque (Steinberg et al., 1989). The recognition that LDL peroxidation may be involved in the initiation of atherosclerosis suggests that antioxidants such as vitamin E may be beneficial in preventing or treating this disease and thereby preventing its serious complications, coronary thrombosis and stroke.

circulation, thereby lowering the plasma cholesterol concentration. The effects of the P/S ratio of dietary fat on plasma lipids are discussed further in Chapter 41.

REGULATION OF GENE EXPRESSION

Polyunsaturated fatty acids regulate the expression of many genes that are involved in lipid metabolism. Saturated and monounsaturated fat do not affect the transcription of these genes. Transcriptional effects are produced by both the ω3 and ω6 polyunsaturated fatty acid classes. Dietary studies with corn oil and fish oil indicate that Δ6-desaturation must occur before a polyunsaturated fatty acid is active; in other words, linoleate (9,12-18:2) is inactive, but its derivatives such as arachidonate (5,8,11,14-20:4) that have undergone Δ6-desaturation are effective (Clarke et al., 1997). Table 15–3 lists some of the genes that are regulated in this manner.

The regulatory mechanism involves a group of nuclear transcription factors called peroxisome proliferator-activated receptors (PPAR). Three PPAR have been identified, PPAR α, δ, and γ. When an activating substance binds to a PPAR, it forms a heterodimer with a second nuclear receptor, the retinoid X receptor (see Chapter 26). The heterodimer binds to a response element called peroxi-

NUTRITION INSIGHT

Olive Oil in the Treatment of Hypercholesterolemia

Recent studies indicate that substitution of olive oil for saturated fat reduces plasma low density lipoprotein (LDL) cholesterol. Olive oil contains large amounts of oleate, the main monounsaturated fatty acid in plasma and tissues. Thus, the effect of olive oil is similar to that of the plant oils that are rich in ω6 polyunsaturated fatty acids, which include corn, sunflower seed, and safflower oils. The interpretation is that the cholesterol-lowering effect of dietary fat modification results from a reduction in the saturated fatty acid intake rather than from any specific effect of polyunsaturated fatty acids. Because of concerns about increasing the susceptibility of LDL to lipid peroxidation, there is an increasing tendency to recommend diets rich in olive oil rather than linoleate when the aim is to reduce the patient's plasma LDL cholesterol concentration.

TABLE 15–3

Representative Genes Regulated by Essential Fatty Acids or Their Metabolic Products

Gene	Function
Acyl CoA synthase	Synthesis of acyl CoA
Acyl CoA oxidase	Peroxisomal fatty acid oxidation
Trifunctional enzyme	Peroxisomal fatty acid oxidation
Medium-chain acyl CoA dehydrogenase (MCAD)	Mitochondrial fatty acid oxidation
Cytochrome P450(4A6)	Fatty acid omega-oxidation
Liver fatty acid binding protein (L-FABP)	Intracellular fatty acid binding
Stearoyl CoA desaturase	Acyl CoA Δ9-desaturation
Adipocyte P2 (aP2)	Fatty acid binding in adipocytes
Malic enzyme	Production of NADPH
Glucose 6-phosphate dehydrogenase	Production of NADPH

some proliferator response element (PPRE), which is contained in the promoter region of certain genes. Exposure of cells to unsaturated fatty acids activates PPARs, and both fatty acids and metabolites of fatty acids have been shown to bind to PPARs. Recent studies indicate that unsaturated fatty acids, especially C18 unsaturated fatty acids, bind to PPARs. Some products of arachidonate also bind. LTB$_4$ and 8-HETE, lipoxygenase products formed from arachidonate, activate PPARα, and the prostaglandin metabolite 15-deoxy-PGJ$_2$ activates PPARγ (Forman, 1997; Krey et al., 1997).

Although PPARs are part of the molecular mechanism that mediates the increased capacity to utilize fatty acids, this nuclear receptor family does not appear to be part of the process that downregulates fatty acid synthase, a key gene in the biosynthetic pathway. Therefore, more than one molecular mechanism must be involved in the regulation of fatty acid metabolism by polyunsaturated fatty acids.

REFERENCES

Brossard, N., Croset, M., Normand, S., Pousin, J., Lecerf, J., Laville, M., Tayot, J. L. and Lagarde, M. (1997) Human plasma albumin transports [^{13}C]docosahexaenoic acid in two lipid forms to blood cells. J Lipid Res 38:1571–1582.

Buettner, G. R. (1993) The pecking order of free radicals and antioxidants: Lipid peroxidation, α-tocopherol, and ascorbate. Arch Biochem Biophys 300:535–543.

Clarke, S. D., Turini, M. and Jump, D. (1997) Polyunsaturated fatty acids regulate lipogenic and peroxisomal gene expression by independent mechanisms. Prostaglandins Leukot Essent Fatty Acids 57:65–69.

Connor, W. E., Neuringer, M. and Reisbeck, S. (1992) Essential fatty acids: The importance of n-3 fatty acids in the retina and brain. Nutr Rev 50:21–29.

Delton-Vanderbroucke, I., Grammas, P. and Anderson, R. E. (1997) Polyunsaturated fatty acid metabolism in retinal and cerebral microvascular endothelial cells. J Lipid Res 38:147–159.

DeWitt, D. L. (1991) Prostaglandin endoperoxide synthase: Regulation of enzyme expression. Biochim Biophys Acta 1083:121–134.

Downing, D. T. (1992) Lipid and protein structures in the permeability barrier of mammalian epidermis. J Lipid Res 33:301–313.

Dyerberg, J. and Bang, H. O. (1979) Haemostatic function and platelet polyunsaturated fatty acids in Eskimos. Lancet ii:433–435.

Forman, B.M., Chen, J. and Evans, R. M. (1997) Hypolipidemic drugs, polyunsaturated fatty acids, and eicosanoids are ligands for peroxisome proliferator-activated receptors α and δ. Proc Natl Acad Sci USA 94:4312–4317.

Geiger, M., Mohammed, B. S., Sankarappa, S. and Sprecher, H. (1993) Studies to determine if rat liver contains chain-length-specific acyl-CoA 6-desaturase. Biochim Biophys Acta 1170:137–142.

Krey, G., Braissant, D., L'Horset, F., Kalkhoven, E., Perroud, M. and Parker, M. G. (1997) Fatty acids, eicosanoids, and hypolipidemic agents identified as ligands of peroxisome proliferator-activated receptors by coactivated-dependent receptor ligand assay. Mol Endocrinol 11:779–791.

Litman, B. J. and Mitchell, D. C. (1996) A role for phospholipid polyunsaturation in modulating membrane protein function. Lipids 31:S193–S197.

Martinez, M. (1996) Docosahexaenoic acid therapy in docosahexaenoic acid-deficient patients with disorders of peroxisomal biogenesis. Lipids 31:S145–S152.

Mohammed, B. S., Sankarappa, S., Geiger, M. and Sprecher, H. (1995) Reevaluation of the pathway for the metabolism of 7,10,13,16-docosatetraenoic acid to 4,7,10,13,16-docosapentaenoic acid in rat liver. Arch Biochem Biophys 317:179–184.

Moore, S. A., Yoder, E., Murphy, S., Dutton, G. R. and Spector, A. A. (1991) Astrocytes, not neurons, produce docosahexaenoic acid (22:6ω-3) and arachidonic acid (20:4ω-6). J Neurochem 56:518–524.

Moore, S. A., Hurt, E., Yoder, E., Sprecher, H. and Spector, A. A. (1995) Docosahexaenoic acid synthesis in human skin fibroblasts involves peroxisomal retroconversion of tetracosahexaenoic acid. J Lipid Res 36:2433–2443.

Mustad, V. A., Etherton, T. D., Cooper, A. D., Mastro, A. M., Pearson, T. A., Jonnalagadda, S. S. and Kris-Etherton, P. M. (1997) Reducing saturated fat intake is associated with increased levels of LDL receptors on mononuclear cells in healthy men and women. J Lipid Res 38:459–468.

North, J. A., Spector, A. A. and Buettner, G. R. (1994) Cell fatty acid composition affects free radical formation during lipid peroxidation. Am J Physiol 267:C177–C188.

Reaven, P. D., Parthasarathy, S., Grasse, B. J., Miller, E.,

Steinberg, D. and Witztum, J. (1993) Effects of oleic acid-rich and linoleic acid-rich diets on the susceptibility of low density lipoprotein to oxidative modification in mildly hypercholesterolemic subjects. J Clin Invest 91:668–676.

Scott, B. L. and Bazan, N. J. (1989) Membrane docosahexaenoate is supplied to the developing brain and retina by the liver. Proc Natl Acad Sci USA 86:2903–2907.

Sprecher, H. W., Baykousheva, S. P., Luthria, D. L. and Mohammed, B. S. (1995) Differences in the regulation of biosynthesis of 20- and 22-carbon polyunsaturated fatty acids. Prostaglandins Leukot Essent Fatty Acids 52:99–104.

Steinberg, D., Parthasarathy, S., Carew, T. E., Khoo, J. C. and Witztum, J. L. (1989) Beyond cholesterol: Modifications of low-density lipoprotein that increase its atherogenicity. N Engl J Med 320:917–924.

Uauy, R. D., Birch, E. E., Birch, D. G. and Peirano, P. (1992) Visual and brain function measurements of ω3 fatty acid requirements in infants. J Pediatr 120S:168–180.

Voss, A., Reinhart, M., Sankarappa, S. and Sprecher, H. (1991) The metabolism of 7,10,13,16,19-docosapentaenoic acid to 4,7,10,13,16-docosahexaenoic acid in rat liver is independent of 4-desaturase. J Biol Chem 266:19995–20000.

Yerram, N. R., Moore, S. A. and Spector, A. A. (1989) Eicosapentaenoic acid metabolism in brain microvessel endothelium: Effect on prostaglandin formation. J Lipid Res 30:1747–1757.

RECOMMENDED READINGS

Bracco, U. and Deckelbaum, R. J. (eds.) (1992) Polyunsaturated Fatty Acids in Human Nutrition, pp. 1–243. Raven Press, New York.

Burns, C. P. and Spector, A. A. (1994) Biochemical effects of lipids on cancer therapy. J Nutr Biochem 5:114–123.

Jump, D. B., Clarke, S. D., Thelen, A., Liimatta, M., Ren, B. and Badin, M. (1996) Dietary polyunsaturated fatty acid regulation of gene transcription. Prog Lipid Res 35:227–241.

Schoonjans, K., Staels, B. and Auwerx, J. (1996) Role of peroxisome proliferator-activated receptor (PPAR) in mediating the effects of fibrates and fatty acids on gene expression. J Lipid Res 37:907–925.

Sprecher, H., Luthria, D. L., Mohammed, B. S. and Baykousheva, S. P. (1995) Reevaluation of the pathways for the biosynthesis of polyunsaturated fatty acids. J Lipid Res 36:2471–2477.

CHAPTER 16

◆ ◆

Regulation of Fuel Utilization

Malcolm Watford, D.Phil., and Alan G. Goodridge, Ph.D.

OUTLINE

FUELS

The macronutrients—carbohydrates, lipids, and proteins—are the sources of energy in the diet. Although the protein requirement is based on the need to maintain protein synthesis, and all macronutrients are involved in numerous biosynthetic functions, the bulk of macronutrients consumed each day are catabolized for energy production. A metabolic fuel may be defined as a circulating compound that is taken up by tissues for energy production. The major fuels are glucose, free fatty acids, triacylglycerols in lipoprotein complexes, ketone bodies, and amino acids. Lactate, glycerol, and alcohol also serve as fuels. Not all fuels are available at the same time, and their replenishment from exogenous (dietary) or endogenous (body) sources must be balanced and regulated in order to maintain homeostasis.

Constraints on Fuel Utilization

Organisms may be confronted with a supply of macronutrients that is inadequate to meet current needs with respect to total calories or specific nutrients. One solution potentially available to any mobile organism is to move to another location that has an adequate supply of nutrients. In many cases, this is not feasible, and nature has provided a number of alternative strategies. Regulation of the uptake and metabolism of nutrients provides the basis for adjustments. Prokaryotes and unicellular eukaryotes, such as yeast, can induce a new set of enzymes that takes advantage of other nutrients in the existing environment. Alternatively, many prokaryotes can sporulate; growth and metabolic rates in bacterial spores are reduced to very low levels and nutrient requirements are minimal. Such spores then await the development of conditions more propitious to growth.

Both cold-blooded (poikilothermic) and warm-blooded (homeothermic) vertebrates that hibernate have a solution that, in principle, is analogous to sporulation; they lower their energy requirements by lowering their body temperatures. Hibernation does not provide as long-term a potential for survival as sporulation, but it does allow the organism to survive extended periods of unfavorable conditions. Most homeothermic vertebrates, however, cannot hibernate. Furthermore, lowering body temperature is not always a feasible strategy by which poikilothermic animals can survive periods of food deprivation. Vertebrates deal with the inevitable periods of food deprivation by storing fuel when food is available and using the stored fuel during times of deprivation.

Birds and mammals are homeothermic animals, which means that they maintain a constant body temperature irrespective of the ambient temperature (within limits). Homeotherms have minimal (resting) metabolic rates that are related to their respective rates of heat loss. From the mouse to the elephant, minimal heat loss and basal metabolic rate are proportional to surface area. Small animals have much higher surface area to body weight ratios than do large animals, and they have higher rates of heat loss and hence higher energy utilization per unit of volume than do larger animals. It is this energy turnover, plus that resulting from physical activity and a small component for the thermic effect of food, that must be balanced with an adequate source of energy, as discussed in more detail in Chapters 17 through 19. Energy consumed must equal energy utilized or changes in body energy stores will result:

Changes in Body Energy Stores =
    Energy Intake − Energy Expenditure

When food is abundant, calories in excess of current energy needs are stored, first as glycogen and then as triacylglycerol. When food is unavailable, the stored energy is used for current needs. Because the nature and amounts of fuels provided by the diet are not identical to those of fuels consumed or stored by the body, the synthesis, oxidation, and storage of each of the individual macronutrients must be regulated.

Tissue-Specific Metabolism of Fuels

Perhaps the most important concept for understanding metabolism is tissue specificity; different tissues show different and characteristic patterns of fuel utilization, storage, and release (Table 16–1). In this respect, the brain and other structures of the central nervous system are important tissues to consider. The brain must receive a constant supply of fuel, but it is only capable of using glucose and ketone bodies. In key regions of the brain the blood–brain barrier limits the rate of transfer of long-chain fatty acids. Thus, the rate of oxidation of long-chain fatty acids is limited so that even when their level in the circulation rises they do not contribute significantly as a

fuel for the brain (Vannucci and Hawkins, 1983). Similarly, although many amino acids undergo a variety of interconversions within the brain, they do not play a major role in overall energy supply.

Under most conditions the brain utilizes glucose, which it oxidizes completely. There is some evidence that under extreme pathological conditions the brain can take up lactate, but normally lactate levels are not high enough for this to occur. Similarly, the use of ketone bodies is usually minimal because the level of circulating ketones is low in the healthy, fed individual. However, after a few days of starvation, and during some pathological conditions, the levels of ketone bodies rise, and the brain oxidizes them in preference to glucose. Even when ketone bodies are available, parts of the brain still require glucose. Although some glucose is still completely oxidized, the metabolism of most glucose is restricted to glycolysis, with a resultant release of lactate, when ketone bodies are being used. This regulation of brain energy metabolism is very important, because the brain is unable to obtain sufficient glucose to maintain function at glucose levels of less than 3 mmol/L (54 mg/100 mL of plasma). To maintain blood glucose levels above this minimum, particularly in starvation when the only sources of glucose are endogenous (hepatic glycogen breakdown and gluconeogenesis), it is important to provide alternative fuels, such as fatty acids and ketone bodies, in order to decrease the body's need for glucose.

Skeletal muscle makes up most of the lean body mass and accounts for much of the daily energy metabolism, although this varies greatly depending on the amount of physical work performed. Different types of muscle can, and do, use different fuels, but in general skeletal muscle is capable of using glucose, fatty acids (including those derived from circulating and intra-tissue triacylglycerols), ketone bodies, and the branched-chain amino acids (leucine, isoleucine, and valine). In addition, skeletal muscle takes up and stores considerable amounts of glucose (stored as glycogen) and free fatty acids (stored as triacylglycerol) for later use during contraction. Not all these fuels are completely oxidized in skeletal muscle; considerable amounts of

TABLE 16–1
Tissue-Specific Metabolism

Tissue	Fuel Used	Fuel Released
Brain	Glucose Ketone bodies	Lactate (only in prolonged starvation; the brain can utilize lactate under some pathological conditions)
Skeletal muscle	Glucose Free fatty acids Triacylglycerols Branched-chain amino acids	Lactate Alanine Glutamine
Heart	Free fatty acids Triacylglycerols Ketone bodies Glucose Lactate	
Liver*	Amino acids (partial oxidation) Free fatty acids Lactate Glycerol Glucose Alcohol	Glucose Ketone bodies Lactate (during absorptive phase) Triacylglycerols
Intestine†	Glucose Glutamine	Lactate Alanine
Red blood cells	Glucose	Lactate
Kidney	Glucose Free fatty acids Ketone bodies Lactate Glutamine	Glucose (renal gluconeogenesis important only in prolonged starvation)
Adipose tissue	Glucose Triacylglycerols	Lactate Glycerol Free fatty acids

*The liver is also the site of galactose and fructose metabolism.

†The small intestine also releases dietary glucose, galactose, fructose, amino acids, and lipids.

lactate may be released from glucose metabolism. Furthermore, the breakdown of branched-chain amino acids and some other amino acids in the muscle results in the formation and release of alanine and glutamine. Muscle glycogen is used as a local fuel store and is not able to contribute directly to the circulating glucose supply because muscle lacks glucose 6-phosphatase. Heart muscle represents a special case because it is constantly working. It is highly aerobic and largely dependent on fatty acid oxidation for its energy requirements; at times of glucose excess the heart will oxidize glucose, and it may even take up and oxidize lactate when circulating lactate levels rise. Further discussion of fuel utilization by muscle during rest and exercise can be found in Chapter 39.

The liver plays a major regulatory role because, in effect, it monitors the intake of nutrients. It takes up glucose and other monosaccharides and stores them as glycogen to be released later as glucose. It takes up lactate, amino acids, and glycerol and converts them to glucose 6-phosphate, either to be stored as glycogen or released directly as glucose (gluconeogenesis); and it takes up fatty acids either for reesterification or for β-oxidation and ketone body production. In addition, alcohol is metabolized exclusively in the liver. Although the liver has the capacity to oxidize completely each of the macronutrients, this is probably not a major fate of most macronutrients. Indeed, partial oxidation of dietary amino acids (protein) alone would provide more than enough energy for the liver. Thus, hepatic amino acid metabolism conserves most of the carbon skeletons as glucose; hepatic fatty acid oxidation is limited mainly to the production of ketone bodies; and hepatic glucose metabolism results in net lactate release across the liver in the absorptive period. In theory, the liver could utilize excess carbohydrate and amino acids for de novo fatty acid synthesis. Based on measurements, however, net synthesis of fat is not of quantitative importance for energy storage in humans consuming typical Western diets (>30% of calories as fat). Indeed, excess dietary carbohydrate and protein are normally oxidized before dietary fat is catabolized (Horton et al., 1995; see Chapter 18 also).

In addition to the liver, the kidneys are the only organs capable of gluconeogenesis. Renal gluconeogenesis is probably of quantitative importance only during prolonged starvation or metabolic acidosis. This issue is uncertain because certain cells in the kidney utilize glucose at high rates at the same time that other cells are producing glucose. Although the kidneys account for less than 0.5% of body mass, they account for about 10% of total oxygen consumption at rest, indicating their quantitative importance in energy metabolism. The kidneys are very heterogeneous, and different cells show marked differences in metabolism of specific fuels; different renal cells have differing capacities to use glucose, lactate, fatty acids, ketone bodies, and certain amino acids, especially glutamine.

Another metabolically active tissue, accounting for 20% of resting oxygen consumption, is the intestinal tract, where dietary glutamine and glutamate and circulating glutamine are major respiratory fuels for the absorptive epithelial cells. Glucose is utilized and, if available, free fatty acids and ketone bodies are used. Within enterocytes, glucose is not oxidized completely; partially metabolized glucose carbons are released as lactate. Glutamine also undergoes partial oxidation; the carbon skeleton is probably partially conserved as the 3-carbon compounds lactate, pyruvate, and alanine. In addition, the metabolism of glutamine in these cells results in the production of ammonia, proline, and citrulline. The colonic mucosa demonstrates a specific and unique metabolism in that colonocytes derive most of their energy from the oxidation of butyrate produced during the fermentation of dietary fiber and resistant starch by the microflora in the lumen of the colon (Roediger, 1982).

A few tissues contain obligatory glycolytic cells: they are able to obtain energy only from the metabolism of glucose to lactate (with a little via the pentose phosphate pathway). The best known example is the mammalian red blood cell, which, lacking mitochondria, is unable to extensively oxidize any fuels because the principal oxidative pathways are intramitochondrial and dependent upon oxygen as a terminal electron acceptor. This group of tissues also includes the retina and the renal medulla. Although these cells always require some glucose as an obligatory fuel, they produce lactate as the end product. This lactate then returns to the liver to be converted back into glucose; this cycling of lactate and glucose between tissues and liver is known as the Cori cycle (see Chapter 9).

Although adipose tissue can be the largest tissue mass in the body, its role in energy metabolism is primarily to store and release fatty acids. In the fed state, circulating triacylglycerols are hydrolyzed by lipoprotein lipase in the adipose tissue capillary bed, and the fatty acids are taken up by the adipocytes to be stored as triacylglycerol. Because adipose tissue lacks glycerol kinase activity, the glycerol 3-phosphate required for reesterification is derived from glucose or glycolytic intermediates. During starvation, the stored triacylglycerols are hydrolyzed intracellularly by hormone-sensitive lipase, and the free fatty acids and glycerol are released into the circulation. One important aspect of adipose tissue metabolism is that anatomically different depots show different rates of metabolism and responsiveness to hormones and other signals. In general, intraabdominal adipose tissue is more active metabolically than subcutaneous adipose tissue (Leibel et al., 1989).

Other tissues have various specialized patterns of metabolism but are not generally considered to be of quantitative importance. However, the mammary gland during lactation, the fetus and placenta during gestation, various organs during certain pathological conditions such as hypercatabolic states, or large tumors can have major effects on whole-body energy metabolism.

THE METABOLIC FATE OF MACRONUTRIENTS

There are two sources of fuels for the body: (1) exogenous, those that are derived directly from the diet, and (2) endogenous, those that arise from tissues either directly from fuel stores (such as glycogen or triacylglycerol) or from the metabolism of other fuels (such as lactate or ketone bodies). Most individuals eat discrete meals, and the macronutrients are absorbed, processed, and stored during the absorptive phase after a meal. (The stores of fuel are listed in Table 18–1 of Chapter 18.) The size of the carbohydrate store is limited (~350 g in an adult), and a purely storage form of protein does not exist. On the other hand, triacylglycerol stores appear to be without limit. In the late 1960s, Cahill (1970) studied a group of obese men undergoing therapeutic starvation for 6 weeks. This work led to the concept that glucose homeostasis could be divided into different stages (Fig. 16–1). In this model of glucose homeostasis, the body maintains circulating glucose levels through five major phases, using different physiological mechanisms to regulate glucose production and utilization and providing alternative fuels (Cahill, 1970; Ruderman et al., 1976). The following section briefly outlines the fate of macronutrients in a typical meal and how the body adapts to maintain glucose homeostasis as starvation progresses in subsequent phases. Details of the pathways and specific regulatory mechanisms are provided in Chapters 9 through 14.

The Absorptive or Postprandial Phase

The macronutrients in a standard meal of 90 g of carbohydrate, 30 g of protein, and 20 g of fat (27% of the calories as fat) will be utilized by the body in a characteristic manner. Dietary glucose is taken up from the intestinal lumen into the enterocyte by the sodium-linked glucose transporter SGLT1. A small amount of glucose is utilized by these cells for glycolysis with resultant lactate production, but most passes out of the cell down a concentration gradient via the facilitative hexose transporter GLUT2 and into the portal vein. Although dietary carbohydrate also may be absorbed into the portal system as galactose or fructose, these two sugars normally are probably exclusively metabolized by the liver (see Chapter 9) and hence are not considered part of peripheral carbohydrate metabolism.

The absorption of dietary carbohydrate causes a rise in circulating glucose level, which together with other signals triggers release of insulin. Although insulin does not stimulate hepatic glucose transporters directly, it is required for the uptake and utilization of

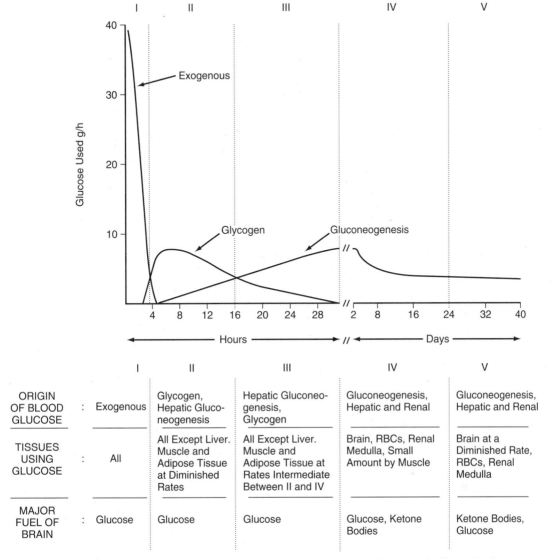

Figure 16–1. *Glucose utilization versus time in the five phases of glucose homeostasis. Stage I refers to the absorptive or postprandial period; II, to the postabsorptive period; III, to early starvation; IV, to intermediate starvation; and V, to prolonged starvation. (From Ruderman, N. B., Aoki, T. T. and Cahill, G. F., Jr. [1976] Gluconeogenesis and its disorders in man. In: Gluconeogenesis: Its Regulation in Mammalian Species [Hanson, R. W. and Mehlman, M. A., eds.]. John Wiley & Sons, New York. Copyright 1976, Wiley Interscience.)*

glucose by the liver. During this phase, the level of glucose in the portal vein rises considerably (up to 15 mmol/L). The liver appears to be able to sense the glucose concentration difference between the portal vein and the hepatic artery (liver receives ~80% of its blood supply via the portal vein and only ~20% via the artery), and the liver shows only net glucose uptake when a large portal to arterial glucose gradient exists together with an elevated level of insulin (Stumpel and

Jungerman, 1997). The liver is able to take up considerable amounts of glucose because it possesses a unique isozyme of hexokinase, hexokinase IV or glucokinase. Glucokinase has a much lower affinity for glucose (and other hexoses) than the other hexokinases, being half saturated at about 5 mmol/L of glucose. In addition, unlike the other hexokinases, glucokinase is not subject to inhibition by physiological levels of glucose 6-phosphate.

These differences in glucokinase kinetics enable the liver to take up glucose and store it as glycogen when glucose is abundant even as the levels of intracellular glucose 6-phosphate increase. Thus the liver takes up glucose, and perhaps as much as 20 g of the glucose in a meal is deposited as glycogen. In addition, the liver may partially catabolize some glucose and may demonstrate net lactate release at this time. However, there also is evidence of lactate uptake by some liver cells, and some glycogen synthesis (perhaps as much as 30% to 40%) may occur via the gluconeogenic (indirect) pathway from the carbon skeletons of lactate and amino acids (Shulman and Landau, 1992).

The remaining glucose (70 g) passes through the liver, causing peripheral plasma glucose levels to rise to 6 to 7 mmol/L. Over the next 2 h, the brain will take up approximately 15 to 20 g of glucose to be oxidized directly as a fuel (Fig. 16–2). The obligatory glycolytic cells will use some glucose (2 to 3 g per h), and when circulating glucose levels are high and those of free fatty acids are low (e.g., as in the absorptive phase), all tissues capable of using glucose probably will be using it as fuel. Most of the glucose, however, will be taken up in an insulin-dependent manner (facilitative transporter GLUT4; see Chapter 9) by skeletal muscle (45 g) and adipose tissue (2 g). In skeletal muscle, approximately half will be oxidized and half stored as glycogen. In adipose tissue, most will be used for the synthesis of glycerol 3-phosphate for triacylglycerol synthesis, and a small quantity may be metabolized to lactate. During the absorptive phase, there is evidence that the net production of lactate by the liver and other tissues provides an important fuel for the kidneys, heart, and possibly colon.

The ingestion of 100 g of protein/day presents the body with a problem because amino acids must be used for protein synthesis or degraded. After a meal, a large surge of amino acids (30 g) enters the circulation, generating signals for increased protein synthesis. About 10 g will be converted to protein, but this leaves 20 g to be catabolized because the body lacks a purely storage form of protein (Fig. 16–3). Much of the glutamine, glutamate, and aspartate in the meal (4 g) will be metabolized by the intestine, with resultant production of alanine, proline, citrulline, ammonia, and lactate. The remaining amino acids are mainly absorbed unmodified and cause a rise in amino acid levels in portal blood that, in turn, stimulates their catabolism in the liver. The branched-chain amino acids, which comprise just over 25% of dietary protein (8 g of those in the meal), are not catabolized by the liver; after about 4 g have been used for protein synthesis, the remaining 4 g will be catabolized in extrahepatic tissues such as skeletal muscle with lesser roles played by the kidneys and adipose tissue. Thus about 40% to 50% of the amino acid load is catabolized by the liver, with the resulting

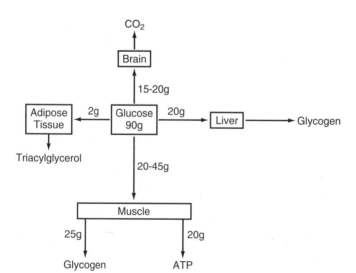

Figure 16–2. *Fate of dietary carbohydrate (glucose) from one meal during the absorptive phase (~2 h). Glucose provides the glycerol moiety for triacylglycerol synthesis. In addition to the fates shown, 2 to 3 g of glucose are required by the obligatory glycolytic cells.*

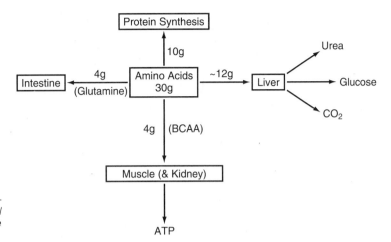

Figure 16–3. *Fate of dietary protein (amino acids) from one meal during the absorptive phase (~2 h).*

synthesis of about 7 to 9 g of glucose (stored as glycogen). Jungas and colleagues (1992) calculated that the complete oxidation of the amino acids from dietary protein could result in excessive ATP production in the liver, and they proposed that the synthesis of glucose (glycogen) and urea, and perhaps even protein, from dietary amino acids could be viewed as mechanisms to regenerate ADP and so allow continued degradation of amino acids by the liver. This analysis suggests that the liver does not oxidize amino acids completely in vivo, and that in the fed/absorptive state the major energy source for synthesis of ATP in the liver is the partial oxidation of amino acids.

Dietary fats are perhaps the simplest to describe in terms of their immediate fate after a meal. Although the digestion, processing, and storage of fats require repeated cycles of hydrolysis and resynthesis of triacylglycerols (see Chapters 7, 13, and 14), most of the fat in a meal will be deposited, mainly in adipose tissue (with limited amounts in liver and skeletal muscle), and stored for utilization at a later time. During the postabsorptive period, the level of free fatty acids in the circulation is low because lipids are transported to tissues as triacylglycerols in lipoproteins. Although dietary fatty acids may undergo some modification, the profile of fatty acids laid down in adipose tissue triacylglycerol is essentially the same as that in the diet.

Synthesis of fatty acids de novo is a minor pathway of energy storage in humans consuming Western diets (>30% of calories as fat)

(Hellerstein et al., 1996). Based on calorimetry studies, even in subjects eating hypercaloric, very low-fat (3% of calories as fat), high-carbohydrate diets, glycogen accumulates up to 1 kg, and net fatty acid synthesis in excess of fatty acid oxidation is detectable only after 5 days of such an extreme regimen (Acheson et al., 1988). However, calorimetry is limited in that it cannot detect de novo fatty acid synthesis directly. Studies with stable isotopes demonstrated de novo fatty acid synthesis in subjects consuming low-fat diets (10% of calories as fat), although it was not in excess of fatty acid oxidation (Hudgins et al., 1996). Furthermore, de novo fatty acid synthesis was not detectable in subjects consuming a more standard diet (40% of energy as fat). Most people find it difficult to maintain a hypercaloric, low-fat/high-carbohydrate diet for more than a few days. Thus, the role of de novo fatty acid synthesis in energy storage and weight gain in the normal population is minimal. However, in the study of subjects consuming 10% of calories as fat in whom de novo fatty acid synthesis was detected, the low-fat/high-carbohydrate diet did result in an increase in circulating triacylglycerols and, perhaps more significantly, in an increase in the degree of saturation of those triacylglycerols, because de novo fatty acid synthesis produces saturated fatty acids, predominantly palmitate (Hudgins et al., 1996).

During the absorptive phase, about 40 g of glucose is taken out of the circulation per hour. This occurs because insulin stimulates glucose uptake and metabolism in skeletal muscle and to a lesser extent in adipose tissue, because insulin stimulates glycogen synthesis in liver, and because most other tissues use glucose as a fuel. Thus 2 to 3 hours after the meal, about one third of the glucose has been stored, and the rest has been oxidized. A third of the amino acids has been used for protein synthesis, and most other amino acids have undergone catabolism, providing the major energy source of the liver together with some storage of the carbon skeletons as glycogen. Lipids have been absorbed more slowly, and have been transported in the circulation as triacylglycerols in lipoproteins, limiting their availability and oxidation. The majority of the fatty acids from dietary lipids will be stored in adipose tissue depots for future use.

Postabsorptive or Fasting Glucose Homeostasis

Once the nutrients in a meal have been absorbed, the body relies on endogenous sources for its energy. The brain requires about 120 g of glucose per day, and the glycolytic tissues will use another 50 to 60 g. Blood glucose levels must be maintained to allow brain function, so the body responds in a coordinated and tissue-specific manner to regulate provision and utilization of fuels. Falling blood glucose levels (Fig. 16–4) cause decreased insulin secretion and increased glucagon secretion (Fig. 16–5). At physiological levels in humans, glucagon is known only to act on the liver, where one of its prime actions is to stimulate the breakdown of glycogen. Because liver contains glucose 6-phosphatase, it releases glucose 6-phosphate derived from glycogenolysis into the circulation as free glucose and so maintains glucose levels. However, if all tissues continued to use glucose as the major fuel, the reserves of liver glycogen would not last very long. Thus, as hepatic glycogen is mobilized, some tissues switch to alternative fuels, decreasing use of glucose and prolonging the availability of liver glycogen. Insulin is a very strong inhibitor of lipolysis in adipose tissue, and the fall in circulating insulin levels relieves such inhibition. A simultaneous rise in catecholamines stimulates lipolysis in adipose tissue. The combined effects of the fall in insulin and rise in

catecholamine concentrations result in a rise in the level of free fatty acids in the circulation (Fig. 16–4).

Tissues such as skeletal muscle have a defined hierarchy for the fuels that they oxidize. When free fatty acids are available, skeletal muscle oxidizes them in preference to glucose. Thus the decrease in circulating glucose and insulin results in an increased availability of free fatty acids, which are then used as a fuel instead of glucose. This is known as the glucose–fatty acid cycle or the Randle cycle (Fig. 16–6) (Randle et al., 1963). The oxidation of fatty acids (and ketone bodies) occurs within the mitochondrial matrix and generates large amounts of acetyl CoA, NADH, ATP, and citrate. Elevated levels of these compounds inhibit glucose metabolism through feedback inhibition of pyruvate dehydrogenase and allosteric inhibition of 6-phosphofructo-1-kinase (see Chapter 9).

During the postabsorptive phase, circulating glucose is maintained by the breakdown of liver glycogen. The brain accounts for 50% of glucose utilization. Although other tissues are still using glucose, it is at a reduced rate, and they are beginning to substitute other fuels. This glucose-sparing effect of fat-derived fuels means that as starvation develops, less glucose is used by the body.

Liver glycogen stores are not limitless, and eventually (after about 24 h of starvation), they become depleted. Once this has occurred, the only source of glucose is gluconeogenesis (the synthesis of glucose from noncarbohydrate precursors). Therefore, as liver glycogen stores begin to decline, gluconeogenesis becomes more important and is the only source of blood glucose after ~24 h of starvation. Gluconeogenesis, however, is very costly in terms of substrate. The only substrates for gluconeogenesis during starvation are lactate (and pyruvate), glycerol, and amino acids. The body is not able to make glucose from the 2-carbon units released during fatty acid oxidation, and hence fatty acids are not gluconeogenic substrates. Also important is the fact that gluconeogenesis does more than just provide "new" glucose for the brain to oxidize but also is involved in the recycling of lactate and alanine carbons back to glucose.

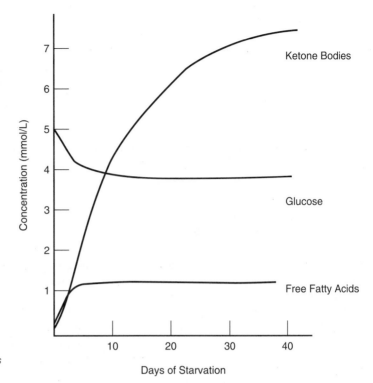

Figure 16–4. Plasma concentrations of fuels during prolonged starvation.

Throughout starvation the obligatory glycolytic tissues continue to utilize glucose, but they conserve the carbon skeleton as lactate, which is recycled into glucose (Cori cycle). Thus these tissues do not represent a drain on the circulating glucose pool, but they do demand continuing gluconeogenesis from lactate in liver. The energy for the synthesis of glucose within the liver is provided from the partial oxidation of fatty acids. Similarly, although alanine is quantitatively the most important amino acid taken up by the liver for glucose synthesis, the carbon skeleton of this alanine is derived primarily from glucose me-

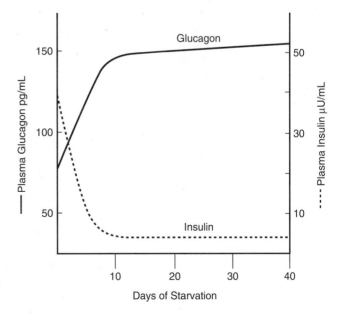

Figure 16–5. Plasma levels of insulin and glucagon during prolonged starvation.

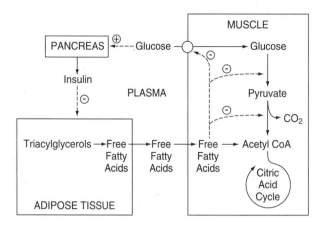

Figure 16–6. The glucose–fatty acid (Randle) cycle. A rise in plasma glucose stimulates insulin release by the pancreas. When plasma glucose levels decrease, insulin levels will also decrease. This results in increased mobilization of free fatty acids from adipose tissue; the fatty acids are then utilized in tissues such as muscle with a resultant inhibition of glucose utilization. (The production of ketone bodies by the liver and their resultant utilization in peripheral tissues spare glucose oxidation in a similar manner. Overall, this is known as the glucose-sparing effect of fat-derived fuels.)

tabolism in peripheral tissues and likewise simply recycles glucose carbon via the glucose-alanine cycle (see also Chapters 9 and 11). Thus, recycled glucose cannot contribute to the net amount of glucose required by the brain, because net use of glucose from this pool would compromise the metabolism of a number of tissues and lead to hypoglycemia. Therefore the brain relies on gluconeogenesis to provide "new" glucose synthesized from glycerol and amino acids. The amount (~18 g/day) of glucose synthesized from glycerol is relatively small and remains fairly constant throughout starvation. The major gluconeogenic substrates providing "new" glucose are amino acids that are derived from the net breakdown of body protein. Initially, the principal source may be hepatic proteins, but within a few hours the bulk of amino acids will be derived from increased net proteolysis in skeletal muscle. Not all amino acid carbon will yield glucose; on average, 1.6 g of amino acids is required to synthesize 1 g of glucose. Thus, to keep the brain supplied with glucose at a rate of 110 to 120 g/day, the breakdown of 160 to 200 g of protein, or close to 1 kg of muscle tissue, would be required. This is clearly undesirable, and the body limits glucose utilization to reduce the need for gluconeogenesis and so spare body protein.

High levels of fatty acids in the circulation result in their partial oxidation in the liver and the resultant production of ketone bodies. The ketone bodies are released into the circulation during starvation, and their concentration rises (see Fig. 16–4). Many tissues, including the brain, use ketone bodies as fuels; this spares glucose metabolism via a mechanism similar to the sparing of glucose by oxidation of fatty acids as an afternative fuel. The use of ketone bodies therefore replaces some of the glucose required by the brain. In addition, it decreases glucose oxidation in the brain by limiting some glucose metabolism to glycolysis to lactate. Thus, after 4 to 6 days of starvation, utilization of blood glucose has decreased to 1 to 2 g/h for oxidation in the brain and perhaps a similar amount for the Cori and glucose-alanine cycles in other tissues.

The high levels of ketone bodies in the circulation produce a metabolic acidosis and also result in excretion of considerable quantities of ketone bodies in the urine. The loss of some energy in the urine seems to be a price that is paid in order to provide the brain with an alternative substrate. In response to the ketoacidosis, both to maintain pH and to limit excretion of inorganic anions, the kidneys produce large amounts of ammonia and bicarbonate and excrete ammonium ions (NH_4^+). The substrate for renal ammonia production is glutamine (derived from muscle proteolysis), and the carbon skeleton of glutamine is recovered as glucose through renal gluconeogenesis. Thus, during the ketoacidotic phase of starvation, the kidney becomes a major gluconeogenic organ; this occurs at a time when the liver has decreased its rate of gluconeogenesis considerably.

Thus in long-term starvation (Fig. 16–7), the brain is the only tissue that completely oxidizes glucose. However, the brain's consumption of glucose occurs at a reduced rate,

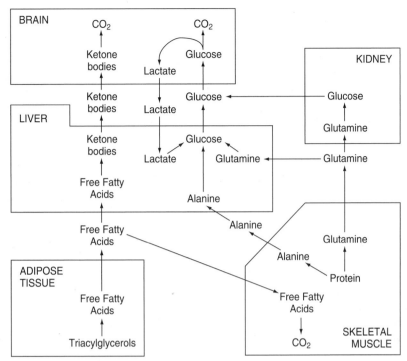

Figure 16–7. *Fuel utilization during prolonged starvation. The only tissues utilizing glucose are the brain and the obligatory glycolytic tissues (omitted for clarity). Fatty acids have become the major fuel for tissues such as liver and muscle, and ketone bodies have replaced a considerable amount of the brain's glucose utilization. In addition, the brain has restricted some of its glucose utilization to glycolysis with the release of lactate, thus reducing glucose oxidation to extremely low rates.*

with ketone bodies providing most of the fuel to the brain. Glucose use in other tissues is limited to glycolysis to lactate (or alanine), which conserves the gluconeogenic potential. The liver derives most of its energy from the partial oxidation of fatty acids, and most other tissues are using either fatty acids or ketone bodies as the major fuel.

HORMONAL SIGNALS FOR REGULATION OF FUEL UTILIZATION

The coordinated regulation of metabolism illustrated by the maintenance of glucose homeostasis described earlier requires key signals that can communicate the state of alimentation of the body to the tissues. Substrate supply (e.g., glucose uptake by the liver at high portal glucose levels or use of free fatty acids and ketone bodies only when they are available) can and does play a very important role. However, the main circulating signaling agents are hormones, especially in-

sulin, glucagon, catecholamines, glucocorticoids, and thyroid hormones. A number of other hormones and circulating factors, together with paracrine and autocrine agents, also participate in the regulation of tissue metabolism.

Hormones and Their Actions in the Regulation of Fuel Metabolism

Insulin is a polypeptide hormone synthesized and secreted by the β cells of the islets of Langerhans in the pancreas. It is secreted in response to changes in circulating glucose; a change of as little as 2 mg/100 mL of plasma can be detected by the pancreas. Insulin release also can be stimulated in response to certain amino acids in the circulation. Other important signals for insulin secretion include gut hormones and nervous stimulation.

Insulin has many effects in a variety of tissues. The insulin-stimulated uptake of glucose in skeletal muscle and adipose tissue involves the transporter GLUT4 and is well characterized (see Chapter 9). However, even in the liver where glucose transport is not directly stimulated by insulin, the hormone still signals glucose storage and utilization. Insulin is a major signal in decreasing hepatic glucose output after feeding and in increasing hepatic glucose use for glycogen synthesis and the flux of glucose through glycolysis, pyruvate dehydrogenase, and the citric acid cycle. In adipose tissue, insulin increases fatty acid uptake and triacylglycerol storage via increases in lipoprotein lipase activity and, at the same time, decreases lipolysis by decreasing hormone-sensitive lipase activity. The latter may be one of insulin's strongest actions be-

cause it occurs at very low insulin levels and effectively lowers the levels of free fatty acids in the circulation, thereby decreasing their utilization as a fuel.

In addition, insulin brings about other changes, including stimulation of amino acid transport and protein synthesis and a decrease in protein degradation in a variety of tissues. Insulin also regulates the expression of a number of genes; for example, expression of glucokinase (glucose utilization) in the liver is increased by insulin whereas expression of phosphoenolpyruvate carboxykinase (glucose production) is decreased. Some actions of insulin, particularly those seen at very

---

CLINICAL CORRELATION

Diabetes Mellitus

Diabetes mellitus is a chronic disease that results from a lack of secretion of insulin in sufficient amounts or in a lack of insulin stimulation of its target cells. Diabetes mellitus is often diagnosed by an elevated fasting blood glucose level, by excretion of glucose in the urine, or by an abnormal glucose tolerance test. Diabetes mellitus is the third leading cause of death in the United States, following heart disease and cancer.

Diabetes mellitus occurs in two major forms: (1) type I, insulin-dependent, juvenile-onset diabetes mellitus, and (2) type II, noninsulin-dependent, maturity-onset diabetes mellitus. In insulin-dependent diabetes (IDDM), the pancreas lacks or has defective β cells and secretes no or essentially no insulin. Onset is thought to occur when 80% or more of the pancreatic β cells have been destroyed by the immune system. Because the patients do not synthesize or secrete insulin, daily insulin injections are essential.

Noninsulin-dependent diabetes mellitus (NIDDM) is a more complex disease that may be present for many years prior to diagnosis and that has a strong genetic component. NIDDM accounts for the majority (>80%) of the diagnosed cases of diabetes. It usually occurs after age 40 years and is often (>80%) associated with obesity. NIDDM patients exhibit varying levels of plasma insulin, but their tissues are resistant to its actions. Prior to the onset of diabetes, the bodies of these patients probably maintained blood glucose homeostasis by increasing the release of insulin in response to a glucose load. Ultimately, as insulin resistance develops, the pancreas is not able to secrete sufficient insulin to maintain blood glucose levels. Insulin resistance means that insulin fails to control key functions in liver, skeletal muscle, and adipose tissue. Changes in diet, together with a loss of weight and increased physical activity, or the use of drugs that enhance insulin secretion and action often can control NIDDM without the need for exogenous insulin administration.

Thinking Critically

1. In untreated NIDDM, the plasma glucose level is high due to both reduced clearance of glucose from the plasma and increased release of glucose into the plasma. Explain how a reduced response to insulin might decrease the removal of glucose from, and increase glucose release into, the circulation.

2. In what ways are the fuel supply and hormonal signals similar in untreated diabetes mellitus and starvation? In what ways are they dissimilar?

3. Untreated IDDM is associated with high levels of ketone bodies in the circulation. Explain.

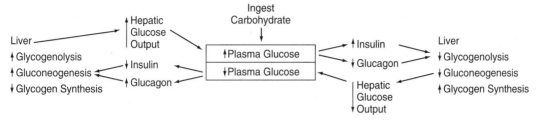

Figure 16–8. *Insulin and glucagon regulate hepatic glucose output. Insulin also lowers plasma glucose levels by increasing uptake into skeletal muscle and adipose tissue.*

high concentrations, may be related to its structural similarity to growth factors; these actions include an increase in DNA synthesis and an overall increase in cell growth. Insulin is an anabolic hormone in that it increases storage of glycogen and triacylglycerols; decreases glycogenolysis, gluconeogenesis, and lipolysis; and generally stimulates net protein synthesis. As insulin stimulates the removal of blood glucose into the tissues, circulating levels of glucose drop and insulin secretion consequently slows; thus insulin and glucose effectively form a negative feedback loop (Fig. 16–8).

Glucagon is a polypeptide hormone secreted by the α cells of the islets of Langerhans in the pancreas. Glucagon secretion is inhibited by high blood glucose, and, therefore, regulation of its concentration is usually opposite to that for insulin. However, glucagon secretion also is increased by some amino acids. These two hormones tend to have opposite effects on fuel metabolism, and it is common to read of the insulin:glucagon ratio. Although a useful concept, this term should not be taken to mean that there is any direct competition of insulin and glucagon for the same receptors. In humans, glucagon acts only on the liver, where it works through a

cyclic AMP (cAMP)-dependent mechanism to increase hepatic glucose output by stimulation of glycogen breakdown and gluconeogenesis. It also stimulates β-oxidation, proteolysis, amino acid transport and catabolism, and urea synthesis. Long-term effects of glucagon include increased expression of the phosphoenolpyruvate carboxykinase gene and of the genes encoding the urea cycle enzymes. By increasing hepatic glycogen breakdown and gluconeogenesis, glucagon causes an increase in blood glucose levels (Fig. 16–8).

Adrenergic hormones are catecholamines secreted by the adrenal medulla (mainly epinephrine, which is also called adrenaline) and from the sympathetic nervous system (norepinephrine, which is also called noradrenaline). Synthesis of catecholamines is discussed in Chapters 11 and 23; see Fig. 11–24). Epinephrine is released into the circulation at times of stress, the fight or flight response, and during starvation. In contrast, the neurological release of norepinephrine occurs directly at nerve endings in the tissues to provide a very localized signal. The actions of the catecholamines largely depend on the type of receptor(s) present on the cell surface, as detailed in Table 16–2.

TABLE 16–2

Adrenergic Receptors

	Receptor Type		
	β	α₁	α₂
Second messenger	cAMP	Ca²⁺	Decrease of cAMP
Effects	Glycogenolysis Vasodilation	Glycogenolysis Lipolysis Vasoconstriction	Inhibition of lipolysis Vasoconstriction

Modified from Frayn, K. N. (1996) Metabolic Regulation: A Human Perspective, p. 100. Portland Press, London.

Broadly, adrenergic receptors can be classified into two α (α_1, α_2) and three β (β_1, β_2, and β_3) types (Frayn, 1996; Lafontan and Berlan, 1993). All three β-receptors signal increased lipolysis, glycogenolysis, and gluconeogenesis, and α_1-receptors are involved in stimulating glycogenolysis. In contrast, α_2-receptors inhibit lipolysis. It is interesting that there are marked tissue differences in the expression of adrenergic receptors. Subcutaneous adipose tissue usually has relatively more α_2-receptors whereas intraabdominal adipose tissue has relatively more β-receptors. This could account for the observation that intraabdominal lipid stores are more rapidly lost than subcutaneous stores during caloric restriction. Despite the somewhat contradictory actions of catecholamines, the elevated levels observed during starvation result in net increases in lipolysis and in hepatic glucose output. Adrenergic hormones also have marked effects on the circulation: β-adrenergic actions include increased heart rate and blood vessel dilation, whereas binding of catecholamines to both types of α-adrenergic receptors generally causes constriction of blood vessels.

Glucocorticoids, predominantly cortisol (Fig. 16–9), are steroid hormones synthesized by the adrenal cortex, and although their levels do not change markedly during starvation or after feeding, they do appear to be essential for the action of a number of other hormones, especially those involving changes in specific gene expression. Glucocorticoids are often termed permissive, in that the action of other hormones is compromised if cortisol levels are low. In general, cortisol stimulates hepatic glucose output and expression of hepatic genes encoding gluconeogenic enzymes. Glu-

cocorticoids are also involved in maintaining elevated rates of proteolysis in skeletal muscle in conditions of net protein breakdown.

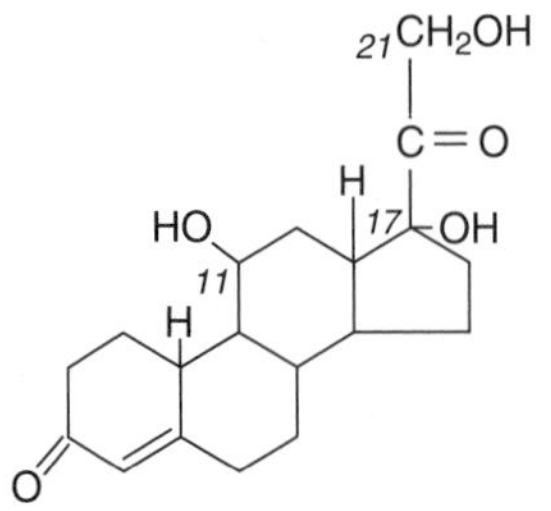

The thyroid hormones, triiodothyronine (T_3, active form) and thyroxine (T_4), are synthesized in the thyroid gland and by conversion of T_4 to T_3 in other tissues as described in Chapter 33. (See Fig. 33–1 for hormone structures.) The level of T_3 falls in starvation, whereas the concentration of an inactive form, reverse T_3, rises. The thyroid hormones regulate metabolism in a long-term manner by changing gene expression and by modulating the effects of other hormones. For example, although the rise in circulating epinephrine during starvation would be expected to increase the rate of metabolism, this does not occur, perhaps because lower levels of thyroid hormones decrease the rate of metabolism.

Mechanisms of Hormone Action

Hormones initiate their actions by binding to receptors. The presence, abundance, and specificity of certain receptors in a given tissue determine its responsiveness to these hormones. The actual physiological responses depend upon various signal transduction mechanisms or upon changes in gene expression or protein synthesis.

There are two general types of hormone receptors in mammalian cells: (1) those on the cell surface that bind the hormone and then transmit the signal to the inside of the cell via a second messenger, and (2) those that bind the hormone inside the cell such that the ligand-receptor complex is the intracellular signaling agent, often acting in the nucleus. Glucagon, insulin, and the catecholamines (adrenergic hormones) are examples of the first type; glucocorticoids and thyroid hormones are examples of the second type.

Glucagon, insulin, and catecholamines bind to specific receptors on the cell membrane. Such receptors contain an extracellular domain that binds the hormone and transmembrane and intracellular domains that anchor the receptor in the membrane and transmit the signal to the inside of the cell. The glucagon receptor and the β- and α-adrenergic receptors share some common mechanisms, including use of cAMP as the intracel-

Figure 16–9. *Structure of cortisol, a glucocorticoid hormone.*

lular messenger. The initial intracellular event after hormone binding is interaction of the receptor with a specific guanosine triphosphate (GTP)–binding protein (called a G-protein) located on the inner surface of the plasma membrane (Fig. 16–10). There are a variety of G-proteins, but classes important in signal transduction via regulation of cAMP production are G_s, stimulatory proteins, and G_i, inhibitory proteins. G-proteins are composed of three subunits: G_α, G_β, and G_γ. The specificity resides mainly in the α subunit of these heterodimeric proteins.

Effects mediated by glucagon or β-adrenergic receptors involve G_s-proteins. As shown in Figure 16–10, when glucagon or β-adrenergic receptors are activated by hormone binding, $G_{s\alpha}$ binds GTP in exchange for guanosine diphosphate (GDP) with simultaneous dissociation of the α subunit from the β,γ complex. The dissociated $G_{s\alpha}$-GTP subunit then interacts with and activates adenylate cyclase, which is also located on the inner surface of the membrane. This results in synthesis of cAMP from ATP as long as the $G_{s\alpha}$-GTP/adenylate cyclase complex exists. $G_{s\alpha}$ also has a low level of GTPase activity that slowly hydrolyzes GTP to GDP. This renders $G_{s\alpha}$ inactive, and $G_{s\alpha}$-GDP recomplexes with the β,γ subunits to form the inactive heterodimer. The cycle can proceed only in the direction indicated because activation involves an exchange of GDP for GTP, whereas inactivation involves hydrolysis of GTP to GDP.

In contrast to the glucagon or β-adrenergic receptors, which interact with G_s-proteins, effects of catecholamines are mediated through α_2-adrenergic receptors that involve inhibitory G- or G_i-proteins. The GTP-GDP exchange and association-disassociation of subunits proceeds as described for the stimulatory G-proteins. In this case, however, the GTP-bound, activated form of $G_{i\alpha}$ inhibits the activity of adenylate cyclase and results in a decrease in cAMP concentration.

Adenylate cyclase catalyzes the synthesis of cAMP, which is a second messenger within the cell. The level of cAMP regulates the activity of protein kinase A (cAMP-dependent protein kinase). When the level of cAMP is low, the kinase exists as an inactive heterotetrameric complex containing two regulatory subunits (R) and two catalytic subunits (C). When cAMP binds to the regulatory subunits, the catalytic subunits are released in an active form:

$$R_2C_2 + 4\ cAMP \rightarrow R_2(cAMP)_4 + 2\ C$$

Protein kinase A is responsible for the phosphorylation and consequent activation or inactivation of a variety of proteins involved in glycogen, glucose, lipid, and amino acid metabolism. Other targets of protein kinase A include transcription factors that regulate expression of metabolically important enzymes. The levels of cAMP in the cell also are regulated by the rate of hydrolysis of cAMP to AMP by phosphodiesterase.

Catecholamines also may react with α_1-adrenoreceptors that act via association with a G-protein (e.g., G_q) to activate phospholipase C. This occurs via a mechanism similar to that for activation of adenylate cyclase by G_s-proteins. As shown in Figure 16–11, phospholipase C hydrolyzes phosphatidylinositol 4,5-bisphosphate (PIP$_2$), a minor component of the inner leaflet of the plasma membrane and mainly the species 1-stearoyl-2-arachidonyl-*sn*-glycerol, to inositol 1,4,5-triphosphate (IP$_3$) and diacylglycerol. IP$_3$ acts as a water-soluble second messenger; it opens a Ca^{2+} transport channel and thereby stimulates the release of Ca^{2+} from the endoplasmic reticulum into the cytosol. The rise in intracytosolic Ca^{2+} stimulates various processes via binding to calmodulin. The diacylglycerol released by phospholipase C acts as a second messenger within the plasma membrane by activating protein kinase C in the presence of Ca^{2+} and phosphatidylserine. Protein kinase C phosphorylates and thereby modulates the activities of several proteins, including glycogen synthase. The diacylglycerol may be further degraded in some tissues to yield arachidonate as substrate for eicosanoid synthesis, as discussed in Chapter 15. Other agents or processes that regulate calcium levels include vasopressin and muscle contraction; the latter is very important in coordinating glycogen breakdown with ATP generation in muscle.

The insulin receptor is composed of two α and two β subunits linked by disulfide bonds (Fig. 16–12) (Kahn, 1994). The extracel-

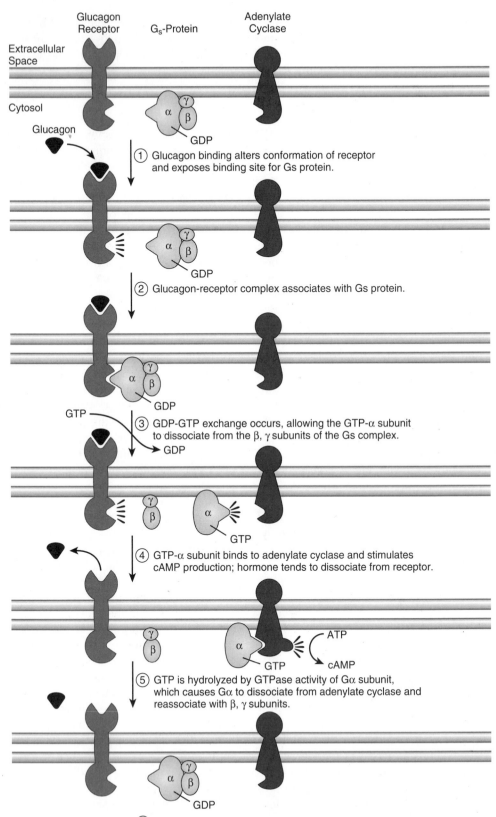

① Glucagon binding alters conformation of receptor and exposes binding site for Gs protein.

② Glucagon-receptor complex associates with Gs protein.

③ GDP-GTP exchange occurs, allowing the GTP-α subunit to dissociate from the β, γ subunits of the Gs complex.

④ GTP-α subunit binds to adenylate cyclase and stimulates cAMP production; hormone tends to dissociate from receptor.

⑤ GTP is hydrolyzed by GTPase activity of Gα subunit, which causes Gα to dissociate from adenylate cyclase and reassociate with β, γ subunits.

⑥ Activation of Gs and of adenylate cyclase may be repeated by reassociation of glucagon with receptor.

Figure 16–10 See legend on opposite page

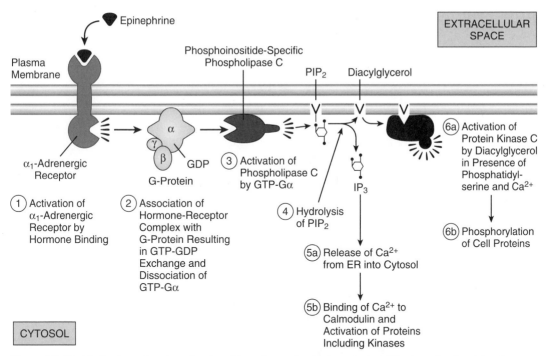

Figure 16–11. *Mechanism of action of epinephrine via α₁-adrenergic receptors. Binding of epinephrine to an α₁-adrenergic receptor is coupled via a G-protein to activation of phospholipase C. Phospholipase C catalyzes the hydrolysis of phosphatidylinositol 4,5-bisphosphate (PIP₂) in the membrane to release inositol 1,4,5-triphosphate (IP₃) and diacylglycerol. Biological effects in the cell result from the stimulation by IP₃ of Ca²⁺ release from the endoplasmic reticulum (ER) into the cytosol and from the activation of protein kinase C by diacylglycerol.*

lular domain is composed of the α subunit, which binds insulin, and the N-terminal end of the β subunit. The β subunit contains a single transmembrane domain that transmits the signal to the cytosol. The intracellular domain of the β subunit possesses a tyrosine kinase activity. Insulin binding to the receptor activates this tyrosine kinase activity, which first autophosphorylates specific tyrosyl residues on the β subunit. This autophosphorylation in turn activates the β subunit tyrosine kinase so it is able to phosphorylate cytosolic protein substrates, such as insulin receptor substrate 1, which, in turn, bind to and activate other proteins. A variety of different signal transduction cascades are involved in mediating the actions of insulin in the cell.

Thyroid hormones and steroid hormones such as the glucocorticoids are very lipophilic

and circulate bound to specific carriers. They enter cells, probably by diffusion, and then bind to specific receptors that may be located in the nucleus (T_3) or the cytosol (glucocorticoid). The glucocorticoid-receptor complex is translocated from the cytosol to the nucleus. The activated ligand-receptor complexes then bind to specific sites on the chromosomes and regulate (enhance or repress) the rate of transcription of specific genes. (Further discussion of the action of hormones that are ligands for nuclear receptors can be found in Chapters 26, 27, and 33.)

REGULATION AND CONTROL OF FUEL UTILIZATION

The tissue-specific metabolism mentioned in the previous sections is clearly regulated. Not

Figure 16–10. *Mechanism of glucagon action and of epinephrine action via β-adrenergic receptors. The role of a G$_s$-protein in stimulating adenylate cyclase activity (cAMP production) in response to glucagon is illustrated. Epinephrine acts in a similar mechanism via β-adrenergic receptors. Epinephrine also works via α₂-receptors, which are coupled to G$_i$-proteins and result in inhibition of adenylate cyclase activity and lower levels of cAMP.*

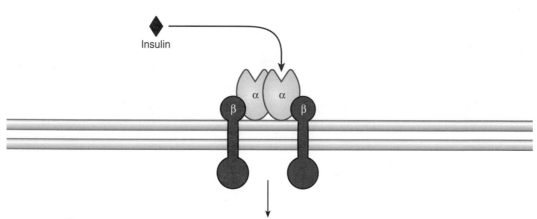

(1) Binding of insulin to the insulin receptor activates the tyrosine kinase activity of the cytosolic domains of the receptor's β subunits, which causes autophosphorylation of tyrosyl residues of the receptor's cytosolic domains.

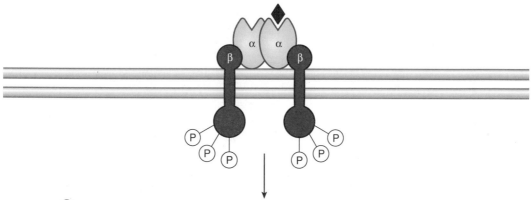

(2) Receptor tyrosine kinase phosphorylates cytosolic "relay" proteins (such as insulin receptor substrate 1, IRS-1), which then bind and activate other proteins. A number of different signal transduction cascades result in changes in cellular physiology and/or patterns of gene expression via serine/threonine phosphorylation/dephosphorylation.

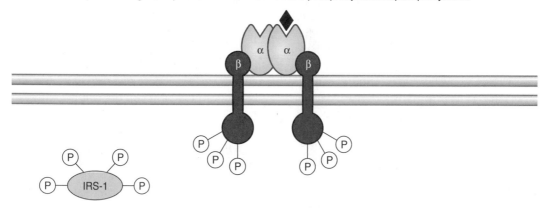

Figure 16–12. *Mechanisms of insulin action. Insulin binding to the insulin receptor results in receptor tyrosine kinase activity of the β subunits of the insulin receptor, which first autophosphorylates specific tyrosyl residues on the β subunits. This autophosphorylation, in turn, activates the β subunit tyrosine kinase so it is able to phosphorylate cytosolic protein substrates, such as insulin receptor substrate 1 (IRS-1). IRS-1 then binds and activates other proteins, eventually bringing about its biological effects as a result of serine/threonine phosphorylation.*

all pathways are operating in all tissues at all times. Tissue-specific metabolism is often due to the expression, or lack of expression, of genes encoding enzymes of different pathways, but this is a crude method of control that does not allow rapid regulation of flux. As explained in the previous sections, blood glucose levels are regulated, and regulation can be defined as a systemic property. Control, however, is a local property and is defined as the power to change the state of metabolism in response to an external signal. Thus control is measurable as the degree of influence that an external factor has on the system. It can be said that insulin and glucagon regulate blood glucose levels by control of metabolism in various tissues.

When regulation and control are considered, it is important to remember that metabolic pathways do not exist independently in the body. A beginning and end of a pathway is usually defined for convenience. In reality, even glycolysis in red blood cells, which appears to begin with glucose and end with lactate, actually requires the continued provision (from the intestine or liver) of glucose into the plasma and the continued removal of the lactate by the liver. Although this scheme is an oversimplification, it illustrates how a very simple pathway extends to other tissues and processes; the utilization of glucose by red blood cells is directly linked to the control of such processes as hepatic glycogen metabolism and gluconeogenesis.

Characteristics of Regulatory Enzymes

One of the major goals of the study of intermediary metabolism is to understand regulation and control. Although there has been a somewhat conventional paradigm in this area, it has become apparent that the traditional explanations have many limitations, and more quantitative methods are being developed. A number of terms have been introduced in an effort to aid in the identification and description of control; these included rate-limiting step, pacemaker, and flux-generating step. Although these concepts have been useful, they do not always accurately describe the physiological aspects of regulation and control and, unfortunately, often give the impression that

control rests with a single enzyme. A brief consideration follows of qualities that are characteristic of regulation and control, and of some of the problems encountered with traditional explanations of regulation. A full description of the theories and problems of quantitative control analysis can be found in a recent monograph by Fell (1996).

The rate of flux through a metabolic pathway is controlled by regulatory enzymes and transporters. A regulatory enzyme is defined as one whose activity is controlled by external factors, not simply by substrate supply, and as one whose activity controls some pathway function. It is useful to define two types of regulatory enzymes: (1) those that stabilize (control) metabolite concentrations and maintain homeostasis, and (2) those that change or control flux through the pathway. Both are regulatory, but not all regulatory enzymes are flux-controlling enzymes. The two types of control often occur at different steps in a given pathway.

A number of properties have been described that are claimed to be characteristic of regulatory enzymes, but no property by itself can be taken as direct evidence that an enzyme is regulatory or controlling. Enzymes that catalyze reactions near the beginning of a pathway make teleological sense as sites of control, because regulation at this point would avoid the buildup of intermediates and prevent the waste of valuable cofactors. However, when flux in most pathways is changed, there is no major change in the levels of intermediates along the pathway. For example, when the rate of glycolysis in skeletal muscle changes by over 1000-fold, the levels of intermediates change by less than 10-fold, and most changes are trivial (Fell, 1996). Because such small changes in metabolite concentrations would result only in minor changes in flux through subsequent enzymes, the results indicate that the activity of more than one enzyme has been changed by external factors. Similarly, the argument has been made that the enzyme with the lowest maximal activity, as determined in vitro, would be easiest to control. At times this seems to have been interpreted as the enzyme with the lowest activity in vivo, but this is not valid because all enzymes in a pathway must be operating at the same rate in vivo, otherwise large excesses (and deficits) of intermediates would arise. In practice, all enzymes in most pathways show activities in vitro that are many times the maximal flux of the pathway in vivo. For example, the capacities of the enzymes of glycolysis in heart muscle are all at least ten times the maximal flux measured in the intact organ.

Another property used to identify regulatory enzymes is that they catalyze reactions that are far removed from equilibrium in the cell (i.e., enzymes that catalyze unidirectional reactions). The levels of metabolic intermediates in a cell are usually at a steady state, and there is no noticeable change with time. Even when there is a change in flux in the pathway, a new steady state is achieved relatively quickly. In part, this is due to the fact that most enzymes catalyze reactions in two directions, and the overall reaction will be close to equilibrium if the forward and back reactions are proceeding at nearly equal rates. In practice, this means that changing the activity in one direction will also change the activity in the other direction, with little net effect on overall flux; therefore, a change in activity of a reversible reaction is of little regulatory value.

However, some enzymatic reactions are effectively irreversible in the cell because the back reaction is very slow or nonexistent. These reactions exhibit very large negative changes in free energy (ΔG) (i.e., they are far removed from equilibrium). The position of the equilibrium is a thermodynamic property of the system; enzymes can speed up the rate at which equilibrium is achieved, but they cannot change the position of an equilibrium. Enzymes that catalyze nonequilibrium reactions in the cell are considered good candidates for regulation, because changes in activity in one direction are not immediately negated by changes in the rate of the back direction. However, it is not always easy to determine whether an enzyme catalyzes a nonequilibrium reaction in vivo, and even when there is clear evidence that it does, this cannot be interpreted as definitive evidence that the enzyme controls flux in the pathway. Finally, even the existence of a well-defined regulatory mechanism of whatever type cannot be taken as proof that the enzyme is regulatory.

Although all the foregoing criteria are useful in identifying potential regulatory enzymes, definitive conclusions can be drawn only from quantitative analysis of the entire pathway. Normally, hormones and other agents have effects on numerous enzymes in a pathway and in related pathways. For example, in the liver, glucagon will increase phosphorylation of pyruvate kinase and 6-phosphofructo-2-kinase, resulting in decreased flux in glycolysis, while at the same time increasing synthesis of the gluconeogenic enzyme phosphoenolpyruvate carboxykinase and thus bringing about a net increase in gluconeogenesis. However, glucagon also regulates hepatic glycogen metabolism so that the glucose 6-phosphate produced via gluconeogenesis is not stored as glycogen. Thus in order to change gluconeogenic flux, glucagon controls the activities of many enzymes, some of which are not directly linked to the pathway, and all of these play some role in the ultimate metabolic change. Therefore, modern quantitative methods are designed to address the question, how much does flux in the pathway change if the activity of a specific enzyme is changed? The experimental evidence points to multiple points of control in a pathway, with the degree of importance of different steps often changing with the physiological state.

Mechanisms of Enzyme Control

Control of enzymatic activity can be conveniently split into two models: (1) short-term and (2) long-term. As their names imply, they are distinguished by the length of time required for bringing about changes, but this distinction does not apply absolutely. In reality, these two terms refer to two distinct mechanisms of regulation. Short-term control refers to changes in the specific activity of an enzyme, with no change in its concentration. Long-term control refers to changes in the amount of enzyme, with no change in kinetic properties. The two mechanisms are not exclusive, and some enzymes are subject to both short-term and long-term control in response to the same stimulus. In some cases, a short-term response can take as long as a long-term response; control of protein concentration is highly dependent on the half-life of the protein (see the following information and Chapter 10). All regulatory mechanisms must be reversible if they are to be of physiological importance.

Short-term control can be brought about by a variety of mechanisms. Many specific examples are given in Chapters 9, 11, 13, and 14. Short-term regulation is often related to small changes in the levels of key intermediates such as ATP and NADH. Often this is due simply to changes in cosubstrate or coenzyme supply. For example, a change in NADH concentration will usually be mirrored by an opposite change in NAD$^+$, and a change in acyl CoA concentration will result in an opposite change in the free CoASH concentration. Any change in these ratios will affect flux through reactions catalyzed by enzymes utilizing one of these couplets. Both allosteric activation and inhibition are important short-term mechanisms that involve the binding of a regulatory molecule to a distinct site on an enzyme. Several examples of short-term control can be seen in the pathway for glycolysis. For example, ATP is a strong inhibitor of 6-phospho-fructo-1-kinase, and this inhibition can be relieved by a second allosteric factor, such as fructose 2, 6-bisphosphate in liver or AMP in muscle. Other enzymes in glycolysis, such as hexokinase, which is inhibited by glucose 6-phosphate, and hepatic pyruvate kinase, which is stimulated by fructose 1,6-bisphosphate and inhibited by alanine, also are allosterically regulated. In addition, hepatic pyruvate kinase is subject to covalent modification and is phosphorylated by cAMP-dependent protein kinase (e.g., in response to glucagon); this makes it more sensitive to allosteric inhibition.

Reversible covalent modification of enzymes is an important short-term regulatory mechanism. A number of covalent modifications have been described (Lehninger et al., 1993), but the most common type is phosphorylation-dephosphorylation. Since the first description of activation of an enzyme (glycogen phosphorylase) by phosphorylation, there have been numerous reports of protein phosphorylation. Such phosphorylations usually occur on seryl, threonyl, or tyrosyl residues. Phosphorylation results in activation of some

---

 NUTRITION INSIGHT

Alcohol Consumption and Hypoglycemia

Alcohol is metabolized in the liver by alcohol dehydrogenase, which catalyzes the oxidation of ethanol to acetaldehyde:

$$CH_3CH_2OH + NAD^+ \rightarrow CH_3CHO + NADH + H^+$$

Consumption of alcohol, especially by an undernourished individual, can cause hypoglycemia. Drinking alcohol after strenuous exercise can have the same effect. This hypoglycemia can be quite dangerous, especially because a person may be thought to be inebriated when, in fact, he or she is suffering from hypoglycemia that may lead to irreversible damage to the central nervous system.

Thinking Critically

1. What is the normal source of glucose for maintenance of normoglycemia between meals? How might this source of glucose be affected by fasting/starvation or by strenuous exercise? What role would this play in the development of hypoglycemia subsequent to alcohol consumption?

2. Metabolism of ethanol to acetaldehyde is accompanied by the conversion of NAD$^+$ to NADH and a potentially dramatic increase in the ratio of NADH to NAD$^+$ in the cytosol of liver cells. Considering the role of NAD$^+$ in ethanol and pyruvate/lactate metabolism, how would gluconeogenesis from pyruvate (alanine) or lactate be affected by alcohol consumption? What role might this play in development of hypoglycemia?

enzymes and in inhibition of others. Many cases of protein phosphorylation have been reported that do not change the kinetic properties of the enzyme and therefore are of unknown function.

Important examples of enzymes that are controlled by phosphorylation-dephosphorylation include hormone-sensitive lipase in adipose tissue (activated by phosphorylation in response to catecholamines and inactivated by dephosphorylation in response to insulin), glycogen synthase (inactivated by phosphorylation in response to glucagon in liver), and 6-phosphofructo-2-kinase (a bifunctional enzyme, which loses kinase activity while its fructose 2,6-bisphosphatase activity is enhanced in response to glucagon in liver). Another very important phosphorylation is that of pyruvate dehydrogenase, which is inactivated by phosphorylation catalyzed by a specific kinase bound to the enzyme complex. Phosphorylation (inactivation) of pyruvate dehydrogenase is stimulated by acetyl CoA and NADH and inhibited by high CoA, NAD$^+$, or pyruvate. Dephosphorylation (activation) of the enzyme is stimulated by insulin. This is a crucial step in maintaining the body's glucose reserves, because inhibition of the oxidative decarboxylation of pyruvate (3 carbons) to acetyl CoA (2 carbons) conserves the gluconeogenic potential; the body lacks a mechanism to reverse this reaction.

A somewhat different form of short-term control is the physical movement of proteins within a cell. A well-known example of this is the insulin-regulated movement of GLUT4 glucose transporters to the cell surface of skeletal muscle and adipocytes, which increases the glucose transport capacity of these cells. Another example is the movement and activation of glucokinase and glycogen synthase within the liver in response to hormones, a process that results in the enzymes becoming physically close to or removed from their substrates (Agius and Peak, 1997).

Changes in the amount of enzyme protein (long-term control) are brought about by changes in the synthesis and/or degradation of the protein and consequently are rather slow, often taking days or hours to occur. However, some enzymes can show these long-term changes within relatively short time periods (<1 h), whereas some short-term covalent modifications can take almost as long. The steady-state concentrations of proteins (enzymes) are functions of the rates of their synthesis and degradation. Enzyme synthesis is a zero-order reaction: the rate is linear with time and can be described by a constant k_s. However, enzyme degradation follows first-order reaction kinetics, meaning that the actual rate is dependent on the amount of enzyme present (e.g., when enzyme synthesis decreases, the degradation rate will decrease exponentially with time). The rate of enzyme degradation can be described as the product of the enzyme concentration at time zero, E, and a degradation constant, k_d, so that the rate of enzyme degradation is E•k_d. Therefore, it is not meaningful to describe degradation in absolute rates, because the absolute rate changes depending on the amount of enzyme present. Instead, either the k_d or the apparent half life is typically used to describe the rate of protein degradation. Half life ($t_{1/2}$) can be defined as the time taken for 50% of the original enzyme to be degraded. Different proteins exhibit half lives that range from a few minutes to many days. Proteins with very short half lives not only will be degraded rapidly, but they also will respond rapidly to changes in the synthesis or degradation rate and so are able to establish new steady-state concentrations much more quickly than proteins with long half lives. Such proteins are ideal candidates for regulation (Schimke, 1973; Walker, 1983).

An example of a highly regulated key enzyme of glucose metabolism is phosphoenolpyruvate carboxykinase in liver. This enzyme has a half life of about 6 h and is regulated exclusively by long-term mechanisms. Most of this regulation is brought about by changes in the rate of transcription of the phosphoenolpyruvate carboxykinase gene. During starvation, one of the initial hormonal signals is increased glucagon, which increases glycogenolysis in liver via the second messenger cAMP. The increase in cAMP stimulates transcription of the phosphoenolpyruvate carboxykinase gene and results in higher rates of synthesis of the enzyme protein and hence higher enzyme activity. Thus as starvation slowly develops and as liver glycogen stores are gradually depleted, the liver is synthesizing new phosphoenolpyruvate carboxykinase and so increasing its capacity to carry out gluconeogenesis. Such a mechanism is highly suited to a situation such as starvation in which changes in metabolism occur over several hours. On the other hand, this mechanism would not be suitable for rapid responses such as muscle contraction during which short-term mechanisms such as allosterism allow responses in fractions of a second. Although changes in phosphoenolpyruvate carboxykinase level are largely the result of changes in transcription of the gene, changes in phosphoenolpyruvate carboxykinase protein level also can occur through changes in its mRNA turnover or changes in the rate of degradation of the enzyme protein itself.

As with all reports of regulation, evidence that an enzyme is itself regulated, even via long-term changes in the amount of enzyme protein, cannot be taken to indicate changes in flux in the pathway or to imply that such changes in the enzyme activity are in any way regulatory. They may be simply adaptive in nature; many such changes occur long after flux through the pathway has changed in response to more rapid control at various points in the pathway. In the final analysis, any theory of metabolic regulation and control must be compatible with the evidence for changes in flux in vivo.

REFERENCES

Acheson, K. J., Schutz, Y., Bessard, T., Anantharaman, K., Flatt, J. P. and Jequier, E. (1988) Glycogen storage capacity and de novo lipogenesis during massive carbohydrate overfeeding in man. Am J Clin Nutr 48:240–247.

Agius, L. and Peak, M. (1997) Binding and translocation of glucokinase in hepatocytes. Biochem Soc Trans 25:145–150.

Cahill, G. F., Jr. (1970) Starvation in man. N Engl J Med 282:668–675.

Fell, D. (1996) Understanding the Control of Metabolism. Portland Press, London.

Frayn, K. (1996) Metabolic Regulation: A Human Perspective, pp. 87–102. Portland Press, London.

Hellerstein, M. K., Schwarz, J.-M. and Neese, R. A. (1996) Regulation of hepatic de novo lipogenesis in humans. Annu Rev Nutr 16:523–557.

Horton, T. J., Drougas, H., Brachy, A., Reed, G. W., Peters, J. C. and Hill, J. O. (1995) Fat and carbohydrate overfeeding in humans: Different effects on energy storage. Am J Clin Nutr 62:19–29.

Hudgins, L. C., Hellerstein, M., Seidman, C., Neese, R., Diakun, J. and Hirsch, J. (1996) Human fatty acid synthesis is stimulated by a eucaloric low fat, high carbohydrate diet. J Clin Invest 97:2081–2091.

Jungas, R. L., Halperin, M. L. and Brosnan, J. T. (1992) Quantitative analysis of amino acid oxidation and related gluconeogenesis in humans. Physiol Rev 72:419–448.

Kahn, C. R. (1994) Insulin action, diabetogenes, and the cause of type II diabetes. Diabetes 43:1066–1084.

Lafontan, M. and Berlan, M. (1993) Fat cell adrenergic receptors and their control of white and brown fat cell function. J Lipid Res 34:1057–1091.

Lehninger, A. L., Nelson, D. L. and Cox, M. M. (1993) Principles of Biochemistry, pp. 233–235. Worth Publishers, New York.

Leibel, R. L, Edens, N. K. and Fried, S. K. (1989) Physiological basis for the control of body fat distribution in humans. Annu Rev Nutr 9:417–443.

Randle, P. J., Garland, P. B., Hales, C. N. and Newsholme, E. A. (1963) The glucose fatty acid cycle. Its role in insulin sensitivity and the metabolic disturbances of diabetes mellitus. Lancet i:785–794.

Roediger, W. E. (1982) Utilization of nutrients by isolated epithelial cells of the rat colon. Gastroenterology 83:424–429.

Ruderman, N. B., Aoki, T. T. and Cahill, G. F., Jr. (1976) Gluconeogenesis and its disorders in man. In: Gluconeogenesis: Its Regulation in Mammalian Species (Hanson, R. W. and Mehlman, M. A., eds.), pp. 515–532. Wiley Interscience, New York.

Schimke, R. (1973) Control of enzyme levels in mammalian tissues. Adv Enzymol 37:135–187.

Shulman, G. I. and Landau, B. R. (1992) Pathways of glycogen repletion. Physiol Rev 72:1019–1035.

Stumpel, F. and Jungerman, K. (1997) Sensing by intrahepatic muscarinic nerves of a portal-arterial glucose concentration gradient as a signal for insulin-dependent glucose uptake in the perfused rat liver. FEBS Lett 406:119–122.

Vannucci, S. and Hawkins, R. (1983) Substrates for energy metabolism of the pituitary and pineal glands. J. Neurochem 41:1718–1725.

Walker, R. (1983) The Molecular Biology of Enzyme Synthesis: Regulatory Mechanisms of Enzyme Adaptation. Wiley Interscience, New York.

RECOMMENDED READINGS

DeFronzo, R. A. (1997) Pathogenesis of type 2 diabetes: Metabolic and molecular implications for identifying diabetes genes. Diabetes Rev 5:177–269.

Frayn, K. N. (1996) Metabolic Regulation: A Human Perspective. Portland Press, London.

Halperin, M. L. and Rolleston, F. S. (1993) Clinical Detective Stories. Portland Press, London.

Moran, L. and Scrimgeour, G. (1994) Biochemistry, Chapters 14 and 23. Neil Patterson Press, Carborro, North Carolina.

Newsholme, E. A. and Leech, A. R. (1986) Biochemistry for the Medical Sciences. John Wiley and Sons, Chichester, United Kingdom.

Randle, P. J. (1986) Fuel selection in animals. Biochem Soc Trans 14:799–806.

Energy

◆ ◆

Energy is defined as the capacity for doing work. In the biological world, the various types of work that require energy include mechanical work, chemical work, and osmotic and electrical work. In animals and humans, the energy that sustains the various forms of biological work is derived from the carbohydrates, lipids, and proteins of the diet; this energy initially came from the sun and was stored by plants during photosynthesis at the beginning of the food chain. Some of the food energy is stored in the body as specific fuel reserves, mainly as glycogen and triacylglycerol, for use during the absence of food intake.

All forms of energy may be described as consisting of either potential or kinetic

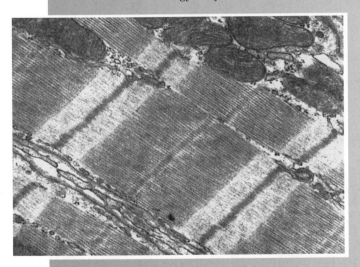

energy. For people, food is a source of potential energy. In the catabolism of carbohydrates, proteins, and lipids, some of this potential energy is stored or conserved in forms in which it can be used to support various energy-utilizing reactions. The first law of thermodynamics states that energy can neither be created nor destroyed. Some of the chemical energy available in glucose can be converted in the process of catabolism to another form of chemical energy, adenosine 5'-triphosphate (ATP). In skeletal and cardiac muscle, chemical energy involved in the energy-rich phosphate bonds of ATP may be converted to mechanical energy during the process of muscle contraction. The energy involved in the proton gradient produced across the inner mitochondrial membrane during electron transport is converted to chemical energy when the proton gradient is used to drive ATP synthesis. Ultimately, most of the potential energy taken in as food is converted to and lost from the body as heat.

The second law of thermodynamics states that all processes tend to progress toward a situation of maximum entropy (disorder or randomness). Entropy can be viewed as the energy in a system that is unavailable to perform useful work. The

Electron Micrograph of Muscle; Courtesy of Cornell Integrated Microscopy Center, Cornell University, Ithaca, NY.

portion of the total energy in a system that is available for useful work is called the free energy and is usually denoted by G. Reactions with positive free-energy changes (endergonic reactions) may be coupled to and driven by reactions that have negative free-energy changes (exergonic reactions); the sum of the ΔG values for individual reactions in a pathway must be negative in order for a metabolic sequence to be thermodynamically feasible.

Most biological work is mediated by hydrolysis of energy-rich bonds, particularly by hydrolysis of so-called high-energy phosphate bonds. Whereas hydrolysis of simple phosphate esters, such as glucose 6-phosphate and glycerol 3-phosphate has $\Delta G^{\circ\prime}$ values in the range of 1 to 3 kcal/mol, hydrolysis of phosphoric acid anhydrides such as the β- and γ-phosphates of ATP, of enol phosphates such as phosphoenolpyruvate, and of thiol esters such as acetyl CoA is associated with $\Delta G^{\circ\prime}$ values of about -7.3, -14.8, and -7.7 kcal/mol, respectively. These high-energy phosphate esters retain the energy in the structural, chemical, electrostatic, and resonant properties of the molecules. They release or transfer large amounts of free energy upon hydrolysis of the phosphate ester bonds because hydrolysis results in formation of products that are more stable (i.e., have more resonant forms or less electrostatic repulsion) than the high-energy phosphate substrate.

Adenosine 5′-triphosphate plays a central role in linking energy-producing and energy-utilizing pathways. Potential ATP "units" or "equivalents" are often counted as a means of expressing the amount of available energy, the rate at which energy can be produced and/or utilized, or the amount of energy that can be obtained from storage depots. In the cell, the hydrolysis of ATP must be balanced with the phosphorylation of adenosine diphosphate (ADP). During macronutrient catabolism, some ATP equivalents are formed as a result of substrate-level phosphorylation, but most ATP is formed in the final stages of fuel catabolism in the mitochondria, i.e., by the transfer of reducing equivalents to oxygen via the electron transport chain and oxidative phosphorylation driven by the proton gradient. Because of the central role of oxidative phosphorylation in conservation of chemical energy in ATP, the production of reducing equivalents, such as $NADH + H^+$ or $FADH_2$, by catabolic pathways and the transfer of these hydrogens (electrons and protons) to oxygen as the terminal acceptor are closely linked to overall energy expenditure by the body.

In this unit, energy nutrition is considered largely from a whole body perspective. Nutritionists have traditionally considered the energy requirement or expenditure as being constituted by three major categories: energy for support of the normal processes of growth and maintenance (called basal metabolism), energy for the assimilation or use of dietary fuels (called specific dynamic action or thermic effect of food), and energy for activity. For maintenance of body weight, energy intake and energy expenditure must be balanced. If energy intake is greater than energy expenditure, excess energy will be stored as triacylglycerol in adipose tissue and lead to obesity. If energy intake is less than energy expenditure, this will result in loss of body weight and, if severe, can lead to protein-energy malnutrition.

◆ ◆

Martha H. Stipanuk

CHAPTER 17

Cellular and Whole-Animal Energetics

Adamandia D. Kriketos, Ph.D., John C. Peters, Ph.D., and James O. Hill, Ph.D.

OUTLINE

Metabolic Sources of Heat Production
Oxidative Phosphorylation
Oxidation of Fuel Molecules
Efficiency of Energy Conservation from
    Fuel Oxidation

Substrate Cycling
Measurement of Energy Expenditure
Components of Energy Expenditure
Determinants of Resting Metabolic Rate

COMMON ABBREVIATIONS

ADP (adenosine diphosphate)
ATP (adenosine triphosphate)
BAT (brown adipose tissue)
EE_{act} (energy expenditure due to activity)
FFM (fat-free mass)
RMR (resting metabolic rate)
RQ (respiratory quotient)
TEF (thermic effect of food)
UCP (uncoupling protein)

Total-body energy utilization is the sum of the myriad of energy-utilizing and energy-producing reactions occurring within individual cells and organ systems throughout the body. The various metabolic reactions that serve to sustain life are fueled by the energy released from the biological oxidation of energy-yielding nutrients in the food we consume. A fraction of the energy released from biological oxidation processes is captured in so-called "high energy" molecules, namely ATP (adenosine triphosphate), which is the main energy currency of the cell, and a few other specialized molecules such as creatine phosphate. These energy carriers fuel the various biochemical processes within cells that support basal metabolism, growth, and other essential functions. Chemical bond energy not captured in ATP synthesis is released as heat, which helps maintain body temperature.

METABOLIC SOURCES OF HEAT PRODUCTION

Current research suggests that heat production within cells has three components: essential, obligatory, and regulatory (Fig. 17–1). Essential heat production is associated with the heat released during the reactions associated with the anabolic and catabolic cycles responsible for tissue turnover, primarily via the utilization and resynthesis of ATP molecules. Obligatory heat production originates from a variety of energy-utilizing molecular transport mechanisms. Examples of these obligatory processes include reactions involved in the absorption, digestion, and storage of nutrients, the Na^+,K^+-pump located in the cell membrane, and the proton pump located within the mitochondrial membrane. In homeothermic organisms (i.e., those that maintain a constant body temperature), regulatory heat production comprises a third component of cellular heat production.

Many neural and endocrine factors affect these various heat-producing reactions within cells (Fig. 17–1). Thyroid hormone, for example, increases oxygen consumption and stimulates the metabolism of all warm-blooded animals. Thyroid hormone affects several components of the electron transport chain, the cell membrane Na^+,K^+-ATPase pump, and fat, carbohydrate, and protein metabolism. The effects of thyroid hormone on energy metabolism are discussed in more detail in Chapter 33.

Quantitatively, the energy expended in fueling various molecular transport mechanisms, many of which are responsible for

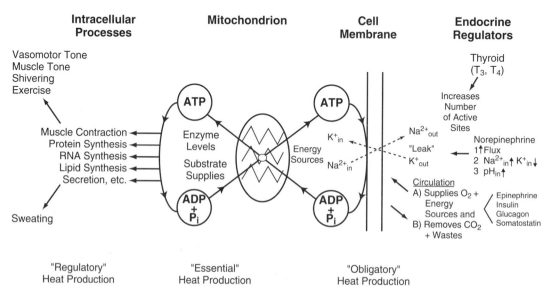

Figure 17–1. Nature of biochemical pathways for heat production. (From Goldman, R.F. [1980] Effect of environment on metabolism. In: Assessment of Energy Metabolism in Health and Disease [Kinney, J. M., ed.], pp. 117–121. Report of the First Ross Conference on Medical Research. Ross Laboratories, Columbus, OH.)

maintaining essential electrochemical gradients across membranes, is responsible for a significant fraction of whole-body energy expenditure at rest. For example, it has been estimated that the Na^+,K^+-ATPase reaction, which is coupled to transport of Na^+ into cells and movement of K^+ out, accounts for 20% to 40% of whole-body resting energy expenditure (resting metabolic rate, or RMR) (McBride and Kelly, 1990). In highly metabolically active cell types, such as hepatocytes (liver cells), proton pumping across the mitochondrial membrane may represent up to 30% of the energy utilization of the cell (McBride & Kelly, 1990). Numerous other processes that transport amino acids, glucose, and nucleic acids, as well as reactions responsible for macromolecular synthesis/degradation (e.g., membrane protein and phospholipid turnover), also contribute substantially to cellular and whole-body energy utilization.

Regulatory heat production, an essential function in homeotherms, is needed to maintain a constant body temperature in the face of fluctuating environmental temperature. Shivering, which is triggered in response to cold exposure, can involve a substantial increase in skeletal muscle contraction, which results in a significant increase in ATP turnover and subsequently increased heat production. Conversely, exposure of the individual to increased environmental temperature stimulates sweat production, which helps cool the body through the heat loss associated with evaporation. The processes of modulating heat production confer tremendous flexibility to many species so that they may survive in many different environmental conditions.

OXIDATIVE PHOSPHORYLATION

The coupling of fuel molecule oxidation to heat production and ATP synthesis is localized within the mitochondria of mammalian cells. The specialized proteins and enzymes required for the oxidative phosphorylation chain of reactions are specifically localized on the inner mitochondrial membrane. Oxidative phosphorylation is the process by which a molecule of inorganic phosphate is condensed with ADP (adenosine diphosphate) to form ATP, a process driven by the step-by-step transfer of electrons along a chain of electron carriers, as illustrated in Figure 17–2. The rate of ATP synthesis is governed or regulated by the availability of ADP. ADP is the "spent" end product of ATP-requiring reactions and is regenerated into ATP. Thus, ATP production is directly coupled to ATP utilization through the generation and phosphorylation of the ADP intermediate.

The synthesis of ATP during oxidative phosphorylation is linked to the release of electrons carried by flavin and pyridine nucleotides to proteins of the electron transfer chain. Hydrogen ions are pumped out of the mitochondrial matrix across the inner mitochondrial membrane at three sites along the electron transport chain to create an electrochemical gradient. This proton gradient is subsequently dissipated as protons are allowed back through the membrane by the ATP synthase, which couples this process to ATP synthesis. Sufficient free energy may be collected at three sites along the electron transport chain (levels of Complexes I, III, and IV, as shown in Figure 17–2) to allow phosphorylation of ADP to ATP. A maximum of three molecules of ATP can be generated from each nucleotide molecule of NADH oxidized (by donating its pair of electrons to the electron transfer chain). The oxidation of $FADH_2$ occurs at a later step in the electron transport chain, and a maximum of only two molecules of ATP can be generated from each $FADH_2$ molecule. A thorough description of the electron transport chain can be found in most biochemistry textbooks; also see Figure 20–7 in Chapter 20.

The oxidation of fuel molecules utilizes molecular oxygen, especially as the terminal electron acceptor at the end of the electron transport chain, and the energy yield or heat production generated by these biochemical processes can be determined by measuring oxygen consumption. A frequently used index of the efficiency of oxidative phosphorylation is the P:O ratio. It is defined as the number of molecules of inorganic phosphate incorporated into organic form per atom of oxygen consumed (Murphy and Brand, 1987). At maximal biological efficiency, the complete oxidation of NADH yields 3 ATP molecules,

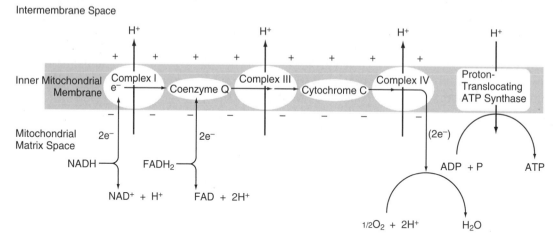

Figure 17–2. *A general scheme for mitochondrial electron transport and oxidative phosphorylation. The transport of electrons from nicotinamide adenine dinucleotide, reduced form (NADH), and flavin adenine dinucleotide, reduced form (FADH₂) is accomplished by specific carrier molecules that constitute the electron transport chain. The terminal electron (and proton) acceptor is oxygen, and water is formed as a product of electron transport. The generation of the proton gradient by pumping protons out of the mitochondrial matrix is also shown. Dissipation of this proton gradient by the ATP synthase is coupled to ATP synthesis.*

and so the ratio observed for this process is 3. For the complete oxidation of FADH₂, the P:O ratio is 2. Few direct attempts to determine the P:O ratio in intact cells have been made because of difficulties encountered in trying to determine the rapid turnover of ATP molecules involved in the maintenance of a cell's metabolic activities without disturbing the cell's internal milieu. Nevertheless, the physiological P:O ratio is almost certainly somewhat less than the maximal values of 3 and 2 that are commonly used as a basis for calculating "ATP equivalents" of NADH and FADH₂, respectively.

OXIDATION OF FUEL MOLECULES

Free energy for the synthesis of ATP within cells comes from the oxidation of energy-yielding molecules in food, which include predominantly carbohydrate, fat, protein, and also alcohol if consumed (Flatt, 1985). The ATP yield per gram of glucose (from glycogen), fatty acid, or amino acid oxidized differs in proportion to the oxidation state of the different molecules. A molecule of glucose,

for example, is more highly oxidized than a fatty acid molecule, and thus less energy per gram is released in its complete oxidation to CO_2 than is released by complete oxidation of a fatty acid.

Net ATP yield depends on the amount of energy (ATP) the body must expend in the complete metabolism of the energy-yielding molecule as well as on that produced via substrate-level phosphorylation and oxidative phosphorylation. For example, the complete oxidation of 1 molecule of glucose via glycolysis, pyruvate dehydrogenase, and the citric acid cycle (as described in Chapter 9) results in synthesis of 40 ATPs, the expenditure of 2 ATPs, and a net yield of 38 ATPs. If we further consider the oxidation of fuels already stored in the body, so that the inefficiencies or costs of digestion, absorption, and assimilation are not factors, we can consider examples of how net ATP yield may vary with the tissue and particular pathway (sequence of reactions) by which the fuel is catabolized.

For example, if liver glycogen were released as glucose and the glucose were taken up and completely oxidized by muscle, the net ATP yield from the oxidation of this glu-

NUTRITION INSIGHT

Physiological Fuel Values

Physiological fuel value is a term used to connote the energy value of a food obtained by subtracting energy lost in the excreta (feces and urine) from the total energy value of the food. Atwater and his associates at the Connecticut (Storrs) Agriculture Experiment Station determined the digestibility and fuel values of a number of food materials in the late 1800s/early 1900s and proposed the general physiological fuel equivalents of 4.0, 8.9, and 4.0 kcal/g of dietary protein, fat, and carbohydrate, respectively, for application to the mixed American diet. In the years following the publication of Atwater's work, the 4, 9 (rounded), and 4 factors came into widespread usage in estimating the caloric value of foods. These factors are still widely used today, a century later.

One should note that factors for carbohydrate, fat, or protein in specific foods may vary considerably owing to differences in digestibility or chemical composition. The general factors are intended for application to mixed diets. The carbohydrate factor is applied to total food carbohydrate, which includes nondigestible carbohydrate that is now referred to as dietary fiber. Also, the derivation of the factors attributed all the energy lost in the urine to excretion of protein nitrogen as urea; this is not strictly correct, but errors in calculation of energy value of foods by application of Atwater's protein factors to diets have been estimated to be small.

More recently, the data and values of Atwater were checked and confirmed by 108 digestion experiments conducted by Merrill and Watt (1973) at the United States Department of Agriculture. The available energy of the diets, determined from gross energy values of food, feces, and urine, showed close agreement with calculations based on the application of average energy factors to the protein, fat, and carbohydrate in the diet. Merrill and Watt also recalculated Atwater's general factors for protein, fat, and carbohydrate, based on a typical American mixed diet in 1949. They obtained average values of 4.0, 8.9, and 3.9, which were essentially the same as the general factors Atwater reported in 1899.

cose derived from liver glycogen stores would be 38 mol of ATP per mole of glucose. On the other hand, if muscle glycogen were the source of the glucose, with breakdown of glycogen to glucose 1-phosphate, the complete metabolism of this glucose phosphate within the muscle could generate 39 ATP per mole of glucose phosphate; one less ATP would be expended because ATP-dependent phosphorylation of glucose was not required. Under anaerobic conditions, muscle might convert plasma glucose to lactate (with a net yield of 2 mol of ATP per mole of glucose), but the conversion of lactate back to glucose by liver (with a net cost of 6 mol of ATP per 2 mol of lactate), followed by its complete oxidation to $CO_2 + H_2O$) (net release of 38 ATP per mole of glucose) would result in the net generation of 34 mol of ATP per mole of glucose completely oxidized with intermediate cycling to lactate and back to glucose.

Not all the free energy of dietary fuel molecules is available to the body. Some energy is lost due to incomplete digestion and absorption of fuel molecules. In general, a small amount (usually no more than 5% to 10%) of the gross energy content of food is lost in feces due to incomplete digestion and absorption. The fate of absorbed fuel energy is shown in Figure 17–3. Once absorbed, an additional 5% to 10% of the energy in the food molecules is expended in the processes of transport, storage, and biochemical conversion of different fuels into appropriate storage forms (e.g., glucose is converted to glycogen, fatty acids are esterified to form triacylglycerol, and amino acids are utilized for tissue protein synthesis) (Acheson et al., 1984). Additionally, some energy is lost within the body as heat during the oxidation of fuel molecules, while the rest of the energy is conserved in the high-energy phosphate bonds of ATP. Some absorbed energy is lost in the urine or via the bile/feces due to excretion of incompletely

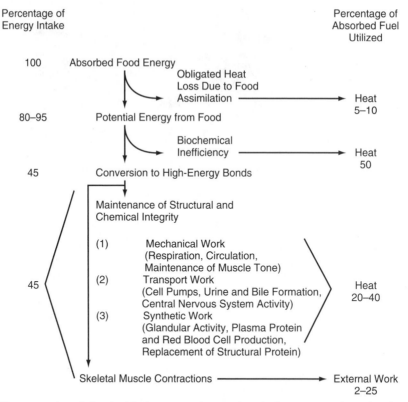

Figure 17–3. The conversion of absorbed fuel energy to heat and work. Some energy from the absorption of food is lost to the processes involved in digestion, whereas the remaining food energy is used for the maintenance of metabolic processes.

oxidized metabolites. In particular, the excretion of urea as a waste product of amino acid oxidation results in a loss of about 20% of the potential energy that could have been derived from amino acid oxidation. Thus, the efficiency of energy capture from the processes of digestion, storage, and metabolism of fuel molecules determines the amount of ATP available for the body's use.

Roughly half the total energy released from oxidation of metabolic fuel is lost as heat to the environment without formation of ATP; this stems from the inherent inefficiency of converting the molecular bond energy in fuel molecules to ATP bond energy. The remaining energy that is captured in the form of ATP is used to fuel both internal (e.g., mechanical, transport, and synthetic) and external (skeletal muscle contraction) work. Some energy is also lost as heat when ATP is hydrolyzed for work.

EFFICIENCY OF ENERGY CONSERVATION FROM FUEL OXIDATION

The efficiency of energy conservation or the efficiency of the coupling of electron transfer to ATP synthesis can be affected by different pharmacological agents, such as dinitrophenol, caffeine, nicotine, and amphetamines. These agents dissipate the proton-motive force across the inner mitochondrial membrane, which is essential for driving ATP synthesis; so, while electron transport from NADH and $FADH_2$ to oxygen proceeds normally, ATP synthesis is disrupted. This loss of respiratory control leads to increased oxygen consumption and more rapid oxidation of NADH and $FADH_2$ that is not dependent on the regeneration of ATP from ADP (Himms-Hagen, 1989).

In contrast to the uncoupling caused by pharmacological agents, the physiological uncoupling of oxidative phosphorylation can be useful in generating heat to maintain body temperature in hibernating animals, in some newborn animals (including humans), and in mammals adapted to cold climates (Himms-Hagen, 1989). Newborn infants have a significant amount of brown adipose tissue (BAT), but by adulthood only an insignificant amount of this specialized tissue is present in the body. The inner mitochondrial membrane of BAT contains thermogenin, also known as the uncoupling protein 1 (UCP1), which permits the reentry of protons into the mitochondrion independently of the synthesis of ATP so that the potential energy represented by the proton gradient is lost as heat.

Recently, two other uncoupling proteins (UCP2 and UCP3) were identified in many tissues of the human body. UCP2 and UCP3, unlike UCP1, are not solely affected by exposure to cold (Vidal-Puig et al., 1997). In rats fed a high-fat diet, UCP2 expression increased, suggesting it may be involved in regulating energy expenditure in response to excess caloric intake. The genetic expression of some uncoupling proteins has been linked to obesity, although there is no direct evidence to date that they play a significant role in the etiology of obesity. The UCP2 gene, for example, maps to regions of human chromosome 11 and mouse chromosome 7 that have been linked to hyperinsulinemia and obesity. It is possible that alterations in function or expression of the genes regulating these "energy-wasting" proteins may contribute to an underlying susceptibility to obesity stemming from increased energetic efficiency (Wolf, 1997).

SUBSTRATE CYCLING

Substrate cycling denotes a situation in which a key enzyme in a metabolic pathway is opposed by another enzyme that catalyzes the reverse reaction and that may act simultaneously. Because ATP is consumed in these enzyme-catalyzed reactions but there is no net change in reactant or product concentrations, these reactions are often termed "futile cycles." The ATP hydrolysis used to fuel these reactions contributes to heat production but is not coupled to net metabolic or external

work. Changes in the rate of substrate cycling within cells may be one means by which the efficiency of energy utilization can be increased or decreased, leading to changes in the overall efficiency of metabolism and energy utilization by the whole body (Newsholme and Parry-Billings, 1992). One such enzyme/reaction couple is the interconversion of fructose 6-phosphate and fructose 1,6-bisphosphate by 6-phosphofructo-1-kinase and fructose 1,6-bisphosphatase. In this cycle, as in all futile cycles, ATP is expended but no net metabolism is accomplished. Other potentially important substrate cycles include interconversions of glucose and glucose 6-phosphate, of protein and amino acids, and of fatty acids and triacylglycerols (Newsholme and Parry-Billings, 1992).

MEASUREMENT OF ENERGY EXPENDITURE

Energy expenditure (heat production), whether in cells, tissues, or the whole body, is most often measured using the methods of direct and indirect calorimetry. Direct calorimetry measures the heat released from the cell, tissue, or body by directly measuring changes in the temperature of the environment surrounding the organism (usually a carefully controlled, closed environmental chamber) (Jequier and Schutz, 1983). Indirect calorimetry measures oxygen consumption as a surrogate for heat production. This is valid, because in aerobic organisms most heat production originates from metabolic oxidation reactions, which utilize molecular oxygen in specific amounts depending on the substrate (or mixture of substrates) oxidized. For example, the oxidation of glucose yields the following stoichiometry:

$$C_6H_{12}O_6 + 6\ O_2 =$$
$$6\ H_2O + 6\ CO_2 + 673\ kcal$$

The energy yield per mole of O_2 utilized has been determined experimentally for the main oxidative substrates, and these factors can be used to calculate heat production from the quantity of oxygen consumed (Table 17–1).

Energy expenditure is measured increas-

TABLE 17–1
Energy and Respiratory Equivalent of Body Fuels

Food	Energy (kcal/g)			Respiratory Equivalent		
	Complete oxidation of food component in bomb calorimeter	"Complete oxidation" of absorbed or stored fuel in body*	Physiological fuel value of consumed foodstuff†	O_2 (kcal/liter)	CO_2 (kcal/liter)	RQ‡ (V_{CO_2}/V_{O_2})
Carbohydrate	4.1	4.1	4	5.05	5.05	1.00
Protein	5.4	4.2	4	4.46	5.57	0.80
Fat	9.3	9.3	9	4.74	6.67	0.71
Alcohol	7.1	7.1	7	4.86	7.25	0.67
Average				4.83	5.89	0.82

*N is excreted as urea, which has an energy content of 5.4 kcal/g N. All energy in urine is attributed to N excretion in the calculation of fuel values, and the correction factor is 7.9 kcal/g N, or 1.25 kcal/g protein.
†Values are further adjusted for digestibility (incomplete absorption).
‡RQ, respiratory quotient.

ingly by the combination of indirect calorimetry and tracer techniques in order to study details of substrate oxidation in tissues and in the whole body (Romijn et al., 1993). Because, in general, tracers are administered into and sampled from the blood compartment, they can trace the kinetics of blood-borne substrates, whereas calorimetry estimates whole-body (blood plus tissues) oxidation. Oxidation of tissue substrates that do not pass through the blood stream in their pathways to oxidation is included when metabolic rate is measured by indirect calorimetry (precisely to the extent that their combustion consumes O_2 and releases CO_2), but it may not be detectable by changes in the concentration of a labeled tracer amount of the substrate in the blood. Thus, in principle, the difference between calorimetric and tracer estimates of substrate oxidation should reflect phenomena that occur entirely at the tissue level (Wolfe, 1992).

The O_2 consumption of individual tissues in vivo can be estimated by making measurements of the arteriovenous concentration difference of oxygen across a tissue in conjunction with measurement of blood flow. Although muscle is the largest tissue in the adult whole body, accounting for about 40% of adult body weight, its estimated RMR is relatively low (about 10 to 15 kcal · kg^{-1} · day^{-1}), so its contribution to the total energy expenditure of the body is about 20% to 25%.

In a resting subject consuming an average diet providing roughly 35% fat, 12% protein, and 53% carbohydrate (as percentages of total energy intake), who is studied in the postabsorptive state, about 4.83 kcal are expended for every liter of O_2 consumed. In other words:

Metabolic rate (kcal · h^{-1}) =
4.83 kcal · (liter O_2 consumed)$^{-1}$ · h^{-1}

Although different amounts of oxygen are consumed during the biological oxidation of different energy-yielding foodstuffs, the foregoing equation will estimate heat production to within about 8% of the actual value regardless of which nutrients are being oxidized.

In practice, direct calorimetry is not often used, in part because of the long delay between heat production and release of the heat to the surrounding environment. This delay occurs because the body has a large capacity for heat storage. A delay between heat production and release necessitates long measurement times and makes it difficult to associate particular metabolic events with heat production measured within a particular time frame.

Because the body's oxygen store is very small, measurement of oxygen consumption by indirect calorimetry can provide a rapid measure of heat production that is in close temporal association with metabolic energy utilization. An additional advantage of indirect calorimetry is the ability to measure substrate (fuel molecule) oxidation rates. The amount of heat released per liter of O_2 consumed depends on the type of nutrient being oxidized (i.e., protein, carbohydrate, or fat) (Kinney, 1992). By measuring CO_2 production and urinary nitrogen excretion in addition to O_2 consumption, it is possible to determine the proportion of the different nutrients that are oxidized and thus to calculate the heat released from each nutrient class (Table 17–1).

In recent years, another indirect method has been developed for measuring total energy expenditure in free-living individuals over periods of 10 to 14 days (Schoeller and Hnilicka, 1996). This newer method uses water doubly labeled with the isotopes ^2H (deuterium) and ^{18}O. The principle behind the doubly labeled water method is based on the fact that ^2H from the body's labeled water pool leaves as water whereas the ^{18}O equilibrates with CO_2 (via $H_2CO_3 \rightleftharpoons CO_2 + H_2O$) and leaves the body as both water and CO_2. The difference in the disappearance rates of the two isotopes and a measure of the size of the body water pool provide an estimate of unlabeled CO_2 production from oxidation of fuels (Fig. 17–4). Oxygen consumption can then be calculated from an estimate of the respiratory quotient (RQ = CO_2 produced/O_2 consumed) of the diet; RQ can be measured or estimated from diet composition and tabled values.

COMPONENTS OF ENERGY EXPENDITURE

The measurement of oxygen consumption in the whole animal represents, under ideal conditions, the sum of all oxidative processes occurring within the body. Energy expenditure has several components (Ravussin et al., 1986). The largest contribution to daily energy expenditure is referred to as resting metabolic rate (RMR) and reflects the energy requirements for sustaining basic metabolic functions of an awake individual at rest. Resting metabolic rate is usually measured in the morning in a subject who has fasted overnight and who has been lying quietly for 30 to 60 minutes. Energy expenditure is then measured, typically for 30 to 60 minutes using indirect calorimetry. Values for RMR are generally 5% to 15% greater than would be values for the so-called basal metabolic rate (BMR). BMR conceptually represents the minimal energy requirements of the organism but is impractical to measure; RMR is measured in an awake individual. The difference in resting versus basal energy expenditure largely reflects the energy cost of arousal; e.g., increased brain

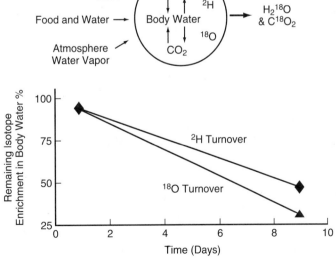

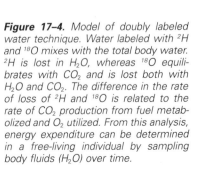

Figure 17–4. Model of doubly labeled water technique. Water labeled with ^2H and ^{18}O mixes with the total body water. ^2H is lost in H_2O, whereas ^{18}O equilibrates with CO_2 and is lost both with H_2O and CO_2. The difference in the rate of loss of ^2H and ^{18}O is related to the rate of CO_2 production from fuel metabolized and O_2 utilized. From this analysis, energy expenditure can be determined in a free-living individual by sampling body fluids (H_2O) over time.

activity and maintenance of muscle tone for posture. Resting metabolic rate accounts for 60% to 75% of total daily energy expenditure in an average sedentary individual. The other components of daily energy expenditure include the thermic effect of food (TEF) and the thermic effect of physical activity (EE_{act}).

The TEF is the increase in O_2 consumption and energy expenditure, above the RMR, which occurs over several hours following the ingestion of food (Jequier and Schutz, 1988). The increased O_2 consumption accompanying food ingestion reflects the metabolic cost of digestion, absorption, and processing of nutrients (e.g., conversion of glucose to glycogen) and typically amounts to 7% to 10% of the energy content of the food consumed. Thus, consumption of a 500-kcal mixed meal generates a thermic effect of approximately 35 to 50 kcal.

The magnitude of the TEF is directly related to total energy ingested, and different macronutrients produce different thermic effects. Protein is generally found to produce a TEF of about 15% to 30%. That is, 15% to 30% of the bond energy in the protein is spent in the process of utilizing the constituent amino acids (either oxidizing them or incorporating them into body proteins during normal protein turnover). The metabolic cost of either oxidizing carbohydrate or storing it as glycogen is 6% to 8% (Flatt, 1992). The theoretical cost of converting excess carbohydrate to fat is about 20%. Recent studies in humans have shown that net conversion of carbohydrate to fat occurs only in rare situations of massive sustained carbohydrate overfeeding (Hellerstein et al., 1996). The net metabolic cost of either oxidizing or storing ingested fat is only 2% to 3% of the energy consumed.

Characteristics of both the diet (amount and composition of food ingested) and of individuals (e.g., body composition and gender) influence TEF. The overall contribution of differences in total energy balance between individuals due to differences in TEF is considered to be small.

Energy expended in physical activity, or EE_{act}, represents the energy cost of the external work performed and is the most variable component of total daily energy expenditure. Estimating the energy expended in physical activity is very difficult in free-living individuals owing to the range of different activities possible and the difficulty in accurately measuring the duration and intensity of each. The amount of work performed is the major determinant of EE_{act} (e.g., a moderate activity level accounts for 30% and a heavy activity accounts for 50% of total daily energy expenditure, respectively), but EE_{act} is also influenced by the cost of the activity (i.e., the work efficiency). EE_{act} may range from near zero to greater than three to four times resting energy requirements. The energy cost of a given activity depends on body mass, so that increases or decreases in body mass will alter the cost of weight-bearing activity. In addition, there may be individual differences in work efficiency that are not related to body size. However, it is likely that between-subject differences in work efficiency contribute much less to differences in EE_{act} than between-subject differences in amount of physical activity performed. Some differences between individuals may be related to differences in spontaneous motor activity. In experimental studies of individuals confined to a small room, spontaneous motor activity varied from 200 to 900 kcal/day. This suggests that a significant fraction of the variation in total energy expenditure (and potentially body weight) between individuals may be related to differences in spontaneous activity, even when the environment is similar.

Typically, activity is estimated using an activity diary or a mechanical motion-sensing device worn on the body. These indirect measures of activity are then used in conjunction with accurately determined energy expenditure values for various activities measured in subjects using indirect calorimetry under carefully controlled conditions. The recent development of the doubly labeled water technique for determining total body energy expenditure has provided a valuable tool for assessing physical activity patterns among free-living individuals.

The partitioning of total body energy production at rest among the various body organ systems is shown in Figure 17–5 (Elia, 1992). Brain, liver, kidney, and heart are the most metabolically active organs within the body at rest and comprise over half the RMR, although they account for only 5% to 6% of body

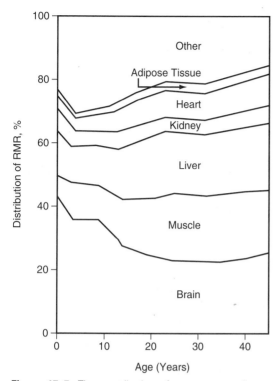

Figure 17–5. *The contribution of energy expenditure by different organs to resting metabolic rate. Area is calculated from the product of the organ (tissue) weight and organ (tissue) metabolic rate. (Adapted from Elia, M. [1992] Organ and tissue contribution to metabolic rate. In: Energy Metabolism: Tissue Determinants and Cellular Corollaries [Kinney, J.M. and Tucker, H.N., eds.], pp. 61–79. Raven Press Ltd., New York.)*

weight. The contribution to total metabolic rate of these organs is proportional to the blood flow to these tissues. These tissues have a metabolic rate that is 15 to 40 times greater than an equivalent mass of resting muscle and 50 to 100 times greater than adipose tissue. Skeletal muscle also represents a significant fraction of resting energy expenditure because of its large total mass, but on a per gram basis, skeletal muscle is much less active than these other organs. Of course, the contribution of muscle tissue to total energy expenditure increases markedly during physical activity (Elia, 1992).

The metabolic rate per unit of organ weight appears to change little throughout life (solid squares in Figure 17–6). In infants, the brain is the largest contributor to metabolic rate, due to its exaggerated size per unit of body weight. RMR (per unit of body weight)

decreases with age primarily owing to the reduction in proportion of body weight contributed by the main metabolic organs over time. Throughout adulthood, the size and metabolic activity of these organs remain stable, and hence the RMR per unit of body weight remains constant in the adult years (solid circles in Figure 17–6).

DETERMINANTS OF RESTING METABOLIC RATE

The majority (83%) of variance in RMR and 24-hour energy expenditure is accounted for by fat-free mass (FFM); age and gender contribute modestly (Ravussin and Bogardus, 1989). Figure 17–7 shows a strong tendency for 24-hour energy expenditure to aggregate closely within families compared with between families. This familial trait suggests, but does not prove, that metabolic rate is genetically determined (Bogardus et al., 1986). Bouchard and colleagues have studied the heritability of RMR in monozygotic and dizygotic twins and showed higher correlations in monozygotic twins than in dizygotic twins, whether RMR is expressed per kilogram of body weight or of FFM (Bouchard et al., 1989). These investigators suggest that the more genes are shared, the more similar the metabolic rate, independent of body size and composition.

As mentioned earlier, the body relies on the generation of ATP to supply free energy to drive metabolic processes. The pathways involved in whole body and cellular energy utilization and metabolism are under the control of neuronal factors, as well as hormones, substrate availability, and enzyme activities (Bray, 1987). Table 17–2 gives a brief summary of neuronal and hormonal factors regulating energy utilization, the most notable being the hormones epinephrine, norepinephrine, insulin, glucagon, and thyroid hormone. Like the activity of the nervous system, hormone secretion is adjusted in response to various internal and external stimuli and significantly affects the cellular metabolic rate.

Activation of the sympathetic nervous system causes the release of the catecholamines epinephrine and norepinephrine from the ad-

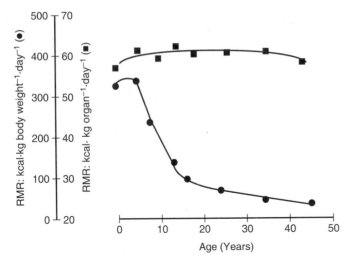

Figure 17–6. Changes in resting metabolic rate during growth and development. The whole body RMR per kg of body weight is shown along with the metabolic rate for liver, kidney, brain, and heart combined per kg of organ weight. (Organ weight refers to the sum of the weights of liver, kidney, brain, and heart.) (Adapted from Elia, M. [1992] Organ and tissue contribution to metabolic rate. In: Energy Metabolism: Tissue Determinants and Cellular Corollaries [Kinney, J. M. and Tucker, H.N., eds.], pp. 61–79. Raven Press Ltd., New York.)

renal medulla. Activation of this system occurs predominantly in response to stress and is accompanied by the secretion of other hormones. These hormones act together to increase the metabolic rate of cells by altering the rate of numerous biochemical processes. The pancreatic hormones insulin and gluca-gon affect the rates of utilization of carbohydrate and fat metabolism predominantly via activation of transporters, whereas thyroid hormone affects the expression of specific proteins by altering nuclear transcription rates, thus affecting metabolic rate and heat production.

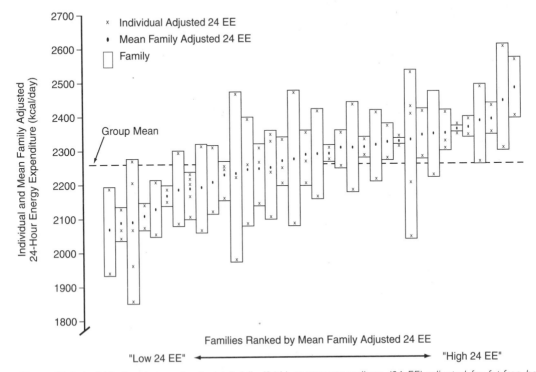

Figure 17–7. Individual and mean family total daily (24-h) energy expenditure (24 EE) adjusted for fat-free body mass, fat mass, age, and sex. (Redrawn from Bogardus, C., Lillioja, S., Ravussin, E., Abbott, W., Zawadzki, J.K., Young, A., Knowler, W.C., Jacobowitz, R. and Moll, P.P. [1986] Familial dependence of the resting metabolic rate. N Engl J Med 315:96–100. Copyright 1986 Massachusetts Medical Society. All rights reserved.)

TABLE 17–2
Neuronal and Endocrine Factors Affecting Substrate Oxidation

Source	Hormone	Action
Anterior pituitary	Growth hormone	Mobilizes fatty acids for energy and inhibits carbohydrate metabolism
	Prolactin	Mobilizes fatty acids
	Endomorphins	Affects feeding, released during stress
Adrenal cortex	Cortisol/corticosterone	Promotes use of fatty acids and protein catabolism
Adrenal medulla	Epinephrine/norepinephrine	Facilitates sympathetic activity, increases glycogen catabolism and fatty acid release; release stimulated by stress
Thyroid	Thyroid hormones: T_3 and T_4	Stimulate metabolic rate; regulated by whole-body metabolism
Pancreas	Insulin	Promotes carbohydrate, fatty acid, and amino acid transport into cells and increases carbohydrate catabolism
	Glucagon	Promotes release of glucose from liver to blood, increases fat metabolism, decreases amino acid levels
Ovaries	Estrogen and progesterone	Increases fat deposition
Testes	Testosterone	Decreases body fat

Physiological stresses include injury, fever, surgery, renal failure, burns, infections, and even starvation or malnutrition (Elia, 1992). In these cases, characteristically catecholamine and hormone levels increase, RMR increases, and glucose and free fatty acid concentrations rise in the blood. Studies examining patients with severe illnesses accompanied by fever have shown up to a 13% increase in metabolic rate for each degree Celsius of increase in body temperature (Beisel et al., 1980). During fever, there is an increase in the production and utilization of the metabolizable, energy-yielding substrates made available to cells, and this is primarily an increased utilization of glucose as a result of accelerated rates of glycogenolysis and gluconeogenesis.

An accelerated cellular uptake of thyroid hormones, especially T_3, occurs in many infections. An increase in thyroid hormone promotes an increase in the metabolic rate of all cells, but, unlike for catecholamines, the effect of an increased level of thyroid hormone occurs over a period of days to weeks. In the situation of a patient suffering from severe burns, the body requires an increased metabolic rate to ensure a stable body temperature when much of the body's insulation is lost by the injury to skin. In addition, in most illnesses increased energy is required as a result of the increased production of immune response agents such as cytokines and the subsequent energy-requiring processes associated with their actions.

Whole-body energy utilization is complex, reflecting different pathways in different cell types and tissues (Elia, 1992). Pathways of energy utilization are affected by a variety of internal (e.g., presence of disease) and external (e.g., environmental temperature) stimuli that modify total-body energy expenditure. The biochemical and genetic bases for differences in efficiency of different pathways are emerging as new tools of molecular biology become available. Likewise, the advent of new tools to measure energy expenditure in free-living people (e.g., doubly labeled water) makes it possible to study determinants of whole-body energy expenditure, which reflect the cumulative contribution of all the different cells and tissues in the body. Differences among individuals in the efficiency of energy utilization by cellular biochemical pathways may underlie differences in susceptibility to obesity and other disorders of energy balance.

REFERENCES

Acheson, K. J., Ravussin, E., Wahren, J. and Jequier, E. (1984) Thermic effect of glucose in man: Obligatory and facultative thermogenesis. J Clin Invest 74:1572–1580.

Beisel, W. R., Wannemacher, R. W., Jr. and Neufeld, H. A. (1980) Relation of fever to energy expenditure. In: Assessment of Energy Metabolism in Health and Disease (Kinney, J. M., ed.), pp. 144–150. Report of the First Ross Conference on Medical Research. Ross Laboratories, Columbus, OH.

Bogardus, C., Lillioja, S., Ravussin, E., Abbott, W., Zawadzki, J. K., Young, A., Knowler, W. C., Jacobowitz, R. and Moll, P. P. (1986) Familial dependence of the resting metabolic rate. N Engl J Med 315:96–100.

Bouchard, C., Tremblay, A., Nadeau, A., Despres, J-P., Theriault, G., Boulay, M. R., Lortie, G., Leblanc, C. and Fournier, G. (1989) Genetic effect in resting and exercise metabolic rates. Metabolism 38: 364–370.

Bray, G. (1987) Overweight is risking fate: Definition, classification, prevalence, and risks. In: Human Obesity (Wurtman R. J. and Wurtman J. J., eds.). Ann NY Acad Sci 499:14–28.

Elia, M. (1992) Organ and tissue contribution to metabolic rate. In: Energy Metabolism: Tissue Determinants and Cellular Corollaries. (Kinney, J. M. and Tucker, H. N., eds.), pp. 61–79. Raven Press Ltd., New York.

Flatt, J. P. (1985) Energetics of intermediary metabolism. In: Substrate and Energy Metabolism (Garrow, J. S. and Halliday, D., eds.), pp. 58–69. John Libbey, London.

Flatt, J. P. (1992) The biochemistry of energy expenditure. In: Obesity (Bjorntorp, P. and Brodoff, B., eds.), pp.100–116. J. B. Lippincott, Philadelphia.

Hellerstein, M. K., Schwarz, J.-M. and Neese, R. A. (1996) Regulation of hepatic de novo lipogenesis in humans. Annu Rev Nutr 16:523–557.

Himms-Hagen, J. (1989) Brown adipose tissue thermogenesis and obesity. Prog Lipid Res 28:65–115.

Jequier, E. and Schutz, Y. (1983) Long-term measurements of energy expenditure in humans using a respiration chamber. Am J Clin Nutr 38:989–998.

Jequier, E. and Schutz, Y. (1988) Energy expenditure in obesity and diabetes. Diabetes Metab Rev 4:583–593.

Kinney, J. M. (1992) Overview: Indirect calorimetry: Theory and practice. In: Energy Metabolism: Tissue Determinants and Cellular Corollaries (Kinney, J. M. and Tucker, H. N., eds.), pp. 113–121. Raven Press Ltd., New York.

McBride, B. W. and Kelly, J. M. (1990) Energy cost of absorption and metabolism in the ruminant gastrointestinal tract and liver: A review. J Anim Sci 68:2997–3010.

Merrill, A. L. and Watt, B. K. (1973) Energy Values of Foods; Basis and Derivation. USDA Agriculture Handbook #74 (revised). United States Department of Agriculture, Washington, D.C.

Murphy, M. P. and Brand, M. D. (1987) Variable stoichiometry of proton pumping by the mitochondrial respiratory chain. Nature 329:170–172.

Newsholme, E. A. and Parry-Billings, M. (1992) Some evidence for the existence of substrate cycles and their utility in vivo. Biochem J 285:340–341.

Ravussin, E. and Bogardus, C. (1989) Relationship of genetics, age, and physical fitness to daily energy expenditure and fuel utilization. Am J Clin Nutr 49: 968–975.

Ravussin, E., Lillioja, S., Anderson, T. E., Christin, L. and Bogardus, C. (1986) Determinants of 24-hour energy expenditure in man: Methods and results using a respiratory chamber. J Clin Invest 78:1568–1578.

Romijn, J. A., Coyle, E. F., Sidossis, L. S., Gastaldelli, A., Horowitz, J. F., Endert, E. and Wolfe, R. R. (1993) Regulation of endogenous fat and carbohydrate metabolism in relation to exercise intensity and duration. Am J Physiol 265:E380–E391.

Schoeller, D. A. and Hnilicka, J. M. (1996) Reliability of the doubly labeled water method for the measurement of total daily energy expenditure in free-living subjects. J Nutr 126:348S–354S.

Vidal-Puig, A., Solanes, G., Grujic, D., Flier, J. S. and Lowell, B. B. (1997) UCP3: An uncoupling protein homologue expressed preferentially and abundantly in skeletal muscle and brown adipose tissue. Biochem Biophys Res Commun 235:79–82.

Wolf, G. (1997) A new uncoupling protein: A potential component of the human body weight regulation system. Nutr Rev 55:178–179.

Wolfe, R. R. (1992) Assessment of substrate cycling in humans using tracer methodology. In: Energy Metabolism: Tissue Determinants and Cellular Corollaries (Kinney, J. M. and Tucker, H. N., eds.), pp. 495–523. Raven Press Ltd., New York.

RECOMMENDED READINGS

Bray, G. (1987) Overweight is risking fate: Definition, classification, prevalence, and risks. In: Human Obesity (Wurtman, R. J. and Wurtman, J. J., eds.). Ann NY Acad Sci 499:14–28.

Flatt, J. P. (1985) Energetics of intermediary metabolism. In: Substrate and energy metabolism (Garrow, J. S. and Halliday, D., eds.), pp. 58–69. John Libbey, London.

Jequier, E. and Schutz, Y. (1988) Energy expenditure in obesity and diabetes. Diabetes Metab Rev 4:583–593.

Ravussin, E. and Bogardus, C. (1989) Relationship of genetics, age, and physical fitness to daily energy expenditure and fuel utilization. Am J Clin Nutr 49:968–975.

CHAPTER **18**

◆ ◆

Control of Energy Balance

John C. Peters, Ph.D., Adamandia D. Kriketos, Ph.D., and James O. Hill, Ph.D.

O U T L I N E

C O M M O N   A B B R E V I A T I O N S

BMR (basal metabolic rate)
EE$_{act}$ (energy expenditure of physical activity)
FFM (fat-free mass)
RMR (resting metabolic rate)
TEF (thermic effect of food)

BASIC CONCEPTS

A typical adult human who consumes 2500 kcal per day will ingest nearly 1,000,000 kcal of energy in a single year. This energy is used to fuel obligatory metabolic processes (internal work) and to provide fuel for physical activity (external work). For an individual to maintain energy balance, therefore, the one million ingested kilocalories must be balanced by an equivalent energy expenditure. Failure to do so results in either an increase or decrease in body energy stores.

Given the widespread occurrence of obesity in developed countries, it might seem that the precision of whatever system is operating to maintain energy balance is rather poor. On the contrary, even accounting for the prevalence of obesity, the precision is quite remarkable. An error of only 1% (considered respectable for most mechanical devices), 10,000 kcal/year, would represent the equivalent of 2.8 pounds of body fat. If such a positive energy balance persisted over a single 10-year period, this would lead to an accumulation of 28 pounds, enough body fat to account for the "middle-age spread" that occurs over several decades in many individuals. Clearly, the error between energy intake and expenditure in the majority of people is much less than this.

How does the body balance energy intake and energy expenditure so precisely? Is energy balance itself controlled or is the precision of energy balance a byproduct of precise control of something else? In this chapter, basic concepts of energy and nutrient balance are described and what is known about con-trol of energy intake and expenditure and the way in which the two interact to influence energy balance is reviewed.

Energy Balance

Energy balance, by definition, is a condition in which energy intake and energy expenditure are equivalent over the time period of observation. Energy balance is positive and net body energy gain occurs when energy intake exceeds energy expenditure. Conversely, when energy expenditure exceeds energy intake, negative energy balance occurs, and net body energy is lost.

The Energy Balance Equation

Change in body energy stores =
    energy intake − energy expenditure

Total body energy stores are substantial (Table 18–1). When an individual is at energy balance, these stores remain stable. Energy to fuel resting metabolism and everyday activity is provided by energy-yielding nutrients in food. Short-term energy needs (e.g., between meals) are met by utilization of tissue glycogen reserves and some fat. Glycogen reserves and energy-yielding substrates in the circulation represent a very small storage depot and normally are exhausted within 24 hours during a fast. During prolonged fasting or during energy restriction for weight loss, significant protein is also degraded and used for energy in addition to substantial fat utilization. Although most of the triacylglycerol stored in adipose tissue is available to the body during a prolonged fast, not all energy contained in

---

TABLE 18–1
Energy Stores in a 30-kg Child and a 70-kg Adult Male

Energy Form	Storage Site	30-kg Child*		70-kg Adult Male†	
		kg	*kcal*	*kg*	*kcal*
Triglyceride	Adipose tissue	4.5	31,500	15	115,000
Protein	Muscle	1.5	6250	6	25,000
Glycogen	Liver and muscle	0.13	500	0.35	1400
Glucose or lipid	Body fluids	0.011	40	0.025	100

*Data from Rosenbaum and Leibel (1988).
†Data from Cahill (1970) and Frayn (1996).

body protein is available for use as fuel. Body proteins serve important structural and functional purposes and therefore cannot be depleted without affecting survival of the organism.

The magnitude of change in body energy that occurs when there is an imbalance between energy intake and expenditure, of course, depends on the length of time over which the energy imbalance occurs. Because total daily energy needs in most individuals range between 1500 and 3000 kcal, given the large size of body energy reserves, short-term imbalances such as occur meal to meal or day to day would not be expected to lead to significant changes in body energy (body weight). Conversely, sustained imbalances that occur over several days, weeks, or months can lead to substantial changes in body energy, and hence changes in body weight.

Gain or loss of significant amounts of body energy in turn affects other components of the energy balance equation, because weight gain or loss is associated with gain or loss of active metabolic tissue mass, and this is associated with an increase or decrease in total energy expenditure, accordingly. Likewise, alterations in body mass usually affect energy intake, because food intake normally is proportional to energy expenditure. Thus, when a prolonged imbalance occurs between energy intake (E_{in}) and energy expenditure (E_{out}), the resulting change in body energy (and body weight) is not a linear function of the energy excess or deficit, but depends on the composition of the tissue mass lost or gained and the effects of those specific changes on energy expenditure and energy intake.

Nutrient Balance

In a practical sense, people do not eat pure energy; they eat nutrients in the form of food

---

NUTRITION INSIGHT

What Is the Energetic Equivalent of Body Tissues? Implications for Weight Loss

The energetic equivalent of a given amount of body mass either gained or lost depends on its composition. Lean tissue such as muscle is about 80% water, with the remaining 20% being largely protein with smaller amounts of fat and carbohydrate. In contrast, adipose tissue is only about 15% water, the remainder (85%) being storage lipid with a very small amount of protein contributing to the cell structure and intracellular enzymes. Given these differences in the composition of body tissues, the amount of energy represented by a kilogram of body weight will differ accordingly.

For example, the body energy lost when a kilogram of muscle is lost would be roughly 1120 kcal (200 g × 5.6 kcal/g for protein). Only about 800 kcal of this energy would be net energy available to supply the body's fuel needs; the remaining 320 kcal would be required to metabolize the nitrogen derived from the breakdown of the amino acids in the protein to the excretory product, urea.

Loss of a kilogram of adipose tissue (85% lipid) represents a body energy loss of about 7905 kcal (850 g × 9.3 kcal/g). In contrast to protein, essentially all of the energy represented by stored fat can contribute to net fuel energy. Thus, a kilogram of body fat represents nearly 10 times (7905 kcal/kg fat ÷ 800 kcal/kg lean) the energy for fuel represented by a kilogram of lean tissue.

These figures provide some perspective on weight loss claims appearing in the popular press. Take the example of a claim touting a 2.5-kg weight loss in a week by simply following a new diet (i.e., no exercise involved). If the weight loss were really adipose tissue, as hoped by the dieter, the loss would represent 41,995 kcal of body energy. For the average sedentary individual only about 2500 kcal are needed each day to maintain body weight, or 17,500 kcal per week. It is therefore impossible to lose 2.5 kg of fat in a week by dieting alone—in order to lose 2.5 kg of fat, the individual would have to eat nothing for 16.5 days!

and the nutrients are oxidized by the body to provide energy. The predominant energy-yielding nutrients in the human diet are the macronutrients: protein, carbohydrate, and fat (and alcohol). Because there is little net conversion of either protein or carbohydrate into fat under most typical dietary conditions, achieving balance between energy intake and energy expenditure in an adult really requires achieving balance of each macronutrient (Flatt, 1995). Nutrient and energy balance in the adult occurs when the intake of protein, carbohydrate, and fat (and alcohol) are equivalent to the body's oxidation of each.

When energy and nutrient balance are achieved

Protein Intake = Protein Oxidized
Carbohydrate Intake = Carbohydrate Oxidized
Fat Intake = Fat Oxidized
Alcohol Intake = Alcohol Oxidized

If one of these energy-yielding nutrients is consumed in excess of the amount of that nutrient oxidized by the body in the short term, the excess is stored. As is discussed later in this chapter, the body appears to have metabolic priorities that dictate how much of a given nutrient is oxidized versus stored and the form in which the excess energy is stored. The form (e.g., glycogen, fat) in which the excess energy is stored in the short term, such as after a meal, can have an important influence on the long-term fate of that excess energy, which ultimately influences body weight and body composition.

Is Energy Balance or Nutrient Balance Regulated?

Body weight and body composition remain quite stable over long periods of time (years) in most individuals. This might suggest that body weight, body composition, or perhaps energy balance itself, is regulated, much like other homeostatic systems in biology, such as blood glucose concentration. Alternatively, stability of these variables may result merely from regulation of other processes.

Body Weight as a Set-Point. The concept of a body weight set-point came from the observation that experimental animals tended to defend a particular body weight under a variety of conditions of energy deficit or energy surfeit (Keesey and Corbett, 1984). If, for example, an animal was food restricted so that it lost 20% of its body weight, the animal would, upon cessation of food restriction, return to its prerestriction body weight. Subsequent studies showed that in order to alter this apparent body weight set-point under a given set of conditions, a change in the fundamental mechanisms regulating food intake and energy expenditure was required. Destruction of the ventromedial hypothalamus in the brain, the so-called satiety center, caused animals to overeat and reach a new higher body weight, which the animal then defended (i.e., a new set-point). Alternatively, destruction of the lateral hypothalamus, the so-called feeding center, resulted in reduced food intake, weight loss, and a new lower body weight or set-point that was defended. A variety of studies and years of clinical experience have shown that once a stable body weight is achieved under a given set of circumstances, humans also tend to defend a given body weight (Leibel et al., 1995).

Defense of body weight appears strongest in situations that would lead to loss of existing body energy stores. Substantial clinical experience in treating obese individuals using hypocaloric weight-loss programs has shown that, although a high percentage of subjects can successfully achieve weight loss, about 90% regain the weight once they discontinue the weight-management program.

The relative strength of the body's defense against a gain in body energy stores appears to be weaker than that protecting against energy deficit. This is apparent in the growing problem of obesity among both adults and children. Today, roughly a third of the United States population is obese, up from 25% just a decade ago (Kuczmarski et al., 1994). The relatively weak defense against positive energy balance appears to exist whether the energy gain is provoked by increased energy intake, decreased physical activity, or both. In experimental overfeeding studies, it has been shown that the body has a limited capacity to burn off excess energy, and most of the excess is stored (Horton et al., 1995). Furthermore, in population studies, decreases in physical activity are strongly associated with increases

RDAs for Energy Across the Life Cycle

	Average Energy Allowance	
	(kcal/day)	*(kcal·kg⁻¹·day⁻¹)*
Infants, 0–0.5 yr	650	108
0.5–1.0 yr	850	98
Children, 1–3 yr	1300	102
4–6 yr	1800	90
7–10 yr	2000	70
Males, 11–14 yr	2500	55
15–18 yr	3000	45
19–50 yr	2900	37–40
51+ yr	2300	30
Females, 11–14	2200	47
15–50 yr	2200	36–40
51+ yr	1900	30
Pregnant	(+300 in 2nd and 3rd trimesters)	
Lactating	(+500)	

The RDAs for energy are estimates of average amounts required for growth of children, for maintenance of body weight in adults with an assumption of light to moderate activity, and for the added demands of pregnancy and lactation. Requirements of individuals will vary with activity level and body size (primarily, lean body mass).

From the National Research Council (1989) Recommended Dietary Allowances, 10th ed., p. 33. National Academy Press, Washington, D.C.

in body weight and fat content (Lissner and Heitmann, 1995). Considering that humans evolved largely in a subsistence environment, it should not be surprising that there is a bias toward efficiently storing excess dietary energy and defending body energy. Indeed, in evolutionary terms, a biological defense against storing excess energy when it is available would not appear to confer a natural selection advantage.

Body Weight as Settling Point. Body weight and body composition do not remain fixed throughout the adult life of most individuals, despite periods of many years during which relative constancy is achieved. The general increase in body weight and body fat that occurs in most adults between the ages of 30 and 60 years and the frequent increase in body weight that occurs in many women following pregnancy and childbirth are two common situations in which a new stable higher body weight is achieved and defended. A sub-

stantial change in either the internal (e.g., hormonal) or external (e.g., activity level) environment can produce a substantial change in the level of body weight defended.

In view of the available evidence, it seems appropriate to refer to a particular body weight and composition that an individual might temporarily defend as a settling point, rather than a set-point. This concept seems more accommodating than the term set-point because it takes into account that most people defend several different body weights over the course of a lifetime. These different settling points are determined by the different physiological, psychological, and environmental circumstances the individual may be experiencing during that period of life. For example, declining levels of physical activity, which in the United States are often associated with the transition from adolescence to adult life, encourage positive energy balance, weight gain, and a new, higher settling point.

CONTROL OF ENERGY INTAKE

Dietary energy is provided predominately by the macronutrients: protein, carbohydrate, and fat (and alcohol). Results from the first phase of the third National Health and Nutrition Examination Survey (McDowell, et al., 1994) show that adult women and men consume, on average, between 1500 and 3000 kcal/day, depending on age and sex (Table 18–2). Of this total energy intake, the current typical American diet consists of approximately 15% of energy from protein, 49% from carbohydrate, and 34% from fat (Table 18–2). An additional 2% of energy is consumed from alcohol. On a population basis, these values do not vary considerably as a function of age, sex, or ethnicity.

Energy intake is controlled by a complex system involving both behavioral and biological components. These components are interrelated in as much as food intake itself is a behavior and the biological components of the system must respond to, and indeed may be forced to adapt to, the consequences of this behavior. Ultimately, eating behavior involves the interaction/integration of genetics, metabolism, learning history, and the current context in which eating is taking place.

Behavioral Aspects of Energy Intake

Human eating behavior is a learned habitual behavior (Rodin, 1992). Food intake under any given circumstance is influenced by the learning history of the individual as it relates

TABLE 18–2
Dietary Energy and Macronutrient Intakes in the United States

Sex and Age	Energy (kcal/day)	Protein g/day	Protein % kcal	Carbohydrate g/day	Carbohydrate % kcal	Fat g/day	Fat % kcal	Alcohol g/day	Alcohol % kcal
Females									
All ages	1732	64	15.2	217	51.1	67	33.9	5	1.6
2–11 months	850	25	11.2	112	52.4	35	37.6	0	0.0
1–2 years	1236	45	14.9	163	53.0	47	34.0	0	0.0
3–5	1516	54	14.3	204	54.4	57	33.1	0	0.0
6–11	1753	63	14.5	229	52.9	68	34.2	0	0.0
12–15	1838	62	13.5	243	54.4	72	33.7	0	0.0
16–19	1958	67	14.1	254	52.4	77	34.4	2	0.6
20–29	1957	69	14.5	241	50.0	75	34.0	9	3.0
30–39	1883	70	15.3	228	49.7	75	34.2	8	2.4
40–49	1764	67	15.8	213	49.0	70	34.9	5	1.8
50–59	1629	64	16.1	199	49.8	63	33.8	5	2.1
60–69	1578	64	16.6	199	51.1	59	32.8	4	1.5
70–79	1435	58	16.6	185	52.4	53	32.3	2	0.9
80 years/over	1329	52	15.9	179	54.5	47	31.3	1	0.6
Males									
All ages	2478	92	15.1	299	49.2	96	34.1	12	3.1
2–11 months	903	27	11.8	119	52.7	37	36.9	0	0.0
1–2 years	1339	50	15.0	176	53.2	51	33.5	0	0.0
3–5	1663	59	14.3	225	54.8	62	32.8	0	0.0
6–11	2036	71	14.2	272	53.5	78	33.9	0	0.0
12–15	2578	89	14.2	346	54.0	97	33.1	0	0.0
16–19	3097	111	14.4	381	49.6	120	34.6	13	2.6
20–29	3025	110	14.6	353	47.6	116	34.0	23	4.9
30–39	2872	106	15.1	335	47.4	113	34.6	18	4.3
40–49	2545	96	15.6	298	46.9	98	33.9	18	4.9
50–59	2341	93	16.1	266	46.3	95	35.7	12	3.4
60–69	2110	84	16.4	253	48.7	80	33.3	11	3.2
70–79	1887	74	16.0	231	49.4	73	33.8	7	2.7
80 years/over	1776	69	16.0	225	51.2	67	33.3	4	1.5

Data from McDowell, M. A., Briefel, R. R., Alaimo, K., et al. (1994). Energy and macronutrient intakes of persons ages 2 months and over in the United States: Third National Health and Nutrition Examination Survey, Phase 1, 1988–91. National Center for Health Statistics, Centers for Disease Control and Prevention, U.S. Department of Health and Human Services, Publication no. 255.

to that circumstance. Learning begins in early childhood, at which time the child develops food preferences through experience with different foods. Properties of the food itself (e.g., orosensory properties), as well as the social and cultural context in which the food is consumed, can be associated with the metabolic effects of the food to form the basis of a learned, conditioned response. This associative learning is important for controlling food and energy intake in a sociocultural environment in which food is typically eaten only at particular times. This is because there is a temporal separation between the orosensory stimulus and context in which food is eaten (which occur immediately) and the metabolic consequences of the food (which may take many hours to complete).

The taste (e.g., sweet, sour), energy density, and variety of foods offered to children have been found to shape children's food preferences (Birch, 1992). Infants and young children display an innate preference for the sweet taste (Drewnowski, 1997). In addition, studies in young children show that they will condition preferences for foods that are energy dense (Kern et al., 1993). Offering children a wide variety of foods to choose from increases the spectrum of foods they come to prefer. All of these factors appear to contribute to ensuring that the child consumes adequate energy and sufficient essential nutrients to support good growth and development. As the child grows older, learned food acceptance patterns and eating habits are continually reinforced and extended such that, by adulthood, there is a rich experiential background that affects eating behavior at any given meal.

At any given eating occasion, the amount and composition of food an individual consumes is affected by the immediate context of consumption superimposed on the underlying biology (e.g., hunger drive) and the learning history. The cost of food acquisition, the variety of foods present, the number of other people present, and the time of day are just a few of the factors that have been shown to affect short-term food intake and selection (Rolls et al., 1981; de Castro and de Castro, 1989).

Beyond these immediate environmental and nutritional conditions, cognitive factors such as body awareness, self-image, and beliefs about particular foods can influence both short- and long-term food intake. The prevalence of eating disorders such as anorexia and bulimia nervosa among teenage girls is an example of how cognitive factors can override the biology and learning history, leading to inappropriate food and energy intake (Brownell and Fairburn, 1995).

Biological Aspects of Energy Intake Control

Underlying these complex behavioral elements are the biological mechanisms that control energy intake to meet energy needs. Control of energy intake is often viewed as part of a homeostatic system. In this homeostatic system, some aspect of body energy is the parameter considered to be maintained between some specified limits, and food intake and energy expenditure are considered as mechanisms for adding energy or removing energy from the body energy pool to maintain homeostasis.

The homeostatic model assumes that what is being regulated is not energy intake per se, but rather body energy stores and potentially the distribution of energy within the various stores (e.g., glycogen, fat). Energy intake is controlled to maintain tissue energy stores, a scheme that also ensures that energy expenditure needs are met. The advantage of this system is that it does not rely on mechanisms that monitor short-term energy intake and expenditure, but it is more geared toward long-term integration of energy input and output and their net effect on body energy stores over time. Failure in the long-term to consume sufficient energy to meet energy expenditure needs would result in a change in tissue energy stores of the organism, which would in turn stimulate a response to restore energy stores.

The system that controls energy intake in relation to energy needs has several elements. It has a central controlling element, the brain, where all information is integrated and which directs a coordinated response to input stimuli. There are controlled systems for food ingestion, absorption, nutrient interconversion, metabolism, and storage. Additionally, the system has both input (afferent) and output (efferent) signaling capabilities to and from the brain.

Afferent signals can be neural or humoral, and both serve as elements of a feedback loop that informs the brain about events in the periphery (e.g., sensory properties of available food or amount and composition of food eaten). Efferent signals are the output of the brain and are signals that drive motor function involved in food acquisition and ingestion, as well as signals that ensure that the appropriate hormonal environment exists to process incoming nutrients from the food ingested. These afferent and efferent signal pathways constitute the essential elements of a feedback scheme, conceptually similar to the functional elements of a common household heating system in which a temperature sensor is linked to a system that adjusts heat output in order to maintain temperature at a specified level.

Afferent Signals Involved in Short-Term Control of Energy Intake. Short-term signals involved in control of energy intake include preabsorptive and postprandial signals. Afferent signals are generated from the ingestion, absorption, and metabolism of nutrients (Table 18–3). The sight, smell, and taste of food are all important sensory signals that can affect the quantity and composition of food and energy ingested. Neural pathways transmit this information directly to the brain, where it is processed by the brain centers involved in control of food intake. These brain centers can elicit efferent signals (e.g., neural stimulation of insulin secretion) that serve to prime the metabolic machinery to process ingested food.

Following food ingestion, gastrointestinal signals provide information to the brain about the quantity and quality (composition) of food ingested. Stretch receptors in the stomach signal the brain via neural pathways about meal size, while a variety of gastrointestinal peptides secreted into the circulation following meal ingestion signal the brain directly or indirectly via stimulation of peripheral neural pathways (Morley, 1990). Certain of these peptides are secreted in response to specific nutrients. For example, products of fat and protein digestion (e.g., fatty acids or amino acids) stimulate release of the peptide cholecystokinin (CCK) into the circulation. CCK activates vagal afferent nerves that signal the brain to reduce subsequent food intake (Smith et al., 1985).

Signals from the absorbed nutrients themselves (e.g., glucose and amino acids), apart from the neural and hormonal mechanisms, have been suggested to embody the signals that control appetite and food intake. The glucostatic (Mayer, 1953) and aminostatic (Mellinkoff, 1957) theories of food intake control are based on the idea that either the blood or tissue concentration or rate of utilization of glucose and amino acids serve as a feedback signal to the brain to modulate food intake.

Afferent Signals Involved in Long-Term Control of Energy Intake. Long-term signals are signals from body energy stores (Table 18–3). The concept that regulation of food intake may be tied to the size of the fat mass and may be responsive to signals from adipose tissue was first introduced by Kennedy (1953) several decades ago. Advances in molecular biology recently led to the discovery

---

TABLE 18–3
Afferent Signals Involved in Food Intake Control

Sensory Signals
  Sight
  Smell
  Taste

Gastrointestinal Signals
  Cholecystokinin
  Bombesin
  Gastric inhibitory peptide
  Enterostatin

Metabolic Signals
  Nutrient-derived signals
    Glucose
    Amino acids
    Fatty acids
  Signals derived from or associated with
    metabolism or energy storage
    depots
    Insulin
    Glucagon
    Ketone bodies
    Leptin

of a peptide called leptin, which may serve as the long-anticipated signal that links adipose energy stores and brain mechanisms that regulate energy intake and expenditure.

Leptin, the protein product of the leptin or OB gene, is synthesized and secreted by adipose tissue in direct proportion to the size of fat stores (Flier, 1997). Systemic or intracerebroventricular injection of leptin into genetically obese mice reduces food intake and increases energy expenditure, resulting in reduction of body fat. Extremely high doses of leptin also reduce food intake in nonobese animals. Leptin exerts its effect on food intake and energy expenditure by binding to a specific leptin receptor present in many tissues, including brain (Tartaglia, 1997). Despite these pronounced effects in animals, the role of leptin in the regulation of energy balance in humans is less clear. Circulating leptin concentrations and the protein itself are not abnormal in obese individuals, suggesting that any involvement in disordered energy balance (e.g, obesity) might involve changes at the leptin receptor level. Although a complete understanding of leptin's role in control of energy homeostasis in humans is still emerging, it has been proposed that the main role for leptin in humans is to signal the brain whether body fat stores are sufficient to support growth and reproduction (Chehab et al., 1997; Rosenbaum et al., 1997).

Brain Mechanisms Involved in Control of Energy Intake. The hypothalamus is the key brain structure involved in the control of food and energy intake (Grossman, 1975). Animal studies have demonstrated that the ventromedial hypothalamus (VMH) is involved in suppression of feeding. Within the VMH, the paraventricular nucleus (PVN) is the anatomical structure that integrates satiety signals (Schwartz and Seeley, 1997; Levine and Billington, 1997). Conversely, the lateral hypothalamus (LH) is the brain center involved in stimulation of feeding. Damage or ablation of the VMH results in overeating and body weight gain, whereas destruction of the LH results in reduced food intake and body weight loss (Grossman, 1975).

A number of different neuromodulators (amino acids, monoamines, and peptides) are involved in the central control of feeding behavior in animals (Blundell, 1991). These molecules act in discrete brain centers to either stimulate or inhibit feeding (Table 18–4).

Efferent Signals Involved in Control of Energy Intake. Efferent signals include both the neuronal outputs that coordinate the various motor functions involved in food acquisition and ingestion, as well as signals that are associated with changes in food intake and body nutrient stores. The sympathetic and parasympathetic systems act in reciprocal fashion in the control of food intake and associated metabolism (Bray, 1991). The activity of the sympathetic nervous system (SNS) appears to be inversely related to food intake, at least in animals. Administration of an appetite suppressant such as an amphetamine decreases food intake and increases sympathetic activity. Conversely, ventromedial hypothalamic lesions increase food intake and decrease sympathetic activity. Ingestion of food activates the parasympathetic nervous system, which stimulates the peripheral release of insulin, the predominant anabolic hormone associ-

---

TABLE 18–4
Neuromodulators that Stimulate or Inhibit Food Intake

Neuromodulators that Inhibit Food Intake

Neurotransmitters	*Peptide Hormones*
Serotonin	Neurotensin
Dopamine	Cholecystokinin
Norepinephrine	Somatostatin
Epinephrine	Enterostatin
γ-aminobutyrate	Anorectin
	Bombesin
	Glucagon
	Calcitonin
	Arginine vasopressin
	Corticotropin-releasing · hormone

Neuromodulators that Stimulate Food Intake (when injected into the brain in satiated animals)

Neurotransmitters	*Neuropeptides*
Serotonin	Opioids
Growth hormone-releasing hormone	Galanin
	Neuropeptide Y
γ-aminobutyrate	Peptide YY
Norepinephrine	β-endorphin
	Kephalins
	Pancreatic polypeptide
	Dynorphin

ated with metabolic processing of ingested nutrients.

CONTROL OF ENERGY EXPENDITURE

Total daily energy expenditure reflects the total amount of nutrient oxidized to meet the body's energy needs. For measurement purposes, total energy expenditure may be subdivided into three major components: (1) resting metabolic rate (RMR), (2) the thermic effect of food (TEF), and (3) the energy expended in physical activity (EE_{act}). These components and a further explanation of their contribution to daily energy expenditure can be found in Chapter 17.

Over- and Underfeeding

Over- and underfeeding produce changes in total energy expenditure, which act to oppose changes in body energy stores. The magnitude and duration of these changes is generally small in relation to the perturbation of energy balance and is not sufficient to prevent changes in body energy stores.

During food restriction, TEF and EE_{act} decline, as would be expected from reduced food intake and a reduction in total body mass. Resting metabolic rate, however, declines more rapidly than would be expected from the loss of body mass and from the decline in spontaneous physical activity due to general fatigue. In one study in which subjects were fed an energy-restricted diet for 24 weeks, subjects lost 23% of their initial body weight (Keys et al., 1950). Concurrent with this, RMR declined by 36% and muscle mass was reduced by 40%. In relative terms, RMR per unit of fat-free mass decreased by 14%, suggesting an increase in metabolic efficiency of the remaining body tissue. This adaptive reduction in RMR may be a defense against further loss of body energy stores. It has been suggested that this adaptive reduction in RMR may be mediated by altered neuroendocrine status (e.g., reduced circulating thyroid hormone) or reduced activity of the sympathetic nervous system (Danforth, 1984; Young and Landsberg, 1977).

During overfeeding, the adaptive increase in energy expenditure is generally modest and may be nutrient specific. For example, a 50% increase in total energy intake coming exclusively from carbohydrate has been observed to increase total daily energy expenditure by about 10%, whereas the same level of fat overfeeding produced only a 3% increase in energy expenditure (Horton, et al., 1995). As with underfeeding, these adaptive alterations in energy expenditure are believed to be mediated by changes in neuroendocrine status and the activity of the sympathetic nervous system.

Changes in Body Composition

Because RMR is influenced by body composition, changes in body composition can affect RMR. It has been suggested that one way to increase energy expenditure in order to combat obesity is to increase RMR by increasing muscle mass and decreasing fat mass. Although it is difficult to estimate contribution of muscle mass per se to RMR, the contribution of fat-free mass (FFM) (which is largely muscle) can be estimated. Each one kilogram increase in FFM increases RMR by about 22 kcal/day. Thus, it would be necessary to increase FFM by 4.5 kg in order to increase daily energy expenditure by 100 kcal. Increasing FFM, therefore, is not a practical means to increase energy expenditure in order to bring about a shift in energy balance.

Aging. Total daily energy expenditure declines with aging (see Chapter 17, Fig. 17–5). FFM also declines with aging, and because RMR is highly correlated with FFM, a decline in RMR is expected. There is no convincing evidence that TEF changes with aging, and there is no strong theoretical reason why this would be expected. Additionally, people often become more sedentary as they age, which reduces EE_{act}. Remaining physically active can prevent much of the decline in RMR with aging, largely due to preservation of lean tissue mass (Poehlman and Horton, 1990).

Physical Activity

The amount of physical activity performed is the factor most capable of modifying total daily energy expenditure. Energy expenditure can be increased by 100 kcal/day with only 20 to 30 min of walking at about 2 miles/hour. With other moderate aerobic activities such as cycling, tennis, or swimming, the additional caloric expenditure above RMR can range from 125 to 350 kcal/30 min (Table 18–5).

Thus, although total daily obligatory energy expenditure (i.e., RMR) can be altered in the short term by severe alterations in energy intake or in the longer term by changes in body composition, the magnitude of possible changes is relatively small. In contrast, substantial alterations in total daily energy expenditure can be produced by as little as 30 min of physical activity.

Composition of Energy Expenditure

The fuel for energy expenditure is supplied by protein, carbohydrate, and fat (and alcohol).

TABLE 18–5
Energy Cost of Various Forms of Physical Activity

Mild to Moderate Exercise	kcal burned per hour*
Walking 2 to 2.5 miles per hour (mph)	185–255
Bicycling or stationary cycling (5.5 mph)	245
Golf (walking with clubs)	270
Aerobic exercise (low impact)	275
Ballroom dancing	300
Strength training	300
Hiking (3 mph, with 20 lb backpack)	400
Treadmill walking (4 mph)	345
Tennis	425
Rowing machine (easy)	300

Moderate to Intense Exercise	kcal burned per hour*
Rope jumping	660
Swimming	540
Walking (5 mph)	555
Bench-stepping class	610
Jogging (5.5 mph)	655
Bicycling or stationary cycling (13 mph)	655
Stair climbing machine	680
Running (7.2 mph)	700
Cross-country skiing (5 mph)	600
Rowing machine (higher intensity)	655

*Values are kcal/h above resting metabolic rate for an average 70 kg subject.

Data calculated from Ainsworth, B. E., Haskell, W. L., Leon, A. S., et al. (1993). Compendium of physical activities: Classification of energy costs of human physical activities. Med Sci Sport Exerc 25:71–80.

This fuel can be supplied by the diet or by endogenous energy storage depots in the body. The relative contributions of these dietary fuels to the fuel mixture burned by the body appears to follow a hierarchy that is consistent with (1) the storage capacity of the body for each macronutrient in relation to its intake, (2) the energy cost of converting the ingested nutrient into a form with a greater storage capacity, and (3) the specific fuel needs of specific body tissues. In this metabolic hierarchy, the priorities for substrate oxidation are alcohol > protein > carbohydrate > fat.

Alcohol has highest priority for oxidation because there is no body storage pool and it can be toxic if it accumulates in body tissues. Amino acids are next in the oxidative hierarchy. Again, there is no specific storage pool in the body for excess amino acids; body proteins are functional in nature. Carbohydrate is third in the oxidative hierarchy. Carbohydrate can be stored as glycogen, but storage capacity is limited. Glycogen stores in a typical adult range from 200 to 500 g (predominantly in muscle and liver) and are only enough to supply a single day of energy needs. Conversion of carbohydrate to fat is energetically expensive, requiring investment of adenosine triphosphate (ATP) equivalent to 20% of the energy contained in the carbohydrate (Flatt, 1992); oxidation of excess glucose is more energetically efficient than is its conversion to fat. Carbohydrate is somewhat unique in that it is an obligatory fuel for certain tissues, including the central nervous system and red blood cells. In contrast to the other macronutrients, there is a virtually unlimited storage capacity for fat, largely in adipose tissue. Storage of dietary fat in adipose tissue is very efficient (97% to 98%) and, unlike carbohydrate, fat is not a unique fuel source for any body tissue.

Because of the oxidative priority of alcohol and protein (amino acids), the body has an exceptional ability to maintain balances of these nutrients across a wide range of intakes of each. In addition, because body carbohydrate stores are not significantly larger than daily carbohydrate intake and because net de novo lipogenesis from carbohydrate does not occur under normal circumstances, carbohydrate oxidation also closely matches carbohydrate intake, and carbohydrate balance is maintained across a wide range of carbohydrate intake. By contrast, fat does not promote its own oxidation, and the amount of fat oxidized is not proportional to intake but comprises the difference between total energy needs and oxidation of the other priority fuels.

$$\text{Fat Oxidation} = \text{Total Energy Expenditure} -$$
$$(\text{Protein Oxidation} +$$
$$\text{Carbohydrate Oxidation})$$

The low metabolic priority for fat oxidation and the large storage capacity of the body for fat in relation to daily fat intake may weaken the precision of the body to regulate energy balance when the diet is rich in fat. The precision of regulation is likely to be poor under conditions of limited physical activity, because increased activity is the most efficient means to increase fat oxidation.

INTEGRATION OF ENERGY INTAKE AND EXPENDITURE

Although we have discussed energy and nutrient intake and expenditure as separate components of the energy balance relationship, the two are inextricably linked with each influencing the other. The body's ability to maintain energy and nutrient balance reflects the existence of a complex regulatory system involving integration of neural and hormonal inputs and outputs from the hypothalamic brain centers that regulate energy intake and expenditure. This system allows the body to achieve a steady state of energy and nutrient balance and to defend that steady state against challenges. Most adults maintain a relatively constant body weight and body composition over long periods of time and defend against disruptions to the state of energy balance. For example, an increase in energy intake above energy expenditure disrupts energy balance. If the increased energy intake is sustained, body weight increases and is accompanied by increases in energy expenditure. Body weight stabilizes and energy balance is achieved when energy expenditure is increased to the level of energy intake. Conversely, a decrease in energy intake disrupts energy balance and produces a loss of body weight, accompanied by a reduction in energy expenditure. Body weight stabilizes when energy expenditure declines to the level of energy intake.

Recent work highlighting the importance of nutrient balance in addition to total energy balance has improved understanding of the body weight regulatory system. As discussed earlier, acute changes in intake of alcohol, protein, or carbohydrate are rapidly balanced by changes in oxidation of each. In contrast, fat oxidation is not tightly linked to fat intake. As a consequence, positive or negative energy balance are largely conditions of positive or negative fat balance. The point at which a stable body weight and body composition is reached and defended, therefore, is that point at which fat balance is achieved (settling point).

For a given individual, the major factors that influence fat balance are the amount and composition of food eaten and the total amount of physical activity. Positive fat balance can be produced by overconsumption of energy or restriction of physical activity. Positive fat balance occurs when diets of any composition are overconsumed. This is because balances of protein, carbohydrate, and alcohol are preferentially achieved at the expense of fat oxidation. During carbohydrate overfeeding, for example, carbohydrate oxidation increases to maintain carbohydrate balance, but because carbohydrate is providing proportionately more fuel for oxidative needs, fat oxidation is providing less than usual, creating positive fat balance (Horton et al., 1995). Diets high in fat are particularly problematic: they increase the palatability and energy density of the food consumed, which contributes to overconsumption of total energy, and the excess energy does not increase fat oxidation and is efficiently stored. The best strategy for avoiding positive fat balance is to avoid overconsumption of energy. This may be facilitated by consuming a low-fat diet.

Restricting the habitual level of physical activity reduces fat oxidation because working muscle is a major contributor to the body's total oxidation of fat. Because fat intake and oxidation are not closely linked, positive fat balance results if the decline in fat oxidation is not offset by an equivalent reduction in fat intake.

Negative fat balance can be brought about by underconsumption of total energy or fat or by an increase in the level of habitual physical activity. During underconsumption of energy, the dietary supply of the priority metabolic fuels carbohydrate and protein are insufficient to meet the body's energy needs. The remaining energy needs must be met by fat oxidation, which comes largely from endogenous fat stores. Similarly, increased oxidation of fat is the predominate mechanism by which energy needs are met when the level of habitual physical activity is increased.

Energy Balance, Fat Balance, and the Settling Point

In most individuals, under most environmental circumstances, maintenance of energy balance is largely a matter of achieving and maintaining fat balance. Given the preceding discussion, one might ask how a new steady state of body weight and body composition is achieved following a positive or negative perturbation in fat balance. There are two mechanisms by which this can occur. First, changes in behavior can lead to adjustments in either intake or oxidation of fat (e.g., altering total energy or fat intake and altering physical activity). Second, in the absence of sufficient behavior changes, fat oxidation is altered following alterations in the body fat mass. As an example of behavioral adjustments, the negative fat balance produced by reducing energy intake could be eliminated totally by a compensatory reduction in physical activity. However, this is not likely to be the typical response, and one would usually expect to see some loss of body mass and the accompanying reduction in energy expenditure. As an example of metabolic adjustments, overconsumption of total energy and fat produces positive energy balance. If the behavioral adjustments are absent or insufficient to subsequently offset the excess intake, increases in the body fat mass result. Increased body fat mass is associated with increased levels of circulating free fatty acids, which elevate total fat oxidation. Thus, a stable body weight is reached at the point where the body fat mass has increased sufficiently so that fat oxidation equals fat intake.

The current environment in the United States is characterized by the wide availability of energy-dense foods, many of which are high in fat, coupled with an increasingly sedentary lifestyle. Under these circumstances, maintenance of a large body fat mass may be a necessary consequence in order to achieve fat balance.

REFERENCES

Ainsworth, B. E., Haskell, W. L., Leon, A. S., Jacobs, D. R. Jr., Montoye, H. J., Sallis, J. F. and Paffenbarger, R.S. Jr. (1993) Compendium of physical activities: Classification of energy costs of human physical activities. Med Sci Sport Exerc 25:71–80.

Birch, L. L. (1992) Children's preference for high-fat foods. Nutr Rev 50:249–255.

Blundell, J. E. (1991) The biology of appetite. Clin Appl Nutr 1:21–31.

Bray, G. A. (1991) Obesity, a disorder of nutrient partitioning: The MONA LISA hypothesis. J Nutr 121:1146–1162.

Brownell, K. D. and Fairburn, G. C. (eds.) (1995) Eating Disorders and Obesity: A Comprehensive Handbook. Guilford Press, New York.

Cahill, G. F. (1970) Starvation in man. N Engl J Med 282:668–675.

Chehab, F. F., Mounzih, K., Lu, R. and M. E. Lim. (1997) Early onset of reproductive function in normal female mice treated with leptin. Science 275:88–90.

Danforth, E. Jr. (1984) The role of thyroid hormones in the control of energy expenditure. Clin Endocrinol Metab 13:581–595.

De Castro, J. and De Castro, E. (1989) Spontaneous meal patterns in humans: Influence of the presence of other people. Am J Clin Nutr 50:237–247.

Drewnowski, A. (1997) Taste preferences and food intake. Annu Rev Nutr 17:237–253.

Flatt, J. P. (1992) The biochemistry of energy expenditure. In: Obesity (Bjorntorp, P. and Brodoff, B., eds.), pp. 100–116. J. B. Lippincott, Philadelphia.

Flatt, J. P. (1995) Diet, lifestyle, and weight maintenance. Am J Clin Nutr 62:820–836.

Flier, J. S. (1997) Leptin expression and action: New experimental paradigms. Proc Natl Acad Sci USA 94:4242–4245.

Frayn, K. (1996) Metabolic Regulation: A Human Perspective, pp. 78–102. Portland Press, London.

Grossman, S. P. (1975) Role of the hypothalamus in the regulation of food and water intake. Psychol Rev 82:200–224.

Horton, T. J., Drougas, H., Brachey, A., Reed, G. W., Peters, J. C. and Hill, J. O. (1995) Fat and carbohydrate overfeeding in humans: Different effects on energy storage. Am J Clin Nutr 62:19–29.

Keesey, R. E. and S. W. Corbett (1984) Metabolic defense of the body weight set point. In: Eating and Its Disorders. (Stunkard, A. J., Stellar, E., eds.), pp. 87–96. Raven Press, New York.

Kennedy, G. C. (1953) The role of depot fat in the hypothalamic control of food intake in the rat. Proc R Soc Lond B Biol Sci 140:578–596.

Kern, D. L., McPhee, L. Fisher, J., Johnson, S. and Birch L. L. (1993) The postingestive consequences of fat condition preferences for flavors associated with high dietary fat. Physiol Behav 54:71–76.

Keys, A., Brozek, J., Henshel, A., Michelson, O. and Taylor, H. L. (1950) The Biology of Human Starvation. University of Minnesota Press, Minneapolis, MN.

Kuczmarski, R. J., Flegal, K. M., Campbell, S. M. and Johnson, C. L. (1994) Increasing prevalence of overweight among U.S. adults: The National Health and Nutrition Examination Surveys, 1960 to 1991. JAMA 272:205–211.

Leibel, R. L., Rosenbaum, M. and Hirsch, J. (1995) Changes in energy expenditure resulting from altered body weight. N Engl J Med 332:621–628.

Levine, A. S. and Billington, C. J. (1997) Why do we eat? A neural systems approach. Annu Rev Nutr 17:597–619.

Lissner, L. and Heitmann, B. L. (1995) Dietary fat and obesity: Evidence from epidemiology. Eur J Clin Nutr 49:79–90.

Mayer, J. (1953) Glucostatic mechanism of regulation of food intake. N Engl J Med 249:13–16.

McDowell, M. A., Briefel, R. R., Alaimo, K., Bischof, A. M., Caughman, C. R., Carroll, M. D., Loria, C. M. and Johnson, C. L. (1994) Energy and macronutrient intakes of persons ages 2 months and over in the United States: Third National Health and Nutrition Examination Survey, Phase 1, 1988–91. National Center for Health Statistics, Centers for Disease Control and Prevention, U.S. Department of Health and Human Services, Publication no. 255.

Mellinkoff, S. (1957) Digestive system. Annu Rev Physiol 19:175–204.

Morley, J. E. (1990) Appetite regulation by gut peptides. Annu Rev Nutr 10:383–395.

National Research Council (1989) Recommended Dietary Allowances, 10th ed., p. 33. National Academy Press, Washington, D.C.

Poehlman, E. T. and Horton, E. S. (1990) Regulation of energy expenditure in aging humans. Annu Rev Nutr 10:255–275.

Rodin, J. (1992) Determination of food intake regulation in obesity. In: Obesity (Bjorntorn, P. and Brodoff, B., eds.), pp. 220–230. J. Lippincott, Philadelphia.

Rolls, B. J., Rowe, E. A., Rolls, E. T., Kingston, B., Megson, A. and Gunary, R. (1981) Variety in a meal enhances food intake in man. Physiol Behav 26:215–221.

Rosenbaum, M. and Leibel, R. L. (1988) Pathophysiology of childhood obesity. Adv Pediatr 35:73–137.

Rosenbaum, M., Leibel, R. L. and Hirsch, J. (1997) Obesity. N Engl J Med 337:396–407.

Schwartz, M. W. and Seely, R. J. (1997) The new biology of body weight regulation. J Am Diet Assoc 97:54–58.

Smith, G. P., Jerome, C. and Norgren, R. (1985) Afferent axons in the abdominal vagus mediate satiety effect of cholecystokinin in rats. Am J Physiol 249:R638–R643.

Tartaglia, L. A. (1997) The leptin receptor. J Biol Chem 279:6093–6096.

Young, J. B. and Landsberg, L. (1977) Suppression of sympathetic nervous system during fasting. Science 196:1473–1475.

RECOMMENDED READINGS

Blundell, J. E. (1991) The biology of appetite. Clin Appl Nutr 1:21–31.

Bray, G. A. (1991) Obesity, a disorder of nutrient partitioning: The MONA LISA hypothesis. J Nutr 121:1146–1162.

Flatt, J. P. (1992) The biochemistry of energy expenditure. In: Obesity (Bjorntorp, P. and Brodoff, B., eds.), pp. 100–116. J.B. Lippincott, Philadelphia.

Rosenbaum, M., Leibel, R. L. and Hirsch, J. (1997) Obesity. N Engl J Med 337:396–407.

Schwartz, M. W. and Seely, R. J. (1997) The new biology of body weight regulation. J Am Diet Assoc 97:54–58.

CHAPTER 19

◆ ◆

Disturbances of Energy Balance

James O. Hill, Ph.D., Adamandia D. Kriketos, Ph.D., and John C. Peters, Ph.D.

OUTLINE

Obesity

Definition
Prevalence of Obesity
Health Consequences of Obesity
Factors Involved in Development of
  Obesity
  Genetic Factors
  Environmental Factors
  Interactions of Genes and Environment
Obesity Management
Methods of Obesity Treatment
  *Behavioral Weight Loss Treatment
    Programs*
  Surgical Treatment
  Pharmacological Treatment
Why Is It Difficult to Maintain a Reduced
  Body Weight?

Starvation

Occurrence, Definition, and Historical
  Perspective
Effects on Energy Balance, Fuel
  Metabolism, and Body Composition
Adaptation to Prolonged Starvation

Protein Energy Malnutrition

Effects of Energy Balance, Fuel
  Metabolism, and Body Composition
Adaptation to Chronic Undernutrition
Long-term Effects of Protein Energy
  Malnutrition

COMMON ABBREVIATIONS

BMI (body mass index)
CVD (cardiovascular disease)
FFM (fat-free mass)
NIDDM (noninsulin-dependent diabetes mellitus)
PEM (protein energy malnutrition)
RMR (resting metabolic rate)
TEF (thermic effect of food)

■ Obesity

Obesity is a disease in which the accumulation of body fat adversely affects health (Pi-Sunyer, 1993). Obesity is closely associated with other diseases, chiefly noninsulin-dependent diabetes mellitus (NIDDM) and cardiovascular disease (CVD) (Despres, 1993). Individuals who accumulate excess body fat in upper body adipose depots, particularly intraabdominal or visceral depots, may be at greater risk of developing negative health consequences of obesity than individuals who accumulate the same amount of excess body fat in the lower body (Pouliot et al., 1994).

DEFINITION

In populations, the body mass index (BMI), calculated as weight (kg) divided by height^2 (m^2), provides the best estimate of the level of obesity, and the waist circumference provides the best estimate of visceral adipose tissue (Pi-Sunyer, 1993). Table 19–1, developed by the World Health Organization (WHO), provides a classification of obesity based on BMI and shows the relative risk of co-morbidities within each BMI category (Pi-Sunyer, 1993). A waist circumference of 39 inches or more for men and 35 inches or more for women indicates visceral obesity, a condition

that further increases risk of co-morbid conditions (WHO, 1997). Most information relating BMI and waist circumference to disease risk has been obtained in white populations. It is likely that ethnic populations differ in the level of risk associated with a particular BMI and waist circumference.

PREVALENCE OF OBESITY

Obesity is increasing at an alarming rate in both developed and developing countries (Pi-Sunyer, 1993; WHO, 1997). Prevalence rates for overweight and obesity in the United States are obtained from the National Health (and Nutrition) Examination Surveys (NHES or NHANES), which have provided prevalence data for obesity since 1960 (Fig. 19–1). In these surveys, overweight was defined as a BMI between 25.0 and 29.2 kg/m^2, and obesity was defined as BMI $\geq$ 30 kg/m^2. Whereas the prevalence of overweight has remained relatively constant since the 1960s, the prevalence of obesity increased dramatically over the past two decades (Flegal et al., 1998).

Based on NHANES III data, the prevalence of overweight was similar in adult white men and women but higher in African-American and Hispanic women than in men from these ethnic groups. The prevalence of overweight was about 50% in African-American and Hispanic women.

Overweight and obesity are more difficult to assess in children than in adults because children are constantly changing their height and weight. However, all indications are that overweight and obesity are also increasing in children. In NHANES III, overweight in children and adolescents was defined as being above the BMI that represented the 85th percentile in the National Health Examination Survey (NHES) conducted from 1963 through 1965 for children ages 6 to 17 years. By definition, 15% of children had a BMI over the 85th percentile in the 1963 through 1965 NHES survey. Figure 19–2 shows that 22% of children and adolescents in the 1988 through 1991 NHANES III survey were above the BMI that represented the 85th percentile in the NHES study (Troiano et al., 1995).

TABLE 19–1
Classification of Obesity Based on Body Mass Index (BMI) and Risk of Co-morbidities

Classification	BMI (kg/m^2)	Risk of Co-morbidities
Underweight	<18.5	Low (but risk of other clinical problems increased)
Normal range	18.5–24.9	Average
Overweight	≥25.0	
Pre-obese	25.0–29.9	Increased
Obese class I	30.0–34.9	Moderate
Obese class II	35.0–39.9	Severe
Obese class III	≥40.0	Very severe

Adapted from World Health Organization (1997) Obesity: Preventing and Managing the Global Epidemic: Report of a WHO Consultation on Obesity. Geneva, June 3–5.

Age-adjusted Prevalence of Overweight (BMI 25-29.9) and Obesity (BMI ≥30)

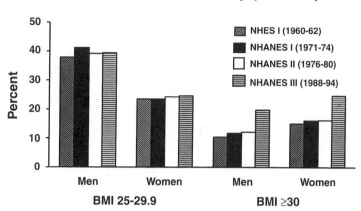

Figure 19–1. Prevalence of overweight and obesity in American adults. Overweight was defined as a body mass index (BMI) of 25.0 to 29.9 kg/m² and obesity as a BMI ≥ 30 kg/m². (Based on data of Flegal, K. M., Carroll, M. D., Kuczmarski, R. J., and Johnson, C. L. [1998] Overweight and obesity in the United States: Prevalence and trends, 1960–1994. Int J Obesity 22:39–47.)

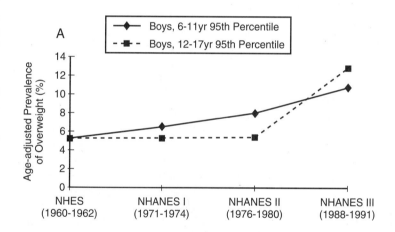

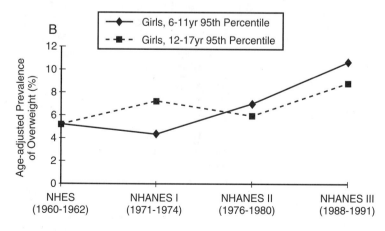

Figure 19–2. Age-adjusted prevalence of overweight in boys (A) and girls (B) aged 6 to 17 years across all races. Data are from national surveys (1963–1991) and are based on use of the 95th percentile cutoff point definition. (Reproduced from Troiano, R. P., Flegal, K. M., Kuczmarski, R. J., Campbell, S. M. and Johnson, C. L. [1995] Overweight prevalence and trends for children and adolescents. Arch Pediatr Adolesc Med 149:1085–1091.)

	TABLE 19–2	
	Frequent Co-Morbidities Associated with Obesity	

Greatly Increased (*Relative Risk* >>3)	**Moderately Increased** (*Relative Risk* ~2–3)	**Slightly Increased** (*Relative Risk* ~1–2)
Diabetes	Coronary heart disease	Cancer (breast cancer in postmenopausal women, endometrial cancer, colon cancer)
Gallbladder disease	Hypertension	Reproductive hormone abnormalities
Dyslipidemia	Osteoarthritis (knees)	Polycystic ovary syndrome
Insulin resistance	Hyperuricemia and gout	Impaired fertility
Breathlessness		Low back pain due to obesity
Sleep apnea		Increased anesthetic risk
		Fetal defects associated with maternal obesity

Adapted from World Health Organization (1997) Obesity: Preventing and Managing the Global Epidemic: Report of a WHO Consultation on Obesity. Geneva, June 3–5.

HEALTH CONSEQUENCES OF OBESITY

Obesity is associated with many physiological and psychosocial risks. Table 19–2 lists the most frequently observed co-morbidities associated with obesity. The risk of developing a co-morbidity is influenced by the extent of obesity, the location of excess body fat, and weight gain over the adult years. In general, obesity-associated morbidity and mortality increase in direct proportion to increases in BMI. This is shown in Figure 19–3, where all-cause mortality (risk of death from any cause) is plotted against BMI. It can be seen that all-cause mortality begins to increase at BMIs nearing 30 and continues to increase in a linear fashion above 30.

Data from many studies suggest that ex-cess fat located in visceral depots is an independent risk factor for NIDDM and CVD (Despres, 1993). For any specific BMI, a high waist circumference is associated with greater risk of impaired health than a low waist circumference. Visceral fat may increase obesity-related co-morbidities because of its proximity to the liver. It is thought that a high concentration of fatty acids released from visceral adipose tissue depots may be taken up by the liver and lead to insulin resistance and dyslipidemia (Despres et al., 1989). The factors that determine the location of storage of excess fat are not well understood, but sex hormones seem to play an important role in regulating body fat distribution (Zamboni et al., 1994).

A third factor influencing risk of obesity-associated disease is weight gain over adulthood. Regardless of BMI, a large weight gain after the age of 18 years is associated with a significantly greater risk of developing NIDDM in both men and women (Colditz, 1995). The current edition of Dietary Guidelines for Americans recommends that weight gain after the age of 18 years be avoided (U.S. Department of Agriculture and U.S. Department of Health and Human Services, 1995).

Visceral obesity is frequently found along with other risk factors for NIDDM and CVD, including impaired glucose tolerance, elevated blood pressure, increased triglyceride and decreased high density lipoprotein (HDL) levels, and insulin resistance. This has led some researchers to propose a metabolic syndrome in which insulin resistance may be the underlying factor (Zavaroni et al., 1994).

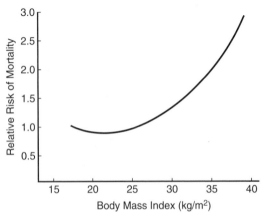

Figure 19–3. *U-shaped relationship of body mass index to excess mortality in adults. Relative risk was defined as 1.0 for adults with BMIs between 20 and 25.*

Accumulation of visceral fat may lead to insulin resistance, which in turn leads to hyperinsulinemia, dyslipidemia and hypertension, and eventually to NIDDM and CVD.

Obese people in Western societies are often subjected to discrimination because of their body size. Some data suggest that obese individuals are less likely than their lean peers to enter desirable professions and that they may make less money (Gortmaker et al., 1993). Overweight and obese children also appear to suffer psychosocial consequences, such as impaired social functioning and, in adolescents, low self-esteem (Gortmaker et al., 1993).

FACTORS INVOLVED IN DEVELOPMENT OF OBESITY

Obesity can occur only when energy ingested exceeds energy expended. However, because of the many genetic and environmental influences on both energy intake and energy expenditure, obesity must be considered to be a heterogeneous disorder with multiple causes. The gene × environment interaction is likely to explain the majority of variation in body weight, and separating the genetic from the environmental determinants of obesity presents a formidable challenge for scientists.

Genetic Factors

Studies in genetically identical twins have shown a strong genetic component to body weight regulation. Identical twins raised in different environments show similarities in body weight and body composition. Furthermore, when pairs of identical twins are overfed or subjected to long-term exercise training, the changes in body weight and body composition are much more similar between identical twins than among twin pairs.

Major advances have occurred in the understanding of the genetic basis of obesity over the past few years. Beginning with the identification of the *ob* gene and its protein product leptin, scientists have now identified five genes whose mutations cause obesity in rodents (Table 19–3). These genes code for proteins that appear to influence both energy intake and energy expenditure. Leptin was the first obesity gene identified, and a deficiency in leptin produces obesity in the *ob/ob* mouse. The genetic defect leads to an inability to manufacture an active form of leptin. Injections of leptin into obese *ob/ob* mice reduce food intake and decrease body weight. Leptin appears to bind to leptin receptors in the brain and to affect food intake through interactions with other brain peptides. Leptin is thought to affect energy intake and body composition differently in response to overfeeding and starvation, as illustrated in Figure 19–4.

Because human obesity involves many genes, it is not clear whether identification of gene products such as leptin will have direct implications for obese humans. Studies in human subjects show that blood leptin levels are positively correlated with body fatness. The

TABLE 19–3
Genetic Mutations in Rodents That Cause Obesity

Gene	Mutation	Gene Product	Rodent Chromosome	Human Homologue	Action
Lep	*ob*	Leptin	6 (mouse)	7q31.3	Central effects resulting in decreased food intake and increased energy expenditure
Lepr	*db*	Leptin receptor	4 (mouse)	1p32	Leptin signal processing, transport, or clearance (?)
	fa		5 (rat)		
Cpe	*fat*	Carboxypeptidase E	8 (mouse)	11p15	Prohormone (including neuropeptide) processing
Tub	*tub*	Phosphodiesterase	7 (mouse)	4q32 (?)	Hypothalamic cellular apoptosis (?)
Agouti	Ay	Agouti signaling protein	2 (mouse)	20q11.2	Blocking of melanocortin-4 receptor

Adapted from Rosenbaum, M., Leibel, R. L. and Hirsch, J. (1997) Obesity. N Engl J Med 337:396–407. Copyright 1997 Massachusetts Medical Society. All rights reserved.

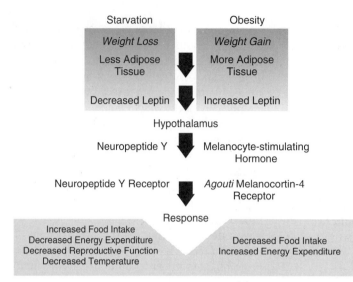

Figure 19–4. A model of the potential role of leptin in the regulation of energy balance. (Adapted from Gura, T. [1997] Obesity sheds its secrets. Science 275:751–753.)

most overweight subjects have the highest leptin levels (Havel et al., 1996). Clearly, a lack of leptin is not a major cause of obesity in humans. The fact that leptin is high in obese humans has led to the notion that obesity may involve a leptin resistance and a problem in getting enough leptin across the blood-brain barrier into the brain. It is hypothesized that the high blood levels of leptin are a physiological response to low leptin levels in the brain. Human trials with leptin are underway and should provide some insight into this hypothesis. Regardless of whether or not leptin can be used to treat human obesity, genetic research will identify metabolic pathways that are affected by obesity genes, and this information should increase our understanding of how obesity develops and help us develop pharmacological interventions to treat the disease.

The influence of genes on obesity must be through their effects on food intake or energy expenditure. Whereas leptin appears to influence food intake, other genes could affect energy expenditure. Individuals with very low energy requirements may be at higher risk for obesity development than individuals with higher energy requirements. Substantial research has been done to identify "defects" in energy expenditure that might contribute to obesity. Although individual differences in energy expenditure have been identified and likely play a role in susceptibil-

ity to obesity, no specific defect in energy expenditure that may explain human obesity has been identified. Nevertheless, several candidate genes have been identified that may contribute to individual differences in energy expenditure among individuals (Bouchard and Pérusse, 1993). These genes code for protein products that are closely linked to energy-utilizing processes in the body. For example, differences in the efficiency of coupling of electron transport to the generation of ATP in the mitochondrion may be responsible for individual differences in energetic efficiency. It is important to note that obese individuals usually have a higher, not a lower, total energy expenditure than do nonobese subjects, because of their larger body mass. Energy expenditure per unit of fat-free mass (FFM) is usually found to be similar between lean and obese subjects.

Environmental Factors

There must be powerful environmental influences on the development of obesity. The large increase in the prevalence of obesity that has occurred in the United States over the past few decades cannot be attributed to genetic causes and suggests that changes in environmental factors are influencing the prevalence of obesity. Furthermore, when populations such as the Japanese or Chinese mi-

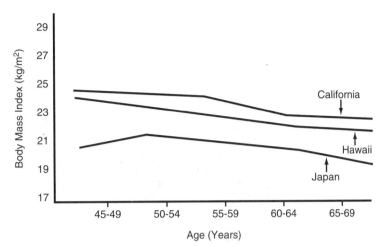

Figure 19–5. Mean body mass index in Japanese men aged 45 to 69 years in Hawaii, California, and Japan in 1965–1968. (Adapted from Curb, J. D. and Marcus, E. B. [1991] Body fat and obesity in Japanese Americans. Am J Clin Nutr 53:1552S–1555S. Copyright American Society for Clinical Nutrition.)

grate to the United States, their BMI increases (Fig. 19–5).

The increasing proportion of fat and the high energy density of the diet, together with reductions in physical activity, are thought to be major contributing factors to the increase in the prevalence of obesity (Pi-Sunyer, 1993). Americans consume diets with an average of 34% to 40% of total energy from fat. When similar diets are fed to laboratory rats, the majority of rats become obese (Pagliassotti et al., 1997). Obesity appears to result both from an increased voluntary energy intake and from the fact that excess dietary fat is stored in the body more efficiently than is excess dietary carbohydrate or protein (Horton et al., 1995). This is discussed in more detail in Chapter 18.

Americans are becoming less physically active and more sedentary. Much of the decline in physical activity can be attributed to modernization, which has made it easier to be sedentary both at work and at home (WHO, 1997). The increasing availability of automobiles and labor-saving devices has substantially reduced the amount of time spent being physically active.

Increasing time spent in sedentary activities such as watching television and video and playing video games is thought to play a role in reducing physical activity in children. The high attractiveness of these sedentary activities makes it difficult to promote more physically active behaviors (WHO, 1997).

It must be noted that although approxi-mately one third of American adults are over-weight or obese, the majority are not. Thus, we must consider factors such as consumption of high-fat diets or physical inactivity not as known causes of obesity but as factors that increase the probability of creating a mismatch between energy intake and energy expenditure. Viewed in this way, it is not surprising that some individuals remain lean while consuming a high-fat diet and being inactive. It is likely that an individual's genotype will help determine whether or not environmental variables such as high-fat diets and inactivity lead to positive energy balance and obesity.

Interactions of Genes and Environment

Obesity is most likely to occur when a genetically susceptible individual encounters an environment conducive to obesity. An example is provided by Pima Indians living in Arizona. This population shows an extremely high prevalence of obesity, about 80%. The high prevalence seems to occur as a result of relatively low energy requirements per unit of FFM, coupled with low levels of physical activity and high intake of an energy-dense diet. Researchers have identified a group of Pima Indians living in northern Mexico who are genetically the same as the Pima Indians living in southern Arizona (Fig. 19–6). The Mexican Pimas are farmers, consuming food that they grow and engaging in high levels of physical activity. The Mexican Pimas are significantly less obese than the Arizona Pimas, demonstrating

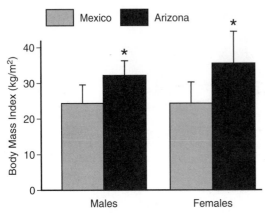

Figure 19–6. *Mean body mass index (± standard deviation) of Pima Indians living in either a traditional lifestyle in Maycoba, Mexico, or a modern lifestyle in Arizona. *In both sexes, BMI was significantly higher (P < 0.0001) in Pimas living in Arizona compared with that of Pimas living in Mexico. (Adapted from Ravussin, E. and Tataranni, P. A. [1997] Dietary fat and human obesity. J Am Diet Assoc 97:S42–S46. Copyright 1997, The American Dietetic Association.)*

the importance of environmental factors on body weight. However, the BMI for the Mexican Pimas is still greater than might be expected for a highly active population consuming a low-fat diet, suggesting that Pima Indians have genes that favor high body weights.

There is currently no consensus about the relative contribution of genetics versus environment to obesity. Some investigators have estimated that genes can explain 25% to 75% of the variation in body weight (Bouchard

and Pérusse, 1993). However, the secular trend toward increased body weight in the United States highlights the importance of the interaction of the genotype with the environment. Because the genotype has not changed during the past decade, nongenetic factors, such as decreased physical activity and increased energy intake, must have made a major contribution to the increased body weight.

OBESITY MANAGEMENT

Figure 19–7 illustrates potential goals for obesity treatment. We now know that most adults are gaining weight over their adult years, and this may be especially true of obese individuals. Thus, prevention of weight gain for both lean and obese individuals should be the first goal in obesity management. Second, we should aim for achieving minor or modest weight loss. Normalization of weight in obese individuals is rare.

Weight loss in obese individuals is associated with improvements in risk factors for NIDDM and CVD. These include reduction in plasma glucose and insulin concentrations, lowering of blood pressure, and normalization of dyslipidemia. Data from a number of studies have shown that modest weight loss (approximately 10%) is associated with substantial improvement in glycemic control, lipid patterns, and blood pressure (Goldstein,

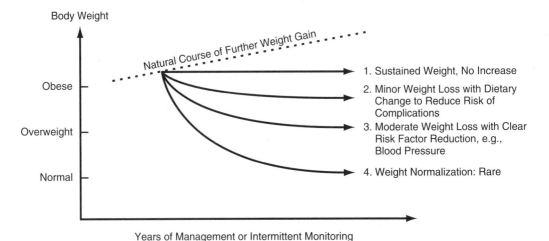

Figure 19–7. *Goals of obesity treatment. (Modified from Rossner, S. [1992] Pregnancy, weight cycling and weight gain on obesity. Int J Obes 16:935–936.)*

1992). Given the difficulty in maintaining large weight reductions, and data suggesting that more modest weight loss can improve health, it is important to set realistic goals for obesity treatment. Because the likelihood of an individual with a BMI of 37 kg/m² achieving a BMI of 25 kg/m² is not great, it may be more realistic for that individual to produce and maintain a 10% body weight reduction. Although a great deal of short-term research (studies over less than a 2-year period) suggests that reducing body weight by 10% will improve health, longer studies are needed to confirm that maintenance of such a body weight reduction will maintain the health benefits. Nonetheless, aiming for a 10% reduction in body weight is a reasonable goal. Once the individual demonstrates the ability to maintain this weight reduction, further weight loss can be attempted.

There have been some reports of increased morbidity and mortality associated with weight loss, but these studies have not been controlled for involuntary weight loss. Studies in which only voluntary weight loss was assessed show that weight loss is associated with reduced morbidity and mortality. However, we need more long-term, carefully controlled studies to better evaluate the potential negative effects of weight loss. Nevertheless, we know that risk factors improve with weight loss, and treating obesity in those at risk for serious health consequences seems appropriate.

METHODS OF OBESITY TREATMENT

Whereas producing weight loss is relatively easy, maintaining a weight loss over a long period of time is difficult. Almost all "diets" work in the sense that they produce weight loss, but once the diet is discontinued the weight is usually regained over time. It is generally believed that the overall success rate in maintaining weight loss over 5 years is less than 5% to 10%. A great deal of research is aimed at understanding why maintaining a weight loss is so difficult and how to improve the success rate.

Behavioral Weight Loss Treatment Programs

The current state-of-the-art program for obesity treatment consists of a behavioral treatment program aimed at modifying diet and physical activity. Such programs help overweight individuals make sustained changes in dietary and physical activity habits. Dietary modification usually involves some energy restriction, ranging from use of very low calorie diets to moderate energy restriction. There is usually an emphasis on reducing the proportion of total daily energy from fat. Participants are also taught to increase physical activity. This has traditionally involved helping subjects engage in regular aerobic activity, but in recent years, resistance training and the combination of aerobic and resistance training has been used. There is also a growing emphasis on increasing lifestyle activity and on increasing daily activity via multiple short bouts of exercise. To increase lifestyle activities, subjects are encouraged to take the stairs instead of the elevator and to park farther away from work or the store to increase walking. Much recent data suggest that increasing physical activity via three 10-minute bouts of exercise is as effective as performing one 30-minute bout. There is increasing emphasis on helping subjects choose physical activities that are enjoyable.

Comprehensive behavioral weight loss programs include staff with expertise in behavioral psychology, nutrition, and exercise physiology. These comprehensive programs have been shown to be more successful than treatments that provide only energy restriction. Very low calorie diets, for example, reliably produce substantial weight loss. This weight loss is better maintained if subjects also are encouraged to exercise and participate in a behavioral program. Overall, even with these methods, most subjects who successfully lose weight in behavioral weight loss programs regain most of that weight within 5 years (Fig. 19–8).

Most behavioral weight loss programs provide active treatment (usually via small groups) for periods of 3 to 6 months. Some also provide a follow-up period with some contact with behaviorists. As behavioral

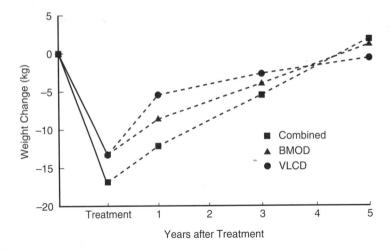

Figure 19–8. Changes in body weight at the end of treatment and during a 5-year follow-up diet period. VLCD, very low calorie diet; BMOD, behavior modification therapy; Combined, both VLCD and BMOD. (Adapted from Wadden, T. A. [1993] Treatment of obesity by moderate and severe caloric restriction. Results of clinical research trials. Ann Intern Med 119:688–693.)

weight loss programs have become longer, subjects have been able to maintain weight losses for longer. This suggests that problems of weight regain begin after subjects leave the active treatment. Better techniques for maintaining weight loss after the conclusion of behavioral weight loss programs are greatly needed.

Surgical Treatment

Gastrointestinal surgery (vertical banded gastroplasty or gastric bypass) is a viable option for many severely overweight subjects (Sugerman, 1993). Most experts believe that subjects should not be considered for surgery unless they have first tried more conventional treatment (behavioral weight loss programs). Furthermore, potential patients should be selected only after careful examination by a multidisciplinary team with medical, surgical, psychiatric, and nutritional expertise. Lifelong medical surveillance after surgery is required. In appropriate patients, surgical treatment appears to produce substantial reductions in body weight, which in many patients are maintained over long periods of time and which often reduce co-morbid conditions associated with obesity.

Pharmacological Treatment

As obesity is becoming recognized not simply as a syndrome of poor will power, but as a disease having strong genetic, biochemical, and metabolic components, interest has increased in the pharmacological treatment of obesity. The approval of the drug dexfenfluramine by the Food and Drug Administration (FDA) in 1996 represented the first approval of an obesity drug in over 20 years. Unfortunately, this drug was withdrawn in 1997 because of previously unrecognized side effects. Pharmacological agents currently under development can be grouped into three general classes: appetite suppressants, drugs that affect nutrient absorption, and drugs that increase energy expenditure.

The appetite suppressant drugs currently under development affect neurotransmitter activity in either the serotonin or norepinephrine systems. Some compounds appear to affect both systems. Drugs in this category reduce voluntary energy intake by reducing appetite. On a cellular level, most of these drugs inhibit reuptake of serotonin and/or increase production of norepinephrine in the brain. Sibutramine, an example of a serotonin reuptake inhibitor, is under review by the FDA.

Appetite suppressants of the newer generation are not addictive and appear to be effective at helping produce moderate weight loss for periods of 1 to 2 years. Because of the newness of these drugs, little information is available about long-term safety and efficacy. It is important to realize that obesity is a chronic condition and that any drug that proves useful in obesity treatment will likely require chronic use. With all available drugs, weight gain occurs when the drug is stopped.

On average, 30% to 50% of subjects taking the currently available appetite suppressants achieve weight reduction of 8% to 10% of initial body weight and maintain these losses over periods of at least 1 year. Reductions in risk factors and co-morbidities of obesity decline with weight loss in these subjects.

Some recent reports have associated increased incidence of primary pulmonary hypertension and valvular heart disease with dexfenfluramine and with the combination of phentermine and fenfluramine. Insufficient data are available to assess the true extent of these adverse effects. However, the possibility of these severe side effects emphasizes that obesity drugs should be used only in those individuals who have an increased risk of co-morbidities due to their obesity and should not be used simply for cosmetic purposes.

Drugs that block the action of digestive enzymes or that block absorption of nutrients (such as fat) from the gastrointestinal (GI) tract are being developed. This serves to reduce total energy available to the body. Among these drugs is the GI lipase inhibitor orlistat, which prevents absorption of dietary fat from the GI tract, resulting in less ingested fat available for metabolism. Weight losses of 9% to 11% of initial body weight have been reported when orlistat is combined with a moderate calorie-restricted diet. These losses have been shown to be maintained up to 2 years and are associated with reductions in risk factors and obesity-associated co-morbidities. Orlistat is currently under review by the FDA.

Among this group of drugs is ephedrine (often used in combination with caffeine or aspirin) and a group of compounds that act on β_3-adrenergic receptors (see Chapter 16) to increase energy expenditure. Although this latter class of compounds has met with great success in animal studies, their effectiveness in humans is only beginning to be assessed. No drugs in this category are currently approved by the FDA for weight loss.

As obesity genes are identified, the protein products of these genes may become the basis of antiobesity drugs. As an example, leptin, the product of the *ob* gene, discussed in the earlier section on Genetic Factors, reduces food intake and body weight in some animal models. Leptin is currently being investigated as an obesity treatment agent.

WHY IS IT DIFFICULT TO MAINTAIN A REDUCED BODY WEIGHT?

Is the difficulty of maintaining a reduced body weight a problem with behavior or with physiology? The two most frequently suggested metabolic changes that occur with weight loss and that may predispose to weight regain are a decrease in energy expenditure and a decrease in daily fat oxidation.

A lower body weight is associated with lower energy requirements. If the level of physical activity does not change, all components of energy expenditure will decline with weight loss. The body mass lost by energy restriction consists of approximately 60% to 70% fat and 30% to 40% FFM. Any decline in FFM would be expected to produce a reduction in resting metabolic rate (RMR). Weight reduction involving energy restriction would also produce a decline in the thermic effect of food (TEF). Finally, as body mass declines, the energy cost of weight-bearing physical activity would decline. The declines in TEF and the energy cost of physical activity would be small in relation to the change in RMR.

A major question is whether the reductions in energy expenditure that occur with weight loss leave the reduced obese person with a lower level of energy expenditure than would be expected from the new body mass. Some investigators have found this to be the case and suggest that this helps explain the high rate of relapse in the reduced obese individual. Not all investigators have found the reduced-obese persons to have lower energy requirements than expected from their body mass. Although there is debate about whether energy requirements of the reduced obese are lower than expected, it is clear that total energy expenditure declines with weight loss (assuming voluntary physical activity is constant). To maintain a reduced body weight, the obese-reduced individual must reduce energy intake and/or increase physical activity compared with baseline levels. Inability to make these permanent changes in lifestyle likely contributes to the high rate of weight regain. Again, gene × environment interactions are likely to be important, with some individuals probably showing greater declines in energy expenditure with weight loss than others. Those with greater declines in energy expenditure would be at higher risk for weight regain because they would be required to make and sustain greater lifestyle changes in order to maintain their reduced body weights.

Some investigators have reported that weight loss in obese individuals is associated with a reduced ability to oxidize fat. When compared with never-obese subjects consuming a similar diet, reduced-obese subjects oxidize less fat over 24 hours. It has been suggested that this reduced ability to oxidize fat may involve reduced sympathetic nervous system activity. A reduced ability to oxidize fat may be a predisposing factor in body fat gain, because any ingested fat that is not oxidized is stored as body fat. At present, fat oxidation has been studied in only a very few reduced-obese subjects. Whether this is a widespread characteristic of reduced-obese subjects and whether a low rate of fat oxidation contributes either to development of obesity or to an inability to maintain a weight reduction awaits further research.

The changes in energy expenditure and substrate oxidation that accompany weight loss make it essential to make permanent changes in lifestyle (e.g., diet and physical activity) in order to maintain a weight loss. Much of the poor success in weight maintenance could simply be because it is difficult for people to make permanent changes in behaviors that have been present for long periods of time. In support of this idea, when children and parents lose weight together, children are more successful in maintaining weight losses over time than their parents. This may be because it is easier for children to make and maintain the necessary lifestyle changes, having not practiced the predisposing lifestyle behaviors for as long a period as adults have.

■ Starvation

In contrast to obesity, starvation can be induced by a reduction in energy intake leading to a decrease in body weight. An adequate energy intake is especially important in children in order to maintain a satisfactory growth rate. Reduced dietary intake leads to declines in growth velocity in the child and reductions in body weight in the adult. When compared with normal individuals of the same stature, age, and gender, undernourished subjects have a reduced lean body mass as well as less fat, whereas the obese have an increase in both.

The response to starvation can best be understood as a protective mechanism in which the body attempts to maintain energy balance and avoid loss of body mass. When energy intake is low, the body relies on endogenous fuel sources, which are mainly adipose tissue triacylglycerols and skeletal muscle proteins. The primary metabolic signals touching off these events are a fall in the plasma level of insulin and an increase in the concentration of glucagon, caused by limited intake of dietary carbohydrate and thus a low plasma glucose concentration. Hypoinsulinemia facilitates mobilization of free fatty acids, starvation ketosis, and net catabolism of skeletal muscle protein to maintain visceral protein synthesis.

OCCURRENCE, DEFINITION, AND HISTORICAL PERSPECTIVE

Lusk in 1928 defined starvation as the deprivation of any element necessary for an organism's nutrition. The term now usually refers to a chronic, inadequate intake of dietary energy, protein, or both. Adaptation to such a low-calorie diet typically includes a decrease in physical activity and a decrease in RMR. When these decreases do not lower the energy output sufficiently to bring energy expenditure into balance with the limited intake, endogenous fuels must be used to balance the equation, resulting in a net loss of body energy stores.

Starvation affects many populations all over the world. It is known that severe food shortages in poor, underdeveloped countries have led to international reports of overwhelming famine and starvation. Starvation can also occur in susceptible elderly populations that do not receive proper nutrition and in some individuals who are hospitalized for long periods of time. These latter populations are susceptible to starvation due to the inability to eat or to the substantial increase in energy expenditure that results from severe trauma or infection.

EFFECTS ON ENERGY BALANCE, FUEL METABOLISM, AND BODY COMPOSITION

Fat is the major storage fuel of animals, and in fasting, the body fat supply appears to determine the length of survival. The survival of a nonobese fasting individual coincides roughly with the predicted time of depletion of fat, approximately 60 days; an obese individual obviously has a greater supply of fat stores. In contrast, carbohydrate is a quantitatively insignificant storage fuel. Although the amount of glycogen in the body is much less than that of fat, glycogen is a rapidly mobilizable energy source that has a rapid turnover rate. Glycogen or glucose can be anaerobically metabolized to lactate, and it is the obligatory fuel for parts of the brain, the red blood cells, and the renal medulla. Protein catabolism provides amino acids that can be used as a fuel and for gluconeogenesis. In contrast to the depletion of fat or glycogen stores, depletion of protein stores causes functional consequences because proteins are particularly important in the structural composition of all cells of the body.

ADAPTATION TO PROLONGED STARVATION

The essential features of the metabolic response to starvation are altered rates and patterns of fuel utilization and protein metabolism, aimed at minimizing fuel needs and limiting lean tissue loss. The nature of the starvation diet determines the pattern of hormone levels and fuel consumption. In total fasting, fat oxidation dominates in a metabolic setting of low insulin levels and ketosis. Fuel utilization by the brain, kidney, and muscle is markedly altered in total fasting. The brain switches from exclusively glucose to predominantly ketone body oxidation. The fuel of resting muscle switches from predominantly fatty acids to ketone bodies, finally returning, after weeks of total fasting, to fatty acid oxidation again. The metabolic acidosis of prolonged fasting induces a compensatory increase in renal production of ammonia in order to increase removal of hydrogen ions from the body as ammonium. This change is associated with augmented renal gluconeogenesis and a somewhat greater loss of body nitrogen than would occur without the acidosis.

Despite the important influence of lack of dietary carbohydrate and of hormone responses on fuel consumption patterns, starvation diets produce an alteration of overall protein metabolism that is characterized by an initial rapid loss of body protein, followed by a prolonged period during which further protein losses are minimized to protect lean body mass. This is associated with a slowed rate of synthesis and breakdown of body protein.

■ Protein Energy Malnutrition

Loss of body energy stores and loss of protein mass are the cardinal features of the group of syndromes collectively referred to as protein energy malnutrition, or PEM. The primary cellular role of protein is to create the functionally active matter of metabolizing cells: enzymes, contractile fibers, and the thousands of other constituents of protoplasm. During periods of negative energy balance, endogenous sources of energy are consumed to provide fuel for metabolic reactions. As the body is depleted of glycogen, fat, and protein, body weight declines and loss of protein-related cellular functions occurs.

Protein deficiency may be due to absolute lack of protein, lack of sufficiently complete protein, and/or imbalance of carbohydrate with protein. Dietary energy and protein deficiencies usually occur together, but sometimes one predominates and, if severe enough, may lead to the clinical syndrome of kwashiorkor (predominantly protein deficiency) or marasmus (mainly energy deficiency). Marasmus is commonly referred to as starvation. Marasmic kwashiorkor is a combination of chronic energy deficiency and chronic or acute protein deficit. Frequently this condition is associated with deficiencies in mineral and vitamin concentrations within the body.

The origin of PEM can be primary, when it is the result of inadequate food intake, or secondary, when it is the result of other diseases that lead to low food ingestion, inadequate nutrient absorption or utilization, increased nutritional requirements, and/or increased nutrient losses. The term malnutrition is usually used in lay language for protein energy malnutrition. PEM is the most important nutritional disease in the developing countries because of its high prevalence and its relationship with child mortality rates, impaired physical growth, and inadequate social and economic development. It is estimated that a half-billion people in the world are impaired due to present or previous periods of PEM. Maternal malnutrition prior to and/or during pregnancy is more likely to produce an underweight newborn baby. This intrauterine malnutrition can be compounded after birth or after weaning by insufficient food to satisfy the infant's needs for catch-up growth, resulting in PEM. In industrialized countries, many weight loss diets and food fads can predispose people to, or actually produce, some degree of PEM.

EFFECTS ON ENERGY BALANCE, FUEL METABOLISM, AND BODY COMPOSITION

Protein energy malnutrition develops gradually over many days or months. This process allows a series of metabolic and behavioral adjustments that result in decreased nutrient demands and alterations in fuel metabolism and body composition, similar to those seen in starvation. Although undernutrition retards growth in all parts of the body, some parts are affected more than others. In severe undernutrition, adipocytes become unrecognizable as cells, the empty space between cells fills with an extracellular gel, and muscle fibers shrink. There is less change in the composition of the

kidneys and heart, and the brain is the least affected.

As the cumulative energy deficit becomes more severe, subcutaneous fat is markedly reduced, and protein catabolism leads to muscular wasting. Visceral protein is preserved longer, especially in the marasmic patient.

ADAPTATION TO CHRONIC UNDERNUTRITION

In marasmus, there is usually an increase in basal oxygen consumption, which then declines as the disease becomes more severe. In kwashiorkor, the severe dietary protein deficit leads to an earlier visceral depletion of amino acids that affects visceral cell function and reduces oxygen consumption, Thus in individuals with kwashiorkor, RMR decreases per unit of lean or total body mass.

Blood glucose concentration usually remains normal, mainly at the expense of gluconeogenic amino acids, but it falls in severe PEM or when complications arise from serious infections due to fasting. The latter change in severe PEM is not so much a reduction of total nitrogen or amino acid turnover but an increase in the proportion of the amino acid pool that is used for resynthesis of protein and a corresponding reduction in the proportion of amino acids that are catabolized with nitrogen excretion and gluconeogenesis.

LONG-TERM EFFECTS OF PROTEIN ENERGY MALNUTRITION

The gradual and inevitable loss of body protein as a result of a long-term dietary protein deficit is primarily a loss of skeletal muscle protein. Some visceral protein is lost in the early development of PEM, but then the amount of visceral protein becomes stable until the nonessential tissue proteins are depleted. Once these less critical tissues are depleted, the loss of visceral protein increases; at this point death may be imminent unless nutritional therapy is successfully instituted.

In adults, mild to moderate PEM results in leanness, with reduction in subcutaneous tissue. The most common change in body composition is a reduction of adiposity below the average 12% and 20% expected in normal, well-nourished men and women, respectively. If undernutrition is imposed early in life, when growth is at its most rapid, then complete recovery in size (height and weight) may never be possible, even though the undernutrition is temporary and plentiful food is supplied thereafter.

REFERENCES

Bouchard, C. and Pérusse L. (1993) Genetics of obesity. Annu. Rev Nutr 13:337–354.

Colditz, G. A., Willett, W. C., Rotnitzky, A. and Manson, J. E. (1995) Weight gain as a risk factor for clinical diabetes mellitus in women. Ann Intern Med 122:481–486.

Despres, J.-P. (1993) Abdominal obesity as an important component of insulin-resistance syndrome. Nutrition 9:452–459.

Despres, J.-P., Nadeau, A., Tremblay, A., Ferland, M., Morrjani, S., Lupien, P. J., Therlault, G., Pinault, S. and Bouchard, C. (1989) Role of deep abdominal fat in the association between regional adipose tissue distribution and glucose tolerance in obese women. Diabetes 38:304–309.

Flegal, K. M., Carroll, M. D., Kuczmarski, R. J. and Johnson, C. L. (1998) Overweight and obesity in the United States: Prevalence and trends, 1960–1994. Int J Obesity 22:39–47.

Goldstein, D. J. (1992) Beneficial health effects of modest weight loss. Int J Obes 16:397–415.

Gortmaker, S. L., Must, A., Perrin, J. M., Sobol, A. M. and Dietz, W. H. (1993) Social and economic consequences of overweight in adolescence and young adulthood. N Engl J Med 329:1036–1037.

Havel, P. J., Kasim-Karakas, S., Mueller, W., Johnson, P. R., Gingerich, R. L. and Stern, J. S. (1996) Relationship of plasma leptin to plasma insulin and adiposity in normal weight and overweight women: Effects of dietary fat content and sustained weight loss. J Clin Endocrinol Metab 81:4406–4413.

Horton, T. J., Drougas, H., Brachey, A., Reed, G. W., Peters, J. C and Hill, J. O. (1995) Fat and carbohydrate overfeeding in humans: Different effects on energy storage. Am J Clin Nutr 62:19–29.

Pagliassotti, M. J., Gayles, E. C. and Hill, J. O. (1997) Fat and energy balance. Ann N Y Acad Sci 827:431–448.

Pi-Sunyer, F. X. (1993) Medical hazards of obesity. Ann Intern Med 119:655–660.

Pouliot, M.-C., Despres, J.-P., Lemieux, S., Moorjani, S., Bouchard, C., Tremblay, A., Nadeau, A. and Lupien, P. J. (1994) Waist circumference and abdominal sagittal diameter: Best simple anthropometric indexes of abdominal visceral adipose tissue accumulation and related cardiovascular risk in men and women. Am J Cardiol 73:460–468.

Sugerman, H. J. (1993) Surgery for morbid obesity. Surgery 114:865–867.

Troiano, R. P., Flegal, K. M., Kuczmarski, R. J., Campbell, S. M. and Johnson, C. L. (1995) Overweight prevalence and trends for children and adolescents. Arch Pediatr Adolesc Med 149:1085–1091.

U.S. Department of Agriculture and U.S. Department of Health and Human Services. Dietary Guidelines for Americans, 4th ed. Washington, D.C., 1995.

World Health Organization (1997) Obesity: Preventing and Managing the Global Epidemic. Report of a WHO Consultation on Obesity. Geneva, June 3–5, 1997.

Zamboni, M., Armellini, F., Turcato, E., de Pergola, G., Todesco, T., Bissoli, L., Bergamo Andreis, I. A. and Bosello, O. (1994) Relationship between visceral fat, steroid hormones and insulin sensitivity in premenopausal obese women. J Intern Med 236:521–527.

Zavaroni, I., Bonini, L., Fantuzzi, M., Dall'aglio, E., Passeri, M. and Reaven, G. M. (1994) Hyperinsulinaemia, obesity, and syndrome X. J Intern Med 235:51–56.

RECOMMENDED READINGS

Kuczmarski, R. J., Flegal, K. M., Campbell, S. M. and Johnson, C. L. (1994) Increasing prevalence of overweight among US adults. JAMA 272:205–211.

Pi-Sunyer, F. X. (1993) Medical hazards of obesity. Ann Intern Med 119:655–660.

World Health Organization (1997) Obesity: Preventing and Managing the Global Epidemic. Report of a WHO Consultation on Obesity. Geneva, June 3–5, 1997.

The Vitamins

◆◆◆◆◆◆◆◆◆◆◆◆◆◆◆◆◆◆◆◆◆◆◆◆◆◆◆◆◆◆

Vitamins are defined as organic compounds that are required in the diet in only small amounts to maintain fundamental functions of the body (growth, metabolism, cellular integrity). This definition distinguishes vitamins from the organic macronutrients because vitamins are not catabolized to CO_2 and H_2O to satisfy part of the energy requirement and are not used for structural purposes; hence, vitamins are required in much smaller amounts than are carbohydrates, proteins, and triacylglycerols. Vitamins are distinguished from the minerals (which also are required in relatively small amounts compared with nutrients used as sources of energy) by their organic rather than inorganic nature.

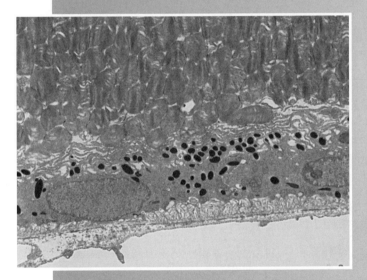

Well before the 20th century, the curative effects of certain foods were recognized. An ancient Egyptian medical treatise recommended eating roast ox liver or black cock's liver to cure night blindness. Early reports indicate that writings as far back as 1500 B.C. record the fact that consumption of liver cured night blindness. It has been known for nearly three centuries that scurvy can be controlled by dietary means. In 1747, Lind, a British physician, hypothesized that various "acidic principles" might have antiscorbutic properties. Lind tested his theory by feeding a variety of acidic substances to sailors suffering from scurvy. The treatments included two oranges or one lemon per day, and these citrus fruits had miraculous curative powers. As early as 1855, beriberi, which was a common affliction among Japanese sailors, was found to be prevented or cured by using meat, milk, and vegetables to supplement the regular polished rice diet of Japanese seamen.

It was during the 20th century, however, that the vitamins were isolated, identified, and chemically synthesized. The first of these essential dietary factors to be isolated and chemically identified was the anti-beriberi substance, which was

Electron Micrograph courtesy of Dr. Joe E. Hollyfield, Cleveland Clinic Foundation, Cleveland, Ohio.

isolated from rice polishings by Funk, a Polish biochemist who was working at the Lister Institute in London. Funk called this factor "vitamine" based on evidence that it was an "amine" that was "vital" for life. In 1912, Funk extended the use of this term and the "vitamine theory" to include those other trace dietary essentials that were missing in individuals with rickets, scurvy, and pellagra as well as in those with beriberi. The name "vitamine" was changed to "vitamin" later as the structures of additional essential organic factors were discovered and it became clear that most were not amines.

The first major subdivision of the vitamins stems from such work as was done by Stepp in Germany, McCollum and Davis at the University of Wisconsin, and Osborne and Mendel at Yale University. Using different solvents to extract growth factors from foods, these investigators found one could separate "fat-soluble" and "water-soluble" factors. Around 1915, McCollum and Davis demonstrated a need for a fat-soluble factor "A" present in butterfat and egg yolk and a heat-labile, water-soluble factor "B" present in wheat germ for growth of young rats. The latter was found to cure beriberi. Ensuing efforts from a number of laboratories led to specific identification of the fat-soluble vitamins as belonging to groups now called A, D, E, and K. Other workers who concentrated on the effects of water-soluble vitamins came to realize that the factor that Holst and Frolick in Oslo had shown in 1907 to be required for guinea pigs to avoid a scurvy-like condition was the antiscorbutic activity associated with lemon juice. Zilva and others at the Lister Institute termed this factor vitamin C. In the search for factors that would prevent beriberi as well as pellagra, it became apparent that "water-soluble B" was not a single substance, as pointed out by Goldberger in the 1920s. The successive efforts of numerous investigators were required to unravel the "B complex." Most of the activity toward the certain identification of the individual B vitamins spanned about 25 years, from the isolation of B_1 (thiamin) in 1926 to the structure determination of B_{12} (cyanocobalamin) in 1955. The chemical synthesis of cyanocobalamin was not accomplished until 1970.

The identification of vitamins over the course of the 20th century resulted in knowledge of 13 vitamins that are dietary essentials for humans. These include eight B vitamins (thiamin, niacin, riboflavin, folate, vitamin B_6, vitamin B_{12}, biotin, and pantothenic acid), vitamin C or ascorbic acid, and the fat-soluble vitamins A, D, E, and K. As vitamins were further characterized, it was found that the activity of a particular vitamin was often found in several closely related compounds known as vitamers. For example, vitamin B_6 is used to refer not only to pyridoxine (pyridoxol), but also to pyridoxal and pyridoxamine, and vitamin A is used to refer to retinol, retinal, and retinoic acid.

Also, as more has been learned about the vitamins, it has become clear that some of the vitamins are not strictly dietary essentials. Vitamin D is synthesized in the skin from an endogenous precursor (7-dehydrocholesterol) upon exposure to sunlight. Niacin-containing coenzymes, and subsequently niacin, are synthesized from the amino acid tryptophan.

Most vitamins are not related chemically, and they differ in their biochemical/physiological roles. The historical water-soluble and fat-soluble classification distinguishes vitamins by their physical solubility in solvents, and this classification also broadly separates the vitamins by some of the types of processes involved in their digestion, absorption, and transport, as well as by some aspects of their functions.

The most common function of vitamins is as essential components of coenzymes. All of the B vitamins, vitamin C, and reduced vitamin K are required as coenzymes or as components of coenzymes that are synthesized from the vitamins. Coenzymes are defined as small, organic molecules that are required by an enzyme and that participate in the chemistry of catalysis. Most coenzymes shuttle back and forth between two (or more) different forms. Coenzymes include ascorbic acid, reduced vitamin K, biotin (covalently bound to enzyme), nicotinamide adenine dinucleotide (NAD) and nicotinamide adenine dinucleotide phosphate (NADP) (niacin-containing), flavin adenine dinucleotide (FAD) and flavin mononucleotide (FMN) (riboflavin-containing), thiamin pyrophosphate, several folate coenzymes, methyl-B_{12} and deoxyadenosyl-B_{12} pyridoxal phosphate and pyridoxamine phosphate (vitamin B_6 coenzymes), and coenzyme A and enzyme-bound 4'-phosphopantetheine (derivatives of pantothenic acid). These coenzymes may be covalently attached to the enzyme protein (biotin, FAD in a few cases, and 4'-phosphopantetheine), tightly associated with specific apoenzymes to form the active holoenzyme (FAD and FMN, B_{12} coenzymes, most folate coenzymes, and B_6 coenzymes), or only weakly associated with their apoenzymes such that the cofactors behave in a manner similar to substrates (NAD and NADP, some folate coenzymes, coenzyme A, ascorbate, and reduced vitamin K). (It should be noted that not all coenzymes are formed from vitamins; for example, coenzyme Q, lipoic acid, dolichol phosphate, and biopterin are synthesized in the body.)

The other functions of vitamins are more varied. Two of the vitamins are required for synthesis of hormones: vitamin D is required for formation of 1,25-dihydroxyvitamin D, and vitamin A is required for formation of all-*trans*-retinoic acid. Vitamin A also acts as a visual pigment in the form of 11-*cis*-retinal. Vitamin E serves as a lipid-soluble antioxidant, and vitamin C also has antioxidant functions. The niacin-containing coenzyme NAD also serves as substrate for adenosine diphosphate (ADP)-ribosylation reactions.

In the following eight chapters, the vitamins are discussed. The details of coenzyme, hormone, and antioxidant function are discussed because these biochemical and physiological functions are the bases of the requirements for these vitamins, and clinical signs of deficiency result from impairment of these functions. Some of the B vitamins have been grouped because they play major roles in particular general areas of metabolism. Niacin, riboflavin, and thiamin are grouped together because these three vitamins play critical roles in the central pathways of metabolism of energy-yielding nutrients. Folate, vitamin B_{12}, and vitamin B_6 are grouped together because amino acids are important substrates for reactions that require the coenzymes formed from these vitamins. Biotin and pantothenic acid are covered in a single chapter because these two vitamins are intimately (but not exclusively) involved in lipid metabolism. Vitamin C, vitamin A, vitamin D, and vitamin E are covered in individual chapters because of their specialized functions in the body.

◆◆◆

Donald B. McCormick

Martha H. Stipanuk

CHAPTER 20

◆ ◆

Niacin, Riboflavin, and Thiamin

Donald B. McCormick, Ph.D.

OUTLINE

COMMON ABBREVIATIONS

FAD (flavin adenine dinucleotide)
FMN (flavin mononucleotide)
NAD (nicotinamide adenine dinucleotide)
NADP (nicotinamide adenine dinucleotide phosphate)
NaMN (nicotinate mononucleotide)
NMN (nicotinamide mononucleotide)
TPP (thiamin pyrophosphate; also called TDP, thiamin diphosphate)

◼ Niacin

Niacin (previously designated as vitamin B₃) is essential for formation of pyridine nucleotide coenzymes (nicotinamide adenine dinucleotide [NAD], nicotinamide adenine dinucleotide phosphate [NADP]) that function indispensably in oxidation-reduction reactions involved in the catabolism of glucose, fatty acids, ketone bodies, and amino acids. These coenzymes ultimately are coupled to electron-to-oxygen transfer systems, which are the terminal connections between energy-yielding metabolic events and molecular oxygen, and also are essential for reductive biosynthetic reactions. In addition, one of the coenzyme forms of niacin (NAD) also serves as the donor of adenosine diphosphate (ADP)-ribose moieties for ADP-ribosylation reactions. Niacin is the first of three B vitamins included in this chapter. The intimate involvement of the coenzymes formed from niacin, riboflavin, and thiamin in the intermediary metabolism of energy-yielding nutrients is the basis for grouping these three vitamins in a single chapter.

NIACIN AND PYRIDINE NUCLEOTIDE COENZYME STRUCTURE AND NOMENCLATURE

The term niacin is chemically synonymous with nicotinic acid (pyridine-3-carboxylic acid), which was prepared in 1867 by oxidation of nicotine, isolated in 1911 from rice polishings, and established in 1937 as a vitamin shown to cure black tongue in dogs. The word niacin now is used as the generic name for the specific compound, nicotinic acid or nicotinate, as well as for nicotinamide (pyridine-3-carboxamide or niacinamide). Because the amino acid tryptophan also may serve as a precursor for synthesis of pyridine nucleotide coenzymes, the term "niacin equivalent" (NE) is used for expression of niacin intakes and requirements. "Niacin activity" and "niacin deficiency" are used in the nutritional literature to refer collectively to nicotinic acid, nicotinamide, and NE from tryptophan. Structures for the two vitaminic forms are shown in Figure 20–1.

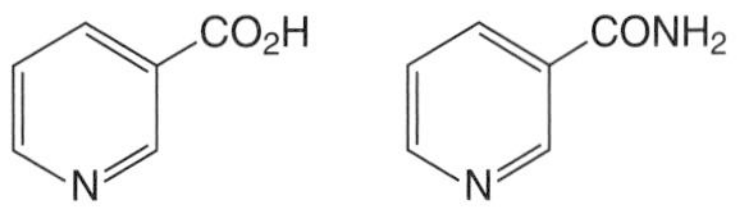

Figure 20–1. *Structures of nicotinic acid and nicotinamide.*

the operational forms derived from these vitamers are pyridine nucleotide coenzymes. Because nicotinamide is a common constituent, current nomenclature for the biologically oxidized forms are nicotinamide adenine dinucleotide (NAD) and nicotinamide adenine dinucleotide phosphate (NADP). NAD was originally known as coenzyme I (CoI) and then diphosphopyridine nucleotide (DPN); NADP was first coenzyme II (CoII), then triphosphopyridine nucleotide (TPN). Structures for the oxidized forms of the two pyridine nucleotide coenzymes are shown in Figure 20–2.

The naming of the biologically reduced forms of pyridine nucleotides, wherein the nicotinamide ring bears an additional hydrogen at position 4, as illustrated in Figure 20–3, has followed two conventions. Because these coenzymes require two equivalents of hydrogen for their reduction, one earlier system was to add the prefix "dihydro" to the written name and indicate such forms with the abbreviations NADH₂ and NADPH₂. Because neutral

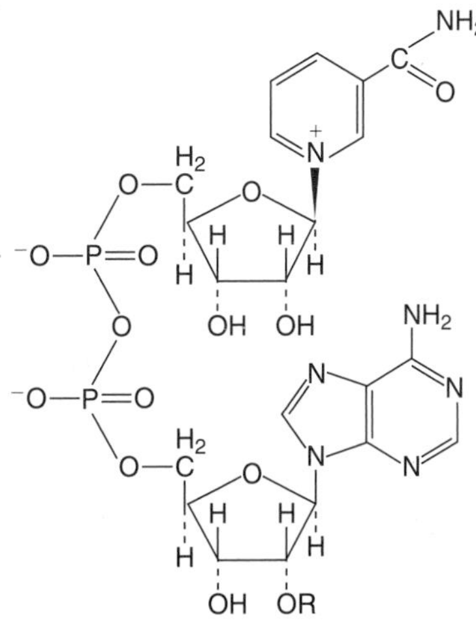

Figure 20–2. *Structures of oxidized pyridine nucleotide coenzymes: NAD⁺, R = H; NADP⁺, R = PO₃⁻².*

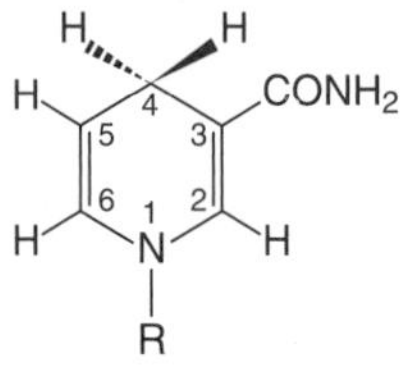

Figure 20–3. *Structure and numbering of the 1,4-dihy-dro-nicotinamide portion of reduced pyridine nucleotide coenzymes. R = ribofuranosyl diphosphoadenosine.*

solutions of these reduced compounds only have one hydrogen, which is abstracted as a hydride ion from substrates that additionally release the second hydrogen as a solvated proton, more appropriate abbreviations for reduced coenzymatic forms are NADH and NADPH. Additionally, the oxidized forms are conventionally indicated with a plus, i.e., NAD$^+$ and NADP$^+$, to reflect the charge on the quaternary pyridinium nitrogen, even though net charges on the coenzyme molecules in neutral or physiological solutions are negative because of pyrophosphoryl and phosphoryl ionizations (see Fig. 20–2). Hence, typical enzyme-catalyzed reactions, with a reduced substrate and an oxidized product, are written as:

Substrate + NAD(P)$^+$ ⇆

Product + NAD(P)H + H$^+$

SOURCES, DIGESTION, AND ABSORPTION

Niacin, predominantly in covalently bound forms, is widely distributed in foods of both plant and animal origin. Good sources of preformed niacin include meats, poultry, fish, legumes, peanuts, and some cereals. Enrichment of grain products with niacin makes enriched flours and grain products good sources as well. In uncooked foods of animal origin, the major forms of niacin are the cellular pyridine nucleotides, NAD(H) and NADP(H). Although these are relatively stable to heat, some niacin undoubtedly is released during food processing by action of tissue pyrophosphatases, phosphatases, and glycohydrolases. In uncooked foods of plant origin, there are even more diverse forms of bound

niacin. Much of the niacin in cereals (largely in the bran) is not readily biologically available because it is esterified to complex carbohydrate (niacin) and to a lesser extent to peptides (niacinogens). Pretreatment of corn with lime water (i.e., calcium hydroxide), as in the traditional preparation of tortillas in Mexico and Central America, releases much of the bound nicotinic acid. Roasting of green coffee beans converts some of the trigonelline (1-methyl nicotinic acid) to nicotinic acid. A portion of the L-tryptophan in proteins can be metabolized in some species (e.g., rats and humans) to produce nicotinic acid mononucleotide (NaMN), an intermediate in the pathway for synthesis of functional pyridine coenzymes from nicotinate, as shown in Figure 20–4.

Recommended Dietary Allowances (RDAs) or Adequate Intakes (AIs) for niacin now are given in terms of NE to include estimates of direct and indirect sources of the vitamin (Institute of Medicine, 1998). An estimated average conversion factor of 60 mg tryptophan to yield 1 mg niacin is used to calculate NE available from tryptophan. Hence, 1 NE is provided by 1 mg of nicotinate, 1 mg of nicotinamide, or 60 mg of tryptophan. The tryptophan content of proteins averages about 1%, and a diet for humans in excess of 100 g protein per day presumably could provide 16 mg NE and meet the RDA without inclusion of preformed niacin.

The major pathway for tryptophan catabolism after 3-hydroxykynurenine results in formation of CO_2 and H_2O, rather than quinolinate or NaMN, so humans convert only about 2.75% of the amino acid to NaMN. At the level of α-amino-β-carboxymuconic ε-semialdehyde, a divergent reaction catalyzed by picolinic carboxylase leads to formation of 2-aminomuconic semialdehyde, which undergoes cyclization to picolinate (2-carboxypyridine). The activity of this so-called carboxylase is relatively high in some animals, such as cats, which are dependent on preformed niacin in their diets. Picolinate carboxylase activity has been shown to be elevated with an induced diabetic state in some species such that the efficiency of conversion of tryptophan to NaMN and subsequently to NAD is impaired. Some steroid hormones (glucocorticoids and

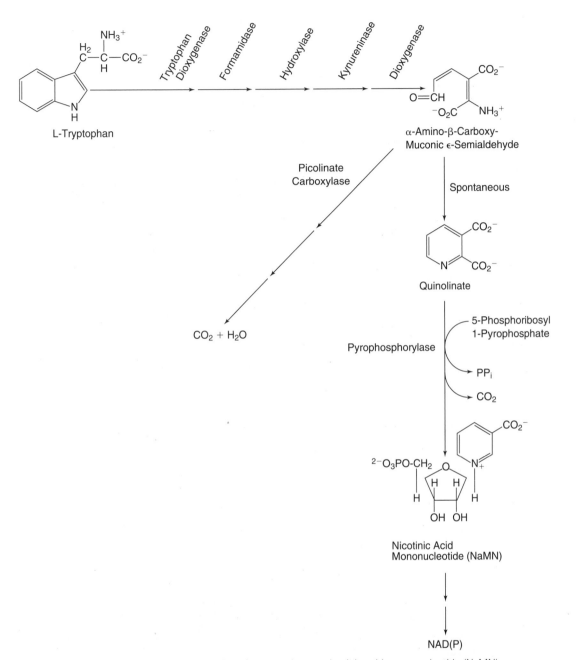

Figure 20–4. *Metabolic conversion of L-tryptophan to nicotinic acid mononucleotide (NaMN).*

estrogens) elevate tryptophan dioxygenase and may increase the yield of pyridine coenzymes (Knox and Piras, 1967). Sensitivity of the pathway to the status of micronutrients, especially B_6, riboflavin, Fe^{2+}, and perhaps Cu^{2+}, relates to their cofactor roles with certain of the enzymes for tryptophan catabolism. (See Chapter 11 for more discussion of tryptophan metabolism.)

The coenzyme forms of niacin in the gastrointestinal tract are rapidly hydrolyzed to nicotinamide mononucleotide (NMN) by nonspecific pyrophosphatases in the intestinal lumen (Gross and Henderson, 1983). Alkaline phosphatase catalyzes further cleavage to nicotinamide riboside, from which nicotinamide slowly is released. Additionally, NAD glycohydrolase (NADase) within mucosal cells may

Food Sources of Preformed Niacin

- Meat, poultry, and fish
- Peanuts
- Enriched grain products

RDAs Across the Life Cycle
(1 Niacin Equivalent [NE] = 1 mg niacin or 60 mg tryptophan)

	mg NE/day
Infants, 0–5 mo	2 (AI)
6–11 mo	3 (AI)
Children, 1–3 yr	6
4–8 yr	8
9–13 yr	12
Males, >13 yr	16
Females, >13 yr	14
Pregnant	18
Lactating	17

Enriched grain products contain fully available free niacin, but much of the naturally occurring niacin in cereals is bound and as little as 30% may be available. In addition to foods that contain preformed niacin, all sources of protein are sources of NE. On average, 1 g of dietary protein provides 10 mg tryptophan or 0.17 mg NE. Normally, tryptophan is more important than preformed niacin in meeting requirements for NE.

From Institute of Medicine. (1998) Dietary Reference Intakes for Thiamin, Riboflavin, Niacin, Vitamin B_6, Folate, Vitamin B_{12}, Pantothenic Acid, Biotin, and Choline. National Academy Press, Washington, D.C.

NUTRITION INSIGHT

Enrichment of Grain Products with B Vitamins

Milling of grains results in loss of vitamins and minerals, which are concentrated in the outer layers of the kernels (bran and aleuerone layer) and in the germ. Beginning in the early 1940s, the American government established standards for enrichment of flour and other grain products. These standards are targeted at restoring the levels of thiamin, riboflavin, niacin, and iron to the levels found in whole-grain products. For example, the standards for enrichment of flour are 2.9 mg thiamin, 1.8 mg riboflavin, 24.0 mg niacin, and 20 mg iron per pound of flour. Beginning in 1998, enriched-grain products also have been fortified with folate. Hence, products labeled "enriched" are good sources of these four vitamins and iron. Whole-grain products are good sources of these nutrients as well as a number of other vitamins and minerals, which also are lost in milling but are not added as part of the enrichment program.

contribute to the breakdown of the coenzymes to nicotinamide.

Both nicotinic acid and its amide are absorbed from the small intestine by a sodium (Na^+)-dependent saturable process as well as by passive diffusion that continues to increase at higher nonphysiological concentrations (Bechgaard and Jespersen, 1977). Absorption of nicotinic acid also occurs by passive diffusion in the stomach.

TRANSPORT AND CONVERSION OF NIACIN TO COENZYMES

Facilitated and simple diffusion of niacin followed by formation and metabolic trapping of the nucleotides accounts for uptake of niacin from plasma by tissues. The facilitated diffusion of niacin into erythrocytes involves an anion transport protein as carrier. Both red cells and liver rapidly remove and convert niacin to NAD by the biosynthetic (Preiss-Handler) pathway. Intracellular NAD glycohydrolases then release nicotinamide, which circulates to other tissues as precursor to pyridine nucleotide coenzymes.

Pyridine nucleotide formation from nicotinate and nicotinamide occurs widely in tissues, as summarized in Figure 20–5. The Preiss-Handler pathway involves a phosphoribosyl transferase–catalyzed conversion of nicotinate and phosphoribosylpyrophosphate (PRPP) to nicotinate mononucleotide (NaMN) with release of pyrophosphate. NaMN also arises from tryptophan metabolism via quinolinate, which undergoes decarboxylation during the phosphoribosyl transferase reaction. NaMN is adenylylated to form dea-

mido-NAD in an ATP-requiring reaction catalyzed by NAD pyrophosphorylase. The conversion of the deamido intermediate to NAD is accomplished by an ATP-requiring NAD synthetase reaction in which the amide of glutamine is transferred to NaMN. Although nicotinamidase catalyzes hydrolysis of some nicotinamide to nicotinate that can be reutilized for NAD synthesis by the Preiss-Handler pathway, nicotinamide also is used directly for NAD synthesis. The Dietrich pathway couples PRPP with nicotinamide to form NMN, which with ATP directly forms NAD. Some NAD is phosphorylated by ATP and a kinase to form NADP.

NAD is turned over to regenerate nicotinamide and release the adenosine diphosphoribose (ADP-ribose) moiety in reactions catalyzed by glycohydrolases or ADP-ribosyl transferases. NAD glycohydrolases responsible for this can use water in simple hydrolysis, or they can transfer the ADP-ribose to another base. ADP-ribosyl transferases can add the ADPR moiety to specific protein bases. The poly-ADP-ribosylations that are catalyzed by poly(ADP-ribose) polymerase (synthetase) may account for the relatively rapid turnover of NAD in human cells (Rechsteiner et al., 1976).

NIACIN CATABOLISM AND EXCRETION

There is little loss of niacin into urine when intake is modest, because both vitamers are actively reabsorbed from glomerular filtrates. Rather, several metabolites that are formed enzymatically, primarily in liver, appear in urine. The N^1-methyl derivatives result primar-

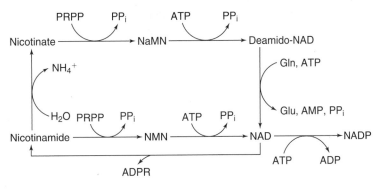

Figure 20–5. Interconnections of vitaminic and coenzymatic forms of niacin. Glu, glutamate; Gln, glutamine; NaMN, nicotinate mononucleotide; NAD(P), nicotinamide adenine dinucleotide (phosphate); PP$_i$, inorganic pyrophosphate; PRPP, phosphoribosyl pyrophosphate.

ily from *S*-adenosylmethionine-dependent *N*-methyltransferase activity, but some N^1-methyl nicotinate also arises from food and bacterial methylation of niacytin (esterified nicotinic acid). The 2- and 4-pyridone oxidation products of N^1-methylnicotinamide arise from the action of aldehyde oxidase. Their quantities vary with species, as do such oxidation products as the *N*-oxide and 6-hydroxy compounds (Mrochek et al., 1976; McCreanor and Bender, 1986). Conjugation of nicotinic acid with glycine to form nicotinuric acid becomes increasingly significant as the quantity of nicotinic acid ingested increases toward pharmacological levels.

FUNCTIONS OF PYRIDINE NUCLEOTIDE COENZYMES IN METABOLISM

The pyridine nucleotide coenzymes function in numerous oxidoreductase systems, usually of the dehydrogenase/reductase type, which include such diverse reactions as the conversion of alcohols (often sugars and polyols) to aldehydes or ketones, hemiacetals to lactones, aldehydes to acids, and certain amino acids to keto acids. The common mechanism of operation (generalized in Figure 20–6) involves the stereospecific abstraction of a hydride ion (H^-) from the substrate, with *para* addition to one (A) or the other (B) side of carbon 4 in the pyridine ring of the nucleotide coenzyme (Creighton and Murthy, 1990). The second hydrogen of the substrate group oxidized is concomitantly removed as a proton (H^+), which in solution exists as the hydronium ion.

Most dehydrogenases using NAD or NADP function reversibly. Glutamate dehydrogenase, for example, favors the oxidative direction, whereas others, such as glutathione reductase, catalyze preferential reduction. A

further generality is that most NAD-dependent enzymes are involved in catabolic reactions, whereas NADP-dependent systems are more common to biosynthetic reactions. For example, NAD-dependent enzymes (e.g., 3-hydroxyacyl CoA dehydrogenase, 3-hydroxybutyrate dehydrogenase, glyceraldehyde 3-phosphate dehydrogenase, and branched-chain keto acid dehydrogenase) catalyze steps in the β-oxidation of fatty acyl CoAs, the oxidation of ketone bodies, the degradation of carbohydrates, and the catabolism of amino acids. NADPH serves as an important reducing agent for the synthesis of fats and steroids (e.g., reactions catalyzed by 3-ketoacyl reductase, enoyl reductase, and HMG CoA reductase). See Chapters 9, 11, and 13 for more examples of NAD- and NADP-dependent reactions in carbohydrate, amino acid, and lipid metabolism.

For the pyridine nucleotide coenzymes to continue to react catalytically, they must cycle by coupling with oxidation-reduction sequences. This may occur by coupling dehydrogenation reactions with hydrogenation reactions (i.e., the coupling of glyceraldehyde 3-phosphate dehydrogenase and lactate dehydrogenase in anaerobic glycolysis or the coupling of NADPH production by the pentose phosphate pathway [hexose monophosphate shunt] with fatty acid synthesis) or by coupling the dehydrogenation reactions with electron transport as found in mitochondria.

Both NAD and NADP serve as parts of the intracellular respiratory mechanism of all cells; they assist in the stepwise transfer of electrons or reducing equivalents from various energy substrates to the cytochromes, which in turn transfer the electrons (and H^+) to oxygen to form water. Reduced NAD (NADH) usually donates its electrons to a flavin coenzyme in the mitochondrial electron transport chain responsible for ATP production. These reactions are outlined in Figure 20–7. The role

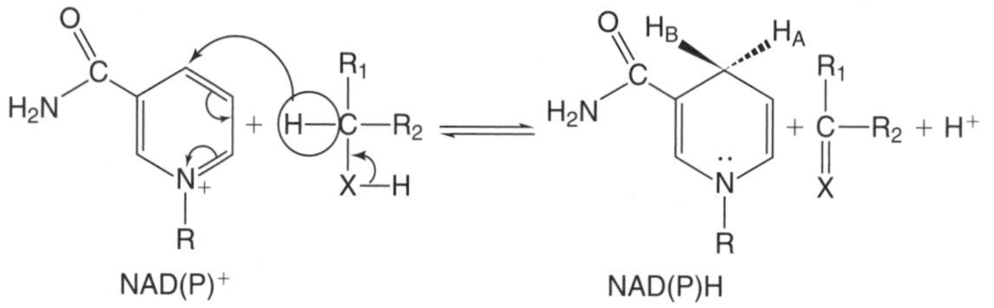

NAD(P)⁺   NAD(P)H

Figure 20–6. *Mechanism for substrate oxidation by pyridine nucleotide coenzymes. Typically, X is an electronegative atom, e.g., oxygen, and the subscript A and B on prochiral hydrogens reflect stereospecificity.*

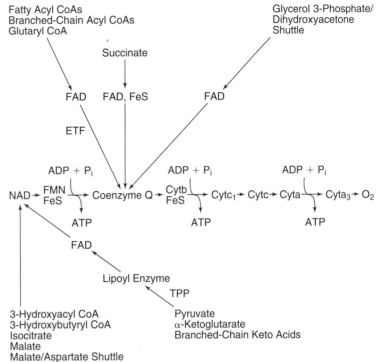

Figure 20–7. Role of pyridine nucleotides and flavocoenzymes in the funneling of reducing equivalents to the mitochondrial respiratory chain. Major sources of reducing equivalents generated in the mitochondria are shown. The main extramitochondrial source is NADH formed in glycolysis; these reducing equivalents are carried into the mitochondria by the malate-aspartate or the glycerol phosphate-dihydroxyacetone shuttles. Cyt, cytochrome; ETF, electron transfer flavoprotein; FAD, flavin adenine dinucleotide; FeS, iron-sulfur protein; FMN, flavin mononucleotide; TPP, thiamin pyrophosphate.

of NADPH and cytochrome P450 in the hydroxylation of steroids (for biosynthesis of steroid hormones from cholesterol) is illustrated in Figure 20–8. Cytochrome P450 hydroxylase

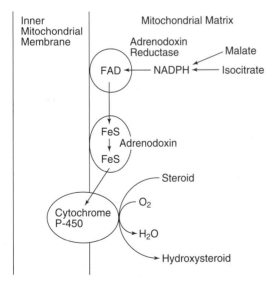

Figure 20–8. Mitochondrial cytochrome P450 monoxygenase system. FeS, iron-sulfur protein (adrenodoxin). Note that because NADP(H) cannot penetrate the mitochondrial membrane, sources of reducing equivalents are confined to substrates such as malate and isocitrate for which there are intramitochondrial NADP-specific dehydrogenases. FAD, flavin adenine dinucleotide.

(monooxygenase) systems also exist in the endoplasmic reticulum (ER) of cells. These monooxygenase systems in the ER use reducing equivalents of NADH and NADPH and are involved in metabolism of drugs such as phenobarbital. (See Chapter 40 for more discussion of detoxification systems.)

Because NAD and NADP do not cross the inner mitochondrial membrane, the cytosolic and mitochondrial pools do not mix. However, tissues that have mitochondria have systems capable of "shuttling" reducing equivalents across the inner mitochondrial membrane from the cytosol to the mitochondrial compartment. Reducing equivalents (NADH) formed during oxidative metabolism in the cytosol are carried into the mitochondria by the glycerol phosphate and malate-aspartate shuttles. Additionally, reducing equivalents may be carried out of the mitochondria during periods of active fatty acid biosynthesis (via citrate, which can be dehydrogenated by cytosolic NADP-linked isocitrate dehydrogenase to generate NADPH) or during active gluconeogenesis (via aspartate, which is converted to fumarate via the urea cycle, to malate by cytosolic fumarase, and then to oxaloacetate by NAD-dependent malate dehydrogenase, generating NADH). The sequential actions of cytosolic citrate lyase, NAD-dependent malate dehydrogenase, and NADP-dependent malic enzyme convert cytosolic NADH to cytosolic NADPH for use in lipid synthesis.

NONCOENZYMATIC FUNCTIONS OF NIACIN

Nicotinamide coenzymes also participate in other (nonredox) biological reactions that involve ADP-ribosylations. In these reactions, NAD serves as a substrate rather than as a coenzyme. The ADP-ribose moiety of NAD is transferred to the acceptor molecule, and free nicotinamide is released. In mammals, poly-ADP-ribosylated proteins appear to function in DNA repair, DNA replication, and cell differentiation. Increased activity of poly(ADP-ribose) polymerase in mammalian cells appears to be a response to DNA fragmentation in the nucleus (increased excision-repair activity in response to DNA-damaging agents) (Schraufstatter et al., 1986; Junod et al., 1989). This enzyme adds mostly mono(ADP-ribose) to chromatin proteins, but also it can add homopolymeric chains of ADP-ribose. The activity of poly(ADP-ribose) polymerase is sufficiently large to cause a depletion of intracellular NAD following environmentally induced DNA damage.

Nicotinic acid has been suggested to be a structural component of a biologically active form of chromium, called the glucose tolerance factor, that exhibits an insulin-potentiating effect by increasing glucose tolerance. (See Chapter 36 for more discussion of glucose tolerance factor.)

Pharmacological doses of nicotinic acid (but not nicotinamide) reduce serum cholesterol and triacylglycerol concentrations in man, decrease the concentrations of very low density lipoproteins (VLDL) and low density lipoproteins (LDL) but increase the concentration of high density lipoproteins (HDL) in plasma, and reduce the recurrence rate of nonfatal myocardial infarction (DiPalma and Thayer, 1991). These metabolic changes appear to result from an antilipolytic effect, but the mechanism is unknown. Use of large doses of nicotinic acid, but not large doses of nicotinamide, causes release of the vasodilator histamine. Hence, flushing of the face is a common side effect of nicotinic acid administration. Long-term use may cause gastrointestinal irritation, possible liver damage, and other adverse effects. Large doses of both vitaminic forms of niacin have stimulatory effects on the central nervous system. These effects are clearly unrelated to the vitamin function of niacin.

NIACIN DEFICIENCY

Pellagra ("rough skin") is a niacin-deficiency disease. Its occurrence has been associated with diets in which corn or sorghum was a staple item, including diets in the United States and Southern Europe in the early 1900s. Pellagra is still encountered in India and in parts of China and Africa.

The reasons for the association of pellagra with corn-based diets have been the subject of much research over the years and still are not completely understood. Much of the niacin in corn is bound in an unavailable form, but the tryptophan content of corn is also low, and corn products are relatively more deficient in tryptophan than in niacin. Degermination of corn could have played a role in the occurrence of pellagra in the past, because the milling removed much of the niacin and tryptophan in the corn. The fact that traditional Central American diets do not cause pellagra, even though they contain a large amount of corn, has been attributed to the cooking in lime that the corn receives in tortilla preparation; this alkaline treatment makes niacin more available, but also results in substantial loss of niacin in the washings. The absence of pellagra in Central and South American countries where the staple is maize has also been attributed to widespread consumption of coffee. Although the occurrence of pellagra also has been related to the presence of high levels of leucine in foods, a clear role of leucine in the cause of pellagra has not been supported by most recent studies.

Development of pellagra is often associated with poor diets and increased energy requirements. Pellagra also can develop in patients who are receiving certain drugs (e.g., isoniazid used in treatment of tuberculosis, which depletes the pyridoxal phosphate coenzyme essential for tryptophan conversion to NAD), in patients with malignant carcinoid in whom tryptophan is diverted mainly to serotonin with a reduction in its conversion to quinolinate or NAD, in individuals with chronic alcoholism, and in individuals with certain genetic disorders (e.g., Hartnup's disease, which affects intestinal transport and renal tubular reabsorption of tryptophan and other neutral amino acids, or a defect in the hydroxylation of kynurenine). See Chapters 6 and 11 for more discussion of Hartnup's disease and serotonin synthesis.

Symptoms of pellagra or niacin deficiency include (1) functional changes in the gastrointestinal tract that are manifested as an absence of normal response to histamine, diminished secretion of HCl in the gastric juice, and an impaired absorption of vitamin B_{12}, fat, glucose, and D-xylose; and (2) nonspecific lesions of the central nervous system. The first symptoms of pellagra usually are weakness, lassitude, anorexia, and indigestion. These are followed by the classic "three Ds": *dermatitis, diarrhea, and dementia*. The dermatitis has a characteristic appearance on those parts of the body exposed to sunlight, heat, or mild trauma (such as mechanical stress) such as the face, neck, and surfaces of the hands, feet, and elbows. These lesions usually are bilaterally symmetrical. Diarrhea does not develop in all cases; it may be accompanied by vomiting, dysphagia, and a severe inflammation of the mouth and other mucous membranes. The mental symptoms develop in untreated cases and include irritability, headaches, sleeplessness, loss of memory, and emotional instability.

BIOCHEMICAL ASSESSMENT OF NIACIN NUTRITURE

Biochemical assessment of niacin nutritional status is usually based on measurement of urinary metabolites (McCormick and Greene, 1999). Measurements of *N*-methylnicotin-

---

CLINICAL CORRELATION

Case Study of Pellagra in an Adult Woman

Oakley and Wallace (1994) reported a case involving a young woman in New Zealand who presented with pellagra. She had a variety of neurological and dermal symptoms consistent with a diagnosis of pellagra. She did not have diarrhea. Her symptoms were precipitated by prolonged lactation and increased activity. She had breast-fed her daughter for 3 years, and had been particularly active while building her own home. Dietary intake of niacin equivalents was within a normal range. Her total excretion of urinary amino acids was abnormally high (77 mmol/L compared with a reference range of 2 to 36 mmol/L). Chromatography of urinary amino acids revealed elevated loss of tryptophan and other large neutral amino acids (alanine, serine, threonine, valine, methionine, isoleucine, tyrosine, phenylalanine). Taurine, glycine, ornithine, lysine, arginine, and aspartate were present in urine in normal amounts. Her symptoms resolved with oral nicotinamide plus other B vitamins.

Thinking Critically

1. From the information given, what underlying metabolic abnormality was probably responsible for the development of pellagra in this woman with a normal intake of niacin?

2. Pellagra secondary to inherited disorders usually presents in childhood. Why would periods of rapid growth or of prolonged lactation, as in this case, precipitate the appearance of pellagra? Why might increased activity precipitate the appearance of pellagra?

amide, the 2-pyridone, the sum of these two metabolites, and the ratio of these two metabolites have been used as indicators of niacin status. Results usually are better when determinations are made following administration of a test dose of nicotinate or nicotinamide.

NIACIN REQUIREMENTS

Because both the availability of niacin from bound niacin and the conversion of tryptophan to niacin vary, it is difficult to predict the niacin status of populations on the basis of analysis of diets for tryptophan and niacin. Current estimates of the average niacin requirement are based primarily on the intakes that corresponded to urinary excretion of the niacin metabolite N'-methylnicotinamide at levels above 1.0 mg/day (Institute of Medicine, 1998). The Estimated Average Requirement (EAR) is 12 mg of NE/day for men and 11 mg of NE/day for women.

Currently, the RDA for adults is 14 mg of NE for women and 16 mg of NE for men (Institute of Medicine, 1998). About 75 g of high-quality protein will provide about 15 mg of NE from its tryptophan content, and most mixed diets supply more than 5 mg of preformed niacin. The RDA is relatively easy to meet, with typical intakes in the United States of 25 to 40 mg of NE per day, but it should be recognized that tryptophan rather than niacin is the major source of NE in typical diets. Tryptophan content of proteins ranges from about 0.6% for corn to 1.5% for animal products. One should note that food composition tables usually do not take into account the bioavailability of niacin (from cereals) and do not include an estimate of NE available from tryptophan in the food.

Pregnant women and women taking contraceptive steroids or steroid hormones appear to have some differences in tryptophan metabolism as compared with nonpregnant females. There is some question of whether the increased urinary excretion of tryptophan degradation products represents increased flux through the pathway leading to increased NAD synthesis, or a decrease in kynureninase activity that results in increased excretion of tryptophan catabolites (and less NAD synthe-

sis) as does a vitamin B_6 deficiency (see Chapter 11). Despite the lack of consensus about changes in tryptophan metabolism in pregnant women, an increased intake of NE is recommended during pregnancy and lactation because of the increased energy requirements and needs for growth in maternal and fetal compartments and for secretion in the milk (Institute of Medicine, 1998).

■ Riboflavin

Like niacin, riboflavin (also known as vitamin B_2) is essential for synthesis of coenzymes that function indispensably in oxidation-reduction reactions involved in the catabolism of glucose, fatty acids, ketone bodies, and amino acids. These flavocoenzymes (FAD, FMN) are coupled ultimately to electron-to-oxygen transfer systems, which are the terminal connections between energy-yielding metabolic events and molecular oxygen and also are essential for reductive biosynthetic reactions.

RIBOFLAVIN AND FLAVOCOENZYME STRUCTURE AND NOMENCLATURE

Riboflavin is the common name for vitamin B_2, which is chemically specified as 7,8-dimethyl-10-(1'-D-ribityl)isoalloxazine. "Ribo" refers to the ribityl side chain, and "flavin" is now synonymous with any substituted isoalloxazine. The structure for this yellow, fluorescent, water-soluble compound is shown in Figure 20–9.

The physiologically functional flavo-

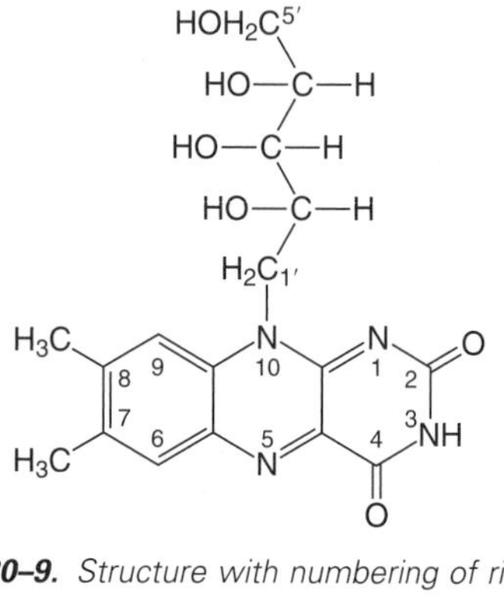

Figure 20–9. *Structure with numbering of riboflavin.*

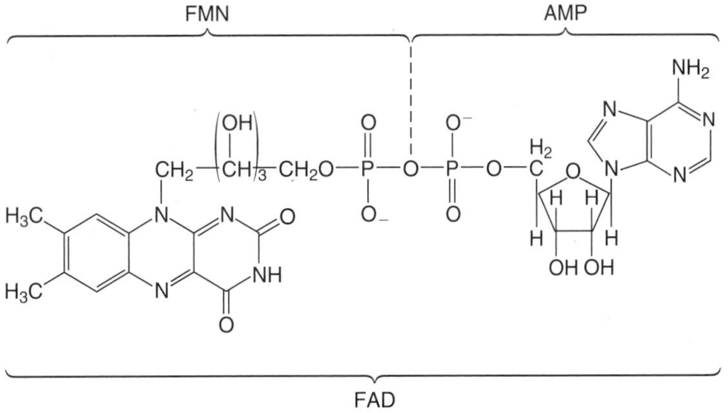

Figure 20–10. Structure of common flavocoenzymes indicating that FAD is comprised of FMN plus an AMP moiety.

coenzymes derived from the vitamin are riboflavin 5′-phosphate, commonly called flavin mononucleotide (FMN), and flavin-adenine dinucleotide (FAD). This latter, most widespread coenzyme is shown with its component parts of FMN and 5′-adenylate (AMP) in Figure 20–10.

Although most flavin coenzymes are noncovalently associated (ionic, hydrophobic) with the apoenzymic proteins, some are covalently bound. In the case of humans, only a few covalent flavoproteins are known. These are the 8α-*N*(3)-histidyl(peptide)-FADs of the dehydrogenases for succinate, sarcosine (*N*-methylglycine) and N,N-dimethylglycine that are in mitochondrial inner membranes, and the 8α-*S*-cysteinyl(peptide)-FAD of monoamine oxidase found in mitochondrial outer membranes. Structures for these mammalian types of covalent flavins are illustrated in Figure 20–11. Another covalently bound flavocoenzyme of uncertain linkage occurs in lysosomal pipicolate oxidase.

Flavocoenzymes are involved in oxidation-reduction reactions in which the ring portion of the flavocoenzyme involving nitrogens 1 and 5 and carbon 4α undergoes sequential addition or loss of hydrogens and electrons. Of nine chemically discernible forms (three levels of redox and three species for acidic, neutral, and basic conditions), five have biological relevance because of pH considerations. These biological forms are summarized in Figure 20–12.

SOURCES, DIGESTION, AND ABSORPTION

Riboflavin within foods is mainly in coenzymatic forms, with over two thirds typically as FAD, except for milk and eggs, where relatively large amounts of riboflavin per se occur. It has been estimated that at least a third of the adult RDA for riboflavin is supplied in the American diet by milk and dairy products (Block et al., 1985). Certainly meats, especially liver, and green vegetables supply much of the rest. Although cereals are rather poor sources, enriched flour and breakfast cereals contribute significant amounts of riboflavin. Covalently bound flavins present in food (approximately 5% to 10% of total naturally occurring flavocoenzymes) are unavailable as nutritional sources of the vitamin, because the 8α-(amino acid)-riboflavins obtained from digestion cannot be used for resynthesis of coenzymes (Chia et al., 1978).

Although riboflavin and its phosphate (FMN) are relatively stable to heat in slightly acidic and neutral conditions, they become more labile in base. Cleavage of the ribityl side chain with loss of vitaminic activity occurs when solutions that contain riboflavin are exposed to light. Such photo-products as lumichrome and lumiflavin are the result.

Following ingestion, flavocoenzymes are released from noncovalent attachment to proteins during gastric acidification and subsequent proteolysis. Nonspecific action by pyrophosphatases (nucleotidohydrolases) and phosphomonoesterase (alkaline phosphatase) on the coenzyme forms occurs in the upper small intestine. A small amount of 8α-(amino acid)-riboflavins and traces of other ring and side-chain substituted flavins also are released during digestion.

Riboflavin and traces of other free flavins primarily are absorbed in the proximal small intestine by a saturable, Na$^+$-dependent trans-

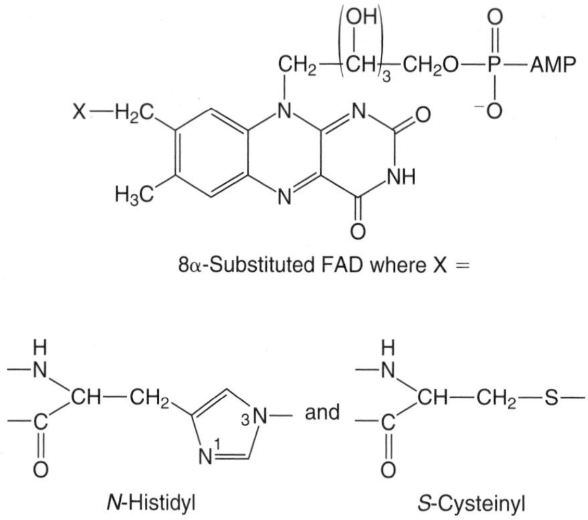

8α-Substituted FAD where X =

N-Histidyl   S-Cysteinyl

Figure 20–11. *Representative covalent flavins in mammals where 8α-attachment is to such electronegative atoms as N or S within amino acid residues of enzymes.*

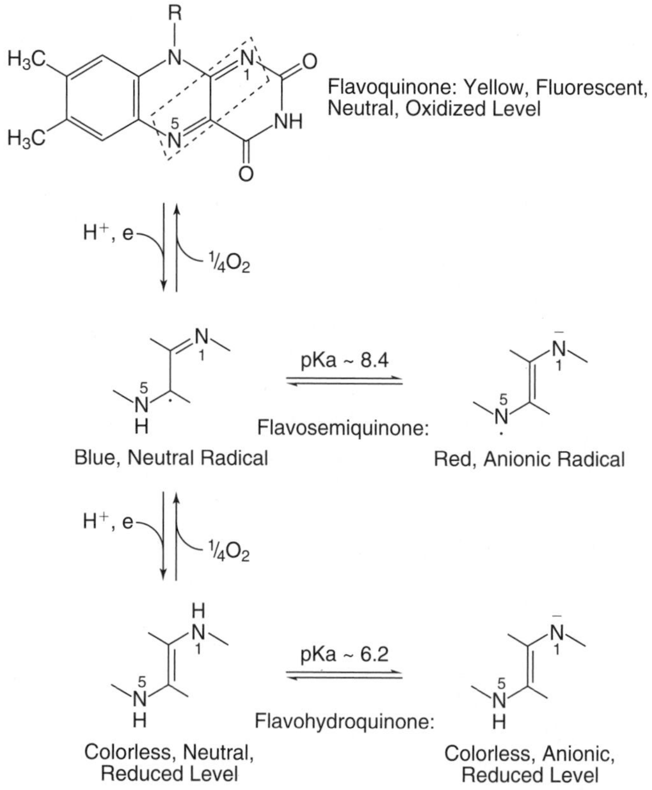

Flavoquinone: Yellow, Fluorescent, Neutral, Oxidized Level

H⁺, e⁻ / ¼O₂

pKa ~ 8.4

Flavosemiquinone:

Blue, Neutral Radical   Red, Anionic Radical

H⁺, e⁻ / ¼O₂

pKa ~ 6.2

Flavohydroquinone:

Colorless, Neutral, Reduced Level   Colorless, Anionic, Reduced Level

Figure 20–12. *Physiologically relevant states of flavocoenzymes.*

Food Sources of Riboflavin

- Milk and dairy products
- Meats, especially organ meats, and eggs
- Broccoli, spinach, mushrooms
- Fortified, ready-to-eat breakfast cereals

RDAs Across the Life Cycle

	mg riboflavin/day
Infants, 0–5 mo	0.3 (AI)
6–11 mo	0.4 (AI)
Children, 1–3 yr	0.5
4–8 yr	0.6
9–13 yr	0.9
Males, >13 yr	1.3
Females, 14–18 yr	1.0
>18 yr	1.1
Pregnant	1.4
Lactating	1.6

From Institute of Medicine. (1998) Dietary Reference Intakes for Thiamin, Riboflavin, Niacin, Vitamin B_6, Folate, Vitamin B_{12}, Pantothenic Acid, Biotin, and Choline. National Academy Press, Washington, D.C.

port process. The uptake that occurs with physiological concentrations of riboflavin intake is facilitated transport, but passive diffusion also occurs up to the limits imposed by the modest solubility of this vitamin. In the adult human, intake and apparent absorption increase proportionately up to about 27 mg in a single dose, but there is little or no further absorption at higher intakes (Zempleni et al., 1996a). Bile salts appear to facilitate uptake. There is very little enterohepatic circulation of riboflavin in humans.

TRANSPORT AND CONVERSION OF RIBOFLAVIN TO COENZYMES

Some of the riboflavin circulating in blood plasma is loosely associated with albumin, although significant amounts complex with other proteins, notably immunoglobulins (Whitehouse et al., 1991). Estrogen induction of distinct plasma riboflavin-binding proteins in mammals suggests sequestration for fetal uptake in a manner that corresponds to the marked increase in riboflavin-binding protein in plasma and eggs of laying hens.

As with most water-soluble vitamins, up-take of riboflavin from plasma by tissues involves facilitated and simple diffusion, followed by metabolic trapping. The facilitated diffusion may well involve a carrier such as the protein that binds riboflavin in the plasma membrane of hepatocytes (Nokubo et al., 1989). Metabolic trapping as riboflavin 5′-phosphate (FMN) reflects the role of flavokinase (Aw et al., 1983; Bowers-Komro and McCormick, 1987). There is an active, Na^+-dependent efflux of riboflavin from the choroid plexus in the brain and from renal tubular cells.

Flavocoenzymes are formed by a sequential pathway that involves two cytosolic enzymes, flavokinase and FAD synthetase, which are widely distributed in tissues. This two-step process is shown in Figure 20–13. Both steps require ATP, with Zn^{2+} preferred in the γ-phosphate exchange catalyzed by flavokinase (Na-

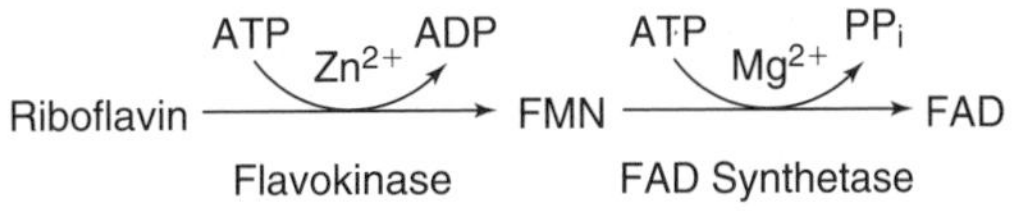

$$\text{Riboflavin} \xrightarrow[\text{Flavokinase}]{\overset{\text{ATP} \quad \text{ADP}}{Zn^{2+}}} \text{FMN} \xrightarrow[\text{FAD Synthetase}]{\overset{\text{ATP} \quad PP_i}{Mg^{2+}}} \text{FAD}$$

Figure 20–13. *Enzymatic steps in flavocoenzyme formation.*

kano and McCormick, 1991) and Mg^{2+} used in the adenylylation effected by the FAD synthetase (Oka and McCormick, 1987). Production of flavocoenzymes is sensitive to changes in flavokinase activity, which decreases during a deficiency of riboflavin (Lee and McCormick, 1983) and is induced by riboflavin repletion (Merrill et al., 1978). Thyroid hormone increases flavokinase activity by conversion of the enzyme from a less-active to a more-active form (Lee and McCormick, 1985). The FAD synthetase step may serve to downregulate flavocoenzyme formation in that FAD synthetase is inhibited by its product, FAD (Yamada et al., 1990). In the covalent attachment of FAD, the apoenzyme itself catalyzes the flavinylation (Decker, 1993).

RIBOFLAVIN CATABOLISM AND EXCRETION

There is varied but not extensive catabolism of riboflavin in mammalian species, and many of the products that have been found in excreta, particularly urine, reflect the action of microflora in the gut and the effects of photodegradation (Chastain and McCormick, 1991). Because there is little storage of riboflavin as such, the urinary excretion of flavins ($\sim$300 μg/day in normal adults) reflects dietary intake. For normal adults eating varied diets, riboflavin accounts for 60% to 70% of urinary flavin. Other urinary flavins are the 7-hydroxymethyl metabolite, 10% to 15%; 8α-sulfonylriboflavin, 5% to 10%; 8-hydroxymethylriboflavin, 4% to 7%; riboflavinyl peptide ester, 4% to 5%; 10-(2'-hydroxyethyl)flavin, 1% to 3%; traces of lumiflavin and varyingly 10-formylmethylflavin and the carboxymethylflavins (Chastain and McCormick, 1987, 1988; Roughead and McCormick, 1991). Both 7- and 8-hydroxymethylriboflavin are the result of the action of microsomal mixed-function oxidases. Side-chain degradation products, such as lumichrome, 10-formylmethylriboflavin, and the 10-hydroxyethylflavin, may result largely from the action of intestinal microorganisms. Both lumichrome and lumiflavin are photodecomposition products. The 8α-flavin peptides and their catabolites are formed from dietary and endogenous covalently linked flavins. Traces of 5'-riboflavinyl glucoside also have been found.

Secretion of flavin into milk is a significant process given the importance of milk as a food source. For milk from both cows (Roughead & McCormick, 1990a) and humans (Roughead & McCormick, 1990b), the flavin in highest concentration other than the free vitamin is FAD, which can account for over a third of total flavin. Much of the FAD in cow's milk is hydrolyzed to FMN during pasteurization. Significant quantities of 10-(2'-hydroxyethyl)flavin and the 10-formylmethylflavin from which it is derived are secreted in milk, and 10-(2'-hydroxyethyl)flavin may reach 10% to 12% of the flavin in cow's milk. Because these catabolites have antivitaminic activities, as reflected in competitive inhibition both of cellular uptake and subsequent flavokinase-catalyzed phosphorylation of riboflavin, the presence of 10-(2'-hydroxyethyl)-flavin in cow's milk subtracts from the biological activity of this food. Several percent of both 7- and 8-hydroxymethylriboflavins are also present, with more of the former. The 7-hydroxymethyl compound, also named 7α-hydroxyriboflavin, is the major flavin catabolite that appears in human plasma after oral administration of riboflavin (Zempleni et al., 1996b). Smaller amounts of other catabolites, including the 10-formylmethylflavin and lumichrome, account for most of the rest of the flavin in milk.

FUNCTIONS OF FLAVOCOENZYMES IN METABOLISM

Flavocoenzymes participate in oxidation-reduction reactions in numerous pathways and in energy production via the respiratory chain (see Figures 20–7 and 20–8). Flavoproteins function in either one- or two-electron transfer reactions. Those involved in one-electron transfers cycle through the radical semiquinone, which can exist as either a neutral or anionic species (see Figure 20–12). A further electron can lead to a fully reduced hydroquinone, again either neutral or anionic. The FMN portion of the microsomal NADPH-cytochrome P450 reductase uses reduced FAD as a one-electron donor and cytochrome P450 as acceptor; it cycles between neutral semiquinone and fully reduced hydroquinone. The FAD in the electron-transferring flavoprotein, which mediates electron flow from fatty acyl CoA to the mitochondrial electron transport chain, cycles between oxidized quinone and anionic semiquinone. Additionally, a single-step, two-electron transfer from substrate can occur in nucleophilic reactions. Such cases as hydride ion transfer from reduced pyridine nucleotide (e.g., with dihydroorotate dehydrogenase) or the carbanion generated by base abstraction of a substrate proton (e.g., with D-amino acid oxidase) may lead to attack at the flavin N-5 position; some species such as activated molecular oxygen add at the C-4α position to generate a transient hydroperoxide (e.g., with microsomal FAD-containing mono-oxygenase). These and other examples have been summarized along with a discussion of putative mechanisms (Merrill et al., 1981).

In these oxidation-reduction reactions, the ring portion of the flavocoenzyme involving nitrogens 1 and 5 and carbon 4α undergoes sequential addition or loss of hydrogens and electrons as shown in Figure 20–14. Flavocoenzymes are varyingly able to catalyze both one- and two-electron redox reactions. In some cases an enzyme (e.g., NADPH-cytochrome P450 reductase that contains both FAD and FMN) can catalyze both one and two-electron redox reactions. In most cases, however, a given flavoprotein probably catalyzes its natural reaction, not fully understood for all cases, by a one- or two- electron transfer mechanism.

In a manner analogous to that of the

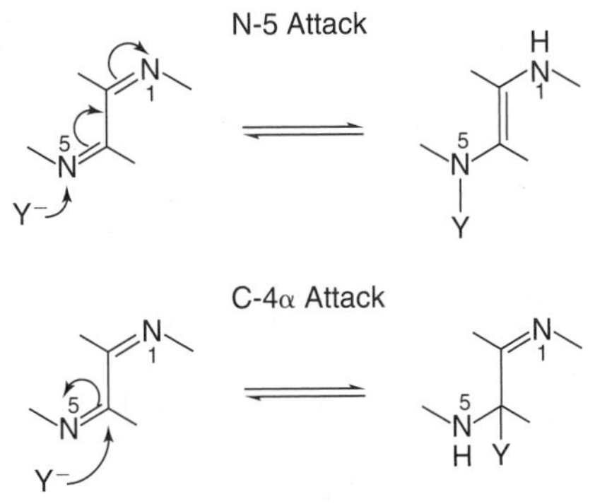

Figure 20–14. *Reaction types encountered with flavoquinone coenzymes and natural nucleophiles (Y⁻).*

pyridine nucleotide-dependent dehydrogenases, the transfer of hydrogen can take place at either face (*re* or *si*) of the isoalloxazine ring system. A number of flavoproteins have now been categorized on this steric basis (Creighton and Murthy, 1990).

Flavoprotein-catalyzed dehydrogenations include both pyridine nucleotide-dependent and independent reactions in which the pyridine nucleotides act as electron donors or acceptors, reactions with sulfur-containing compounds, hydroxylations, oxidative decarboxylations, dioxygenations, and reduction of O_2 to hydrogen peroxide. The intrinsic abilities of flavins to be altered in their oxidation-reduction potentials upon differential binding to proteins, to participate in both one- and two-electron transfers, and in reduced (1,5-dihydro) form to react rapidly with oxygen permit them to function in a wide range of reactions.

RIBOFLAVIN DEFICIENCY

The physiological responses to inadequate dietary intake of riboflavin are numerous and can be severe. In ariboflavinosis, growth typically is stunted and a variety of skin lesions appear. Clinical features of riboflavin deficiency include seborrheic dermatitis; soreness and burning of the lips, mouth, and tongue; photophobia; burning and itching of the eyes; superficial vascularization of the cornea; cheilosis; angular stomatitis; glossitis; anemia; and neuropathy. The similar skin lesions observed in riboflavin and vitamin B_6 deficiencies appear to reflect impaired collagen formation and, in the case of riboflavin, may be due to decreased activity of pyridoxine (pyridoxamine) 5'-phosphate oxidase, which requires FMN as a cofactor for the conversion of pyridoxamine 5'-phosphate (PMP) to pyridoxal 5'-phosphate (PLP). Riboflavin and its coenzyme derivatives are light sensitive. Newborn infants with hyperbilirubinemia who are treated by phototherapy commonly require additional riboflavin during treatment.

Enzymatic alterations occur in riboflavin deficiency. Flavokinase, which is unstable in the absence of its riboflavin substrate, decreases in activity, and there is an increase in

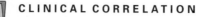

CLINICAL CORRELATION

Multiple Acyl CoA Dehydrogenase Disorders and Riboflavin

Multiple acyl CoA dehydrogenase disorders or glutaric acidemia type II result in excretion of a variety of organic acids (including glutaric, 2-hydroxyglutaric, adipic, suberic, ethylmalonic, and other dicarboxylic acids; and isovaleric, 2-methylbutyric, isobutyric, and other metabolites of branched-chain amino acids) along with esters of fatty acids with glycine or carnitine in the urine. The ω-oxidation of fatty acids to dicarboxylic acids and the transesterification of acyl groups with carnitine and glycine are the result of alternative pathways of metabolism for substrates whose normal catabolic pathways are blocked.

Cultured skin fibroblasts from patients with multiple acyl CoA dehydrogenase deficiency have a severely reduced capacity for oxidation of a variety of organic acyl CoAs, including short-, medium-, and long-chain fatty acyl CoAs; glutaryl CoA (from lysine or tryptophan); isovaleryl CoA (from leucine); 2-methylbutyryl CoA (from isoleucine); and isobutyryl CoA (from valine). Although the oxidation of these metabolites requires several different dehydrogenases, each specific for its substrate, this group of dehydrogenases share a common oxidizing agent, an electron transfer flavoprotein (ETF) that contains tightly bound FAD. The ETF-FADH$_2$ is reoxidized by ETF dehydrogenase with reduction of coenzyme Q (ubiquinone); this connects the flow of electrons to the electron transport chain and eventually to oxygen, with formation of water and generation of ATP. Multiple acyl CoA dehydrogenase deficiency has been attributed to a defect of either ETF or ETF dehydrogenase.

Multiple acyl CoA dehydrogenation disorders usually present in infancy with failure to thrive and repeated episodes of vomiting, lethargy, and coma with dicarboxylic aciduria and hypoketotic hypoglycemia. Mild or late-onset forms of multiple acyl CoA dehydrogenase disorders are rarer, and the clinical picture is variable.

Recently, diagnosis of multiple acyl CoA dehydrogenase deficiency was made in a 62-year-old man who was admitted to the hospital because of easy fatigue in his legs during walking (Araki et al., 1994). He had also experienced fatigue of his neck muscles from holding his head erect. Biopsied muscle samples showed excessive lipid accumulation. The muscle free carnitine concentration was at the lower end of the normal range, and the acylcarnitine to free carnitine ratio in skeletal muscle was elevated above the normal range. The concentrations of lactate and pyruvate in the blood were within the normal range in the resting state, but were markedly increased after a 7.5-minute walk. Riboflavin therapy resulted in a dramatic improvement in both clinical and biochemical parameters.

Thinking Critically

1. In this adult patient, how could you explain the excessive lipid storage in muscle? The muscle fatigue?

2. In this adult patient, a defect in FAD binding to ETF dehydrogenase was suspected. Why?

3. What dietary recommendations would you make for children with multiple acyl CoA dehydrogenase deficiency in terms of fat, carbohydrate, and protein intake? Would energy production via aerobic oxidation of glucose be affected in these patients? Explain.

4. Secondary carnitine deficiency has been diagnosed in a number of cases, as in this adult patient. Plasma free carnitine is typically low or undetectable, but acylcarnitine is present in plasma. Marked clinical improvements have been observed in patients following carnitine supplementation. What is a possible basis for the carnitine deficiency or the accumulation of acylcarnitine?

FAD synthetase activity. These changes may explain the relatively greater decrease in hepatic FMN than in FAD levels that occurs in riboflavin deficiency. Marked decreases in the activities of FMN- and FAD-requiring enzymes, such as xanthine oxidase and glutathione reductase, occur in tissues from riboflavin-deficient animals.

Negligible amounts of riboflavin are excreted in the urine during riboflavin deficiency; this suggests that the body may be capable of reutilizing much of the riboflavin released by its own catabolic processes. Despite an apparent ability to conserve some riboflavin, the daily need to replace tissue turnover in the adult appears to remain greater than 0.5 mg.

BIOCHEMICAL ASSESSMENT OF RIBOFLAVIN NUTRITURE

Currently, the most commonly used method for assessing riboflavin status is the determination of glutathione reductase activity in freshly lysed erythrocytes (McCormick and Greene, 1999). The augmentation in activity after incubation with FAD in vitro has been used to assess riboflavin nutrition both in experimental animals and in humans. A low absolute activity of erythrocyte glutathione reductase and an elevated fractional stimulation of that activity by addition of FAD are indicative of riboflavin deficiency. Urinary riboflavin excretion (24 hr) of less than 10% of that ingested also may reflect inadequate nutrition. The red blood cell concentration of riboflavin also has been used as an indicator of riboflavin status, with values less than 15 μg/100 mL of erythrocytes considered as low or deficient.

RIBOFLAVIN REQUIREMENTS

Riboflavin requirements have been related to protein allowances, lean body mass, metabolic body size, and energy intake. All of these are in themselves related; not surprisingly, allowances calculated by the various methods do not differ significantly. Urinary excretion of riboflavin is low in adults and children who consume less than 0.5 mg/1000 kcal and rises sharply as dietary riboflavin is increased to 0.75 g/1000 kcal and higher. Lesions of riboflavin deficiency have been seen in subjects receiving approximately 0.35 mg/1000 kcal. FAD stimulation of erythrocyte glutathione reductase activity was in a normal range in adults with riboflavin intakes of 0.6 mg or more per 1000 kcal. Based on intakes that prevent clinical and biochemical signs of deficiency, the Institute of Medicine (1998) set the Estimated Average Requirement (EAR) for riboflavin at 1.1 mg/day for men and 0.9 mg/day for women.

The current RDA for riboflavin is 1.3 mg/day for men and 1.1 mg/day for women (Institute for Medicine, 1998). Increments for pregnancy ($+0.3$ mg per day) and for lactation ($+0.5$ mg per day) are recommended. Riboflavin has a low toxicity. No cases of riboflavin toxicity in humans have been reported. This may be due to its low solubility or to the ready excretion of unbound riboflavin in the urine.

■ Thiamin

Thiamin (also known as vitamin B_1) is required for formation of its coenzyme, thiamin pyrophosphate (TPP). Thiamin pyrophosphate functions in prime interconversions of sugar phosphates and in decarboxylation reactions with energy production from α-keto acids and their acyl CoA derivatives, which are catabolically derived from carbohydrates and amino acids.

THIAMIN AND THIAMIN COENZYME STRUCTURE AND NOMENCLATURE

Thiamin (vitamin B_1) is a pyrimidyl-substituted thiazole [3-(2-methyl-4-aminopyrimidinyl)methyl-4-methyl-5-(β-hydroxyethyl)thiazole], as illustrated in Figure 20–15. The vitamin usually is isolated or synthesized and handled as a solid thiazolium salt (e.g., thiamin chloride hydrochloride.

The principal if not sole coenzyme form of thiamin is the pyrophosphate ester called

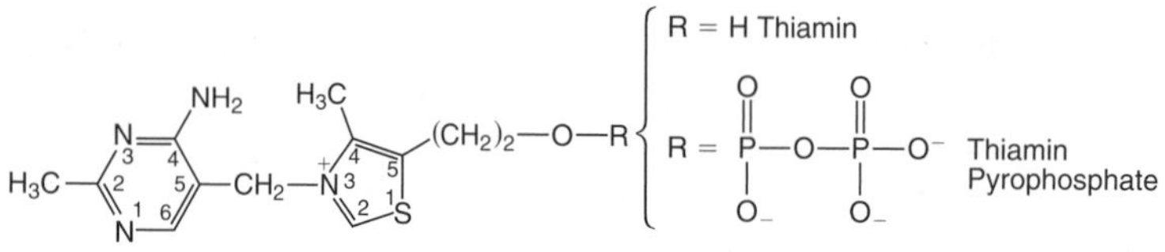

Figure 20–15. *Structures and numbering of thiamin and its pyrophosphate coenzyme.*

TPP or thiamin diphosphate (TDP), also shown in Figure 20–15. Mono- and triphosphate esters occur naturally as well, and the triphosphate has been implicated in nerve function.

SOURCES, DIGESTION, AND ABSORPTION

Thiamin occurs in natural foods mainly as the phosphorylated derivatives. More abundant sources are unrefined cereal germs and whole grains, meats (especially pork), nuts, and legumes. Enriched flours and grain products in the United States contain added thiamin, as well as niacin and riboflavin (Gubler, 1991).

Elevation of temperature, especially in aqueous media above neutral pH, leads to rapid loss of thiamin activity. The thiazole ring is subject to base attack at carbon 2, followed by ring opening to an acyclic sulfide. Under oxidizing conditions, thiamin can form disulfides intermolecularly or thiochrome intramolecularly. Rupture of the methylene bridge to the thiazole nitrogen also occurs readily when thiamin is exposed to sulfite, which is formed during preservation of foods with sulfur dioxide.

Following release of thiamin during digestive hydrolysis catalyzed by pyrophosphatase and phosphatase in the upper small intestine, the vitamin is readily absorbed by an active transport process that is probably carrier mediated at intakes less than 5 mg/day for adults (McCormick and Greene, 1999). At higher intakes, passive diffusion increasingly contributes to absorption. Pyrophosphorylation catalyzed by thiamin pyrophosphokinase (thiaminokinase) takes place in the jejunal mucosal cells to yield TPP, a process of metabolic trapping that seemingly relates to the facilitation of uptake. The exit of thiamin from the mucosal cell on the basolateral side is Na^+-dependent and coupled to ATPase.

TRANSPORT AND CONVERSION OF THIAMIN TO COENZYME

Thiamin is carried by the portal circulation to the liver and from there to the general circulation. The free vitamin occurs in the plasma, but TPP predominates in the cellular components. Leukocytes have a 10-fold higher concentration than erythrocytes. Thiamin transport into cells seems to occur by a similar saturable carrier in various tissues, but there is a marked variation of transport capacity among tissues. For example, transport capacity is high in hepatocytes as in enterocytes, but much lower in erythrocytes. This suggests that the number or efficiency of carrier sites may differ according to the type of tissue or its function (Rindi, 1992).

There is not much storage, perhaps 30 mg, of this water-soluble vitamin and its phosphates in the body. About half is in muscle and the rest in heart, liver, kidneys, and nervous tissues. Approximately 80% is as the pyrophosphate, 10% as the triphosphate, and the rest as thiamin and its monophosphate.

The three main enzymes that participate in the formation and interconversions of thiamine and its phosphate esters are noted in Figure 20–16. A pyrophosphokinase catalyzes formation of the coenzyme TPP. Some of this is routed to the mono- and triphosphates by a TPP-ATP phosphoryltransferase activity shown to be attributable to cytosolic adenylate kinase (Kawasaki, 1992). This enzyme can reversibly catalyze the conversion of two moles of the diphosphate (ADP or TPP) to form one of triphosphate (ATP or TTP) and one of monophosphate (AMP or TMP). There are tissue phosphatases that can hydrolyze TMP to release thiamin. A membrane-associated triphosphatase, mainly in nervous tissue, and pyrophosphatases also contribute to the interconversions of free and phosphorylated forms of thiamin (Ogawa and Sakai, 1982).

Food Sources of Thiamin

- Enriched grain products
- Meats, especially pork
- Nuts

RDAs Across the Life Cycle

	mg thiamin/day
Infants, 0–0.5 yr	0.2 (AI)
0.5–1 yr	0.3 (AI)
Children, 1–3 yr	0.5
4–8 yr	0.6
9–13 yr	0.9
Males, >13 yr	1.2
Females, 14–18 yr	1.0
>18 yr	1.1
Pregnant	1.4
Lactating	1.5

From Institute of Medicine. (1998) Dietary Reference Intakes for Thiamin, Riboflavin, Niacin, Vitamin B_6, Folate, Vitamin B_{12}, Pantothenic Acid, Biotin, and Choline. National Academy Press, Washington, D.C.

THIAMIN CATABOLISM AND EXCRETION

Thiamin much in excess of tissue needs is rapidly excreted in the urine. At least 50 metabolites have been reported to occur in the urine from rats and humans (Neal, 1970), but six of these have been identified to reflect the main catabolic events. These major urinary catabolites of thiamin are thiamin acetic acid, 2-methyl-4-amino-5-formylaminomethylpyrimidine, 4-methyl-5-(2-hydroxyethyl)thiazole, 2-methyl-4-amino-pyrimidine-5-carboxylic acid, 2-methyl-4-amino-5-hydroxymethylpyrimidine, and 4-methylthiazole-5-acetic acid. Additionally, small amounts of the thiamin disulfide and thiochrome have been identified. Thiaminase II, present in intestinal bacteria, leads to formation of the pyrimidine and thiazole portions that are in part further oxidized in their hydroxymethyl functions to yield substituted pyrimidine carboxylates and thiazole carboxylates. Cleavage into the rings also occurs, as noted from the formation of the formylmethylaminopyrimidine. As with some urinary flavins, several of the numerous metabolites of thiamin arise from action of symbiotic microflora in the gut.

FUNCTIONS OF COENZYMATIC THIAMIN IN METABOLISM

There are two general types of reactions in which TPP functions as the Mg^{2+}-coordinated coenzyme for so-called active aldehyde transfers, which involve attack of carbonyl metabolites by the carbanion generated at carbon 2 on the thiazole moiety of TPP, as shown in Figure 20–17. First, in decarboxylation of α-keto acids, the condensation of the thiazole moiety of TPP with the α-carbonyl carbon on the acid leads to loss of CO_2 and production of a resonance-stabilized carbanion. Proto-

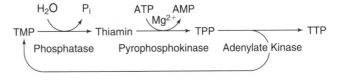

Figure 20–16. *Interconversions of thiamin and its mono- (TMP), di- (TPP), and tri- (TTP) phosphates.*

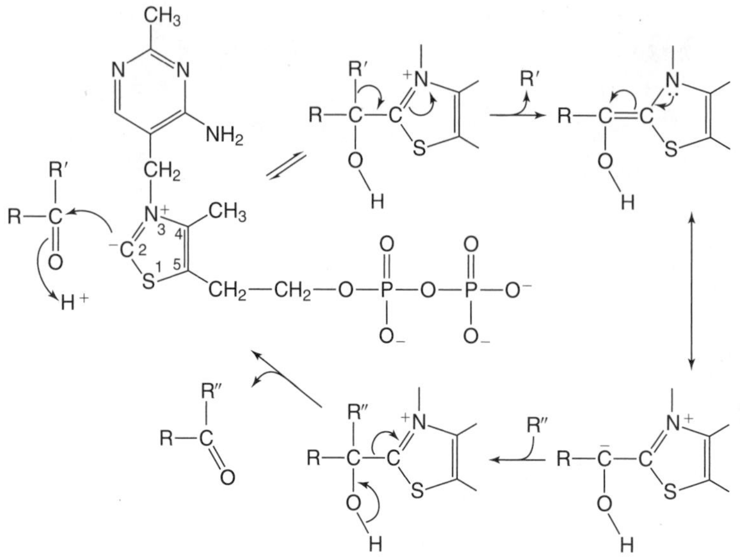

Figure 20–17. *Function of the thiazole moiety of TPP in α-keto acid decarboxylations (where R' is a carboxylate lost as CO_2 and R″ is a proton generating an aldehyde) and in ketolations (where R' is a carbohydrate moiety releasing a glycose and R″ is a different glycose generating a new carbohydrate).*

nation and release of aldehyde (acetaldehyde from pyruvate) occur in fermentative organisms such as yeast, which have only the TPP-dependent decarboxylase. However, in higher eukaryotes, including humans, the TPP-dependent decarboxylases exist as part of multienzymic dehydrogenase complexes. These enzyme complexes transfer the α-hydroxyalkyl group from TPP to a covalently linked lipoic acid prosthetic group with oxidation of the hydroxyalkyl carbanion to an acyl group with the concomitant reduction of the lipoyl disulfide bond, transfer of the acyl group from the lipoyl prosthetic group to coenzyme A to form the respective acyl CoA, the reduction of FAD to $FADH_2$ with reoxidation of the dihydrolipoyl group to disulfide form, and the oxidation of $FADH_2$ back to FAD by conversion of NAD^+ to NADH. These TPP- (and FAD- and NAD-) dependent α-ketoacid dehydrogenase complexes are used to catalyze the oxidative decarboxylation of pyruvate to acetyl CoA, α-ketoglutarate to succinyl CoA, and the α-ketoacids from branched-chain amino acids to their respective acyl CoAs. The pyruvate and branched-chain amino acid dehydrogenase complexes also convert α-ketobutyrate to propionyl CoA.

The other general reaction involving TPP is the transformation of α-ketols (ketose phosphates). Although specialized phosphoketolases in certain bacteria and higher plants can split ketose phosphates to simpler, released products, the reactions of importance to humans and most animals are transketolations. Transketolase is a TPP-dependent enzyme found in the cytosol of many tissues, especially liver and blood cells, in which the pentose phosphate pathway (also called the hexose monophosphate shunt or 6-phosphogluconate pathway) of glucose metabolism exists. Transketolase catalyzes the reversible transfer of a glycoaldehyde moiety (α,β-dihydroxyethyl-TPP) from the first two carbons of a donor ketose phosphate (D-xylulose 5-phosphate or D-sedoheptulose 7-phosphate) to the aldehyde carbon of an aldose phosphate (D-ribose 5-phosphate or D-erythrose 4-phosphate). These sugar rearrangements are essential for synthesis of ribose and for funneling the 5-carbon sugar phosphate back into the glycolytic/gluconeogenic pathways as triose or hexose phosphates.

Altogether, there are interconnecting pathways from metabolism of carbohydrates and amino acids that have steps critically dependent upon TPP, as summarized in Figures 20–18 and 20–7. Additional discussion of reactions requiring TPP can be found in Chapters 9 and 11; see Figures 9–17, 9–19, 11–19, 11–21, and 11–28.

Although thiamin as its pyrophosphate contributes to nervous system function in such essential reactions as energy production

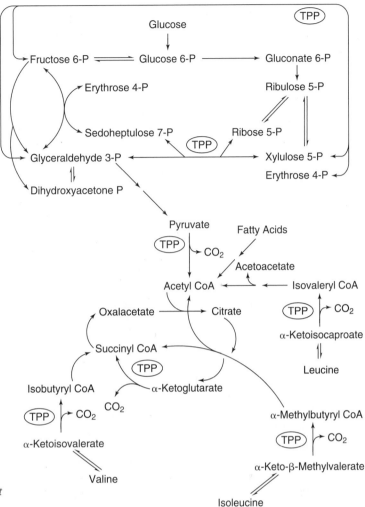

Figure 20–18. *Pathways dependent on coenzymatic TPP.*

and biosynthesis of lipids and acetylcholine, it appears that there is another incompletely understood role, particularly for the triphosphate (Bender, 1992; Haas, 1988). Electrical stimulation of nerves leads to hydrolysis and release of both di- and triphosphates of thiamin from axonal membranes, which also have relatively high activities of enzymes that cause formation and breakdown of TTP.

THIAMIN DEFICIENCY

Beriberi is the name (Indonesian) given to the disease resulting from thiamin deficiency (McCormick and Greene, 1999). The causes for deficiency include inadequate intake due to diets largely dependent on milled, nonen-riched grains such as rice and wheat or to the ingestion of raw fish that contain microbial thiaminases, which hydrolytically destroy the vitamin in the gastrointestinal tract. Tea may contain antithiamin factors that also have been detected in certain other plant extracts. Chronic alcoholism is a common contributor to deficiency in that there is not only a low intake of thiamin (and other B vitamins), but also impaired absorption and storage. There are several thiamin-responsive inborn errors of metabolism; these include a megaloblastic anemia of unknown mechanism, lactic acidosis due to low or defective pyruvate decarboxylase, branched-chain ketoaciduria with poor activity of the branched-chain keto acid dehydrogenase system, and subacute necrotizing encephalomyelopathy associated with a lack of thiamin triphosphate in neural tissues. Therapeutic doses of 5 to 20 mg of thiamin daily have proved beneficial in some cases. Finally, other at-risk patients are those undergoing long-term renal dialysis or intravenous feeding and even those with chronic febrile infections.

Clinical signs primarily involve the nervous and cardiovascular systems. In the adult, symptoms most frequently observed are mental confusion, anorexia, muscular weakness, ataxia, peripheral paralysis, paralysis of the motor nerves of the eye, edema (wet beriberi), muscle wasting (dry beriberi), tachycardia, and an enlarged heart. In infants, symptoms appear suddenly and severely, often involving cardiac failure and cyanosis (bluish coloration of skin and mucous membranes due to deficient oxygenation of the blood). Commonly, the distinction between wet (cardiovascular) and dry (neuritic) manifestations of beriberi relate to duration and severity of the deficiency, the degree of physical exertion, and caloric intake. The wet or edematous condition results from severe physical exertion and high carbohydrate intake, whereas the dry or polyneuritic form stems from relative inactivity with caloric restriction along with chronic thiamin deficiency. The three major physiological derangements that involve the cardiovascular system are peripheral vasodilatation that leads to a high cardiac output state, biventricular myocardial failure, and retention of sodium and water that leads to edema. Nervous system involvement includes peripheral neuropathy, Wernicke's encephalopathy, and the amnesic psychosis of Korsakoff's syndrome.

BIOCHEMICAL ASSESSMENT OF THIAMIN NUTRITURE

Numerous methods have been used to assess the state of thiamin nutrition in man (McCormick and Greene, 1999). The most common of these are (1) the measurement of the activity of erythrocyte transketolase, a thiamin pyrophosphate-requiring enzyme; (2) the measurement of blood or urinary levels of thiamin using various chemical, microbiological, and chromatographic techniques; and (3) the measurement of blood levels of pyruvate and α-ketoglutarate. The measurement of whole blood or erythrocyte transketolase activity (basal level) and the enhancement of enzymatic activity with added TPP is considered to be the most reliable method; TPP stimulation of greater than 16% indicates possible deficiency. Symptoms of beriberi (such as peripheral neuropathy and cardiac abnormalities) usually do not appear until the TPP stimulation of erythrocyte transketolase is about 40%.

THIAMIN REQUIREMENTS

The RDAs for thiamin are 1.2 mg of thiamin/day for men and 1.1 mg/day for women. EARs for thiamin are based on the relation between thiamin intake and appearance of clinical signs of deficiency, on excretion of thiamin and its metabolites, and on erythrocyte transketolase and TPP effects; these estimates are 1.0 mg of thiamin/day for men and 0.9 mg/day for women (Institute of Medicine, 1998).

The RDAs have been increased by 0.3 mg for pregnant women and by 0.4 mg for lactating women to cover the estimated requirements for growth in maternal and fetal compartments, secretion in the milk, and small increases in energy utilization. Recommendations for infants are based on the thiamin content of human breast milk and on caloric intake; the Adequate Intake (AI) for infants is 0.03 mg/kg or 0.2 mg/day up to 5 months and then 0.3 mg/day. Recommendations for children are extrapolated from adult values with consideration of body size and needs for growth.

Thiamin requirements appear to be elevated in individuals with elevated caloric intakes, especially when calories are derived primarily from carbohydrates, in individuals consuming ethanol, in renal patients undergoing long-term dialysis, in patients fed intravenously for long periods, and in patients with chronic febrile infections. Folate deficiency appears to depress thiamin absorption. The depression of thiamin absorption observed in alcoholics may be secondary to a folate deficiency. Individuals deplete body stores of thiamin rapidly during starvation or semistarvation.

Thiamin requirements and metabolism

NUTRITION INSIGHT

Alcoholism and Genetics as Factors in Thiamin Deficiency Disorders

In Western countries, symptomatic thiamin deficiency is usually associated with alcoholism. The majority of individuals with Wernicke-Korsakoff syndrome have a history of chronic alcohol abuse. Wernicke's encephalopathy is characterized by disturbances in ocular motility and by ataxia with tremors. Korsakoff's psychosis is characterized by confusion and severe impairment of memory, especially for recent events. A poor diet with low thiamin intake, sustained caloric intake from alcohol, and possible impairments in thiamin absorption and utilization play a role in the development of Wernicke-Korsakoff disease. It also appears that an inborn error or genetic variant predisposes some individuals to thiamin deficiency diseases. Fibroblast cultures from patients with Wernicke-Korsakoff disease show an elevated K_m of transketolase for TPP or, in other words, poor binding of coenzyme TPP to the apoenzyme transketolase to form active holoenzyme. Hence, alcohol consumption along with a genetic predisposition both may be factors in development of thiamin deficiency diseases. Symptoms respond to parenterally administered thiamin, but not all patients recover completely.

may be altered by various thiaminases and thiamin antagonists such as caffeic acid, tannic acid, and heme-containing animal tissues. Thiaminases are found in viscera of some freshwater fish and shellfish and in several microorganisms. Thiamin antagonists may be found in coffee, tea, rice bran, and other sources. Thiamin deficiency has been associated with consumption of large amounts of raw fish or large amounts of tea.

Some thiamin-responsive inborn errors of metabolism can be treated with pharmacological doses of thiamin. Some patients with inborn errors that result in low activity of the branched-chain keto acid dehydrogenase complex respond to treatment with 10 to 1000 times the RDA for thiamin. Another thiamin-responsive inborn error is thiamin-responsive lactic acidosis, which is due to low activity of the pyruvate dehydrogenase complex in the liver.

Thiamin produces a variety of pharmacological effects and even death due to depression of the respiratory center when administered in doses thousands of times larger than those required for optimal nutrition. No toxic effects of thiamin administered by mouth have been reported in man. Thiamin is readily cleared by the kidneys. Injection of doses up to 200 times the daily maintenance dose generally has not led to toxic effects, but some individuals appear to develop a hypersensitivity to thiamin.

REFERENCES

Araki, E., Kobayashi, R., Kohtake, N, Goto, I. and Hashimoto, T. (1994) A riboflavin-responsive lipid storage myopathy due to multiple acyl CoA dehydrogenase deficiency: An adult case. J Neurol Sci 126:202–205.

Aw, T. Y., Jones, D. P. and McCormick, D. B. (1983) Uptake of riboflavin by isolated rat liver cells. J Nutr 113:1249–1254.

Bechgaard, H. and Jespersen, S. (1977) Gastrointestinal absorption of niacin in humans. J Pharm Sci 66:871–872.

Bender, D. A. (1992) Vitamin B_1: Thiamin. In: Nutritional Biochemistry of the Vitamins, pp. 128–155. Cambridge University Press, Cambridge.

Block, G., Dresser, C. M., Hartman, A. H. and Carroll, M. D. (1985) Nutrient sources in the American diet: Quantitative data from the NHANES survey. Am J Epidemiol 122:13–26.

Bowers-Komro, D. M. and McCormick, D. B. (1987) Riboflavin uptake by isolated rat kidney cells. In: Flavins and Flavoproteins (Edmondson, D. E. and McCormick D. B., eds.), pp. 449–453. Walter de Gruyter, Berlin.

Chastain, J. L. and McCormick, D. B. (1987) Flavin catabolites: Identification and quantitation in human urine. Am J Clin Nutr 46:830–834.

Chastain, J. L. and McCormick, D. B. (1988) Characterization of a new flavin metabolite from human urine. Biochem Biophys Acta 967:131–134.

Chastain, J. L. and McCormick, D. B. (1991) Flavin metabolites. In: Chemistry and Biochemistry of Flavins (Müller, F., ed.), vol. I, pp. 195–200. CRC Press, Boca Raton, FL.

Chia, C. P., Addison, R. and McCormick, D. B. (1978) Absorption, metabolism, and excretion of 8α-(amino acid)riboflavins in the rat. J Nutr 108:373–381.

Creighton, D. J. and Murthy, N. S. R. K. (1990) Stereochemistry of enzyme-catalyzed reactions at carbon. In: The Enzymes (Sigmon, D. S. and Boyer, P. D., eds.), vol. 19, pp. 323–421. Academic Press, San Diego.

Decker, K. F. (1993) Biosynthesis and function of enzymes with covalently bound flavin. Annu Rev Nutr 13:17–41.

DiPalma, J. R. and Thayer, W. S. (1991) Use of niacin as a drug. Annu Rev Nutr 11:169–187.

Gross, C. J. and Henderson, L. M. (1983) Digestion and absorption of NAD by the small intestine of the rat. J Nutr 113:412–420.

Gubler, C. J. (1991) Thiamin. In: Handbook of Vitamins (Machlin, L. H., ed.), 2nd ed., pp. 233–281. Marcel Dekker, New York.

Haas, R. H. (1988) Thiamin and the brain. Annu Rev Nutr 8:483–515.

Institute of Medicine. (1998) Dietary Reference Intakes for Thiamin, Riboflavin, Niacin, Vitamin B_6, Folate, Vitamin B_{12}, Pantothenic Acid, Biotin, and Choline. National Academy Press, Washington, D.C.

Junod, A. J., Jornot, L. and Petersen, H. (1989) Differential effects of hyperoxia and hydrogen peroxide on DNA damage, polyadenosine diphosphate-ribose polymerase activity, and nicotinamide adenine dinucleotide and adenosine triphosphate contents in cultured endothelial cells and fibroblasts. J Cell Physiol 140:177–185.

Kawasaki, T. (1992) Thiamin triphosphate synthesis in animals. In: Proceedings of the 1st International Congress on Vitamins and Biofactors in Life Sciences (Kobayashi, T., ed.), pp. 383–386. Center for Academic Publications Japan, Tokyo.

Knox, W. E. and Piras, M. M. (1967) Tryptophan pyrrolase of liver. J Biol Chem 242:2959–2965.

Lee, S.-S. and McCormick, D. B. (1983) Effect of riboflavin status on hepatic activities of flavin-metabolizing enzymes in rats. J Nutr 113:2274–2279.

Lee, S.-S. and McCormick, D. B. (1985) Thyroid hormone regulation of flavocoenzyme biosynthesis. Arch Biochem Biophys 237:197–201.

McCormick, D. B. and Greene, H. L. (1999) Vitamins. In: Tietz Textbook of Clinical Chemistry (Burtis, C. A. and Ashwood, E. R., eds.), 3rd ed., pp. 999–1029. W. B. Saunders, Philadelphia.

McCreanor, G. M. and Bender, D. A. (1986) The metabolism of high intakes of tryptophan, nicotinamide and nicotinic acid in the rat. Br J Nutr 56:577–586.

Merrill, A. H., Jr., Addison, R. and McCormick, D. B. (1978) Induction of hepatic and intestinal flavokinase after oral administration of riboflavin to riboflavin-deficient rats. Proc Soc Exp Biol Med 158:572–574.

Merrill, A. H., Jr., Lambeth, J. D., Edmondson, D. E. and McCormick, D. B. (1981) Formation and mode of action of flavoproteins. Annu Rev Nutr 1:281–317.

Mrochek, J. E., Jolley, R. L., Young, D. S. and Turner, W. J. (1976) Metabolic responses of humans to ingestion of nicotinic acid and nicotinamide. Clin Chem 22:1821–1827.

Nakano, H. and McCormick, D. B. (1991) Stereospecificity of the metal·ATP complex in flavokinase from rat small intestine. J Biol Chem 266:22125–22128.

Neal, R. A. (1970) Isolation and identification of thiamin catabolites in mammalian urine; isolation and identification of some products of bacterial catabolism of thiamin. In: Methods in Enzymology, vol. 18, part A (McCormick, D. B. and Wright, L. D., eds.), pp. 133–140. Academic Press, New York.

Nokubo, M., Ohta, M., Kitani, K. and Zs-Nagy, I. (1989) Identification of protein-bound riboflavin in rat hepatocyte plasma membrane as a source of autofluorescence. Biochim Biophys Acta 931:303–308.

Oakley, A. and Wallace, J. (1994) Hartnup disease presenting in an adult. Clin Exp Dermatol 19:407–408.

Ogawa, K. and Sakai, M. (1982) Recent findings on ultra cytochemistry of thiamin phosphatases. In: Thiamin: Twenty Years of Progress (Sable, H. Z. and Gubler, C. J., eds.), vol. 378, pp. 188–214. Ann NY Acad Sci, New York.

Oka, M. and McCormick, D. B. (1987) Complete purification and general characterization of FAD synthetase from rat liver. J Biol Chem 262:7418–7422.

Rechsteiner, M., Hillyard, D. and Olivera, B. M. (1976) Turnover of nicotinamide adenine dinucleotide in cultures of human cells. J Cell Physiol 88:207–218.

Rindi, G. (1992) Some aspects of thiamin transport in mammals. In: Proceedings of the 1st International Congress on Vitamins and Biofactors in Life Sciences (Kobayashi, T., ed.), pp. 379–382. Center for Academic Publications Japan, Tokyo.

Roughead, Z. K. and McCormick, D. B. (1990a) Qualitative and quantitative assessment of flavins in cow's milk. J Nutr 120:382–388.

Roughead, Z. K. and McCormick, D. B. (1990b) Flavin composition of human milk. Am J Clin Nutr 52:854–857.

Roughead, Z. K. and McCormick, D. B. (1991) Urinary riboflavin and its metabolites: Effects of riboflavin supplementation in healthy residents of rural Georgia (USA). Eur J Clin Nutr 45:299–307.

Schraufstatter, I. U., Hinshaw, D. B., Hyslope, P. A., Spragg, R. G. and Cochrane, C. G. (1986) Oxidant injury of cells. J Clin Invest 777:1312–1320.

Whitehouse, W. S. A., Merrill, A. H., Jr. and McCormick, D. B. (1991) Riboflavin-binding protein. In: Chemistry and Biochemistry of Flavins (Müller, F., ed.), vol. I, pp. 287–292. CRC Press, Boca Raton, FL.

Yamada, Y., Merrill, A. H., Jr. and McCormick, D. B. (1990) Probable reaction mechanisms of flavokinase and FAD synthetase from rat liver. Arch Biochem Biophys 278:125–130.

Zempleni, J., Galloway, J. R. and McCormick, D. B. (1996a) Pharmacokinetics of orally and intravenously administered riboflavin in healthy humans. Am J Clin Nutr 63:54–66.

Zempleni, J., Galloway, J. R. and McCormick, D. B. (1996b) The identification and kinetics of 7α-hydroxyriboflavin (7-hydroxymethylriboflavin) in blood plasma from humans following oral administration of supplements. Int J Vitam Nutr Res 66:151–157.

RECOMMENDED READINGS

Bender, D. A. (1992) Niacin. In: Nutritional Biochemistry of the Vitamins, pp. 184–222. Cambridge University Press, Cambridge.

Bender, D. A. (1992) Vitamin B_1: Thiamin. In: Nutritional Biochemistry of the Vitamins, pp. 128–155. Cambridge University Press, Cambridge.

Gubler, C. J. (1991) Thiamin. In: Handbook of Vitamins, 2nd ed. (Machlin, L. H., ed.), pp. 233–281. Marcel Dekker, New York.

McCormick, D. B. (1989) Two interconnected B vitamins: Riboflavin and pyridoxine. Physiol Rev 69:1170–1198.

CHAPTER **21**

◆ ◆

Folic Acid, Vitamin B₁₂, and Vitamin B₆

Barry Shane, Ph.D.

OUTLINE

COMMON ABBREVIATIONS

AdoHcy (S-adenosylhomocysteine)
AdoMet (S-adenosylmethionine)
Cbl (cobalamin, vitamin B_{12})
$H_4PteGlu$ (tetrahydropteroylglutamate)
$H_4PteGlu_n$ (tetrahydropteroylpolyglutamate, n indicating the number of glutamyl residues)
IF (intrinsic factor)
PL (pyridoxal)
PLP (pyridoxal 5'-phosphate)
PM (pyridoxamine)
PMP (pyridoxamine 5'-phosphate)
PN (pyridoxine or pyridoxol)
PNP (pyridoxine 5'-phosphate)
PteGlu (pteroylglutamate or folic acid)
TC (transcobalamin)

■ FOLATE

Folate was initially investigated as a dietary factor that prevented megaloblastic anemia of pregnancy and as a growth factor present in green leafy vegetables (foliage), hence its name. Folate and vitamin B_{12} deficiency lead to an identical and indistinguishable megaloblastic anemia in which blood cells are enlarged due to a derangement of DNA synthesis, and it has been known for many years that the pernicious anemia that results from defects in vitamin B_{12} availability is caused by induction of a secondary folate deficiency. Because of the role of folate coenzymes in the synthesis of DNA precursors, folate antagonists have found widespread clinical use as anticancer and antimicrobial agents. More recently, the observation that periconceptional supplementation with folate reduces the incidence of neural tube defects and possibly other birth defects has generated considerable clinical and public health interest and has led to fortification of the American food supply with folate.

CHEMISTRY OF FOLATE

Folic acid (pteroylmonoglutamic acid, PteGlu) consists of a 2-amino-4-hydroxy-pteridine (pterin) moiety linked via a methylene group at the C-6 position to a p-aminobenzoylglutamic acid moiety (Fig. 21–1). Folate metabolism involves the reduction of the pyrazine ring of the pterin moiety to the coenzymatically active tetrahydro form, the elongation of the glutamate chain by the addition of L-glutamate residues in an unusual γ-peptide linkage, and the acquisition and oxidation or reduction of one-carbon units at the N-5 and/or N-10 positions (Fig. 21–1). Folate is used as a generic name for all these derivatives, whereas folic acid is usually used to refer specifically to either pteroylmonoglutamic acid or its ionized form. Folate coenzymes function as acceptors and donors of one-carbon moieties in reactions involving nucleotide and amino acid metabolism, which is known as one-carbon metabolism. Over 95% of tissue folates are polyglutamate species, primarily with glutamate chain lengths between 5 and 8. The polyglutamates are more effective substrates than pteroylmonoglutamates with most folate-dependent enzymes, and they usually exhibit greatly increased affinities for these enzymes. The polyanionic nature of the polyglutamate chain, coupled with intracellular protein binding, allows tissues to retain and concentrate these forms of the vitamin, whereas the monoglutamate species are the transport forms.

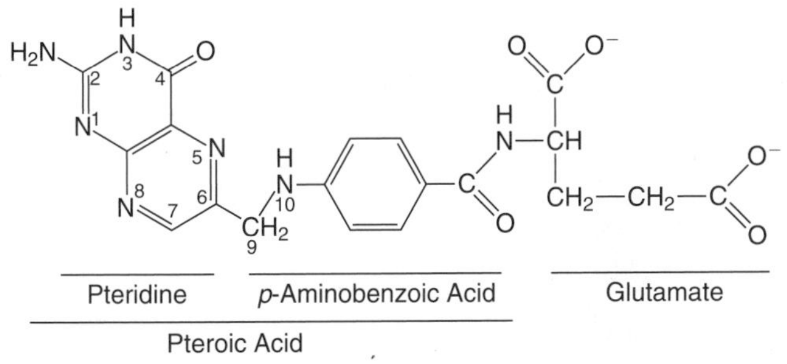

Folic Acid, Pteroylglutamate (PteGlu)

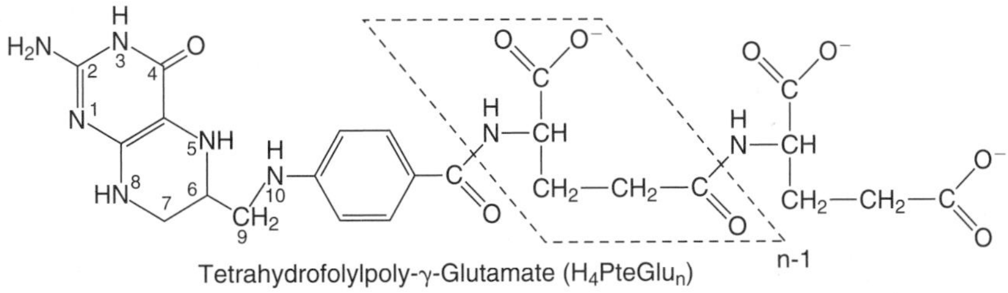

Tetrahydrofolylpoly-γ-Glutamate ($H_4PteGlu_n$)

One Carbon Substituent		Position	Oxidation State
Methyl	$—CH_3$	N-5	Methanol
Methylene	$—CH_2—$	N-5, N-10	Formaldehyde
Methenyl	—CH=	N-5, N-10	Formate
Formyl	—CHO	N-5 or N-10	Formate
Formimino	HN=CH—	N-5	Formate

Figure 21–1. *Structure of folic acid (PteGlu) and tetrahydrofolylpoly-γ-glutamate ($H_4PteGlu_n$). One-carbon substituents can be at the N-5 and/or N-10 positions of the reduced folate molecule.*

SOURCES OF FOLATE

Folates are synthesized by microorganisms and plants as the 7,8-dihydrofolate form, and all naturally occurring folates are reduced derivatives. Fully oxidized folic acid is found in the diet only when foodstuffs are fortified with folic acid or when dietary folates are oxidized. Reduced folates are less stable than folic acid, and their stability varies depending on the one-carbon substitution. Large losses of food folate can occur during food preparation such as heating, particularly under oxidative conditions. Additional losses can also occur by the leaching out of folate during food preparation.

BIOAVAILABILITY AND ABSORPTION OF FOLATE

Most dietary folates are polyglutamate derivatives, and the polyglutamates are hydrolyzed by a brush border membrane γ-glutamylhydrolase activity in the small intestine to yield the monoglutamate forms that are absorbed across the intestinal mucosa. Absorption is via a saturable carrier-mediated process, but at high folate concentrations a diffusion-like process also occurs. The intestinal transporter, which is encoded by the reduced folate carrier gene (RFC-1), is a transmembrane protein that is expressed in most, if not all, tissues; the specificity of this transporter for various folates differs among tissues and between the apical and basolateral membranes of cells such as enterocytes. Affinities for reduced folates are in the low micromolar range, whereas affinities for folic acid are similar in some tissues such as the intestine but can be 100-fold lower in other tissues. These differences may reflect tissue-specific differences in posttranslational modification of the reduced folate carrier protein.

The mechanism by which folate crosses

Food Sources of Folate

- Fortified cereals
- Vegetables
- Bread and bread products
- Citrus fruits and juices
- Meat, poultry, and fish

RDAs Across the Life Cycle

	μg folate/day
Infants, 0–5 mo	65 (AI)
6–11 mo	80 (AI)
Children, 1–3 y	150
4–8 y	200
9–13 y	300
Males, > 13 y	400
Females, >13 y	400
Pregnant	600*
Lactating	500

*Higher levels may be required to minimize the risk of birth defects. The recommendation for women of child-bearing age, who are capable of becoming pregnant, is to take 400 μg of folic acid per day, derived from supplements and/or fortified food, in addition to their normal food folate intake.

From Institute of Medicine (1998) Dietary Reference Intakes: Thiamin, Riboflavin, Niacin, Vitamin B$_6$, Folate, Vitamin B$_{12}$, Pantothenic Acid, Biotin, and Choline. National Academy Press, Washington, D.C.

the mucosal cell and is released across the basolateral membrane into the portal circulation is not well understood. Some metabolism of folate, primarily to 5-methyl-H$_4$PteGlu, can occur during this process, but metabolism is not required for transport. The degree of metabolism in the intestinal mucosa is dependent on the folate dose given. When pharmacological doses of various folates are given, most of the transported vitamin appears unchanged in the portal circulation.

The bioavailability of folic acid when given as a supplement or in fortified food is high (Jackson et al., 1997). However, the bioavailability of food folate is less than 50% and may be significantly lower than this because recent studies have suggested that methods commonly used for the analysis of folate in foodstuffs may have underestimated the folate content. Pharmacological doses of folate are well absorbed, but most of the vitamin is not retained in the body due to a

limited capacity of tissues to retain large amounts of folate.

TRANSPORT AND TISSUE ACCUMULATION OF FOLATE

Pteroylmonoglutamates, primarily 5-methyl-H$_4$PteGlu, are the circulating forms of folate in plasma, and mammalian tissues cannot transport polyglutamates with chains of more than two glutamyl residues. After folate absorption into the portal circulation, much of this folate can be taken up by the liver via the reduced folate carrier. In the liver, it is metabolized to polyglutamate derivatives and retained, or it may be released into blood. Some folate is secreted in bile, but this can be reabsorbed in the intestine via an enterohepatic circulation. The plasma folate concentration in humans is usually in the 10 to 30 nmol/L range. The predominance of 5-methyl-

H$_4$PteGlu in plasma probably reflects that this is the major cytosolic folate in mammalian tissues. The extent of release of short-chain folylpolyglutamates from tissues is unknown. Plasma contains a soluble γ-glutamylhydrolase activity, and any polyglutamate released into plasma would be hydrolyzed to the monoglutamate.

Some plasma folate is bound to low-affinity protein binders, primarily albumin. Plasma also contains low levels of a high-affinity folate-binding protein. The levels of the high-affinity binder are increased in pregnancy and are very high in some leukemia patients, although the physiological significance of this is unclear. The high-affinity binder is a soluble form of a second membrane–associated folate transporter known as folate-binding protein, or the folate receptor. There are at least three distinct folate-binding protein genes, and the encoded protein is usually attached to the plasma membrane of cells via a glycosylphosphatidylinositol anchor. High levels of folate-binding protein are expressed in the choroid plexus, kidney proximal tubes, and placenta and in a number of human tumors, whereas lower levels have been found in a variety of other tissues. Folate-binding protein effects reabsorption of folate in the kidney by a receptor-mediated endocytotic process and is believed to play a similar role in folate transport in other tissues. The function of the soluble form of folate-binding protein, which is expressed at high levels in milk, is not understood, but it may also play a role in folate transport.

Red blood cells contain higher levels of folate (normally 0.5 to 1 μmol/L) than does plasma. Mature red cells do not transport or accumulate folate; their folate stores are formed during erythropoiesis and are retained, probably due to binding to hemoglobin, through the 120-day life span of the human red cell. Red cell folate levels are often used as a measure of long-term folate status. Fasting plasma folate levels also are an indicator of status, but plasma levels also can be influenced by recent dietary intake.

INTRACELLULAR METABOLISM AND TURNOVER OF FOLATE

The interconversion of folate one-carbon forms is intertwined with the metabolic roles of folate and is outlined later. Folate coenzymes are found primarily in the mitochondria and cytosol of the cell, and accumulation of folate in these compartments requires the conversion of folates to polyglutamates, which is catalyzed by the enzyme folylpolyglutamate synthetase (Shane, 1989).

$$MgATP + Folate(glu_n) + Glutamate \rightarrow$$
$$MgADP + Folate(glu_{n+1}) + P_i$$

Folylpolyglutamate synthetase is encoded by a single human gene, and cytosolic and mitochondrial isozymes are generated by alternative transcription start sites for the gene and by alternative translational start sites for its mRNA. Tetrahydrofolate and its polyglutamate forms are the preferred substrates for folylpolyglutamate synthetase, whereas 5-substituted folates such as 5-methyl-H$_4$PteGlu are poor substrates. Because 5-methyl-H$_4$PteGlu is the major folate transported into most tissues, the extent of folate accumulation is dependent on a tissue's ability to metabolize 5-methyl-H$_4$PteGlu to H$_4$PteGlu via the methionine synthase reaction (Figs. 21–2, 21–3). Rapid efflux of unmetabolized 5-methyl-H$_4$PteGlu from the tissue to plasma occurs.

The mitochondrial folate transporter has not been well characterized but is specific for reduced folates. The major hepatic mitochondrial folates are 10-formyl-H$_4$PteGlu$_n$ and H$_4$PteGlu$_n$, and much of the latter is bound to two folate enzymes, dimethylglycine dehydrogenase and sarcosine dehydrogenase. A large proportion of the major cytosolic folate in liver, 5-methyl-H$_4$PteGlu$_n$, is bound to glycine N-methyltransferase, whereas much of the H$_4$PteGlu$_n$ is bound to 10-formyltetrahydrofolate dehydrogenase.

Tissues contain a soluble lysosomal γ-glutamylhydrolase activity, sometimes called folate conjugase, that may be involved in the hydrolysis of folylpolyglutamates with their subsequent release from the tissue. However, the major route of folate turnover and catabolism appears to involve the degradation of folate coenzymes to pterin derivatives and aminobenzoylpolyglutamates via oxidative cleavage at the C-9, N-10 bond. Recent studies suggest that the enzyme responsible for this cleavage is specific for 5-formyl-H$_4$PteGlu$_n$. The aminobenzoylpolyglutamates generated are

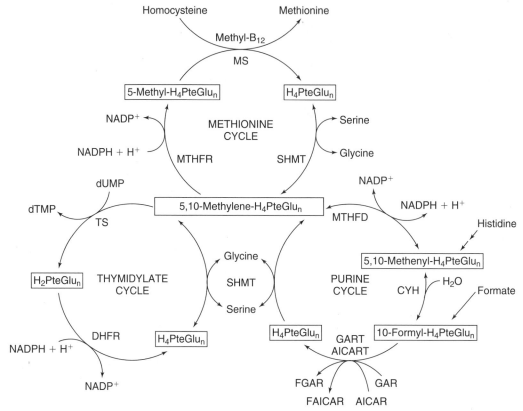

Figure 21–2. *The major metabolic cycles of folate-dependent one-carbon metabolism in the cytoplasm of cells. SHMT, serine hydroxymethyltransferase; MTHFR, methylenetetrahydrofolate reductase; MS, methionine synthase; TS, thymidylate synthase; DHFR, dihydrofolate reductase; MTHFD, methylenetetrahydrofolate dehydrogenase; CYH, methenyltetrahydrofolate cyclohydrolase; GAR, glycinamide ribonucleotide; GART, GAR formyltransferase; AICAR, 5-amino-4-imidazolecarboxamide ribonucleotide; AICART, AICAR formyltransferase; dUMP, 2-deoxyuridine 5'-phosphate; dTMP, 2-deoxythymidine 5'-phosphate.*

hydrolyzed to aminobenzoylglutamate by lyso-somal γ-glutamylhydrolase and *N*-acetylated, at least in liver, and the *N*-acetyl-aminoben-zoylglutamate is excreted in the urine. In humans, only very small amounts of intact folate are found in urine, and cleavage products represent the bulk of the excretion.

METABOLIC FUNCTIONS OF FOLATE

Folate coenzymes act as acceptors or donors of one-carbon units in a variety of reactions involved in amino acid and nucleotide metabolism in mammalian tissues. The various metabolic cycles of one-carbon metabolism in the cytosol and mitochondria of mammalian tissues are shown in Figures 21–2, 21–3, and 21–4.

Folate and One-Carbon Metabolism

Although the major pathways of methionine, thymidylate, and purine synthesis occur in the cytosol, extensive folate metabolism occurs in the mitochondria; mitochondrial folate metabolism plays an important role in glycine metabolism and in providing one-carbon units for cytosolic one-carbon metabolism. Folate coenzymes act as co-substrates in these reactions. Consequently, folate metabolism and its regulation are interwoven with the regulation of the synthesis of products of one-carbon metabolism, and factors that regulate any one cycle of one-carbon metabolism would be expected to influence folate availability for the other cycles of one-carbon metabolism. The C-3 of serine is the major source of one-carbon units for folate metabolism. Additional

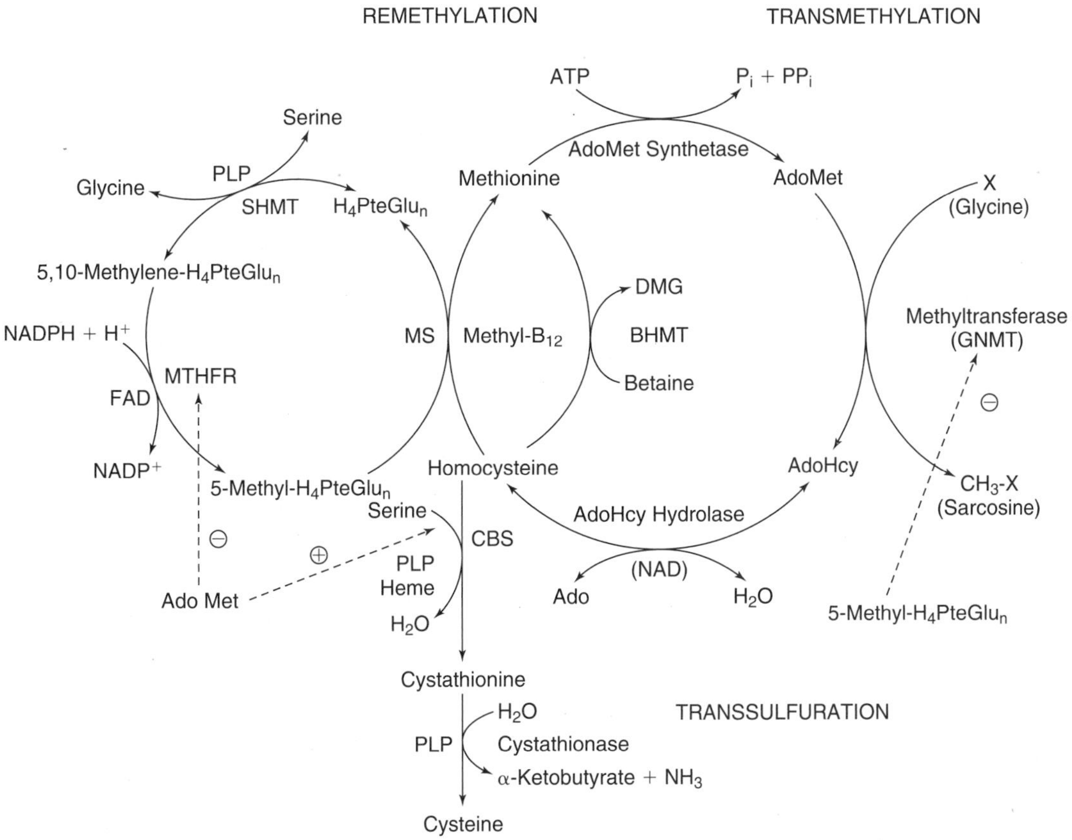

REMETHYLATION   TRANSMETHYLATION

Figure 21–3. *The folate-dependent methionine resynthesis cycle and its relationship to transmethylation and transsulfuration cycles in tissues. SHMT, serine hydroxymethyltransferase; MTHFR, methylenetetrahydrofolate reductase; MS, methionine synthase; BHMT, betaine homocysteine methyltransferase (liver-specific); DMG, dimethylglycine; GNMT, glycine N-methyltransferase (primarily liver and kidney); AdoMet, S-adenosylmethionine; AdoHcy, S-adenosylhomocysteine; X, methyl acceptor; CBS, cystathionine β-synthase.*

sources include formate, much of which is derived from serine metabolism in the mitochondria, and the imidazole ring C-2 of histidine.

Folates in mammalian tissues are metabolized to polyglutamates of chain lengths considerably longer than the triglutamate form required for folate retention. For most folate-dependent enzymes, the major kinetic advantages are achieved by elongation of the glutamate chain to the triglutamate. Longer polyglutamate forms are required for the enzymes involved in the methionine resynthesis cycle. Many of the enzymes involved in folate metabolism are multifunctional, with multiple catalytic sites on a single protein, or are part of multiprotein complexes. For some of these complexes, the longer polyglutamate derivatives allow channeling of substrates between active sites without release of intermediate products from the complex. The polyglutamate tail is believed to be "anchored" to a site on the complex. Channeling of substrates between active sites prevents the accumulation of intermediate products in bulk cell water and increases the efficiency of metabolic pathways.

Amino Acid Metabolism

Interconversion of Serine and Glycine. Serine hydroxymethyltransferase, a PLP-containing enzyme, catalyzes the reversible transfer of formaldehyde from serine to $H_4PteGlu_n$ to generate 5,10-methylene-$H_4PteGlu_n$ and glycine (see Fig. 21–2; also described in Chapter 11, Fig. 11–18):

Serine + $H_4PteGlu_n$ ↔
    Glycine + 5,10-Methylene-$H_4PteGlu_n$

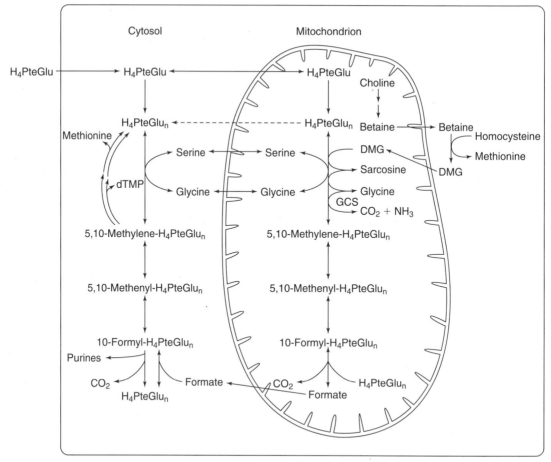

Figure 21–4. *Compartmentalization of folate-dependent one-carbon metabolism. Mitochondrial choline degradation is restricted primarily to liver, whereas the mitochondrial glycine cleavage system (GCS) is primarily present in liver and kidney. DMG, dimethylglycine.*

Mammalian cells contain two serine hydroxy-methyltransferase isozymes, one cytosolic and one mitochondrial, encoded by separate genes. The cytosolic enzyme is the predominant species in liver, although the mitochondrial form predominates in cultured cells. Serine hydroxymethyltransferase is an abundant protein in liver, and the C-3 of serine is the major source of one-carbon units for folate metabolism. The 5,10-methylene-$H_4PteGlu_n$ formed in this reaction plays a central role in one-carbon metabolism because its one-carbon moiety can be directed into the three cytosolic one-carbon cycles of methionine, de novo purine, and thymidylate synthesis (see Fig. 21–2).

The directionality of the serine hydroxymethyltransferase reactions in the cytosol and mitochondria is not well understood. Serine,

a nonessential amino acid, may be derived from glucose or obtained from the diet. Some tissues are net producers of glycine whereas others, such as kidney, are net producers of serine from glycine. Mammalian cell mutants that lack mitochondrial serine hydroxymethyltransferase activity but have normal levels of cytosolic activity require exogenous glycine for growth. Serine and glycine are rapidly transported across the mitochondrial membrane, whereas transport of reduced folate occurs at a much slower rate. Although this suggests that the mitochondrial isozyme is required for net glycine synthesis, it is possible that the cytosolic enzyme is associated with the enzymes of cytosolic one-carbon metabolism and that the serine to glycine flux in the cytosol is regulated by the needs for one-carbon units for the various cycles of one-carbon metabolism. Glycine is a gluconeogenic amino acid, which suggests that, in liver and kidney at least, the net flux through one of the hydroxymethyltransferase isozymes will be in the direction of serine synthesis under normal conditions of net gluconeogenesis.

The major pathway of glycine catabolism is via the glycine cleavage system (Fig. 21–4), a reaction in which an additional one-carbon moiety is supplied to the folate pool:

$$\text{Glycine} + \text{H}_4\text{PteGlu}_n + \text{NAD}^+ \rightarrow$$
$$\text{5,10-Methylene-H}_4\text{PteGlu}_n + \text{NADH}$$
$$+ \text{CO}_2 + \text{NH}_4{}^+$$

The mitochondrial glycine cleavage system, which is present in high concentrations in liver and kidney, is a multienzyme complex with four components. P-protein, which contains PLP, catalyzes glycine decarboxylation and transfer of methylamine to lipoic acid on H-protein. The lipoic acid is reduced, and the carbon moiety from glycine is oxidized to the level of formaldehyde. T-protein catalyzes the transfer of formaldehyde to H$_4$PteGlu$_n$, and the reduced lipoate on H-protein is reoxidized by NAD$^+$ in a reaction catalyzed by L-protein. Although potentially reversible, the glycine cleavage system does not appear to play a role in the synthesis of glycine. Coupling of the serine hydroxymethyltransferase and glycine cleavage systems provides a mechanism for the synthesis of serine from glycine. One molecule of serine can arise by reversal of the hydroxymethyltransferase, with the 5,10-methylene-H$_4$PteGlu$_n$ required arising from oxidative decarboxylation of an additional molecule of glycine via the cleavage system.

Serine hydroxymethyltransferase also catalyzes the conversion of 5,10-methenyl-H$_4$PteGlu$_n$ to 5-formyl-H$_4$PteGlu$_n$. 5-Formyl-H$_4$PteGlu$_n$ is a potent inhibitor of some folate-dependent enzymes, including serine hydroxymethyltransferase, and is the substrate for the folate catabolism enzyme; it is not used directly as a substrate in one-carbon transfer reactions. 5-Formyl-H$_4$PteGlu$_n$ can be reconverted to 5,10-methenyl-H$_4$PteGlu$_n$ by methenyltetrahydrofolate synthetase:

$$\text{5-Formyl-H}_4\text{PteGlu}_n + \text{MgATP} \rightarrow$$
$$[\text{5,10-Methenyl-H}_4\text{PteGlu}_n]^+ + \text{MgADP} + \text{P}_i$$

5-Formyl-H$_4$PteGlu is used clinically and experimentally as a source of reduced folate because it is more stable than other reduced folates.

Methionine Cycle. A major cytosolic cycle of one-carbon utilization involves the reduction of 5,10-methylene-H$_4$PteGlu$_n$ to 5-methyl-H$_4$PteGlu$_n$, followed by the transfer of the methyl group to homocysteine to form methionine and regenerate H$_4$PteGlu$_n$ (see Fig. 21–3).

5,10-Methylene-H$_4$PteGlu$_n$ reduction is catalyzed by the flavoprotein methylenetetrahydrofolate reductase:

$$\text{5,10-Methylene-H}_4\text{PteGlu}_n + \text{NADPH} + \text{H}^+ \rightarrow$$
$$\text{5-Methyl-H}_4\text{PteGlu}_n + \text{NADP}^+$$

The reaction is irreversible under in vivo conditions and is the committed step in methionine synthesis.

The next enzyme in this cycle, methionine synthase, is one of only two B$_{12}$-dependent mammalian enzymes, and it catalyzes the transfer of the methyl group from 5-methyl-H$_4$PteGlu$_n$ to homocysteine:

$$\text{5-Methyl-H}_4\text{PteGlu}_n + \text{Homocysteine} \rightarrow$$
$$\text{H}_4\text{PteGlu}_n + \text{Methionine}$$

The methionine synthase reaction is the only reaction in which the methyl group of 5-methyl-H$_4$PteGlu$_n$ can be metabolized in mammalian tissues. Although methionine is an essential amino acid, the methionine synthase reaction plays a major role in methyl group metabolism because it allows the reutilization of the homocysteine backbone as a carrier of methyl groups derived primarily from the C-3 of serine. The enzyme contains tightly bound cob(I)alamin, and the reaction proceeds via a methylcob(III)alamin intermediate, described later in this chapter.

Homocysteine is not found in the diet but arises from hydrolysis of S-adenosylhomocysteine (AdoHcy), the product of S-adenosylmethionine (AdoMet)-dependent methylation reactions (see Fig. 21–3). Homocysteine can be metabolized to cysteine in reactions catalyzed by two pyridoxal 5′-phosphate (PLP)-dependent enzymes, cystathionine β-synthase and cystathionase. This transsulfuration pathway is described in Chapter 11. Alternatively, homocysteine can be converted back to methionine via the folate-dependent methionine synthase reaction described earlier or by betaine-homocysteine methyltransferase, which catalyzes the transfer of one of the methyl groups of betaine to homocysteine to generate methionine and dimethylglycine. Betaine arises from choline oxidation in liver mitochondria (Fig. 21–4). The cytosolic betaine methyltransferase does not contain bound cobalamin and does not use a folate coenzyme as a substrate. It is present in high concentrations in liver, but its physiological significance in terms of methionine and methyl group status is not clear. The dimethylglycine product of the methyltransferase reaction is converted to glycine in the mitochondria. The folate-dependent mitochondrial flavoproteins dimethylglycine dehydrogenase and sarcosine dehydrogenase catalyze the oxidative demethylation of dimethylglycine to sarcosine and sarcosine to glycine, respectively, with the generation of 5,10-methylene-H_4PteGlu$_n$.

The extent of homocysteine remethylation or transsulfuration is tissue-dependent, and many tissues export homocysteine and cystathionine into the circulation. Tissue levels of homocysteine are normally low; increased homocysteine causes increased levels of AdoHcy, an inhibitor of many methylation reactions. Kidney and liver are thought to be important organs for homocysteine remethylation and for transsulfuration.

Remethylation is also dependent on the methyl group status of the tissue. The major regulator of the folate-dependent methionine cycle is AdoMet, which is a potent allosteric inhibitor of methylenetetrahydrofolate reductase (see Fig. 21–3). Liver contains a high K_m AdoMet synthetase, and hepatic levels of AdoMet reflect methionine status. High levels of AdoMet inhibit the reductase, reducing remethylation of homocysteine, and activate cystathionine β-synthase, stimulating transsulfuration of homocysteine to cysteine. Conversely, when AdoMet is low, remethylation of homocysteine is favored and transsulfuration is inhibited.

Liver and kidney also contain a major cytosolic protein, glycine N-methyltransferase, that acts as a sink for excess methyl groups. This enzyme catalyzes the AdoMet-dependent methylation of glycine to sarcosine. Although folate is not a substrate for this enzyme, 5-methyl-H_4PteGlu$_n$ is a potent inhibitor, and the protein is a major cytosolic folate-binding protein. When AdoMet levels are high, methylenetetrahydrofolate reductase is inhibited, reducing 5-methyl-H_4PteGlu$_n$ formation and relieving inhibition of glycine methyltransferase, thus allowing removal of excess methyl groups. At low AdoMet concentrations, methylenetetrahydrofolate reductase is more active, 5-methyl-H_4PteGlu$_n$ accumulates, and glycine methyltransferase is inhibited. Excess methionine, which can be toxic, results in an elevated level of sarcosine, some of which is excreted in urine.

Although methylenetetrahydrofolate reductase is the major regulatory enzyme in the methionine cycle, the significant proportion of methylfolates in tissues suggests that the methionine synthase reaction is also an important rate-limiting step in the metabolic cycles of one-carbon metabolism. Both methylenetetrahydrofolate reductase and methionine synthase are low-abundance proteins and are present at considerably lower concentrations than most of the other enzymes involved in the metabolism of folate coenzymes.

5-Methyl-H_4PteGlu is the major form of folate taken up by tissues. Removal of the methyl group, via the methionine synthase reaction, is required before the entering folate can be utilized in other reactions of one-carbon metabolism or metabolized to polyglutamates that are retained by cells. As the entering monoglutamate has to compete with the preferred 5-methyl-H_4PteGlu$_n$ substrates, incorporation of exogenous folate by tissues is repressed by high intracellular folate or by expansion of the 5-methyl-H_4PteGlu$_n$ pool.

Histidine Catabolism. The C-2 of the imidazole ring of histidine provides one-carbon units at the oxidation level of formate for one-carbon metabolism. Cytosolic formiminoglutamate formiminotransferase catalyzes the transfer of a formimino group from formiminoglutamate, an intermediate in the histidine catabolism pathway, to H_4PteGlu$_n$, as follows:

NUTRITION INSIGHT

New Recommendations for Choline Intake

Choline is formed in vivo by the synthesis and degradation of phosphatidylcholine, which occurs mainly in the liver. Adenosylmethionine serves as the methyl group donor for the three methylations involved in the conversion of phosphatidylethanolamine to phosphatidylcholine. Degradation of phosphatidylcholine gives rise to free choline. The free choline, which can also come from the diet, can be reconverted to phosphatidylcholine via formation of phosphocholine and CDP-choline and addition of phosphocholine to diacylglycerol, but this is a quantitatively less important pathway than the pathway for phosphatidylcholine synthesis from phosphatidylethanolamine. In addition to being a component of phospholipids, choline is required for synthesis of acetylcholine, a neurotransmitter, and serves as a precursor of betaine, which can donate a methyl group to homocysteine to reform methionine. Clearly, choline metabolism is related to overall methyl group metabolism and requirements because adenosylmethionine is a donor of methyl groups in the endogenous synthesis of choline and because betaine, derived from choline, can be a source of preformed methyl groups for synthesis of methionine and hence adenosylmethionine.

Choline is present as part of phospholipids in foods such as eggs, liver, and soybeans and as free choline in certain vegetables such as cauliflower. In addition, lecithin (phosphatidylcholine) is added to some processed foods as an emulsifying agent. Betaine is present in some foods such as beets. Average daily intake of choline in the United States is estimated to be about 400 to 900 mg. Choline is usually added to infant formulas in amounts that approximate the choline content of human milk.

Although dietary choline has been considered an important component of animal diets for a number of years, human needs for dietary choline are not well defined. Choline needs can be met at least partially by endogenous synthesis, and it is not clear whether a dietary supply of choline is needed at any or all stages of the life cycle. A single dietary depletion study in healthy adult men demonstrated an increase in plasma alanine aminotransferase levels, which may have suggested abnormal liver function. The Food and Nutrition Board of the National Academy of Sciences, Institute of Medicine (1998) recently set Adequate Intakes (AIs) for choline based on or extrapolated from the intakes required to maintain normal aminotransferase levels in these subjects.

Adequate Intakes for Choline Across the Life Cycle

	mg choline/day
Infants, 0–5 mo	125
6–11 mo	150
Children, 1–3 y	200
4–8 y	250
9–13 y	375
Males, > 13 y	550
Females, 14–18 y	400
> 18 y	425
Pregnant	450
Lactating	550

Formiminoglutamate + H$_4$PteGlu$_n$ →
    5-Formimino-H$_4$PteGlu$_n$ + Glutamate

The formimino moiety is converted to 5,10-methenyl-H$_4$PteGlu$_n$ in a formiminotetrahydrofolate cyclodeaminase catalyzed reaction:

5-Formimino-H$_4$PteGlu$_n$ + H$^+$ →
    [5,10-Methenyl-H$_4$PteGlu$_n$]$^+$ + NH$_3$

Formiminotransferase and cyclodeaminase activities reside on a single bifunctional protein. In folate deficiency, formiminoglutamate catabolism is impaired, and it is excreted in elevated amounts in urine.

Nucleotide Synthesis

Thymidylate Cycle. Folates are not involved in the de novo synthesis of the pyrimidine ring (described in Chapter 11, Fig. 11–15). However, folate is required for the synthesis of thymidylate (see Fig. 21–2). Thymidylate synthase catalyzes the transfer of formaldehyde from folate to the 5-position of deoxyuridylate:

$$5,10\text{-Methylene-}H_4PteGlu_n + dUMP \rightarrow$$
$$H_2PteGlu_n + dTMP$$

$H_4PteGlu_n$ provides the reducing component for reduction of the transferred methylene moiety to a methyl group and is oxidized to $H_2PteGlu_n$ in the process. $H_2PteGlu_n$ is inactive as a coenzyme and has to be reduced back to $H_4PteGlu_n$, in a reaction catalyzed by dihydrofolate reductase, before it can play a further role in one-carbon metabolism:

$$H_2PteGlu_n + NADPH + H^+ \rightarrow$$
$$H_4PteGlu_n + NADP^+$$

Dihydrofolate reductase also catalyzes the reduction of pharmaceutical folic acid to dihydrofolate, although folic acid is a poorer substrate than is dihydrofolate. The major role of dihydrofolate reductase is the reduction of $H_2PteGlu_n$ formed during thymidylate synthesis, and it also reduces dietary $H_2PteGlu$.

Thymidylate synthase activity is expressed only in replicating tissues, and expression of the synthase and dihydrofolate reductase mRNA is highest during the S phase of the cell cycle. Folate antagonists that inhibit these enzymes have been used extensively as anticancer agents. Methotrexate, a 4-aminofolic acid analog, is a potent inhibitor of dihydrofolate reductase. Treatment of rapidly growing cells with this drug causes trapping of folate in the nonfunctional dihydrofolate form. Slowly growing tissues, which have negligible or low levels of thymidylate synthase activity, do not convert reduced folate to the dihydrofolate form as rapidly, so are less affected by a dihydrofolate reductase inhibitor.

Clinical resistance to drugs such as methotrexate often develops. Mechanisms for resistance include a decrease in the level of, or a mutation in, the reduced folate carrier resulting in decreased methotrexate uptake; amplification of the dihydrofolate reductase gene resulting in an increase in the level of enzyme activity; and a decrease in folylpolyglutamate synthetase activity which reduces accumulation of the drug by the tissue.

Purine Cycle. $10\text{-Formyl-}H_4PteGlu_n$ is used in two steps of de novo cytosolic purine biosynthesis (see Chapter 11, Fig. 11–14). The C-8 and C-2 positions of the purine ring are derived from $10\text{-formyl-}H_4PteGlu_n$ in reactions catalyzed by glycinamide ribonucleotide (GAR) transformylase and 5-amino-4-imidazolecarboxamide ribonucleotide (AICAR) transformylase (see Fig. 21–2):

$$10\text{-Formyl-}H_4PteGlu_n + GAR \rightarrow$$
$$H_4PteGlu_n + \text{Formyl-GAR}$$

$$10\text{-Formyl-}H_4PteGlu_n + AICAR \rightarrow$$
$$H_4PteGlu_n + \text{Formyl-AICAR}$$

$10\text{-Formyl-}H_4PteGlu_n$ is formed by the oxidation of $5,10\text{-methylene-}H_4PteGlu_n$, which is catalyzed reversibly by methylenetetrahydrofolate dehydrogenase and methenyltetrahydrofolate cyclohydrolase (see Fig. 21–2):

$$5,10\text{-Methylene-}H_4PteGlu_n + NADP^+ \leftrightarrow$$
$$[5,10\text{-Methenyl-}H_4PteGlu_n]^+ + NADPH$$

$$[5,10\text{-Methenyl-}H_4PteGlu_n]^+ + H_2O \leftrightarrow$$
$$10\text{-Formyl-}H_4PteGlu_n + H^+$$

Alternatively, $10\text{-formyl-}H_4PteGlu_n$ can be obtained by the direct formylation of $H_4PteGlu_n$ (Fig. 21–4), catalyzed by formyltetrahydrofolate synthetase:

$$\text{Formate} + MgATP + H_4PteGlu_n \rightarrow$$
$$10\text{-Formyl-}H_4PteGlu_n + MgADP + P_i$$

The dehydrogenase, cyclohydrolase and synthetase are associated on a single trifunctional protein in mammalian tissues that is called C_1 synthase. The synthase consists of two separate domains: one contains the dehydrogenase and cyclohydrolase activities and the other the synthetase activity.

Mitochondria can also interconvert 5,10-methylene-H_4PteGlu$_n$ and 10-formyl-H_4PteGlu$_n$, and this is thought to be catalyzed by a mitochondrial C_1 synthase (Fig. 21–4). Mitochondria convert the folate one-carbon to formate, which can then leave the mitochondria and be used for cytosolic purine biosynthesis. A separate bifunctional 5,10-methylenetetrahydrofolate dehydrogenase-cyclohydrolase that uses NAD^+ rather than $NADP^+$ as the acceptor has also been described. This mitochondrial enzyme activity is found in embryonic, undifferentiated, and transformed tissues and cells. One suggested role for this enzyme is to increase the one-carbon flux into purine biosynthesis and away from other one-carbon cycles such as methionine synthesis.

Disposal of One-Carbon Units

One-carbon moieties are oxidized to CO_2 in a reaction catalyzed by 10-formyltetrahydrofolate dehydrogenase (Fig. 21–4):

$$10\text{-Formyl-}H_4\text{PteGlu}_n + NADP^+ + H_2O \rightarrow$$
$$H_4\text{PteGlu}_n + CO_2 + NADPH + H^+$$

The purified enzyme also catalyzes the hydrolysis of 10-formyl-H_4PteGlu$_n$ to H_4PteGlu$_n$ and formate. In liver, the metabolic flux through this reaction may be regulated by the 10-formyl-H_4PteGlu$_n$/H_4PteGlu$_n$ ratio rather than by the tissue concentration of 10-formyl-H_4PteGlu$_n$, because the concentrations of these folates are in excess of their K_m and K_i values for the enzyme under physiological conditions. The physiological role of this protein would appear to be to regulate the proportion of folate present in the H_4PteGlu$_n$ form, presumably to make it available for other reactions of one-carbon metabolism.

FOLATE DEFICIENCY: SYMPTOMS AND METABOLIC BASES

Folate deficiency is usually due to a dietary insufficiency, although it can arise from other causes such as malabsorption syndromes or drug treatment. A number of cases of increased requirement due to genetic heterogeneity recently have been identified, including some individuals who require increased folate in early pregnancy to reduce the risk of birth defects. As might be expected from its metabolic roles, the clinical effects of deficiency are related to defects in DNA synthesis, particularly in fast-growing tissues, and in methyl group metabolism. The classical symptom is a megaloblastic anemia reflecting deranged DNA synthesis in erythropoietic cells. Folate deficiency is also associated with increased risk for vascular disease (Rimm et al., 1998) and an increased incidence of some cancers. Depression and a polyneuropathy have also been reported, although the evidence linking folate deficiency to neurological disease is not conclusive. However, in frank genetic diseases, involving rare cases of severe defects in various folate-dependent enzymes, neurological symptoms have been clearly documented, with many cases of mental retardation.

Megaloblastic Anemia

Megaloblastic anemia is characterized by enlarged red cells and hypersegmentation of the nuclei of circulating polymorphonuclear leukocytes with reduced cell number. Megaloblastic changes also occur in other tissues, but the condition is usually detected clinically by the anemia. The megaloblastic anemia of folate deficiency is identical to that observed in vitamin B_{12} deficiency. Folate deficiency anemia was not observed, in a single study, in subjects with red cell folate levels above 140 ng/mL (320 nmol/L). Megaloblastic cells have almost two-fold the normal content of DNA, and the cells are arrested in the G2 phase of the cell cycle just prior to mitosis, preventing cell division. The DNA contains breaks suggesting a defect in DNA synthesis or repair. If cell division occurs, the cells undergo apoptosis (programmed cell death).

These defects are thought to be caused by defective thymidylate synthesis coupled with an enlarged deoxyuridine triphosphate (dUTP) pool that results in uracil misincorporation into DNA. Damaged reticulocytes and red cells are normally removed by the spleen. Splenectomized subjects with low red cell folate levels have an increased uracil content and double-strand breaks in their DNA, and folate supplementation reverses these abnormal findings (Blount et al., 1997). Uracil in DNA normally arises from deamination of cytosine, which constantly occurs at a slow rate. Since uracil behaves exactly as thymidine in DNA, cytosine deamination to uracil can lead to a mutagenic change from a cytosine-guanine (C-G) base pair to a uracil (thymine)-adenine [U(T)-A] base pair during replication. Normally, this potential damage is repaired by uracil-DNA glycosylase, which removes the uracil base. A few additional bases are removed on either side of the damage, and the DNA is repaired by complementary base pairing, with a C being reinserted opposite the G. Tissues also contain a dUTPase, which hydrolyzes dUTP to dUMP and keeps dUTP levels very low. Uracil misincorporation in place of thymidine during DNA synthesis or repair is normally minimized by competition between the small dUTP pool and the larger deoxythymidine triphosphate (dTTP) pool. If uracil is misincorporated in place of T (opposite an A), the glycosylase removes the uracil and a T is reinserted. In folate deficiency, thymidylate pools are depressed and dUTP pools are increased, leading to increased uracil incorporation instead of dTTP. Increased repair by the glycosylase would lead to more transient single-strand breaks. In addition, repair of the damage by reinsertion of thymidine is inefficient due to the lower thymidylate pools, and the probability of uracil being reinserted by mistake is higher, which leads to prolongation of the single-strand breaks. If uracil is misincorporated on both DNA strands in close proximity, a double-strand break, which cannot be repaired, can occur during the uracil-DNA glycosylase-mediated repair.

Cancer

Epidemiological studies have suggested that folate deficiency is associated with increased risk for certain types of cancer, including colon cancer. The mechanism behind this has not been ascertained, but uracil misincorporation arising from defective thymidylate synthesis has been hypothesized as one possibility. Transcription of many genes is turned off during development by methylation of their promoter regions, and changes in gene methylation have been observed in tumors. As folate deficiency impairs the remethylation of homocysteine to methionine and alters AdoMet/AdoHcy ratios, it has also been proposed that the increased cancer risk in folate deficiency may be due to hypomethylation of DNA. It has been demonstrated that methionine deficiency causes hypomethylation of DNA. However, a clear demonstration that folate deficiency results in DNA hypomethylation remains to be carried out.

The increased cancer risk in folate-deficient subjects is reduced in subjects homozygous for a common polymorphism in methylenetetrahydrofolate reductase (Ma et al., 1997, also see later). This polymorphism causes decreased enzyme activity and presumably impaired conversion of 5,10-methylene-H_4PteGlu$_n$ to 5-methyl-H_4PteGlu$_n$. It is thought that this allows a redirection of more of the folate one-carbons into the cycles of nucleotide biosynthesis in these subjects.

Cancer Treatment

Folate antagonists that are inhibitors of thymidylate synthase, dihydrofolate reductase, and de novo purine biosynthetic enzymes have been used extensively for the treatment of a variety of cancers. These metabolic poisons, which cause a functional folate deficiency, generally show a selective toxicity for rapidly growing tumors because of the increased rates of DNA synthesis in these tumors. In experimental animals, toxicity and drug effectiveness are reduced by the provision of purines and thymidine. Uracil misincorporation and apoptosis have been demonstrated as the mechanism for cell death. Uracil misincorporation is also potentially mutagenic, and successful treatment with antifolates, or with many other drugs used for cancer chemotherapy, for that matter, carries the risk of further cancers after 10 to 20 years.

Hyperhomocysteinemia and Vascular Disease

It has long been known that severe genetic conditions that result in homocystinuria and a very marked hyperhomocysteinemia are associated with a variety of clinical symptoms, including early-onset occlusive cardiovascular and cerebrovascular disease. These genetic diseases include deficiencies of methylenetetrahydrofolate reductase and cystathionine β-synthase, enzymes involved in the homocysteine remethylation and transsulfuration pathways, respectively. Elevated homocysteine increases proliferation of smooth muscle cells and inhibits proliferation of endothelial cells by a mechanism that is not understood. Many potential reasons for the adverse effects of homocysteine have been described. These include effects on transcription factors involved in regulation of cell growth, disulfide bond formation with proteins such as apolipoprotein B-100, modulation of nitric oxide (NO) synthase activity, and increased cellular AdoHcy levels. It has not been established whether any of these potential adverse changes is responsible for vascular disease.

Recently, it has been recognized that chronic mild hyperhomocysteinemia is a major risk factor for occlusive vascular disease (Refsum et al., 1998). Plasma homocysteine concentrations in patients with vascular disease are about 30% higher than in controls, and carotid artery stenosis is positively correlated with plasma homocysteine concentrations over the entire range of normal and abnormal homocysteine values (Selhub et al., 1995). Prospective assessment of vascular disease risk in men with higher homocysteine concentrations indicated that plasma homocysteine levels only 12% above the upper limit of normal levels are associated with a threefold increase in acute myocardial infarction. (See Chapter 41 for more discussion of risk factors for cardiovascular disease.)

Elevated plasma homocysteine levels are responsive to increased folate intake. Fasting homocysteine levels have been inversely correlated with both plasma folate and food folate intake. Increased folate intake lowers the mean homocysteine of groups, with the greatest effect on those with the highest plasma homocysteine levels. A common polymorphism [alanine (ala) to valine (val)] in methylenetetrahydrofolate reductase that results in a "heat-labile" enzyme and decreased enzyme activity in tissues has been implicated as one

reason for the folate-responsiveness of a subset of hyperhomocysteinemic subjects (Frosst et al., 1995). The incidence of the val/val homozygote (around 10% in most populations) is significantly greater in subjects with higher homocysteine levels. Although the contribution of this polymorphism to elevated homocysteine levels has varied from study to study, and the incidence of the polymorphism varies among different population groups, the val/val polymorphism may at most contribute to or be associated with 30% of hyperhomocysteinemia. About 50% of the general population is heterozygous or homozygous for this polymorphism, and it is particularly interesting that a simple nutritional intervention may ameliorate at least some of the adverse effects of a potentially deleterious genetic trait. Although elevated homocysteine increases vascular disease risk, and increased folate intake decreases plasma homocysteine levels (Selhub et al., 1993), it remains to be determined whether increased folate intake reduces vascular disease risk.

B$_{12}$- and PLP-dependent enzymes are also involved in homocysteine metabolism. Impaired vitamin B$_{12}$ status also has been associated with higher concentrations of fasting plasma homocysteine in the general population, but B$_{12}$ is quantitatively a less important risk factor than is folate for hyperhomocysteinemia (Selhub et al., 1993). Improved vitamin B$_6$ status has little effect on fasting homocysteine levels but attenuates the increase in plasma homocysteine following a methionine load or a meal. The locus of the B$_6$ effect is believed to be the PLP-dependent cystathionine β-synthase, but a role for the PLP-dependent serine hydroxymethyltransferase cannot be excluded.

Birth Defects

Neural tube defects, including most forms of spina bifida, are the most common types of birth defect in humans, affecting about 0.1% of births. The recurrence rate for this condition is about 5%. The observation that periconceptual folate supplementation with folic acid reduced the incidence of these defects by about two thirds has led to fortification of the United States food supply with folic acid

NUTRITION INSIGHT

Genetic Heterogeneity and Vitamin Requirements; Methylenetetrahydrofolate Reductase Polymorphism and Homocysteinemia as an Example

Subjects who are homozygous for a common polymorphism in the methylenetetrahydrofolate reductase gene (C677T in the mRNA, resulting in an alanine to valine substitution) have lower lymphocyte methylenetetrahydrofolate reductase levels, higher plasma homocysteine levels, and a higher risk for vascular disease. Depending on the population, anywhere from 5% to 25% are homozygous and up to 50% heterozygous for this polymorphism, but the adverse effects are seen only in the homozygous val/val variant. The ala to val change in the protein lowers the affinity of the enzyme for its FAD cofactor but does not affect the affinity of the enzyme for its substrates. Apoprotein lacking FAD is unstable, and the metabolic effects of this polymorphism are due to lower amounts of enzyme rather than an abnormal enzyme activity. Folate stabilizes the enzyme by decreasing the rate of loss of FAD.

Among subjects with poor folate status, homozygotes for this polymorphism would be expected to display lower enzyme activity. Improved folate status would stabilize the protein, thus reducing the difference in enzyme level compared with control subjects. Although it is expected that metabolic and adverse effects of this polymorphism would primarily affect people with poorer folate status and may also be influenced by riboflavin status, the level of folate intake at which differences between the val/val and ala/ala variants become insignificant currently is not known. An important question that remains to be answered is whether the present RDA for folate is sufficient to normalize enzyme levels in val/val subjects or whether these individuals have a requirement that is higher than the RDA as set for the general population. It is likely that genetic polymorphisms, particularly common ones such as this, are responsible for much of the variation in nutrient requirements among individuals. As more information becomes available, RDAs may eventually be set based on the genotypes of individuals.

A genetic defect in an enzyme complicates the interpretation of normal measures of nutrient status. Although a general folate deficiency can be detected by impairments in a variety of folate status indicators, not all indicators will suggest impaired status when the impairment is due to a genetic change. The val/val variant in methylenetetrahydrofolate reductase impairs homocysteine remethylation but may redirect more of the folate one-carbon flux into nucleotide synthesis; this may explain why some studies have demonstrated a reduced risk of colon cancer in subjects with this polymorphism. Although reduced folate status may be indicated in val/val subjects by higher plasma homocysteine levels, the deoxyuridine suppression test, which measures folate-dependent thymidylate synthesis, may suggest improved folate status.

(Scott et al., 1990). The neural tube closes in the fourth week of gestation, and supplementation is useful only if given very early in pregnancy, at a time when many women do not realize they are pregnant. Although folate status affects the risk for neural tube defects, this condition is not thought to be a result of folate deficiency per se. It appears to be a genetic disease, possibly multigenetic, with a phenotype that can be modified by increased folate in the subset of individuals who are folate-responsive. As the mechanism behind the disease is not known, there is currently no screening technique to identify individuals at risk.

A defect in homocysteine metabolism has been proposed as a mechanism, although the evidence supporting this proposal can be considered only very preliminary. Plasma homocysteine levels are slightly higher in affected mothers, and homocysteine can cause teratogenic effects in embryo culture. An increased incidence of the homozygous ala to val polymorphism in methylenetetrahydrofolate reductase was reported that could account for at most 15% of neural tube defects. An epidemiological study suggested that vitamin B_{12} status is an independent risk factor for neural tube defects, which would implicate methionine synthase as a possible locus of

LIFE CYCLE CONSIDERATION

Folate and Birth Defects

The observation that periconceptual supplementation with folic acid reduces the incidence of neural tube defects—the major type of birth defects in humans—by greater than 70% is quite remarkable. Research in this area has focused on potential genetic causes, such as polymorphisms in genes encoding folate-dependent enzymes, and on potential environmental causes, such as reduced folate status, but the mechanism for the efficacy of increased folate intake is currently unknown. It is likely that these birth defects result from a combination of genetic and environmental factors. Experimental animals do not develop neural tube defects when placed on a folate-deficient diet during pregnancy. Although a number of mouse models of neural tube defects have been described and the causative genetic defect is known for some of these, none of the known defects appears to be responsible for human birth defects.

The risk of human neural tube defects is minimized by 400 μg/day of supplemental folic acid in addition to normal dietary folate intake. Lower levels of folic acid may be as effective, but this is not known. The additional folic acid is required in the first 3 weeks of pregnancy, a period when many women would not realize that they are pregnant. Furthermore, many women at risk may not be aware of, or be responsive to, the need for additional folate. Consequently, the American food supply is now fortified with sufficient folic acid to provide, on average, an additional 100 μg of folate, as folic acid, per day. This level of fortification was chosen to balance the potential benefits of increased folic acid on prevention of birth defects with the potential adverse effects of increased folate intake on masking symptoms of vitamin B$_{12}$ deficiency. Women of childbearing age would need to take an additional 300 μg of folic acid daily, either as a supplement or as increased intake of fortified food, to meet current recommendations.

Although fortification of the American food supply with folic acid has been instigated only recently, initial evaluations of the folate status of the United States population suggest that the current level of fortification has had a major impact. Significant elevations of plasma folate and decreases in plasma homocysteine levels have already been observed. Information on the extent to which this level of fortification protects against birth defects should be obtained in the next few years in this grand experiment on 250 million Americans.

the defect. The human methionine synthase gene has recently been cloned. However, no polymorphisms or mutations in this gene that track with neural tube defects have been identified thus far.

The folate intervention trials that established the protective effect of folic acid, coupled with other surveys, have indicated that 400 μg of supplemental folic acid, in addition to customary dietary folate intake, is sufficient to provide the maximum benefit in reducing the incidence of folate-responsive birth defects. It is not known whether lower levels of supplementation would be as effective, nor whether disease risk could be reduced by dietary folate alone, as food folate is less bioavailable than folic acid. The recent implementation of fortification of the American food supply with folic acid is designed to

provide an average intake of 100 μg of supplemental folic acid in addition to normal dietary folate intake. This represents a compromise between the needs of the relatively small population at risk for birth defects and the relatively larger population at risk for masking of symptoms of vitamin B$_{12}$ deficiency by high folate (see later). Preliminary studies have suggested that folate supplementation may also have a beneficial effect on other pregnancy outcomes, although one of the intervention trials that demonstrated the protective effect of folate for neural tube defects also noted an increased spontaneous abortion rate in supplemented subjects.

Although the fortification of the food supply with folic acid has just started, an additional potential benefit has been the reduction of plasma homocysteine levels in the

United States population. It remains to be seen whether this has a positive effect on vascular disease incidence.

Malabsorption Syndromes

Diseases of the intestinal tract, such as tropical sprue and nontropical sprue (gluten enteropathy), lead to general malabsorption syndromes, including folate deficiency. Folate is normally absorbed in the jejunum. In some sprue cases, the malabsorption in the jejunum is partially alleviated by increased absorption farther down in the small intestine.

Assay and Detection of Deficiency

As described previously, folate status is most commonly assessed by plasma or red cell folate levels. This can be measured by microbiological assay using *Lactobacillus casei* as the test organism, but this test can be confounded if the subject is on antibiotic treatment. The most widely used clinical test is a competitive radioassay procedure for plasma or red cell folate that uses milk folate–binding protein as the protein binder. Although simpler than the microbiological method, it is less precise. The levels of metabolites such as urinary formiminoglutamate and plasma homocysteine can also be used to assess folate status, but, as indicated later, the levels of these metabolites are also abnormal under conditions of vitamin B_{12}, and in some cases, vitamin B_6, deficiency.

FOLATE REQUIREMENTS

The current RDA for adults is 400 μg of folate/day. An intake of 600 μg/day is recommended for pregnant women; higher levels may be required to minimize the risk of birth defects. The recommendation for women of childbearing age, who are capable of becoming pregnant, is to take 400 μg of folic acid/day, derived from supplements and/or fortified food, in addition to their normal food folate intake. Recommended folate intakes for infants are set as Adequate Intakes (AIs) and are based on the folate content of milk of well-nourished mothers. Increases in dietary intake of folate do not affect maternal milk folate levels.

FOLATE TOXICITY

No toxicity of high doses of folate has been reported. However, large doses of folic acid can produce a hematological response in subjects with megaloblastic anemia caused by vitamin B_{12} deficiency. When folate was first isolated, and prior to the isolation of vitamin B_{12}, many pernicious anemia patients were treated with large quantities of folic acid. Folate does not correct the severe neurological symptoms of vitamin B_{12} deficiency, and some studies suggested that folate treatment of B_{12}-deficient subjects may have exacerbated the development of neurological defects. Because large doses of folate may mask the development and diagnosis of anemia in vitamin B_{12}-deficient subjects and increase the risk that these subjects are recognized only when they develop irreversible neurological symptoms, megadose levels of folate should be avoided. An upper level of intake of folic acid from supplements plus fortified foods has been proposed to be set at 1 mg. There is no evidence of any adverse effect of high intakes of food folate per se.

■ VITAMIN B₁₂

A megaloblastic anemia was described in the 19th century that appeared to be associated with degenerative disease of the stomach. It was called pernicious anemia because of its invariably fatal outcome. In the 1920s, Minot and Murphy described the first effective treatment of this disease, 1 pound of raw liver a day, for which they received a Nobel prize. It soon became apparent that normal gastric juice contained a factor (intrinsic factor) that was required for the utilization of a dietary component (extrinsic factor, vitamin B_{12}) that was needed to prevent the anemia. Because of the identical anemia that arises from folate or B_{12} deficiency, it was originally thought that extrinsic factor was folic acid, and folic acid was used to treat pernicious anemia patients when it was isolated in the 1940s. With the isolation of vitamin B$_{12}$ a few years later, it became clear that pernicious anemia was due to a B$_{12}$ deficiency.

CHEMISTRY OF VITAMIN B$_{12}$

Vitamin B$_{12}$ (cobalamin) consists of a central cobalt atom surrounded by a hemelike planar corrin ring structure (Fig. 21–5), with the four pyrrole nitrogens coordinated to the cobalt. It contains a phosphoribo-5,6-dimethylbenzimidazolyl side group, with one of the nitrogens linked to the cobalt by coordination at the "bottom" position. When bound to enzymes, this lower axial ligand is usually replaced by an active site histidyl residue. The "upper" axial position can be occupied by a number of different ligands, including methyl, hydroxyl, and 5'-deoxyadenosyl groups (Fig. 21–6). In what is commonly known as vitamin B$_{12}$, the upper ligand is a cyano group (cyanocobalamin); cyanocobalamin is rarely found naturally but arises as an artifact formed by extraction of trace amounts of cyanide during purification of the vitamin from natural sources. Vitamin B$_{12}$ is a complex molecule, and a Nobel prize was awarded for the determination of its structure. Metal-carbon bonds are rare in nature, and this molecule is the only example of a cobalt-carbon bond.

In cyanocobalamin and the naturally occurring hydroxy (or aqua) cobalamin forms, the cobalt atom is trivalent Co^{3+}, the most oxidized form. Cob(III)alamin is an electrophile, cob(II)alamin is a radical, and cob(I)alamin is a very strong nucleophile (Glusker, 1995). The coenzyme forms of the vitamin are the unliganded, fully reduced Co^{1+} derivative or cob(I)alamin, 5'-deoxyadenosylcob(III)alamin, also known as coenzyme B$_{12}$, and methylcob(III)alamin. These forms of the vitamin are very sensitive to oxidation and photolysis.

SOURCES OF VITAMIN B$_{12}$

Vitamin B$_{12}$ is synthesized by some anaerobic microorganisms. Most higher organisms do not use vitamin B$_{12}$ as a coenzyme and neither have a requirement for it nor synthesize the vitamin. Except for some algae, such as seaweed, plant sources do not contain vitamin B$_{12}$. The major dietary sources for humans are meat, dairy products, and some seafoods. B$_{12}$

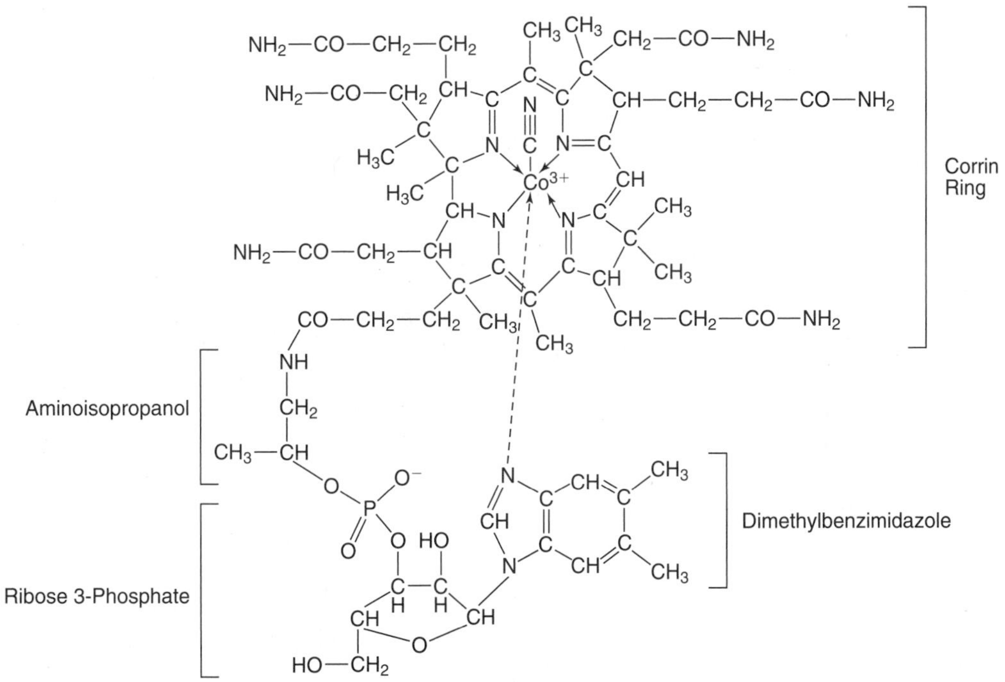

Figure 21–5. Structure of vitamin B$_{12}$ (cyanocobalamin).

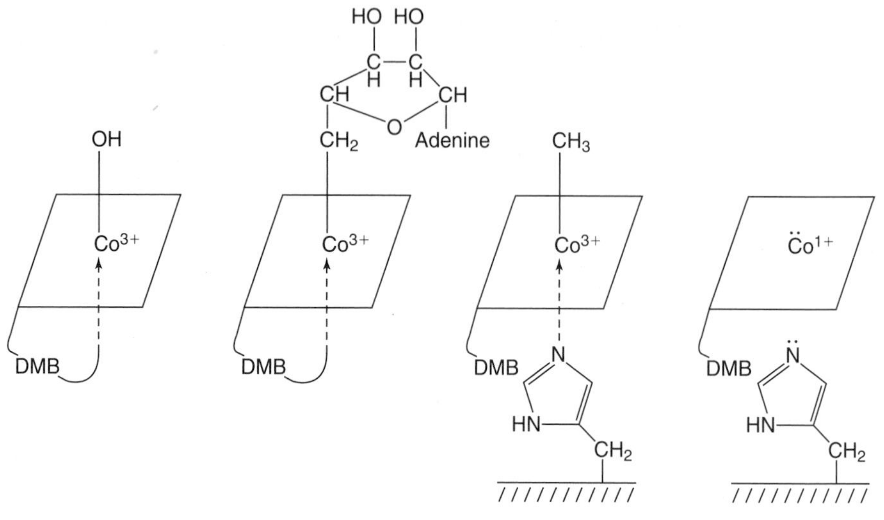

Hydroxycobalamin   5'-Deoxyadenosylcobalamin   Methylcobalamin   Cob(I)alamin
(Coenzyme B_{12})   (Protein-bound)

Figure 21–6. Intracellular forms of B_{12}. In B_{12} enzymes, the ligand to the lower axial position of the cobalt atom is an imidazole nitrogen of a histidyl residue on the protein instead of the dimethylbenzimidazolyl (DMB) side group of B_{12}; this is shown for methylcobalamin bound to methionine synthase. The lower axial position is unliganded (base-off form) in the cob(I)alamin-enzyme derivative.

can also be obtained from fortified cereals and supplements. A strictly vegetarian diet provides very low levels of the vitamin, which can come from algal sources and possibly bacterial contamination associated with plant roots. Vegetarians tend to have low plasma vitamin B_{12} levels. Despite this, nutritional deficiency of vitamin B_{12} due to inadequate intake is rare. Instead, most problems of inadequate vitamin B_{12} status arise from defects in vitamin absorption.

BIOAVAILABILITY AND ABSORPTION OF VITAMIN B_{12}

The bioavailability of food vitamin B_{12} varies depending on the amount of B_{12} in the diet but normally averages around 50%. The mechanism of absorption is complex and is outlined in Figure 21–7. Vitamin B_{12} in food is bound to protein and is released in the stomach by the acid environment and by proteolysis of binders by pepsin. The released vitamin B_{12} initially binds to R-binders, which are dietary proteins that have affinity for vitamin B_{12}. The stomach contains specialized parietal

cells that contain the H^+, K^+-ATPase that produces gastric acid. In humans, these cells also secrete a glycoprotein called intrinsic factor (IF) that can bind vitamin B_{12}. As the vitamin B_{12}-R-binder complexes pass through the small intestine, the R-binders are hydrolyzed by pancreatic proteases, and the freed vitamin B_{12} binds to IF. Sufficient IF is released following a meal to bind 2 to 4 μg of vitamin B_{12}. Vitamin B_{12} is absorbed via receptors located at the distal ileum at the end of the small intestine. The receptor recognizes the IF-B_{12} complex, not vitamin B_{12}. In the presence of Ca^{2+}, the IF-B_{12} complex binds to the IF receptor, and the complex is internalized by a receptor-mediated endocytotic process. The endosomes fuse with lysosomes, and the IF is degraded and the vitamin B_{12} is released into the cytosol. Vitamin B_{12} is released from the gut epithelial cells as a complex bound to a 38-kDa glycoprotein called transcobalamin II (TC-II). This process of absorption across the gut epithelium takes about 3 to 4 h. The 460-kDa IF receptor is also expressed in the kidney and in the yolk sac of animals and has recently been cloned, although the reason why it should be expressed in the kidney is not

Food Sources of Vitamin B$_{12}$

- Meat, poultry, fish
- Milk
- Shellfish
- Fortified cereals

RDAs Across the Life Cycle

	μg vitamin B$_{12}$/day
Infants, 0–5 mo	0.4 (AI)
6–11 mo	0.5 (AI)
Children, 1–3 y	0.9
4–8 y	1.2
9–13 y	1.8
Males, > 13 y	2.4*
Females, > 13 y	2.4*
Pregnant	2.6
Lactating	2.8

*Because of the high incidence of malabsorption of food B$_{12}$ by elderly people, the recommendation for elderly people (over 50 years) is that they derive their B$_{12}$ requirement primarily from crystalline vitamin B$_{12}$ in fortified foods and/or supplements.

From Institute of Medicine (1998) Dietary Reference Intakes: Thiamin, Riboflavin, Niacin, Vitamin B$_6$, Folate, Vitamin B$_{12}$, Pantothenic Acid, Biotin, and Choline. National Academy Press, Washington, D.C.

clear. There is a suggestion that the receptor may also bind other protein ligands in the kidney.

Vitamin B$_{12}$ can also be absorbed by a diffusion-like process, but this is very inefficient: less than 1% of a vitamin B$_{12}$ dose can be absorbed by this process.

TRANSPORT OF VITAMIN B$_{12}$

The TC-II-B$_{12}$ complex carries newly absorbed vitamin B$_{12}$ around the body and provides tissues with vitamin B$_{12}$. TC-II-B$_{12}$ is transported into tissues by receptor-mediated endocytosis, in this case via a receptor that recognizes TC-II. The TC-II-B$_{12}$ complex is degraded in the lysosome, and the free vitamin B$_{12}$ is transported out of the lysosome to the cytosol (Fig. 21–8). The lysosomal vitamin B$_{12}$ transporter has not been characterized. A rare human genetic disease involving a defect in this transporter has been described in which vitamin B$_{12}$ accumulates in the lysosome.

The half life of the TC-II-vitamin B$_{12}$ complex in plasma is about 6 min. Plasma contains two additional vitamin B$_{12}$–binding proteins or R-binders called transcobalamin I (TC-I) and transcobalamin III (TC-III). Plasma turnover of these transcobalamins is much slower than that of TC-II. Although newly absorbed vitamin B$_{12}$ is associated with TC-II, about 80% of the plasma vitamin B$_{12}$ is associated with TC-I. The role of TC-I is not entirely clear, but this 60-kDa glycoprotein may be involved in transfer of vitamin B$_{12}$ to the liver. Liver contains a nonspecific asialoglycoprotein receptor that can mediate uptake of TC-I and TC-III.

Most of the body store of vitamin B$_{12}$, estimated at about 2 to 3 mg, is in the liver. 5′-Deoxyadenosylcobalamin is the major form of the vitamin in liver, whereas methylcobalamin is the major form in plasma. The vitamin is excreted via the urine and via the bile. Normally, the enterohepatic circulation results in effective reuptake, via the IF receptor, of biliary vitamin B$_{12}$. Turnover rates of whole-body vitamin B$_{12}$ have been estimated at about 0.1%/day.

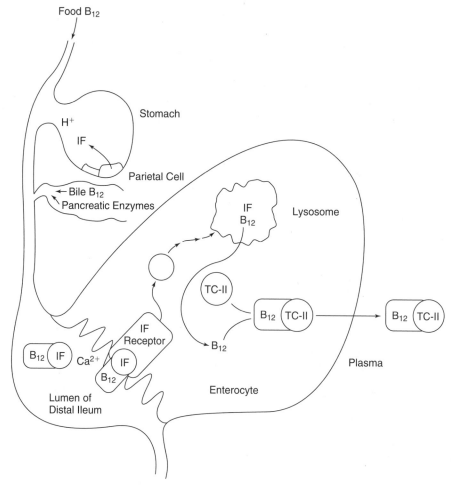

Figure 21–7. *Absorption and processing of dietary B$_{12}$. IF, intrinsic factor; TC-II, transcobalamin II.*

INTRACELLULAR METABOLISM OF VITAMIN B$_{12}$

Mammals need vitamin B$_{12}$ as a cofactor for two enzymes, cytosolic methionine synthase, which utilizes methylcob(III)alamin as the cofactor, and mitochondrial methylmalonyl CoA mutase, which uses 5′-deoxyadenosylcob(III)-alamin as its cofactor. Vitamin B$_{12}$ is released into the cytosol of cells as hydroxycob(III)-alamin and is reduced to cob(I)alamin. Cob-(I)alamin is then methylated to methylcob(III)-alamin after binding to methionine synthase. Alternatively, vitamin B$_{12}$ can be transported into the mitochondria and reduced, and the 5′-deoxyadenosyl ligand added from ATP in a reaction catalyzed by a deoxyadenosyltrans-ferase (Fig. 21–8). Rare human genetic defects

in many of these steps in vitamin B$_{12}$ metabolism have been described.

METABOLIC FUNCTIONS OF VITAMIN B$_{12}$

The reduced vitamin B$_{12}$ coenzymes are highly reactive and are capable of catalyzing very aggressive chemistry. Bacteria use 5′-deoxy-adenosylcob(III)alamin as a cofactor for many reactions in which carbon-carbon bonds are cleaved by a mechanism that involves free radicals. During catalysis, the cobalt-carbon bond of the coenzyme is split, and a free radical is formed on the coenzyme, which can be transferred to an amino acid residue on the enzyme and then to the substrate.

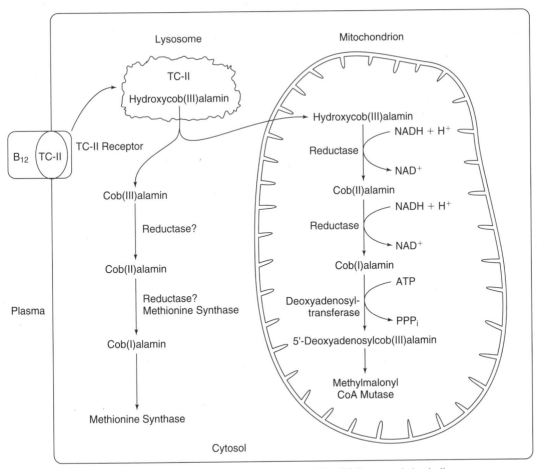

Figure 21–8. *Tissue uptake and metabolism of B_{12}. TC-II, transcobalamin II.*

Methionine Synthase

Methylcobalamin is a cofactor for the previously described folate-dependent methionine synthase involved in homocysteine remethylation (see Figs. 21–2, 21–3, and 21–9). Methionine synthases are large, monomeric Zn metalloproteins (about 140 kDa) and consist of three domains: a catalytic domain containing the binding sites for 5-methyl-$H_4PteGlu_n$ and homocysteine, a B_{12} domain in which the B_{12}-cofactor binds, and an accessory protein domain. Most of the methionine synthase in mammalian tissues is normally present as the holoenzyme form, containing a tightly bound B_{12} cofactor. The cob(I)alamin cofactor is methylated by 5-methyl-$H_4PteGlu_n$, generating enzyme-bound methylcob(III)alamin and releasing $H_4PteGlu_n$, and then methylcob(III)-alamin transfers its methyl group to homocysteine to generate methionine. Heterolytic cleavage of the cobalt-carbon bond regenerates the enzyme-bound cob(I)alamin cofactor. The cofactor is occasionally oxidized to the nonfunctional cob(II)alamin form during catalysis. The enzyme is reactivated by one or several poorly characterized accessory proteins that catalyze the AdoMet and NADPH-dependent reductive methylation of enzyme-bound cob(II)alamin to methylcob(III)alamin. Bacteria possess two methionine synthase accessory proteins, one a flavodoxin, that use NADH, FAD, and FMN as cofactors. The gene for a single human methionine synthase reductase protein that contains binding sites for NADPH, FAD and FMN has recently been cloned.

Methionine synthase can also catalyze the reduction of the anesthetic gas nitrous oxide to nitrogen. During this process, a hydroxyl radical is formed, which can lead to destruction of the polypeptide backbone of

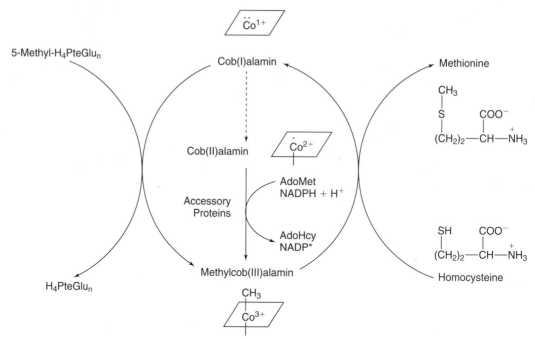

Figure 21–9. *Remethylation of homocysteine via the methionine synthase reaction. Enzyme-bound cob(I)alamin can be methylated by 5-methyl-$H_4PteGlu_n$ to generate the methylcob(III)alamin intermediate, or it can be oxidized to the nonfunctional cob(II)alamin form. Cob(II)alamin is reduced and methylated via the action of accessory proteins that interact with methionine synthase.*

the protein and inactivation of the enzyme. Nitrous oxide is sometimes used to inactivate methionine synthase in experimental animals to generate a model for the metabolic effects of vitamin B_{12} deficiency.

The many organisms that do not use B_{12} cofactors possess a B_{12}-independent methionine synthase that catalyzes the 5-methyl-$H_4PteGlu_n$–dependent methylation of homocysteine to methionine. This enzyme, which is not found in mammalian tissues, is absolutely specific for a folylpolyglutamate substrate. Many bacteria express the B_{12}-dependent enzyme when cultured in the presence of cobalamin, whereas the B_{12}-independent enzyme is induced in the absence of cobalamin. A question that arises is why have some organisms, such as mammals, retained the B_{12}-dependent enzyme, which necessitates a very complex process for vitamin B_{12} transport and metabolism and makes the organism susceptible to all the problems that can be caused by defects in these processes (see later), rather than simply using the B_{12}-independent methionine synthase expressed by many other organisms? The answer is not obvious but may be

related to the very poor catalytic activity of the B_{12}-independent enzyme. In organisms such as yeast, or bacteria cultured in the absence of cobalamin, the B_{12}-independent enzyme is induced to very high levels to compensate for its poor catalytic activity, and it is one of the major proteins expressed by these organisms. The more catalytically effective B_{12}-dependent enzyme is a low-abundance protein.

Methylmalonyl CoA Mutase

Mitochondrial β-oxidation of dietary odd-chain fatty acids produces propionyl CoA in addition to acetyl CoA. Propionyl CoA is converted to D-methylmalonyl CoA in a reaction catalyzed by the biotin-dependent propionyl CoA carboxylase (Fig. 21–10). Propionyl CoA and methylmalonyl CoA can also arise during catabolism of isoleucine, valine, methionine, and threonine (Chapter 11; Figs. 11–19, 11–21, and 11–28). A racemase converts D-methylmalonyl CoA to L-methylmalonyl CoA, and the 5′-deoxyadenosylcobalamin–dependent methylmalonyl CoA mutase catalyzes the conversion of L-methylmalonyl CoA to succinyl

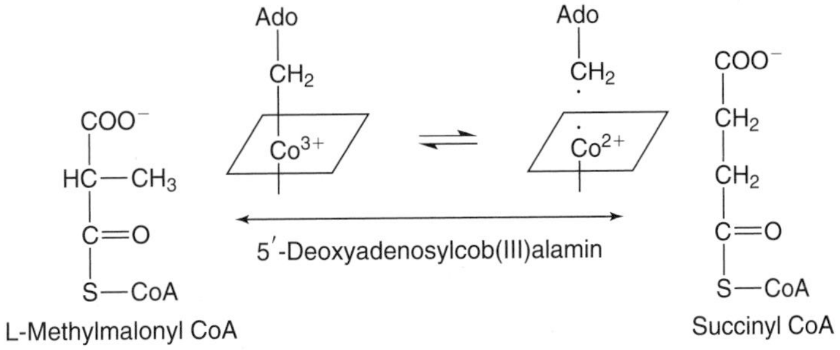

Figure 21–10. The methylmalonyl CoA mutase reaction. The mutase catalyzes the homolytic cleavage of coenzyme B$_{12}$ to generate an adenosyl radical, which interacts with the substrate, and a B$_{12}$ cofactor radical.

CoA. The mutase reaction involves the breakage and migration of a carbon-carbon bond. All these reactions occur in the mitochondria, and the succinyl CoA formed has several potential fates, including entry into the citric acid cycle and heme biosynthesis. In liver, conversion of propionyl CoA to succinyl CoA allows the carbon skeletons of some amino acids, as well as propionyl CoA from odd-chain fatty acid metabolism, to be used for gluconeogenesis.

VITAMIN B$_{12}$ DEFICIENCY: SYMPTOMS AND METABOLIC BASES

Vitamin B$_{12}$ deficiency is rarely caused by a dietary insufficiency and most commonly arises from a defect in vitamin B$_{12}$ absorption. The classical manifestations are pernicious anemia, which is a megaloblastic anemia identical to that observed with folate deficiency, and severe and often irreversible neurological disease called subacute combined degeneration of the spinal cord, which is characterized by demyelination and peripheral neuropathy. Memory loss and dementia have also been observed. Although the development of anemia often precedes the neurological disease and allows the detection and treatment of B$_{12}$ deficiency prior to the development of neurological damage, this is not always the case, and some patients present with neurological disease in the absence of anemia. Neurological symptoms occur in 75% to 90% of patients with clinical B$_{12}$ deficiency and may be the only symptom in 25%. The reason for this is not clear. Because the anemia is due to induction of a functional folate deficiency, it has been speculated that B$_{12}$-deficient subjects who have high folate intakes, such as vegetarians or individuals taking folate supplements, may be more likely to develop neurological symptoms without developing anemia, but firm evidence in support of this hypothesis is lacking.

Vitamin B$_{12}$ Malabsorption

Defects in vitamin B$_{12}$ absorption affect a significant proportion of elderly people. Classical pernicious anemia is caused by an inability to absorb vitamin B$_{12}$ as a result of lack of production of IF. The disease is age-related and is usually due to destruction of the parietal cells in the stomach, which is caused by an autoimmune disease in which antibodies to the H$^+$,K$^+$-ATPase or to IF are produced. Because body vitamin B$_{12}$ stores are usually ample at the onset of the disease and the turnover of body stores is slow, it can take many years before deficiency symptoms become apparent. Whole-body turnover is increased owing to an inability to reabsorb biliary vitamin B$_{12}$ as well as dietary vitamin B$_{12}$. The destruction of the parietal cells decreases acid production, which also impairs release of dietary vitamin from protein binders. The prevalence of untreated pernicious anemia in elderly people has been estimated to be about 2%. About 3% of elderly people test positive for IF autoantibodies, which may suggest a somewhat higher incidence of untreated pernicious anemia (Carmel, 1996). The Schilling test is sometimes used clinically to verify a diagnosis of pernicious anemia. In this test, the absorption of labeled vitamin B$_{12}$, as measured by its appearance in urine, is defective in pernicious anemia patients but becomes normal if IF is given together with the labeled vitamin B$_{12}$ dose.

Although absorption of vitamin B$_{12}$ by diffusion potentially could overcome the loss of the IF-mediated transport of dietary vitamin B_{12}, this would require extremely high intakes of vitamin B_{12} because diffusion is very inefficient (less than 1%), and additional high doses would be required to make up for the failure to reabsorb biliary losses. The disease is easily treated by monthly intramuscular injections of 1 mg of vitamin B_{12}.

Malabsorption of dietary vitamin B_{12} also can arise from any condition of decreased acid production or pancreatic insufficiency. The prevalence of atrophic gastritis in subjects 50 years and older has been estimated at 10% to 30%, and many elderly people suffer from *Helicobacter pylori* infection. These conditions result in an impairment of food vitamin B_{12} absorption because of an impaired ability to release the vitamin from protein binders, while absorption of vitamin B_{12} in the absence of food is unimpaired. This condition can be detected by a modified Schilling test in which the absorption of food B_{12} is compared with that of crystalline vitamin B_{12}. Bacterial overgrowth in the gut also can compete for vitamin B_{12} and reduce the amount of vitamin available for absorption. Problems with bacterial overgrowth can be treated with antibiotics. Surgical stomach resection, a procedure that is sometimes used for the treatment of obesity, can also lead to decreased acid and IF production. Vitamin B_{12} absorption also can be impaired in general malabsorption syndromes, such as sprue and ileitis.

Megaloblastic Anemia

The reason for the identical megaloblastic anemia that results from folate and vitamin B_{12} deficiency is best explained by the methyl trap hypothesis (Shane and Stokstad, 1985). The two vitamins are cofactors for the methionine synthase reaction. In pernicious anemia patients, methionine synthase activity in bone marrow is reduced over 85%, and most of the protein is present in the apoenzyme form. This causes an accumulation of cellular folates in the 5-methyl-H_4PteGlu$_n$ form, and this is essentially the only form of folate found in the cytosol of experimental animals in which methionine synthase has been inactivated. 5-Methyl-H_4PteGlu$_n$ can be metabolized only via the methionine synthase reaction and is func-

tionally unavailable unless converted to H_4PteGlu$_n$. The trapping of folate in this form results in lack of folate coenzymes for other reactions of one-carbon metabolism, including thymidylate and purine synthesis. Consequently, the symptoms are identical to those seen in folate deficiency, which is a megaloblastic anemia. Megaloblastic changes occur in the blood profiles of subjects treated with the anesthetic nitrous oxide due to destruction of methionine synthase. After treatment, enzyme levels gradually return to normal owing to synthesis of new protein.

Tissue accumulation of folate is also grossly impaired. Because 5-methyl-H_4PteGlu is the major form of folate transported into tissues, and because its conversion to polyglutamates and retention by tissues requires its metabolism to H_4PteGlu, the block in methionine synthase activity results in an inability of tissues to accumulate exogenous folate such that most of the transported 5-methyl-H_4PteGlu is released back into the circulation. This reduction in the ability of tissues to accumulate folate, coupled with turnover of tissue folate pools, leads to a reduction in tissue folate levels, and an absolute tissue folate deficiency ensues on top of the functional deficiency caused by the methyl trap. In experimental animals placed on a vitamin B_{12}-deficient diet, or in animals treated with nitrous oxide to inhibit methionine synthase activity, plasma folate levels initially increase because of the inability of tissues to retain entering folate, but eventually drop to low levels because of an inability to retain folate in the body.

The complex regulation of the folate and vitamin B_{12}-dependent methionine synthesis cycle has been discussed previously. It appears that no mechanisms exist that can compensate for impaired B_{12} availability.

Subacute Combined Degeneration

The mechanism behind the neurological symptoms of vitamin B_{12} deficiency is not understood. Most experimental animals do not develop neurological symptoms when placed on a vitamin B_{12}-deficient diet, in part because it is difficult to eliminate gut bacterial synthesis of vitamin B_{12} as a source of the vitamin. Although rarely used as a model, the South

CLINICAL CORRELATION

Megaloblastic Anemia: A Common Complication of Folate and Vitamin B$_{12}$ Deficiency

Megaloblastic anemia, a manifestation of defective DNA synthesis in hematopoietic cells, can arise from impaired folate or vitamin B$_{12}$ status. Folate-deficiency megaloblastic anemia is almost always a nutritional disease caused by inadequate folate in the diet, and its incidence is increased in pregnancy. Vitamin B$_{12}$-deficiency megaloblastic anemia, which is more common than that due to folate deficiency in the American population, is rarely due to inadequate dietary vitamin B$_{12}$ but usually arises from malabsorption of the vitamin, a condition that affects a significant proportion of elderly people. An elevated folate intake can correct the anemia due to depressed B$_{12}$ status but not the other symptoms of vitamin B$_{12}$ deficiency. As a result of concerns about this masking effect of folate, the amount of folic acid added to fortified foods in the US has been restricted.

Although rare, many cases of inborn errors of B$_{12}$ metabolism have been described. Studies with cultured skin fibroblasts from patients with these inborn errors have indicated 7 complementation groups that may correspond to defects in 7 different genes. Some patients exhibiting megaloblastic anemia have defects in proteins involved in B$_{12}$ transport or coenzyme synthesis, whereas others have defects in methionine synthase. Recently, a null human mutant in methionine synthase was described in whom enzyme activity was completely blocked. This infant had very severe megaloblastic anemia. The ability of this patient to survive gestation was surprising as the methionine synthase gene knockout in the mouse is embryonically lethal, which again illustrates that experimental animal models for human disease do not always faithfully mimic the human condition.

Thinking Critically

An infant presents with severe megaloblastic anemia and hyperhomocysteinemia but normal plasma folate and methylmalonic acid. Assays of methionine synthase extracted from fibroblasts from this patient suggest close to normal activity.

(1) What would you diagnose as a likely cause of this condition?

(2) How might you treat this patient?

African fruit bat does display neurological abnormalities when made vitamin B$_{12}$-deficient, as do nonhuman primates.

As mammals have only two B$_{12}$-dependent enzymes and methionine synthase is the locus of the defect causing anemia, attention has been focused on the role of methylmalonyl CoA mutase in the etiology of the neurological defects. Vitamin B$_{12}$ deficiency causes accumulation of methylmalonyl CoA in the mitochondria, an elevation in circulating methylmalonate, acidosis, and elevated methylmalonate excretion. The accumulation of mitochondrial methylmalonyl CoA depletes the CoA pool available for other mitochondrial enzymes and metabolites, and the increased propionyl CoA can be incorporated into long-chain fatty acids in place of acetyl CoA. A role for the accumulation of unusual

fatty acids in myelin as a reason for the demyelination has been proposed, but evidence for this is not convincing. However, humans with severe genetic impairment of the *mut* locus encoding the mutase suffer from a variety of severe clinical conditions and metabolic abnormalities but do not develop subacute combined degeneration of the spinal cord or megaloblastic anemia, indicating that demyelination is not caused by a block in mutase activity.

Monkeys treated with nitrous oxide develop neurological disease similar to that observed in humans, and these symptoms are prevented by methionine supplementation, suggesting that the neurological disease of B$_{12}$ deficiency may also result from a defect in methionine synthesis (in this case, because of the impairment in methionine synthesis). In the few known cases of genetic defects in methionine synthase or in the enzymes responsible for methylcobalamin synthesis, the patients exhibit the expected megaloblastic anemia and some also exhibit demyelination. Similarly, some patients with defects in methylenetetrahydrofolate reductase exhibit the same neurological symptoms as are observed in B_{12} deficiency. These patients do not exhibit megaloblastic anemia, because a defect in the reductase prevents the formation of 5-methyl-H_4PteGlu$_n$ and increases folate coenzyme availability for nucleotide synthesis. Although the mechanism responsible for the neurological disease of B_{12} deficiency is not understood, current evidence supports the hypothesis that it is related to defective methionine synthesis and that the locus of the defect is methionine synthase. A mouse "knockout" model for methionine synthase has recently been developed. The homozygous deletion appears to be embryonically lethal, as might be predicted because of the expected derangement in DNA synthesis. The heterozygote may prove to be a useful animal model for elucidating the development of neurological disease resulting from B_{12} deficiency.

Hyperhomocysteinemia

The relationship of hyperhomocysteinemia to vascular disease risk was described earlier. Plasma homocysteine is elevated in pernicious anemia because of the block in methionine synthase activity. In population studies, subjects with the lowest deciles of plasma vitamin B_{12} had the highest plasma homocysteine values (Selhub et al., 1993). Although a slight correlation was observed between dietary vitamin B_{12} and homocysteine levels, it was less marked, reflecting that defects in absorption rather than dietary vitamin content play a greater role in the development of impaired vitamin B_{12} status.

Assay and Detection of Vitamin B_{12} Deficiency

Total plasma vitamin B_{12} can be measured by microbiological assay. These tests sometimes also measure B_{12} analogs that have no vitamin activity in humans. The most widely used clinical test is a competitive radioassay procedure for plasma vitamin B_{12} that uses IF as the protein binder. IF will not bind B_{12} analogs, and this test is specific for biologically active forms of the vitamin. A plasma level below 200 ng/mL is considered indicative of deficiency. However, plasma levels above 200 ng/mL are often seen in subjects who, by other criteria such as vitamin malabsorption tests, are at risk for developing deficiency symptoms. Because plasma B_{12} is not a very sensitive indicator of status, other tests, such as the degree of saturation of TC-II by vitamin B_{12} have been proposed as more sensitive indicators of status but are not routinely used.

Because B_{12} deficiency induces a folate deficiency, many of the biochemical effects of B_{12} deficiency are identical to those seen in folate deficiency. Although plasma folate is initially raised, as the deficiency progresses plasma and red cell folate concentrations are reduced, plasma homocysteine is elevated, and urinary formiminoglutamate excretion is increased. Using these biochemical tests, it is not possible to distinguish whether an individual is folate- or vitamin B_{12}-deficient or both. A low plasma B_{12} level would be indicative of B_{12} deficiency, whereas a normal plasma B_{12} coupled with low plasma or red cell folate would suggest folate deficiency. An increase in plasma or urinary methylmalonate would also be a specific indicator of impaired vitamin B_{12} status. Although folate status does not affect methylmalonate levels, a high-fiber diet may result in elevated methylmalonate levels. Fermentation of fiber in the colon can generate propionate, which is absorbed and metabolized to methylmalonate.

A diagnosis of megaloblastic anemia can be confirmed by the appearance and size of blood cells. Because of the severe and sometimes irreversible nature of the neurological disease in untreated B_{12} deficiency, early detection of neurological impairment is critical. Using a tuning fork to check for an absent vibration sensation is a simple neurological test that can detect early stages of impairment.

VITAMIN B_{12} REQUIREMENTS

The current RDA for the adult is 2.4 μg of vitamin B_{12}/day. An intake of 2.6 μg/day is recommended for pregnant women. Because of the high incidence of malabsorption of food vitamin B$_{12}$ in elderly people, it is recommended that subjects older than 50 years meet the RDA by taking foods fortified with B$_{12}$ or by taking a supplement. Recommendations of Adequate Intakes (AIs) for infants are based on the vitamin B$_{12}$ content of milk of well-nourished mothers.

VITAMIN B$_{12}$ TOXICITY

No toxicity of high doses of vitamin B$_{12}$ have been reported, and milligram doses are used to treat pernicious anemia with no apparent side effects.

■ VITAMIN B$_6$

Vitamin B$_6$ was originally isolated as an anti-dermatitis and antianemia factor for animals. The classical clinical symptoms of vitamin B$_6$ deficiency are a seborrheic dermatitis, microcytic anemia, epileptiform convulsions, and depression and confusion. Microcytic anemia is a reflection of decreased hemoglobin synthesis. More recently, interest in vitamin B$_6$ status has centered on its role in decreasing circulating homocysteine, a risk factor for vascular disease.

CHEMISTRY OF VITAMIN B$_6$

Vitamin B$_6$ compounds are 4-substituted 2-methyl-3-hydroxy-5-hydroxymethylpyridine compounds (Fig. 21–11). There are six major derivatives with vitamin activity: pyridoxal (PL), the 4-formyl derivative; pyridoxine (PN), the 4-hydroxymethyl derivative; pyridoxamine (PM), the 4-aminomethyl derivative; and their respective 5′-phosphate derivatives (PLP, PNP, and PMP). The major forms in animal tissues are the coenzyme species PLP and PMP. PN is usually the major form in plant foods, and a large proportion of the PN in plants can be present as a glucoside derivative. PN is the form of the vitamin normally present in supplements or fortified foods. The major excre-

tory form of vitamin B$_6$ is the 4-carboxylate derivative 4-pyridoxic acid.

Vitamin B$_6$ compounds, and in particular PL and PLP, are light sensitive. Large losses in food vitamin B$_6$ can occur during heating and by leaching of the vitamin during food preparation.

SOURCES OF VITAMIN B$_6$

Cereals, meat, fish, poultry, and noncitrus fruits are the major contributors of vitamin B$_6$ in the American diet. Rich sources are highly fortified cereals, beef liver, and other organ meats.

BIOAVAILABILITY AND ABSORPTION OF VITAMIN B$_6$

Vitamin B$_6$ is absorbed in the small intestine by a nonsaturable passive diffusion mechanism. The 5′-phosphate derivatives are hydrolyzed by a phosphatase prior to transport. PN glucoside is normally deconjugated by a mucosal glucosidase. In humans, some PN glucoside is absorbed intact and can be hydrolyzed to PN in various tissues.

The bioavailability of vitamin B$_6$ supplements is greater than 90%. Bioavailability of nonglucoside forms of the vitamin in foods is greater than 75%, whereas the bioavailability of PN glucoside in food is about half as much. Vitamin B$_6$ in a mixed diet, which would typically contain about 15% PN glucoside, is about 75% bioavailable (Jackson et al., 1997). Pharmacological doses of vitamin B$_6$ compounds are well absorbed, but most of the absorbed vitamin is eliminated in the urine at high doses.

TRANSPORT, METABOLISM, AND TISSUE ACCUMULATION OF VITAMIN B$_6$

Most of the absorbed nonphosphorylated B$_6$ is taken up by the liver and metabolized to PLP, the major coenzymatic form (Fig. 21–11). PN, PL, and PM are converted to their respective 5′-phosphate derivatives by the enzyme

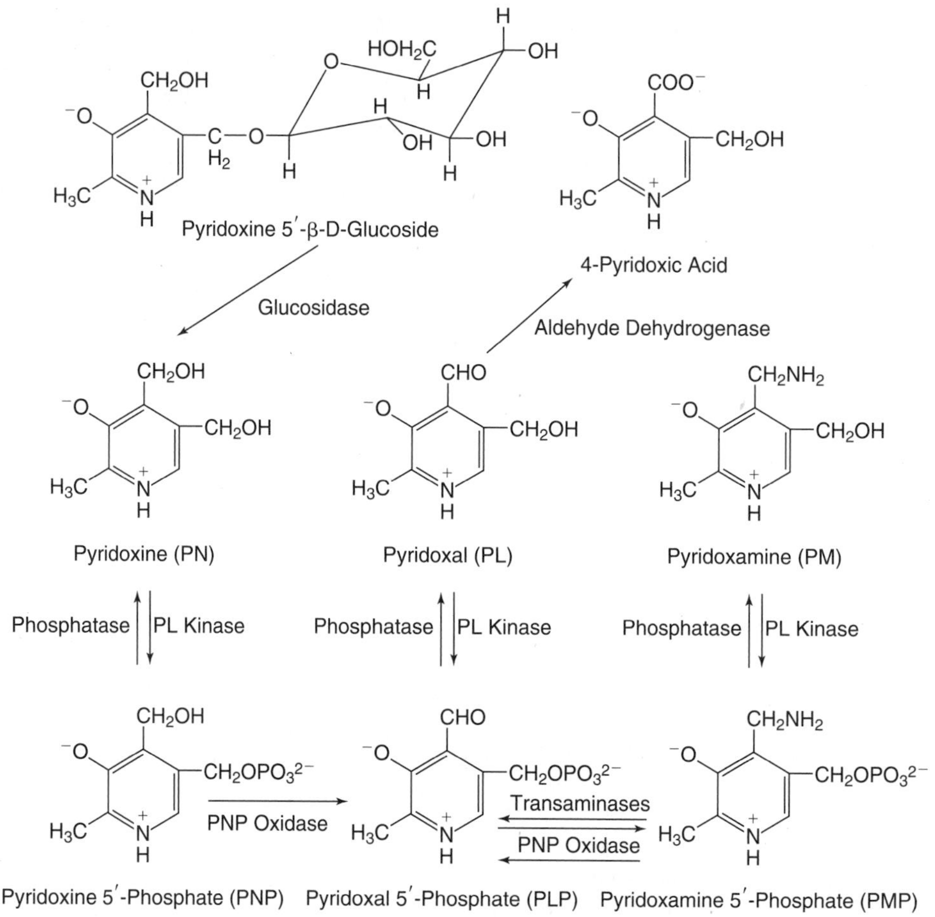

Figure 21–11. *Vitamin B$_6$ compounds and their interconversion and metabolism.*

PL kinase. PL kinase is present in all tissues, including the red blood cell. PNP, which is normally found only at very low concentrations in tissues, and PMP are oxidized to PLP by the flavoprotein PNP oxidase. PMP can also be converted to PLP by transamination reactions. PLP is distributed in various subcellular compartments, but most is in the cytosol and mitochondria. Most of the PL kinase activity is found in the cytosol, and the mechanism by which PLP gets into the mitochondria is unclear.

PLP binds to proteins and PLP-dependent enzymes via Schiff base formation with the ε-amino group of specific lysyl residues (Fig. 21–12). PLP itself is not thought to cross membranes. However, protein-bound PLP is in equilibrium with free PLP, and free PLP can be hydrolyzed to PL by various phosphatases and released by the tissue; protein binding

protects PLP from the action of these phosphatases. Conditions of increased phosphatase activity, both in tissues and in plasma, can lead to increased hydrolysis of PLP. Tissue protein capacity for binding PLP limits tissue accumulation of vitamin B$_6$. At high intakes of vitamin B$_6$, tissue-binding capacity is exceeded, and the free PLP is rapidly hydrolyzed to the nonphosphorylated PL, which is released by the liver and other tissues into the circulation. At pharmacological doses of B$_6$, the high PLP-binding capacities of proteins in muscle (phosphorylase), plasma (albumin), and red blood cells (hemoglobin) allow them to accumulate high levels of PLP when other tissues are saturated.

PL in liver can be oxidized to the inactive excretory metabolite pyridoxic acid by a flavoprotein aldehyde dehydrogenase. On normal diets, urinary pyridoxic acid excretion

Food Sources of Vitamin B$_6$

- Meat, poultry, fish
- Fortified cereals
- Starchy vegetables
- Noncitrus fruits and juices

RDAs Across the Life Cycle

	mg vitamin B$_6$/day
Infants, 0–5 mo	0.1 (AI)
6–11 mo	0.3 (AI)
Children, 1–3 y	0.5
4–8 y	0.6
9–13 y	1.0
Males, 14–50 y	1.3
>50 y	1.7
Females, 14–18 y	1.2
19–50 y	1.3
>50 y	1.5
Pregnant	1.9
Lactating	2.0

From Institute of Medicine (1998) Dietary Reference Intakes: Thiamin, Riboflavin, Niacin, Vitamin B$_6$, Folate, Vitamin B$_{12}$, Pantothenic Acid, Biotin, and Choline. National Academy Press, Washington, D.C.

accounts for about half the vitamin B$_6$ compounds excreted. With large doses of vitamin B$_6$, the proportion of unmetabolized vitamin excreted increases and, at very high doses of PN, much of the dose is excreted unchanged in the urine. Vitamin B$_6$ is also excreted in feces, but this may be due to biosynthesis in the lower gut.

Plasma PLP, a major form of the vitamin in plasma, is derived from liver as a PLP-albumin complex. Because plasma PLP reflects liver PLP levels (and stores), plasma PLP is a sensitive indicator of tissue vitamin B$_6$ status. Circulating nonphosphorylated forms of the vitamin can be transported into tissues and blood cells. Plasma PLP is also a source of tissue vitamin, but it must dissociate from albumin and be hydrolyzed to PL before it is available.

Estimates of total body vitamin B$_6$ stores in healthy adults range from about 400 μmole to 1000 μmole (60 to 170 mg), and 80% to 90% of this is in muscle, primarily bound to phosphorylase. The overall body half life of vitamin B$_6$ is about 25 days, with a daily fractional turnover rate of less than 3%.

METABOLIC FUNCTIONS OF VITAMIN B$_6$

PLP serves as a coenzyme for more than 100 enzymes, which primarily include enzymes involved in amino acid metabolism, such as aminotransferases, decarboxylases, aldolases, racemases, and dehydratases (see Chapter 11). The carbonyl group of PLP binds to proteins as a covalent Schiff base with the ε-amine of a lysyl residue in the active site. For practically all PLP enzymes, the initial step in catalysis involves displacement of the protein lysyl residue by the amino group of the entering amino acid, which forms a new Schiff base with the coenzyme (Fig. 21–12). The coenzyme is no longer covalently attached to the enzyme, but the aldimine derivative remains tightly bound. Electron movement and labilization of the different bonds around the α-carbon of the amino acid can result in transamination, decarboxylation, racemization, α,β-elimination/addition, or R-group elimination/addition. The catabolism of nearly all amino acids involves transfer of their amino groups to α-keto acids. The major amino

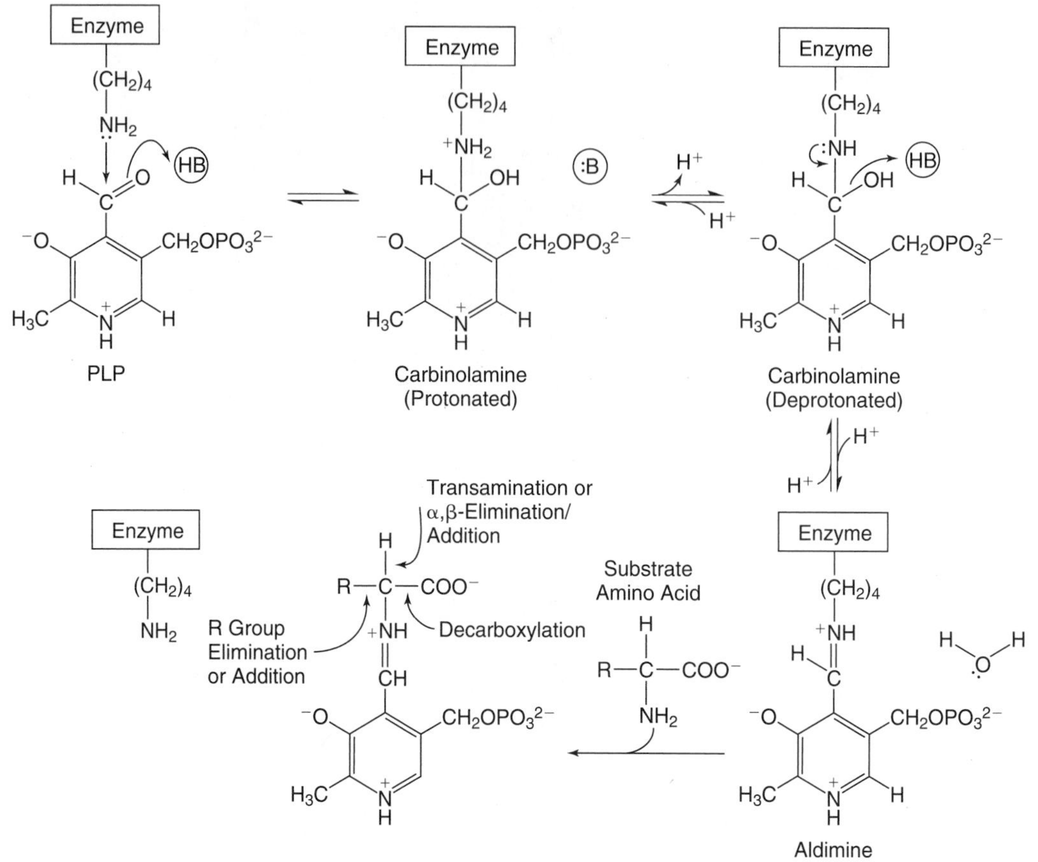

Figure 21–12. *Schiff base formation between PLP and the ε-amino group of a lysyl residue at the active site of an enzyme. (HB, residue on the enzyme that acts as an acid-base catalyst.) An entering amino acid substrate displaces the lysyl residue and forms a Schiff base with the coenzyme. The coenzyme remains tightly bound to the protein via electrostatic interactions through its 5'-phosphate. Labilization of the various bonds around the α-carbon of the amino acid can result in elimination, addition, transamination, or decarboxylation reactions.*

group acceptors are α-ketoglutarate and pyruvate; transamination with these keto acids results in formation of glutamate and alanine, respectively, while the amino acid substrate is converted to its respective keto acid (see Chapter 11).

These transamination reactions proceed via a ketimine intermediate and initially generate the keto acid of the amino acid and PMP (Fig. 21–13). Reversal of this reaction using α-ketoglutarate or pyruvate as the entering keto acid generates glutamate or alanine. Aminotransferase reactions normally result in the transfer of the α-amino group of an amino acid to a keto acid. However, the PMP that is formed in the first part of the reaction sometimes dissociates from the enzyme before the keto acid can interact, which results in a slow conversion of PLP to PMP. A PMP-enzyme

intermediate is not formed in other PLP-enzyme–catalyzed reactions.

Decarboxylases are involved in many areas of metabolism, including the formation of a number of hormones and neurotransmitters, such as epinephrine, serotonin, and dopamine. Elimination of CO_2 from a compound results in a large drop in free energy, and decarboxylase reactions are essentially irreversible.

PLP is a cofactor for mitochondrial δ-aminolevulinate synthase, which catalyzes the first and rate-limiting step in heme biosynthesis in liver (Fig. 21–14). Labilization of the R group of glycine and addition of succinate generates the transient intermediate α-amino-β-ketoadipate, which is rapidly decarboxylated to δ-aminolevulinate. Two molecules of δ-aminolevulinate condense to form porpho-

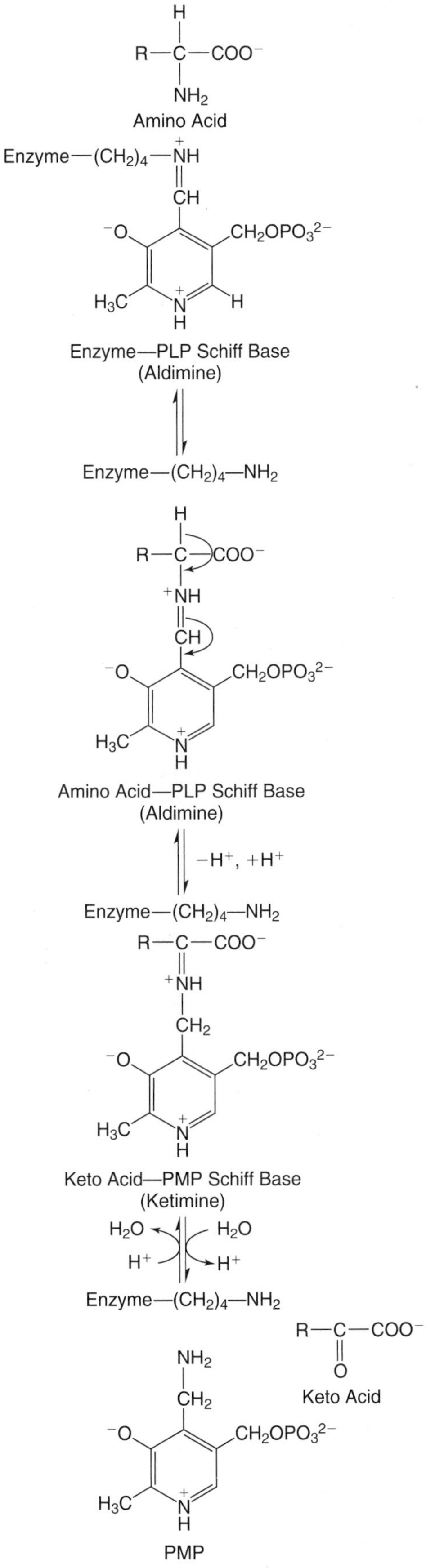

Figure 21–13. *Intermediates in the transamination of an amino acid to a keto acid. Reversal of these steps converts a second keto acid to an amino acid and regenerates the PLP cofactor bound to the enzyme.*

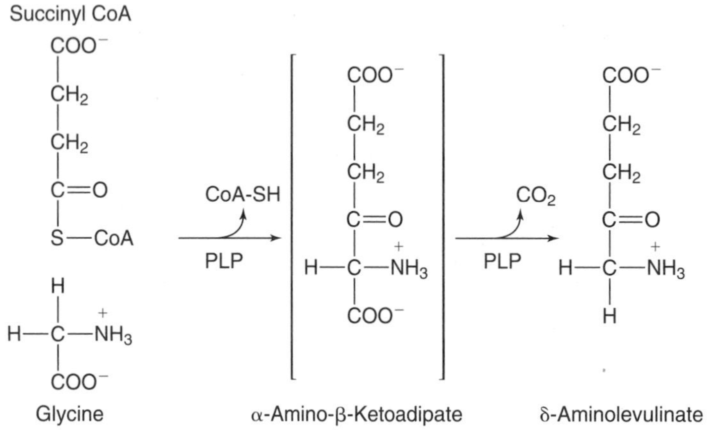

Succinyl CoA

Figure 21–14. The δ-aminolevulinate synthase reaction.

Glycine   α-Amino-β-Ketoadipate   δ-Aminolevulinate

bilinogen, and further condensation and metabolism yields heme. The synthesis of δ-aminolevulinate synthase is regulated by heme.

As described previously, PLP is a cofactor for serine hydroxymethyltransferase, cystathionine β-synthase and cystathionase, which are enzymes involved in the metabolism of homocysteine (see Fig. 21–3).

PLP enzymes are also involved in lipid and carbohydrate metabolism. PLP is a cofactor in the muscle glycogen phosphorylase reaction, but in this reaction the 5′-phosphate group, rather than the 4-carbonyl group, is directly involved in catalysis. Most of the PLP in the body is associated with muscle phosphorylase. PLP is a cofactor for serine palmitoyl transferase, an enzyme involved in sphingolipid synthesis.

Some recent studies have shown that PLP modifies the properties of the glucocorticoid receptor, and it has been suggested that PLP may play a role in steroid hormone action. Similarly, PLP has been shown to affect the transcription rate of some genes. High levels of PLP were used in both studies, and it has not been established that these observations have physiological relevance. PLP at high levels can form Schiff bases with nonspecific lysyl residues on proteins.

VITAMIN B₆ DEFICIENCY: SYMPTOMS AND METABOLIC BASES

Vitamin B₆ deficiency can lead to a seborrheic dermatitis, microcytic anemia, convulsions, depression, and confusion. Electroencephalogram abnormalities have also been reported in controlled studies of B₆ depletion. With the exception of the anemia, the exact mechanisms behind these clinical abnormalities have not been established.

Microcytic Anemia

Microcytic anemia is a reflection of decreased hemoglobin synthesis. Replication of the erythroid cell is regulated by its heme content, and reticulocyte cell division stops when the hemoglobin protein concentration reaches about 20%. Cells that are defective in heme biosynthesis continue to replicate; cell number can increase, but the cells are small (microcytic) and total blood concentration of hemoglobin is reduced (anemia). The role of PLP as a cofactor for δ-aminolevulinate synthase, the first enzyme in heme biosynthesis, can entirely explain this vitamin B₆ deficiency syndrome.

Convulsions and Electroencephalographic Abnormalities

PLP is a cofactor for decarboxylases that are involved in neurotransmitter synthesis; reduced activity of some of these enzymes could explain the convulsions and electroencephalographic (EEG) abnormalities, but this has not been proved. It has also been proposed that the convulsions are caused by abnormal tryptophan metabolites that accumulate in the brain in vitamin B₆ deficiency. A widespread outbreak of convulsions occurred in the 1950s in infants who were fed a formula that contained a very low vitamin B$_6$ content, and these convulsions did respond to PN administration. Although occasional cases of convulsions in breast-fed infants of mothers with poor vitamin B$_6$ status have been reported since then, these are quite rare, and the possibility that other factors were responsible for the convulsions has not been eliminated.

Hyperhomocysteinemia

As described earlier, plasma concentrations of homocysteine are influenced by vitamin B$_6$ and folate and, to a lesser extent, vitamin B$_{12}$ intakes. The increase in plasma homocysteine following a methionine load or a meal is responsive to, and primarily affected by, vitamin B$_6$ status, reflecting the ability of PLP-dependent cystathionine β-synthase to catalyze the transsulfuration and removal of homocysteine (see 21–3).

Alcohol

Alcoholics tend to have low plasma PLP levels and a decreased vitamin B$_6$ status that is independent of poor diet and of defects in metabolism caused by liver damage. Acetaldehyde, the oxidation product of ethanol, decreases cellular PLP levels and is thought to displace PLP from proteins, making PLP more susceptible to hydrolysis by phosphatases.

Assay and Detection of Deficiency

A variety of biochemical indicators have been used to assess vitamin B$_6$ status. Plasma PLP is a reflection of liver PLP and thus tissue stores, and it generally correlates with other indices of B$_6$ status. It is normally measured by an enzymatic assay using apotyrosine decarboxylase. A plasma PLP level of less than 20 nmol/L is considered to reflect adverse vitamin status in the adult. Clinical symptoms of vitamin B$_6$ deficiency and abnormal EEG patterns have been observed in some vitamin-depleted subjects when their plasma PLP levels fall to 10 nmol/L. Plasma PLP values decrease slightly with increased protein intake. They are high in the fetus and the neonate

and decrease gradually throughout the life span.

The stimulation of red blood cell aspartate aminotransferase or alanine aminotransferase activities by PLP has been used to evaluate vitamin B$_6$ status. These tests assess the amount of enzyme in the apoenzyme versus holoenzyme form, the proportion of which increases with B$_6$ depletion. The excretion of tryptophan catabolites following a loading dose of tryptophan has also been used to assess vitamin B$_6$ status. The urinary excretion of xanthurenate, which is normally a minor tryptophan catabolite, is increased in vitamin B$_6$ deficiency. Although tryptophan is catabolized primarily to CO_2 (see Chapters 11 and 20), a number of branch points in this pathway can lead to the synthesis of quantitatively minor metabolites such as NAD and xanthurenate. The activity of one of the enzymes in tryptophan catabolism, the PLP-dependent kynureninase, is reduced in vitamin B$_6$ deficiency, which causes a diversion of the metabolic flux into the xanthurenate synthesis pathway. Urinary excretion of xanthurenate can be a nonspecific test, however, because the first enzyme in the tryptophan catabolic pathway, tryptophan dioxygenase, may be induced by steroid hormones and kynureninase itself is decreased during pregnancy. Xanthurenate, as well as other tryptophan catabolites, is elevated in pregnancy and in high-dose oral contraceptive users, in the absence of a vitamin B$_6$ deficiency. An increase in plasma homocysteine levels following a methionine challenge dose is a fairly specific test of vitamin B$_6$ status.

VITAMIN B$_6$ REQUIREMENTS

The RDA for vitamin B$_6$ is 1.3 mg/day for adults (19 to 50 years) and 1.9 mg/day for pregnant women. For adults over 50 years, the RDA is 1.5 mg/day for women and 1.7 mg/day for men. Adequate Intakes (AIs) for infants are based on the vitamin B$_6$ content of milk of well-nourished mothers. Clinical symptoms of vitamin B$_6$ deficiency have never been observed in experimental subjects receiving intakes of 0.5 mg/day. Because of the role of PLP as a coenzyme for many enzymes involved in amino acid metabolism, it has been proposed that vitamin B_6 requirements are influenced by protein intake and that the RDA should be based on protein intake. However, not all studies have demonstrated a relationship between protein intake and requirement. The median intake in the United States of vitamin B_6 from food sources is about 2 mg for men and about 1.5 mg for women; intakes are higher in supplement users.

VITAMIN B_6 TOXICITY

A severe sensory neuropathy has been described in subjects taking very large doses of PN (1 to 6 g/day) for the treatment of conditions such as carpal tunnel syndrome, premenstrual syndrome, asthma, and sickle cell disease. The reason for the sensory neuropathy is not known, but PLP modification of proteins may be involved in the development of this condition. Although the efficacy of PN megadoses for treatment of these conditions has little scientific rationale, the toxic effects of megadoses have been clearly demonstrated. Because few studies have specifically looked for adverse effects of high doses of vitamin B_6, the lowest safe dose is not known. Some evidence for toxicity has been reported for daily doses of 500 mg, whereas the absence of adverse effects has been rigorously documented in subjects taking daily doses of 100 mg or 300 mg of PN. A safe upper level of 100 mg/day has recently been recommended; 100 mg of PN is approximately equal to total body stores in healthy individuals.

REFERENCES

Blount, B. C., Mack, M. M., Wehr, C. M., MacGregor, J. T., Hiatt, R. A., Wang, G., Wickramasinghe, S. N., Everson, R. B. and Ames, B. N. (1997) Folate deficiency causes uracil misincorporation into human DNA and chromosomal breakage: Implications for cancer and neuronal damage. Proc Natl Acad Sci USA 94:3290–3295.

Carmel, R. (1996) Prevalence of undiagnosed pernicious anemia in the elderly. Arch Intern Med 156:1097–1100.

Frosst, P., Blom, H. J., Milos, R., Goyette, P., Sheppard, C.

A., Matthews, R. G., Boers, G. J., den Heijer, M., Kluitmans, L. A., van den Heuvel, L. P. and Rozen, R. (1995) A candidate genetic risk factor for vascular disease: A common mutation in methylenetetrahydrofolate reductase. Nat Genet 10:111–113.

Glusker, J. P. (1995) Vitamin B_{12} and the B_{12} coenzymes. Vitam Horm 50:1–76.

Institute of Medicine (1998) Dietary Reference Intakes: Thiamin, Riboflavin, Niacin, Vitamin B_6, Folate, Vitamin B_{12}, Pantothenic Acid, Biotin, and Choline. National Academy Press, Washington, D.C.

Jackson, J. J., Fairweather-Tait, S. J., van der Berg, H. and Cohn, W. (1997) Assessment of the bioavailability of micronutrients. Eur J Clin Nutr 51: Suppl. 1.

Ma, J., Stampfer, M. J., Giovannucci, E., Artigas, C., Hunter, D. J., Fuchs, C., Willett, W. C., Selhub, J., Hennekens, C. H. and Rozen, R. (1997) Methylenetetrahydrofolate reductase polymorphism, dietary interactions, and risk of colorectal cancer. Cancer Res 57:1098–1102.

Refsum, H., Ueland, P. M., Nygard, O. and Vollset, S. E. (1998) Homocysteine and vascular disease. Annu Rev Med 49: 31–62.

Rimm, E. B., Willett, W. C., Hu, F. B., Sampson, L., Colditz, G. A., Manson, J. E., Hennekens, C. and Stampfer, M. J. (1998) Folate and vitamin B_6 from diet and supplements in relation to risk of coronary heart disease among women. JAMA 279: 359–364.

Scott, J. M., Kirke, P. N. and Weir, D. G. (1990) The role of nutrition in neural tube defects. Annu Rev Nutr 10:277–295.

Selhub, J., Jacques, P. F., Wilson, P. W. F., Rush, D. and Rosenberg, I. H. (1993) Vitamin status and intake as primary determinants of homocysteinemia in an elderly population. JAMA 270:2693–2698.

Selhub, J., Jacques, P. F., Bostom, A. G., D'Agostino, R. B., Wilson, P. W. F., Belanger, A. J., O'Leary, D. H., Wolf, P. A., Schaefer, E. J. and Rosenberg, I. H. (1995) Association between plasma homocysteine concentrations and extracranial carotid-artery stenosis. N Engl J Med 332: 286–291.

Shane, B. (1989) Folylpolyglutamate synthesis and the regulation of one carbon metabolism. Vitam Horm 45:263–335.

Shane, B. and Stokstad, E. L. R. (1985) Vitamin B_{12}–folate interrelationships. Annu Rev Nutr 5:115–141.

RECOMMENDED READINGS

Bailey, L. B. (ed.) (1995) Folate in Health and Disease. Marcel Dekker, New York.

Blakley, R. L. and Benkovic, S. J. (eds.) (1984) Folates and Pterins, Vol. 1: Chemistry and Biochemistry of Folates. Wiley, New York.

Blakley, R. L. and Whitehead, V. M. (eds.) (1986) Folates and Pterins, Vol. 3: Nutritional, Pharmacological, and Physiological Aspects. Wiley, New York.

Machlin, L. J. and Rucker, R. (eds.) (1999) Handbook of the Vitamins; Nutritional, Biochemical, and Clinical Aspects, 3rd ed. Marcel Dekker, New York.

Scriver, C. R., Beaudet, A. L., Sly, W. S. and Valle, D. (eds.) (1995) The Metabolic and Molecular Bases of Inherited Disease, 7th ed. McGraw-Hill, New York.

CHAPTER **22**

◆ ◆

Pantothenic Acid and Biotin

Lawrence Sweetman, Ph.D.

O U T L I N E

C O M M O N   A B B R E V I A T I O N S

CoA (coenzyme A)
ACP (acyl carrier protein)

■ PANTOTHENIC ACID

Pantothenic acid (vitamin B₅) was discovered in the 1930s as a factor in tissue extracts that prevented an experimental deficiency disease in fowl, characterized by skin lesions. Pantothenic acid is metabolized to two major enzyme cofactors: acyl carrier protein (ACP) and coenzyme A (CoA). These cofactors contain a sulfhydryl group (—SH) that is directly involved in biochemical reactions, forming "high-energy" thioesters with carboxylic acids. CoA forms thioesters with a very wide range of metabolic intermediates. ACP and CoA both are essential for the synthesis of fatty acids, and CoA has additional important roles in fatty acid oxidation, in ketone body metabolism, in oxidative metabolism of pyruvate via pyruvate dehydrogenase and the citric acid cycle, and in the metabolism of a wide variety of organic acids, including those formed in the catabolism of many amino acids. Figure 22–1 outlines the cellular location and the interrelationships of these major areas of metabolism. These reactions include the formation of CoA thioesters, the transfer or condensation of the acyl group of the acyl CoA with another compound with the release of CoA, the requirement for CoA thioesters as substrates and products of dehydrogenation and dehydration reactions, and acyl group exchange reactions that do not involve the release of free CoA.

MICROBIAL SYNTHESIS AND STRUCTURE OF PANTOTHENIC ACID

Microorganisms synthesize pantoate (pantoic acid) from α-ketoisovalerate, the keto acid derived from the amino acid valine. A hydroxymethyl group is attached to α-ketoisovalerate and the keto group is reduced to a hydroxy group to form pantoate. Beta-alanine produced by the decarboxylation of the amino acid aspartate is condensed with pantoate to form pantothenate (pantothenic acid). This synthesis does not occur in humans. Pantothenic acid is fairly widely distributed in foods, giving rise to its name (from Greek *pant-*, meaning all or every). Liver, meats, milk, whole-grain cereals, and legumes are good sources. Pantothenic acid is contained in foods in various bound forms, including CoA and CoA esters, ACP, and as a glucoside in tomatoes.

ABSORPTION, TRANSPORT, AND EXCRETION OF PANTOTHENIC ACID

CoA and acyl carrier protein from the diet are enzymatically degraded in the intestine to release free pantothenic acid. Uptake of pantothenic acid is mediated by a saturable sodium (Na⁺)-dependent transporter, utilizing the Na⁺ electrochemical gradient for active transport with the highest rate of transport in the jejunum (Fenstermacher and Rose, 1986). Pantetheine also is absorbed by the intestine but is hydrolyzed to pantothenic acid in the intestinal cells. CoA, dephospho-CoA, and phosphopantetheine are not absorbed by the intestine and must be digested to pantothenic acid before absorption (Shibata et al., 1983). The absorbed pantothenic acid is transported by the blood, primarily as bound forms in red blood cells. How this is made available to tissues is unclear, and it may be that the low concentration of free pantothenic acid in plasma (0.06 to 0.08 mg/L as compared with 1.0 to 1.8 mg/L in whole blood) is the form taken up by tissues.

Pantothenic acid (pantothenate) is transported into cells by a saturable Na⁺-dependent mechanism with a high degree of specificity (Tahiliani and Beinlich, 1991). The transport across the blood-brain barrier also is saturable but does not appear to be Na⁺-dependent. In the kidney tubules, pantothenic acid largely is reabsorbed at physiological concentrations by an Na⁺-dependent process. At higher concentrations, there is tubular secretion of pantothenic acid (excretion of a higher concentration in the urine than is present in the plasma). As a result, there is a positive correlation between dietary intake of pantothenic acid and its excretion in the urine. There are no known catabolites of pantothenic acid; only pantothenic acid is excreted in urine.

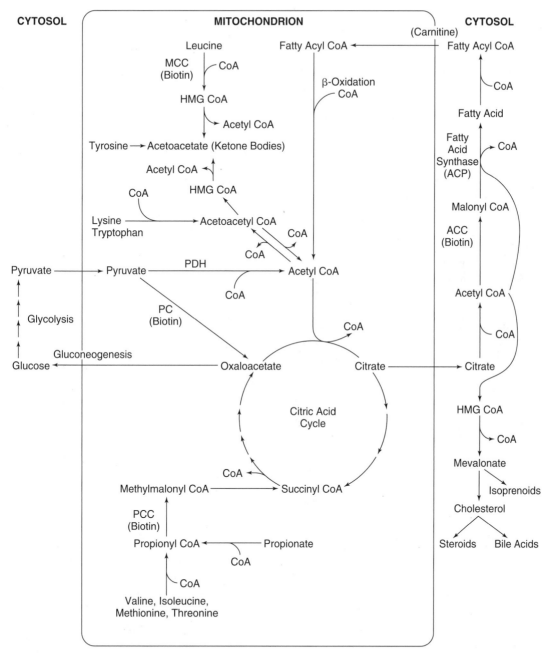

Figure 22–1. Roles of coenzyme A (CoA), acyl carrier protein (ACP), and biotin in cellular metabolism. The major steps of cellular metabolism in which pantothenic acid is involved as ACP in fatty acid synthase and as CoA in other reactions are summarized. The steps catalyzed by the four biotin-containing carboxylases (ACC, acetyl CoA carboxylase; PCC, propionyl CoA carboxylase; MCC, 3-methylcrotonyl CoA carboxylase; PC, pyruvate carboxylase) also are shown. Other abbreviations are PDH, pyruvate dehydrogenase; HMG CoA, 3-hydroxy-3-methylglutaryl CoA.

COENZYME A AND ACYL CARRIER PROTEIN SYNTHESIS AND DEGRADATION

Coenzyme A Synthesis

Within cells, pantothenic acid is metabolized to CoA in the cytosol (Fig. 22–2). The initial reaction is phosphorylation of the hydroxyl group of the pantoic acid portion of pantothenic acid with adenosine triphosphate (ATP), catalyzed by pantothenate kinase, to form 4'-phosphopantothenate. This is the rate-limiting step for synthesis of CoA and regulation of pantothenate kinase activity controls the rate of CoA synthesis. The activity of pantothenate kinase is inhibited by the intermediates 4'-phosphopantothenate and dephospho-CoA, by the end product CoA, and by the acetyl-, propionyl-, and malonyl-esters of CoA (acyl CoAs). Carnitine protects from the inhibition by CoA and acyl CoA by competing with them for their binding of pantothenate kinase.

The next step in the synthesis of CoA is catalyzed by 4'-phosphopantothenoylcysteine synthetase, which couples ATP hydrolysis with formation of an amide bond between the carboxyl of 4'-phosphopantothenate and the amino group of the sulfur amino acid, cysteine. The product, 4'-phosphopantothenoyl cysteine is decarboxylated by a specific decarboxylase to form 4'-phosphopantetheine. A specific adenylyltransferase adds the adenosine 5'-monophosphate (AMP) group of ATP to the 4'-phospho group of 4'-phosphopantetheine to form dephospho-CoA. The final step in the synthesis of CoA is the phosphorylation of the 3'-hydroxyl of dephospho-CoA, catalyzed by dephospho-CoA kinase and utilizing ATP. All of the enzymes in the CoA biosynthetic pathway are present in the cytosol, but the last two enzymes are also present in mitochondria. Notable features of the structure of CoA are the 3'-phosphoadenosine 5'-diphosphate (3'-phospho-ADP) moiety linked with the pantoate portion, and the reactive sulfhydryl group at the end of the long, flexible chain derived from β-alanine and cysteine. Coenzyme A, or CoA, is often abbreviated as CoASH to illustrate this reactive sulfhydryl group, and thioesters of organic acids with CoASH are often abbreviated as acyl-SCoA.

The majority of the CoA in cells is found within the mitochondria, with about 75% of liver CoA in mitochondria and 95% of heart CoA in mitochondria. This is consistent with the mitochondria being the major cellular organelle involved in fatty acid oxidation and in the final oxidative steps in the catabolism of all fuels; CoA plays a major role in these processes. Because the mitochondria represents only a small fraction of the cellular volume, the concentration of CoA in mitochondria (2.2 mmol/L) is 40 to 150 times the concentration of CoA in the cytosol (0.015 to 0.05 mmol/L). This large concentration difference is maintained by the transport of the negatively charged CoA into the mitochondria, which is driven by the membrane electrical gradient (Tahiliani, 1989). CoA is also involved in the oxidation of very-long-chain fatty acids in peroxisomes, but little is known about how it enters these organelles. In the cytosol, CoA also is used for the synthesis of the ACP domain of the fatty acid synthase enzyme, which catalyzes fatty acid synthesis.

Acyl Carrier Protein Synthesis

There are several acyl carrier proteins known in yeast and bacteria, but the ACP domain of fatty acid synthase is the most important and best studied. Fatty acid synthase is the only mammalian enzyme complex containing the ACP domain that has been well characterized. ACP is synthesized as an enzymatically inactive apoprotein that lacks the prosthetic group, but after covalent attachment of the phosphopantetheine group, it becomes the enzymatically active holoacyl carrier protein. This attachment reaction, catalyzed by holoacyl carrier protein synthetase, uses CoA to form a phosphoester bond between the 4'-phosphopantetheine portion of CoA and a specific seryl residue of the ACP, with release of the 3'-phospho-AMP moiety of CoA (Fig. 22–3). Note that as in CoA, the reactive sulfhydryl group of acyl carrier protein is at the end of the long chain derived from β-alanine and cysteine. There is an acyl carrier protein hydrolase that releases 4'-phosphopantetheine from holo-ACP to reform apo-ACP. Interestingly, the combined action of the acyl carrier protein hydrolase and synthetase results in the

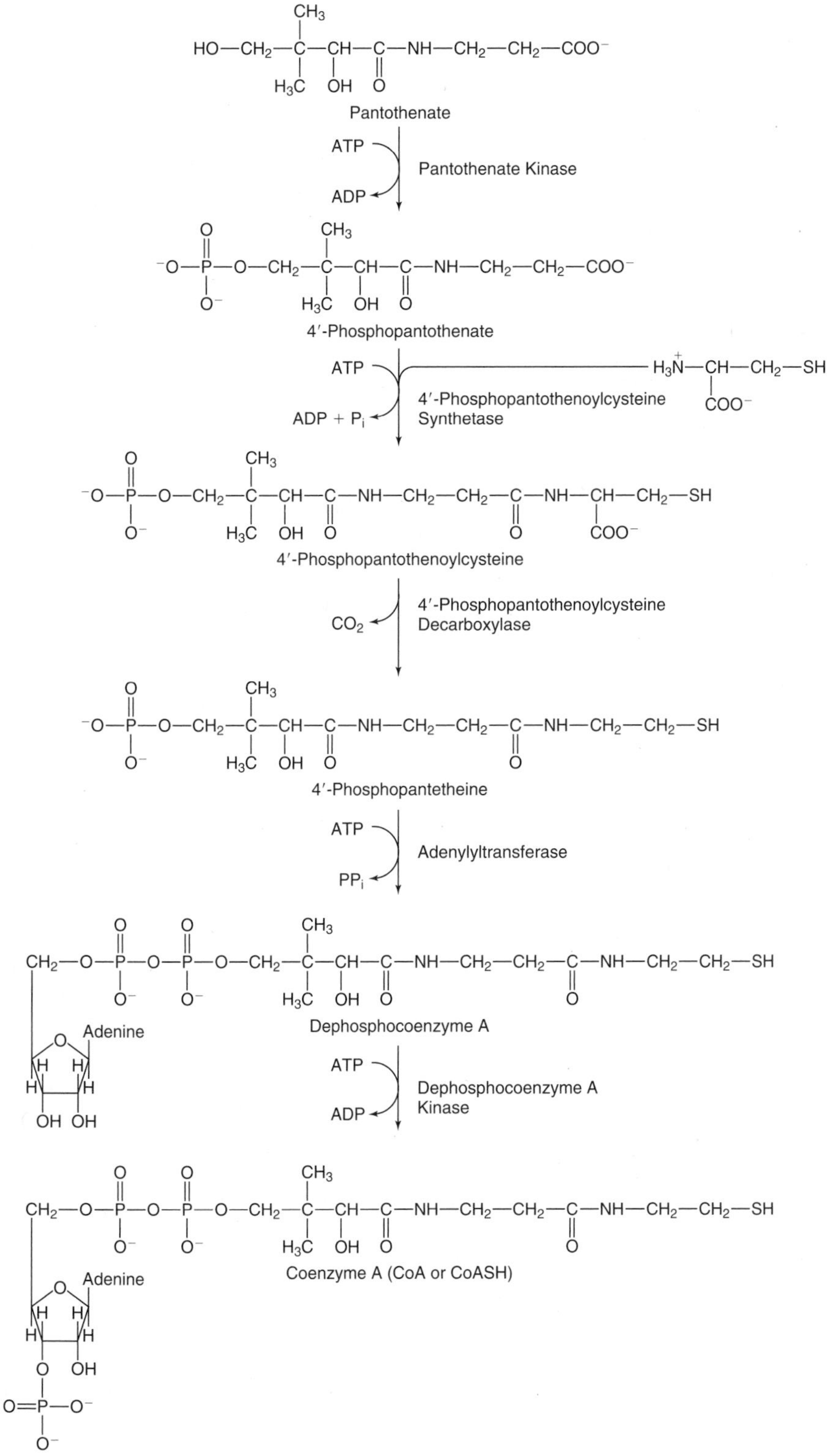

Figure 22–2. *Coenzyme A synthesis and structure. CoA is synthesized from pantothenic acid, the amino acid cysteine, and ATP in mammalian cells.*

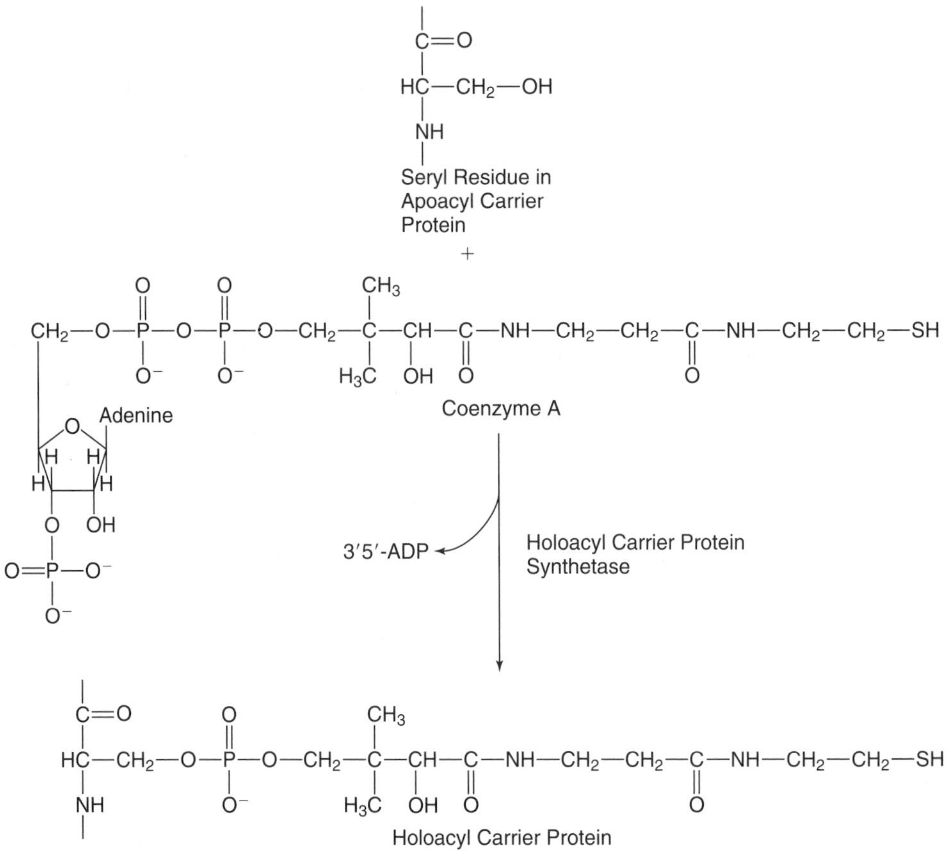

Figure 22–3. *Acyl carrier protein synthesis. CoA is cleaved to form 3', 5'-ADP with attachment of 4'-phosphopante-theine, as a phosphate ester, to the hydroxyl group of a seryl residue in apoACP to form holoACP, a component of fatty acid synthase.*

rapid turnover of the 4'-phosphopantetheine of acyl carrier protein with a half-life measured in hours compared to the half-life of the fatty acid synthase, which is measured in days in rat tissues (Tweto et al., 1971).

Coenzyme A and 4'-Phosphopantetheine Degradation

The degradation of CoA essentially is the reverse of its synthesis. CoA does not appear to be degraded in the mitochondria, but in the lysosomes the 3'-phosphate group is removed by nonspecific phosphatases to form dephospho-CoA. This is degraded to 4'-phosphopantetheine and AMP by a nucleotide pyrophosphatase located in the plasma membrane fraction. CoA also is degraded by this enzyme, but at a much lower rate and with a much higher K_m. Surprisingly, acyl CoAs also are readily degraded to 4'-phosphopantetheine.

Whether 4'-phosphopantetheine is derived from the degradation of CoA or the turnover of ACP, the phosphate is removed by phosphatases to give pantetheine. This is hydrolyzed to pantothenic acid and cysteamine by pantetheinase, which is found in both the microsomal (endoplasmic reticulum) and lysosomal fractions of rat liver and kidney. The pantothenic acid can be excreted or used for resynthesis of CoA. The cysteamine is oxidized to hypotaurine and further oxidized to taurine, which is excreted in the urine.

ROLES OF COENZYME A AND ACYL CARRIER PROTEIN IN METABOLISM

CoA has many functions in metabolism, including its role in the formation of acyl carrier protein. Both CoA and acyl carrier protein are used to form thioesters with carboxylic acid

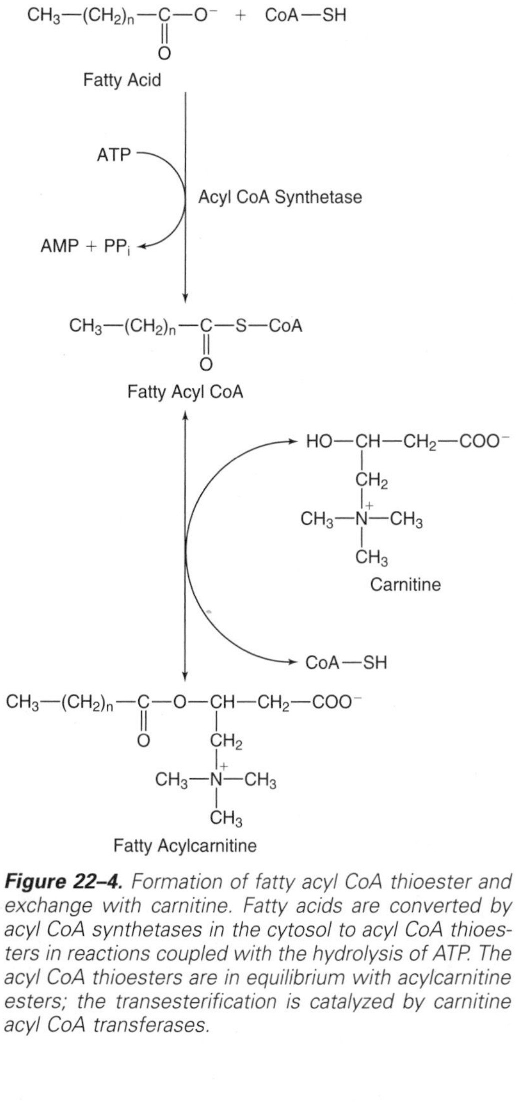

Figure 22–4. *Formation of fatty acyl CoA thioester and exchange with carnitine. Fatty acids are converted by acyl CoA synthetases in the cytosol to acyl CoA thioesters in reactions coupled with the hydrolysis of ATP. The acyl CoA thioesters are in equilibrium with acylcarnitine esters; the transesterification is catalyzed by carnitine acyl CoA transferases.*

groups of fatty acids and other compounds, as shown in Figure 22–4. Much of the metabolism of fatty acids and certain amino acid derivatives, as well as a number of amphibolic steps in metabolism, occur using CoA thioester substrates and producing CoA thioester products.

Coenzyme A and Acyl Carrier Protein in Fatty Acid Synthesis

Both CoA and ACP are essential for the synthesis of fatty acids in the cytosol (see Fig. 22–1; see also Chapter 13). Acetyl CoA, the substrate for fatty acid synthesis in the cytosol, is generated in the mitochondria from the oxidative decarboxylation of pyruvate by py-

ruvate dehydrogenase. Pyruvate itself is generated from cytosolic metabolism of glucose or gluconeogenic substrates and then is transported into the mitochondria. Because the acetyl CoA generated in the mitochondria cannot cross the mitochondrial membrane, the carbon for fatty acid synthesis leaves the mitochondria in the form of citrate after condensation with oxaloacetate. Citrate is transported to the cytosol, where it is cleaved by citrate lyase (in an ATP- and CoA-requiring reaction) to regenerate the oxaloacetate and the acetyl CoA that serves as substrate for fatty acid synthesis in the cytosol. Acetyl transacylase transfers the acetyl group from acetyl CoA to the pantetheine sulfhydryl of ACP, releasing free CoA in the process; these two carbons from acetyl CoA form the methyl end of the fatty acid that will be synthesized. A biotin-containing enzyme, acetyl CoA carboxylase, uses bicarbonate and ATP to convert acetyl CoA to malonyl CoA. Fatty acid synthase utilizes this malonyl CoA to sequentially add two-carbon units to the acetyl- or acyl-ACP, with the liberation of the third carbon of malonyl CoA as CO_2. This process results in the synthesis of even-numbered fatty acids of 16 or 18 carbons. When the synthesis of a fatty acid is complete, a thioesterase hydrolyzes the ACP-fatty acid thioester, releasing the fatty acid and regenerating the ACP sulfhydryl. The rate of fatty acid synthesis is regulated primarily by the concentration of malonyl CoA, which is determined by regulation of the activity of acetyl CoA carboxylase, as is described later in this chapter.

Coenzyme A in Oxidative Decarboxylation Reactions Catalyzed by α-Keto Acid Dehydrogenase Complexes

A key role for CoA in fuel metabolism is its function in α-keto acid dehydrogenase complexes that catalyze the oxidative decarboxylation of keto acids. In the metabolism of carbohydrates, the end product of the glycolytic pathway for glucose is the simple, three-carbon α-keto acid pyruvate. In order for pyruvate to be completely oxidized via the citric acid cycle and oxidative phosphorylation, the pyruvate is oxidatively decarboxylated to acetyl CoA (with release of CO_2 and reduction of NAD) by the pyruvate dehydrogenase complex. This complex reaction involves five coenzymes (four of them derived from vitamins): TPP, NAD, FAD, lipoate, and CoA (see Chapters 9 and 20; Fig. 9–17). In the decarboxylation of pyruvate, the two-carbon aldehyde unit is attached to TPP, oxidized, transferred to a lipoyl enzyme, and then transferred to CoA to form acetyl CoA. Acetyl CoA is a central compound in metabolism, having several catabolic as well as anabolic fates. The CoA eventually is released as free CoA as further metabolism of acetyl CoA progresses (see Chapter 9, Figs. 9–16 and 9–18).

Two other enzyme complexes that catalyze the oxidative decarboxylation of keto acids with formation of acyl CoA products include the α-ketoglutarate dehydrogenase complex and the branched-chain α-keto acid dehydrogenase complex. The α-ketoglutarate dehydrogenase complex converts α-ketoglutarate to succinyl CoA; this reaction is part of the citric acid cycle and is required for the oxidation of the carbon chains of several amino acids, including glutamate, proline, arginine, and histidine. The CoA is released from succinyl CoA in the next step of the citric acid cycle. The branched chain α-keto acid dehydrogenase complex, again in a series of reactions analogous to those of pyruvate dehydrogenase, catalyzes the first committed step in the catabolic pathway for the branched-chain amino acids. The α-keto acids from transamination of valine, isoleucine, and leucine are oxidatively decarboxylated to form branched-chain acyl CoA products with one less carbon in the chain. These are metabolized in a number of different steps as CoA esters and ultimately yield simple acyl CoA products such as acetyl CoA and propionyl CoA, which enter central pathways of metabolism. (See Chapter 11 for details of amino acid metabolism, including the role of coenzyme A.)

Coenzyme A in Fatty Acid β-Oxidation

CoA plays a major role in the β-oxidation of fatty acids in the mitochondria, which may result in the complete degradation of fatty acids to acetyl CoA, which can be further oxidized in the citric acid cycle (see Fig. 22–1; see also Chapter 13, Figs. 13–9 and 13–10). Most of the fatty acids consumed in dietary triacylglycerols or obtained from adipose stores have chains of 16 or more carbons. These long-chain fatty acids require a carrier system for their transport from the cytosol into the mitochondria. In the cytosol, the free, long-chain fatty acids are activated to CoA thioesters by acyl CoA synthetases that couple ATP hydrolysis with thioester formation. These fatty acyl CoAs are transesterified to carnitine to form "energy-equivalent" acylcarnitines, which are transported across the mitochondrial inner membrane. On the outer mitochondrial membrane, the enzyme carnitine palmitoyltransferase I (CPT I) converts the fatty acyl CoA to acyl carnitine and free CoA. A carnitine acylcarnitine-translocase moves the acylcarnitines into the mitochondria and free carnitine out of the mitochondria. Carnitine palmitoyltransferase II (CPT II) on the inner mitochondrial membrane regenerates fatty acyl CoA in the mitochondria.

In the β-oxidation, two-carbon segments of the fatty acyl CoA are sequentially removed as acetyl CoA. The series of reactions for each cycle are dehydrogenation to the unsaturated acyl CoA, hydration to 3-hydroxyacyl CoA, dehydrogenation to the 3-ketoacyl CoA, and thiolytic cleavage by CoA to release acetyl CoA and a fatty acyl CoA with two less carbons. There are multiple dehydrogenases with overlapping chain-length specificities that favor acyl CoAs with very long, long, medium, or short chains. Reducing equivalents generated in the various dehydrogenation steps are funneled into the electron transport chain. Most tissues use fatty acids as a fuel. Cardiac muscle is particularly dependent on fatty acid oxidation for energy, and many abnormalities of fatty acid oxidation can cause cardiomyopathy.

The rate of fatty acid oxidation is controlled by the rate of transport of fatty acids into the mitochondria. The rate of transport is controlled largely by the activity of CPT I, which is strongly inhibited by malonyl CoA. When fatty acid synthesis is increased by activation of acetyl CoA carboxylase to produce more malonyl CoA as substrate for fatty acid synthase (see Chapter 13, Fig. 13–2), the increased malonyl CoA inhibits CPT I, decreasing fatty acid transport into the mitochondria and thus preventing the reoxidation of newly synthesized fatty acids. When the plasma concentration of free fatty acids is elevated as in the starved state, acetyl CoA carboxylase is inhibited, decreasing the synthesis of malonyl CoA and decreasing malonyl CoA inhibition of CPT I so that fatty acids enter the mitochondria for β-oxidation.

Coenzyme A in Ketone Body Synthesis and Oxidation

Ketone bodies are an important source of fuel derived from fat metabolism when glucose is limiting, as in starvation (see Fig. 22–1; also see Chapter 13, Figs. 13–14 and 13–15). Acetoacetate and its reduction product, 3-hydroxybutyrate, were called ketone bodies because some acetoacetate is spontaneously decarboxylated to acetone, a ketone. Ketone bodies are synthesized in the liver from acetoacetyl CoA and acetyl CoA produced via β-oxidation of fatty acids (see Fig. 22–1). Acetoacetyl CoA is condensed with acetyl CoA to form 3-hydroxy-3-methylglutaryl CoA and free CoA by mitochondrial 3-hydroxy-3-methylglutaryl CoA (HMG CoA) synthetase. This is then cleaved by HMG CoA lyase to form free acetoacetate and acetyl CoA. The net result of this cycle is the conversion of acetoacetyl CoA to acetoacetate and free CoA, but there is no enzyme that directly catalyzes this hydrolysis. Acetoacetate and 3-hydroxybutyrate are interconverted by NAD(H)-dependent 3-hydroxybutyrate dehydrogenase with 3-hydroxybutyrate being the major form.

Acetoacetate and 3-hydroxybutyrate are released from the liver into the blood and then are taken up by other tissues that are able to use them as fuels. In the extrahepatic tissues, the acetoacetate is converted to a CoA ester using succinyl CoA as the CoA donor. The acetoacetyl CoA can then be metabolized to acetyl CoA (last step of β-oxidation) and further oxidized by the citric acid cycle and oxidative phosphorylation.

Additional Roles of Coenzyme A in Amino Acid and Organic Acid Catabolism

In addition to its major role in fatty acid synthesis and oxidation, in oxidative decarboxyl-ation of α-keto acids, and in the citric acid cycle, CoA also is involved in the mitochondrial metabolism of a large number of other carboxylic acids as CoA thioesters. The catabolism of many amino acids involves the removal of the amino group, leaving a carboxyl group that can be esterified to CoA for further metabolism. As described earlier, the branched-chain α-keto acids derived from valine, isoleucine, and leucine are decarboxylated to form acyl CoA derivatives. These are oxidized to unsaturated acyl CoAs in the same manner as the fatty acid acyl CoAs. 3-Methylcrotonyl CoA derived from leucine is carboxylated by a biotin-containing carboxylase and eventually converted to HMG CoA, which is cleaved to acetoacetate (a ketone body) and acetyl CoA by the lyase involved in ketone body synthesis. Valine and isoleucine are metabolized via pathways involving acyl CoAs to form propionyl CoA and propionyl CoA plus acetyl CoA, respectively. In addition, the amino acids threonine and methionine also are metabolized via oxidative decarboxylation of α-ketobutyrate to propionyl CoA intermediates. Propionyl CoA is then carboxylated by a biotin-containing enzyme, as will be described later in this chapter, to form succinyl CoA. The amino acids lysine, hydroxylysine, and tryptophan are catabolized to α-ketoadipate, which is oxidatively decarboxylated to form glutaryl CoA and ultimately two molecules of acetyl CoA.

Other Metabolic Roles of Coenzyme A

Acyl CoAs are involved in many synthetic reactions. The CoA ester of HMG CoA, formed in the cytosol, is the starting material for the synthesis of isoprenoids, cholesterol, and steroids. Isoprenoids include ubiquinone (which functions as coenzyme Q in the electron transport chain of mitochondria) and dolichol (which is involved in glycoprotein synthesis); steroids include cholesterol and steroid hormones derived from cholesterol. Acetyl CoA is a substrate for the acetylation of amino and hydroxyl groups of many compounds. Another role for CoA is the detoxification of drugs and other exogenous compounds. A well-known example is the conversion of benzoate to hippurate, which is excreted. Benzoyl CoA is synthesized in an ATP-requiring reaction, and the benzoyl group is then transferred to the amino group of glycine to form hippurate (benzoylglycine). Aspirin similarly is metabolized via a CoA ester to form the acylglycine salicylurate for excretion.

COENZYME A AND CARNITINE INTERRELATIONS

The esters of CoA and carnitine have very similar energy contents. They are maintained in equilibrium by carnitine acyl CoA transferases. The carnitine palmitoyl CoA transferases and their role in transporting long-chain fatty acids into mitochondria for β-oxidation have already been described in this chapter and also in Chapter 13. In addition, carnitine acetyl CoA transferase catalyzes the interconversion of a number of short-chain carnitine esters and CoA thioesters. Additional transferases are involved in transport of medium-chain fatty acids. Free carnitine and carnitine esters act as a buffer to maintain free CoA and acyl CoA levels. If acyl CoAs accumulate, as occurs in inherited disorders of fatty acid oxidation or metabolism of some organic acids, free CoA could be depleted below the levels needed for its essential roles in metabolism. The conversion of some acyl CoAs to acylcarnitines frees up CoA and maintains a more normal ratio of free to esterified CoA. In addition, acyl CoAs are inhibitors of a number of enzymes, and decreasing their concentra-tion by converting them to acylcarnitines reduces this inhibition. The acylcarnitines also can be translocated out of the mitochondria, enter the blood circulation, and be excreted by the kidneys as a means of removing accumulated esters of CoA that may be toxic. A side effect of this is that, in inherited disorders in which acylcarnitines are excreted in large amounts, carnitine itself may become depleted in tissues and this, in turn, decreases the transport of fatty acids into the mitochondria (see Chapters 13 and 20).

DIETARY SOURCES, RECOMMENDED INTAKES, AND DEFICIENCY SYMPTOMS

Pantothenic acid is widely distributed in plant and animal sources, existing both free and bound as ACP and CoA. Total pantothenic acid in foods is determined by hydrolysis of the bound forms to free pantothenic acid and quantitation of the released pantothenic acid by microbiological growth assays or radioimmunoassays. There is considerable loss of pantothenic acid in highly processed food. The average dietary intake of pantothenic acid is about 5 to 6 mg/day, with somewhat lower intake in the elderly and young children (Hoppner et al., 1978). From studies of dietary intake and urinary excretion, it is estimated that only about 50% of dietary pantothenic acid is available. Because of the wide distribu-

CLINICAL CORRELATION

Carnitine Treatment of Fatty Acid Oxidation Disorders

A secondary deficiency of carnitine can occur in patients with inherited deficiencies of dehydrogenases involved in the β-oxidation of fatty acids (Roe and Coates, 1995). An example is medium-chain acyl CoA dehydrogenase (MCAD) deficiency, in which the oxidation of the medium-chain length octanoyl CoA is decreased. MCAD deficiency is a relatively common inherited disorder with a frequency as high as 1 in 10,000 in populations of Irish, English, or German descent. With a deficiency of MCAD, octanoyl CoA accumulates and is converted to octanoylcarnitine, resulting in increased plasma levels of octanoylcarnitine and increased excretion of octanoylcarnitine in the urine. Over a period of time, this increased loss of carnitine from the body as octanoylcarnitine in the urine can result in abnormally low levels of free carnitine in plasma and tissues. Administration of oral carnitine, usually 100 mg per kg body weight daily in four divided doses, raises the blood carnitine levels to normal and leads to increased excretion of octanoylcarnitine. This may help to dispose of the toxic accumulations of octanoate.

tion of panthothenic acid in foods, no spontaneous deficiency has been reported. Adequate Intakes (AIs) for panthothenic acid have been set based primarily on amounts needed to replace urinary excretion with an assumed bioavailability of 50% (Institute of Medicine, 1998). Urinary excretion of adults consuming typical American diets is approximately 2.6 mg/day, and the AI for adults is 5 mg/day. Pantothenic acid is included in most multivitamin supplements, generally in the amount of 10 mg.

Pantothenic acid deficiency has been induced in a small number of human volunteers via a pantothenic acid-free diet. There were no clinical symptoms at 9 weeks, even though urinary excretion of pantothenic acid had decreased by 75%, but the volunteers appeared listless and complained of fatigue (Fry et al., 1976). Other volunteers fed a diet deficient in pantothenic acid together with an antagonist (ω-methylpantothenic acid) to block pantothenic acid utilization developed headaches, fatigue, and a sensation of weakness (Bean and Hodges, 1954; Hodges et al., 1958). Additional symptoms included personality changes, sleep disturbances, impaired motor coordination, and gastrointestinal disturbances. All symptoms were reversed by stopping the antagonist and giving pantothenic acid.

■ BIOTIN

Biotin was discovered in the 1920s and 1930s as a factor that prevented dermatitis, hair loss, and neurological abnormalities caused by feeding a diet high in raw egg white to rats. The protein avidin in raw egg white binds biotin with a very high affinity and prevents the intestinal absorption of biotin, causing a deficiency of biotin that leads to the clinical symptoms. Biotin is covalently attached as a coenzyme to form several enzymes that function as carboxylases. Three of the four enzymes that contain biotin are carboxylases that act on CoA ester substrates in fatty acid metabolism and amino acid catabolism, as shown in Figure 22–1. The fourth enzyme carboxylates pyruvate.

BIOTIN SYNTHESIS

Biotin contains two five-membered rings that consist of a ureido group attached to a tetrahydrothiophene ring; a side chain (valeric acid) of five carbons ending with a carboxyl group is attached to the tetrahydrothiophene ring (Fig. 22–5). Biotin is synthesized by bacteria, yeast, algae, and some plant species from pimelate, a seven-carbon dicarboxylic acid, and

Food Sources of Pantothenic Acid

- Meat, fish, poultry (especially liver)
- Milk and yogurt
- Legumes and whole-grain cereals

Adequate Intakes Across the Life Cycle

	mg/day
Infants, 0–5 mo	1.7
6–11 mo	1.8
Children, 1–3 y	2
4–8 y	3
9–13 y	4
Males, >13 y	5
Females, > 13 y	5
Pregnant	6
Lactating	7

From The Institute of Medicine. (1998) Dietary Reference Intakes for Thiamin, Riboflavin, Niacin, Vitamin B_6, Folate, Vitamin B_{12}, Pantothenic Acid, Biotin, and Choline. National Academy Press, Washington, D.C.

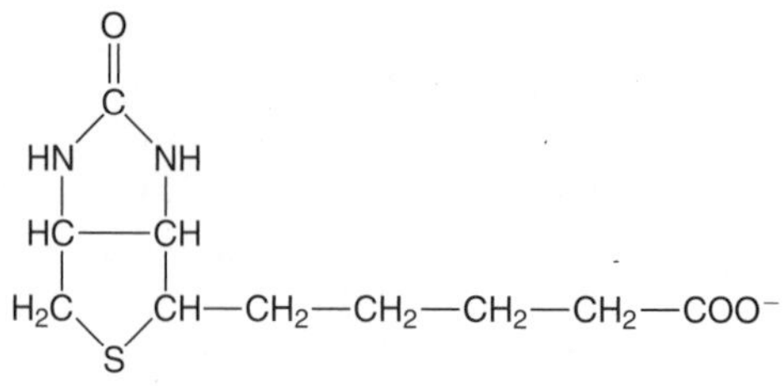

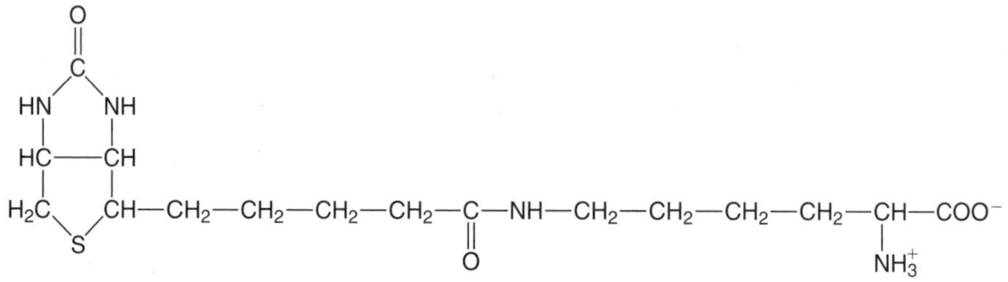

Figure 22–5. Biotin and biocytin structures. Biotin has a 5-carbon valeric acid side chain attached to a five-membered ring containing a ureido group and a second ring of tetrahydrothiophene. The ureido group is involved in the reactions of carboxylases and is the portion of the molecule to which the protein avidin binds. In biocytin (N-biotinyl-L-lysine), the carboxyl group of biotin is linked by an amide bond to the ε-amino group of lysine. Biocytin is derived from the proteolytic degradation of biotin-containing carboxylase enzymes.

the amino acids alanine and cysteine. The natural isomer has the D-(+) configuration. Because biotin functions as a cofactor covalently bound to proteins called carboxylases, the biotin in the cell and in food sources may be attached in an amide bond to the ε-amino group of a lysyl residue in enzyme proteins.

BIOTIN ABSORPTION, TRANSPORT, EXCRETION, AND DEGRADATION

In the digestion of dietary proteins and peptides that contain covalently bound biotin, the proteolytic enzymes and peptidases do not cleave the biotinyl-lysine amide bond. Upon digestion, the lysine and small lysine-containing peptides with covalently attached biotin are released. The released lysine with biotin covalently attached is called biocytin (Fig. 22–5). Biocytin and biotinyl-lysyl peptides are hydrolyzed, to release free biotin and lysine or lysyl-containing peptides, by a specific hydrolase called biotinidase, present in the pancreatic digestive secretions.

Free biotin from the diet or that produced by digestion of proteins and the action of biotinidase is transported across the intestine by a carrier-mediated, Na$^+$-dependent proc-

ess. Biocytin is not actively transported, and although it can be absorbed from the intestine by passive diffusion, its uptake is much slower than the active transport of biotin (Said et al., 1993).

In the blood, 80% of biotin is free in the plasma, with the rest bound reversibly or covalently to plasma proteins (Mock and Malik, 1992). Biotin enters cells by diffusion and Na$^+$-dependent transport. Biotin is actively transported across the blood-brain barrier, with cerebrospinal fluid concentrations being about 2.5 times the plasma concentrations (Lo et al., 1991). In the kidney, biotin is reabsorbed by a carrier-mediated, Na$^+$-dependent transport system; the renal clearance is about 40% of that of creatinine.

Most earlier studies of biotin excretion assumed that the assays for biotin, either the microbiological growth assays or avidin-binding assays, were specific for biotin. Using chromatographic separations followed by avidin-binding assays, it was shown that a number of biotin degradation products are excreted and that biotin accounts for about 43% of the total excretion (Mock et al., 1993). The major metabolic degradation product (about 30% of the avidin-binding material) is bisnorbiotin (the biotin ring structure with a 3-carbon side chain) formed by the β-oxidation shortening of the 5-carbon valerate side chain by two carbons. The other degradation product (about 11% of the total) is biotin sulfoxide, in which the thiophene ring sulfur has been oxidized to a sulfoxide. Similarly, biotin was found to account for only about half of the avidin-binding material in serum (Mock et al., 1995). Recently, small amounts of three additional metabolites of biotin, biotin sulfone, bisnorbiotin methylketone, and tetranorbiotin sulfoxide, were identified in urine (Zempleni et al., 1997).

HOLOCARBOXYLASE SYNTHETASE

The only known function of biotin in humans and other mammals is as a prosthetic group in four carboxylases. These enzymes are synthesized as enzymatically inactive apocarboxylase proteins, and become active holocarboxylases after the covalent attachment of biotin. Holocarboxylase synthetase attaches the biotin to the apocarboxylases in two sequential reactions (Fig. 22–6). First, biotin is activated with ATP to form biotinyladenylate. This then reacts with the ε-amino group of a specific lysyl residue, which is flanked by methionyl residues, in the active site of the apocarboxylases to form an amide bond between the carboxyl of the biotin side chain and the ε-amino group of the lysyl residue (i.e., the linkage present in biotinyl-lysine or biocytin); the AMP moiety of the biotinyladenylate is released. Note that the side chain of biotin coupled to the side chain of lysine puts the reactive ring portion of biotin at the end of a long, flexible chain in the holocarboxylase proteins.

Holocarboxylase synthetase is present in both the cytosol and the mitochondria. Acetyl CoA carboxylase is a cytosolic enzyme, and the apocarboxylase is biotinylated in the cytosol. The other three carboxylases are present in the mitochondria. It is not known whether their apoenzymes normally are biotinylated by cytosolic holocarboxylase synthetase and then transported into the mitochondria as holoenzymes, or whether the carboxylases are transported into the mitochondria as apoenzymes and then biotinylated to form the holo-

carboxylases. In experimental biotin deficiency in rats or cultured human fibroblasts, the apocarboxylases do accumulate in the mitochondria, and these mitochondrial apocarboxylases are converted rapidly to holocarboxylases when biotin is added to the diet or culture media, demonstrating that biotinylation can occur in the mitochondria.

BIOTIN-CONTAINING CARBOXYLASES

The role of biotin in the carboxylases is to serve as a CO_2 carrier and carboxyl donor to substrates. There are four unique biotin-containing carboxylases in mammalian tissues, which are summarized in Figure 22–7.

Carboxylase Mechanism

The carboxylases use energy from the hydrolysis of ATP to dehydrate HCO_3^- (bicarbonate) to CO_2 (carbon dioxide) forming ADP and carboxyphosphate. As shown in Figure 22–8, the carboxyphosphate then carboxylates the one-nitrogen of biotin, with release of phosphate, to form N-1 carboxybiotinyl-enzyme, which then acts as the CO_2 carrier and donor. These two steps allow HCO_3^-, which is present at a higher concentration in the cell fluid than is CO_2, to be used for formation of bound CO_2, which is more chemically reactive than HCO_3^- in the nucleophilic attack of the substrate in carboxylation reactions (Knowles, 1989).

In carboxylation reactions, the carboxyl group of carboxy-biotinyl-enzyme is transferred, via formation of CO_2 and abstraction of a proton from an enolizable carbon of the acceptor to form a nucleophile that attacks the CO_2, resulting in the carboxylated product (Fig. 22–8). The reaction also involves the metal ions magnesium and potassium. In the carboxylases, the active site for carboxylation of biotin, using HCO_3^- and ATP, and the active site for the transfer of the carboxyl group to the substrate are adjacent. The side chain of biotin provides the necessary flexibility to allow the biotinyl coenzyme to be carboxylated in one site and used as a CO_2 donor at a second site.

The substrates for all four mammalian

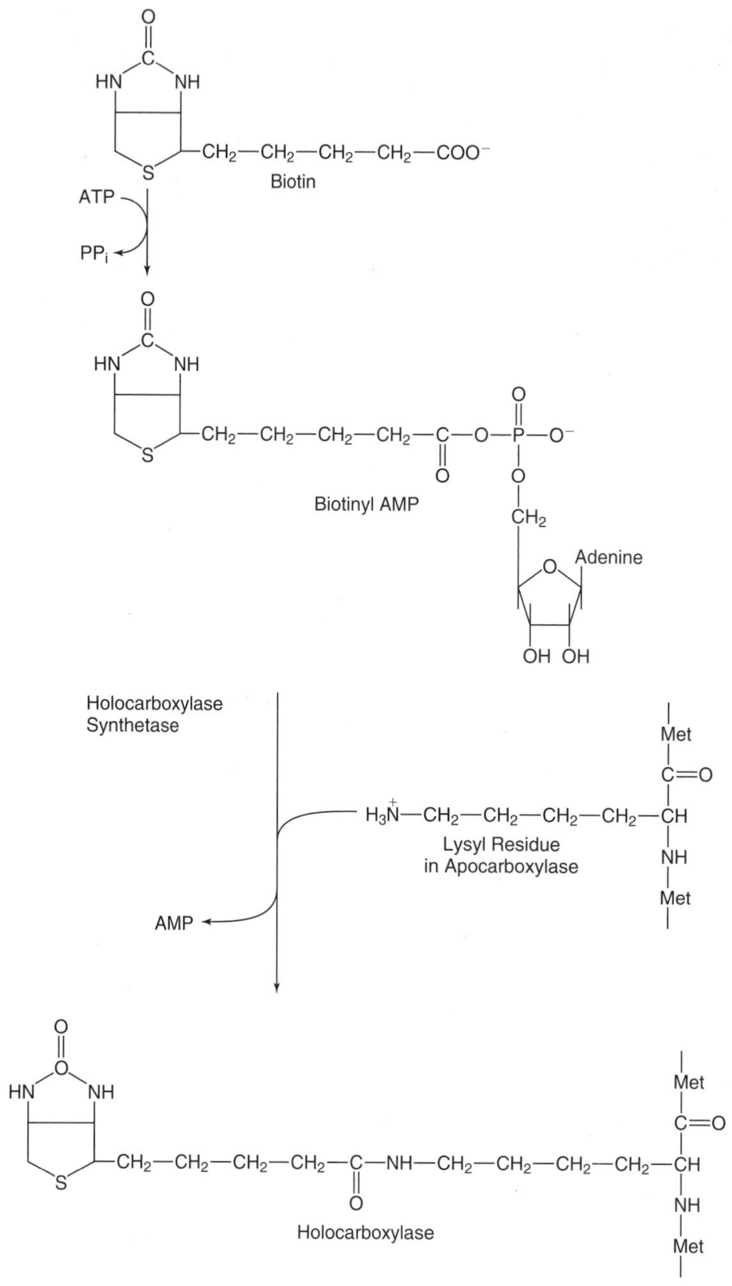

Figure 22–6. *Holocarboxylase synthetase reaction. The formation of holocarboxylase involves two sequential reactions that are catalyzed by holocarboxylase synthetase: formation of biotinyl-AMP from biotin and ATP, followed by formation of an amide bond of biotin with a specific lysyl residue in an apocarboxylase to form a holocarboxylase with release of AMP.*

carboxylases are monocarboxylic acids themselves, and the products are dicarboxylic acids. Pyruvate, the substrate for pyruvate carboxylase, has an α-keto group that is easily enolized to activate the 3-carbon of pyruvate for participation in the carboxylation reaction to form oxaloacetate (which could also be called 3-carboxypyruvate). 3-Methylcrotonyl CoA derived from leucine catabolism is the substrate for 3-methylcrotonyl CoA carboxyl-

ase. It has an α,β-double bond conjugated with the thioester bond of CoA, making it reactive for carboxylation at the 4 position to form the product 3-methylglutaconyl CoA. The other two acids that are substrates for carboxylases do not have an easily enolizable carbon, but the 2-carbon of these short-chain fatty acids is made more reactive by employing their CoA thioester derivatives. Thus, acetyl CoA is carboxylated at the 2-carbon by

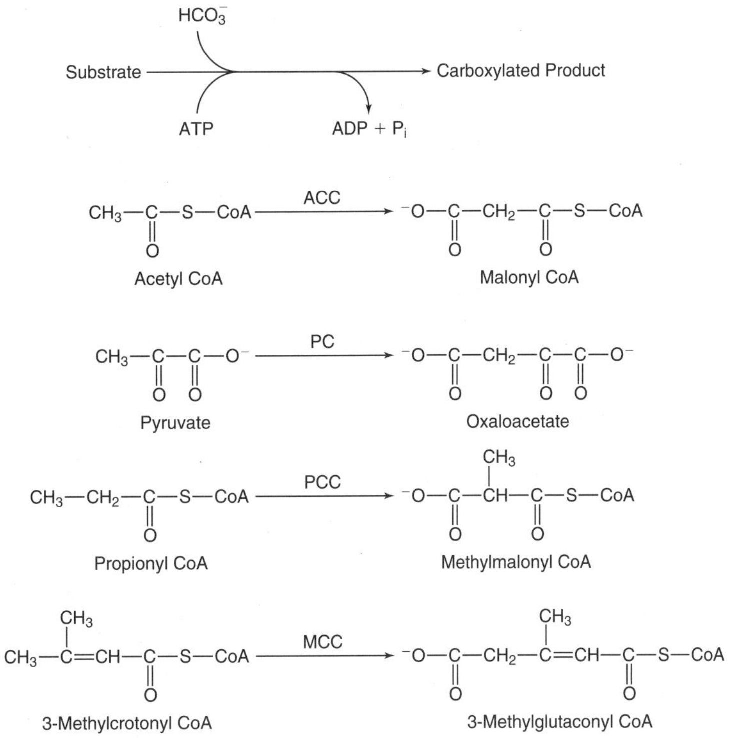

HCO₃⁻ → HCO_3^-

Substrate ⟶ Carboxylated Product

ATP   ADP + Pᵢ

$$CH_3-\overset{O}{\underset{}{\overset{\|}{C}}}-S-CoA \xrightarrow{ACC} {}^-O-\overset{O}{\overset{\|}{C}}-CH_2-\overset{O}{\overset{\|}{C}}-S-CoA$$

Acetyl CoA — Malonyl CoA

$$CH_3-\overset{O}{\overset{\|}{C}}-\overset{O}{\overset{\|}{C}}-O^- \xrightarrow{PC} {}^-O-\overset{O}{\overset{\|}{C}}-CH_2-\overset{O}{\overset{\|}{C}}-\overset{O}{\overset{\|}{C}}-O^-$$

Pyruvate — Oxaloacetate

$$CH_3-CH_2-\overset{O}{\overset{\|}{C}}-S-CoA \xrightarrow{PCC} {}^-O-\overset{O}{\overset{\|}{C}}-\overset{CH_3}{\underset{}{CH}}-\overset{O}{\overset{\|}{C}}-S-CoA$$

Propionyl CoA — Methylmalonyl CoA

$$CH_3-\overset{CH_3}{\underset{}{C}}=CH-\overset{O}{\overset{\|}{C}}-S-CoA \xrightarrow{MCC} {}^-O-\overset{O}{\overset{\|}{C}}-CH_2-\overset{CH_3}{\underset{}{C}}=CH-\overset{O}{\overset{\|}{C}}-S-CoA$$

3-Methylcrotonyl CoA — 3-Methylglutaconyl CoA

Figure 22–7. Carboxylase substrates and products. The substrates and products of the four mammalian biotin-containing carboxylases are shown. Bicarbonate becomes a carboxyl group of the products, and the reaction is driven by energy released from the coupled hydrolysis of ATP. ACC, acetyl CoA carboxylase; MCC, 3-methylcrotonyl CoA carboxylase; PC, pyruvate carboxylase; PCC, propionyl CoA carboxylase.

acetyl CoA carboxylase to form malonyl CoA, and propionyl CoA is carboxylated at the 2-carbon by propionyl CoA carboxylase to form methylmalonyl CoA.

No inherited genetic deficiency of acetyl CoA carboxylase has been documented, probably reflecting the very essential role for this enzyme in fatty acid synthesis such that its absence would be incompatible with life. In contrast, rare, inherited genetic deficiencies of each of the three mitochondrial carboxylases are known, and studies of the perturbed biochemistry in these subjects has contributed to our knowledge of the important roles of biotin-containing carboxylases in normal metabolism. Patients with any one of these isolated deficiencies of carboxylases do not respond biochemically or clinically to treatment with large doses of biotin because their defects are in the apocarboxylase protein rather than in the holocarboxylase synthetase that attaches biotin to the carboxylases. Even if a patient had a defect in an apocarboxylase at the site of attachment for biotin, higher concentrations of biotin would not be expected to increase the ability of normal holo-

carboxylase synthetase to covalently attach biotin to the apocarboxylase.

Acetyl CoA Carboxylase

The role of acetyl CoA carboxylase in the formation of malonyl CoA as the rate-limiting step for synthesis of fatty acids has been described already. The reaction catalyzed is shown in Figure 22–7. This cytosolic enzyme exists as a very large polymer with a molecular mass in the millions of daltons when it is active, and the enzyme is inactivated by dissociation into its protomer units. Citrate activates acetyl CoA carboxylase by increasing polymerization. CoA itself activates acetyl CoA carboxylase by lowering the K_m for acetyl CoA. The enzyme is inhibited by the products of fatty acid synthesis, the long-chain acyl CoAs, which act to depolymerize the enzyme. In addition, acetyl CoA carboxylase activity is regulated by covalent modification (phosphorylation) in response to the hormones insulin and glucagon; a high insulin-to-glucagon ratio favors dephosphorylation of the enzyme to an active form, whereas a low insulin-to-

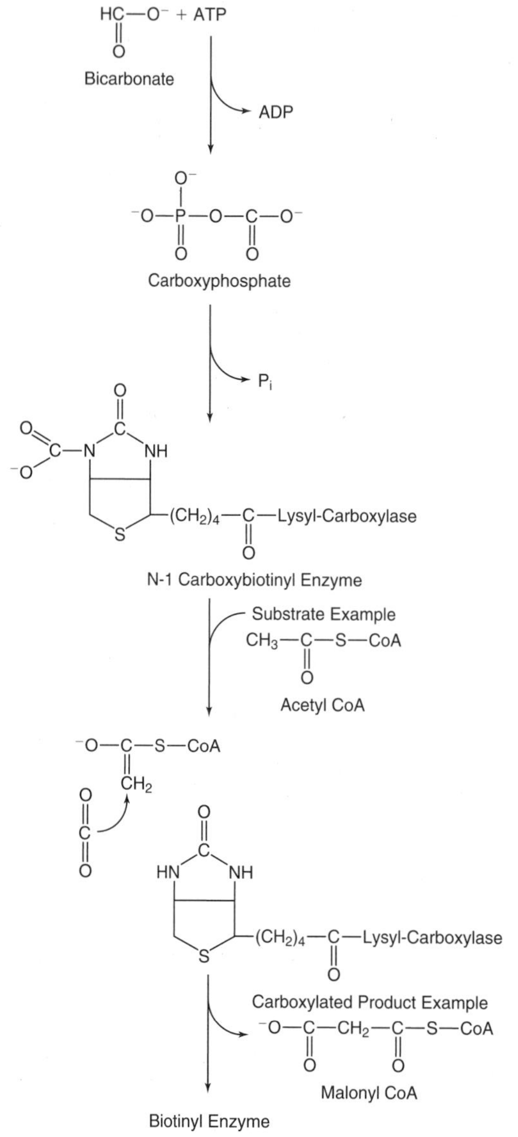

HC—O⁻ + ATP

Bicarbonate

ADP

$$^-O—\overset{O^-}{\underset{O}{P}}—O—\overset{O}{C}—O^-$$

Carboxyphosphate

P_i

N-1 Carboxybiotinyl Enzyme

—(CH₂)₄—C—Lysyl-Carboxylase

Substrate Example

CH₃—C—S—CoA

Acetyl CoA

—O—C—S—CoA

Carboxylated Product Example

⁻O—C—CH₂—C—S—CoA

Malonyl CoA

Biotinyl Enzyme

Figure 22–8. *Mechanism of carboxylation by biotinyl enzymes. With energy provided by the hydrolysis of ATP, bicarbonate is attached to biotin to form N-1 carboxybiotin. The carboxyl group is then transferred to an enolizable carbon in the substrate to form the carboxylated product. The carboxylation of acetyl CoA to malonyl CoA is shown as an example.*

glucagon ratio favors phosphorylation to the inactive form. The amount of acetyl CoA carboxylase protein also is affected by dietary, nutritional, and hormonal changes. Thus, the regulation of acetyl CoA carboxylase activity is complex, as one might expect for an enzyme that catalyzes the rate-limiting step of fatty acid synthesis and the production of a compound (malonyl CoA) that regulates fatty

acid oxidation by controlling the transport of fatty acids into the mitochondria.

Pyruvate Carboxylase

Pyruvate carboxylase is a mitochondrial enzyme that catalyzes the synthesis of the citric acid cycle intermediate, oxaloacetate, from pyruvate, as shown in Figure 22–7. In all tissues, pyruvate carboxylase has an important anaplerotic role in maintaining the levels of oxaloacetic and other intermediates of central pathways of fuel metabolism, including the citric acid cycle. Anaplerosis refers to the replenishment of intermediates in a metabolic cycle that may be depleted by removal from the cycle. Carboxylation of pyruvate to oxaloacetate is an essential step in the utilization of precursors such as pyruvate, lactate, and many amino acids for gluconeogenesis. (See Chapters 9 and 11 for more details of these pathways.)

Pyruvate carboxylase shows allosteric activation by its substrate pyruvate and also by the allosteric activator acetyl CoA, which is a product of pyruvate dehydrogenase and of fatty acid oxidation and an indicator of fuel availability in the mitochondria. The amount of pyruvate carboxylase protein in liver is also increased in diabetes and in hyperthyroidism.

A genetic deficiency of pyruvate carboxylase results in accumulation of pyruvate. Pyruvate is reduced to lactate, resulting in elevated levels of lactate in blood. Blood or plasma lactate levels commonly are measured in clinical laboratories. Pyruvate is also transaminated, resulting in an elevated concentration of alanine in the blood. In the A form of pyruvate carboxylase deficiency, the patient presents in the first few months of life with mild or moderate lactic acidemia and psychomotor retardation. Most children die within the first few years, and the survivors have severe mental retardation. Interestingly, the majority of the A form deficiency occurs in Native Americans from the Algonkian linguistic group. In the more severe B form of pyruvate carboxylase deficiency, symptoms occur shortly after birth with severe lactic acidemia and elevated blood ammonia concentrations; death usually occurs before 3 months of age.

Propionyl CoA Carboxylase

Propionyl CoA carboxylase catalyzes the carboxylation of propionyl CoA to methylmalonyl CoA in the mitochondria, as shown in Figure 22–7. The methylmalonyl CoA is isomerized by a vitamin B_{12} coenzyme-containing mutase to succinyl CoA, and succinyl CoA then can be metabolized by the citric acid cycle enzymes. Sources of propionyl CoA include the propionyl CoA formed from catabolism of the amino acids valine, isoleucine, threonine, and methionine; the propionyl CoA formed in the final step in the β-oxidation of odd-numbered fatty acids; the propionyl CoA released as a byproduct of bile acid synthesis from cholesterol; and a significant amount of propionate produced by the intestinal microflora. The sequential reactions of propionyl CoA carboxylase and methylmalonyl CoA mutase provide a path for the conversion of these propionate precursors to oxaloacetate, a central intermediate in glucose and amino acid metabolism and an intermediate in the citric acid cycle. Propionyl CoA carboxylase is not rate limiting in the metabolism of propionyl CoA, the enzyme activity is not subject to regulation by effector molecules, and the levels of propionyl CoA carboxylase protein are not altered by dietary or hormonal changes.

Propionic acidemia is caused by an inherited deficiency of propionyl CoA carboxylase. Patients have repeated, life-threatening episodes of severe ketosis and metabolic acidosis, often beginning in the neonatal period. Symptoms include vomiting, dehydration, and lethargy, progressing to coma and death if not treated. Frequent neurological complications include developmental delay, seizures, cerebral atrophy, and electroencephalogram (EEG) abnormalities. The elevated concentrations of propionyl CoA result in formation of elevated levels of diagnostically characteristic metabolites. These include methylcitrate, which is continuously elevated in urine, and 3-hydroxypropionate, propionylglycine, and a variety of other metabolites that are elevated during severe metabolic decompensation. A severe secondary elevation of blood ammonia also occurs during episodes. Propionyl CoA is in equilibrium with propionylcarnitine, which is excreted in the urine;

loss of propionylcarnitine can lead to a secondary deficiency of carnitine. Therefore, treatment includes giving carnitine to prevent a carnitine deficiency and to promote the conversion of propionyl CoA to propionylcarnitine, which restores CoA concentrations and facilitates excretion of the nonmetabolizable propionate.

The most important treatments for propionic acidemia is the restriction of dietary protein in order to limit the amino acid precursors of propionate and the use of special formulas that have very low levels of isoleucine, valine, methionine, and threonine, which are the amino acid precursors of propionate. The required intake of these essential amino acids is met by addition of natural proteins with careful calculation of the intake of each amino acid. Clinical management requires continuous careful nutritional assessment because the amino acids that are restricted in these diets are essential amino acids that must be given in amounts sufficient for protein synthesis and normal growth, but not in excess, which would lead to their catabolism and increased propionate production.

3-Methylcrotonyl CoA Carboxylase

3-Methylcrotonyl CoA carboxylase has a single function in the catabolic pathway for leucine. It catalyzes the carboxylation of 3-methylcrotonyl CoA to 3-methylglutaconyl CoA, as shown in Figure 22–7. 3-Methylglutaconyl CoA subsequently is hydrated to 3-hydroxy-3-methylglutaryl CoA, which is cleaved to acetoacetate and acetyl CoA by the same lyase involved in ketone body metabolism. 3-Methylcrotonyl CoA carboxylase is not regulated by small molecules or by dietary or hormonal factors.

The inherited deficiency of 3-methylcrotonyl CoA usually presents with episodes of vomiting, severe metabolic acidosis, extremely low plasma glucose concentrations, and very low levels of carnitine in plasma. The elevated 3-methylcrotonyl CoA is metabolized to relatively nontoxic metabolites, with the major one being 3-hydroxyisovalerate. The abnormal metabolites, 3-methylcrotonylglycine and 3-hydroxyisovalerylcarnitine, also are excreted. Treatment with carnitine to correct and prevent carnitine deficiency and moderate restriction of protein in the diet to limit leucine intake generally result in normal development. A few relatives of affected patients have been found to have the same enzyme deficiency but no clinical symptoms.

HOLOCARBOXYLASE SYNTHETASE DEFICIENCY

The inherited deficiency of holocarboxylase synthetase activity results in decreased activities of all four of the biotin-containing carboxylases: acetyl CoA, pyruvate, propionyl CoA, and 3-methylcrotonyl-CoA carboxylases. The occurrence of multiple carboxylase deficiencies due to a genetic error in coding for one protein, the holocarboxylase, is strong evidence for the role of a single holocarboxylase in the formation of all four holocarboxylases. Multiple carboxylase deficiency results in clinical symptoms related to the roles of all four carboxylases in metabolism. Symptoms usually occur shortly after birth in patients with a more severe enzyme deficiency and include severe ketoacidosis, seizures, lethargy, and coma. Death can occur if these symptoms are not treated. Some patients, who have a milder form of holocarboxylase deficiency and who usually present at several months of age, also show symptoms of hair loss (alopecia) and an erythematous skin rash, which are typical symptoms of biotin deficiency in experimental animals. Elevated urinary excretion of the metabolites characteristic of each of the individual deficiencies are seen collectively in the urine of individuals with multiple carboxylase deficiency. The most elevated metabolite is 3-hydroxyisovalerate from deficiency of 3-methylcrotonyl CoA carboxylase. Also elevated are methylcitrate due to propionyl CoA carboxylase deficiency and lactate from the deficiency of pyruvate carboxylase. Treatment with large oral doses of biotin, ranging from 10 to 60 mg of biotin per day, usually gives dramatic normalization of the biochemical abnormalities, clearing of any skin rash, and regrowth of hair. There is clinical improvement, provided irreversible neurological damage had not occurred during an acute episode. Many patients who were diagnosed during their first episode and subsequently maintained on pharmaco-

logical doses of biotin are clinically well, although some continue to excrete moderately elevated amounts of abnormal metabolites. Because of the biotin-responsiveness, dietary treatment such as protein restriction generally is unnecessary.

When the kinetic properties of the mutant holocarboxylase synthetase in fibroblasts from patients are determined, the K_m for biotin generally is found to be highly elevated. Additionally, the enzyme activity usually is significantly above zero, approaching normal for some patients, when activity is assayed at high concentrations of biotin. The mechanism by which treatment with pharmacological doses of biotin is believed to operate is the elevation of tissue levels of biotin far above normal and into the range of the K_ms of the mutant holocarboxylase synthetase. Thus, even with considerably lower activity of holocarboxylase synthetase than normal, the apocarboxylase are adequately converted to active holocarboxylases, effectively correcting the multiple carboxylase deficiencies. A complete absence of holocarboxylase synthetase activity, which would mean no activity of all four carboxylases, would probably be incompatible with life.

Holocarboxylase synthetase deficiency has been diagnosed prenatally and treated in utero by giving the pregnant mother 10 mg of biotin per day. The newborn had no biochemical abnormalities and no clinical symptoms and has remained healthy, treated with 10 mg of biotin per day.

BIOTINIDASE DEFICIENCY

Another inherited disorder of biotin metabolism is the deficiency of biotinidase, the enzyme required to release biotin from biocytin or biotinyl-lysine-containing peptides derived from the proteolytic digestion of holocarboxylases in the normal turnover of the carboxylases and in the digestion of foods. Biotinidase is present in most cells, in plasma, and in pancreatic secretions. Patients generally do not present with symptoms for some time after birth, because sufficient biotin had been available in utero from the mother for full biotinylation of their carboxylases. The concentration of biotin in the cord blood of normal babies is higher than in the maternal blood, and newborns have higher plasma biotin levels than do older children. The plasma biotin concentration decreases after the second week of life, even though the biotin content of breast milk usually is increasing at this time. Biotinidase-deficient patients develop a clinically observable deficiency of biotin after weeks, months, or even years of life; due to the failure to cleave biocytin, they develop symptoms of seizures, hypotonia, ataxia, developmental delay, hearing loss, optic atrophy, skin rash, and hair loss. The variable age of onset of symptoms probably is related to the relative amounts of available free biotin in the diet compared to the unusable protein-bound biotin (biocytin) and also to the amount of residual biotinidase activity found in a particular patient. The abnormal metabolite excretions are similar to those of holocarboxylase synthetase (multiple carboxylase) deficiency, but the metabolite concentrations in the urine generally are not as elevated.

The effect of treatment of biotinidase deficiency with pharmacological doses of biotin (10 mg per day) is dramatic, with prompt correction of the metabolic acidosis and disappearance of abnormal metabolites, followed by clearing of the skin rash and regrowth of hair. There may be a catch up in development, but the hearing loss and optic atrophy are not reversible. The rapid response to treatment results from the fact that biotinidase deficiency basically results in a deficiency of biotin. As soon as biotin is administered, the already synthesized inactive apocarboxylases are converted rapidly to active holocarboxylases, leading to normalization of metabolism. Although the usual treatment is with large doses of biotin, typically 10 mg per day, a more moderate intake of free biotin would probably be sufficient once the tissue levels of biotin have been raised to normal. However, there appears to be increased renal loss of biotin in biotinidase deficiency, as well as increased excretion of biocytin and biotinyl-peptides, so several hundred micrograms of biotin per day may be required.

Because of the wide variability of the symptoms among patients, biotinidase defi-ciency can be difficult to diagnose clinically. The incidence of biotinidase deficiency of 1 in 112,000 newborns is relatively high for an inborn error of metabolism, and treatment with biotin is very effective and inexpensive. Therefore, inexpensive screening tests have been developed to determine biotinidase deficiency in newborn screening programs using the same filter papers with dried blood spots that are used for screening for phenylketonuria (PKU) and other inherited disorders. In the United States, however, relatively few states perform routine newborn screening for biotinidase deficiency. Administration of the vitamin biotin to patients who are identified by newborn screening as deficient in biotinidase prevents all clinical symptoms.

DIETARY SOURCES, RECOMMENDED INTAKES, AND DEFICIENCY SYMPTOMS

Biotin is widely distributed in foods, existing both as free biotin, biocytin, or as biotin covalently bound to lysyl residues in biotinyl-proteins. Total biotin generally has been determined by microbiological growth assays or avidin-binding assays after hydrolysis of bound forms to free biotin. There is very little information about the relative amounts of free biotin, biocytin, and protein-bound biotin in foods. Liver, egg yolks, and cooked cereals are relatively high in biotin. The daily intake of biotin in Canadian diets was calculated to be 60 µg per day (Hoppner et al., 1978). Biotin also is produced by intestinal flora, but this may be relatively unavailable for absorption because the urinary excretion of biotin approximates that of the dietary intake, whereas fecal excretion is much higher. Because of insufficient information about biotin requirements, only Adequate Intakes (AIs) have been set for biotin based on average dietary intakes (Institute of Medicine, 1998). The AI for adults is 30 µg of biotin/day. Multivitamin preparations generally contain 20 to 40 µg of biotin.

Because of the wide distribution of biotin in foods, a dietary deficiency is very rare. However, with an abnormal diet low in biotin and high in raw egg white, a deficiency with clinical symptoms of hair loss, dermatitis, and

Food Sources of Biotin

- Liver
- Whole-grain cereals
- Nuts and legumes, peanut butter

Adequate Intakes Across the Life Cycle

	µg/day
Infants, 0–5 mo	5
6–11 mo	6
Children, 1–3 y	8
4–8 y	12
9–13 y	20
Males, 14–18 y	25
>18 y	30
Females, 14–18 y	25
>18 y	30
Pregnant	30
Lactating	35

From The Institute of Medicine. (1998) Dietary Reference Intakes for Thiamin, Riboflavin, Niacin, Vitamin B₆, Folate, Vitamin B₁₂, Pantothenic Acid, Biotin, and Choline. National Academy Press, Washington, D.C.

neurological symptoms can occur. Raw egg white contains the protein avidin, which binds biotin with a very high affinity, preventing its uptake from the intestine. A diet high in avidin has been given to human volunteers for 11 weeks to induce biotin deficiency (Sydenstricker et al., 1942). All subjects developed dermatosis, muscle pains, localized loss of sensation, anorexia, nausea, and weight loss. All symptoms were reversed rapidly by treatment with biotin.

Biochemical abnormalities and clinical symptoms of biotin deficiency can occur even when plasma biotin levels are in the normal range. A better indicator of biotin deficiency appears to be the elevation of 3-hydroxyisovalerate in urine, which is a measure of the low activity of 3-methylcrotonyl CoA carboxylase caused by abnormally low levels of intracellular biotin. A recent study of indicators of biotin deficiency involved 10 volunteers given a diet high in raw egg white for 20 days (Mock et al., 1997). The mean urinary excretion of 3-hydroxyisovalerate was significantly elevated by 3 days and above normal for all subjects by 14 days, continuing to increase until 20 days, when the study ended. Mean urinary excretion of biotin was significantly decreased by 3 days. In contrast, the mean level of biotin in the plasma did not decrease significantly, even at 20 days on the diet.

More information about indicators of biotin deficiency has resulted from the chronic use of anticonvulsants. Patients with epilepsy who received long-term therapy with the anticonvulsants phenytoin, primidone, phenobarbital, or carbamazepine, either alone or in combinations, had reduced plasma biotin levels and excreted elevated amounts of 3-hydroxyisovalerate and other organic acids characteristic of biotin deficiency in their urine (Krause et al., 1984). Patients who received sodium valproate did not have these abnormalities. The mechanism by which the anticonvulsants affect biotin status is unclear.

Severe protein-energy malnutrition can result in marasmus or kwashiorkor. Many patients with severe malnutrition have clinical symptoms similar to those of biotin deficiency: dermatitis, alopecia, hypotonia, ataxia, and developmental delay. In studies of children with marasmus or kwashiorkor, Velazquez et al. (1988) found significantly lower levels of biotin in plasma, even though the urinary biotin concentration expressed relative to creatinine was elevated. Assays of the carboxylases in lymphocytes obtained from these patients showed they had partial deficiencies of propi-

CLINICAL CORRELATION

Total Parenteral Nutrition and Biotin Deficiency

In the 1980s, a number of infants with intestinal malabsorption problems who received total parenteral nutrition (TPN) for extended periods developed clinical signs of biotin deficiency, including hypotonia, developmental delay, hair loss, and skin rash (Mock et al., 1985). The skin rash resembled that caused by zinc deficiency, and zinc deficiency was the initial diagnosis for these patients. Although plasma zinc was low in several patients, supplementation with zinc did not correct the rash. A deficiency of essential fatty acids also can cause a similar skin rash, but the patients were receiving adequate fatty acids in the parenteral feedings. When investigated biochemically, the patients were found to have abnormal excretions of urinary organic acids characteristic of biotin deficiency or of the inherited disorders of biotin metabolism, holocarboxylase synthetase and biotinidase deficiencies. Urinary excretion of biotin was below normal, but several patients had normal levels of biotin in plasma. Treatment with biotin dramatically corrected the clinical and biochemical symptoms, confirming that the patients were deficient in biotin. This disorder resulted from not including biotin among the vitamins given with the long-term TPN. These findings indicating biotin deficiency in infants and other patients on long-term TPN have led to the inclusion of biotin in the current vitamin therapy for long-term TPN.

Thinking Critically

1. Would you expect the amount of 3-hydroxyisovalerate to be normal or elevated in urine of patients receiving long-term TPN that lacked biotin? Would the amount change with biotin treatment?

2. What would be the expected clinical and biochemical response to treatment of biotin deficiency due to TPN with either large pharmacological amounts or smaller, normal intake amounts of biotin?

onyl CoA carboxylase and pyruvate carboxylase and a more severe deficiency of 3-methylcrotonyl CoA carboxylase, indicating biotin deficiency. Supplementation with biotin increased the carboxylase levels (Velazquez et al., 1995). It was concluded that decreased activities of the carboxylases in lymphocytes was a better indicator of biotin deficiency in malnutrition than were plasma levels of biotin. The biotin deficiency in malnutrition could result from a dietary deficiency of biotin, impaired intestinal absorption, or increased renal losses of biotin. In patients recovering from severe malnutrition, the biotin and carboxylase levels returned to normal.

REFERENCES

Bean, W. B. and Hodges, R. E. (1954) Pantothenic acid deficiency induced in human subjects. Proc Soc Exp Biol Med 86:693–698.

Fenstermacher, D. K. and Rose, R. C. (1986) Absorption of pantothenic acid in rat and chick intestine. Am J Physiol 250:G155–G160.

Fry, P. C., Fox, H. M. and Tao, H. G. (1976) Metabolic response to a pantothenic acid deficient diet in humans. J Nutr Sci Vitaminol 22:339–346.

Hodges, R. E., Ohlson, M. A. and Bean, W. B. (1958) Pantothenic acid deficiency in man. J Clin Invest 37:1642–1657.

Hoppner, K., Lampi, B. and Smith, D. C. (1978) An appraisal of the daily intakes of vitamin B_{12}, pantothenic acid and biotin from a composite Canadian diet. Can Inst Food Sci Technol J 11:71–74.

Institute of Medicine. (1998) Dietary Reference Intakes for Thiamin, Riboflavin, Niacin, Vitamin B_6, Folate, Vitamin B_{12}, Pantothenic Acid, Biotin, and Choline. National Academy Press, Washington, D.C.

Knowles, J. R. (1989) The mechanism of biotin-dependent enzymes. Annu Rev Biochem 58:195–221.

Krause, K. H., Kochen, W., Berlit, P. and Bonjour, J. P. (1984) Excretion of organic acids associated with biotin deficiency in chronic anticonvulsant therapy. Int J Vitam Nutr Res 54:217–222.

Lo, W., Kadlecek T. and Packman, S. (1991) Biotin transport in the rat central nervous system. J Nutr Sci Vitaminol 37:567–572.

Mock, D. M., Baswell, D. L., Baker, H., Holman, R. T. and Sweetman, L. (1985) Biotin deficiency complicating parenteral alimentation: Diagnosis, metabolic repercussions, and treatment. J Pediatr 106:762–769.

Mock, D. M., Lankford, G. L. and Cazin, J. Jr. (1993) Biotin and biotin analogs in human urine: Biotin accounts for only half of the total. J Nutr 123:1844–1851.

Mock, D. M., Lankford, G. L. and Mock, N. I. (1995) Biotin accounts for only half of the total avidin-binding substances in human serum. J Nutr 125:941–946.

Mock, D. M. and Malik, M. (1992) Distribution of biotin in human plasma: Most of the biotin is not bound to protein. Am J Clin Nutr 56:427–432.

Mock, N. I., Malik, M. I., Stumbo, P. J., Bishop, W. P. and Mock, D. M. (1997) Increased urinary excretion of 3-hydroxyisovaleric acid and decreased urinary excretion of biotin are sensitive early indicators of decreased biotin status in experimental biotin deficiency. Am J Clin Nutr 65:951–958.

Roe, C. R. and Coates, P. M. (1995) Mitochondrial fatty acid oxidation disorders. In: The Metabolic and Molecular Bases of Inherited Disease (Scriver, C. R., Beaudet, A. L., Sly, W. S. and Valle, D., eds.), 7th ed., vol. 1, pp. 1501–1533. McGraw-Hill, New York.

Said, H. M., Thuy, L. P., Sweetman, L. and Schatzman, B. (1993) Transport of the biotin derivative biocytin (N-biotinyl-L-lysine) in rat small intestine. Gastroenterology 104:75–80.

Shibata, K., Gross, C. J. and Henderson, L. M. (1983) Hydrolysis and absorption of pantothenate and its coenzymes in the rat small intestine. J Nutr 113:2207–2215.

Sydenstricker, V. P., Singal, S. A., Briggs, A. P., DeVaughn, N. M. and Isbell, H. (1942) Observations on the "egg white injury" in man. JAMA 118:1199–1200.

Tahiliani, A. G. (1989) Dependence of mitochondrial coenzyme A uptake and the membrane electrical gradient. J Biol Chem 264:18426–18432.

Tahiliani, A. G. and Beinlich, C. J. (1991) Pantothenic acid in health and disease. Vitam Horm 46:165–228.

Tweto, J., Liberati, M. and Larrabee, A. R. (1971) Protein turnover and 4-phosphopantetheine exchange in rat liver fatty acid synthetase. J Biol Chem 246:2468–2471.

Velazquez, A., Martin-del-Campo, C., Baez, A., Zamudio, S., Quiterio, M., Aguilar, J. L., Perez-Ortiz, B., Sanchez-Ardines, M., Guzman-Hernandez, J. and Casanueva, E. (1988) Biotin deficiency in protein-energy malnutrition. Eur J Clin Nutr 43:169–173.

Velazquez, A., Teran, M., Baez, A., Gutierrez, J. and Rodriguez, R. (1995) Biotin supplementation affects lymphocyte carboxylases and plasma biotin in severe protein-energy malnutrition. Am J Clin Nutr 61:385–391.

Zempleni, J., McCormick, D. B. and Mock, D. M. (1997) Identification of biotin sulfone, bisnorbiotin methyl ketone and tetranorbiotin-1-sulfoxide in human urine. Am J Clin Nutr 65:508–511.

RECOMMENDED READINGS

Dakshinamurti, K. and Bhagavan, H. N. (eds.) (1985) Biotin. (Ann NY Acad Sci vol. 447). New York Academy of Sciences, New York.

Knowles, J. R. (1989) The mechanism of biotin-dependent enzymes. Annu Rev Biochem 58:195–221.

Mock, D. M. (1996) Biotin. In: Present Knowledge in Nutrition (Ziegler, E. E. and Filer, J. L. J., eds.), 7th ed., pp. 220–235. International Life Sciences Institutes—Nutrition Foundation, Washington, D. C.

Tahiliani, A. G. and Beinlich, C. J. (1991) Pantothenic acid in health and disease. Vitam Horm 46:165–228.

Wolf, B. (1995) Disorders of biotin metabolism. In: The Metabolic and Molecular Bases of Inherited Disease (Scriver, C. R., Beaudet, A. L., Sly, W. S. and Valle, D., eds.), 7th ed., vol. 2, pp. 3151–3177. McGraw-Hill, New York.

CHAPTER 23

Vitamin C

*Mark Levine, M.D., Steven C. Rumsey, Ph.D.,
Yaohui Wang, M.D., Jae B. Park, Ph.D., and
Rushad Daruwala, Ph.D.*

OUTLINE

NOMENCLATURE, STRUCTURE, FORMATION, CHEMICAL CHARACTERISTICS, AND DEGRADATION OF VITAMIN C

Ascorbic acid (ascorbate, vitamin C) is a 6-carbon lactone synthesized from glucose by many animals (Fig. 23–1). Most mammals synthesize ascorbate in liver, and synthesis occurs in kidney in birds and reptiles. However, several species are unable to synthesize ascorbate, including humans, nonhuman primates, guinea pigs, Indian fruit bats, bulbuls, and some fish. Humans and primates lack gulonolactone oxidase, the terminal enzyme in the biosynthetic pathway. The DNA encoding for the enzyme has undergone substantial mutation so that no protein is produced (Nishikimi et al., 1994). As a consequence, animals unable to synthesize ascorbate must ingest it to survive, and hence ascorbic acid is a vitamin.

Ascorbic acid is an electron donor (reducing agent) (Fig. 23–2), and probably all of its biochemical and molecular functions can be accounted for by this function. Two electrons from the double bond at C2-C3 are avail-

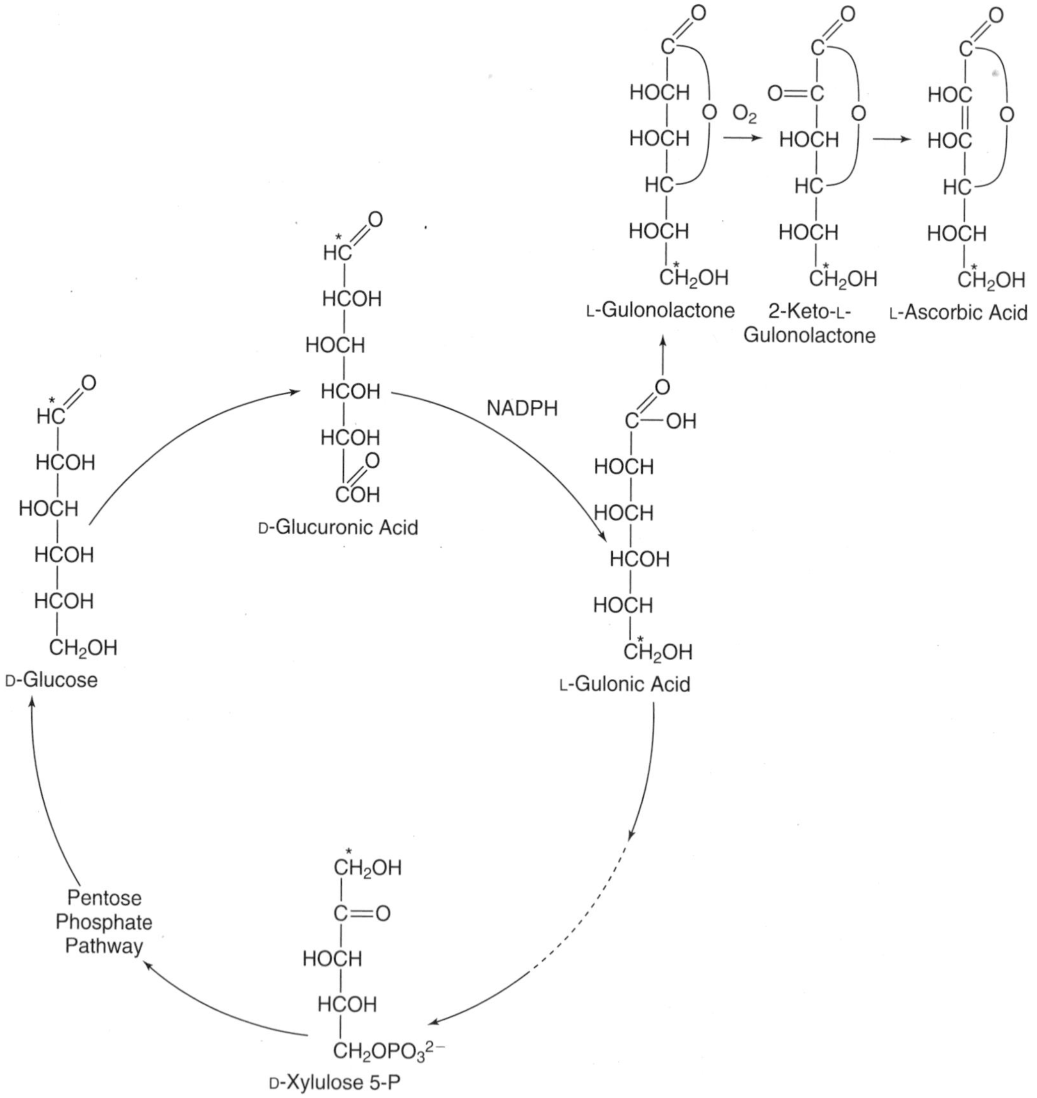

Figure 23–1. Pathway for biosynthesis of ascorbic acid from glucose in mammals. Humans lack gulonolactone oxidase and cannot convert L-gulonolactone to 2-keto-L-gulonolactone.

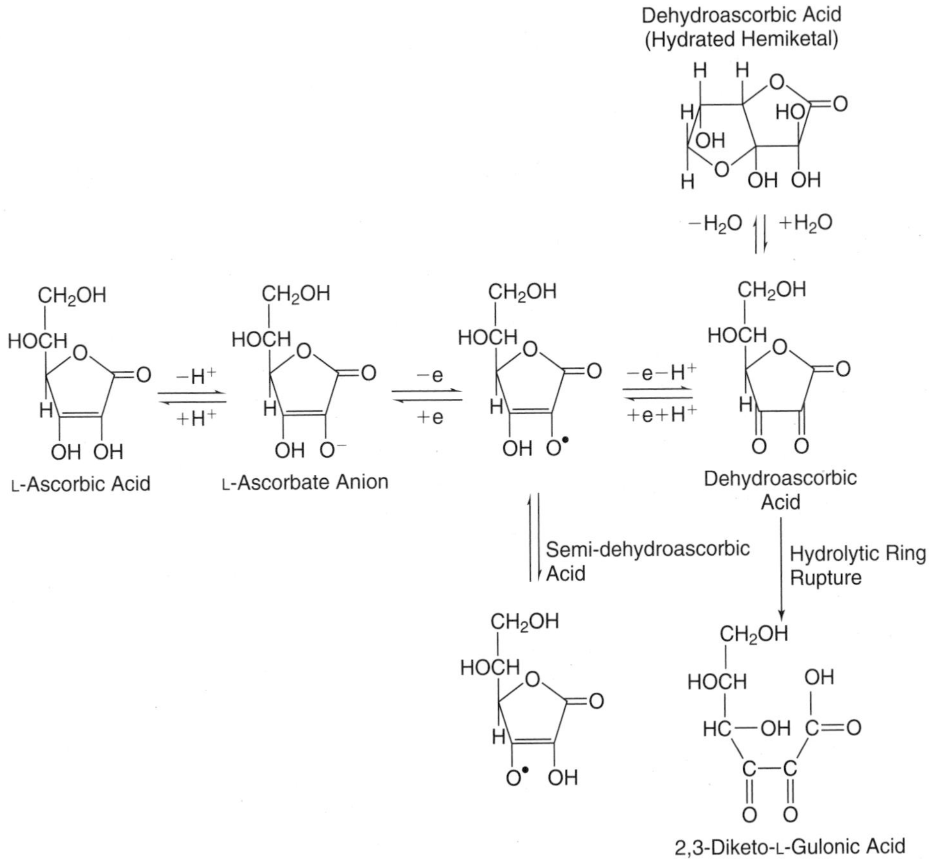

Figure 23–2. Ascorbic acid and its oxidation products. Ascorbic acid at physiological pH is present as the ascorbate anion. Dehydroascorbic acid exists in more than one form, and only two are shown here for simplicity. The hydrated hemiketal is believed to be the favored form in aqueous solutions (Tolbert and Ward, 1982), but it is uncertain which form is present in biological systems. Semidehydroascorbic acid may also have other configurations, which are omitted for simplicity (Lewin, 1976). Formation of 2,3-diketogulonic acid by hydrolytic ring rupture is probably irreversible. (From Washko, P. W., Welch, R. W., Dhariwal, K. R., Wang, Y. and Levine, M. [1992] Ascorbic acid and dehydroascorbic acid analyses in biological samples. Anal Biochem 204:1–14.)

able. The redox couple dehydroascorbic acid/ascorbate is approximately +0.06 volt under standard conditions (Lewin, 1976). The standard redox potential is based on the following relationship:

Electron Acceptor + Electron(s) →
Electron Donor

The redox couple dehydroascorbic acid/ascorbic acid reflects donation of 2 electrons by ascorbate. However, it is likely that electrons from ascorbate are lost sequentially, with formation of the intermediate free radical semidehydroascorbic acid (monodehydroascorbic acid, ascorbate free radical) (Fig. 23–2). Compared with other free radicals, ascor-

bate free radical is stable (10^{-5} sec), does not react well with other compounds to form potentially harmful free radicals, and can be reversibly reduced to ascorbate (Buettner, 1993). These properties suggest that ascorbate may be an ideal electron donor.

The redox potential of ascorbate free radical/ascorbate is approximately +0.3 volt under standard conditions. Based only on standard redox potentials, ascorbate would not appear to be a good electron donor. However, the overall propensity of redox couples to donate or accept electrons is the reduction potential. In addition to standard redox potential, the reduction potential as defined by the Nernst equation accounts for the concentrations of electron acceptor and electron donor.

Standard conditions assume that concentrations are equal at 1 mol/L. However, the reduction potential can be markedly affected when there are different concentrations of electron donor and acceptor. Under conditions in which ascorbate concentration is in excess of ascorbate free radical, ascorbate acts as an electron donor, and ascorbate free radical is formed. In fact, the expected physiological condition is that ascorbate will be in great excess compared with ascorbate free radical. Once ascorbate free radical forms, the Nernst equation predicts that the second electron will also be lost to form dehydroascorbic acid. Thus, the redox potential for the dehydroascorbic acid/ascorbic acid couple actually reflects the sum of the dehydroascorbic acid/ascorbate free radical and ascorbate free radical/ascorbate couples.

Dehydroascorbic acid is the first stable product formed from ascorbate oxidation. Dehydroascorbic acid is formed from ascorbate by a wide variety of oxidants found in biological systems, such as molecular oxygen, molecular oxygen plus trace metal (iron, copper), superoxide, hydroxyl radical, and hypochlorous acid. Although dehydroascorbic acid is stable in relation to the ascorbate free radical half life of 10^{-5} sec, dehydroascorbic acid stability is still only minutes at physiological pH. At pH less than 4, dehydroascorbic acid stability improves markedly. Dehydroascorbic acid may exist in one of multiple forms (Tolbert and Ward, 1982). It is possible that the predominant form in vivo is the hydrated hemiketal. Although the term dehydroascorbic acid is used widely in the scientific literature, dehydroascorbic acid is probably not an acid in vivo, and the designation "dehydroascorbate" is incorrect.

Dehydroascorbic acid has two fates: it is either hydrolyzed irreversibly to 2,3-diketogulonic acid or reduced to ascorbate, presumably via the ascorbate free radical intermediate (Fig. 23–2). Formation of 2,3-diketogulonic acid is a result of hydrolytic ring rupture, which is why the reaction is irreversible. Dehydroascorbic acid reduction occurs either chemically or enzymatically. Chemical reduction can be mediated in vitro or in vivo by reducing agents with favorable redox potentials. Chemical reduction is mediated in vivo

by glutathione with formation of glutathione disulfide (Winkler et al., 1994). Enzymatic reduction is mediated in vivo by at least two proteins. One of these proteins is glutaredoxin (thioltransferase). Reduction of dehydroascorbic acid by glutaredoxin is at least 10- to 20-fold faster than chemical reduction and is glutathione dependent (Park and Levine, 1996). A second protein isolated from red blood cells also mediates dehydroascorbic acid reduction (Maellaro et al., 1994). This protein has been purified but not yet identified. It also requires glutathione for maximal activity. A third protein, protein disulfide isomerase, has dehydroascorbic acid reductase activity as a pure protein, but its contribution to reduction in vivo is not clear (Wells et al., 1990).

Diketogulonic acid as the product of irreversible ascorbate oxidation has several potential fates. Resulting compounds may include xylose, xylonate, lyxonate, and oxalate (Lewin, 1976). Although carbons from ascorbate were reported to be expired as carbon dioxide in animals, this probably does not occur in humans (Baker et al., 1975). Of all metabolites, the only one of clinical significance is oxalate, discussed later.

FOOD SOURCES, ABSORPTION, AND BIOAVAILABILITY OF VITAMIN C

Ascorbate is found in many fruits and vegetables. Fruits high in vitamin C include cantaloupe, kiwi, strawberries, lemons, and oranges. Good vegetable sources are broccoli, red pepper, cauliflower, spinach, tomatoes, Brussels sprouts, and asparagus. Fruit and vegetable juices that are good sources of the vitamin are orange, grapefruit, and tomato juices. Many foods, such as breakfast cereals and fruit drinks, are fortified with vitamin C. Foods low in vitamin C include meat, poultry, eggs, dairy products, and unfortified grains.

It is conceivable that both ascorbate and dehydroascorbic acid are present in foods. The data show that ascorbate predominates, accounting for 80% to 90% of the total vitamin content, with dehydroascorbic acid accounting for 10% to 20% (Vanderslice and Higgs, 1991). There is little information concerning

Food Sources of Vitamin C

- Fruits (especially cantaloupe, kiwi, oranges, strawberries, and watermelon)
- Vegetables (especially broccoli, red pepper, cauliflower, Brussels sprouts, asparagus, potatoes, cabbage, collard greens, green peas, and carrots)
- Fruit juices (especially orange and grapefruit)
- Vegetable juices (especially tomato)

RDAs Across the Life Cycle

	mg vitamin C/day
Infants, 0–0.5 y	30
0.5–1.0 y	35
Children, 1–3 y	40
4–10 y	45
Males, 11–14 y	50
15–51+ y	60
Females, 11–14 y	50
15–51+ y	60
Pregnant	70
Lactating, 1st 6 mo	95
2nd 6 mo	90

Ingestion of at least 100 mg of vitamin C per day is suggested for smokers.

From National Research Council (1989) Recommended Dietary Allowances, 10th ed., National Academy Press, Washington, D. C.

the relationship between food aging and progressive ascorbate oxidation and/or dehydroascorbic acid formation, but increased oxidation is expected as food ages.

The ascorbate epimer erythorbic acid (D-isoascorbic acid, D-araboascorbic acid)is used as a food additive. It is added as a preservative to smoked or cured meats and some beverages. Erythorbic acid has no antiscorbutic activity. There is potential for erythorbic acid to give false elevations of plasma ascorbate concentrations. For this to occur, plasma samples would have to be taken within a few hours after erythorbate-containing foods were eaten. Because erythorbic acid is cleared from plasma within 12 hours, potential interference from erythorbic acid is easily avoided by taking plasma samples after an overnight fast (Sauberlich et al., 1996).

Ascorbic acid in guinea pigs is absorbed in the ileum and probably in the jejunum of the small intestine. In animal intestine experimental systems, ascorbate absorption is Na+ dependent, and ascorbate absorption in humans probably occurs by a similar mecha-

nism (Stevenson, 1974). Guinea pigs specifically have been studied because, like humans, they must obtain ascorbate from the diet.

Bioavailability is a measure of the amount of substance absorbed. Bioavailability can be relative or absolute (Rowland and Tozer, 1989). Relative bioavailability compares absorption of two or more forms of a dose. Relative bioavailability experiments for vitamin C are fairly straightforward to perform (Melethil et al., 1986), but they do not provide direct information about the absolute amount of dose absorbed. The absolute amount of a dose absorbed is its true bioavailability. True bioavailability is determined from oral and intravenous administration of a dose when a subject is at steady state (equilibrium for the dose). Once a subject is at steady state for the dose under study, that dose is administered orally, and the change in plasma concentration from the dose is measured by serial sampling. When the data are displayed as a function of time, an area under the curve and above baseline reflects the increment from the oral dose. The same dose is then administered intravenously, the change in plasma concentration is again determined by serial sampling, and the area under this curve is calculated. True bioavailability is the area under the curve from oral absorption divided by the area under the curve from intravenous administration, expressed as a percentage. One hundred percent bioavailability represents complete absorption. Because of the necessity for steady-state conditions and repeated serial sampling, true bioavailability data for vitamin C have not been available until recently. These new data indicate that true bioavailability is nearly 100% for vitamin C doses of between 15 and 200 mg (Graumlich et al., 1997; Levine et al., 1996a). Bioavailability declines for higher doses and is approximately 50% for a dose of 1250 mg.

Based on guinea pig studies, dehydroascorbic acid is also absorbed in the jejunum of the small intestine (Rose et al., 1988). Dehydroascorbic acid absorption appears to be Na^+ independent. Once absorbed, dehydroascorbic acid is probably reduced to ascorbate (see ascorbate recycling later). Dehydroascorbic acid prevents scurvy in guinea pigs, but much higher doses are needed than for ascorbate (Otsuka et al., 1986). Although dehydroascorbic acid is probably absorbed by humans and reduced to ascorbate, the data are difficult to interpret because of assay imprecision and artifacts. There are no true bioavailability studies for dehydroascorbic acid in humans.

TRANSPORT OF ASCORBATE INTO CELLS

Ascorbate is found in plasma of humans and animals. Because it is water soluble and not protein bound, it can be assumed that ascorbate also distributes into the extracellular space. The ascorbate concentrations in many tissues are 5- to 100-fold higher than that of plasma, and therefore ascorbate must be transported against a concentration gradient. Cells and tissues that accumulate ascorbate include adrenal cortex, adrenal medulla, pituitary (anterior, intermediate, and posterior lobes), neutrophils, lymphocytes, monocytes, platelets, fibroblasts, osteoblasts, chondro-

cytes, endothelial cells, liver, spleen, brain, lung, kidney, testes, ovaries, lens, cornea, retina, bone marrow, pancreas, and heart (Rumsey and Levine, 1998).

Until recently, the mechanisms of ascorbate accumulation were uncertain. Two major possibilities were unresolved and were believed to be mutually exclusive. One was transport of ascorbate as such, and the other was transport of oxidized ascorbate as dehydroascorbic acid, with subsequent intracellular reduction to ascorbate. For many years, ascorbate and dehydroascorbic acid transport experiments were both confusing and controversial. Prior to 1980, ascorbate and dehydroascorbic acid measurements were often difficult to interpret because the methods were insensitive, nonspecific, subject to interference and artifacts, and unable to account for instability of the substances measured (Washko et al., 1992). These measurement (assay) difficulties permeated nearly all biochemical and clinical aspects of vitamin C biology in addition to transport. Many ascorbate assay problems were solved by methods that used high performance liquid chromatography (HPLC), although problems remain for dehydroascorbic acid as discussed later. With these assays, new data provided solutions to some of the transport problems and revealed exciting separate mechanisms of ascorbate and dehydroascorbic acid transmembrane transport.

Ascorbate is transported by a carrier protein that is Na^+-dependent, saturable, and energy-dependent. Transporter activity has been found in most tissues that concentrate ascorbate. Ascorbate analogs selectively inhibit ascorbate transport (Welch et al., 1995). The ascorbate transporter has been expressed using the *Xenopus laevis* (frog oocyte) expression system (Dyer et al., 1994), but to date the protein has not been isolated or cloned.

In distinct contrast to ascorbate, dehydroascorbic acid transport is Na^+- and energy-independent. Dehydroascorbic acid transport is at least 10- to 20-fold faster than ascorbate transport (Welch et al., 1995). Dehydroascorbic acid is transported by the Na^+-independent glucose transporter isoforms GLUT1 and GLUT3 (Rumsey et al., 1997). The isoform GLUT4 may also transport dehydroascorbic acid but much less efficiently. Dehydroascorbic acid is not transported by other Na^+-independent sugar transporter isoforms (GLUT2 and GLUT5) nor by the Na^+-dependent sugar transporter SGLT1. Ascorbate is not transported by any of the glucose transporters. Although not proved, it is likely that many of the cell types that have Na^+-dependent ascorbate transport activity also transport dehydroascorbic acid. After dehydroascorbic acid is transported intracellularly, it is reduced (Rumsey et al., 1997; Washko et al., 1993; Welch et al., 1995). It is likely that internal reduction is immediate and complete under physiological conditions. Although residual dehydroascorbic acid has been detected in some tissues, it is uncertain whether dehydroascorbic acid was truly present intracellularly or whether the measurement reflected an artifact (oxidation) from sample preparation (Washko et al., 1992).

Once dehydroascorbic acid reduction to ascorbate occurs, ascorbate efflux is probably negligible. Continued dehydroascorbic acid transport is driven by subsequent ascorbate reduction, so that reduction would always be expected to be complete. If reduction were incomplete, internal dehydroascorbic acid would efflux via glucose transporters. The mechanisms of dehydroascorbic acid reduction, discussed earlier, are tissue dependent. In some tissues, reduction may be mediated chemically by glutathione alone, although this is controversial (Maellaro et al., 1994; Park and Levine, 1996; Winkler et al., 1994). In neutrophils, the glutathione-dependent protein glutaredoxin mediates reduction, whereas in red cells, reduction may be mediated by either glutaredoxin or an unidentified 31-kDa protein or both (Maellaro et al., 1994). Reduction mechanisms in other tissues remain to be determined.

To understand ascorbate and dehydroascorbic acid transport, it is necessary to consider continued measurement difficulties for dehydroascorbic acid (Washko et al., 1992). Ascorbate is detected directly by ultraviolet (UV) or electrochemical detection. In contrast, there is no useful direct detection system for dehydroascorbic acid. Electrochemical detection of dehydroascorbic acid has not been successful, and UV detection

is very insensitive. Dehydroascorbic acid is usually detected indirectly, via ascorbate assays. Sample ascorbate is measured, the sample is reduced, and ascorbate is measured again. The difference between the reduced and unreduced sample is taken as dehydroascorbic acid. Difficulties with this approach are obvious. Inadvertent oxidation can cause large errors. Because ascorbate is usually detected in great excess compared with dehydroascorbic acid, dehydroascorbic acid is determined by subtracting a large number from a large number. It may be impossible to determine whether a sample has 1% to 2% dehydroascorbic acid versus no dehydroascorbic acid. These problems will be solved if a direct detection method for dehydroascorbic acid becomes available.

Ascorbate and dehydroascorbic acid transport depend on substrate availability. Taking into account the assay difficulties for dehydroascorbic acid, ascorbate is probably the predominant if not exclusive substrate in the human circulation under normal conditions (Dhariwal et al., 1991b). If dehydroascorbic acid were to form in blood, it would be expected to be transported immediately into red blood cells or neutrophils and trapped by reduction, and it should remain undetectable in plasma. Outside the circulation, ascorbate is the expected extracellular substrate under nonoxidizing conditions. Under such conditions, it is likely most ascorbate accumulation is mediated by the ascorbate transporter. Thus, ascorbate transport can be considered constitutive because the substrate ascorbate is continuously available.

Once oxidants are generated, however, dehydroascorbic acid is formed, transported into cells, and reduced to ascorbate. Dehydroascorbic acid transport can be considered substrate-induced transport, because the substrate is present only when oxidants cause its formation from ascorbate. Once dehydroascorbic acid is available, it is transported intracellularly and immediately reduced to ascorbate. This cycle of extracellular ascorbate oxidation and subsequent intracellular reduction is called ascorbate recycling (Washko et al., 1993; Welch et al., 1995) (Fig. 23–3). Ascorbate recycling is most likely to occur during the time that diffusible oxidants

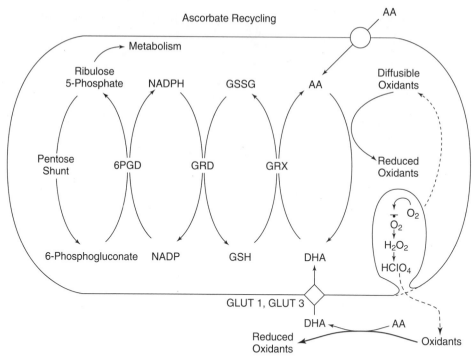

Figure 23–3. *Ascorbate recycling in human neutrophils. Ascorbate and dehydroascorbic acid are transported differently. The putative ascorbate transporter (open circle) transports ascorbate and probably maintains millimolar concentrations of ascorbate within neutrophils. With activation, neutrophils secrete reactive oxygen species, which may oxidize ascorbate to dehydroascorbic acid. The dehydroascorbic acid is rapidly transported by glucose transporter isoforms GLUT1 and GLUT3 (open diamond). Intracellular dehydroascorbic acid is immediately reduced to ascorbate. In neutrophils, glutaredoxin is responsible for the majority of intracellular reduction. Glutaredoxin activity is glutathione-dependent and probably requires the enzymes shown. Although dehydroascorbic acid is transported by GLUT1 and GLUT3, it is unknown whether one or both isoforms are responsible for dehydroascorbic acid entry in neutrophils. Ascorbate recycling may also occur in other cell types as a function of oxidants produced and extracellular ascorbate oxidation. AA, ascorbate; DHA, dehydroascorbic acid; GRD, glutathione reductase; GRX, glutaredoxin; GSH, glutathione; GSSG, glutathione disulfide; 6-PGD, 6-phosphogluconate dehydrogenase.*

are present and increased intracellular ascorbate could be utilized for oxidant quenching. Ascorbate recycling thus allows cells to increase intracellular ascorbate concentrations rapidly and is therefore a potentially protective mechanism. Ascorbate recycling and Na^+-dependent ascorbate transport together provide a comprehensive explanation of ascorbate accumulation in tissues (Fig. 23–3).

Regulation of ascorbate transport could have significant and exciting implications for humans. Accumulation could be regulated in response to concentrations in the small intestine, extracellular substrate availability after absorption, utilization by enzymes requiring ascorbate, or oxidation of ascorbate by free radicals. Transport regulation could occur at any of the steps shown in Figure 23–3: extracellular ascorbate and/or dehydroascorbic acid concentrations; ascorbate transporter

synthesis, recruitment, or activity; glucose transporter recruitment, membrane insertion, or recycling; control of proteins responsible for enzymatic reduction (i.e., glutaredoxin) at the transcriptional, translational, or posttranslational level; and regulation of glutathione concentrations. The contributions of each of these mechanisms to ascorbate accumulation in tissues and to absorption in the small intestine are just beginning to be explored. Answers to these issues will probably have a major impact on dietary recommendations for vitamin C consumption in humans (Institute of Medicine, 1994).

ENZYMATIC FUNCTIONS OF ASCORBATE

Vitamin C acts as an electron donor for 11 enzymes (England and Seifter, 1986; Levine,

1986) (Fig. 23–4). Three enzymes are found in fungi and are involved in reutilization pathways for pyrimidines or the deoxyribose moiety of deoxynucleosides (Stubbe, 1985; Wondrack et al., 1978). Because they are not known to be involved in mammalian reactions, they will not be discussed further here. Of the 8 mammalian enzymes, 3 enzymes participate in collagen hydroxylation (Kivirikko and Myllyla, 1985; Peterkofsky, 1991; Prockop and Kivirikko, 1995) and 2 in carnitine biosynthesis (Dunn et al.,1984; Rebouche, 1991). Of the remaining 3 enzymes, one is necessary for biosynthesis of the catecholamine norepinephrine (Kaufman, 1974; Levine et al., 1991), one is necessary for amidation of peptide hormones (Eipper et al., 1992; Eipper et al., 1993), and one is involved in tyrosine metabolism (Englard and Seifter, 1986; Lindblad et al., 1970).

Enzymes that require ascorbate have either monooxygenase or dioxygenase activity. The monooxygenases dopamine β-hydroxylase and peptidyl-glycine α-monooxygenase incorporate a single oxygen atom into a substrate, either dopamine or a peptide with a terminal glycine. The remaining enzymes are dioxygenases, which incorporate molecular oxygen (O_2), with each oxygen atom being incorporated in a different way. The enzyme 4-hydroxyphenylpyruvate dioxygenase incorporates 2 oxygen atoms into different loca-

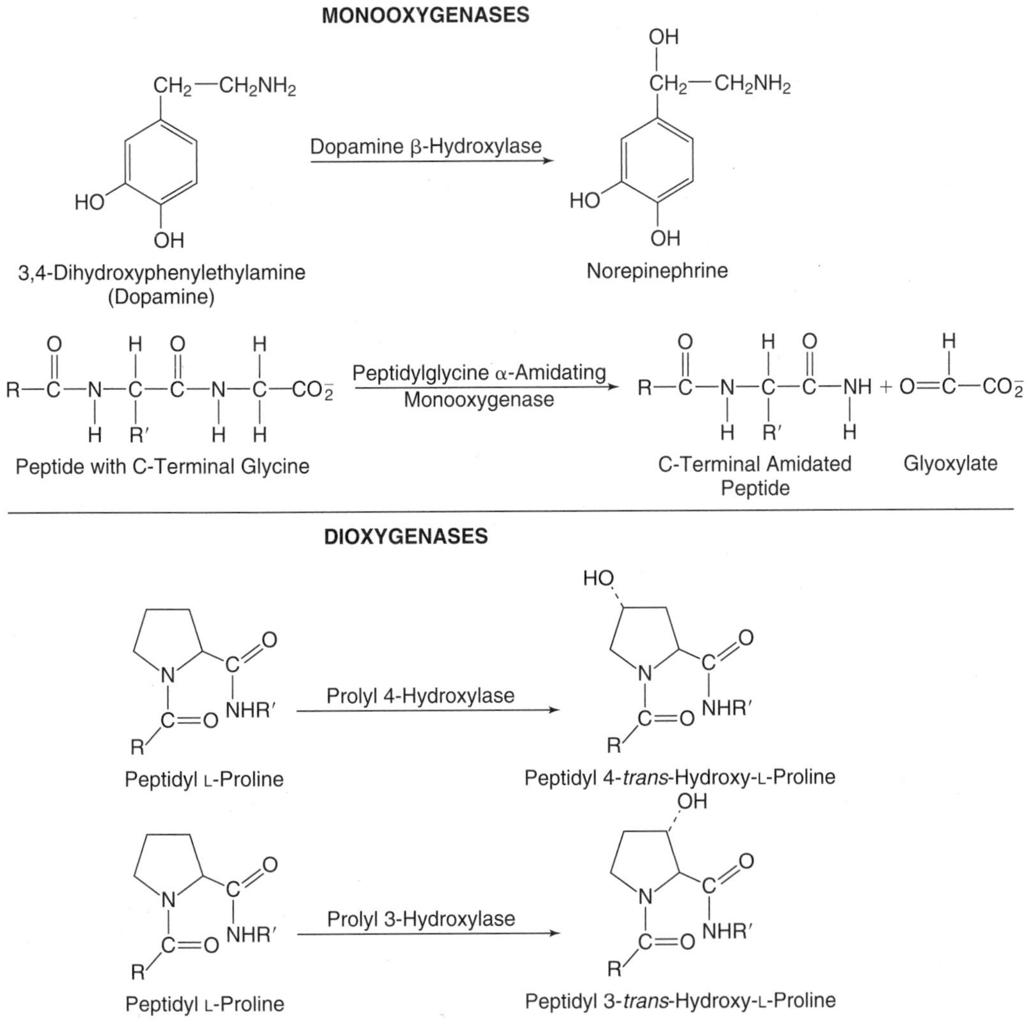

Figure 23–4.

Illustration continued on following page

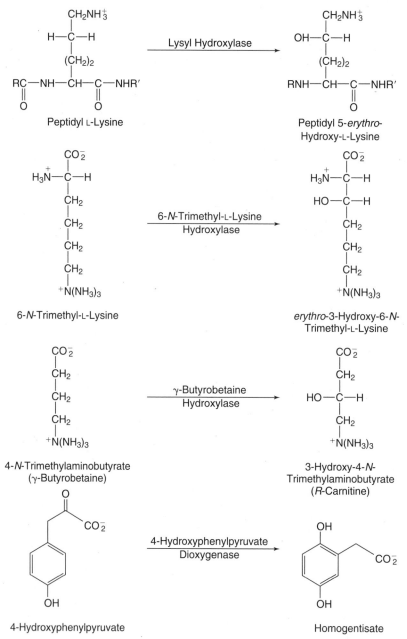

Figure 23–4. *Classification of enzymatic reactions that utilize ascorbate. All the dioxygenase reactions shown except the one catalyzed by 4-hydroxyphenylpyruvate dioxygenase require α-ketoglutarate as a co-substrate. Also see Figures 23–7 and 23–9. (Modified with permission from Englard, S. and Seifter, S. [1986] The biochemical functions of ascorbic acid. Annu Rev Nutr 6:365–406. © 1986 by Annual Reviews.)*

tions of one product. The other dioxygenases incorporate 1 atom of oxygen into α-ketoglutarate to form succinate and the other atom of oxygen into the enzyme-specific substrate.

Monooxygenases

Dopamine β-hydroxylase. This enzyme is necessary for hydroxylation of dopamine for synthesis of the catecholamine norepinephrine in peripheral neurons, central neurons, and adrenal medulla. Because of its abundance, enzyme from adrenal medulla has been characterized in detail. The enzyme is a tetrameric glycoprotein, with subunits arranged as pairs of disulfide-linked monomeric species. There are both membrane-bound and soluble enzyme forms, which probably differ in subunit composition (Fleming and Kent, 1991). The enzyme is believed to contain 2 copper atoms per subunit.

The isolated enzyme requires molecular oxygen, a substrate to be hydroxylated, and ascorbate as the preferred electron donor. Catalase is added to isolated enzyme assays to scavenge the hydrogen peroxide that forms. Under these conditions, enzyme activity is easily measured, and ascorbate is consumed

stoichiometrically 1:1 in relation to consumption of oxygen and to formation of product. The enzyme receives single electrons sequentially from 2 ascorbate molecules, with formation of ascorbate free radical as an intermediate (Fleming and Kent, 1991; Kaufman, 1974).

In intact tissue, enzyme action is more complex and intriguing (Levine et al., 1991) (Fig. 23–5). Both soluble and membrane-bound enzyme forms are localized exclusively in neurosecretory vesicles of neurons and in secretory vesicles (chromaffin granules) of the adrenal medulla. Ascorbate is found within vesicles and in cell cytosol, but ascorbate itself is not transported across vesicles. Instead, electrons from cytosolic ascorbate are transferred in sequential one-electron steps to cytochrome b_{561} in the vesicle membrane (Fleming and Kent, 1991; Kent and Fleming, 1987). Single electrons accepted by cytochrome b_{561} undergo transmembrane electron transfer. Within vesicles, semidehydroascorbic acid accepts these electrons with ascorbate formation (Dhariwal et al., 1991a). Intravesicular semidehydroascorbic acid is formed by action of dopamine β-hydroxylase and ascorbate. To summarize, semidehydroascorbic acid generated by enzyme action within vesicles is re-

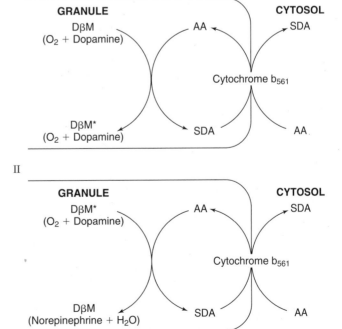

Figure 23–5. Transmembrane electron transfer and dopamine β-hydroxylase reduction in chromaffin granules. Intragranular ascorbic acid reduces dopamine β-hydroxylase by single electron transfer, with formation of semidehydroascorbic acid. In the presence of external (cytosolic) ascorbic acid, intragranular semidehydroascorbic acid is reduced by transmembrane electron transfer via cytochrome b_{561}. There are two steps, indicating that dopamine β-hydroxylase is reduced twice, each time by a single electron. Although oxygen and dopamine are shown associated with the enzyme during its reduction, the precise interaction is unknown. The enzyme catalyzes the hydroxylation of dopamine and the reduction of $\frac{1}{2}O_2$ to H_2O. AA, ascorbate; SDA, semidehydroascorbic acid; DβM, dopamine β-monooxygenase (-hydroxylase); DβM*, reduced dopamine β-monooxygenase (-hydroxylase).

duced to ascorbate by transmembrane electron transfer from external ascorbate. Without extravesicular ascorbate, intact vesicles will synthesize norepinephrine from dopamine using intravesicular ascorbate until it is consumed (Levine et al., 1991). With extravesicular ascorbate, intravesicular ascorbate is maintained by transmembrane electron transfer.

The kinetics for ascorbate in norepinephrine biosynthesis were determined in situ, meaning in intact animal tissue (Levine et al., 1991). The K_m of dopamine β-hydroxylase for intravesicular ascorbate in intact vesicles was approximately 0.5 mmol/L, similar to that of isolated enzyme (Kaufman, 1974). Just as for isolated enzyme, the stoichiometry of the overall reaction in intact tissue is 1:1 for ascorbate consumption to norepinephrine biosynthesis. Because intact vesicles contain 10 to 15 mmol/L of ascorbate, the reaction proceeds at close to V_{max} with respect to ascorbate. The K_m of transmembrane electron transfer for cytosolic ascorbate was approximately 0.3 mmol/L. Because cytosolic ascorbate is at least ten times this value, transmembrane electron transfer also proceeds at V_{max}, with respect to ascorbate in intact animal tissue. These studies demonstrate that kinetics for a vitamin can be determined in situ. The corresponding kinetic parameters in human tissue are not known.

Why is ascorbate utilization by dopamine β-hydroxylase coupled to transmembrane electron transfer? One possibility is that this is a protective mechanism for synthesis of an essential hormone in the event of vitamin C deficiency. If deficiency occurs, intravesicular ascorbate will remain until it is consumed. Because intravesicular ascorbate concentrations permit hydroxylation to proceed at V_{max}, and cytosolic concentrations allow electron transfer to proceed at V_{max}, dopamine hydroxylation should continue even as cytosolic concentrations decline in the event of deficiency. It is unknown how intragranular ascorbate enters secretory vesicles. Because cytosolic ascorbate is also at millimolar concentration, it is possible that cytosolic ascorbate is trapped in vesicles during vesicle assembly.

Peptidylglycine α-Amidating Monooxy-genase. Biologically active peptides act as hormones or paracrine signaling agents and are often synthesized from inactive precursors by posttranslational modification. To confer activity to many bioactive peptides, a carboxy-terminal α-amide group must be added by a process called α-amidation. α-Amidation is mediated by peptidylglycine α-amidating monooxygenase (PAM) (Eipper et al., 1992; Eipper et al., 1993). Amidated peptide hormones include thyrotropin-releasing hormone, gonadotropin-releasing hormone, oxytocin, vasopressin, cholecystokinin, gastrin, calcitonin, substance P, and neuropeptide Y. Precursors to α-amidated peptides have a glycine residue that immediately follows the residue to be α-amidated. Unless the site is at the extreme carboxyl terminus of the precursor peptide, the α-amidation site must be exposed by endoproteolytic cleavage; the signal for cleavage is either x-glycine-basic amino acid-basic amino acid or x-glycine-basic amino acid. In α-amidation, the signal carboxy-terminal glycine is cleaved to release glyoxylate, leaving the amino acid residue "x" as "x-NH$_2$." Peptides have been isolated with x represented by every amino acid except aspartic acid.

PAM is actually a bifunctional enzyme and itself contains two distinct monofunctional domains linked by a protease-sensitive linker (Eipper et al., 1992; Eipper et al., 1993). The two domains are peptidylglycine α-hydroxylating monooxygenase (PHM) and peptidyl-α-hydroxyglycine α-amidating lyase (PAL). The amidation reaction is a two-step reaction, with each reaction mediated by the component monofunctional subunit (Fig. 23–6). The first-step reaction mediated by PHM results in hydroxylation of the peptidylglycine residue with formation of peptidylhydroxyglycine. In the second step, the peptidylhydroxyglycine moiety is cleaved into glyoxylate and the amidated peptide, as mediated by PAL.

The first-step reaction mediated by PHM is rate-limiting. PHM is similar to dopamine β-hydroxylase in several respects. Both enzymes are monooxygenases. As does dopamine β-hydroxylase, PHM requires ascorbate, oxygen, and copper (Eipper et al., 1992; Eipper et al., 1993). The stoichiometry is that 1 mole of ascorbic acid is consumed as 1 mole

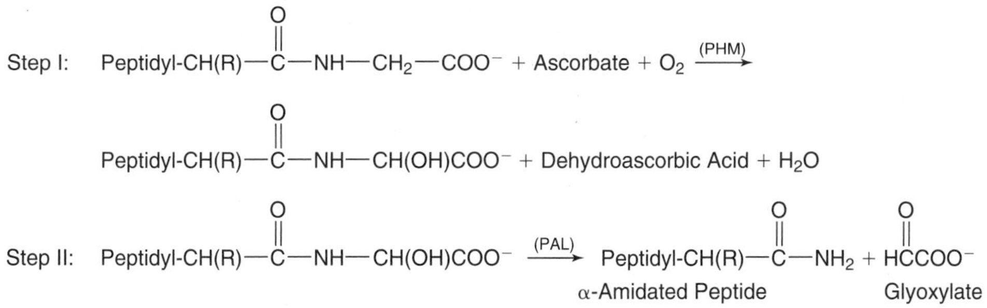

Step I: Peptidyl-CH(R)—C(=O)—NH—CH$_2$—COO$^-$ + Ascorbate + O$_2$ $\xrightarrow{\text{(PHM)}}$

Peptidyl-CH(R)—C(=O)—NH—CH(OH)COO$^-$ + Dehydroascorbic Acid + H$_2$O

Step II: Peptidyl-CH(R)—C(=O)—NH—CH(OH)COO$^-$ $\xrightarrow{\text{(PAL)}}$ Peptidyl-CH(R)—C(=O)—NH$_2$ + HCCOO$^-$

α-Amidated Peptide   Glyoxylate

Figure 23–6. *Mechanism of peptide amidation by peptidyl-glycine α-amidating monooxygenase (PAM). PAM is a bifunctional enzyme consisting of peptidylglycine α-hydroxylating monooxygenase (PHM) and peptidyl-α-hydroxyglycine α-amidating lyase (PAL). (Modified with permission from Eipper, B., Stoffers, D. A. and Mains, R. E. [1992] The biosynthesis of neuropeptides: Peptide alpha amidation. Annu Rev Neurosci 15:57–85. © 1992 by Annual Reviews.)*

of peptidylglycine is converted to product. Copper is essential for activation of molecular oxygen. PHM and dopamine β-hydroxylase share significant amino acid sequence similarity, indicating that these enzymes are evolutionarily linked. The enzymes have 28% identity extending through a common catalytic domain of approximately 270 residues (Eipper et al., 1992; Eipper et al., 1993).

PAM is localized to secretory vesicles. A transmembrane tail close to the carboxyl terminus anchors PAM to the vesicle membrane, and the carboxyl terminus itself is on the cytosolic or extravesicular side of the vesicle membrane (Eipper et al., 1992; Eipper et al., 1993). The monofunctional domains PHM and PAL are localized to the intravesicular space.

Ascorbate utilization by dopamine β-hydroxylase and PAM (PHM) are similar (Eipper et al., 1992; Eipper et al., 1993). Ascorbic acid within granules is utilized by PHM with formation of semidehydroascorbic acid. Cytochrome b$_{561}$ accepts single electrons from cytosolic ascorbate, with reduction of intravesicular semidehydroascorbic acid produced during peptide amidation (Kent and Fleming, 1987). Thus, as for dopamine β-hydroxylase, cytosolic ascorbate maintains intravesicular ascorbate concentrations. Just as for catecholamine-containing vesicles, it is unknown how ascorbate enters peptide secretory vesicles.

In contrast to dopamine β-hydroxylase, which requires ascorbate in situ (Levine et al., 1991), PAM can accept electrons from alternate donors other than ascorbate (Eipper et al., 1992; Eipper et al., 1993). Some amidation occurs in the complete absence of ascorbate.

For example, catecholamines can provide electrons in some cell systems to support peptide amidation.

Dioxygenases

Prolyl 4-Hydroxylase, Prolyl 3-Hydroxylase, and Lysyl Hydroxylase. One of the cardinal symptoms of vitamin C deficiency is poor wound healing, which provided an early clue that vitamin C may be involved in collagen biosynthesis (Crandon et al., 1940; Lind, 1753). We have learned subsequently that the involvement of vitamin C in collagen synthesis is complex, involving both regulation of collagen synthesis at a pretranslational level and distinct regulation of posttranslational processing. These issues will be discussed separately.

Effects of vitamin C on posttranslational modification of procollagen are believed to be enzymatically mediated (Peterkofsky, 1991). Collagen is a protein formed from procollagen polypeptides (Kivirikko and Myllyla, 1985; Prockop and Kivirikko, 1995). The precursors are preprocollagen and procollagen, which must be processed for secretion and stability. Preprocollagen is synthesized on polysomes bound to the rough endoplasmic reticulum. The signal peptide is cleaved, and the resulting procollagen is transported through the Golgi apparatus. Procollagen must be modified before it is secreted. The procollagen polypeptide is composed of variations of the tripeptide sequence x-proline-glycine. In some collagens proline is replaced by lysine. Hydroxylation is influenced by the amino acid in the x position and by adjacent amino acids. After hydroxylation of prolyl or lysyl residues occurs along the length of procollagen polypeptides, 3 procollagen polypeptides self-associate into a triple helix. Some of the hydroxylysyl residues undergo further modification, with O-galactosyl or O-galactosyl-β-glycosyl substitution. Once hydroxylation of procollagen occurs within cells, the triple helix forms and rapid secretion occurs. After secretion, extracellular procollagen is further modified at the amino and carboxyl termini, such that the procollagens can themselves associate into fibrils. The fibrils are then enzymatically modified for formation of stable intermolecular cross-links. (See Chapter 2 for further discussion of the posttranslational modification of procollagen.)

Vitamin C acts with prolyl 3-hydroxylase, prolyl 4-hydroxylase, and lysyl hydroxylase for procollagen hydroxylation (Kivirikko and Myllyla, 1985; Peterkofsky, 1991; Prockop and Kivirikko, 1995). These enzymes are α-ketoglutarate-dependent dioxygenases that require reduced (ferrous) iron. The enzymes require a reducing agent in vitro, and ascorbate is most effective. With isolated prolyl hydroxy-

lase, ascorbate was observed to be consumed nonstoichiometrically. The reaction continued for several cycles in the absence of ascorbate but eventually ceased, and ascorbate was necessary to regenerate enzyme activity. These data are accounted for by the action of ascorbate with enzyme-bound iron. When hydroxylation of prolyl or lysyl residues occurs coupled with the oxidative decarboxylation of α-ketoglutarate to succinate, the enzyme-bound iron is believed to remain reduced as ferrous iron (Fe^{2+}) (Fig 23–7). However, an uncoupled reaction can occur in which α-ketoglutarate and oxygen form succinate and carbon dioxide without hydroxylation of the prolyl or lysyl residue. In this case the iron moiety is oxidized to Fe^{3+}, and ascorbate is required as the specific reducing agent that can reduce the iron moiety back to Fe^{2+}.

The data concerning stoichiometry of ascorbate and enzymatic hydroxylation reactions are hampered by the ascorbate assays used. Many of these experiments were performed before HPLC/electrochemical assays for ascorbate were available. There are no stoichiometric data for hydroxylation in cell systems. In the absence of ascorbate in cell

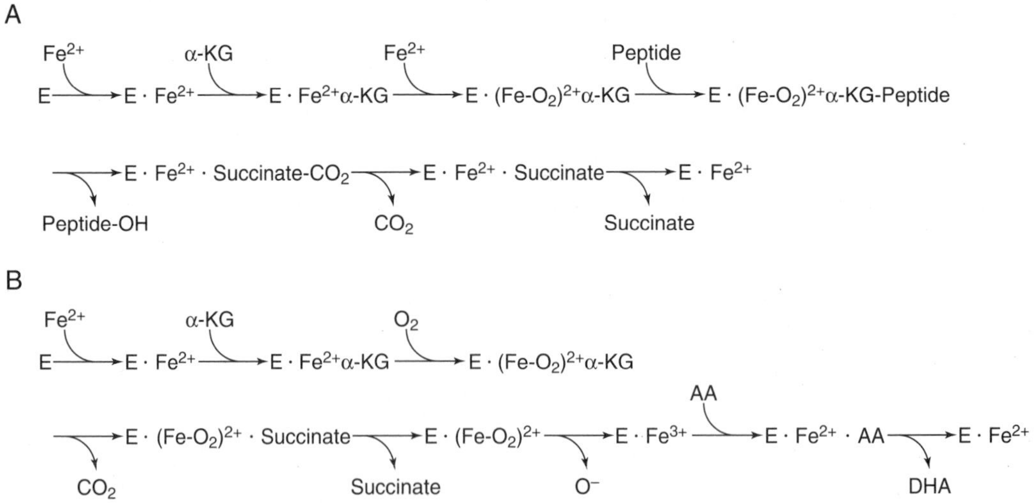

A

$$E \xrightarrow{Fe^{2+}} E \cdot Fe^{2+} \xrightarrow{\alpha\text{-KG}} E \cdot Fe^{2+}\alpha\text{-KG} \xrightarrow{Fe^{2+}} E \cdot (Fe\text{-}O_2)^{2+}\alpha\text{-KG} \xrightarrow{Peptide} E \cdot (Fe\text{-}O_2)^{2+}\alpha\text{-KG-Peptide}$$

$$\xrightarrow{} E \cdot Fe^{2+} \cdot Succinate\text{-}CO_2 \xrightarrow{} E \cdot Fe^{2+} \cdot Succinate \xrightarrow{} E \cdot Fe^{2+}$$
Peptide-OH CO_2 Succinate

B

$$E \xrightarrow{Fe^{2+}} E \cdot Fe^{2+} \xrightarrow{\alpha\text{-KG}} E \cdot Fe^{2+}\alpha\text{-KG} \xrightarrow{O_2} E \cdot (Fe\text{-}O_2)^{2+}\alpha\text{-KG}$$

$$\xrightarrow{} E \cdot (Fe\text{-}O_2)^{2+} \cdot Succinate \xrightarrow{} E \cdot (Fe\text{-}O_2)^{2+} \xrightarrow{} E \cdot Fe^{3+} \xrightarrow{AA} E \cdot Fe^{2+} \cdot AA \xrightarrow{} E \cdot Fe^{2+}$$
CO_2 Succinate O^- DHA

Figure 23–7. *Mechanisms of prolyl 4-hydroxylase and lysyl hydroxylase. (A), The probable mechanism for the complete hydroxylation reaction. The order of binding of O_2 and the peptide substrate are uncertain as is the order of release of the hydroxylated peptide and CO_2. (B), The reaction in the absence of the peptide, in which the enzymes catalyze an uncoupled decarboxylation of α-ketoglutarate. Some peptides that do not become hydroxylated can increase the rate of the uncoupled decarboxylation. In the uncoupled reaction, the reactive iron-oxo complex is probably converted to Fe^{3+} and O^- and ascorbate is needed to reactivate the enzyme by reducing Fe^{3+} to Fe^{2+}. E, enzyme; α-KG, α-ketoglutarate; Peptide-OH, hydroxylated peptide; AA, ascorbate (ascorbic acid); DHA, dehydroascorbic acid. (Modified from Kivirikko, K. I. and Myllyla, R. [1985] Post-translational processing of procollagens. Ann NY Acad Sci 460:187–201.)*

systems, procollagen secretion declines (Peterkofsky, 1991). Procollagen is probably less stable than hydroxylated protein. However, in the complete absence of ascorbate there is substantial residual prolyl residue hydroxylation, which may be as much as 50% of that seen with ascorbate. The alternative electron donors in cells under these conditions are unknown. In some cells a microsomal (endoplasmic reticulum) protein with a cysteinyl-cysteine active site may act as an alternative electron donor, so that ascorbate is not required for prolyl hydroxylation (Peterkofsky, 1991).

There are other effects of ascorbate on collagen synthesis independent of procollagen hydroxylation. Collagen biosynthesis is decreased in scorbutic animals, but this is independent of hydroxylation reactions (Peterkofsky, 1991). This effect is mediated by an effect of scurvy on insulin-like growth factor-1 (IGF-1). When scurvy occurs, excess IGF-1-binding proteins are synthesized, and their binding sites are unsaturated. As a consequence of excess IGF-1-binding sites, free IGF-1 is decreased in scorbutic animals compared with normal controls. Thus, decreased free IGF-1 mediates reduced collagen biosynthesis independently of hydroxylation (Gosiewska et al., 1994).

Other data also indicate that ascorbate stimulates collagen synthesis independently of hydroxylation (Geesin et al., 1988; Sullivan et al., 1994). These effects are seen in cells incubated with ascorbate in culture medium for 24 to 72 h. Incubation with ascorbate for more than 24 h increases collagen mRNA synthesis as much as eight-fold. Because ascorbate in the culture medium oxidizes during this time, the effect on collagen synthesis may be indirect. Ascorbate oxidation under some conditions induces lipid peroxidation. Inhibition of lipid peroxidation by α-tocopherol also prevents the ascorbate-mediated increase in collagen production. The lipid peroxidation product malondialdehyde stimulates collagen production and increases procollagen mRNA, mimicking the effect of ascorbate (Houglum et al., 1991).

It is not known whether the effect of ascorbate on increasing collagen synthesis in cell culture also occurs in vivo. The lipid peroxidation that occurs in cell culture may be a result of culture conditions and may not occur in vivo at all, or it may occur at a substantially slower rate. On the other hand, collagen can be denatured by oxidants such as superoxide (Mukhopadhyay and Chatterjee, 1994). There is animal and clinical evidence that topical ascorbate might protect collagen from oxidant damage (Darr et al., 1992).

There has been tremendous variability and confusion in the scientific literature about the effects of ascorbate on hydroxylation and collagen synthesis (Englard and Seifter, 1986; Ronchetti et al., 1996). Some of the confusion may be due to differences in animal cell lines and primary cultures of human fibroblasts; growth conditions, especially different effects of serum; cell density effects; the type of collagen synthesized; the supply of amino acid substrates; and effects of peptide feedback on collagen synthesis. It remains worthwhile to solve these problems, because of the potential of ascorbate to regulate wound healing in vivo.

Trimethyllysine Hydroxylase and γ-Butyrobetaine Hydroxylase. L-Carnitine, a zwitterionic quaternary amino acid, is required as part of fatty acid metabolism for formation of acyl carnitine derivatives (Englard and Seifter, 1986; Rebouche, 1991). Acylcarnitines are needed for transport of long-chain fatty acids into mitochondria for subsequent oxidation and ATP formation, as described in Chapter 13 (see Fig. 13–9). Carnitine palmitoyltransferase and carnitine palmitoylcarnitine translocase can be involved in the disposal of short-chain organic acids from mitochondria, particularly when blocks in the complete metabolism of these organic acids are present. The formation of acylcarnitines presumably helps maintain a supply of nonesterified coenzyme A, which is required for oxidative metabolism of a variety of compounds.

Human needs for carnitine are met in two ways. Dietary sources of carnitine include poultry, meat, fish, and dairy products. Free carnitine is absorbed almost completely. Carnitine is also synthesized de novo from the essential amino acids lysine and methionine. The proportion of total carnitine accounted for by de novo synthesis is dependent on many factors, especially dietary carnitine and the coexistence of disease states such as renal failure, diabetes mellitus, malignancy, alcohol abuse, and myocardial ischemia.

In the pathway for de novo carnitine synthesis, the 4-carbon chain of carnitine is derived from carbons 3 to 6 of lysine, and the methyl groups of carnitine are provided by S-adenosylmethionine (Fig. 23–8). In mammals, certain peptide-bound lysyl residues are methylated by protein-lysyl methyltransferases that use S-adenosylmethionine as the methyl donor. The methylated product is a 6-N-trimethyllysyl residue, and this residue has been found in calmodulin, histones, myosin, and cytochrome c. 6-N-Trimethyllysine released by proteolytic cleavage undergoes a four-step reaction sequence to form carnitine. The first reaction is a hydroxylation resulting in β-hydroxy-N-methyllysine and is mediated by trimethyllysine hydroxylase. In the second reaction, glycine is released with formation of γ-trimethylaminobutyraldehyde. This substrate undergoes dehydrogenation in the third reaction to form γ-butyrobetaine. In the fourth reaction, γ-butyrobetaine is hydroxylated by γ-butyrobetaine hydroxylase, with carnitine as the product (Dunn et al., 1984; Englard and Seifter, 1986; Rebouche, 1991).

The two hydroxylation reactions in the carnitine synthesis pathway are catalyzed by dioxygenases that require iron, α-ketoglutarate, and a reductant (Dunn et al., 1984). The best reductant in vitro is ascorbate. Of the two enzymes, γ-butyrobetaine hydroxylase has been studied more extensively. Its K_m for ascorbate is approximately 5 mmol/L (Englard and Seifter, 1986). It is likely that the mechanism of ascorbate action is to reduce iron, which is oxidized nonstoichiometrically over the course of repeated reactions, as occurs for prolyl and lysyl hydroxylases (Englard and Seifter, 1986).

One of the first clinical effects of vitamin C deprivation is fatigue (Crandon et al., 1940). Investigators have supposed that the mechanism of fatigue in scurvy was in part coupled to decreased carnitine biosynthesis. Decreased carnitine synthesis could lead to decreased oxidation of fatty acids in muscle and liver, with fatigue as a consequence. It is not clear whether carnitine deficiency is the underlying explanation of the fatigue that occurs in patients with scurvy.

Although the two enzyme activities for carnitine biosynthesis are most active in vitro with ascorbate as a reductant, the effects of ascorbate on carnitine biosynthesis in vivo are more complex and confusing (Englard and Seifter, 1986; Rebouche, 1991). In guinea pigs, ascorbate deficiency results in a variable decrease in the carnitine content of several tissues. Ascorbate-deficient guinea pigs have decreased activity of liver γ-butyrobetaine hydroxylase that can be restored by ascorbate injection (Dunn et al., 1984). Ascorbate deficiency decreases the activity of trimethyllysine hydroxylase in kidney but not liver.

The effect of ascorbate deficiency on substrate utilization for carnitine biosynthesis is difficult to study in mammals because the precursor trimethyllysine is not transported from extracellular fluid into tissues. For any given tissue, the likely substrate for trimethyllysine hydroxylase is trimethyllysine synthesized within that particular tissue. The major site in animals for trimethyllysine conversion to carnitine is probably skeletal muscle, because this site is the major reservoir for free and peptide-bound trimethyllysine.

Once trimethyllysine is hydroxylated, hydroxylation of γ-butyrobetaine occurs primarily in liver and kidney. γ-Butyrobetaine hydroxylase activity in liver would be expected to be decreased in ascorbate deficiency, because liver ascorbate concentrations fall to less than 20% of normal in deficient animals. However, there is probably a great excess of γ-butyrobetaine hydroxylase in liver and/or kidney, because carnitine excretion can be increased 30-fold when γ-butyrobetaine is provided in the diet. Therefore, reduced activity of γ-butyrobetaine hydroxylase is not likely to occur in vivo unless ascorbate deficiency is extremely severe.

Recent results suggest that there may be other explanations of carnitine depletion during vitamin C deficiency (Rebouche, 1995). In vitamin C-deficient guinea pigs, excessive urinary excretion of carnitine contributes to carnitine depletion. When vitamin C-deficient guinea pigs were provided with excess substrate as trimethyllysine or γ-butyrobetaine, their rate of carnitine synthesis was restored nearly to normal. These data also indicate that there is excess spare capacity for carnitine synthesis, which is dependent on precursor availability. In animals or humans with vitamin

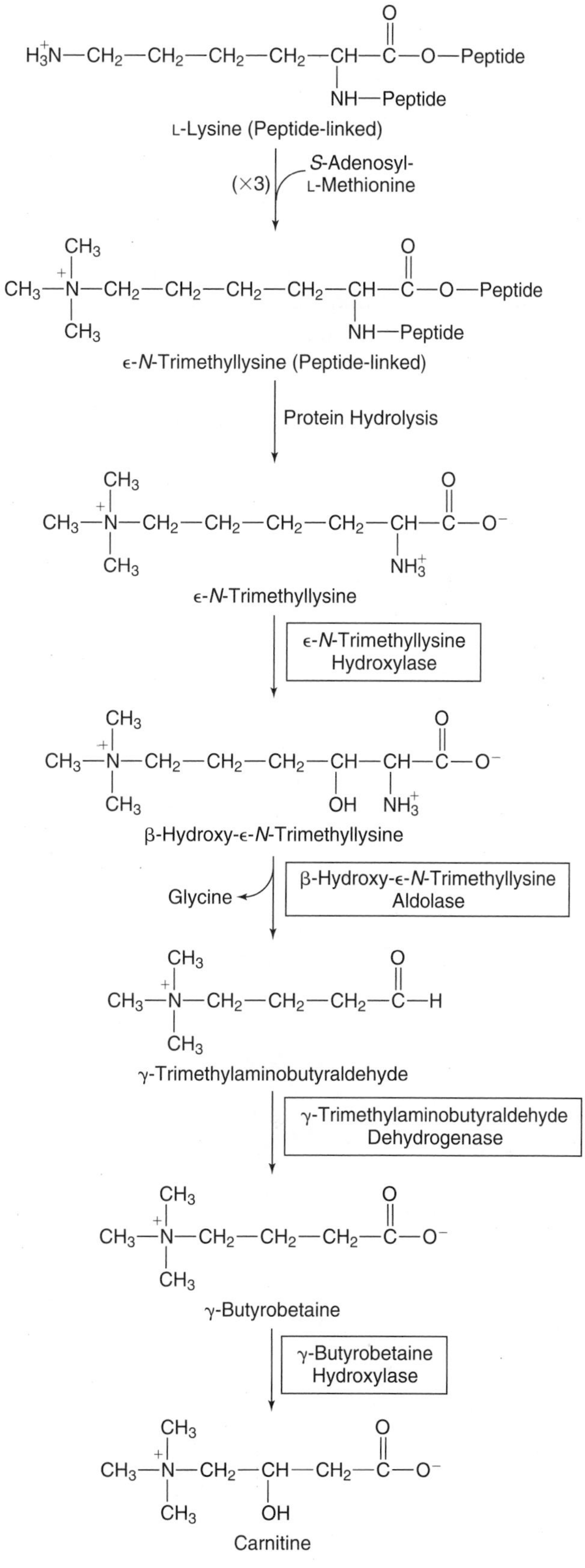

Figure 23–8. Pathway of carnitine biosynthesis in mammals. Trimethyllysine hydroxylase and γ-butyrobetaine hydroxylase are the enzymes that utilize ascorbate (AA). (Redrawn from Rebouche, C. J. [1991] Ascorbic acid and carnitine biosynthesis. Am J Clin Nutr 54:1147S–1152S.)

C deficiency without excess substrate available, carnitine deficiency occurs. It is not certain what percentage of carnitine deficiency is due to decreased biosynthesis versus increased urinary excretion.

4-Hydroxyphenylpyruvate Dioxygenase.
As part of tyrosine catabolism, 4-hydroxyphenylpyruvate dioxygenase catalyzes conversion of 4-hydroxyphenylpyruvate to homogentisate (Fig. 23–9). The enzyme uses molecular oxygen to catalyze coupled oxidations. In the first oxidation, 1 oxygen atom is utilized for oxidative decarboxylation of the pyruvyl moiety, with formation of an acetyl moiety. The second oxygen atom is incorporated into a hydroxyl group replacing the acetyl group, which is shifted to the adjacent carbon (Lindblad et al., 1970) (Fig. 23–9). This latter reaction mechanism is sometimes called "the NIH shift" because it was first characterized by scientists at the National Institutes of Health. Hydroxyphenylpyruvate dioxygenase has been isolated from bacteria and animals, including humans. It appears to be a true dioxygenase and similar to other keto acid–dependent dioxygenases, such as the α-ketoglutarate-dependent dioxygenases described earlier that are involved in prolyl and lysyl hydroxylation and carnitine synthesis. However, the α-keto acid is part of the same molecule that is hydroxylated in the hydroxyphenylpyruvate reaction (Englard and Seifter, 1986), whereas the α-ketoglutarate-dependent dioxygenases oxidatively decarboxylate α-ketoglutarate in addition to hydroxylation of a second substrate molecule. Iron is required by the enzyme, and iron chelators decrease enzyme activity.

Ascorbate is utilized by hydroxyphenylpyruvate dioxygenase as a reducing agent (Lindblad et al., 1970). However, it is not cer-

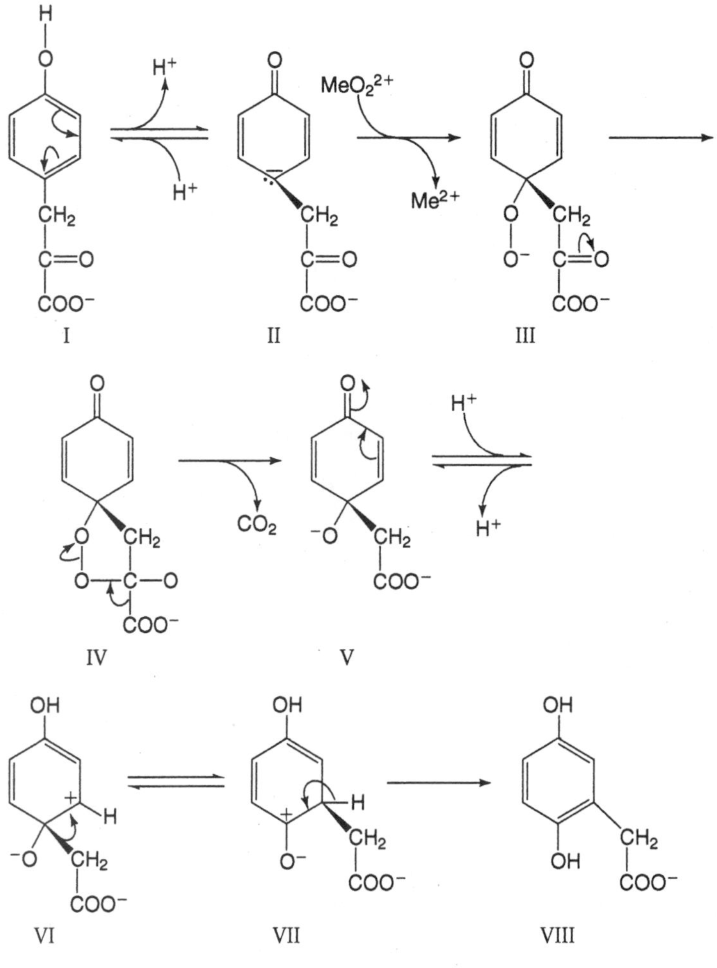

Figure 23–9. Proposed reaction mechanism for the enzymatic formation of homogentisate from p-hydroxyphenyl pyruvate. The reaction of intermediate VI to VII represents the "NIH shift," and Me stands for metal (probably Fe^{2+}). (Redrawn from Lindblad, B., Lindstedt, G. and Lindstedt, S. [1970] The mechanism of enzymic formation of homogentisate from p-hydroxyphenyl pyruvate. J Am Chem Soc 92:7446–7449. Copyright 1970 American Chemical Society.)

tain whether the requirement for a reducing agent is similar to that of the collagen-synthesizing enzymes. The stoichiometry for homogentisate formation and ascorbate consumption is not apparent. Also, other reducing agents are effective in vitro for enzyme activity.

Based on animal studies and clinical trials, there appears to be a relationship between ascorbate deficiency and tyrosine metabolism (Englard and Seifter, 1986; Levine et al., 1941). Scorbutic guinea pigs have excess tyrosine in the circulation (tyrosinemia) and excrete 4-hydroxyphenylpyruvate. Human premature infants display the same pattern. In both guinea pigs and premature infants, ascorbate administration eliminates tyrosinemia and hydroxyphenylpyruvate excretion.

It remains possible that the effect of ascorbate is indirect (Englard and Seifter, 1986). In studies with enzyme isolated from bacteria, the enol form of 4-hydroxyphenylpyruvate is a non-competitive inhibitor of hydroxyphenylpyruvate dioxygenase. Inhibition is relieved by ascorbate and other reducing agents. It is possible that enol-hydroxyphenylpyruvate interacts with enzyme-bound autoxidized iron, with resulting enzyme inhibition. Ascorbate could keep iron in its reduced form, preventing inhibition. If this were the case, the mechanism of ascorbate action on homogentisate formation would be indirect. Whether this mechanism occurs in vivo or in mammalian tissues is not known.

NONENZYMATIC REDUCTIVE FUNCTIONS OF ASCORBATE

Nonenzymatic reductive functions of ascorbate are based on its action as an electron donor in chemical reactions, in which ascorbate is a reducing agent (antioxidant). As a consequence of its redox potential and/or free radical intermediate, ascorbate might act as a chemical reducing agent in many intracellular and extracellular reactions. However, because these are oxidation-reduction reactions, they may not specifically require ascorbic acid as an antioxidant. Chemical reaction conditions used in vitro may not be relevant for reactions that occur in vivo, especially for those reactions that involve iron, copper, or other cat-

ions. Concentrations of iron or copper that will initiate oxidation in vitro may not be physiologically relevant, because these cations are tightly bound to proteins in vivo. The type or amount of oxidant necessary to induce an experimental effect of ascorbate in vitro may also not be relevant in vivo, because that oxidant or its selected concentration might not occur in vivo.

Intracellular Reduction Reactions

Ascorbic Acid and Gene Expression. DNA damage as a result of oxidative metabolism has been postulated to be a contributor to aging, cancer, and other degenerative diseases (Ames et al., 1995). Oxidant damage is repaired efficiently by DNA repair enzymes, but they do not repair all lesions. Other antioxidant defenses include proteins, lipid-soluble antioxidants, and ascorbate. Whether ascorbate specifically protects against oxidant-damaged DNA in vivo remains to be determined.

DNA transcription is regulated by transcription factors, and transcription and transcription factors themselves may be influenced by oxidants. However, the role of ascorbate as a possible transcription factor regulator has not been firmly established. It is possible that the amount of oxidants necessary to influence transcription factor activity experimentally are more than those generated physiologically. The most extensively studied effect of vitamin C on gene expression is the regulation of collagen transcription. The mechanism of this effect may be related to generation of lipid peroxides by prolonged incubation of cells with ascorbate (Houglum et al., 1991). In this case, ascorbate oxidation may actually enhance formation of lipid peroxides, as discussed for prolyl and lysyl hydroxylases in the preceding section. The effect may be an artifact of cell culture conditions, and it is uncertain whether the effect occurs in vivo.

Vitamin C increases acetylcholine receptor amounts in cultured animal cells. Vitamin C specifically increases the mRNA for the acetylcholine receptor α subunit two-fold, but it does not increase mRNA levels for the other 3 subunits of the receptor (Salpeter et al., 1991). There is a delay of approximately 24 h after ascorbate addition for this increase to occur, which is similar to that seen for increased collagen biosynthesis. The mechanism by which α subunit mRNA is increased is unknown. It is possible that the mechanism is coupled to lipid peroxide generation from cell culture conditions, similar to the postulated mechanism of vitamin C effects on collagen biosynthesis.

Ascorbic acid has several effects on proatrial natriuretic peptide. Concomitant with forskolin (an adenylate cyclase activator), ascorbic acid increases proatrial natriuretic peptide mRNA as much as 11-fold (Huang et al., 1993). Ascorbic acid alone does not augment message abundance but increases protein abundance. These mechanisms are therefore independent. The concentration of ascorbic acid needed for increased protein abundance is less than 5 μmol/L. Intracellular concentrations probably would not fall so low even in severe deficiency, so the physiological significance of these findings is not clear.

Ascorbate has effects on other genes, but these effects have not been fully characterized. Ascorbate may affect mRNA transcription of some cytochrome P450 genes and of ubiquitin (Hitomi and Tsukagoshi, 1996). The mechanisms are not clearly understood. Ascorbic acid transiently increases alkaline phosphatase and osteocalcin mRNA in cultured osteoblastic cells by more than 10-fold, but this effect is probably indirect because it is coupled to increased collagen production mediated by ascorbate (Hitomi and Tsukagoshi, 1996). In adipocytes and muscle, effects of ascorbate on gene transcription are also indirect and coupled to synthesis of extracellular matrix (i.e., collagen). Chondrocytes (cartilage cells) increase production of type X collagen mRNA approximately 10-fold in the presence of ascorbate, and this effect is independent of collagen production (Sullivan et al., 1994). Because at least 24 hours of ascorbate exposure is necessary for this effect, it may also be coupled to the generation of lipid peroxides.

Ascorbate and mRNA Translation. In cultured leukemia cells challenged with high concentrations of iron, ascorbate increases ferritin synthesis as much as 50-fold by increasing mRNA ferritin translation (Toth et al., 1995). Ferritin translation is regulated by iron-responsive element-binding proteins. Ascorbate converts these inactive binding proteins in the cytosol to an active form so that ferritin translation is upregulated. The mechanism of this conversion is not certain and could be related to quenching of cytosolic oxidants such as superoxide. It is unknown whether this activation occurs in normal cells, because nonphysiological, high concentrations of iron are required to induce the effect in vitro in tumor cells.

Ascorbate and Intracellular Proteins. Vitamin C has been proposed to protect intracellular proteins from oxidant damage (Delamere, 1996; Sies and Stahl, 1995). This may be relevant in tissues with high oxidant production and/or oxygen concentration, such as neutrophils, monocytes/macrophages, lung, and tissues of the eye exposed to light. Depending on the tissue and the radical generated, ascorbic acid could quench superoxide, hypochlorous acid, singlet oxygen, or hydroxyl radicals. Experimental systems have addressed these issues in vitro. Again, the difficulty is the extrapolation of these data and their relevance to systems operating in vivo.

Vitamin C also has been proposed to accelerate oxidant-mediated protein damage (Delamere, 1996; Stadtman and Berlett, 1997). By quenching superoxide, ascorbate might increase hydrogen peroxide production, but ascorbate does not quench hydrogen peroxide. Ascorbate accelerates free radical production and oxidant damage to proteins in the presence of metals, especially iron and copper. Ascorbate and iron incubation with proteins has been used to demonstrate specific free radical-mediated catabolism of proteins. It is likely that concentrations of free cations in vivo are so low that these reactions do not occur. Ascorbate metabolic products may have other effects on lens proteins of the eye when these are studied in isolated protein systems, but, again, the relevance of these systems to the eye in vivo is uncertain.

Ascorbate and Extracellular Reduction Reactions

Oxidative Reactions Related to Atherogenesis. Just as it has been proposed that it protects against intracellular oxidants, ascorbate has been suggested to have a major role in modulating extracellular oxidants. One of the most widely studied areas is the relationship between ascorbate and low density lipoprotein (LDL) oxidation (Gokce and Frei, 1996; Jialal and Fuller, 1995). An elevated concentration of LDL is a substantial risk factor for development of atherosclerotic cardiovascular disease. LDL appears to be atherogenic only after it is structurally changed. One major pathway of LDL modification may be via oxidative modification via lipid peroxidation. It has been proposed that antioxidants block oxidative modification of LDL. As a water-soluble antioxidant, ascorbate inhibits metal-catalyzed LDL oxidation in vitro in many experimental systems. The mechanism is probably a direct action of ascorbate in quenching of aqueous free radicals. An action of ascorbate in the regeneration of oxidized α-tocopherol has also been proposed, but this mechanism may have less importance for LDL protection. In contrast to its protective effects of LDL in vitro, the effects of ascorbate in vivo are much more difficult to study. The epidemiological data are inconsistent with regard to a possible protective role of ascorbate in heart disease (Gey, 1995; Rimm et al., 1993; Stampfer et al., 1993). Both the metal concentrations used and the time required to induce oxidation in vitro suggest that the observed effects of ascorbate on metal-catalyzed LDL oxidation in vitro are not likely to be representative of ongoing events in vivo in the vascular wall.

Extracellular ascorbate could have other effects on the atherosclerotic process (Weber et al., 1996). Monocyte adhesion to endothelium is an early event in atherogenesis. Ascorbate inhibits leukocyte adhesion to endothelium in animals exposed to cigarette smoke. This effect could be mediated by ascorbate-scavenging of aqueous radicals. Similar findings were observed with human monocytes from smokers. Leukocyte-platelet aggregation is another inflammatory event in atherosclerosis, and particularly in thrombosis. Leukocyte-platelet aggregation was inhibited by vitamin C, and a similar mechanism of oxidant quenching may be responsible. Unfortunately, at least some of these experiments were not physiological. Extracellular free iron was pres-

ent in culture media and may have been required to detect adhesion and its inhibition. (See Chapter 41 for more discussion of atherogenesis.)

Neutrophils, Macrophages, and Fibroblasts. It is possible that extracellular ascorbate quenches oxidants that leak from activated neutrophils or macrophages. Such oxidants could otherwise damage supporting tissues such as fibroblasts and extracellular collagen (Mukhopadhyay and Chatterjee, 1994). Preliminary data support these contentions, but definitive information is lacking.

Plasma. Ascorbate has been suggested to be the primary antioxidant in plasma for quenching aqueous peroxyl radicals and/or lipid peroxidation products (Frei et al., 1990). Ascorbate is preferentially oxidized before other antioxidants in plasma, including uric acid, tocopherols, and bilirubin. These experiments were performed using the chemical oxidant azobis (2-amidinopropane) hydrochloride at 50 mmol/L, plasma, and selected cells. Whether these conditions reflect in vivo oxidant conditions is not known, and results may reflect the choice of oxidant, cell type, or other experimental conditions. Nevertheless, ascorbate remains an ideal radical scavenger that could offer site-specific antioxidant protection.

Gastrointestinal System. Vitamin C is found in gastric juice at concentrations approximately three-fold above the plasma concentration in normal individuals (Rathbone et al., 1989). Ascorbate has been proposed to be secreted into gastric juice, but the mechanism is uncertain. Ascorbate has been proposed to be protective against gastric cancers (Correa, 1992). High dietary intake of vitamin C correlates with reduced gastric cancer risk (Byers and Guerrero, 1995). As for other epidemiological observations for vitamin C and cancer risk, it is not clear what the protective substances are: either vitamin C itself or other components of vitamin C–rich foods. Vitamin C could quench reactive oxygen metabolites, or it could prevent formation of N-nitroso compounds that are potentially mutagenic (Correa, 1992).

Vitamin C in the intestinal tract promotes

iron absorption (Hallberg, 1987). Absorption of soluble nonorganic iron is enhanced by ascorbate. Ascorbate might chelate iron or simply keep iron reduced, facilitating absorption in the small intestine. Intake of 20 to 60 mg of ascorbate, the amount found in single servings of foods rich in vitamin C, enhances iron absorption. Larger amounts have little increased effect.

Enhanced iron absorption by ascorbate is clinically relevant. Patients with iron deficiency (e.g., pregnant women, women with heavy menses, or patients who have undergone blood loss) are given iron with ascorbate. By contrast, ascorbate supplements can be harmful to patients with hemochromatosis (patients who suffer from iron overload) because ascorbate will promote additional iron absorption in these patients who already have too much iron

ASCORBATE FUNCTION AND TISSUE DISTRIBUTION

As noted in the section on transport, ascorbic acid is concentrated by many cells and tissues to concentrations greater than 1 mmol/L (Rumsey and Levine, 1998). The functions of ascorbate in some of these tissues, such as adrenal medulla, pituitary, fibroblasts, osteoblasts, and chondrocytes, is reasonably clear. For other tissues or cells that concentrate ascorbate, including neutrophils, monocytes/macrophages, lens, retina, cornea, peripheral and central neurons, liver, and endothelial cells, potential roles of ascorbate have been suggested but not proved. Still other tissues or cells, such as lymphocytes, platelets, pancreas, adrenal cortex, testis, and ovary, contain millimolar concentrations of ascorbate but have no known specific functions of ascorbate.

ASCORBATE DEFICIENCY

Scurvy, which is now known as the vitamin C deficiency disease, was first described several thousand years ago. The Scottish physician James Lind noted in 1753 that the disease could be prevented by a diet with limes or other food substances (Lind, 1753). The active protective compound, ascorbic acid, was isolated in 1932 by the laboratories of Szent-Gyorgyi and King (King and Waugh, 1932; Svirbely and Szent-Gyorgyi, 1932). Once the vitamin was identified, its deficiency state was studied more systematically. The British Medical Research Council concluded that healthy men have vitamin C body stores that will prevent scurvy for at least 160 days. These estimates are almost certainly incorrect, however, because they were based on low vitamin C intakes that were not verified (Hodges, 1971). Intakes were probably substantially higher than those calculated at the time of the study.

Two studies of the clinical manifestations of severe vitamin C deficiency were conducted in prisoners housed in a metabolic ward (Baker et al., 1969; Baker et al., 1971). In the first study, other nutrients in addition to vitamin C were probably absent from the diet. This problem was corrected in the second study, and the symptoms and signs of scurvy are based on findings from this latter study of 5 men. Symptoms are what the patient tells the physician subjectively and signs are what the physician finds objectively on examination. The first sign of scurvy was petechial hemorrhage, or small areas of bleeding under the skin. Other signs included coiled hairs, bleeding gums, ecchymoses (larger areas of bleeding under the skin), hyperkeratosis (increased skin cells around hair follicles), arthralgias (joint pain), joint effusions (abnormal amounts of fluid in joints), and shortness of breath. All 5 men developed the sicca syndrome, or Sjögren's syndrome, with symptoms of dry eyes, dry mouth, scaling skin, dental caries, and gum tenderness. These men also had evidence of hypochondriasis and depression on psychological tests (Baker et al., 1971; Hodges, 1971).

Fatigue is an important early symptom in vitamin C deficiency. Although fatigue was not described as a symptom of vitamin C deficiency in the second prisoner study, it was mentioned in the first study and in Lind's classic work (Lind, 1753). Fatigue was the first symptom experienced by a researcher who purposely gave himself scurvy to study the disease course (Crandon et al., 1940). In a recent study at the National Institutes of

Health, healthy volunteers were made vitamin C-deficient but did not develop signs of scurvy. The majority of subjects had fatigue as their only symptom (Levine et al., 1996a). Fatigue was reversed when plasma concentrations exceeded 20 μmol/L of ascorbate. Taken together, the findings show that fatigue is the first symptom of vitamin C deficiency and precedes all other symptoms and signs. A simple mnemonic to remember signs and symptoms of scurvy is "EFGH," representing ecchymoses, fatigue, gum bleeding and tenderness, and hyperkeratosis.

Overt vitamin C deficiency in the United States today is seen in malnourished populations, including those with cancer cachexia, poor intake, malabsorption, alcoholism, or chemical dependency (Case Records of the Massachusetts General Hospital, 1995). Because a substantial fraction of the population ingests less than one serving of fruit or vegetable daily (Basch et al., 1994; Life Sciences Research Office, 1995), subclinical vitamin C deficiency may be much more common than overt deficiency. It may be much more difficult for health professionals to recognize because its only symptom, fatigue, is nonspecific and has myriad causes.

TOXICITY AND ADVERSE EFFECTS OF VITAMIN C

Compared with most vitamins, vitamin C is remarkably nontoxic. The adverse effect of most concern is formation of oxalate kidney stones (Urivetzky et al., 1992). Because oxalate is a product of vitamin C metabolism and because it is excreted by the kidney, there has been concern for many years that excess vitamin C ingestion could cause kidney stones. Unfortunately, most studies conducted before 1986 do not provide helpful information, because they utilized assays that did not account for degradation of excreted vitamin C to oxalate before or during assays. Thus, when subjects ingested high amounts of vitamin C, the excreted urinary vitamin C was inadvertently thought to be oxalate. The most convincing study indicates that a specific group of patients are at risk for excess oxalate excretion, or hyperoxaluria, from high intakes of vitamin C (Urivetzky et al., 1992). These patients have a propensity to develop oxalate kidney stones because they excrete high amounts of oxalate in the urine. When these patients are given vitamin C at two successive doses of 500 mg or above, they excrete increased amounts of oxalate, which might increase their risk of kidney stones. It is quite possible that members of the population at large may not realize they have hyperoxaluria until they develop kidney stones. Thus, these data suggest that safe doses of ascorbate in the general population are less than 1000 mg daily.

There are other possible adverse effects of ascorbic acid. It is possible that uric acid excretion in the urine is increased by ascorbate doses of 1000 mg or more (Levine et al., 1996a). It is unknown whether this excretion will cause uric acid kidney stones. Iron absorption in the gastrointestinal tract is increased by ascorbic acid, as noted earlier. Patients who absorb excess iron or who have excess iron stores should avoid ascorbate supplements. These include patients with hemochromatosis, sideroblastic anemia, or thalassemia major (Nienhuis, 1981). Ascorbate ingestion of 250 mg or more can cause false-negatives on tests of occult bleeding in the gastrointestinal tract (Levine et al., 1996b). Patients who are to be screened for occult blood loss in the gastrointestinal tract should avoid ascorbate supplements before this testing is performed. Gram doses of ascorbate taken at one time can cause diarrhea or abdominal bloating (Levine et al., 1996b). Gram doses of ascorbic acid can cause high levels of oxalate in the blood of dialysis patients (Balcke et al., 1984). Finally, patients with glucose 6-phosphate dehydrogenase deficiency can have massive hemolysis if ascorbate is given in gram doses either orally or intravenously (Rees et al., 1993). Despite all these caveats, intakes of ascorbic acid at doses of less than 1 g daily appear to be safe for most people.

RECOMMENDED INGESTION

The current Recommended Dietary Allowance (RDA) for vitamin C is 60 mg daily for healthy adults, based on three criteria (Baker et al., 1969; Baker et al., 1971; Hodges, 1971; National Research Council, 1980, 1989). First, prior intake of 60 mg daily was believed to protect against signs and symptoms of scurvy for at least 1 month if vitamin C ingestion were suddenly to cease. Second, the threshold for urinary excretion of vitamin C was believed to indicate that body stores were close to saturation, and the threshold dose for vitamin C urinary excretion was believed to be 60 mg daily. Third, 60 mg daily was believed to provide adequate body stores of vitamin C

and to compensate for metabolic losses. Most studies of vitamin C requirements have been done with men, and there are limited data on vitamin C requirements for infants, children, and women.

Based on recent evidence, it is clear that 60 mg daily will not protect against symptoms of scurvy for 1 month if vitamin C ingestion were to suddenly cease (Levine et al., 1996a). Until recently, there were no data to support the contention that the threshold of urinary excretion was a suitable indicator of body stores of vitamin C. In fact, new data show

 NUTRITION INSIGHT

Proposed Criteria for Determination of Recommended Intakes of Vitamin C

Levine and coworkers believe that the following 8 criteria should be used to determine recommended intakes for vitamin C (Institute of Medicine, 1994; Levine et al., 1996a, 1996b).

- Vitamin biochemical and molecular function in relation to vitamin concentration
- Availability of the vitamin in the diet
- Steady-state vitamin concentration in plasma as a function of dose
- Steady-state vitamin concentration in tissues as a function of dose
- Vitamin bioavailability (absorption)
- Vitamin excretion
- Vitamin safety and adverse effects
- Beneficial effects in relation to dose: direct effects and epidemiological observations.

Answers are far from complete for all these criteria. Nevertheless, new clinical data are available with regard to many of them (Graumlich et al., 1997; Levine et al., 1996a). These data show that the relationship between the dose of vitamin C and its plasma concentration is sigmoidal, that the current RDA is on the lower third of the steep portion of this curve, and that the first dose beyond the sigmoid part of the curve is 200 mg daily. Cells and tissues saturate at daily doses of 100 mg of vitamin C. Bioavailability at steady state is virtually complete for doses less than or equal to 200 mg. True bioavailability at steady state was 70% for a 500-mg dose and less than 50% for a 1250-mg dose. For these higher doses, that part of the dose that was absorbed was entirely excreted. The dose at which ascorbate first appeared in urine (the threshold dose for urinary excretion) was 100 mg daily. At doses of 1000 mg daily, urinary uric acid and oxalate excretion were increased, which has the potential for increasing kidney stone risk (Urivetzky et al., 1992).

Five servings of fruits and vegetables contain ~220 to 280 mg of ascorbate. Five or more servings of fruits and vegetables daily are protective against cancers of the gastrointestinal tract, although the protective agents are unknown (Byers and Guerrero, 1995). It has been estimated that a plasma concentration of vitamin C above 50 μmol/L may be protective against stroke and cardiovascular disease (Gey, 1995). Using these criteria and combining the biochemical, clinical, and epidemiological evidence, Levine and coworkers suggest that the RDA for vitamin C should be increased to 200 mg daily, and that vitamin C should be obtained from five servings of fruits and vegetables (Levine et al., 1996a, 1996b). Additionally, they suggest that these criteria for determining recommended ingestion of vitamin C may be applicable to other water-soluble vitamins.

that the threshold for urinary excretion is 100 mg daily, not 60 mg daily, and that vitamin C saturation does not occur until intakes are 500 mg daily (Levine et al., 1996a). The calculations suggesting that 60 mg daily would compensate for metabolic losses were based on data obtained in deficient patients. Vitamin C metabolism probably changes as a function of depletion or repletion, which makes it questionable to calculate metabolism for the general population based on data from deficient subjects. Current vitamin C recommendations are not based on function of the vitamin or on providing ideal amounts to maintain health (Levine, 1986).

The Institute of Medicine staff have recently recognized the problems with the current RDA for vitamin C and other dietary antioxidants and are working on new recommendations for vitamin C intake (Institute of Medicine, 1994).

REFERENCES

Ames, B. N., Gold, L. S. and Willett, W. C. (1995) The causes and prevention of cancer. Proc Natl Acad Sci USA 92:5258–5265.

Baker, E. M., Halver, J. E., Johnsen, D. O., Joyce, B. E., Knight, M. K. and Tolbert, B. M. (1975) Metabolism of ascorbic acid and ascorbic-2-sulfate in man and the subhuman primate. Ann N Y Acad Sci 258:72–80.

Baker, E. M., Hodges, R. E., Hood, J., Sauberlich, H. E. and March, S. C. (1969) Metabolism of ascorbic-1-^{14}C acid in experimental human scurvy. Am J Clin Nutr 22:549–558.

Baker, E. M., Hodges, R. E., Hood, J., Sauberlich, H. E., March, S. C. and Canham, J. E. (1971) Metabolism of ^{14}C- and ^{3}H-labeled L-ascorbic acid in human scurvy. Am J Clin Nutr 24:444–454.

Balcke, P., Schmidt, P., Zazgornik, J., Kopsa, H. and Haubenstock, A. (1984) Ascorbic acid aggravates secondary hyperoxalemia in patients on chronic hemodialysis. Ann Intern Med 101:344–345.

Basch, C. E., Syber, P. and Shea, S. (1994) 5-a-day:Dietary behavior and the fruit and vegetable intake of Latino children. Am J Public Health 84:814–818.

Buettner, G. R. (1993) The pecking order of free radicals and antioxidants: Lipid peroxidation, alpha-tocopherol, and ascorbate. Arch Biochem Biophys 300:535–543.

Byers, T. and Guerrero, N. (1995) Epidemiologic evidence for vitamin C and vitamin E in cancer prevention. Am J Clin Nutr 62:1385S–1392S.

Case Records of the Massachusetts General Hospital (1995) Case 39–1955: A 72 year old man with exertional dyspnea, fatigue, and extensive ecchymoses and purpuric lesions. N Engl J Med 333:1695–1702.

Correa, P. (1992) Human gastric carcinogenesis: A multistep and multifactorial process. First American Cancer Society Award Lecture on Cancer Epidemiology and Prevention. Cancer Res 52:6735–6740.

Crandon, J.H., Lund, C.C. and Dill, D.B. (1940) Experimental human scurvy. N Engl J Med 223:353–369.

Darr, D., Combs, S., Dunston, S., Manning, T. and Pinnell, S. (1992) Topical vitamin C protects porcine skin from ultraviolet radiation-induced damage. Br J Dermatol 127:247–253.

Delamere, N.A. (1996) Ascorbic acid and the eye. In: Ascorbic Acid: Biochemistry and Biomedical Cell Biology (Harris, J.R. ed.), Subcellular Biochemistry, Vol. 25, pp. 313–329. Plenum Press, New York.

Dhariwal, K.R., Black, C.D. and Levine, M. (1991a) Semidehydroascorbic acid as an intermediate in norepinephrine biosynthesis in chromaffin granules. J Biol Chem 266:12908–12914.

Dhariwal, K.R., Hartzell, W.O. and Levine, M. (1991b) Ascorbic acid and dehydroascorbic acid measurements in human plasma and serum. Am J Clin Nutr 54:712–716.

Dunn, W.A., Rettura, G., Seifter, E. and England, S. (1984) Carnitine biosynthesis from gamma-butyrobetaine and from exogenous protein-bound 6-N-trimethyl-L-lysine by the perfused guinea pig liver. Effect of ascorbate deficiency on the in situ activity of gamma-butyrobetaine hydroxylase. J Biol Chem 259:10764–10770.

Dyer, D.L., Kanai, Y., Hediger, M.A., Rubin, S.A. and Said, H.M. (1994) Expression of a rabbit renal ascorbic acid transporter in Xenopus laevis oocytes. Am J Physiol 267:C301–C306.

Eipper, B., Milgram, S.L., Husten, E.J., Yun, H. and Mains, R.E. (1993) Peptidylglycine alpha amidating monooxygenase: A multifunctional protein with catalytic, processing, and routing domains. Protein Sci 2:489–497.

Eipper, B., Stoffers, D.A. and Mains, R.E. (1992) The biosynthesis of neuropeptides: Peptide alpha amidation. Annu Rev Neurosci 15:57–85.

Englard, S. and Seifter, S. (1986) The biochemical functions of ascorbic acid. Annu Rev Nutr 6:365–406.

Fleming, P.J. and Kent, U.M. (1991) Cytochrome b$_{561}$, ascorbic acid, and transmembrane electron transfer. Am J Clin Nutr 54:1173S–1178S.

Frei, B., Stocker, R., England, L. and Ames, B.N. (1990) Ascorbate: The most effective antioxidant in human blood plasma. Adv Exp Med Biol 264:155–163.

Geesin, J.C., Darr, D., Kaufman, R., Murad, S. and Pinnell, S.R. (1988) Ascorbic acid specifically increases type I and type III procollagen messenger RNA levels in human skin fibroblast. J Invest Dermatol 90:420–424.

Gey, K.F. (1995) Cardiovascular disease and vitamins. Concurrent correction of suboptimal plasma antioxidant levels may, as an important part of optimal nutrition, help to prevent early stages of cardiovascular disease and cancer, respectively. Bibl Nutr Dieta 52:75–91.

Gokce, N. and Frei, B. (1996) Basic research in antioxidant inhibition of steps in atherogenesis. J Cardiovasc Risk 3:352–357.

Gosiewska, A., Wilson, W., Kwon, D. and Peterkofsky, B. (1994) Evidence for an in vivo role of insulin-like growth factor binding proteins 1 and 2 as inhibitors of collagen gene expression in vitamin C deficient and fasted guinea pigs. Endocrinology 134:1329–1339.

Graumlich, J., Ludden, T.M., Conry-Cantilena, C., Cantilena, L.R., Wang, Y. and Levine, M. (1997) Pharmacokinetic model of ascorbic acid in humans during depletion and repletion. Pharmaceut Res 14:1133–1139.

Hallberg, L. (1987) Wheat fiber, phytates and iron absorption. Scand J Gastroenterol (Suppl.) 129:73–79.

Hitomi, K. and Tsukagoshi, N. (1996) Role of ascorbic acid in modulation of gene expression. In: Ascorbic Acid: Biochemistry and Biomedical Cell Biology (Harris, J.R., ed.), Subcellular Biochemistry, Vol. 25, pp. 41–56. Plenum Press, New York.

Hodges, R.E. (1971) What's new about scurvy? Am J Clin Nutr 24:383–384.

Houglum, K.P., Brenner, D.A. and Chojkier, M. (1991) Ascorbic acid stimulation of collagen biosynthesis independent of hydroxylation. Am J Clin Nutr 54:1141S–1143S.

Huang, W., Yang, Z., Lee, D., Copolov, D.L. and Lim, A.T. (1993) Ascorbic acid enhances forskolin-induced cyclic AMP production and pro-ANF mRNA expression of hypothalamic neurons in culture. Endocrinology 132:2271–2273.

Institute of Medicine (1994) How Should the Recommended Dietary Allowances Be Revised? National Academy Press, Washington, D.C.

Jialal, I. and Fuller, C.J. (1995) Effect of vitamin E, vitamin C, and beta-carotene on LDL oxidation and atherosclerosis. Can J Cardiol 11:97G–103G.

Kaufman, S. (1974) Dopamine-beta-hydroxylase. J Psychiatr Res 11:303–316.

Kent, U. and Fleming, P.J. (1987) Purified cytochrome b_{561} catalyzes transmembrane electron transfer for dopamine beta-hydroxylase and peptidyl glycine alpha-amidating monooxygenase in reconstituted systems. J Biol Chem 262:8174–8178.

King, C.C. and Waugh, W.A. (1932) The chemical nature of vitamin C. Science 75:357–358.

Kivirikko, K.I. and Myllyla, R. (1985) Post-translational processing of procollagens. Ann N Y Acad Sci 460:187–201.

Levine, M. (1986) New concepts in the biology and biochemistry of ascorbic acid. N Engl J Med 314:892–902.

Levine, M., Conry-Cantilena, C., Wang, Y., Welch, R.W., Washko, P.W., Dhariwal, K.R., Park, J.B., Lazarev, A., Graumlich, J., King, J. and Cantilena, L.R. (1996a) Vitamin C pharmacokinetics in healthy volunteers: Evidence for a Recommended Dietary Allowance. Proc Natl Acad Sci USA 93:3704–3709.

Levine, M., Dhariwal, K. R., Washko, P.W., Butler, J.D., Welch, R.W., Wang, Y.H. and Bergsten, P. (1991) Ascorbic acid and in situ kinetics: A new approach to vitamin requirements. Am J Clin Nutr 54:1157S–1162S.

Levine, M., Rumsey, S., Wang, Y., Park, J.B., Kwon, O., Xu, W. and Amano, N. (1996b) Vitamin C. In: Present Knowledge in Nutrition (Filer, L.J. and Ziegler, E.E., eds.), pp. 146–159. International Life Sciences Institute, Washington, D.C.

Levine, S.Z., Gordon, H.H. and Marples, E. (1941) A defect in the metabolism of tyrosine and phenylalanine in premature infants: Spontaneous occurrence and eradication by vitamin C. J Clin Invest 20:209–219.

Lewin, S. (1976) Vitamin C: Its Molecular Biology and Medical Potential. Academic Press, London.

Life Sciences Research Office, Interagency Board for Nutrition Monitoring and Related Research (1995) Third Report on Nutrition Monitoring in the United States. U.S. Government Printing Office, Washington, D.C.

Lind, J. (1753) A Treatise on the Scurvy. A. Millar, London.

Lindblad, B., Lindstedt, G. and Lindstedt, S. (1970) The mechanism of enzymic formation of homogentisate from p-hydroxyphenyl pyruvate. J Am Chem Soc 92:7446–7449.

Maellaro, E., Del Bello, B., Sugherini, L., Santucci, A., Comporti, M. and Casini, A.F. (1994) Purification and characterization of glutathione-dependent dehydroascorbate reductase from rat liver. Biochem J 301:471–476.

Melethil, S.L., Mason, W.E. and Chiang, C. (1986) Dose dependent absorption and excretion of vitamin C in humans. Int J Pharm 31:83–89.

Mukhopadhyay, C.K. and Chatterjee, I.B. (1994) Free metal ion-independent oxidative damage of collagen. Protection by ascorbic acid. J Biol Chem 269:30200–30205.

National Research Council (1980) Recommended Dietary Allowances, 9th ed., pp. 72–81. National Academy Press, Washington, D.C.

National Research Council (1989) Recommended Dietary Allowances, 10th ed., pp. 115–124. National Academy Press, Washington, D.C.

Nienhuis, A.W. (1981) Vitamin C and iron [editorial]. N Engl J Med 304:170–171.

Nishikimi, M., Fukuyama, R., Minoshima, S., Shimizu, N. and Yagi, K. (1994) Cloning and chromosomal mapping of the human nonfunctional gene for L-gulono-gamma-lactone oxidase, the enzyme for L-ascorbic acid biosynthesis missing in man. J Biol Chem 269:13685–13688.

Otsuka, M., Kurata, T. and Arakawa, N. (1986) Antiscorbutic effect of dehydro-L-ascorbic acid in vitamin C–deficient guinea pigs. J Nutr Sci Vitaminol (Tokyo) 32:183–190.

Park, J.B. and Levine, M. (1996) Purification, cloning, and expression of dehydroascorbic acid reduction activity from human neutrophils: Identification as glutaredoxin. Biochem J 315:931–938.

Peterkofsky, B. (1991) Ascorbate requirement for hydroxylation and secretion of procollagen: Relationship to inhibition of collagen synthesis in scurvy. Am J Clin Nutr 54:1135S–1140S.

Prockop, D.J. and Kivirikko, K.I. (1995) Collagens: Molecular biology, diseases, and potential for therapy. Annu Rev Biochem 64:403–434.

Rathbone, B.J., Johnson, A.W., Wyatt, J.I., Kelleher, J., Heatley, R.V. and Losowsky, M.S. (1989) Ascorbic acid: A factor concentrated in human gastric juice. Clin Sci 76:237–241.

Rebouche, C.J. (1991) Ascorbic acid and carnitine biosynthesis. Am J Clin Nutr 5:1147S–1152S.

Rebouche, C.J. (1995) The ability of guinea pigs to synthesize carnitine at a normal rate from epsilon-N-trimethyllysine or gamma-butyrobetaine in vivo is not compromised by experimental vitamin C deficiency. Metabolism 44:624–629.

Rees, D.C., Kelsey, H. and Richards, J.D. (1993) Acute haemolysis induced by high dose ascorbic acid in glucose-6-phosphate dehydrogenase deficiency. Br Med J 306:841–842.

Rimm, E.B., Stampfer, M.J., Ascherio, A., Giovannucci, E., Colditz, G.A. and Willett, W.C. (1993) Vitamin E consumption and the risk of coronary heart disease in men. N Engl J Med 328:1450–1456.

Ronchetti, I.P., Quaglino, D.J. and Bergamini, G. (1996) Ascorbic acid and connective tissue. In: Ascorbic Acid: Biochemistry and Biomedical Cell Biology (Harris, J.R., ed.), Subcellular Biochemistry, Vol. 25, pp. 249–262. Plenum Press, New York.

Rose, R.C., Choi, J.L. and Koch, M.J. (1988) Intestinal transport and metabolism of oxidized ascorbic acid (dehydroascorbic acid). Am J Physiol 254:G824–G828.

Rowland, M. and Tozer, T.N. (1989) Clinical Pharmacokinetics: Concepts and Applications. Lea and Febiger, Philadelphia.

Rumsey, S.C., Kwon, O., Xu, G., Burant, C.F., Simpson, I. and Levine, M. (1997) Glucose transporter isoforms GLUT1 and GLUT3 transport dehydroascorbic acid. J Biol Chem 272:18982–18989.

Rumsey, S.C. and Levine, M. (1998) Absorption, transport, and disposition of ascorbic acid in humans. J Nutr Biochem 9:116–130.

Salpeter, M.M., Liu, E.C., Minor, R.R., Podleski, T.R. and Wootton, J.A. (1991) Acetylcholine receptor regulation in L5 muscle cells is independent of increases in collagen secretion induced by ascorbic acid. Am J Clin Nutr 54:1184S–1187S.

Sauberlich, H.E., Tamura, T., Craig, C.B., Freeberg, L.E. and Liu, T. (1996) Effects of erythorbic acid on vitamin C metabolism in young women. Am J Clin Nutr 64:336–346.

Sies, H. and Stahl, W. (1995) Vitamins E and C, beta carotene, and other carotenoids as antioxidants. Am J Clin Nutr 62:1315S–1321S.

Stadtman, E.R. and Berlett, B.S. (1997) Reactive oxygen-mediated protein oxidation in aging and disease. Chem Res Toxicol 10:485–494.

Stampfer, M.J., Hennekens, C.H., Manson, J.E., Colditz, G.A., Rosner, B. and Willet, W.C. (1993) Vitamin E consumption and the risk of coronary disease in women. N Engl J Med 328:1444–1449.

Stevenson, N.R. (1974) Active transport of L-ascorbic acid in the human ileum. Gastroenterology 67:952–956.

Stubbe, J.A. (1985) Identification of two alpha keto glutarate dependent dioxygenases in extracts of *Rhodotorula glutinis* catalyzing deoxyuridine hydroxylation. J Biol Chem 260:9972–9975.

Sullivan, T.A., Uschmann, B., Hough, R. and Leboy, P.S. (1994) Ascorbate modulation of chondrocyte gene expression is independent of its role in collagen secretion. J Biol Chem 269:22500–22506.

Svirbely, J.L. and Szent-Gyorgyi, A. (1932) The chemical nature of vitamin C. Biochem J 26:865–870.

Tolbert, B.M. and Ward, J.B. (1982) Dehydroascorbic acid. In: Ascorbic Acid: Chemistry, Metabolism, and Uses (Seib, P.A. and Tolbert, B.M., eds.), pp. 101–123. American Chemical Society, Washington, D.C.

Toth, I., Rogers, J.T., McPhee, J.A., Elliott, S.M., Abramson, S.L. and Bridges, K.R. (1995) Ascorbic acid enhances iron-induced ferritin translation in human leukemia and hepatoma cells. J Biol Chem 270:2846–2852.

Urivetzky, M., Kessaris, D. and Smith, A.D. (1992) Ascorbic acid overdosing: A risk factor for calcium oxalate nephrolithiasis. J Urol 147:1215–1218.

Vanderslice, J.T. and Higgs, D.J. (1991) Vitamin C content of foods: Sample variability. Am J Clin Nutr 54:1323S–1327S.

Washko, P.W., Wang, Y. and Levine, M. (1993) Ascorbic acid recycling in human neutrophils. J Biol Chem 268:15531–15535.

Washko, P.W., Welch, R.W., Dhariwal, K.R., Wang, Y. and Levine, M. (1992) Ascorbic acid and dehydroascorbic acid analyses in biological samples. Anal Biochem 204:1–14.

Weber, C., Erl, W., Weber, K. and Weber, P.C. (1996) Increased adhesiveness of isolated monocytes of endothelium is prevented by vitamin C. Circulation 93:1488–1492.

Welch, R.W., Wang, Y., Crossman, A., Jr., Park, J.B., Kirk, K.L. and Levine, M. (1995) Accumulation of vitamin C (ascorbate) and its oxidized metabolite dehydroascorbic acid occurs by separate mechanisms. J Biol Chem 270:12584–12592.

Wells, W.W., Xu, D.P., Yang, Y. and Rocque, P.A. (1990) Mammalian thioltransferase (glutaredoxin) and protein disulfide isomerase have dehydroascorbate reductase activity. J Biol Chem 265:15361–15364.

Winkler, B.S., Orselli, S.M. and Rex, T.S. (1994) The redox couple between glutathione and ascorbic acid: A chemical and physiological perspective. Free Radic Biol Med 17:333–349.

Wondrack, L.M., Hsu, C.A. and Abbott, M.T. (1978) Thymine 7-hydroxylase and pyrimidine deoxyribonucleoside 2′-hydroxylase activities in *Rhodotorula glutinis*. J Biol Chem 253:6511–6515.

RECOMMENDED READINGS

Englard, S. and Seifter, S. (1986) The biochemical functions of ascorbic acid. Annu Rev Nutr 6:365–406.

Harris, J.R., ed. (1996) Ascorbic Acid: Biochemistry and Biomedical Cell Biology. Subcellular Biochemistry, Vol. 25. Plenum Press, New York.

Rumsey, S.C. and Levine, M. (1998) Absorption, transport, and disposition of ascorbic acid in humans. J Nutr Biochem 9:116–130.

CHAPTER **24**

◆◆◆◆◆◆◆◆◆◆◆◆◆◆◆◆◆◆◆◆◆◆◆◆◆◆◆◆◆◆◆◆◆

Vitamin K

John W. Suttie, Ph.D.

O U T L I N E

C O M M O N   A B B R E V I A T I O N S

Gla (γ-carboxyglutamate)
Glu (glutamate)
MK (menaquinone)

VITAMIN K, AN ANTIHEMORRHAGIC FACTOR

In the early 1930s, Danish nutritional biochemist Henrich Dam was attempting to demonstrate that cholesterol was a dietary essential. He fed chicks a diet he had formulated to be low in fat and deficient in cholesterol, and noted that the chicks developed a hemorrhagic syndrome. Addition of cholesterol to the diet did not cure the syndrome, and Dam (1934) soon realized that, in removing cholesterol from the diet, he had also removed another essential factor.

The hemorrhagic condition could be cured by the addition of alfalfa meal to the diet or by the administration of a lipid extract of green plants. Efforts were then directed toward isolating and characterizing the factor exhibiting this response. By 1939, a series of investigations led by Dam in Denmark, Almquist at Berkeley, and Doisy at St. Louis University had established that the form of the vitamin found in alfalfa, now called vitamin K_1 or phylloquinone, was 2-methyl-3-phytyl-1,4-naphthoquinone. Bacterial forms of the vitamin, a series of multiprenyl menaquinones with an unsaturated side chain that were originally called vitamin K_2, subsequently were characterized. These investigations led to the sharing of the Nobel Prize in Medicine by Dam and Doisy in 1941. The hemorrhagic condition that resulted from the dietary lack of vitamin K originally was thought to be due solely to a lowered concentration of the plasma clotting factor prothrombin (factor II), but it was later shown that the synthesis of clotting factors VII, IX, and X was also depressed in the deficient state.

The biochemical events involved in the production of the vitamin K-dependent proteins were not elucidated for another 30 years. The 4-hydroxycoumarins were identified in the 1940s as vitamin K antagonists. They were found to be useful as rodenticides and also became widely used clinical anticoagulants. The use of warfarin and other 4-hydroxycoumarins to experimentally regulate the production of vitamin K-dependent proteins was an important tool in studies of vitamin K action. The lack of a general understanding of the mechanism of protein biosynthesis prevented serious experimental approaches to the cellular and molecular mechanisms involved in the synthesis of vitamin K-dependent proteins until the mid 1960s. By the early 1970s, it had been shown that the vitamin was one of the substrates required for a microsomal enzyme involved in the intracellular conversion of inactive precursors of the vitamin K-dependent proteins to their active forms. The enzyme catalyzed the conversion of specific glutamyl residues to γ-carboxyglutamyl (Gla) residues in these proteins. The biochemical role of vitamin K was therefore analogous to that of a coenzyme derived from one of the water-soluble vitamins. By the early 1990s, the enzyme using vitamin K as a cofactor had been isolated and characterized.

NOMENCLATURE OF VITAMIN K ACTIVE COMPOUNDS

Compounds with vitamin K activity are 2-methyl-1,4-naphthoquinones with a hydrophobic substituent at the 3-position (Fig. 24–1). Phylloquinone, originally called vitamin K_1, is the form isolated from green plants, and it has a phytyl group at the 3-position of the naphthoquinone ring. The bacterially synthesized forms of the vitamin originally were called vitamin K_2 and are now more properly designated as menaquinones. These forms of the vitamin have an unsaturated multiprenyl group at the 3-position. Although a wide range of menaquinones (abbreviated as MK-n) are synthesized by bacteria, long-chain menaquinones with 6 to 10 isoprenoid groups in the side chain (MK-6 to MK-10) are the most common. The synthetic compound menadione (2-methyl-1,4-naphthoquinone) was shown very early to have vitamin K activity and commonly is used as a source of the vitamin in animal feeds. Menadione itself is now known not to be a substrate for the vitamin K-dependent carboxylase, but it is alkylated to an active form, MK-4, in mammalian liver. Phylloquinone, available as a tablet or dispersed in a detergent for parenteral use, is the form of the vitamin available for human use.

SOURCES OF VITAMIN K

Reliable estimates of the vitamin K content of foods have been available only recently.

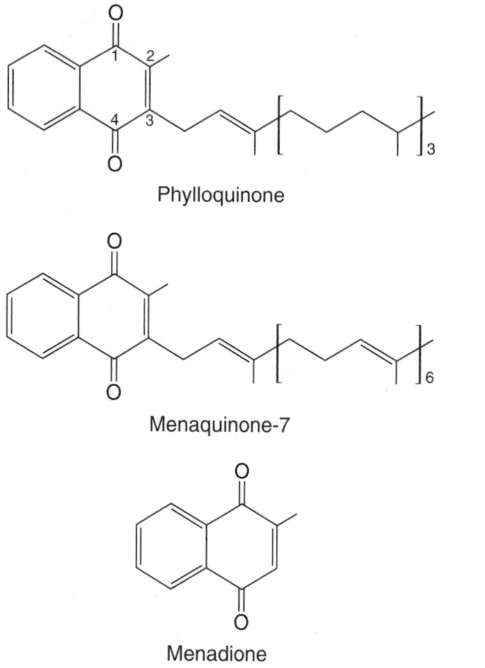

Phylloquinone

Menaquinone-7

Menadione

Figure 24–1. *Structures of compounds with vitamin K activity. Phylloquinone synthesized in plants is the main dietary form of vitamin K. Menaquinone-7 is one of a series of menaquinones produced by intestinal bacteria, and menadione is a synthetic compound that can be converted to menaquinone-4 by animal tissues.*

Available data that have previously been summarized in various nutrition texts and reviews were obtained from chick biological assays of the vitamin K content of foods before a suitable standard was available and should be used with a great deal of caution. Methodology for the analysis of foods for their vitamin K content by lipid extraction followed by high-performance liquid chromatography (HPLC) is now available. A large number of foods and edible oils have been analyzed by these modern methods, and good estimates of the vitamin K content of a wide range of foods are now available (Table 24–1). In general, green vegetables are the major source of phylloquinone in the diet, and foods such as kale, spinach, broccoli, Brussels sprouts, cabbage, and lettuce are excellent sources of the vitamin. These foods contain in excess of 100 μg of phylloquinone per 100 g of fresh weight, whereas the more commonly consumed green vegetables, such as peas and green beans, furnish between 10 and 50 μg/100 g fresh weight. Some cooking oils, chiefly soy-

bean, rapeseed (canola), and to a lesser extent olive oil, also are good sources and are major contributors to the total daily intake of vitamin K. Liver provides a significant dietary intake of menaquinones, but except for liver and a few specialized fermented foods and cheese products, the major form of vitamin K in the diet is phylloquinone of plant origin.

The "normal" intake of vitamin K in the human diet often has been assumed to be in the range of 300 to 500 μg/day. More recent studies using newer data (Booth et al., 1996) have shown that this is a rather high estimate and that the intake of most adults is more likely in the range of 70 to 100 μg/day. Ingestion of high doses of phylloquinone, the natural form of the vitamin, has no toxic effect. Menadione, a synthetic form of the vitamin, was administered to infants at one time but was shown to be associated with hemolytic anemia and liver toxicity. Phylloquinone now is administered routinely to infants to prevent hemorrhagic disease of the newborn.

Intestinal anaerobes such as *Escherichia coli* and *Bacteroides fragilis* produce menaquinones, and the human gut contains large quantities of bacterially produced vitamin K. Early studies indicated that germ-free animals had an increased vitamin K requirement, but the nutritional significance for the human of menaquinones produced in the lower bowel is not yet clear. The extent of, or mechanism of, absorption of menaquinones from the lower bowel has not been clearly established, although human liver does contain significant quantities of menaquinones. There are a large number of case reports of patients exhibiting a vitamin K-responsive hypoprothrombinemia after antibiotic administration. These episodes usually have been assumed to be the result of an influence of the antibiotic on menaquinone synthesis, but the limited data available would indicate that most antibiotics do not negatively influence menaquinone production. Many of the case reports may simply reflect very low dietary intakes of vitamin K due to limited food intake in severely ill patients and hematological responses to various underlying illnesses.

The historical difficulty in producing a vitamin K deficiency in human subjects has been a second factor that suggests to investi-

TABLE 24–1
Vitamin K Content of Some Common Foods*

μg Phylloquinone/100 g of Edible Portion

Vegetables		Grains		Fruits	
Kale	817	Bread	3	Avocado	40
Spinach	400	Oatmeal	3	Grapes	3
Endive	231	White rice	1	Cantaloupe	1
Broccoli	205	Wheat flour	0.6	Bananas	0.5
Brussels sprouts	177	Dry spaghetti	0.2	Apples	0.1
Cabbage	147	Nuts, Oils, Seeds		Oranges	0.1
Lettuce	122	Soybean oil	193	Meat & Dairy	
Green beans	47	Rapeseed oil	141	Ground beef	0.5
Peas	36	Olive oil	49	Chicken	0.1
Cucumbers	19	Safflower oil	11	Pork	<0.1
Tomatoes	6	Sunflower oil	9	Tuna	<0.1
Carrots	5	Corn oil	3	Butter	7
Cauliflower	5	Dry soybeans	47	Cheddar cheese	3
Beets	3	Dry kidney beans	19	3.5% fat milk	0.3
Onions	2	Dry navy beans	2	Skim milk	<0.1
Potatoes	0.8				
Sweet corn	0.5				

*Values are median values based on a compilation of published determinations of vitamin K by HPLC assays.
From data of Booth, S. L., Sadowsky, J. A., Weihrauch, J. L. and Ferland, G. (1993) Vitamin K_1 (phylloquinone) content of foods: A provisional table. J Food Comp Anal 6:109–210.

gators that menaquinones synthesized in the lower bowel are of nutritional importance. The total hepatic pool of menaquinones in humans is about 10 times that of phylloquinone, and this source of vitamin K appears to be at least to some extent utilizable. The high concentration in liver may reflect a slow turnover of this form of the vitamin. Limited data obtained from a rat model suggest that when a typical long-chain bacterial menaquinone, MK-9, is present in liver at concentrations similar to those of phylloquinone, it is not as effectively used as phylloquinone. The current data, therefore, suggest that menaquinones provide some, but only a minor portion of the vitamin K needed to satisfy the human requirement.

ABSORPTION, TRANSPORT, AND METABOLISM OF VITAMIN K

Dietary phylloquinone is absorbed from the gut into the lymphatic system, and any conditions that result in a general impairment of lipid absorption will also adversely influence vitamin K absorption. Following incorporation into chylomicrons in the mucosa of the duodenum and jejunum, the vitamin is secreted into the lymph and enters the liver, associated with chylomicron remnant particles. Circulating phylloquinone is found in the high density (HDL), low density (LDL), and very low density (VLDL) lipoprotein fractions, and its concentration is increased in hyperlipidemic patients. Apolipoprotein E (apo E) genotype is known to influence plasma lipoprotein clearance and has also been demonstrated to influence circulating phylloquinone concentrations. The concentration of phylloquinone in plasma is low, and good values were not available until the early 1980s. Advances in separation techniques using HPLC and development of new methods of detection of the vitamin in column effluents now have improved analysis, and reproducible measurements of both phylloquinone and menaquinones in plasma and tissues are available. Circulating phylloquinone concentrations are very dependent on recent dietary intake, and even postabsorptive values cover a wide range. Plasma phylloquinone concentrations in the normal population (Sadowski et al., 1989) appear to be about 1 nmol/L, with a range from 0.3 to 2.5 nmol/L (0.15 to 1.15 ng/mL). The plasma phylloquinone concentration of the healthy newborn is only about 0.05 nmol/L. Early studies did not detect circulating menaquinones in plasma, but more recently, measurable concentrations of some of the long-chain menaquinones, mainly MK-7 and MK-8, have been reported (Suttie, 1995).

Measurements of human liver vitamin K content also are available. Values reported have been in the range of 2 to 20 ng of phylloquinone/g of liver (Usui et al., 1990). A broad spectrum of bacterially produced long-chain menaquinones (MK-7 through MK-10) also is found in human liver, and the total concentration of menaquinones appears to be about 10-fold higher than that of phylloquinone (Suttie, 1995). Both forms of the vitamin are rapidly concentrated in liver of experimental animals following ingestion. In contrast to the other fat-soluble vitamins, which have a significant tissue storage pool, phylloquinone has a very rapid turnover in liver. The relatively high concentration of menaquinones found in human liver compared to the main dietary source of vitamin K, phylloquinone, may reflect a slower turnover of long-chain menaquinones relative to phylloquinone as has been demonstrated in animal models.

Phylloquinone predominantly is excreted in feces via the bile, but significant amounts also are excreted in the urine. Very little dietary phylloquinone is excreted unmetabolized, but the major metabolites are not well characterized. They appear to represent the stepwise oxidation of the side chain at the 3-position followed by glucuronide conjugation. The biochemical role of the vitamin as a substrate for the liver microsomal γ-glutamyl carboxylase results in the conversion of the vitamin to its 2,3-epoxide. This metabolite appears to be subject to the same general pathways of oxidative degradation as is the parent vitamin. Very limited information suggests that the pathway of degradative metabolism of menaquinones is similar to that of phylloquinone.

FUNCTION OF VITAMIN K IN THE SYNTHESIS OF SPECIFIC PROTEINS

Vitamin K is required for the posttranslational modification of a limited number of proteins during their synthesis. Vitamin K is involved as a substrate for an enzyme that converts specifically targeted glutamyl (Glu) residues to γ-carboxyglutamyl (Gla) residues in these proteins. This modification is essential for normal physiological function of these proteins. Continued function of vitamin K in this reaction is dependent on the recycling of oxidized vitamin K (vitamin K epoxide) back to the hydroquinone form (vitamin KH_2).

Vitamin K Is a Substrate for a γ-Glutamyl Carboxylase

Until the early 1970s, the classical vitamin K-dependent clotting factors were the only proteins known to require vitamin K for their activity, and studies of prothrombin production were key to the determination of the metabolic role of vitamin K. Studies in the mid-1960s using whole animals strongly suggested that vitamin K was involved in converting an inactive hepatic precursor of plasma prothrombin to biologically active prothrombin. This hypothesis was strengthened by clinical observations that an immunochemically similar, but biologically inactive, form of prothrombin was present in increased concentrations in the plasma of patients treated with anticoagulants that antagonized vitamin K action. Characterization of this "abnormal prothrombin" isolated from the plasma of cows fed the anticoagulant dicoumarol revealed that it lacked the specific calcium-binding sites present in normal prothrombin and that it did not demonstrate a calcium-dependent association with negatively charged phospholipid surfaces.

The inability of abnormal plasma prothrombin preparations to bind calcium ions (Ca^{2+}) suggested that the function of vitamin K was to modify a liver precursor of this plasma protein to facilitate calcium binding. The action of the vitamin was therefore not at the level of gene transcription, but rather after messenger RNA (mRNA) translation. Acidic peptides were obtained by proteolytic enzyme digestion of prothrombin, and they subsequently were shown to contain Gla, a previously unrecognized acidic amino acid (Stenflo et al., 1974; Nelsestuen et al., 1974). Peptides containing Gla residues could not be obtained by proteolysis of the abnormal prothrombin. All 10 of the glutamyl residues in the first 42 residues of bovine prothrombin subsequently were shown to be posttranslationally γ-carboxylated to form these effective calcium-binding groups.

The discovery of Gla residues in prothrombin led to the demonstration (Esmon et al., 1975) that crude rat liver microsomal preparations (vesicles derived from the endoplasmic reticulum [ER] when cells are disrupted) contained an enzymatic activity that promoted a vitamin K-dependent incorporation of $H^{14}CO_3^-$ into endogenous precursors of vitamin K-dependent proteins present in these preparations. Subsequent studies established that the fixed $^{14}CO_2$ was present in Gla residues. Small peptides containing adjacent Glu-Glu sequences such as Phe-Leu-Glu-Glu-Val were shown to be substrates for the enzyme activity present in detergent-solubilized microsomal preparations, and they were used to study the properties of this unique carboxylase. The rough microsomal fraction (vesicles formed from the rough ER) of liver is highly enriched in carboxylase activity, and lower but significant activity is found in smooth microsomes (vesicles formed from the smooth ER). Mitochondria, nuclei, and cytosol have negligible vitamin K-dependent carboxylase activity. The available data are consistent with the hypothesis that the carboxylation event occurs on the luminal side of the rough endoplasmic reticulum.

The vitamin K-dependent carboxylation reaction does not require adenosine triphosphate (ATP), and the available data are consistent with the view that the energy to drive this carboxylation reaction is derived from the oxidation of the reduced form of vitamin K by O_2 to form vitamin K-2,3-epoxide (Fig. 24–2). The lack of a biotin requirement, and studies of the CO_2/HCO_3^- requirement indicate that carbon dioxide rather than HCO_3^- is the active species in the carboxylation reaction. (See Chapter 22 for the role of biotinyl-enzymes in carboxylation reactions.) Studies of substrate specificity at the vitamin K-binding site of the enzyme have shown that the only important structural features of this substrate are a 2-methyl-1,4-naphthoquinone substituted at the 3-position with a rather hydrophobic group. The 2-ethyl and des-methyl analogs of the vitamin have little activity, and methyl substitution of the benzenoid ring has

little effect or decreases substrate binding. Synthesis and assay of a large number of low molecular weight peptide substrates of the enzyme have failed to reveal any unique sequences surrounding the Glu residue that are needed as a signal for carboxylation. In general, peptides with Glu-Glu sequences are better substrates than those with single Glu residues.

Early studies of the mechanism of action of the carboxylation reaction indicated that the mechanistic role of vitamin K was to abstract the hydrogen on the γ-carbon of the glutamyl residue to allow attack of CO_2 at this position. This was established by using substrates tritiated at the γ-carbon of each Glu residue to demonstrate that the enzyme catalyzed a vitamin KH_2-dependent and O_2-dependent, but CO_2-independent release of tritium from the substrate. At saturating concentrations of CO_2, there is an apparent equivalent stoichiometry between vitamin K-2,3-epoxide formation and Gla formation. At lower CO_2 concentrations, a large excess of vitamin K epoxide is produced. The degree to which these two reactions are coupled in routine incubations is therefore strongly dependent on incubation conditions.

How epoxide formation is coupled to γ-hydrogen abstraction has been an important mechanistic question. One possibility would be through the action of an oxygenated intermediate that would also be a logical intermediate on the pathway to epoxide formation (Fig. 24–2). Hydrogen abstraction is known to be stereospecific, and it is the pro S hydrogen at the γ-position of the Glu residue that is removed. The fate of the activated Glu residue in the absence of CO_2 has been shown to be protonation rather than formation of an adduct with some other component of the incubation that would result in an altered Glu residue. The enzyme has been shown to catalyze a vitamin KH_2- and oxygen-dependent exchange of ^3H from ^3H_2O into the γ-position of a Glu residue, and this exchange reaction is decreased as the concentration of HCO_3^- in the media is increased. There is a close association between epoxide formation, Gla formation, and γ-C-H bond cleavage. The efficiency of the carboxylation reaction, defined as the ratio of Gla residues formed to γ-C-H bonds

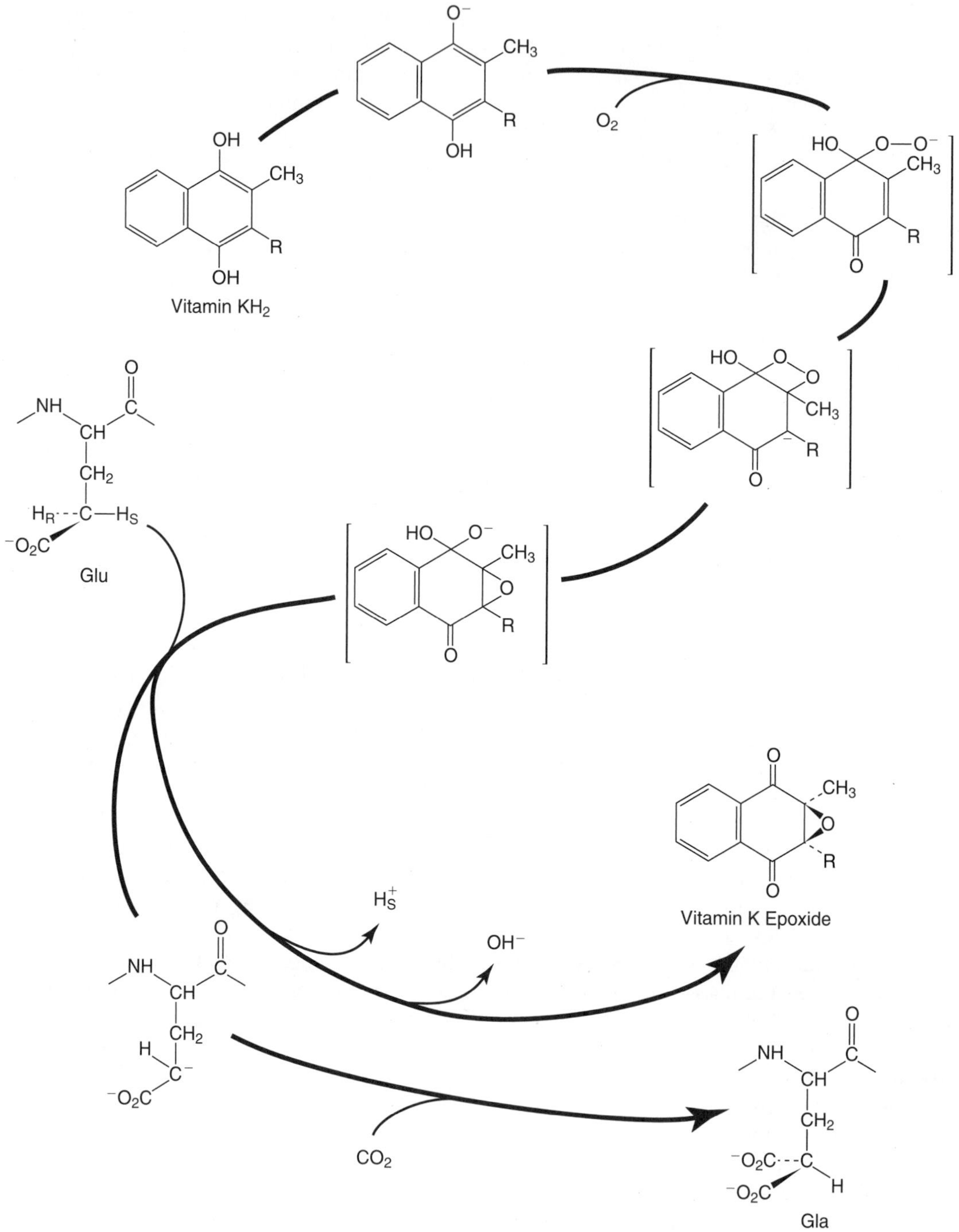

Figure 24–2. The vitamin K-dependent γ-glutamyl carboxylase. The available data support an interaction of O_2 with vitamin KH_2, the reduced (hydronaphthoquinone) form of vitamin K, to form an oxygenated intermediate that is sufficiently basic to abstract the γ-hydrogen of the glutamyl residue (Glu). The products of this reaction are vitamin K-2,3-epoxide and a glutamyl carbanion. Attack of CO_2 on the carbanion leads to the formation of a γ-carboxyglutamyl residue (Gla). The bracketed peroxy, dioxetane, and alkoxide intermediates have not been identified in the enzyme-catalyzed reaction but are postulated based on model organic reactions.

cleaved, is independent of Glu substrate concentration, and the data suggest that this ratio approaches unity at high CO_2 concentrations.

A major gap in an understanding of the mechanism of action of this enzyme has been the assumption that abstraction of a hydrogen from the γ-carbon of glutamic acid would require a strong base (presumably formed from the vitamin), and the lack of evidence for such an intermediate. More recent data (Dowd et al., 1991) have suggested that an initial attack of O_2 at the naphthoquinone carbonyl carbon adjacent to the methyl group results in the formation of a dioxetane ring that generates an alkoxide intermediate. This intermediate is hypothesized to be the strong base that abstracts the γ-methylene hydrogen and leaves a carbanion that can interact with CO_2 (Fig. 24–2). This pathway leads to the possibility that a second atom of molecular oxygen can be incorporated into the carbonyl group of the epoxide product; this activity can be followed by utilization of $^{18}O_2$ in the reaction. This partial dioxygenase activity has been verified by other investigators; although this general scheme is consistent with all of the available data, the mechanism remains a hypothesis at this time.

The physiological role of the vitamin K-dependent carboxylase poses an interesting question in terms of enzyme-substrate recognition. This microsomal enzyme recognizes a small fraction of the total hepatic secretory protein pool and then carboxylates 9 to 12 Glu sites in the first 45 *N*-terminal residues of the vitamin K-dependent plasma proteins. Cloning of these proteins has revealed that the primary gene products contain a very homologous domain between the amino terminus of the mature protein and the signal sequence that targets the polypeptide for the secretory pathway. This "propeptide" region appears to be both a "docking" or "recognition" site for the enzyme and a modulator of the activity of the enzyme by decreasing the apparent K_m of the Glu site substrate. The propeptide domain is undoubtedly of major importance in directing the efficient carboxylation of the multiple Glu sites in these substrates, but it is not known if the enzyme starts at one end of the Gla region and sequentially carboxylates all Glu sites or if the enzyme

carboxylates randomly within this region. Interference with an adequate amount of vitamin K by anticoagulant therapy results in the production of a complex mixture of partially carboxylated forms of prothrombin, and the available data suggest that the most amino-terminal potential Gla residue of these under-γ-carboxylated forms is preferentially carboxylated. This may not be a universal property, as the enzyme preferentially carboxylates the most carboxy-terminal potential Gla site when the des-γ-carboxyl form of a vitamin K-dependent protein in bone is used as an in vitro substrate.

Significant progress toward a detailed understanding of the properties of the enzyme have been limited by the lack of a pure enzyme. An enzyme preparation that has 500 to 1000 times the specific activity of microsomes and can be routinely prepared in 2 days has been available for a number of years. Although this preparation was useful in studying properties of the enzyme, progress in purification to homogeneity was slow. In the early 1990s, two different microsomal proteins, one of 94 kDa and one of 98 kDa, were purified and claimed to be the carboxylase. Using a baculovirus expression system, the 94-kDa protein was expressed in an insect cell line that lacks any endogenous carboxylase activity. The demonstration that microsomal preparations from the transfected insect cells exhibited vitamin K-dependent carboxylase activity established that the 94-kDa protein was the enzyme of interest. (Wu et al., 1991) The role of the 98-kDa protein in the overall carboxylase mechanism, if any, is not known.

Cycling of Vitamin K Between Various Oxidation States

The reactions shown in Figure 24–3 summarize the known major metabolic transformation of vitamin K in rat liver microsomes and point out that three forms of vitamin K [the quinone (K), the hydronaphthoquinone (KH_2), and the 2,3-epoxide (KO)] can feed into a liver vitamin K cycle. The quinone and hydronaphthoquinone forms of the vitamin are interconverted by a number of NAD(P)H-linked reductases, including one that appears to be a microsomal-bound form of the exten-

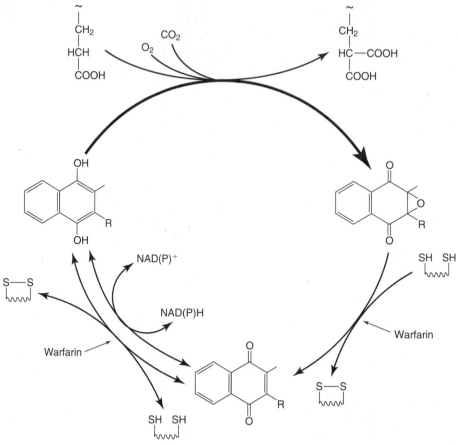

Figure 24–3. *Vitamin K metabolism in rat liver microsomes. Vitamin K epoxide formed in the carboxylation reaction is reduced by a warfarin-sensitive pathway "vitamin K epoxide reductase" that is driven by a reduced dithiol. The quinone form of the vitamin can be reduced to the hydroquinone either by a warfarin-sensitive, dithiol-driven quinone reductase or by one or more of the hepatic NADH or NADPH-linked quinone reductases, which are less sensitive to warfarin.*

sively studied liver NAD(P)H:quinone acceptor oxidoreductase (DT-diaphorase) activity. The quinone form of the vitamin can also be reduced by a dithiol-dependent reductase. Vitamin KH_2 serves as a substrate for the microsomal γ-glutamyl carboxylase/epoxidase that converts the vitamin to its 2,3-epoxide and carboxylates glutamyl to γ-carboxyglutamyl residues. Vitamin K-2,3-epoxide had been shown (Matschiner et al., 1970) to be a major liver metabolite of vitamin K before it was known to be a product of the carboxylase, and it is the substrate for another microsomal enzyme, the 2,3-epoxide reductase. This enzyme uses a sulfhydryl compound as a reductant in vitro, but the physiological reductant has not been identified. In normal liver, the

ratio of vitamin K-2,3-epoxide to the less oxidized forms of the vitamin is about 1:10. Current analytical methods are not capable of distinguishing between the amount of quinone and hydronaphthoquinone form of the vitamin in tissues.

Antagonism of Vitamin K Action by Various Inhibitors

The vitamin K analog 2-chloro-3-phytyl-1,4-naphthoquinone (chloro-K) is an effective inhibitor of the γ-glutamyl carboxylase, and the reduced form of this analog has been shown to be competitive versus the reduced vitamin K site (Fig. 24–4). This compound also has been shown to be an in vivo antagonist, and

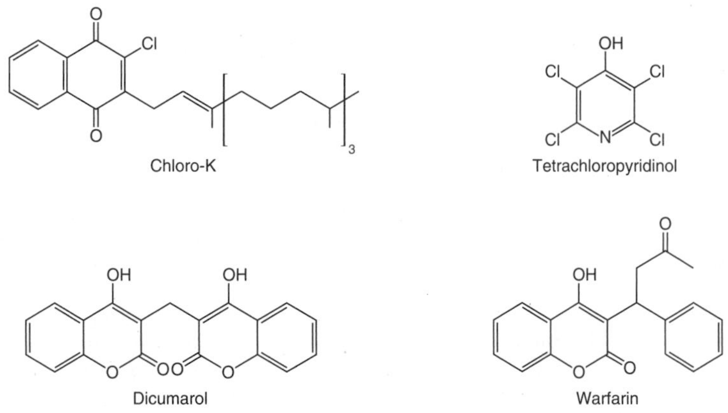

Figure 24–4. *Vitamin K antagonists. Chloro-K and tetrachloropyridinol are inhibitors of the vitamin K-dependent γ-glutamyl carboxylase. The 4-hydroxycoumarins, dicoumarol and warfarin, do not inhibit the carboxylase enzyme, but prevent the recycling of vitamin K-epoxide to the enzymatically active form of the vitamin.*

chloro-K administration results in a hemorrhagic condition. Substitution of a trifluoromethyl group, a hydroxymethyl group, or a methoxymethyl group for the 2-methyl group of vitamin K also results in analogs that are inhibitory compounds. Some compounds not structurally related to vitamin K are also vitamin K antagonists, and tetrachloropyridinol and other polychlorinated phenols have been shown to be strong inhibitors of γ-glutamyl carboxylase.

The most widely used antagonists of vitamin K are the 4-hydroxycoumarins. Dicoumarol (3,3′-methylene bis-[4-hydroxycoumarin]) originally was isolated from moldy sweet clover as the factor responsible for a hemorrhagic disease of cattle that was common in the American Midwest in the early 1930s. A large number of compounds based on this structure have been synthesized, and the most widely used is warfarin (3-[α-acetonylbenzyl]-4-hydroxycoumarin). These compounds are "indirect" vitamin K antagonists in that they do not inhibit the carboxylase (Hildebrandt and Suttie, 1982), but rather block the reduced dithiol conversion of vitamin K-2,3-epoxide to the reduced form of vitamin K (Fig. 24–3). Their use, therefore, creates an acquired deficiency of vitamin K at the active site of the carboxylase and subsequently decreases the synthesis of the vitamin K-dependent plasma clotting factors. Warfarin has been used widely as a rodenticide and is also a very commonly prescribed drug used to treat patients who are at risk of thrombotic events.

PHYSIOLOGICAL ROLES OF VITAMIN K-DEPENDENT PROTEINS

Proteins that depend on vitamin K for their biological activity contain Gla residues and are present in a number of tissues. The most studied and best understood of these are the vitamin K-dependent plasma proteins involved in blood clotting, which are synthesized in the liver.

Proteins Involved in Hemostasis

Prothrombin, also called clotting factor II, is the circulating zymogen of the procoagulant thrombin, and was one of the first plasma proteins isolated. Early investigators demonstrated that prothrombin activity was decreased in plasma obtained from vitamin K-deficient animals. Plasma clotting factors VII, IX, and X (Fig. 24–5) all initially were identified because their activity was decreased in the plasma of a patient with a hereditary bleeding disorder. They subsequently were shown to depend on vitamin K for their synthesis and later shown to contain Gla residues.

The amino-terminal regions (Gla domain) of these proteins are very homologous, and the Gla residues are in essentially the same position as in prothrombin (Fig. 24–6) in all of the vitamin K-dependent clotting factors. Two more Gla-containing plasma proteins with similar homology, protein C and protein S, are involved in a thrombin-initiated inactivation of factor V. They therefore play an anticoagulant rather than a procoagulant role in normal

CLINICAL CORRELATION

Warfarin—Rat Poison and an Effective Clinical Drug

Following discovery of dicoumarol and the synthesis of a large number of analogs, the initial use of these vitamin K antagonists was as a rodenticide. Rats and other rodents can be killed by a large number of toxic agents, but they rapidly become "bait shy." That is, if they ingest a nonlethal dose of a poison, they will refuse to eat bait containing that compound in the future. The turnover time of the circulating vitamin K-dependent clotting factors in plasma is such that they are present at a level that will prevent hemorrhage for 2 or 3 days after their synthesis has been blocked by warfarin ingestion. During this period, the rats continue to eat the poisoned bait and eventually die of internal hemorrhage. These are, therefore, very effective rodenticides. As might be expected, the widespread use of rodenticides containing warfarin has led to the selection of mutant strains that are resistant to this toxic agent. These warfarin-resistant "super rats" are, however, susceptible to other 4-hydroxycoumarins, and the rat poisons commonly available at the present time contain these compounds as the active anticoagulant.

Much lower doses of 4-hydroxycoumarins will not result in hemorrhage but will decrease the rate at which blood clots, and they are prescribed widely as antithrombotic drugs. The oral anticoagulant used in the United States is warfarin, but some of the other 4-hydroxycoumarins, which have somewhat different pharmacokinetic properties, are used widely in other countries. They are used to treat patients who have been diagnosed with deep vein thrombosis, pulmonary embolism, and myocardial infarction in order to prevent the recurrence of thrombosis. They also are given to patients following the insertion of prosthetic heart valves in order to prevent systemic arterial embolism.

There is a rather wide variation in warfarin sensitivity from one patient to another, and the appropriate dose for each individual must be determined by careful monitoring of the "prothrombin time" as the dose is gradually increased to the therapeutic level. Plasma is obtained from blood treated with a Ca^{2+} chelator to prevent coagulation. This test measures the time it takes for the plasma to clot after it has been recalcified and clotting has been initiated by the addition of a crude tissue factor and phospholipid preparation.

Oral anticoagulants such as warfarin are only one of the antithrombotic drugs currently available. Platelet activation plays a key role in the initiation of thrombus formation, and common aspirin is effective as an antithrombotic agent because of its ability to prevent platelet activation. Aspirin has no influence on the formation of fibrin clots mediated by the action of the vitamin K-dependent clotting factors. A third antithrombotic agent, heparin, does block clot formation by interfering with the generation of thrombin. This sulfated polysaccharide activates plasma antithrombin, which then inactivates thrombin and other serine proteases derived from their vitamin K-dependent protein zymogens.

hemostasis. Another Gla-containing plasma protein (protein Z) has been described, but its function is not yet known. All of these proteins play a critical role in hemostasis; because of this, they have been extensively studied, and the complementary DNA (cDNA) and genomic organization of each of them is well documented.

The complex system of blood coagulation (Davie et al., 1991) traditionally is divided into an extrinsic pathway, which involves a tissue factor in addition to blood components, and an intrinsic pathway, which involves components present only in blood. Tissue factor in association with factor VII_a can activate both factor X to X_a and factor IX to IX_a.

The details of the action of the vitamin K-dependent clotting factors are most clearly understood in the case of the "prothrombinase complex." Tissue injury exposes membrane phospholipids, and prothrombin associates with negatively charged phospholipids in a Ca^{2+}-dependent manner that requires the Gla residues. Factor X_a and factor V_a also associate with this complex, and the active serine protease, factor X_a, cleaves prothrombin at two po-

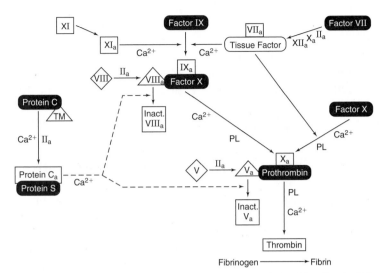

Figure 24–5. Involvement of vitamin K-dependent clotting factors in coagulation. The vitamin K-dependent procoagulants (prothrombin, factor VII, factor IX, and factor X) circulate as zymogens of serine proteases until converted to their active (subscript a) forms. The product of the activation of one factor can activate a second zymogen, and this cascade effect results in the rapid activation of prothrombin to thrombin and the subsequent conversion of soluble fibrinogen to the insoluble fibrin clot. Some of the steps in this activation involve an active protease, a second protein substrate, and a protein cofactor (triangles) to form a Ca^{2+}-mediated association with a phospholipid surface. The other two vitamin K-dependent proteins participate in hemostatic control as anticoagulants, not procoagulants. Protein C is activated by thrombin (II_a) in the presence of an endothelial cell protein called thrombomodulin (TM). Activated protein C functions in a complex with protein S to inactivate factors V_a and VIII_a and to limit clot formation.

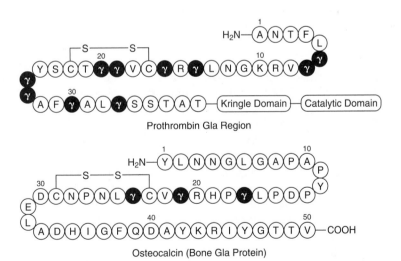

Figure 24–6. Distribution of Gla residues in the Gla domain of prothrombin, and in osteocalcin. All of the 10 Gla residues (closed circles) are located in the first 37 residues, which make up the amino-terminal Gla domain of prothrombin. The remainder of this 71.6-kDa protein does not contain any Gla residues and is composed of the catalytic domain, which generates the serine protease thrombin after activation, and a kringle domain (a sequence that folds into loops stabilized by disulfide bonds). This kringle domain is not found in the other vitamin K-dependent clotting factors, but is found in plasmin, the plasma protein involved in clot lysis. There is little homology between the Gla domain of the plasma vitamin K-dependent clotting factors and the Gla region of the low molecular weight protein osteocalcin.

sitions to form the two chains of thrombin that are attached by a disulfide bond. In a vitamin K deficiency, prothrombin is secreted into the plasma lacking some or all of the Gla residues, and this protein will not form the Ca^{2+}-dependent interaction with negatively charged phospholipids that is essential for rapid thrombin generation and clot formation.

Proteins Found in Bone and Other Tissues

The first vitamin K-dependent protein discovered that was not located in plasma was isolated from bone and contained three Gla residues. It is the second most abundant protein in bone and is called osteocalcin or bone Gla protein (BGP). There is little structural homology (Fig. 24–6) between this protein and the vitamin K-dependent plasma proteins. The demonstration that the level of this osteocalcin in plasma is altered in some metabolic bone diseases has opened possible clinical implications, and often it is measured as a diagnostic tool (Price, 1988). A second protein first isolated from bone (matrix Gla protein) is structurally related to osteocalcin but also is present in other tissues. Like osteocalcin, details of its physiological role are unclear, but both proteins appear to be involved in some manner in the control of tissue mineralization or skeletal turnover. Recent studies with "gene knockout" mice (Ducy et al., 1996; Luo et al., 1997) demonstrated that lack of osteocalcin leads to increased bone formation and that lack of matrix Gla protein results in arterial calcification. The metabolic alterations responsible for these observations are not yet known.

The vitamin K-dependent carboxylase activity is present in most tissues, and a reasonably large number of proteins are subjected to this posttranslational modification. Proteins have been isolated from calcified aorta that seem to be related to, but are different from, osteocalcin, and a vitamin K-dependent protein is present in kidney. Proteins containing Gla residues have been reported in liver mitochondria and in sperm, and more recently vitamin K-dependent cellular proteins with growth factor activity or potential membrane

localization (Kulman et al., 1997) have been identified. Other than the well-established role of the plasma clotting factors, the physiological role of these proteins has not yet been established. The vitamin K-dependent formation of Gla is old on an evolutionary scale, and some sea snails have Gla peptides that are used as potent neurotoxins.

VITAMIN K DEFICIENCY

Although a primary vitamin K deficiency is uncommon in the adult human population, a vitamin K-responsive hemorrhagic disease of the newborn is a rare but long-recognized syndrome. Vitamin K stores of the newborn are low because of poor placental transfer of the vitamin, and the sterile gut precludes any possible production and utilization of menaquinones during early life. These conditions are complicated by a general hypoprothrombinemia in infants caused by the inability of immature liver to synthesize normal levels of clotting factors. The breast-fed infant is at particular risk. The vitamin K content of breast milk is less than that of cow's milk, and a low intake of milk by nursing infants has been shown to be a strong contributing factor in the development of vitamin K deficiency in the newborn. Commercial infant formulas are now routinely supplemented with vitamin K, and the American Academy of Pediatrics (1993) has recommended intramuscular administration of phylloquinone at birth as routine prophylaxis. The practice of oral or intramuscular administration of vitamin K to the newborn is almost universal in developed countries, but hemorrhagic disease remains a potential problem for breast-fed infants in some areas of the world.

The most common condition known to result in a vitamin K-responsive hemorrhagic event in the adult is a low dietary intake of vitamin K by a patient who also is receiving antibiotics. These cases are numerous, which suggests that patients with restricted food intake who also are receiving antibiotics should be closely observed for signs of vitamin K deficiency. These episodes historically have been attributed to an interference of antibiot-

Food Sources of Phylloquinone

- Green leafy vegetables (kale, turnip greens, spinach, broccoli, cabbage, and lettuce)
- Other vegetables and fruits (green beans, peas, and avocados)

RDAs Across the Life Cycle

	µg phylloquinone/day
Infants, 0–0.5 yr	5
0.5–1.0 yr	10
Children, 1–3 yr	15
4–6 yr	20
7–10 yr	30
11–14 yr	45
Males, 15–18 yr	65
19–24 yr	70
25+ yr	80
Females, 15–18 yr	55
19–24 yr	60
25+ yr	65
Pregnant	65
Lactating	65

From National Research Council. (1989) Recommended Dietary Allowances, 10th ed. National Academy Press, Washington, D.C.

ics with the microbial synthesis of menaquinones in the gut, but evidence to substantiate this effect is lacking.

Vitamin K deficiency also has been reported in patients subjected to long-term total parenteral nutrition, and supplementation of the vitamin is advised under these circumstances. Supplementation in the case of biliary obstruction also is advisable, because the impairment of lipid absorption resulting from the lack of bile salts also adversely affects vitamin K absorption. Depression of the vitamin K-dependent coagulation factors frequently has been found in malabsorption syndromes and in other gastrointestinal disorders (e.g., cystic fibrosis, sprue, celiac disease, ulcerative colitis, regional ileitis, Ascaris infection, and short-bowel syndrome) and usually has been observed to respond to vitamin administration.

ASSESSMENT OF VITAMIN K STATUS

Recent advances in methodology have made it possible to routinely measure the plasma or serum phylloquinone concentration, but the factors influencing these concentrations and their relationship to dietary intake have not yet been clarified. Alteration of plasma phylloquinone by dietary restriction of the vitamin now has been reported in a number of studies, and plasma phylloquinone has been reported to be low in a debilitated patient population. However, because of the close relationship of plasma phylloquinone to recent dietary intake, these measurements lack utility for assessing vitamin K status. The clinical "prothrombin time," which is a measure of the rate of thrombin generation in a small sample of plasma, historically has been used to assess the activities of the vitamin K-dependent clotting factors. A major problem in determining a dietary requirement for vitamin K has been the relative insensitivity of the commonly used prothrombin time as a measure of the activity of the vitamin K-dependent plasma proteins.

Assessment of vitamin K status by use of the relatively insensitive clinical prothrombin time has meant that a rather large decrease in vitamin K-dependent clotting factor synthesis was needed to produce an apparent deficiency. More sensitive clotting assays and the ability to immunochemically detect circulating forms of prothrombin that lack some or all of the normal content of Gla residues provide an opportunity to monitor much milder forms of vitamin K deficiency. Recent studies modifying the vitamin K intake of young adults by restriction of foods with a high phylloquinone content have shown that increased concentrations of under-γ-carboxylated prothrombin in plasma and decreased urinary Gla excretion were sensitive criteria of sufficiency. There are a number of reports that vitamin K status may be important in maintaining skeletal health, and in recent studies the extent of under-γ-carboxylation of circulating osteocalcin has been shown to be a very sensitive criterion of vitamin K sufficiency. It is likely that this method will become increasingly important in future studies defining vitamin K status.

RECOMMENDATIONS FOR VITAMIN K INTAKE

The low dietary requirement and the relatively high levels of vitamin K found in most diets prevented an accurate quantitation of the human vitamin K requirement until recent years. In an early study, starved, intravenously fed, debilitated patients were given antibiotics to decrease intestinal vitamin K synthesis, and it was found that daily administration of 1.5 μg/ kg was sufficient to prevent any decreases in the activity of vitamin K-dependent clotting factors. More recent studies, again with limited numbers of subjects, also have suggested that the vitamin K requirement of humans is in the range of 0.5 to 1.0 μg per kilogram per day.

Based on these data, the 10th edition of the Recommended Dietary Allowances (RDA) (National Research Council, 1989) was the first to include an RDA for vitamin K. The intake recommended was 1 μg phylloquinone/kg body weight for adults. An intake of 5 μg of phylloquinone/day for infants during the first 6 months and 10 μg/day from 6 to 12 months was also recommended. In the absence of any specific information about a

unique vitamin K requirement for children, the 1 μg/kg basis used for adults also was applied to children.

REFERENCES

American Academy of Pediatrics. (1993) Controversies concerning vitamin K and the newborn. Pediatrics 91:1001–1003.

Booth, S. L., Sadowski, J. A., Weihrauch, J. L. and Ferland, G. (1993) Vitamin K₁ (phylloquinone) content of foods: A provisional table. J Food Comp Anal 6:109–210.

Booth, S. L., Pennington, J. A. T., and Sadowski, J. A. (1996) Food sources and dietary intakes of vitamin K-1 (phylloquinone) in the American diet: Data from the FDA total diet study. J Am Diet Assoc 96:149–154.

Dam, H. (1934) Haemorrhages in chicks reared on artificial diets: A new deficiency disease. Nature 133:909–910.

Davie, E. W., Fujikawa, K. and Kisiel, W. (1991) The coagulation cascade: Initiation, maintenance, and regulation. Biochemistry 30:10363–10370.

Dowd, P., Ham, S. W. and Geib, S. J. (1991) Mechanism of action of vitamin K. J Am Chem Soc 113:7734–7743.

Ducy, P., Desbois, C., Boyce, B., Pinero, G., Story, B., Dunstan, C., Smith, E., Bonadio, J., Goldstein, S., Gundberg, C., Bradley, A. and Karsenty, G. (1996) Increased bone formation in osteocalcin-deficient mice. Nature 382:448–452.

Esmon, C. T., Sadowski, J. A. and Suttie, J. W. (1975) A new carboxylation reaction: The vitamin K-dependent incorporation of H¹⁴CO₃⁻ into prothrombin. J Biol Chem 250:4744–4748.

Hildebrandt, E. F. and Suttie, J. W. (1982) Mechanism of coumarin action: Sensitivity of vitamin K metabolizing enzymes of normal and warfarin-resistant rat liver. Biochemistry 21:2406–2411.

Kulman, J. D., Harris, J. E., Haldeman, B. A. and Davie, E. W. (1997) Primary structure and tissue distribution of two novel proline-rich γ-carboxyglutamic acid proteins. Proc Natl Acad Sci USA 94:9058–9062.

Luo, G., Ducy, P., McKee, M. D., Pinero, G. J., Loyer, E., Behringer, R. R. and Karsenty, G. (1997) Spontaneous calcification of arteries and cartilage in mice lacking matrix Gla protein. Nature 386:78–81.

Matschiner, J. T., Bell, R. G., Amelotti, J. M. and Knauer, T. E. (1970) Isolation and characterization of a new metabolite of phylloquinone in the rat. Biochim Biophys Acta 201:309–315.

National Research Council (1989) Recommended Dietary Allowances, 10th ed. National Academy Press, Washington, D.C.

Nelsestuen, G. L., Zytkovicz, T. H. and Howard, J. B. (1974) The mode of action of vitamin K: Identification of γ-carboxyglutamic acid as a component of prothrombin. J Biol Chem 249:6347–6350.

Price, P. A. (1988) Role of vitamin K-dependent proteins in bone metabolism. Annu Rev Nutr 8:565–583.

Sadowski, J. A., Hood, S. J., Dallal, G. E. and Garry, P. J. (1989) Phylloquinone in plasma from elderly and young adults: Factors influencing its concentration. Am J Clin Nutr 50:100–108.

Stenflo, J., Fernlund, P., Egan, W. and Roepstorff, P. (1974) Vitamin K dependent modifications of glutamic acid residues in prothrombin. Proc Natl Acad Sci USA 71:2730–2733.

Suttie, J. W. (1995) The importance of menaquinones in human nutrition. Annu Rev Nutr 15:399–417.

Usui, Y., Tanimura, H., Nishimura, N., Kobayashi, N., Okanoue, T. and Ozawa, K. (1990) Vitamin K concentrations in the plasma and liver of surgical patients. Am J Clin Nutr 51:846–852.

Wu, S-M., Morris, D. P. and Stafford, D. W. (1991) Identification and purification to near homogeneity of the vitamin K-dependent carboxylase. Proc Natl Acad Sci USA 88:2236–2240.

RECOMMENDED READINGS

Dowd, P., Ham, S-W., Naganathan, S. and Hershline, R. (1995) The mechanism of action of vitamin K. Annu Rev Nutr 15:419–440.

Link, K. P. (1959) The discovery of dicumarol and its sequels. Circulation 19:97–107.

Suttie, J. W. (1992) Vitamin K and human nutrition. J Am Diet Assoc 92:585–590.

CHAPTER 25

◆ ◆

Vitamin E

Ching K. Chow, Ph.D.

OUTLINE

NOMENCLATURE AND STRUCTURE OF VITAMIN E

Vitamin E was discovered over 70 years ago as a lipid-soluble substance necessary for the prevention of fetal death and resorption in rats that had been fed a rancid lard diet (Evans and Bishop, 1922). Vitamin E is the collective term for all tocopherols and tocotrienols and their derivatives that qualitatively exhibit the biological activity of RRR-α-tocopherol. The term tocopherol is the generic description for all mono-, di-, and trimethyl tocopherols and tocotrienols, and it is not synonymous with the term vitamin E. Four tocopherols and four tocotrienols occur naturally; these differ in the number and position of methyl groups on the chromanol ring (Fig. 25–1). Both the

tocopherols and tocotrienols consist of a chromanol head and a phytyl tail. The structure of a tocotrienol is similar to that of a tocopherol, except the side chain or phytyl tail of a tocotrienol contains double bonds at the 3′, 7′, and 11′ positions. "Tocopherol" is derived from the Greek words *tokos* (childbirth), *phero* (to bring forth), and *ol* (alcohol), and relates to the role of vitamin E in reproduction in animals.

In addition to the naturally occurring isomers, several types of synthetic vitamin E, either in free or ester forms, are available commercially. The tocopherol molecule has three chiral centers in its phytyl tail, making a total of eight stereoisomeric forms possible. The naturally occurring isomer of α-tocopherol (formerly known as d-α-tocopherol) is the 2R,

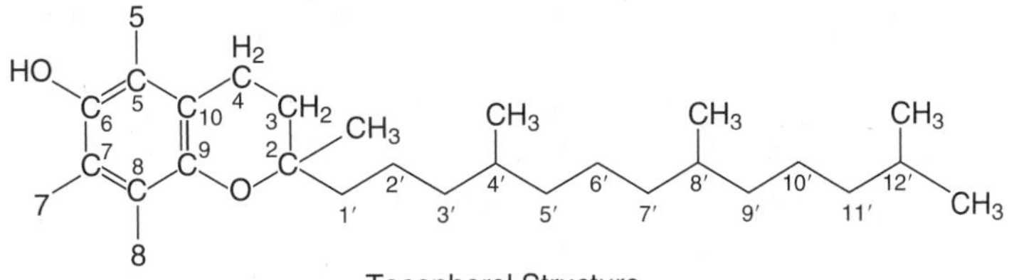

Tocopherol Structure

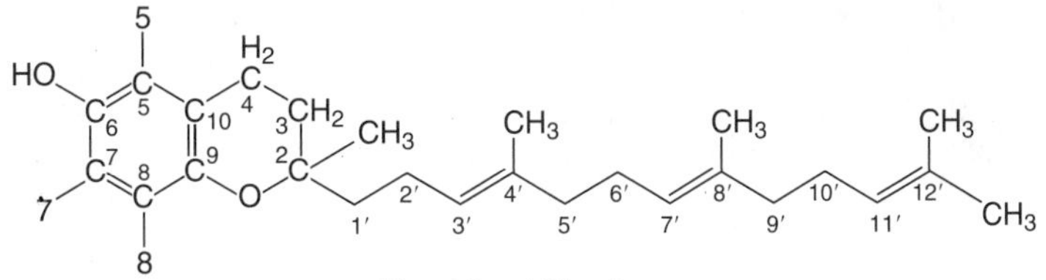

Tocotrienol Structure

Position of Methyls	Tocopherol Structure	Tocotrienol Structure
5,7,8	α-Tocopherol (α-T)	α-Tocotrienol (α-T-3)
5,8	β-Tocopherol (β-T)	β-Tocotrienol (β-T-3)
7,8	γ-Tocopherol (γ-T)	γ-Tocotrienol (γ-T-3)
8	δ-Tocopherol (δ-T)	δ-Tocotrienol (δ-T-3)

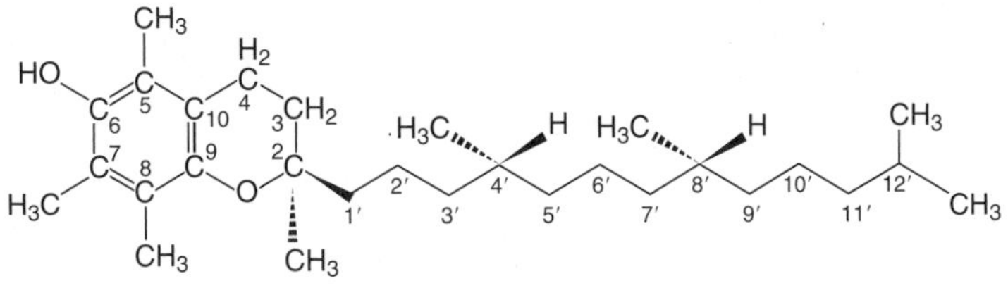

Figure 25–1. Structural formulas of tocopherols and tocotrienols.

2R, 4′R, 8′R-α-Tocopherol

4'R, 8'R isomer, whereas synthetic α-tocopherol consists of a mixture of the eight possible stereoisomers. The tetrahedral arrangement of substituents around each asymmetric center is designated R (from the Latin rectus, meaning right) or S (from the Latin sinister, meaning left). To distinguish the naturally occurring stereoisomer of α-tocopherol from the synthetic mixture, naturally occurring α-tocopherol is designated as RRR-α-tocopherol, and the synthetic mixture of α-tocopherol stereoisomers (previously known as dl-α-tocopherol) is designated as all-racemic (all-rac)-α-tocopherol. Although naturally occurring tocopherols in foods exist primarily as the free or unesterified forms, the ester forms (e.g., α-tocopheryl acetate and α-tocopheryl succinate) of vitamin E are less susceptible to oxidation and are therefore more suitable for food fortification or pharmaceutical applications than the free forms. Esters of tocopherol involve ester linkages between the carboxylate group of a fatty acid or carboxylic acid (i.e., acetate or succinate) and the 6-hydroxyl group on the phenolic ring of the tocopherol.

ABSORPTION, TRANSPORT, AND METABOLISM OF VITAMIN E

The transport and metabolism of vitamin E, like that of many other hydrophobic compounds, follows to some extent the paths of dietary lipid absorption and transport. Vitamin E is absorbed with lipids, incorporated into chylomicrons, and eventually is incorporated into and carried by other circulating lipoproteins. The major route for excretion of vitamin E and its metabolites is biliary and urinary excretion.

Absorption

The process of intestinal absorption of vitamin E is similar to that of lipid components of the diet. Tocopheryl ester, when present, first is hydrolyzed to free tocopherol in the small intestinal lumen. Hydrolysis presumably is catalyzed by pancreatic esterases. Free tocopherol is absorbed, as a part of micelles, by a passive diffusion process from the lumen of the small intestine into the enterocyte. The absorption process is not carrier–mediated and does not require energy. Within the enterocyte, tocopherol is incorporated, along with other lipids, into chylomicrons. The chylomicrons are secreted into the intercellular space, from which they enter the lymphatics and, eventually, the blood stream. The efficacy of tocopherol absorption varies considerably. Generally, the rate of absorption decreases as the amount of tocopherol consumed increases.

In humans, the majority of α-tocopherol taken up by enterocytes enters lymph in chylomicrons, but a small portion of α-tocopherol may enter the blood and be carried to the liver by the portal vein. The absorption of tocopherols other than the α-form is not as well understood. However, there are no major differences in the rates of intestinal absorption of α- and non–α-tocopherols, and an excess of the α-form does not reduce the absorption of non–α-tocopherols (Kayden and Traber, 1993).

Transport and Tissue Uptake

Because of its hydrophobicity, vitamin E requires special transport mechanisms in the aqueous milieu of the body. As described, tocopherols absorbed in the small intestine are incorporated into triacylglycerol-rich chylomicrons, secreted into the intestinal lymph, and eventually delivered to the liver in the chylomicron remnants. Vitamin E taken up by the liver either is stored in the parenchymal cells, incorporated into nascent very low density lipoproteins (VLDL) and secreted into the blood stream, or excreted via the bile.

The mechanisms involved in the uptake of tocopherols by tissues remain unclear. Portions of the vitamin E in association with chylomicrons and VLDL may be transferred to peripheral cells and high density lipoproteins (HDL) during lipolysis by lipoprotein lipase. Lipoprotein lipase bound to the surface of the endothelial lining of capillary walls catabolizes the triacylglycerols in the core of chylomicrons or VLDL and forms chylomicron remnants or low density lipoproteins (LDL). Chylomicron remnants are taken up by the parenchymal cells in the liver via an apo E-mediated mechanism, and LDL are taken up by liver and other tissues via an apo B-100–mediated process. Some free vitamin E is also taken up, along with the free fatty acids, by peripheral tissues during catabolism of lipoproteins by lipoprotein lipase. Recent studies of vitamin E delivery to tissues in transgenic mice overexpressing human lipoprotein lipase in muscle demonstrated enhanced vitamin E uptake by skeletal muscle but not by adipose tissue or brain (Sattler et al., 1996). (See Chapter 14 and Figure 14–1 for an overview of lipoprotein metabolism.)

Plasma Concentration

The secretory pathway via nascent VLDL from liver is critical in maintaining tocopherol concentrations in plasma. During the conversion of VLDL to LDL in the circulation, a portion of tocopherol remains in LDL. As exchange of tocopherol occurs between LDL and HDL, the tocopherol is distributed in all lipoproteins. In humans, the highest concentration of tocopherol is found in LDL and HDL. Tocopherol also is readily exchanged between plasma and red blood cells. Although there is no specific plasma carrier protein for vitamin E, a phospholipid transfer protein that accelerates exchange/transfer of α-tocopherol between lipoproteins and cells is found in human plasma (Kostner et al., 1995). This protein may play a role in determining the concentration of tocopherols present in the circulation and tissues.

Normal plasma vitamin E concentrations in humans range from 11 to 37 μmol α-tocopherol/L (5 to 16 mg/L), 1.6 to 5.4 mmol α-tocopherol/mol lipid (0.8 to 2.7 mg/g) or 2.5 to 8.4 mmol α-tocopherol/mol cholesterol (2.8 to 9.4 mg/g). Approximately 80% to 90% of the total tocopherol in human plasma is the α-form, and the vast majority of the remaining tocopherol is the γ-form. In disorders causing lipid malabsorption (such as in individuals with cystic fibrosis or abetalipoproteinemia), plasma lipids, lipoproteins, and vitamin E concentrations frequently are reduced concurrently (Machlin, 1991).

Tocopherol-Binding Proteins

A tocopherol-binding protein, called α-tocopherol transfer protein, with a molecular mass of 30 to 37 kDa, has been purified from rat and human liver cytosol. This α-tocopherol transfer protein is found only in liver. It has a high degree of specificity for RRR-α-tocopherol, seeming to recognize the three methyl groups and the free hydroxyl group on the chromanol ring and the phytyl tail with RRR stereochemistry (Hosomi et al., 1997). The α-tocopherol transfer protein binds α-tocopherol and enhances its transfer between membranes. In the liver, it brings about the efficient reincorporation of α-tocopherol into the plasma lipoprotein pool by transferring the α-tocopherol returned to the liver via uptake of lipoprotein remnants into VLDL for secretion into the plasma and delivery to peripheral tissues (Traber et al., 1993).

A different α-tocopherol-binding protein, with a molecular mass of 14.2 kDa, has been isolated and purified from rabbit heart and rat liver and heart (Dutta-Roy et al., 1994; Gordon et al., 1995). This protein also specifically binds α-tocopherol, and the binding is rapid, reversible, and saturable. It has been suggested that this binding protein may be involved in intracellular transport and distribution of α-tocopherol in tissues, particularly in its transfer to the membranes of the mitochondria and endoplasmic reticulum (Dutta-Roy et al., 1994).

Hepatic α-tocopherol transfer protein appears to facilitate the incorporation of α-tocopherol into nascent VLDL. By preferentially binding the α-form over the other forms of tocopherols, the binding protein also facilitates the return of α-tocopherols from the liver back to the plasma as VLDL. This leads to the preferential enrichment of LDL and HDL with α-tocopherol, compared with the other forms of tocopherol. The critical role of α-tocopherol transfer protein in regulating plasma tocopherol concentration has been demonstrated in patients with familial isolated vitamin E deficiency (Gotoda et al., 1995; Kayden and Traber, 1993; Ouahchi et al., 1995). These patients have clear signs of vitamin E deficiency (extremely low plasma vitamin E and neurological abnormalities) but have no fat malabsorption or lipoprotein abnormalities. Absence of the transfer or binding protein impairs secretion of α-tocopherol into hepatic lipoproteins (VLDL) and appears

CLINICAL CORRELATION

Familial Isolated Vitamin E Deficiency

Secondary vitamin E deficiency occurs in patients with generalized fat malabsorption caused by disorders such as abetalipoproteinemia, cystic fibrosis, short-bowel syndrome, and cholestatic liver disease. In these patients, prolonged deficiency of vitamin E eventually causes a decrease in the tocopherol content of nervous tissues and results in spinocerebellar dysfunction with progressive ataxia. In contrast, over the past two decades, a number of patients have been documented as having specific inherited forms of vitamin E deficiency. These have been described as familial isolated vitamin E deficiency, or ataxia with isolated vitamin E deficiency. Patients with this autosomal recessive neurodegenerative disease develop symptoms that resemble those of Friedreich's ataxia. These patients have normal gastrointestinal absorption of dietary lipids and α-tocopherol, with normal incorporation of lipids and vitamin E into chylomicrons. They have, however, an impaired ability to incorporate α-tocopherol into VLDL secreted by the liver, a function that apparently allows normal individuals efficiently to reincorporate α-tocopherol obtained from !ipoprotein remnants back into the plasma lipoprotein pool (Traber et al., 1993). Thus, in patients with familial isolated vitamin E deficiency, the absorption and transport of vitamin E to the liver are normal, but the hepatic incorporation of α-tocopherol into VLDL is impaired; this results in a low or undetectable plasma vitamin E concentration and low delivery of vitamin E to tissues.

The α-tocopherol transfer protein (α-TTP) is a cytosolic liver protein with high binding affinity for RRR-α-tocopherol. The physiological function of this enzyme had remained unclear until 1995, even though it was known that this protein transferred α-tocopherol between membranes in vitro. The cDNA for α-TTP was isolated from rats and humans, and the human α-TPP gene was shown to be located at chromosome 8q13 (Arita et al., 1995). Familial vitamin E deficiency mutations had previously been mapped to this same location. Ouahchi et al. (1995) demonstrated α-TTP gene mutations in patients with familial isolated vitamin E deficiency, confirming that mutations of the gene for α-TTP are responsible for isolated vitamin E deficiency. The degree of functionality of the mutant α-TTP seems to be associated with the degree of severity of the neurological damage and age of onset as well as with plasma vitamin E concentration (Gotoda et al., 1995).

High doses of vitamin E can prevent or mitigate the neurological course of this disease. Serum vitamin E concentrations in patients increase when they are treated with large doses of vitamin E, presumably because of the direct transfer of tocopherol from chylomicrons to other circulating lipoproteins.

Thinking Critically

1. The affinity of α-TTP for various forms of vitamin E varies and is highest for RRR-α-tocopherol. There seems to be a linear relationship between the relative binding affinity (RRR-α-tocopherol, 100%; RRR-β-tocopherol, 38%; SRR-α-tocopherol, 11%; RRR-α-tocopherol, 9%; and RRR-δ-tocopherol, 2%) and the known biological activity obtained from the rat resorption-gestation assay (Hosomi et al., 1997). Could the affinity of α-TTP for various tocopherols be one of the determinants of their biological activity? Explain. Do you think the type of tocopherol used as supplements for patients with familial isolated vitamin E deficiency would matter? Explain.

2. Many animal studies have shown that certain vitamin E deficiency symptoms can be partially reversed by other antioxidant compounds, raising questions about the specificity of the vitamin E requirement. What information was obtained from these studies of patients with familial isolated vitamin E deficiency with regard to specific functions of vitamin E?

to be responsible for the low plasma vitamin E status of these patients.

Metabolism

As stated previously, tocopherols can be excreted in the bile and then into the feces. Fecal elimination is the major route of excretion of excess tocopherols or of tocopherols not reincorporated into VLDL in the liver. The excretion of unchanged tocopherols through the biliary route increases as the tocopherol intake increases.

Tocopherols are also metabolized to a number of metabolites. In exerting antioxidant activity, α-tocopherol is first converted to α-tocopheroxyl (tocopheryl chromanoxyl) radical and is then further oxidized to α-tocopheryl quinone (Fig. 25–2). The conversion from α-tocopherol to α-tocopheroxyl radical is reversible, but α-tocopheryl quinone cannot be reduced back to α-tocopherol.

α-Tocopheryl quinone is not excreted as such. It can be reduced to hydroquinone and be further metabolized to α-tocopheronic acid (Chow et al., 1967). Tocopheronic acid is conjugated with glucuronic acid or other compounds and excreted in the urine. Conjugated α-tocopheryl hydroquinone also can be secreted in the bile and eliminated into the feces. Small amounts of the dimer and trimer of α-tocopherol have also been found in rat liver. A conjugated form of 2,5,7,8-tetramethyl-2(2'-carboxyethyl)-6-hydroxy chroman has

been identified as a urinary metabolite of α-tocopherol (Schultz et al., 1995). This metabolite appears to be formed in liver directly from a side-chain degradation of α-tocopherol without oxidative splitting of the chroman ring. Similarly, 2,7,8-trimethyl-2-(2'-carboxyethyl)-6-hydroxy chroman and 2,8-dimethyl-2(2'-carboxyethyl)-6-hydroxy chroman have been identified as urinary metabolites for γ- and δ-tocopherols, respectively (Chiku et al., 1984; Wechter et al., 1996).

BIOLOGICAL FUNCTIONS OF VITAMIN E AND FREE RADICAL–INDUCED LIPID PEROXIDATION

Vitamin E is present in membranes; it protects membrane lipids from oxidative damage. The reaction of α-tocopherol with lipid peroxyl radicals to prevent uncontrolled lipid peroxidation is the best-understood physiological action of vitamin E.

Biological Function

Although many biochemical abnormalities are associated with vitamin E deficiency, the mechanisms by which vitamin E prevents various metabolic and pathological lesions have not yet been elucidated. Vitamin E is the major lipid-soluble, chain-breaking antioxidant found in plasma, red cells, and tissues, and it plays an essential role in maintaining the

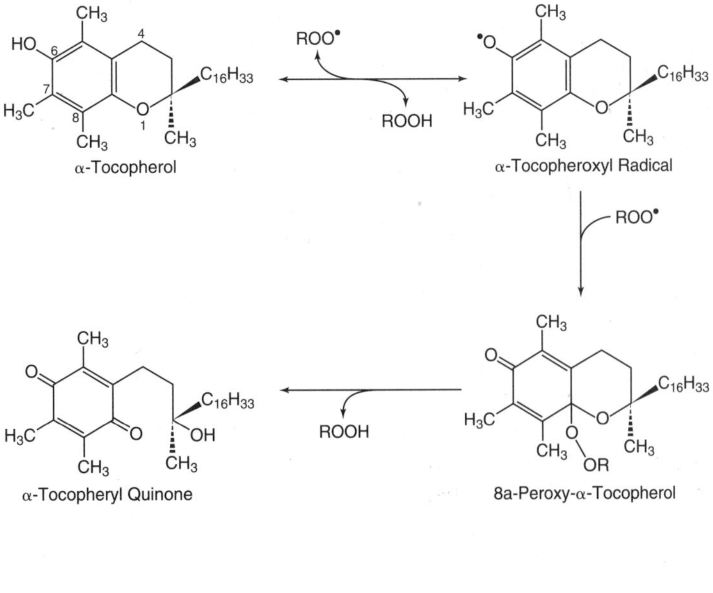

Figure 25–2. *Reactions of α-tocopherol with peroxyl radicals. α-Tocopherol can scavenge two lipid peroxyl radicals (ROO•) as shown with the reaction of one peroxyl radical converting α-tocopherol to α-tocopheroxyl radical, which can react with a second peroxyl radical to form an adduct that is subsequently degraded to α-tocopheryl quinone.*

integrity of biological membranes (Burton and Traber, 1990; Chow, 1985). Among the biological functions proposed for vitamin E, prevention of free radical–initiated lipid peroxidation and the resulting tissue damage is most widely accepted by investigators. The suggestion that vitamin E may play a structural role in the control of membrane permeability and stability is consistent with its role in protection of membrane lipids from oxidative damage.

Several nonantioxidant functions of vitamin E have been suggested. Vitamin E, for example, has been reported to modulate the activities of microsomal (associated with endoplasmic reticulum) enzymes, to downregulate protein kinase C activity and cell proliferation, and to regulate immune response or cell-mediated immunity. Thus vitamin E may function as a biological response modifier by modulating membrane-associated enzyme systems whose effects are amplified by the production of low molecular weight substances (e.g., products of arachidonic acid) that have profound effects at low concentrations in cell regulation and proliferation.

Free Radical–Induced Lipid Peroxidation

The harmful effects resulting from inhalation of a high concentration of oxygen have been attributed to the formation of reactive oxygen species rather than molecular oxygen per se. Superoxide radicals, nitric oxide, lipid alkoxyl, and peroxyl radicals are the most significant reactive oxygen species generated in living systems in aerobic environments. Among them, peroxyl radicals derived from polyunsaturated fatty acids have special significance because of their involvement in lipid peroxidation. Lipid peroxidation is the most common indicator of free radical production in living systems. (See Chapters 15 and 40 for more information on polyunsaturated fatty acids and lipid peroxidation.)

The process of lipid peroxidation (or autoxidation) can be divided into three phases: initiation, propagation, and termination. In the initiation phase (reaction I), carbon-centered lipid radicals (R•) can be produced by proton abstraction from, or addition to, a polyunsaturated fatty acid (RH) when a free radical initi-

ator (I*) is present. During the propagation phrase, the lipid radical reacts readily with molecular oxygen to form a peroxyl radical (ROO•) (reaction II). The peroxyl radical formed can react with another polyunsaturated fatty acid to form a hydroperoxide (ROOH) and a new carbon-centered radical (reaction III). The propagative process can continue until all polyunsaturated fat is consumed or the chain reaction is broken (termination phase). Free radicals can be scavenged and the chain reaction terminated by self-quenching (reaction IV) or by the action of antioxidant (AH) (reaction V), which generates A•. Of the free radical process inhibitors or antioxidants that are known, tocopherols are among the most effective chain-breakers. Tocopherols can react more rapidly with peroxyl radicals than do polyunsaturated fatty acids; therefore, tocopherols are very effective free radical chain-breaking antioxidants.

$$RH \xrightarrow{I^*} R\bullet \qquad \text{(Reaction I)}$$

$$R\bullet + O_2 \rightarrow ROO\bullet \qquad \text{(Reaction II)}$$

$$ROO\bullet + R'H \rightarrow ROOH + R'\bullet \qquad \text{(Reaction III)}$$

$$R\bullet \text{ (or } ROO\bullet) + R'\bullet \rightarrow R\text{-}R' \text{ (or } ROOR') \qquad \text{(Reaction IV)}$$

$$R\bullet \text{ (or } ROO\bullet) + AH \rightarrow RH \text{ (or } ROOH) + A\bullet \qquad \text{(Reaction V)}$$

Antioxidant activity of tocopherols is determined by their chemical reactivity with molecular oxygen, superoxide radicals, or peroxyl radicals, or by their ability to inhibit autoxidation of fats and oils. The action of α-tocopherol in quenching lipid peroxyl radicals is shown in Figure 25–2; the 6-hydroxyl group of the chroman ring is the reactive portion of the tocopherol. The relative antioxidant activity of tocopherols varies considerably depending on the experimental conditions and the assessment method employed (Kamal-Eldin and Appelqvist, 1996). Non–α-tocopherols have been shown to exhibit a higher antioxidant activity than the α-form in a number of in vitro test systems. Also, tocotrienols are more effective than tocopherols in preventing oxidation under certain conditions. Due to the involvement of the 6-hydroxyl group of the chroman ring in the ester linkage, tocopheryl esters are much more stable to oxidation than are free tocopherols; tocopherol esters do not function as antioxidants in vitro and must be hydrolyzed to free tocopherols in vivo before they can act as antioxidants.

Oxidative Damage and Antioxidant Defense

The process of free radical–induced lipid peroxidation has been implicated as a critical initiating event leading to cell injury or organ degeneration. A large variety of conditions are capable of initiating or enhancing oxidative stress within the cellular environment. These conditions include inadequate intake of antioxidants, excess intake of prooxidants, exposure to noxious chemical or physical agents, strenuous physical activities, injury and wounds, and certain hereditary disorders. On the other hand, a large number of enzymatic and nonenzymatic antioxidant systems are present in the cell. Under normal conditions, the metabolic activity of the cell is able to control or prevent most of the adverse effects of oxygen and its reactive intermediates. However, when the antioxidant potential is weakened or oxidative stress is greatly increased, irreversible damage to the cell may occur. The susceptibility of a given organ or organ system to oxidative damage is determined by the overall balance between the extent of oxidative stress and antioxidant capability. Major cellular antioxidant mechanisms include (1) direct interaction with oxidants or oxidizing agents by ascorbic acid, reduced glutathione (GSH), and other reducing agents, (2) scavenging of free radicals and singlet oxygen by vitamin E, ascorbic acid, superoxide dismutase, and other scavengers, (3) reduction of hydroperoxides by GSH peroxidases and catalase, (4) binding or removal of transition metals by ferritin, transferrin, ceruloplasmin, albumin, and other chelators, (5) prevention of reactive oxygen species and other factors from reaching the specific site of action or from reacting with essential cellular components by membrane barriers, and (6) replacement or repair of resulting damage by dietary nutrients and metabolic activities (Chow, 1991).

Various antioxidant systems act at different stages and cellular locations, and vitamin E occupies a key position in the overall antioxidant picture owing to its localization in cell membranes. Approximately one part (by weight) of α-tocopherol is capable of protecting 1000 parts of lipid molecules in biological membranes, and the efficacy of tocopherol is augmented by its interaction with other antioxidant systems. A number of antioxidant systems, including ascorbic acid, GSH, lipoic acid, NADH-cytochrome b_5, and coenzyme Q_{10}, have been shown to be involved in the regeneration of vitamin E (Chow, 1991; Packer et al., 1995). Although the nature of the vitamin E regenerative process in vivo is not entirely clear, it does provide a rational explanation for the fact that it is very difficult to deplete vitamin E in adult animals or human subjects.

FUNCTIONAL INTERACTIONS OF VITAMIN E WITH OTHER NUTRIENTS

The antioxidant function of vitamin E is interrelated with that of other dietary nutrients. In addition to dietary lipids, vitamin E is functionally related to the status of selenium, vitamin C, iron, β-carotene, and sulfur-containing amino acids in the overall antioxidant defense.

Polyunsaturated Lipids

Cell membranes contain a high proportion of polyunsaturated fatty acids, and vitamin E is found predominantly in the membranes. The dietary requirement for vitamin E is related to the degree of unsaturation of the fatty acids in tissue lipids, which can be altered by dietary lipids. The intake of tocopherols generally parallels the intake of polyunsaturated fatty acids. Plant foods that contain high levels of polyunsaturated fatty acids generally are also rich sources of tocopherols. A typical American diet contains approximately 0.5 mg α-tocopherol equivalent (activity equivalent to 0.5 mg of RRR-α-tocopherol) per gram of polyunsaturated fatty acids.

Selenium

Selenium can prevent or reduce the severity of several symptoms of vitamin E deficiency in animals, including necrotic liver degeneration and eosinophilic enteritis in rats and exudative diathesis in chicks. Selenium deficiency in domestic animals is frequently associated with an increased vitamin E requirement, and the situation is often aggravated by the oxidation of vitamin E in feed during storage. The finding that selenium is an integral part of the enzymes glutathione peroxidase and phospholipid hydroperoxide glutathione peroxidase provides a feasible explanation of the metabolic interrelationship between vitamin E and selenium. Selenium complements the antioxidant function of vitamin E via the role of these selenoenzymes in reducing lipid hydroperoxides (ROOH) to the corresponding hydroxy acids (ROH) (reaction VI). This reduction prevents the decomposition of hydroperoxides to form free radicals that may initiate further oxidative reactions. Thus selenium, through its function in glutathione peroxidases, may decrease the requirement of vitamin E. (See Chapter 34 for further discussion of selenium and glutathione peroxidases).

$$\text{ROOH + 2 GSH} \xrightarrow{\text{Glutathione peroxidase}} \text{ROH + GSSG + H}_2\text{O} \quad \text{(Reaction VI)}$$

Vitamin C (Ascorbic Acid)

As an important water-soluble free radical scavenger and reducing agent, vitamin C may complement the function of vitamin E and spare vitamin E requirement. This effect is partly attributable to the involvement of vitamin C in the regeneration of reduced vitamin E. On the other hand, a GSH-dependent dehydroascorbic acid reductase and an NADH-semidehydroascorbic acid reductase appear to be involved in the regeneration of vitamin C.

β-Carotene

In addition to being a precursor of vitamin A, β-carotene is an effective quencher of singlet oxygen and a free radical scavenger. As β-carotene is more effective at low oxygen concentrations and vitamin E is more effective at high oxygen concentrations, these two antioxidants may act complementarily to protect cellular components against oxidative damage.

β-Carotene may also modulate membrane properties important to cell-cell signaling, or possibly serve as an intracellular precursor to retinoic acid. Other carotenoids such as lutein and lycopene may also complement the antioxidant function of vitamin E.

Iron

Removal of transition metal ions, particularly ferrous ion (Fe^{2+}), is of critical importance in preventing generation of hydroxyl radicals (OH•) from hydrogen peroxide (H_2O_2) (reaction VII).

$$H_2O_2 + Fe^{2+} \rightarrow OH^- + OH\bullet + Fe^{3+} \quad \text{(Reaction VII)}$$

Hydroxyl radicals are highly reactive and are capable of initiating oxidative damage. Iron absorbed from the diet or released from ferritin can be sequestered by transferrin, lactoferrin, citrate, and ATP and other phosphate esters. Excess iron absorption/uptake occurs in certain pathological conditions, such as the genetic disease idiopathic hemochromatosis. The effects of iron overload can be lessened by increased vitamin E intake.

Sulfur-Containing Amino Acids

Muscular dystrophy, the condition that occurs in most animal species fed a vitamin E–deficient diet, appears in chicks only when they are fed a diet that is also low in either sulfur amino acids or selenium. This interrelationship of vitamin E with sulfur amino acids appears to be due to a requirement for sulfur amino acids for the synthesis of reduced GSH. GSH is essential for the activity of glutathione peroxidase (reaction VI) and is involved in the regeneration of vitamin E. Oxidized glutathione (GSSG), in turn, is reduced by the activity of GSSG reductase (reaction VIII).

$$\text{GSSG + NADPH + H}^+ \xrightarrow{\text{GSSG reductase}} \text{2 GSH + NADP}^+ \quad \text{(Reaction VIII)}$$

DEFICIENCY, TOXICITY, AND HEALTH EFFECTS OF VITAMIN E

Much of what is known about vitamin E deficiency and toxicity symptoms has come from animal studies. Recent studies of patients with familial vitamin E deficiency have enhanced our understanding of the consequences of a vitamin E deficiency in humans. Recent epidemiological and intervention studies have provided new insights into the effect of vitamin E status on health.

Deficiency Symptoms

A number of species-dependent, tissue-specific vitamin E deficiency symptoms have been reported. The development and severity of certain vitamin E deficiency symptoms are associated with the status of other nutrients, including selenium and sulfur-containing amino acids (Machlin, 1991). For example, the most common deficiency sign is necrotizing myopathy, which occurs in almost all species in the skeletal muscle and in some heart and smooth muscles. Myopathy primarily results from selenium deficiency in domestic animals, but rabbits and guinea pigs develop severe debilitating myopathy when fed a diet deficient in vitamin E but adequate in selenium. On the other hand, rats manifest a relatively benign myopathy when fed a vitamin E-deficient diet, and chickens develop no myopathy unless the diet is depleted of both vitamin E and sulfur-containing amino acids. The reason for the species-dependent and tissue-specific vitamin E deficiency symptoms remains to be delineated.

In humans, lower plasma/serum levels of vitamin E ($<$5 mg/L) are associated with a shorter lifespan of red cells and their increased susceptibility to hemolysis. Vitamin E deficiency is rarely seen in the population of the United States. When it occurs, it is usually a result of lipoprotein deficiencies or lipid malabsorption syndromes. Low plasma vitamin E levels have been observed in patients with a variety of fat malabsorption conditions. Recent studies of children and adults with specific causes of fat/vitamin E malabsorption (such as abetalipoproteinemia, chronic cholestatic hepatobiliary disorder, and cystic fibrosis) have clearly shown that neurologic abnormalities do occur in association with malabsorption syndromes of various etiologies (Machlin, 1991; Kayden and Traber, 1993). The similarity of the neurologic abnor-malities to those that occur in patients with familial isolated vitamin E deficiency suggests that the neurological symptoms are specifically related to the lack of adequate vitamin E in neural tissues.

Toxicity

Both acute and chronic studies with several species of animals have shown that high doses of vitamin E are relatively nontoxic. In humans, a daily dose of 100 to 300 mg of vitamin E (α-tocopherol equivalents) is considered harmless from a toxicological point of view (Kappa and Diplock, 1992). However, high doses of vitamin E supplements may cause increased post-surgery bleeding and may also cause bleeding in patients receiving anticoagulant therapy.

Health Effects

In addition to an increased requirement for vitamin E when polyunsaturated lipid intake is high, increased vitamin E may be needed to provide protection against oxidants and oxidizing agents in the environment (Packer, 1993). Results obtained from a number of recent studies suggest that vitamin E is protective against oxidative stress resulting from exposure to environmental agents, and that increased intake of vitamin E is associated with enhanced immune response and reduced risk of cardiovascular disease, certain cancers, and other degenerative diseases.

Several indexes of immune response, including measures of delayed-type hypersensitivity, antibody production, lymphocyte proliferation, and cytokine production, are influenced by the status of essential nutrients, including vitamin E. Vitamin E supplementation is associated with enhanced production of the cytokine interleukin 2, enhanced lymphocyte proliferation, and decreased production of immunosuppressive prostaglandin E_2. The antioxidant property is likely to play a role in the immunostimulatory effects of vitamin E (Meydani et al., 1990).

Several dietary factors, including decreased vitamin E status, have been implicated in the increased incidence of coronary heart disease. In recent years, several large-scale epidemiological and intervention studies have shown that a higher intake or a higher serum/plasma level of α-tocopherol is associated with a decreased risk of cardiovascular diseases (Stampfer et al., 1993). The ability of vitamin E to prevent LDL oxidation, platelet adhesion, or both may be responsible for the reduced risk of cardiovascular disease. Some recent studies have shown strong associations between serum γ-tocopherol concentrations (but not necessarily α-tocopherol concentrations) and the risk of coronary heart disease (Kushi et al., 1996; Ohrvall et al., 1996).

Vitamin E may reduce cancer risk by reacting directly with mutagens/carcinogens, altering metabolic activation processes, enhancing the immune systems, inhibiting cell proliferation, or other mechanisms. Most of the studies dealing with head/neck, lung, and colorectal cancer suggest a protective effect of vitamin E against cancer risk. However, reports concerning the association between vitamin E intake/status and the risk of breast, bladder, and cervical cancer are not consistent (Chow, 1994).

BIOPOTENCY AND SOURCES OF VARIOUS FORMS OF VITAMIN E

A variety of naturally occurring RRR-tocopherols and tocotrienols is supplied by foods; hence, naturally occurring vitamin E is not the same as the all-*rac*-α-tocopherol used as a vitamin E supplement. The differences in mechanism of action and effectiveness of various forms of vitamin E are not well understood in the context of human nutrition.

Biopotency

Tocopherols differ in their antioxidant and biological activities. The biological activity of tocopherols is assessed in bioassays by determining their relative ability to prevent such deficiency symptoms as fetal resorption and erythrocyte hemolysis in rats. Another measure, the curative myopathy test, is based on the ability of tocopherol to suppress the release of pyruvate kinase from skeletal muscle into the serum of vitamin E–deficient rats.

The biological activity of various forms of vitamin E has been expressed as units of activity in relation to that of all-*rac*-α-tocopheryl acetate, which is a common pharmaceutical or synthetic form of vitamin E. The relative values in the USP Reference Standard units (USP Vitamin E-unit) or international units (IU) per milligram of compound are

> all-*rac*-α-tocopheryl acetate, 1.00
> all-*rac*-α-tocopherol, 1.10
> RRR-α-tocopheryl acetate, 1.36
> RRR-α-tocopherol, 1.49
> all-*rac*-α-tocopheryl succinate, 0.89
> RRR-α-tocopheryl succinate, 1.21

The relative activity of tocopherols based on bioassay methods is shown in Table 25–1.

TABLE 25–1
Vitamin E Activity of Tocopherols

Structure	Resorption-Gestation* (%)	Hemolysis† (%)
RRR-α-tocopherol	100	100
RRR-β-tocopherol	25–50	15–27
RRR-γ-tocopherol	8–19	3–20
RRR-δ-tocopherol	0.1–3	0.3–2
RRR-α-tocotrienol	21–50	17–25
RRR-β-tocotrienol	4–5	1–5
RRR-α-tocopheryl acetate	91	—
All-*rac*-α-tocopherol‡	74	—
All-*rac*-α-tocopheryl acetate‡	67	—

*Based on the fetal development and/or prevention of fetal loss in rats.
†Based on the prevention of hemoglobin liberation from red blood cells.
‡A mixture of 8 stereoisomers.
Data are from Machlin, L. J. (1991) Vitamin E. In: Handbook of Vitamins (Machlin, L. J., ed.), 2nd ed., pp. 99–144. Marcel Dekker, New York; and Pryor, W. A. (1995) Vitamin E and Carotenoid Abstracts, pp. 1–108. VERIS, La Grange, IL.

NUTRITION INSIGHT

Are Non-α-Tocopherols Also Important for Health?

When vitamin E is consumed in the diet, the majority of the tocopherol consumed is RRR-γ-tocopherol, whereas the calculated vitamin E activity (α-tocopherol equivalents) is largely attributed to RRR-α-tocopherol. RRR-α-tocopherol has traditionally been the focus of study because α-tocopherol has the highest potency in bioassays for prevention of deficiency symptoms. Several recent studies have raised questions that need to be considered, particularly with regard to optimal health considerations. Has the importance of dietary γ-tocopherol, other non–α-tocopherols, or tocotrienols been underestimated? Are non–α-tocopherols also important in the prevention of degenerative diseases? Would supplements that better reflect the ratios found in the diet be more useful than preparations of only α-tocopherol?

The Iowa Women's Health Study conducted from 1986 to 1992 was a prospective cohort study of 34,486 postmenopausal women with no evidence of cardiovascular disease (Kushi et al., 1996). In this study, the relationship between dietary antioxidant intake and coronary heart disease mortality was evaluated; 242 subjects died of coronary heart disease during the 6-year study period. Vitamin E intake was inversely associated with risk of death from coronary heart disease, and the relationship was highly significant in a subgroup of 21,809 women who did not take vitamin supplements. Relative risk of death from coronary heart disease was 58% lower in the highest two quintiles of dietary vitamin E intake from food (>7.6 IU per day) than in the lowest quintile (<4.9 IU per day). That vitamin E from foods but not from supplements was inversely associated with mortality from coronary heart disease suggested that vitamin E consumed in food may be a marker for other dietary factors associated with risk of coronary heart disease. However, adjustments for intake of carotenoids, folic acid, vitamin A, vitamin C, fiber, essential fatty acids, meat, and various food groups did not substantially alter the association, whereas intake of vitamin E–rich foods such as nuts and seeds or margarine was inversely associated with risk of death from coronary heart disease.

In a study in Sweden of male patients with coronary heart disease and healthy age-matched reference subjects, the serum α-tocopherol concentrations did not differ significantly between the groups (Ohrvall et al., 1996). However, the coronary heart disease group had a lower mean serum concentration of γ-tocopherol and a higher α-/γ-tocopherol ratio. The findings in this study also suggest that γ-tocopherol may be important, either itself or as a marker for another dietary factor.

Studies with rats fed diets with a constant amount of α-tocopherol (Clement & Bourre, 1997) showed that supplementation of the diet with γ-tocopherol induced increases in the concentrations of both α- and γ-tocopherol in plasma and tissues. These studies suggest that the biopotency of α-tocopherol may be higher when γ-tocopherol is present in the diet.

Additionally, there are differences in the reactivities of α-tocopherol and γ-tocopherol with respect to chemical activity, suggesting that these two tocopherols may complement each other. It has been shown in vitro that γ-tocopherol traps potentially mutagenic electrophiles, such as reactive nitrogen oxide species including peroxynitrite. The 5-position of γ-tocopherol is highly nucleophilic and reactive toward electrophiles such as NO^+ and NO_2^+. In peroxynitrite-induced lipid peroxidation studies, α-tocopherol was converted to α-tocopheryl quinone (2 electron oxidation product), whereas γ-tocopherol was converted to 5-NO_2-γ-tocopherol and its orthoquinone tocored (Christen et al., 1997). It is possible that γ-tocopherol is important for the removal of membrane-soluble electrophilic compounds such as NO_x and hypochlorous acid because of its ability to trap electrophiles as an unreactive carbon-centered adduct. This ability is not shared by α-tocopherol, which has a methyl group on the 5-C on the phenol ring; α-tocopherol may trap the electrophile but is likely to remain chemically reactive.

Thinking Critically

1. Based on what is known or not known about the functions of various forms of vitamin E, what recommendations would you make about vitamin E intake from food or from supplements?

(Note that vitamin E activity is also expressed as α-tocopherol equivalents (α-TE), and that 1 α-TE is equivalent to 1.49 mg all-*rac*-α-tocopheryl acetate.)

Sources

The majority of the tocopherols consumed in the United States are not α-tocopherol. γ-Tocopherol, the predominant form of tocopherols present in soybean oil and corn oil, accounts for over half the estimated total tocopherol intake (Chow, 1985). On the other hand, the majority of tocopherols in cottonseed oil, peanut oil, safflower oil, and olive oil are the α-form. Smaller amounts of β- and δ-tocopherols are present in foods and oils. In addition to cooking oils, significant sources of vitamin E in American diets include regular margarine, regular mayonnaise, and salad dressings, vitamin E–fortified breakfast cereals, vegetable shortenings used for home cooking, peanut butter, eggs, potato chips, whole milk, and tomato products.

REQUIREMENT FOR VITAMIN E AND ASSESSMENT OF VITAMIN E NUTRITIONAL STATUS

Recommendations for vitamin E intake are largely based on customary intakes of vitamin E from the diet. The level of intake from American diets seems to be sufficient to maintain tocopherol concentrations that are adequate for protection of tissue lipids from peroxidation.

Requirement

In 1968, vitamin E was officially recognized as an essential nutrient, and a daily intake of 30 International Units (IU) was recommended for adult men by the National Research Council. Reassessment of dietary fat and tocopherol content in American diets led in 1974 to a revised RDA of 15 IU for adult men. In 1980, the RDA was revised to take into account the dietary contribution of non-α-tocopherols, and the requirement was expressed as α-tocopherol equivalent (α-TE). One α-TE is

---

Food Sources of Vitamin E

- Vegetable oils, margarines, and shortening
- Wheat germ and rice bran
- Nuts and seeds

RDAs Across the Life Cycle

	mg α-TE/day
Infants, 0–0.5 y	3
0.5–1.0 y	4
Children, 1–3 y	6
4–10 y	7
Males, 11+ y	10
Females, 11+ y	8
Pregnant	10
Lactating	11–12

Vitamin E requirements and food content are defined in terms of α-tocopherol equivalents (α-TE). To obtain 1 mg α-TE, one would need to consume 1 mg RRR-α-tocopherol, 1.35 mg all-*rac*-α-tocopherol, 1.49 mg all-rac-α-tocopheryl acetate, or 10 mg RRR-γ-tocopherol. Previously used units for vitamin E were international units (IU), with 1 IU being defined as 1 mg all-*rac*-α-tocopheryl acetate; the conversion between IU and α-TE is 1.49 IU equals 1 mg α-TE. Sunflower, safflower, or cottonseed oil provides ~5 to 7 mg of α-TE per tablespoon (14 g), whereas corn oil and soybean oil provide ~2.0 to 2.5 mg α-TE per tablespoon.

From National Research Council (1989) Recommended Dietary Allowances, 10th ed. National Academy Press, Washington, DC

equal to 1 mg RRR-α-tocopherol, and the amount of other isomers can be converted to α-TE by multiplying the milligram of each isomer by the relative activity factor (i.e., RRR-β-tocopherol, 0.5; RRR-γ-tocopherol, 0.1; all-*rac*-α-tocopherol, 0.74; all-*rac*-α-tocopheryl acetate, 0.67). The 1989 RDA for vitamin E was set at 10 α-TE for adult men and 8 α-TE for adult (nonpregnant, nonlactating) women (National Research Council, 1989). Because 1 IU is defined as 1 mg of all-*rac*-α-tocopheryl acetate, the 1989 RDA is equivalent to 15 IU of vitamin E for the adult man and 12 IU for the adult woman. The normal intake of vitamin E in American diets ranges between 4 and 33 mg α-TE daily in adults not taking vitamin E supplements, with average values of 11 to 13 mg α-TE. This level of intake results in average plasma/serum levels in adults of approximately 10 mg α-tocopherol/L.

Assessment of Vitamin E Nutritional Status

The nutritional status of vitamin E is assessed based on the concentration of tocopherols in the body pool. The tocopherol concentration in plasma/serum, erythrocytes, platelets, or tissues; the degree of erythrocyte hemolysis; and the amount of lipid peroxidation products (e.g., ethane and pentane in exhaled air and malondialdehyde in serum) have been used to assess the nutritional status of vitamin E in humans. The tocopherol concentration in erythrocytes represents past intake (>1 month), whereas the plasma/serum tocopherol concentration reflects recent intake (days). The vitamin E concentration of platelets is more sensitive than that of plasma, erythrocytes, or lymphocytes for measuring dose response to dietary vitamin E. Also, platelet tocopherol concentration is independent of the serum lipid levels, which is an important advantage relative to serum or plasma tocopherol concentrations as an indicator of vitamin E status. Whether these measurements, particularly plasma tocopherol concentrations, accurately reflect body stores of vitamin E has been questioned. Recent studies suggest that plasma tocopherol concentration, in lieu of target tissue concentra-

tions, can be used as a reliable indicator of vitamin E status (Peng et al., 1995).

REFERENCES

Arita, M., Sato, Y., Miyata, A., Tanabe, T., Takahashi, E., Kayden, H. J., Arai, H. and Inoue, K. (1995) Human α-tocopherol transfer protein: cDNA cloning, expression and chromosomal localization. Biochem J 306:437–443.

Burton, G. W. and Traber, M. G. (1990) Vitamin E: Antioxidant activity, biokinetics, and bioavailability. Annu Rev Nutr 10:357–382.

Chiku, S., Hamamura, K. and Nakamura, T. (1984) Novel urinary metabolite of d-δ-tocopherol in rats. J Lipid Res 25:40–48.

Chow, C. K. (1985) Vitamin E and blood. World Rev Nutr Diet 45:133–166.

Chow, C. K. (1991) Vitamin E and oxidative stress. Free Radic Biol Med 11:215–232.

Chow, C. K. (1994) Vitamin E and cancer: An update. In: Nutrition and Disease Update—Cancer (Carroll, K. K. and Kritchevsky, D., eds.), pp. 214–233. AOCS Press, Champaign, IL.

Chow, C. K., Draper, H. H., Csallany, A. S. and Chiu, M. (1967) The metabolism of C14-α-tocopheryl quinone and C14-α-tocopheryl hydroquinone. Lipids 2:390–397.

Christen, S., Woodall, A. A., Shigenaga, M. K., Southwell-Keely, P. T., Duncan, M. W., and Ames, B. N. (1997) γ-Tocopherol traps mutagenic electrophiles such as NO_x and complements α-tocopherol: Physiological implications. Proc Natl Acad Sci USA 94:3217–3222.

Clement, M. and Bourre, J. M. (1997) Graded dietary levels of RRR-γ-tocopherol induce a marked increase in the concentrations of α- and γ-tocopherol in nervous tissues, heart, liver, and muscle of vitamin E–deficient rats. Biochim Biophys Acta 1334:173–181.

Dutta-Roy, A. K., Gordon, M. J., Campbell, F. M., Duthie, G. G. and James, W. P. T. (1994) Vitamin E requirements, transport, and metabolism: Role of α-tocopherol-binding proteins. J Nutr Biochem 5:562–570.

Evans, H. M. and Bishop, K. S. (1922) On the existence of a hitherto unrecognized dietary factor essential for reproduction. Science 56:650–651.

Gordon, M. J., Campbell, F. M., Duthie, G. G. and Dutta-Roy, A. K. (1995) Characterization of a novel α-tocopherol-binding protein from bovine heart cytosol. Arch Biochem Biophys 318:140–146.

Gotoda, T., Arita, M., Arai, H., Inoue, K., Yokota, T., Fukuo, Y., Yazaki, Y., and Yamada, N. (1995) Adult-onset spinocerebellar dysfunction caused by a mutation in the gene for the α-tocopherol-transfer protein. N Engl J Med 333:1313–1318.

Hosomi, A., Arita, M., Sato, Y., Kiyose, C., Ueda, T., Igarashi, O., Arai, H. and Inoue, K. (1997) Affinity for α-tocopherol transfer protein as a determinant of the biological activities of vitamin E analogs. FEBS Lett 409:105–108.

Kamal-Eldin, A. and Appelqvist, L. A. (1996) The chemistry and antioxidant properties of tocopherols and tocotrienols. Lipids 31:671–701.

Kappa, H. and Diplock, A. T. (1992) Tolerance and safety of vitamin E: A toxicological position report. Free Radic Biol Med 13:55–74.

Kayden, H. J. and Traber, M. G. (1993) Absorption, lipoprotein transport, and regulation of plasma concentrations of vitamin E in humans. J Lipid Res 34:343–358.

Kostner, G. M., Oettl, K., Jauhiainen, M., Ehnholm, C. and Esterbauer, H. (1995) Human plasma phospholipid transfer protein accelerates exchange/transfer of α-tocopherol between lipoproteins and cells. Biochem J 305:659–667.

Kushi, L. H., Folsom, A. R., Prineas, R. J., Mink, P. J., Wu, Y. and Bostick, R. M. (1996) Dietary antioxidant vitamins and death from coronary heart disease in postmenopausal women. N Engl J Med 334:1156–1162.

Machlin, L. (1991) Vitamin E. In: Handbook of Vitamins (Machlin, L. J., ed.), 2nd ed., pp. 99–144. Marcel Dekker, New York.

Meydani, S. N., Barklund, M. P., Liu, S., Miller, R. A., Cannon, J. G., Morrow, F. D., Rocklin, R. and Blumberg, J. B. (1990) Vitamin E supplementation enhances cell-mediated immunity in healthy elderly subjects. Am J Clin Nutr 52:557–563.

National Research Council (1989) Recommended Dietary Allowances, 10th ed. National Academy Press, Washington, D.C.

Ohrvall, M., Sundlof, G. and Vessby, B. (1996) Gamma, but not alpha, tocopherol levels in serum are reduced in coronary heart disease patients. J Intern Med 239:111–117.

Ouahchi, K., Arita, M., Kayden, H., Hentati, F., Hamida, M. B., Sokol, R., Arai, H., Inoue, K., Mandel, J.-L. and Koenig, M. (1995) Ataxia with isolated vitamin E deficiency is caused by mutations in the α-tocopherol transfer protein. Nature Genet 9:141–145.

Packer, L. (1993) Vitamin E: Biological activity and health benefits: Overview. In: Vitamin E in Health and Disease (Packer, L. and Fuchs, J., eds.), pp. 977–982. Marcel Dekker, New York.

Packer, L., Witt, E. H. and Trischler, H. J. (1995) Alpha-lipoic acid as a biological antioxidant. Free Radic Biol Med 19:227–250.

Peng, Y.-M., Peng, Y.-S., Lin, Y., Moon, T., Roe, D. J. and Ritenbaugh, C. (1995) Concentrations and plasma-tissue-diet relationships of carotenoids, retinoids, and tocopherols in humans. Nutr Cancer 23:233–246.

Pryor, W. A. (1995) Vitamin E and Carotenoid Abstracts, pp. 1–108. VERIS, La Grange, IL.

Sattler, W., Levak-Frank, S., Radner, H., Kostner, G. M. and Zechner, R. (1996) Muscle-specific overexpression of lipoprotein lipase in transgenic mice results in increased α-tocopherol levels in skeletal muscle. Biochem J 318:15–19.

Schultz, M., Leist, M., Petrzika, M., Gassmann, B. and Brigelius-Flohe, R. (1995) Novel urinary metabolite of α-tocopherol, 2,5,7,8-tetra-2(2′-carboxyethyl)-6-hydroxychroman, as an indicator of an adequate vitamin E supply. Am J Clin Nutr 62:1527S–1534S.

Stampfer, M. J., Henneckens, C. H., Ascherio, A., Giovannucci, E., Colditz, G. A., Rosner, B. and Willett, W. C. (1993) Vitamin E consumption and the risk of coronary disease in men. N Engl J Med 328:1450–1456.

Traber, M. G., Sokol, R. J., Kohlschuetter, A., Yokota, T., Muller, D. P. R., Dufour, R. and Kayden, H. J. (1993) Impaired discrimination between stereoisomers and α-tocopherol in patients with familial isolated vitamin E deficiency. J Lipid Res 34:201–210.

Wechter, W. J., Kantoci, D., Murray, E. D., Jr., D'Amico, D. C., Jung, M. E. and Wang, W.-H. (1996) A new endogenous natriuretic factor: LLU-α. Proc Natl Acad Sci USA. 93:6002–6007.

RECOMMENDED READING

Packer, L. and Fuchs, J., eds. (1993) Vitamin E in Health and Disease. Marcel Dekker, New York.

CHAPTER 26

◆ ◆

Vitamin A

Noa Noy, Ph.D.

OUTLINE

COMMON ABBREVIATIONS

ARAT (acyl CoA:retinol acyltransferase)
CRABP (cellular retinoic acid-binding protein)
CRALBP (cellular retinal-binding protein)
CRBP (cellular retinol-binding protein)
IPM (interphotoreceptor matrix)
IRBP (interphotoreceptor retinoid-binding protein)
LRAT (lecithin:retinol acyltransferase)
RAR (retinoic acid receptor)
RBP (retinol-binding protein)
RPE (retinal pigment epithelium)
RXR (retinoid X receptor)

CHEMISTRY AND PHYSICAL PROPERTIES OF VITAMIN A AND CAROTENOIDS

Vitamin A was initially recognized as an essential growth factor present in foods of animal origin, such as animal fats and fish oils, and this factor was called "fat-soluble A" (McCollum and Davis, 1915; Osborne and Mendel, 1919). It was also observed that some plants displayed the activity of this fat-soluble A factor. Subsequently, it became clear in the early 1930s that some of the plant-derived compounds known as carotenoids display vitamin A activity owing to the ability of animals to convert them to retinol.

Nomenclature

Vitamin A nomenclature has undergone various changes since the discovery of this fat-soluble vitamin. Currently, the term vitamin A is used to generically describe compounds that exhibit the biological activity of retinol, the alcoholic form of vitamin A. The term can thus be applied to many naturally occurring and synthetic derivatives of retinol. Of the more than 600 carotenoids that are known to exist in nature, about 50 display vitamin A activity and are termed provitamin A. More recently, the term retinoids has been coined to describe compounds that share structural similarities with retinol, regardless of their biological activity.

Lability and Limited Solubility of Retinoids in Water

The structures of some physiologically important retinoids as well as the most active provitamin A carotenoid, all-*trans*-β-carotene, are shown in Figure 26–1.

In general, retinoids are composed of three distinct structural domains: they contain a β-ionone ring, a polyunsaturated chain, and a polar end group. The polar end group of naturally occurring retinoids can exist at several oxidation states, varying from the low oxidation state of retinol, to retinal, and to the even higher oxidation state in retinoic acid. Vitamin A is stored in vivo in the form of retinyl esters in which retinol has been esterified with a long-chain fatty acid, with concomitant loss of the polar end group (Fig. 26–1). Retinol can also be converted in vivo to species with larger, more polar end groups (e.g., retinoyl β-glucuronide, Fig. 26–1).

In recent years, a wide array of synthetic analogs of retinoids have been developed. The β-ionone ring has been systematically replaced by multiple hydrophobic groups, the spacer chain has been derivatized to a variety of cyclic and aromatic rings, and the polar end group has been converted into derivatives or precursors of active species. Active synthetic analogs, similar to naturally occurring retinoids, retain an amphipathic nature typified by a hydrophobic moiety and a polar terminus.

The large hydrophobic moiety of retinoids results in a limited solubility of these compounds in water. In addition, the multiple double-bonds of the spacer chain render retinoids susceptible to photodegradation, isomerization, and oxidation. Vitamin A and its analogs are thus stable in a crystalline form or when dissolved in organic solvents under nonoxidizing conditions, but they are labile when exposed to light or in aqueous solutions in the presence of oxygen. The poor solubility and the lability of retinoids in aqueous phases raise important questions regarding their physiology; for example, how do these insoluble compounds transfer across aqueous spaces between different organs, cells, and subcellular locations, and how is their structural integrity retained in vivo when they traverse the aqueous phases of serum and cytosol?

Optical Properties of Retinoids and Carotenoids

Physical methods that have been used to study retinoids include ultraviolet, visible, infrared, and fluorescence spectroscopy; nuclear magnetic resonance and electron spin resonance spectroscopy; and mass spectroscopy. Retinoids have absorption spectra with characteristic maxima in the 320- to 380-nm range. The absorption spectra of carotenoids center in the visible range at around 450 nm. Some retinoids, most notably retinols, are highly fluorescent and display fluorescence emission maxima in the range of 460 to 500 nm.

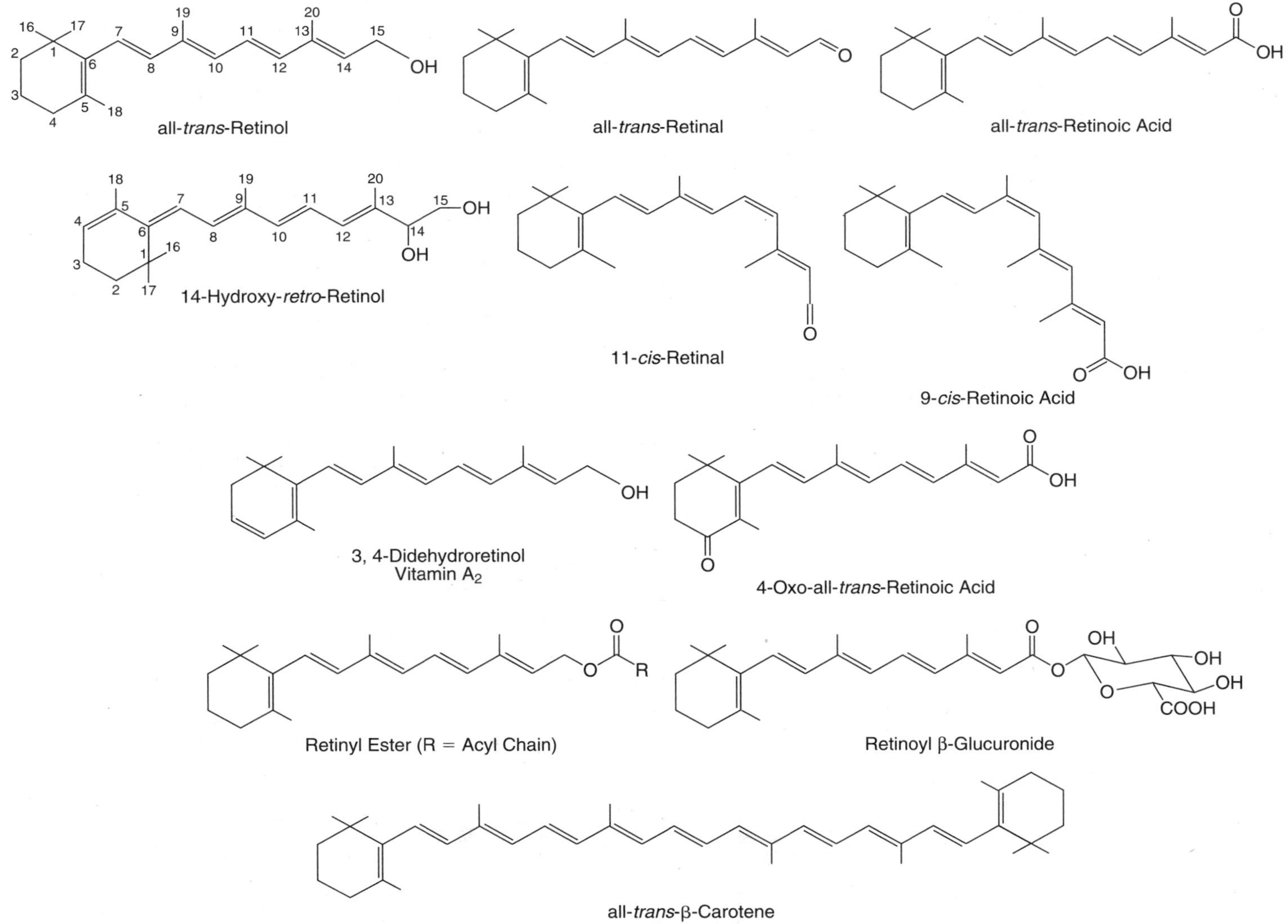

Figure 26-1. *Structures of vitamin A, β-carotene, and some of their biologically active derivatives.*

all-*trans*-Retinoic Acid

9-*cis*-Retinoic Acid

4-Oxo-all-*trans*-Retinoic Acid

Retinoyl β-Glucuronide

all-*trans*-Retinal

11-*cis*-Retinal

3, 4-Didehydroretinol
Vitamin A₂

Retinyl Ester (R = Acyl Chain)

all-*trans*-Retinol

14-Hydroxy-*retro*-Retinol

all-*trans*-β-Carotene

Carotenoids, on the other hand, do not display significant fluorescence at physiologically relevant temperatures. The optical properties of retinoids and, in particular, the environmental sensitivity of the fluorescence of retinols have been widely used to probe their interactions within various compartments in which they are found in cells, such as cellular membranes and binding sites of specific binding proteins.

PHYSIOLOGICAL FUNCTIONS OF VITAMIN A

Vitamin A and its metabolites participate in a wide spectrum of biological functions. They are essential for vision, reproduction, and immune function, and they play important roles in cellular differentiation, proliferation, and signaling. The diverse effects of vitamin A are exerted by several types of retinoids functioning by a variety of mechanisms. The 11-*cis* isomer of retinal participates in visual transduction; retinoic acid and possibly other retinoids are responsible for the effects of vitamin A on gene transcription; and it has recently been suggested that *retro* derivatives of retinol are important for proliferation and activation of lymphocytes. Other retinoid derivatives that are known to be present endogenously display biological activities, but the mechanisms of action of these compounds are not uniformly understood.

Role of 11-*cis*-Retinal in the Visual Function

Light is sensed in the vertebrate eye by rhodopsin, a membrane protein located in the outer segments of photoreceptor cells. Rhodopsin utilizes 11-*cis*-retinal as its chromophore. Two types of photoreceptor cells exist in the human retina: rods, which are stimulated by the weak light of a broad range of wavelengths, and cones, which are responsible for color vision. Absorption of a photon by the 11-*cis*-retinal moiety of rhodopsin triggers a chain of events that culminates in hyperpolarization of the plasma membrane of the cell. As photoreceptor cells form synapses with secondary neurons, the hyperpolarization is communicated further until the visual signal is transmitted to the brain.

The process of the visual signal transduction is a classic example of a signaling cascade and is well characterized (Fig 26–2; Dowling, 1987; Saari, 1994). Absorption of a photon by rhodopsin-bound 11-*cis*-retinal results in isomerization of the chromophore to the all-*trans*-form, a process that induces the protein to undergo several conformational changes through a series of short-lived intermediates. One of the protein intermediates (metarhodopsin II, R* in Fig. 26–2) interacts with another membrane protein named transducin. Transducin is a so-called G-protein; its interaction with R* leads to an exchange of a transducin-bound guanosine diphosphate (GDP) with a guanosine triphosphate (GTP).

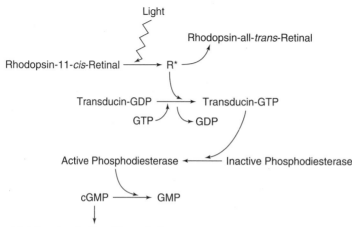

Figure 26–2. Early events in transduction of the visual signal.

In the GTP-bound state, transducin activates an enzyme called phosphodiesterase. Phosphodiesterase catalyzes the breakdown of cyclic guanosine monophosphate (cGMP), which acts to keep the sodium channels of the plasma membranes of rod outer segments in the open state, to an inactive product, GMP. Because the level of cGMP in rod outer segments in the dark is high (about 0.07 mmol/L), the sodium channels under these conditions are open, and the membranes of the cells are depolarized. Activation of phosphodiesterase following illumination results in lower levels of cGMP and leads to closing of the sodium channels and to hyperpolarization of the plasma membrane. The process of visual transduction is regulated further at several levels, including phosphorylation of rhodopsin intermediates, hydrolysis of retinal from rhodopsin, and the ability of a protein known as arrestin to block the interaction of the activated rhodopsin with transducin.

Bleached rhodopsin can be regenerated in the dark by 11-*cis*-retinal freshly supplied to the photoreceptors from retinal pigment epithelium cells (Fig. 26–3), where vitamin A is stored in the form of all-*trans*-retinyl esters. These storage species are enzymatically converted in the pigment epithelium to 11-*cis*-retinal, which is transported across the interphotoreceptor matrix to photoreceptors. The metabolism and transport of retinoids in the eye are discussed later in this chapter.

Regulation of Cell Proliferation and Differentiation by Retinoic Acids

Retinoids have profound effects on the differentiation and growth of a variety of normal and neoplastically transformed cells (Gudas, 1994). One striking example of these effects is the differentiation pattern of cells originating from human promyelocytic leukemia HL-60 cells. These cells differentiate into macrophages when treated with 1,25-dihydroxyvitamin D_3 or with phorbol esters. In contrast, when treated with retinoic acid, HL-60 cells differentiate into granulocytes, followed by an arrest in cell proliferation (Breitman et al., 1980). Other examples include retinoic acid–induced inhibition of the differentiation of fibroblasts into adipocytes and enhancement of differentiation in neuronal cells. Retinoids have also been shown to control the formation of particular patterns, such as digit development during embryogenesis (Hofman and Eichele, 1994). In addition, studies in isolated cells, in animal models, and in human subjects have demonstrated that retinoids can inhibit the process of carcinogenesis and, in some cases, induce transformed cells to revert to the normal phenotype. This last point is well exemplified by the successful treatment of human acute promyelocytic leukemia with retinoic acid (Warrel et al., 1993).

Many of the effects of retinoids on cells are due to the ability of retinoic acid, a vitamin A metabolite, to modulate the expression of a variety of genes that encode for many types of proteins, including growth factors, transcription factors, enzymes, extracellular matrix proteins, proto-oncogenes, and binding proteins. Retinoic acid thus regulates a complex array of metabolic pathways and cellular responses.

Retinoid Nuclear Receptors

The mechanisms underlying the influence of retinoic acid on transcription have become increasingly clear following the identification

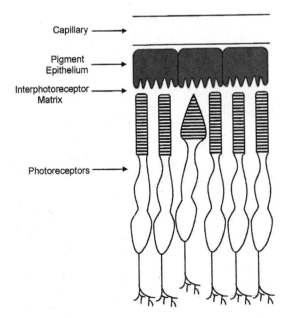

Figure 26–3. Schematic drawing of cells in the retina that are active in utilization and metabolism of retinoids.

of transcription factors that are specifically activated by retinoids. These transcription factors bind to DNA recognition sequences (also called retinoic acid response elements, RARE) in the promoter region of target genes and, upon binding of retinoic acid, activate or repress transcription of these genes (Chambon, 1994; Giguère, 1994; Glass, 1994). Retinoid receptors, which have a molecular weight of about 50 kDa, share a structural similarity with a superfamily of nuclear hormone receptors that are responsive to small hydrophobic ligands such as 1,25-dihydroxyvitamin D_3, thyroid, and steroid hormones. Like the other proteins of this superfamily, retinoid receptors are composed of several functional domains (Fig. 26–4). The N-terminal region of the receptor (A/B domain) is responsible for the basal, i.e., the ligand-independent, activation function. The DNA-binding domain (domain C) contains zinc-finger motifs responsible for the association of the receptor with DNA (see Chapter 32 and Fig. 32–5 for more information on the role of zinc-finger motifs in DNA-binding by proteins). Domain D, known as the hinge region, confers flexibility to the protein molecule. Domain E, termed the ligand-binding domain, contains the ligand-binding pocket and is responsible for the ligand-induced activation function of the receptor. This domain also contains regions that are responsible for protein-protein interactions by retinoid receptors (see later). The C-terminal region of retinoid receptors is termed F and comprises the AF-2 domain, which serves for ligand-dependent association of the receptor with transcriptional co-regulators (Glass et al., 1997).

Two classes of retinoid nuclear receptors, the retinoic acid receptors (RARs) and the retinoid X receptors (RXRs), and several subtypes of each, have been identified to date. The main physiological ligand for RARs is all-*trans*-retinoic acid. Other retinoids that have been reported to bind to and activate RARs include the 4-oxo-derivative of retinoic acid (Pijnappel et al., 1993). RXRs can bind and are activated by the 9-*cis* isomer of retinoic acid, a ligand that can also associate with RARs. However, although 9-*cis*-retinoic acid is a potent activator of RXRs, the metabolic pathway by which 9-*cis*-retinoic acid might be synthesized has not been identified, and 9-*cis*-retinoic acid has not always been detected when tissues have been analyzed for retinoids. Thus, it is unclear at present whether 9-*cis*-retinoic acid is the true physiological ligand of RXRs, and it is possible that a yet unidentified retinoid or a structurally related compound serves as the ligand for these receptors in vivo.

Like other members of the hormone nuclear receptors, RAR and RXR bind to their DNA response elements as dimers. Dimerization, which is strengthened by strong interactions between the ligand-binding domains and by weaker interactions between the DNA-

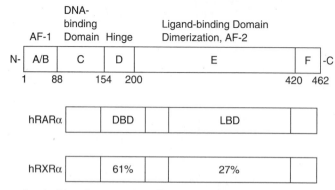

Figure 26–4. *Structure of retinoid nuclear receptors. The amino acid sequence of the hRARα1 is represented by bars and residue numbers (Leid et al., 1992). The receptor is composed of five domains. These include the N-terminal domain, A/B, which contains a basal transactivation function; domain C, which is the DNA-binding region and also participates in dimerization; domain D, which is a hinge region; and domain E, which contains the ligand-binding and dimerization functions. Domain E is also important for ligand-dependent transcriptional activation. The carboxyl terminal domain F serves to link the receptor to transcriptional co-regulator proteins. Homology between the DNA-binding domain and the ligand-binding domains of RARα and RXRα is shown.*

binding domains of the two monomers, serves to increase the specificity of binding of receptors to particular DNA sequences as well as the strength of their interactions with response elements. Mirroring dimer formation by the proteins, DNA response elements for retinoid receptors are usually arranged as two repeats of the same hexameric nucleotide sequence. RXR can bind to DNA and influence rates of transcription of target genes as a homodimer (RXR-RXR). In contrast, RAR homodimers do not readily form. Instead, RAR associates with RXR with a high affinity to form heterodimers, and these heterodimers (i.e., RXR-RAR) are believed to serve as the transcriptionally active species of RAR.

In addition to heterodimerization with RAR, RXRs can also interact with other members of the hormone receptor family; they can form heterodimers with the vitamin D_3 receptor (VDR), with the thyroid hormone receptor (TR), with the peroxisome proliferator-activated receptor (PPAR), which is a nuclear receptor that is activated by long-chain fatty acids and some of their metabolites, and with LXR, which is a receptor that responds to cholesterol. (See Chapters 27 and 15 for more information about transcriptional control by vitamin D and fatty acids, respectively.) RXR has also been reported to form active heterodimers with a few nuclear receptors termed orphan receptors—i.e., proteins that belong to the superfamily of nuclear receptors but for which the ligand is unknown.

Heterodimers of RXR with other nuclear receptors potentially can be responsive to the individual ligands of the two partners, or, in some cases, heterodimerization with RXR may suppress the responsiveness to the partner's ligand. The interactions of RXRs with other members of the hormone receptor superfamily may result in either activation or inhibition of transcription of particular target genes in response to more than one type of ligand. Thus, RXRs seem to function as "master regulators" of several signaling nutrients and hormones as they converge to regulate gene transcription (Fig. 26–5).

Activation of gene transcription by retinoid receptors critically depends on binding of retinoids to these proteins. Recently, the functions of ligand-binding for the activities of the recep-

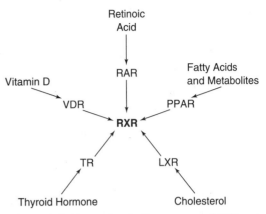

Figure 26–5. *Heterodimerization partners of RXR and their respective ligands.*

tors began to become clear. Binding of ligands to RAR and RXR allows the receptors to associate with accessory proteins that serve as co-activators (Horwitz et al., 1996). It has also been reported that binding of retinoic acid to RAR results in the release of a factor that associates with the unliganded receptor and acts as a co-repressor (Kurokawa et al., 1995; Chen and Evans, 1995; Hörlein et al., 1995). The co-repressor does not associate with RXR, suggesting that ligand-dependent activation of RXR might operate via a different mechanism. Indeed, it was demonstrated that the RXR exists as a tetramer and that binding of 9-*cis*-retinoic acid results in rapid dissociation of protein tetramers to the active species—dimers and monomers (Kersten et al., 1995a–1995c). Ligand-induced dissociation of RXR tetramers thus seems to be the initial step in transcriptional activation mediated by this receptor.

Other Retinoids

In addition to retinal and retinoic acid, other retinoids have been shown to be endogenously present in a variety of tissues. The functions of these derivatives are not completely understood as yet but some of them have been shown to be biologically active. For example, a new class of retinoids termed *retro-retinols* has been implicated in regulating lymphocyte physiology. Vitamin A deficiency in animals and in humans is associated with impaired immune function and results in changes in mass, distribution, morphology,

CLINICAL CORRELATION

Potential Therapeutic Uses of Ligands for Retinoid Nuclear Receptors

By virtue of their ability to modulate the rate of transcription of a variety of genes, retinoids can be potent therapeutic agents. Retinoic acid and synthetic ligands that activate RAR are currently used in therapy and chemoprevention of several types of cancer, including promyelocytic leukemia and head and neck cancers. The ability of RXR to serve as a common partner for several nuclear receptors, such as RAR, VDR, TR, LXR, and PPAR, suggests that retinoid derivatives that are selective toward RXR might be useful in treating a variety of disorders. Indeed, it was recently reported that RXR-selective retinoids enhance sensitivity to insulin and decrease hypertriglyceridemia in mouse models of noninsulin-dependent diabetes and obesity (Mukherjee et al., 1997). It was suggested that this antidiabetic activity is mediated by heterodimers of RXR with PPAR. It was also reported that retinoids increase the expression of apolipoproteins A-I and A-II in a human hepatoblastoma cell line, an activity that was ascribed to RXR-RAR heterodimers (Vu-Dac et al., 1996). Because apolipoproteins A-I and A-II are found in high density lipoproteins, which are known to have a protective effect against coronary artery disease, RXR ligands potentially are of clinical use in protecting against cardiovascular disease.

and properties of lymphocytes. Lymphocyte survival and proliferation critically depend on the presence of retinol, and it has been reported that retinoic acid cannot replace retinol in supporting growth of these cells (Ross and Hammerling, 1994).

The search for the retinol metabolites that are responsible for these effects has recently led to the discovery of *retro*-retinoids, a class of compounds in which the polyene tail is rigidly attached to the β-ionone ring by a double bond, with the remaining double bonds retaining the conjugated system and extending it to the 3,4-double bond within the ring. The most potent retinoid in supporting lymphocyte growth found to date is 14-hydroxy-*retro*-retinol (14-HRR). Another endogenous retinoid with a *retro* configuration, anhydroretinol, was found to function as a competitive inhibitor of 14-HRR, thereby serving as a growth suppressor.

The mechanisms of action of *retro*-retinoids are not known at present. However, these compounds do not associate with any of the known retinoid nuclear receptors, and they seem to function by a signaling pathway distinct from that of retinoic acid. It is likely that *retro*-retinoids influence cellular function at levels other than gene transcription. In addition to immune cell growth, some other physi-

ological needs for vitamin A, such as the requirement for retinol in development of reproductive capacity, cannot be fulfilled by retinoic acid. The growth regulatory properties of *retro*-retinoids raise the possibility that they may be the retinol metabolites responsible for these actions of vitamin A.

Another biologically active retinoid is 3,4-didehydroretinol, also known as vitamin A_2. It is abundant in freshwater fish, in which its metabolite 1l-*cis*-dehydroretinal can serve as a ligand for visual pigments. In the human, 3,4-didehydroretinol was reported to accumulate in tissues of individuals with psoriasis and several other disorders of keratinization (Vahlquist and Torma, 1988). 3,4-Didehydroretinoic acid was found in chick limb buds where it can affect development, presumably by activating retinoid nuclear receptors (Thaller and Eichele, 1990). Oxidized retinoid metabolites such as 4-oxo-retinoic acid were reported to be highly active in determining the positions at which particular digits develop in early embryos and to bind avidly to RARβ (Pijnappel et al., 1993). In addition, it has been demonstrated that some proteins are modified by covalent retinoylation (Takahashi and Breitman, 1991). The addition of a retinoate moiety to proteins seems to represent a novel mechanism by which retinoids can affect cellular physiology. At present, however, the effects of retinoylation on the functions of proteins modified in this fashion are not known.

ABSORPTION, TRANSPORT, STORAGE, AND METABOLISM OF VITAMIN A AND CAROTENOIDS

Two major forms of vitamin A are present in the diet: retinyl esters that are derived from animal sources, and carotenoids, mainly β-carotene, that originate from plant food. Hydrolysis of retinyl esters and the absorption and transport of retinol and carotenoids are closely connected with systems for handling dietary lipids. Retinol and provitamin A carotenoids serve as precursors of the active forms of vitamin A, including 11-*cis*-retinal and all-*trans*-retinoic acid.

Absorption and Metabolism of Vitamin A in the Intestine

Retinyl esters are hydrolyzed in the intestinal lumen to yield free retinol and the corresponding fatty acid (Fig. 26–6). Following hydrolysis, retinol is taken up by the enterocytes. The hydrolysis of retinyl esters requires the presence of bile salts that serve to solubilize

Retinyl Ester (R = Acyl Chain)

Retinol
+
Fatty Acid

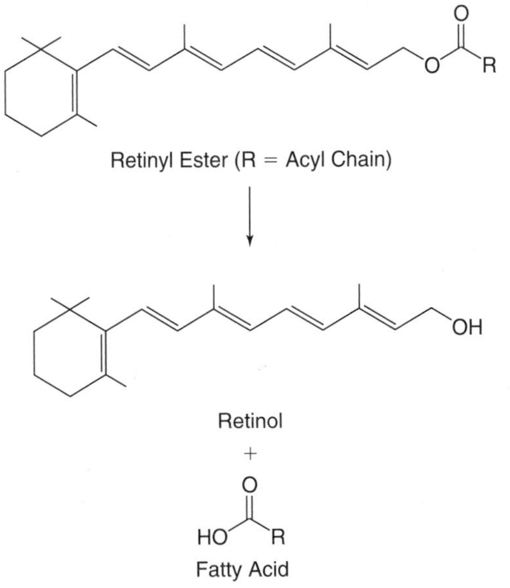

Figure 26–6. Reaction catalyzed by retinyl ester hydrolase.

them in mixed micelles and to activate the hydrolyzing enzymes. Several enzymes that are present in the intestinal lumen may be involved in the hydrolysis of dietary retinyl esters. Some of these enzymes, notably pancreatic lipase and cholesterol esterase, are secreted into the intestinal lumen from the pancreas and were shown in vitro to display retinyl ester hydrolysis activities. In addition, a retinyl ester hydrolase that is intrinsic to the brush border membrane of the small intestine has been characterized in the rat as well as in the human (Rigtrup and Ong, 1992). The different hydrolyzing enzymes are activated by different types of bile salts and have distinct substrate specificities. For example, whereas the pancreatic hydrolases are selective for short-chain retinyl esters, the brush border membrane enzyme preferentially hydrolyzes retinyl esters containing a long-chain fatty acid, such as palmitate or stearate. The brush border retinyl ester hydrolase was shown to be of greater importance in hydrolyzing dietary retinyl esters than the pancreatic enzymes.

Following hydrolysis, retinol enters the absorptive cells of the small intestine. It was recently shown that these cells preferentially take up retinol in the all-*trans* configuration and that uptake can be inhibited by the sulfhydryl reagent *N*-ethylmaleimide (Dew and Ong, 1994). These observations were interpreted to reflect the presence of a plasma membrane transporter that specifically mediates the uptake of all-*trans*-retinol from the intestinal lumen into the absorptive cells.

Intact carotenoids are absorbed by enterocytes at a lower efficiency than that for the absorption of free retinol. Following their uptake, carotenoids are cleaved to yield retinal, which is subsequently reduced to retinol (Fig. 26–7). However, the mechanisms of cleavage of carotenoids and the enzymes responsible for catalysis of these reactions have not been well characterized (Olson, 1989).

The amounts of carotenoids that can pass intact from intestinal cells into blood vary considerably among different species. In the rat, very limited amounts of carotenoids pass into the circulation. On the other hand, in the human and in the ferret, carotenoids are found intact in blood and in various other organs, such as liver and adipose tissue. The

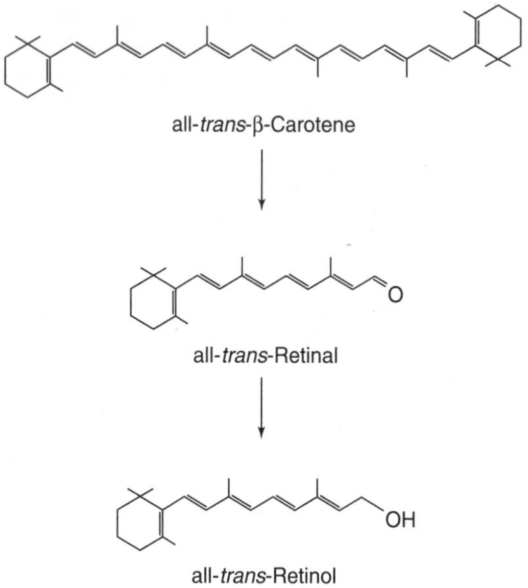

all-*trans*-β-Carotene

all-*trans*-Retinal

all-*trans*-Retinol

Figure 26–7. *Cleavage of β-carotene in intestinal epithelium.*

serum level of carotenoids reflects dietary intake, suggesting that a significant fraction of newly absorbed carotenoids is exported from enterocytes into blood without being metabolically converted within these cells.

It has been suggested that carotenoids may have function(s) other than to serve as precursors for retinol. For example, it has been shown that under some circumstances, β-carotene associated with biological membranes displays an antioxidant activity and can protect membrane lipids from damage by oxygen radicals (Pacifici and Davies, 1991). It should be noted, however, that there is no evidence to suggest that carotenoids are an essential nutrient. Much remains to be clarified regarding the metabolic fate of carotenoids and the physiological roles of these compounds.

Storage and Mobilization of Vitamin A

Storage species of vitamin A are constituted of retinyl esters in which retinol is esterified with a long-chain fatty acid. Esterification is accompanied by loss of the polar end groups of both the retinyl and the fatty acyl moieties and results in exceedingly hydrophobic species, which accumulate within lipid droplets in storage cells. Two classes of enzymes that can cata-

lyze the formation of retinyl esters have been identified (Ross, 1982; MacDonald and Ong, 1988). One of these enzymes utilizes activated fatty acids in the form of fatty acyl CoAs, as shown in Figure 26–8, and is termed acyl coenzyme A:retinol acyltransferase (ARAT).

A second type of retinol-esterifying enzyme that functions independently of the presence of exogenous fatty acyl CoAs is known as lecithin:retinol acyltransferase (LRAT). This enzyme synthesizes retinyl esters by catalyzing the *trans*-esterification of a fatty acyl moiety from the *sn*-1 position of phosphatidylcholine to retinol, as shown in Figure 26–9.

Both ARAT and LRAT are integral membrane proteins and are associated with the microsomal fractions of cells of various tissues. (Microsomes are vesicles derived from the endoplasmic reticulum when cells are disrupted; microsomal is used to describe cellular components associated with the endoplasmic reticulum.) Precise characterization of these enzymes has so far been hampered by the failure to isolate and purify them from the native membranes. It seems, however, that in some tissues the LRAT reaction catalyzes most of the retinol esterification, whereas in other tissues, esterification is catalyzed mainly by ARAT. For example, retinyl esters in plasma and in the liver mainly contain the fatty acyl moieties of palmitate and stearate regardless

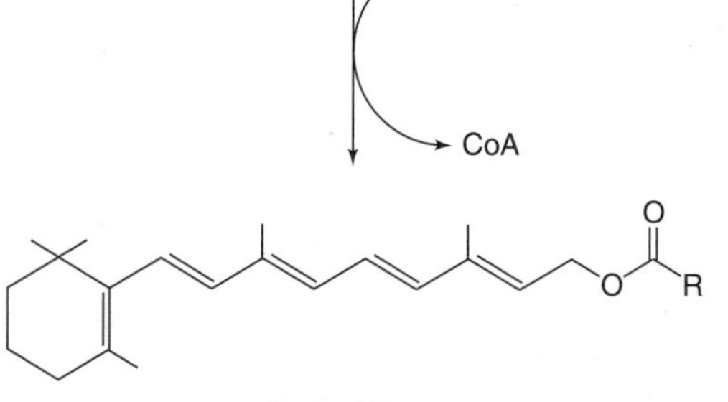

Retinol

$$R-\overset{\overset{\displaystyle O}{\|}}{C}-CoA$$

CoA

Retinyl Ester

Figure 26–8. *Reaction catalyzed by acyl CoA:retinol acyltransferase (ARAT).*

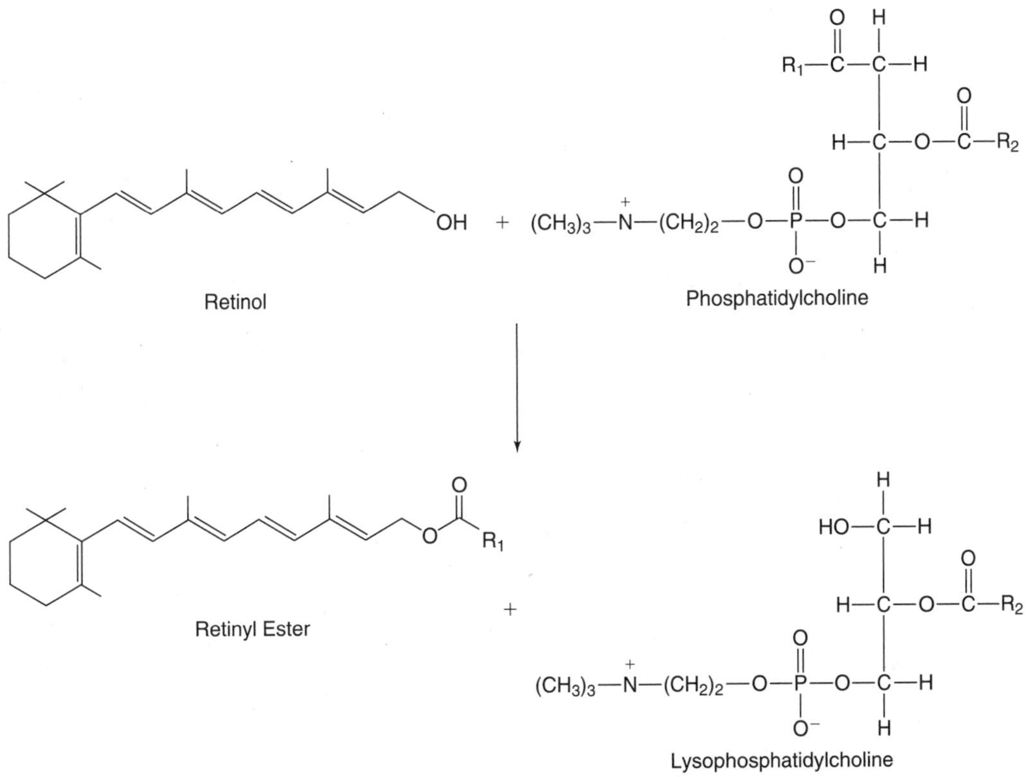

Figure 26–9. *Reaction catalyzed by lecithin:retinol acyltransferase (LRAT).*

of the composition of fatty acids in the diet. The composition of the acyl chains in retinyl esters thus corresponds to the primary species of fatty acids found in the *sn*-1 position of phosphatidylcholines, implicating LRAT as the predominant enzyme in esterification of retinol in the intestine and in liver. On the other hand, it has been reported that esterification in lactating mammary gland is catalyzed mainly by ARAT (Randolf et al., 1991).

Esterification of Retinol in the Intestine. Formation of retinyl esters is the final step of vitamin A absorption in the intestine. The retinyl esters, along with other lipids, are then packaged in chylomicrons and are secreted into the lymphatic system, which serves to deliver them to tissues for storage or use. Activities of both ARAT and LRAT have been noted in intestinal mucosa: the LRAT activity predominates, and ARAT activity significantly contributes to esterification only upon intake of large amounts of retinol.

Delivery of Retinyl Esters to the Liver. The major site of vitamin A storage in the body is the liver. Following their secretion into the lymphatic system and delivery to the blood stream, chylomicrons are processed by lipoprotein lipase. It has been reported that lipoprotein lipase of the adipocyte surface efficiently hydrolyzes retinyl esters, and it has been suggested that this activity may facilitate uptake of retinol by these cells (Blaner et al., 1994). However, a significant fraction of retinyl esters is retained in chylomicron remnants that are cleared from plasma into liver parenchymal cells by receptor-mediated endocytosis.

Hydrolysis and Re-formation of Retinyl Esters. Following uptake of retinyl esters from the circulation by hepatic parenchymal cells, vitamin A is transferred to hepatic stellate cells, where it is stored. The mechanism by which vitamin A is transported between the two cell types is not completely understood. It has been shown, however, that chylomicron retinyl esters are hydrolyzed in the parenchymal cells and that new retinyl esters are formed in the stellate cells, suggesting that

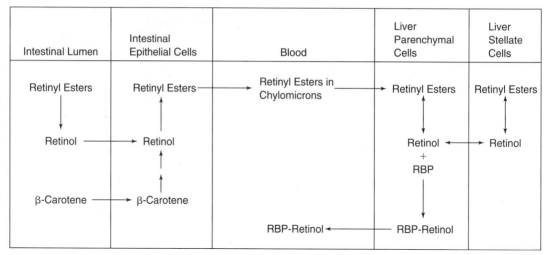

Figure 26–10. *Movement of retinol between different organs and cells involves hydrolysis and formation of retinyl esters.*

vitamin A is transported between the two cell types in the form of free retinol (Blaner and Olson, 1994, and references therein).

The distribution of retinoids between stellate and parenchymal cells has been shown in the rat to depend on the vitamin A status. Under normal dietary conditions, the main fraction of retinyl esters in the liver is found in the stellate cells, where retinyl esters accumulate in lipid droplets. In vitamin A–deficient animals, retinoids are redistributed into parenchymal cells in a process that, again, seems to involve hydrolysis of retinyl esters. Thus, absorption and mobilization of vitamin A between different tissues and cells require continuous hydrolysis and re-formation of retinyl esters (Fig. 26–10).

Several distinct enzymatic activities catalyzing the hydrolysis of retinyl esters have been described in different membrane fractions of both parenchymal and stellate cells of the liver. Some of the retinyl ester hydrolases are activated by bile salts, but the activities of others are independent of bile salts. Re-formation of retinyl esters is catalyzed in the liver by both LRAT and ARAT, with the former pathway predominating under physiological concentrations of retinol.

Though previously little appreciated, it is becoming increasingly clear that, in addition to the liver, extrahepatic tissues play an important role in the overall metabolism and storage of vitamin A. Retinoids are found in extrahepatic organs, including adipose depots, kidney, testis, lung, bone marrow, and eye. These tissues contain significant amounts of retinol and retinyl esters and display esterification as well as retinyl ester hydrolase activities (Blaner and Olson, 1994).

Synthesis of Retinal and Retinoic Acid from Retinol

In analogy with the metabolism of ethanol, retinol can be metabolically converted to the corresponding aldehyde, retinal. Using the same analogy, it is also believed that the corresponding carboxylic acid, retinoic acid, is produced by further oxidation of retinal. As is detailed later, some progress has been made in recent years in identifying the enzymes involved in these reactions. However, in general, it is still not completely clear whether the oxidation of retinol and retinal in vivo is catalyzed by known enzymes with broad specificity for alcohols and aldehydes, or by different enzymes with a narrow selectivity for retinoids.

Conversion to retinal entails the dehydrogenation of retinol and depends on the availability of electron acceptors such as NAD^+ or $NADP^+$. It is known that liver alcohol dehydrogenase, an NAD^+-dependent soluble enzyme with a broad specificity for a variety of alcohols, can catalyze the transformation of retinol to retinal. A different, membrane-bound enzyme termed retinol dehydrogenase, which requires NADP[+], has been identified in liver microsomes and recently has been partially purified and cloned (Chai et al., 1995). In contrast with soluble alcohol dehydrogenases, retinol dehydrogenase is able to metabolize retinol bound to the cellular retinol-binding protein CRBP. It is thus currently believed that retinal formation in vivo occurs mainly by the microsomal retinol dehydrogenase via an NADP[+]-dependent process. Multiple enzymatic activities catalyzing the conversion of retinal to retinoic acid have been observed in the cytosol of various cells (for review, see Blaner and Olson, 1994). Some of these activities were shown to require NAD[+] and thus to reflect the presence of an aldehyde dehydrogenase. In other cases, the conversion is stimulated by NADP[+], which suggests the presence of another enzyme activity.

Other potential pathways for formation of retinoic acid include oxidation of retinal by microsomal cytochrome P450, and direct production by cleavage of β-carotene in a process that might not involve retinol or retinal as intermediates. Retinoic acid is also found in plasma at a concentration on the order of 10 nmol/L, and circulating retinoic acid originating from dietary intake may be an important source of retinoic acid in cells.

Metabolism of Retinoic Acid

Retinoic acid is converted in vivo into several metabolites. The functional significance of these metabolites is not completely understood.

Retinoic Acid Isomers. The most stable isomer of retinoic acid and the predominant species of this compound in vivo is the all-*trans* form. Another isomer, 13-*cis*-retinoic acid, has been reported to be present in blood and in the small intestine. This isomer comprises a significant fraction of retinoic acid at equilibrium and may be present in vivo as a result of nonspecific isomerization. As discussed earlier, another isomer, 9-*cis*-retinoic acid, can bind to nuclear retinoic acid receptors with high affinity and is a powerful modulator of gene transcription. However, the presence of this isomer in vivo has been difficult to demonstrate, and no enzymatic activity that catalyzes the formation of 9-*cis*-retinoic acid has been identified to date.

Polar and Oxidized Metabolites of Retinoids. Several types of polar metabolites of retinoids are formed by the action of "detoxifying" enzymes, which catalyze the conjugation of polar groups onto hydrophobic substrates, thereby enhancing the solubility of the substrate.

Retinoid β-glucuronides are synthesized from either retinoic acid or from retinol in a variety of tissues, including liver, kidney, and intestine. These compounds are also found in blood at concentrations that are comparable to those of retinoic acid. Retinyl and retinoyl glucuronides are formed by microsomal UDP-glucuronyl transferases, which catalyze the conjugation of glucuronic acid to retinol and retinoic acid, respectively. Retinoyl β-glucuronide can be hydrolyzed to yield retinoic acid, a reaction that is catalyzed by lysosomal β-glucuronidase. Retinoyl β-glucuronide has been shown to act as a competent inducer of cell differentiation (Zile et al., 1987), but it does not bind to retinoid nuclear receptors and its mechanisms of action are not known.

Retinoic acid, retinol, and retinal can be metabolized by several forms of the microsomal cytochrome P450 system. The cytochrome P450 reactions, which require NADPH and molecular oxygen, convert these substrates to multiple oxidized metabolites that are found in various tissues, including blood, the small intestine, and the liver. The various endogenously oxidized retinoids have been considered until recently to represent intermediates in retinoid degradation pathways. However, recent observations indicated that some oxidized retinoids, such as the 4-oxo-derivative of retinoic acid, can bind to retinoid nuclear receptors and are highly active in differentiation (Pijnappel et al., 1993; Nikawa et al., 1995). Oxidized retinoid metabolites may thus be directly involved in affecting cellular physiology.

Synthesis of *retro*-Retinoids

As discussed in "Other Retinoids" under Physiological Functions of Vitamin A, it has been suggested that *retro*-derivatives of retinol influence cellular function by a signaling pathway distinct from the activity of retinoic acid. An enzyme that can catalyze the synthesis of the *retro*-retinol growth suppressor anhydroretinol has been identified in the cytosol of insect cells and was named retinol dehydratase (Grün et al., 1995). This enzyme requires the presence of the cofactor 3′-phosphoadenosine 5′-phosphosulfate (PAPS) to catalyze the conversion of retinol to anhydroretinol. Retinol dehydratase shows a homology to a family of enzymes termed sulfotransferases, which participate in signaling pathways by catalyzing the sulfation of a variety of molecules, such as steroid and thyroid hormones and monoamine neurotransmitters. It was hence suggested that a sulfated intermediate is involved in the synthesis of anhydroretinol catalyzed by retinol dehydratase. Retinol dehydratase displays an unusually high affinity for retinol, a property that allows it to efficiently metabolize retinol dissolved in cytosol despite the low physiological concentrations of this hydrophobic substrate in aqueous phases. To date, no mammalian homologue for the insect retinol dehydratase has been identified.

Metabolism of 11-*cis*-Retinoids in the Eye

Synthesis of Retinyl Esters in Retinal Pigment Epithelium. The main vitamin A form that circulates in blood is all-*trans*-retinol. This species is taken up into the eye by retinal pigment epithelium (RPE) (see Fig. 26–3). Retinal pigment epithelium cells contain an unusually high level of enzymatic activity that can convert retinol to retinyl esters. The esterification activity is catalyzed by LRAT and results in formation of all-*trans*-retinyl esters that serve as storage species, as well as precursors for 11-*cis*-retinoids that participate in the visual cycle. LRAT of the RPE cells displays a broad substrate specificity and in the presence of 11-*cis*-retinol can form 11-*cis*-retinyl ester. High levels of these esters have been shown to accumulate in RPE cells in the dark (Sarri, 1994).

Formation of 11-*cis*-Retinoids in Retinal Pigment Epithelium. The reaction by which

all-*trans* retinoids are converted to the 11-*cis* configuration in the eye is a critical part of the visual cycle. This reaction is catalyzed by an isomerase found in RPE microsomal fractions, which is termed all-*trans*-retinyl ester isomerohydrolase. This enzyme utilizes the energy stored in the ester bond of all-*trans*-retinyl esters to produce the 11-*cis* species, as illustrated in Figure 26–11. Retinyl ester hydrolysis is thus coupled with an isomerization reaction to produce 11-*cis*-retinol (Canada et al., 1990).

In RPE cells, 11-*cis*-retinol can also be produced by hydrolysis of 11-*cis*-retinyl esters, a reaction that is catalyzed by a microsomal retinyl ester hydrolase. This enzyme can also hydrolyze retinyl esters in the all-*trans* configuration, but it displays a significantly higher specific activity with the 11-*cis* substrates (Blaner et al., 1987).

The retinoid that supports visual function, 11-*cis*-retinal, is formed by oxidation of 11-*cis*-retinol via a reaction catalyzed by an RPE microsomal 11-*cis*-retinol dehydrogenase. Unlike the liver retinol dehydrogenase, 11-*cis*-retinol dehydrogenase of RPE does not show a significant preference for NAD^+ or $NADP^+$ and can utilize them equally well as electron acceptors. 11-*cis*-Retinol dehydrogenase can also catalyze the reverse reaction, i.e., the reduction of 11-*cis*-retinal to 11-*cis*-retinol, but it is not known whether the reverse reaction is important in vivo. Following its formation, 11-*cis*-retinal is exported from RPE to photorecep-

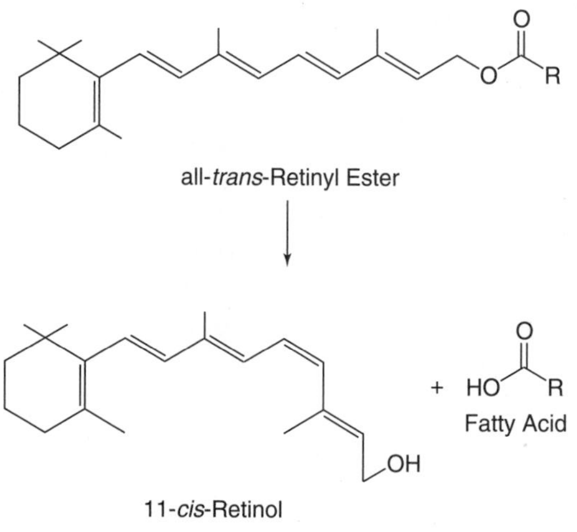

Figure 26–11. *Reaction catalyzed by all-*trans*-retinyl ester isomerohydrolase.*

tor cells, where it serves to regenerate bleached rhodopsin.

Metabolism of Retinal in Photoreceptor Cells. The absorption of a photon by rhodopsin in photoreceptor cells leads to isomerization of rhodopsin-bound 11-*cis*-retinal to the all-*trans* configuration of this retinoid. Photoisomerization initiates visual transduction and is followed by the hydrolysis of the retinal-rhodopsin complex. Free all-*trans*-retinal is then converted by a retinol dehydrogenase to yield all-*trans*-retinol. Thus, the eye contains two types of retinol dehydrogenase activities, one that is located in RPE and is specific for 11-*cis*-retinoids, and a second dehydrogenase that exists in photoreceptor cells and shows specificity for all-*trans*-retinal (Saari, 1994). The preferred reductant for the latter enzyme is NADPH. All-*trans*-retinol produced in photoreceptor cells is transported to the RPE, where it can be converted back to 11-*cis*-retinal. The major metabolic conversions of retinoids in photoreceptor and pigment epithelium cells are shown in Figure 26–12.

RETINOID-BINDING PROTEINS AND TRANSPORT OF RETINOIDS

Due to its amphipathic nature and its poor solubility in water, vitamin A efficiently dissolves in the hydrophobic core of cellular membranes. However, the presence of excess vitamin A in membranes results in disruption of membrane structure and function. In addition, in order to reach their target cells and their sites of action inside cells, retinoids must traverse the oxygen-rich aqueous spaces of plasma and cytosol. Hence, in considering the physiology of vitamin A, it is important to understand how the poorly soluble retinoids are transported through aqueous spaces without loss of structural integrity, and how their concentrations in cellular membranes are retained below membranolytic levels. Partial answers to these questions were provided by the identification of water-soluble proteins that bind physiologically important retinoids. Several retinoid-binding proteins that specifically bind different vitamin A derivatives exist both in the cytosol of cells and in specialized extracellular spaces such as plasma and the interphotoreceptor matrix in the eye (Table 26–1). Thus, in vivo, retinoids are mainly found associated with specific binding proteins. The interactions of retinoids with these proteins retard their degradation, decrease their concentrations in membranes, and increase their concentrations in aqueous spaces.

Retinol-Binding Protein and Transport of Retinol in Blood

Retinol circulates in blood bound to a plasma protein named retinol-binding protein (RBP). This protein is a single polypeptide with a molecular mass of 21 kDa that contains one

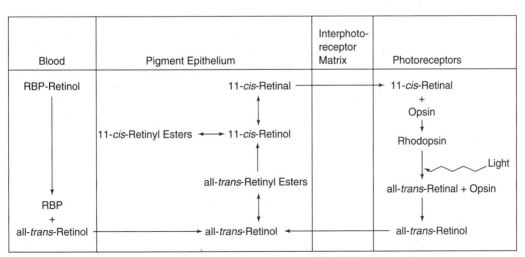

Figure 26–12. Major metabolic conversions of retinoids in the retina.

TABLE 26–1
Retinoid-Binding Proteins

	Molecular Mass (kDa)	Major Ligand(s)	Major Location
Retinol-binding protein (RBP)	21.2	all-*trans*-retinol	Blood
Cellular retinol-binding protein (CRBP)	15.7	all-*trans*-retinol all-*trans*-retinal	Most tissues
Cellular retinol-binding protein II (CRBPII)	15.6	all-*trans*-retinol all-*trans*-retinal	Small intestine, fetal liver
Cellular retinoic acid–binding protein (CRABP)	15.5	all-*trans*-retinoic acid	Most tissues
Cellular retinoic acid–binding protein II (CRABPII)	15.0	all-*trans*-retinoic acid	Skin, ovary, uterus
Cellular retinal-binding protein (CRALBP)	36.0	11-*cis*-retinal 11-*cis*-retinol	Retina
Interphotoreceptor retinoid-binding protein (IRBP)	136.0	11-*cis*-retinal all-*trans*-retinol	Interphotoreceptor matrix

binding site for retinol. The main site of synthesis and secretion of this protein is the liver, which is also the main storage site for vitamin A in the body. Secretion of RBP from the liver is tightly regulated by the availability of retinol (Soprano and Blaner, 1994). In vitamin A deficiency, RBP secretion is inhibited, and the protein accumulates in endoplasmic reticulum. In the presence of retinol, RBP associates with retinol, moves to the Golgi apparatus, and is secreted into blood in the form of the holoprotein. Some extrahepatic tissues, including adipose tissue, kidney, testis, brain, and the digestive tract, were found to synthesize and secrete RBP or to contain mRNA for this protein. It is interesting that it was recently shown that RPE cells in the eye synthesize RBP and secrete it, not into the blood but toward the retina, into the interphotoreceptor matrix (Ong et al, 1994a). These findings indicate that RBP may serve as a carrier protein for retinol in compartments other than plasma.

In plasma, RBP is bound to another protein called transthyretin (TTR), which has a molecular weight of 56 kDa. In addition to associating with RBP, TTR functions as a carrier for thyroid hormones in blood. It is believed that binding of RBP to TTR serves to prevent the loss of the smaller protein (RBP) from the circulation by filtration in the glomeruli. Though TTR is a tetrameric protein composed of four equivalent subunits, it is usually found bound to only one molecule of RBP.

Hence, the protein complex responsible for the plasma transport of retinol is composed of TTR-RBP-retinol at molar ratios of 1:1:1. The concentration of this complex in plasma is kept constant at 1 to 2 μmol/L except in extreme cases of vitamin A deficiency or in disease states.

The retinol-binding site of RBP is a hydrophobic β-barrel that encapsulates the retinol molecule so that the β-ionone ring is buried deep in the barrel, the isoprene chain stretches along the barrel axis, and the hydroxyl end group lies almost at the surface of the protein (Newcomer et al., 1984). Because most physiologically important retinoids differ from retinol only by the composition of their end group, the structure of the RBP-binding site suggests that it may bind other retinoids. Indeed, RBP displays a broad specificity for retinoids. However, in the presence of ligands with polar end groups larger than a hydroxyl, such as the carboxyl group of retinoic acid, the interactions of RBP with TTR are hindered. Consequently, the only retinoid that is found to be associated with RBP in plasma is retinol. In contrast, retinoic acid circulates in plasma bound to serum albumin.

Dissociation of Retinol from Retinol-Binding Protein Prior to Entry into Target Cells

The tight interaction of retinol with the TTR-RBP complex allows this poorly soluble vitamin to circulate in the aqueous plasma. However, target tissues for vitamin A, except perhaps the liver, do not take up the protein complex. Hence, in order to reach the interior of cells, retinol must dissociate from the plasma-binding proteins prior to uptake. There are currently two opposing views of how this process is accomplished.

It has been proposed that a specific receptor for RBP exists in the plasma membranes of target cells. This receptor is postulated to recognize and bind circulating RBP, and to mediate the release of retinol from the protein and its transfer across the plasma membrane to the cytosol. This hypothesis is based on the observations that uptake of radiolabeled retinol by some cells can be inhibited in the presence of RBP complexed with nonlabeled retinol, that plasma membranes of some target cells seem to possess RBP-binding activity, and that a protein that specifically binds RBP has been identified in the eye's RPE cells (e.g., see Bavik et al., 1991; Shingleton et al., 1989). However, it is unknown whether this protein indeed plays a role in retinol uptake or transport.

In contrast, it has been pointed out that because the association of retinol with RBP is reversible, the ligand can spontaneously dissociate from the protein. Because of the hydrophobic nature of retinol, it can also spontaneously associate with cellular membranes. Thus, there might not be a need to postulate the existence of specialized receptors to facilitate the dissociation of the RBP-retinol complex or the movement of retinol across membranes. The measured rates by which retinol spontaneously dissociates from the TTR-RBP complex and traverses membranes were found to be faster than the rates by which retinol is taken up by several target cells, suggesting that the rate of uptake is not limited by the rate of release of retinol from RBP or by events at the plasma membrane (Fex and Johannesson, 1987; Noy and Xu, 1990). It was thus proposed that retinol spontaneously and rapidly equilibrates between binding proteins in plasma and in cytosol, and that the rate of uptake is regulated by the rate of retinol metabolism. This hypothesis is supported by several studies that have failed to detect any RBP-binding activities in plasma membranes

of cells, and by the observations that the uptake of retinol from RBP into target cells proceeded rapidly and did not seem to be a saturable process (Soprano and Blaner, 1994).

Cellular Retinoid-Binding Proteins and Intracellular Retinoid Transport and Metabolism

Multiple types of retinoid-binding proteins exist within cells (see Table 26–1). The nomenclature of these proteins is based on the physiological vitamin A derivative that serves as their main ligand. Cellular proteins that bind retinol, retinal, and retinoic acid have been identified. In addition, the interphotoreceptor matrix, which is the extracellular space between the photoreceptors and RPE cells in the eye (see Fig. 26–3), contains a carrier protein that displays a broad specificity for retinoids. Cellular retinoid-binding proteins are highly conserved across species that are known to utilize vitamin A, implying that they play critical roles in the biology of retinoids. A growing body of evidence indicates that these proteins play multiple roles in retinoid transport and metabolism.

In general, the association of retinoids with cellular binding proteins protects these labile compounds from rapid degradation in aqueous spaces. Binding to proteins also acts to solubilize retinoids in cytosol and to decrease their levels in cellular membranes, thereby protecting the membranes from retinoid-induced lysis. In addition, recent evidence suggests that some cellular retinoid-binding proteins may be involved in retinoid metabolism by directly regulating the activity of enzymes.

Cellular Retinol-Binding Proteins (CRBPs). Two types of cellular retinol-binding proteins—CRBP and CRBPII—have been identified. These proteins have molecular masses of about 15.5 kDa, and they belong to a family of small proteins that bind lipophilic ligands such as retinoids and long-chain fatty acids. CRBP is present in many tissues, including liver, kidney, ovary, testis, lung, eye, spleen, and the small intestine. CRBPII is found almost exclusively in the mucosal epithelium of the small intestine (Ong et al., 1994b). Though they are named for their interactions with retinol, both CRBP and CRBPII also bind retinal. The affinity of CRBP for retinol was reported to be significantly stronger as compared with CRBPII (Li et al., 1991). In contrast, CRBP and CRBPII bind retinal with a similar affinity. The characteristic organ and cellular distribution of the two proteins and their differential affinity for retinol suggest that they play distinct roles in the physiology of vitamin A, but it is believed that both proteins participate in transport and in metabolism of retinol and retinal.

When considering the mechanisms by which retinol-binding proteins may regulate retinoid transport, an important question is whether they play a passive role, or whether they actively mobilize their ligands from one location to another within cells. It has been proposed that the CRBPs participate in the intracellular transport of retinol by extracting retinol directly from the cell surface receptor for RBP. In this scenario, retinol will transfer from the binding site on RBP in blood to the RBP receptor, which will then mediate its transport across the plasma membrane directly to CRBP. Though no experimental evidence for this model exists, it is attractive because it allows for a transport process in which retinol is never exposed to the aqueous phase. In contrast, it has been suggested that CRBP acts as a passive storage compartment in cytosol, and that the protein binds and releases retinol according to concentration gradients of the ligand. In this model, retinol will spontaneously dissociate from RBP and enter its target cell. Once inside the cell, it will bind to CRBP owing to its high affinity for this protein. According to this model, retinol will move from blood into cells as long as CRBP in cytosol is not fully saturated (Noy and Blaner, 1991). Uptake of retinol by particular cells may thus be regulated either by changes in the intracellular concentration of CRBP, or by changes in the rate of metabolism of this ligand. Higher rates of conversion of retinol to metabolites will cause depletion of retinol from intracellular CRBP and will increase the availability of apo-CRBP, which will draw more retinol from the blood into the cell.

CRBP and CRBPII were shown to play important roles in the metabolism of their ligands by protecting them from the activity of some enzymes while allowing them to be metabolized by others. For example, in the intestine, free retinal is efficiently reduced to retinol by a soluble retinol dehydrogenase, but the reaction is inhibited when the substrate is presented to the enzyme bound to CRBPII. In contrast, an intestinal microsomal enzyme can reduce retinal in both the absence and the presence of the binding protein (Kakkad and Ong, 1988). Similarly, esterification of retinol by ARAT of the small intestine is inhibited in the presence of CRBPII, but intestinal LRAT can metabolize both free and CRBPII-bound retinol (Herr and Ong, 1992). Because of the high level of CRBPII in the intestine, most of the retinol in these cells will be bound to CRBPII. The findings of the latter study thus provide an explanation for the predominance of the LRAT-catalyzed over the ARAT-catalyzed reaction in formation of retinyl esters in small intestine.

It was also reported that liver microsomal LRAT can metabolize both free and CRBP-bound retinol, and that this enzyme is inhibited by the addition of apo-CRBP (Herr and Ong, 1992). In contrast, apo-CRBP was found to be an activator of the liver retinyl ester hydrolase (Boerman and Napoli, 1991). The observation that apo-CRBP inhibits the LRAT reaction but activates the hydrolase suggests that the ratio of apo-/holo-CRBP in the liver regulates the homeostasis of retinyl ester formation and hydrolysis. When the concentration of retinol, and thus the level of holo-CRBP, is high, retinyl ester formation will proceed at a fast rate. Conversely, when the availability of retinol decreases, apo-CRBP levels will increase, leading to a lower rate of retinal esterification and an enhanced rate of retinyl ester hydrolysis. Other studies suggested that CRBP can also affect the oxidation of retinol to retinal and the further metabolism of retinal to retinoic acid (Posch et al., 1992).

The mechanisms by which retinol-binding proteins regulate the kinetic properties of enzymes are not clear at present. One question that arises regarding this issue relates to the availability of CRBP-bound ligands to the active sites of enzymes. This question is especially intriguing as retinol is bound to CRBP with the polar end group buried deeply inside the binding pocket (Cowan et al., 1993); it is difficult to envision how any enzyme could gain access to the ligand's end group in such a location. It has been suggested, in regard to this, that protein-protein interactions between the binding protein and specific enzymes may result in movement of the CRBP region that covers the binding site, allowing direct diffusion of retinol into the enzyme's active site (Jamison et al., 1994).

Cellular Retinoic Acid–Binding Proteins (CRABPs).

Two forms of cellular retinoic acid–binding protein, CRABP and CRABPII, have been characterized. These proteins belong to the same family of binding proteins that also includes the CRBPs, and they show a high specificity for retinoic acid. CRABP has been detected in retina and adrenal gland and in reproductive tissues of both male and female animals. CRABPII was found in skin, ovary, and uterus. It is believed that, as with the function of CRBPs, CRABPs participate in transport, metabolism, and sequestration of their ligand. For example, overexpression of CRABP in F9 teratocarcinoma cells diminished the responsiveness of these cells to retinoic acid, suggesting that binding to CRABP decreases the availability of the ligand to its sites of action in the nucleus (Boylan and Gudas, 1991). CRABP may also influence the activities of enzymes that catalyze the metabolism of retinoic acid to polar metabolites (Ong et al., 1994b).

Cellular Retinal-Binding Protein (CRALBP).

The eye and the pineal gland contain a binding protein that is highly specific toward the 11-*cis* isomers of retinal and retinol. CRALBP, which has a molecular mass of about 36 kDa, is not structurally related to CRBPs or CRABPs. The location of CRALBP in the retina and its specificity toward retinoids that function in vision suggest, however, that its roles are similar to those of the retinoid-binding proteins discussed earlier—i.e., that it functions in transport and metabolism of 11-*cis*-retinoids. Indeed, it has been shown that CRALBP can influence the metabolic fate of 11-*cis*-retinol in pigment epithelium cells (Saari et al., 1994). In these cells, 11-*cis*-retinol either can

be oxidized by retinol dehydrogenase to 11-*cis*-retinal and exported to photoreceptor cells for regeneration of rhodopsin or can be esterified by LRAT to form 11-*cis*-retinyl esters (see Fig. 26–12). The presence of CRALBP was found to inhibit the esterification reaction, most likely as a result of sequestration of 11-*cis*-retinol by the protein. In contrast, CRALBP stimulated the reaction catalyzed by 11-*cis*-retinol dehydrogenase, suggesting that direct interactions exist between the binding protein and this enzyme.

Interphotoreceptor Retinoid-Binding Protein (IRBP).

Regeneration of active visual pigments in the eye requires a continuous flux of 11-*cis*-retinal from RPE to photoreceptor cells. Absorption of light by rhodopsin results in conversion of the visual chromophore to all-*trans*-retinol, which is transported back to the RPE for re-isomerization and oxidation (see Fig. 26–12). Thus, the visual cycle includes continuous shuttling of retinoids between photoreceptor and RPE cells via the aqueous space of the interphotoreceptor matrix, which separates the two cell types. The low solubility of retinoids in water and the physiological requirement for their rapid transfer across an aqueous space raise questions regarding the mechanism by which the transport is accomplished.

The main soluble protein component of the interphotoreceptor matrix (IPM) is a highly glycosylated protein, with a molecular mass of 136 kDa, which binds retinoids and other hydrophobic ligands such as long-chain fatty acids. It is believed that this protein, termed the interphotoreceptor retinoid-binding protein (IRBP), serves as a carrier for retinoids between photoreceptor and RPE cells. In contrast with other known retinoid-binding proteins, IRBP possesses three distinct sites for retinoid binding (Chen et al., 1993, 1996). This protein can bind a variety of retinoids but displays a higher binding affinity for retinal in the 11-*cis* configuration and for retinol in the all-*trans* configuration. Thus, the ligand specificity of IRBP corresponds to the physiological need to transport these two particular retinoids across the IPM. Participation of IRBP in shuttling of retinoids in the IPM has also been implied by the observations that the composition of retinoids associated with the protein in the IPM is modulated by light, and that binding of retinoids to IRBP stabilizes them against degradation. It was also reported that IRBP can take up 11-*cis*-retinal from RPE, and that it can efficiently deliver 11-*cis*-retinal to bleached rod outer segments (Saari, 1994; Pepperberg et al., 1993).

However, the exact role of IRBP in the transport process is not known. Theoretically, IRBP could serve simply as a storage compartment for retinoids in the IPM, with the ability to bind and release these ligands according to their concentration gradients. Alternatively, IRBP could function to selectively target specific retinoids to particular locations in the eye by a yet unidentified mechanism. It has been reported that the polyunsaturated fatty acid docosahexaenoic acid (DHA) specifically inhibits binding of the visual chromophore 11-*cis*-retinal to one of the IRBP retinoid-binding sites. DHA is an ω3 fatty acid that comprises about 50% of the acyl chains of phospholipids in photoreceptor cells. Thus, the interrelationships between binding of retinoids and DHA by IRBP may allow IRBP to specifically facilitate movement of 11-*cis*-retinal to photoreceptor cells. More specifically, it was proposed that while IRBP is in the vicinity of the RPE, where the concentration of DHA is low, it will possess a high affinity for 11-*cis*-retinal and associate with it. Movement to the vicinity of photoreceptor cells will expose IRBP to high levels of DHA, resulting in rapid release of 11-*cis*-retinal from the regulated binding site (Chen et al., 1996). This and other models for the function and mechanism of action of IRBP are currently under investigation.

NUTRITIONAL CONSIDERATIONS OF VITAMIN A

The adequacy of vitamin A in the diet is of great concern in many developing countries where vitamin A deficiency is relatively common. Although vitamin A deficiency is uncommon in the United States, there is active interest in dietary vitamin A and carotenoids due to health and toxicity considerations.

Vitamin A Requirements

The current recommendations for vitamin A intake are expressed in terms of equivalents to 1 μg of retinol. Because of the lower availability of β-carotene compared with retinol and the low efficiency of conversion of β-carotene to retinol, the amount of all-*trans*-β-carotene equivalent to 1 μg of retinol was determined to be about 6 μg. In addition, 12 μg of food-derived mixed carotenes are considered equivalent to 1 μg of retinol.

Two sets of recommendations regarding daily intake of vitamin A have been put forward by Expert Committees of the Food and Agriculture Organization and the World Health Organization (FAO/WHO, 1988). Basal intake levels are considered sufficient for fulfilling physiological requirements but not for allowing for any body vitamin A reserves. The basal dietary intakes recommended by FAO/WHO are 180 μg of retinol for infants and 270 μg and 300 μg of retinol for adult women and men, respectively. Higher daily intakes of 350 μg of retinol for infants and 500 and 600 μg retinol for women and men, respectively, were recommended to ensure adequate body reserves to last about 4 months on a vitamin A–deficient diet. The Recommended Dietary Allowances (RDAs) for vitamin A in the United States are, in general, about 25% higher than the daily intakes recommended by the WHO. The RDA (National Research Council, 1989) for women (nonpregnant, nonlactating) is 800 μg of retinol equivalents, and that for men is 1000 μg. It has been cautioned, however, that the lower values may be preferable and that excessive intake of vitamin A, especially during pregnancy, should be avoided (Olson, 1987).

Vitamin A and the Maintenance of Health

A diet rich in vitamin A and carotenoids can play a protective role against several physiological abnormalities. It was reported in early studies that epithelia of vitamin A–deficient organs are histologically similar to neoplastic tissues (Wolbach and Howe, 1925), and a number of epidemiological studies have indicated that consumption of vitamin A and ca-

Food Sources of Vitamin A

Preformed retinol:
• Liver
• Whole and fortified milk
• Eggs
Carotenoids:
• Yellow-orange vegetables and fruits (carrots, sweet potato)
• Dark-green leafy vegetables (spinach, broccoli)

RDAs Across the Life Cycle

	μg retinol equivalents (RE)/day (1 μg RE = 1 μg retinol or 6 μg β-carotene)
Infants, 0–1 y	375
Children, 1–3 y	400
4–6 y	500
7–10 y	600
Males, 11+ yr	1000
Females, 11+ y	800
Pregnant	800
Lactating	1200–1300

Vitamin A in fortified foods and vitamin supplements is in the form of retinyl ester (e.g., retinyl acetate or retinyl palmitate).

From National Research Council (1989) Recommended Dietary Allowances, 10th ed. National Academy Press, Washington, D.C.

rotenoids is inversely correlated with development of several types of cancer. In addition, some studies suggested that retinoids and carotenoids can reverse precancerous oral lesions (Hong and Itri, 1994). Conclusive evidence for the efficacy of dietary preformed vitamin A or of carotenoids in prevention of cancer is still being sought. Dietary vitamin A also plays an important role in enhancing immune responses. It has been reported that even mild vitamin A deficiency can lead to impaired immune response and lymphocyte function, and that vitamin A supplementation of children with no apparent deficiency results in significant reduction in disease mortality (Gerster, 1997). Vitamin A, via its metabolite retinoic acid, is also essential for embryogenesis. Vitamin A deficiency during gestation has been shown to induce fetal malformations in animals and is likely to have similar outcomes in humans. However, specific effects of vitamin A deficiency on fetal development in humans are difficult to discern because vitamin A deficiency is usually accompanied by a general protein/energy

malnutrition. It is of interest that the malformations that have been observed in vitamin A–deficient animals are similar to those that are caused by vitamin A excess (Gerster, 1997).

Excess

Acute vitamin A toxicity has been reported to occur following consumption of polar bear and seal liver by Eskimos and Arctic explorers. Chronic toxicity can occur following routine intake of smaller, but still large, doses of vitamin A over a period of several months and has been observed following daily ingestion exceeding 15,000 μg of retinol. Higher sensitivity is observed in infants and young children, in whom toxic manifestations can occur following daily ingestion of more than 6000 μg of retinol. Both acute and chronic vitamin A toxicity are rare occurrences and are easily reversed by stopping excessive intake. A third type of vitamin A toxicity can occur following ingestion of lower doses during early pregnancy. Under these conditions, vitamin A can have teratogenic effects leading to fetal abnormalities. These effects most likely stem from the effects of the high levels of retinoic acid formed upon excessive intake of vitamin A.

Deficiency

Vitamin A deficiency is manifested by a number of symptoms, the most serious being ocular problems and depressed immune function. Vitamin A deficiency is rare in developed countries where the mean daily intake usually exceeds the RDA. However, in many developing countries in Southern and Southeastern Asia, in Africa, and in Central and South America, vitamin A deficiency is a serious nutritional problem that especially affects preschool-age children. It has been estimated that 1.5 million children worldwide are blind and that vitamin A deficiency is the cause of about 70% of these cases (Underwood, 1994). The initial signs of vitamin A deficiency are night blindness and impaired epidermal integrity manifested by hyperkeratosis. These conditions can be reversed upon supplementation of vitamin A. If left untreated, night blindness is followed by xerophthalmia, a disease associated with structural changes in the cornea.

The first visible structural change is drying of the conjunctiva and the cornea (xerosis) and the development of an opaque area called Bitot's spot. This is followed by development of keratomalacia, which involves irreversible damage to the cornea and leads to blindness (Sommer, 1982).

In addition to keratinization of the cornea, deficiency of vitamin A results in keratinization of tracheal epithelium and in thinning of the intestinal epithelium. Xerophthalmia was reported to be accompanied by upper respiratory infection and diarrhea and to be exacerbated by protein-energy malnutrition (Ganguly, 1989). Vitamin A deficiency is also associated with a lower resistance to infections and with increased mortality in young children (Sommer et al., 1983). Mortality rates in children with night blindness or Bitot's spots were reported to be three- to eight-fold greater compared with children with no visible signs of vitamin A deficiency (Sommer et al., 1983), and supplementation of vitamin A to children in vitamin A–deficient areas was shown to reduce the incidence of mortality significantly (Underwood, 1994). The increased susceptibility to infection associated

---

LIFE CYCLE CONSIDERATION

Vitamin A Supplements in Pregnancy

Studies in animals have shown that retinol can be teratogenic in early pregnancy and lead to fetal abnormalities, including craniofacial, cardiac, thymic, and central nervous system malformations. In humans, the synthetic retinoid isotretinoin, which is used in treatment of severe acne, results in similar malformations. The period of sensitivity in humans is the second to the fifth week of pregnancy. The incidence of birth defects associated with cranial neural crest tissue in babies born to women who consumed more than 4500 μg of retinol per day was reported to be 3.5-fold higher than in babies born to women whose daily consumption of vitamin A was 1500 μg or less (Rothman et al., 1995). The increased incidence of defects was concentrated among babies born to women who consumed high levels of vitamin A prior to the seventh week of gestation.

These observations suggest that intake of vitamin A at doses that are only several-fold higher than the RDA during early pregnancy is associated with a marked increase in the incidence of birth defects. On the other hand, it was recently reported that vitamin A supplements at a total dose exceeding 3000 μg of retinol did not result in a higher incidence of neural crest defects (Lammer et al., 1996). As pointed out by Gerster (1997), it seems prudent at the present time to follow the recommendations of the Teratology Society of the United States: the daily vitamin A dose for pregnant women should never exceed 3000 μg RE, and it is reasonable to replace part of the vitamin A supplement for pregnant women with β-carotene, which has never been shown to be teratogenic either in animals or in humans.

with vitamin A deficiency has been shown both by epidemiological evidence and by studies with laboratory animals to stem from a compromised immune system function (Ross and Hammerling, 1994).

REFERENCES

Bavik, C. O., Eriksson, U., Allen, R. A. and Peterson, P. A. (1991) Identification and partial characterization of a retinal pigment epithelial membrane receptor for plasma retinol-binding protein J Biol Chem 266:14978–14985.

Blaner, W. S., Das, S. R., Gouras, P. and Flood, M. T. (1987) Hydrolysis of 11-*cis* and all-*trans* retinyl palmitate by homogenates of human retinal epithelial cells. J Biol Chem 262:53–58.

Blaner, W. S., Obunike, J. C., Kurlandsky, S. B., Al-Haideri, M.,Piantedosi, R., Deckelbaum, R. J. and Goldberg, I. J. (1994) Lipoprotein lipase hydrolysis of retinyl esters: Possible implications for retinoid uptake by cells. J Biol Chem 269:16559–16565.

Blaner, W. S. and Olson, J. A. (1994) Retinol and retinoic acid metabolism. In: The Retinoids: Biology, Chemistry, and Medicine (Sporn, M. B. Roberts, A. B. and Goodman, D. S., eds.), 2nd ed., pp. 229–255. Raven Press, New York.

Boerman, M. H. E. M. and Napoli, J. L. (1991) Cholate-independent retinyl ester hydrolysis. J Biol Chem 266:22273–22278.

Boylan, J. F. and Gudas, L. J. (1991) Overexpression of the cellular retinoic acid binding-I results in a reduction in differentiation-specific gene expression in F9 teratocarcinoma cells. J Cell Biol 112:965–980.

Breitman, T. R., Selonick, S. E. and Collins, S. J. (1980) Induction of differentiation of the human promyelocytic leukemia cell line (HL-60) by retinoic acid. Proc Natl Acad Sci USA 77:2936–2940.

Canada, F. J., Law, W. C., Rando, R. R., Yamamoto, T., Derguini, F. and Nakanishi, K. (1990) Substrate specificities and mechanism in the enzymatic processing of vitamin A into 11-*cis*-retinol. Biochemistry 29:9690–9697.

Chai, X., Boerman, M. H. E. M., Zhai, Y. and Napoli, J. L. (1995) Cloning of a cDNA for liver microsomal retinol dehydrogenase. J Biol Chem 270:3900–3904.

Chambon, P. (1994) The retinoid signaling pathway: Molecular and genetic analysis. Semin Cell Biol 5:115–125.

Chen, J. D. and Evans, R. M. (1995) A transcriptional corepressor that interacts with nuclear hormone receptors. Nature 377:454–457.

Chen, Y., Saari, J. C. and Noy, N. (1993) Studies on the interactions of all-*trans*-retinol and long-chain fatty acids with interphotoreceptor retinoid-binding protein. Biochemistry 32:11311–11318.

Chen, Y., Houghton, L. A., Brenna, J. T. and Noy, N. (1996) Docosahexaenoic acid modulates the interactions of the interphotoreceptor matrix retinoid-binding protein with 11-*cis*-retinal. J Biol Chem 271:20507–20515.

Cowan, S. W., Newcomer, M. E. and Jones, T. A. (1993) Crystallographic studies on a family of cellular lipophilic transport proteins: The refinement of P2 myelin protein and the structure determination and refinement of cellular retinol-binding protein in complex with all-*trans* retinol. J Mol Biol 230:1225–1246.

Dew, S. E. and Ong, D. E. (1994) Specificity of the retinol transporter of the rat small intestine brush border. Biochemistry 33:12340–12345.

Dowling, J. E. (1987) The Retina: An Approachable Part of the Brain. Harvard University Press, Cambridge, Massachusetts.

Fex, G. and Johannesson, G. (1987) Studies of the spontaneous transfer of retinol from retinol:retinol binding protein complex to unilamellar liposomes. Biochim Biophys Acta 901:255–264.

Food and Agriculture Organization/World Health Organization. (1988) Requirements for vitamin A, iron, folate, and vitamin B_{12}. Report of a joint FAO/WHO Expert Committee. Food and Nutrition Series, Report No. 23. Rome.

Ganguly, J. (1989) Biochemistry of Vitamin A. CRC Press, Inc., Boca Raton, Florida.

Gerster, H. (1997) Vitamin A—functions, dietary requirements, and safety in humans. Int J Vitam Nutr Res 67:71–90.

Giguère, V. (1994) Retinoic acid receptors and cellular binding proteins: Complex interplay in retinoid signaling. Endocrinol Rev 15:61–77.

Glass, C. K. (1994) Differential recognition of target genes by nuclear receptor monomers, dimers, and heterodimers. Endocrinol Rev 15:391–407.

Glass, C. K., Rose, D. W. and Rosenfeld, M. G. (1997) Nuclear receptor coactivators. Curr Opin Cell Biol 9:222–232.

Grün, F., Noy, N., Hammerling, U. and Buck, J. (1995) Purification, cloning, and bacterial expression of retinol dehydratase from *Spodoptera frugiperda*. J Biol Chem 271:16135–16138.

Gudas, L. J. (1994) Retinoids and vertebrate development. J Biol Chem 269:15399–15402.

Herr, F. and Ong, D. E. (1992) Differential interaction of lecithin:retinol acyltransferase with cellular retinoid-binding proteins. Biochemistry 31:6748–6755.

Hofman, C. and Eichele, G. (1994) Retinoids in development. In: The Retinoids: Biology, Chemistry, and Medicine (Sporn, M. B., Roberts, A. B. and Goodman, D. S., eds.), 2nd ed., pp. 387–441. Raven Press, New York.

Hong, W. K. and Itri, L. M. (1994) Retinoids and human cancer. In: The Retinoids: Biology, Chemistry, and Medicine (Sporn, M. B., Roberts, A. B. and Goodman, D. S., eds.), 2nd ed., pp. 597–630. Raven Press, New York.

Hörlein, A. J., Näär, A. M., Heinzel, T., Torchia, J., Gloss, B., Kurokawa, R., Ryan A., Kamei, Y., Söderström, M., Glass, C. K. and Rosenfeld, M. G. (1995) Ligand-dependent repression by the thyroid hormone receptor mediated by a nuclear receptor-co-repressor. Nature 377:397–403.

Horwitz, K. B., Jackson, T. A., Bain, D. L., Richer, J. K., Takimoto, G. S. and Tung, L. (1996) Nuclear receptor coactivators and corepressors. Mol Endocrinol 10:1167–1177.

Jamison, R. S., Newcomer, M. E. and Ong, D. E. (1994) Cellular retinoid-binding proteins: Limited proteolysis reveals a conformational change upon ligand-binding. Biochemistry 33:2873–2879.

Kakkad, B. and Ong, D. E. (1988) Reduction of retinaldehyde bound to cellular retinol-binding protein (type II) by microsomes from rat small intestine J Biol Chem 263:12916–12919.

Kersten, S., Kelleher, D., Chambon, P., Gronemeyer, H. and Noy, N. (1995a) The retinoid X receptor forms tetramers in solution. Proc Natl Acad Sci USA 92:8645–8649.

Kersten, S., Pan, L., Chambon, P., Gronemeyer, H. and Noy, N. (1995b) On the role of ligand in retinoid signaling: 9-*cis* retinoic acid modulates the oligomeric state of the retinoid X receptor. Biochemistry 34:13717–13721.

Kersten, S., Pan, L. and Noy, N. (1995c) On the role of ligand in retinoid signaling. Positive cooperativity in the interactions of 9-*cis* retinoic acid with tetramers of the retinoid X receptor. Biochemistry 34:14263–14269.

Kurokawa, R., Söderström, M., Hörlein, A., Halachmi, S., Brown, M., Rosenfeld, M. G. and Glass, C. K. (1995) Polarity-specific activities of retinoic acid receptors. Nature 377:451–454.

Lammer, E. J., Shaw, G. M., Wasserman, C. R. and Block, G. (1996) High vitamin A intake and risk for major abnormalities involving structures with an embryological cranial neural crest cell component. Teratology 53:91–92.

Leid, M., Kastner, P. and Chambon, P. (1992) Multiplicity generates diversity in the retinoic acid signaling pathways. Trends Biochem Sci 17:427–433.

Li, E., Qian, S. J., Winter, N. S., d'Avignon, A., Levin, M. S. and Gordon, J. I. (1991) Fluorine nuclear magnetic resonance analysis of the ligand-binding properties of two homologous rat cellular retinol-binding proteins expressed in *E. coli*. J Biol Chem 266:3622–3629.

MacDonald, P. N. and Ong, D. E. (1988) A lecithin:retinol acyltransferase activity in human and rat liver. Biochem Biophys Res Commun 156:157–163.

McCollum, E. V. and Davis, M. (1915) The essential factors in the diet during growth. J Biol Chem 23:231.

Mukherjee, R., Davies, P. J. A., Crombie, D. L., Bischoff, E. D., Cesario, R. M., Jow, L., Hamann, L. G., Boehm, M. F., Mondon, C. E., Nadzan, A. M., Paterniti, J. R. and Heyman, R. A. (1997) Sensitization of diabetic and obese mice to insulin by retinoid X receptor agonists. Nature 386:407–410.

National Research Council (1989) Recommended Dietary Allowances, 10th ed. National Academy Press, Washington, D. C.

Newcomer, M. E., Jones, T. A., Aqvist, J., Sundelin, J., Rask, L. and Peterson, P. A. (1984) The three-dimensional structure of retinol-binding protein. EMBO J 3:1451–1454.

Nikawa, T., Schulz, W. A., van den Brink, C. E., Hanusch, M., van der Saag, P., Stahl, W. and Sies, H. (1995) Efficacy of all-*trans*-β-carotene, canthaxanthin, and all-*trans*-, 9-*cis*, and 4-oxoretinoic acids in inducing differentiation of an F9 embryonal carcinoma RARβ-lacZ reporter cell line. Arch Biochem Biophys 316:665–672.

Noy, N. and Blaner, W. S. (1991) Interactions of retinol with binding proteins: Studies with rat cellular retinol-binding protein and with rat retinol-binding protein. Biochemistry 30:6380–6386.

Noy, N. and Xu, Z.-J. (1990) The interactions of retinol with binding proteins: Implications for the mechanism of uptake by cells. Biochemistry 29:3878–3883.

Olson, J. A. (1987) Recommended dietary intake of vitamin A in humans. Am J Clin Nutr 45:704.

Olson, J. A. (1989) Provitamin A function of carotenoids: The conversion of β-carotene into vitamin A. J Nutr 119:105–108.

Ong D. E., Davis, J. T., O'Day, W. T. and Bok, D. (1994a) Synthesis and secretion of retinol-binding protein and transthyretin by cultured retinal pigment epithelium. Biochemistry 33:1835–1842.

Ong, D. E., Newcomer, M. E. and Chytil, F. (1994b) Cellular retinoid-binding proteins. In: The Retinoids: Biology, Chemistry, and Medicine (Sporn, M. B., Roberts, A. B. and Goodman, D. S., eds.), 2nd ed., pp. 283–318. Raven Press, New York.

Osborne, T. B. and Mendel, L. B. (1919) The vitamins in green foods. J Biol Chem 37:187.

Pacifici, R. E. and Davies, K. J. A. (1991) Protein, lipid, and DNA repair systems in oxidative stress: The free-radical theory of aging revisited. Gerontology 37:166–180.

Pepperberg, D. R., Okajima, T-I. L., Wiggert, B., Ripps, H., Crouch, R. K. and Chader, G. J. (1993) The interphotoreceptor retinoid-binding protein. Mol Neurobiol 7:61–85.

Pijnappel, W. W. M., Hendriks, H. F. J., Folkers, G. E., van den Brink, C. E., Dekker, E. J., Edelenbosch, C., van der Saag, P. T. and Durston, A. J. (1993) The retinoid ligand 4-oxo-retinoic acid is a highly active modulator of positional specification. Nature 366:340–344.

Posch, K. C., Burns, R. D. and Napoli, J. L. (1992) Biosynthesis of all-*trans* retinoic acid from retinal. Recognition of retinal bound to cellular retinol-binding protein (type I) as substrate by a purified cytosolic dehydrogenase. J Biol Chem 267:19676–19682.

Randolf, R. K., Winkler, K. E. and Ross, A. C. (1991) Fatty acyl coenzyme A dependent and fatty acyl coenzyme A independent retinol esterification by rat liver and mammary gland microsomes. Arch Biochem Biophys 288:500–508.

Rigtrup, K. M. and Ong, D. E. (1992) A retinyl ester hydrolase activity intrinsic to the brush border membrane of rat small intestine. Biochemistry 31:2920–2926.

Ross, C. A. (1982) Retinol esterification by rat liver microsomes. J Biol Chem 257:2453–2459.

Ross, C. A. and Hammerling, U. (1994) Retinoids and the immune system. In: The Retinoids: Biology, Chemistry, and Medicine (Sporn, M. B., Roberts, A. B. and Goodman, D. S., eds.), 2nd ed., pp. 521–543. Raven Press, New York.

Rothman, K. J., Moore, L. L., Singer, M. R., Nguyen, U.-S. D. T., Mannino, S. and Milunsky, A. (1995) Teratogenicity of high vitamin A intake. N Engl J Med 333:1369–1415.

Saari, J. C. (1994) Retinoids in the photosensitive systems. In: The Retinoids: Biology, Chemistry, and Medicine (Sporn, M. B., Roberts, A. B., and Goodman, D. S., eds.), 2nd ed., pp. 351–385. Raven Press, New York.

Saari, J. C., Bredberg, D. L. and Noy, N. (1994) Control of substrate flow at a branch in the visual cycle. Biochemistry 33:3106–3112.

Shingleton, J. L., Skinner, M. K. and Ong, D. E. (1989) Characteristics of retinol accumulation from serum-binding protein by cultured Sertoli cells. Biochemistry 28:9641–9647.

Sommer, A. (1982) Field guide to the design and control of xerophthalmia, 2nd ed. World Health Organization, Geneva.

Sommer, A., Tarwotjo, I., Hussaini, G. and Susanto, D. (1983) Increased mortality in children with mild vitamin A deficiency. Lancet 2:585–588.

Soprano, D. R. and Blaner, W. S. (1994) Plasma retinol-binding protein. In: The Retinoids: Biology, Chemistry, and Medicine (Sporn, M. B., Roberts, A. B. and Goodman, D. S., eds.), 2nd ed., pp. 257–281. Raven Press, New York.

Takahashi, N. and Breitman, T. R. (1991) Retinoylation of proteins in leukemia, embryonal carcinoma, and normal kidney cell lines: Differences associated with differential responses to retinoic acid. Arch Biochem Biophys 285:105–110.

Thaller, C. and Eichele, G. (1990) Isolation of 3,4-didehydroretinoic acid, a novel morphogenetic signal in the chick wing bud. Nature 345:815–819.

Underwood, B. A. (1994) Vitamin A in human nutrition: Public health considerations. In: The Retinoids: Biology,

Chemistry, and Medicine (Sporn, M. B., Roberts, A. B. and Goodman, D. S., eds.), 2nd ed., pp. 211–227. Raven Press, New York.

Vahlquist, A. and Torma, H. (1988) Retinoids and keratinization; Current concepts. Int J Dermatol 27:81–95.

Vu-Dac, N., Schoonjans, K., Kosykh, V., Dallongeville, J., Heyman, R. A., Staels, B. and Auwerk, J. (1996) Retinoids increase human lipoprotein A-II expression through activation of the retinoid X receptor but not the retinoic acid receptor. Mol Cell Biol 16:3350–3360.

Warrel, R. P., Jr., de The, H., Wang, Z. Y. and Degos, L. (1993) Acute promyelocytic leukemia. N Engl J Med 329:177–189.

Wolbach, S. B. and Howe, P. (1925) Tissue changes following deprivation of fat-soluble A vitamin. J Exp Med 42:753–778.

Zile, M. H., Cullum, M. E., Simpson, R. U., Barua, A. B. and Swartz, D. A. (1987) Induction of differentiation of human promyelocytic leukemia cell line HL-60 by retinoyl glucuronide, a biologically active metabolite of vitamin A. Proc Natl Acad Sci USA 84:2208–2212.

RECOMMENDED READINGS

Blaner, W. S. and Olson, J. A. (1994) Retinol and retinoic acid metabolism. In: The Retinoids: Biology, Chemistry, and Medicine (Sporn, M. B., Roberts, A. B. and Goodman, D. S., eds.), 2nd ed., pp. 229–256. Raven Press, New York.

Mangelsdorf, D. J., Umesono, K. and Evans, R. M. (1994) The retinoid receptor. In: The Retinoids: Biology, Chemistry, and Medicine (Sporn, M. B., Roberts, A. B. and Goodman, D. S., eds.), 2nd ed., pp. 319–350. Raven Press, New York.

Ong, D. E., Newcomer, M. E. and Chytil, F. (1994) Cellular retinol-binding proteins. In: The Retinoids: Biology, Chemistry, and Medicine (Sporn, M. B., Roberts, A. B. and Goodman, D. S., eds.), 2nd ed., pp. 283–318. Raven Press, New York.

Saari, J. C. (1994) Retinoids in photosensitive systems. In: The Retinoids: Biology, Chemistry, and Medicine (Sporn, M. B., Roberts, A. B. and Goodman, D. S., eds.), 2nd ed., pp. 351–385. Raven Press, New York.

CHAPTER **27**

◆ ◆

Vitamin D

Michael F. Holick, Ph.D., M.D.

O U T L I N E

C O M M O N   A B B R E V I A T I O N S

7-DHC (7-dehydrocholesterol)
25-OH-D (25-hydroxyvitamin D; also known as calcidiol)
1,25(OH)₂D (1,25-dihydroxyvitamin D; also known as calcitriol)
VDR (vitamin D receptor)
VDRE (vitamin D response element)

PHOTOBIOLOGY OF VITAMIN D

Vitamin D is not by the strict definition a vitamin because it can be synthesized in the skin by the action of sunlight. Therefore, factors that limit exposure of the skin to sunlight may play a major role in determining a person's vitamin D status.

Photosynthesis of Previtamin D_3 in Human Skin

7-Dehydrocholesterol (7-DHC, provitamin D_3), the immediate precursor of cholesterol, is present in the viable epidermis and dermis. During exposure to sunlight, 7-DHC absorbs sunlight (photons) with energies of between 290 and 315 nm (ultraviolet B radiation, UVB). This process causes a transformation of 7-DHC to previtamin D_3 (Fig. 27–1) (Holick, 1994). After previtamin D_3 is made, it undergoes an internal transformation of its double bonds that is stimulated by the body's temperature to form vitamin D_3 over a period of a few hours (Fig. 27–1). As previtamin D_3 is converted to vitamin D_3, its three-dimensional structure changes, facilitating vitamin D_3's translocation from the skin cell into the blood stream. Once in the blood stream, it is bound to a specific vitamin D–binding protein commonly known as an α_1-globulin.

Sunlight-mediated Regulation of Vitamin D_3 Synthesis in the Skin

It is not possible to make an intoxicating amount of vitamin D_3 in the skin due to prolonged exposure to sunlight. The reason for this is that once previtamin D_3 is photosynthesized in the skin, it can either be converted to vitamin D_3 or, if exposed to sunlight, be degraded into biologically inert photoproducts known as lumisterol and tachysterol (Fig. 27–1) (Holick, 1994). Vitamin D_3 is also exquisitely sensitive to photodegradation by sunlight (Webb et al., 1989). Therefore, if vitamin D_3 does not exit from the skin into the circulation before being exposed to sunlight, it is degraded by sunlight into supersterol I, supersterol II, and 5,6-*trans*-vitamin D_3 (Fig. 27–1).

Effect of Melanin Pigmentation on the Cutaneous Production of Previtamin D_3

Loomis (1967) popularized the theory that melanin pigmentation in humans evolved to protect people who lived at or near the equator from producing excessive, intoxicating amounts of vitamin D_3. He further speculated that as peoples migrated north and south of the equator they lost their skin pigmentation in order to promote an adequate amount of vitamin D_3 synthesis in their skin to protect their bones from developing rickets and osteomalacia. Melanin is an excellent sunscreen that absorbs the ultraviolet radiation from sunlight. Therefore, melanin competes with 7-DHC in the skin for the UVB photons. As a result, increased skin pigmentation decreases the production of previtamin D_3 in the skin (Clemens et al., 1982).

We have previously found that blacks with very dark skin pigmentation require tenfold longer exposure to simulated sunlight to make the same amount of vitamin D_3 in their skin as does a light-skinned white (Clemens et al., 1982). Because sunlight prevents an excessive production of either previtamin D_3 or vitamin D_3 in the skin by causing the photodegradation of excessive amounts of these compounds, it is unlikely that melanin pigmentation evolved for the purpose of preventing vitamin D_3 intoxication due to excessive exposure to sunlight of peoples who live near the equator. It is, however, intriguing to consider the possibility that skin pigmentation gradually disappeared in peoples that migrated north and south of the equator in order to promote an adequate production of vitamin D_3 in the skin. This concept remains a theory and has not been proved. However, it should be noted that blacks who live in Northern Europe, where food is not fortified with vitamin D as it is in the United States, do not suffer from a higher incidence of rickets and osteomalacia caused by vitamin D deficiency when compared with Northern European whites.

Environmental Effects on the Production of Vitamin D_3

The time of day, season of the year, and latitude have dramatic effects on the amount of

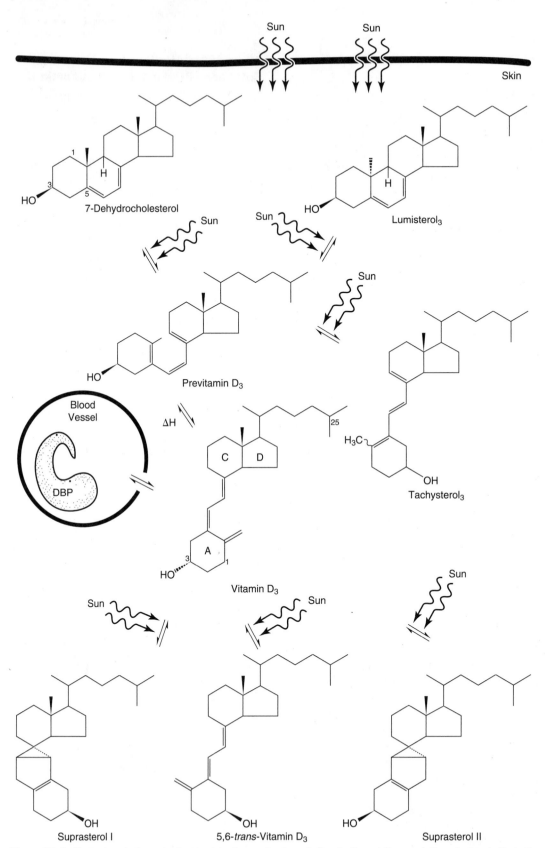

Figure 27–1. Photochemical events that lead to the production of vitamin D_3 and the regulation of vitamin D_3 in the skin. DBP, vitamin D binding protein. (Adapted from Holick, M. F. [1994] Vitamin D: New horizons for the 21st century. Am J Clin Nutr 60:619–630. Used with permission of the American Society for Clinical Nutrition.)

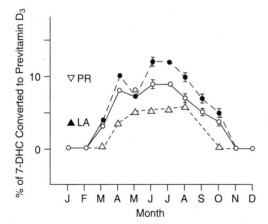

Figure 27–2. *Photosynthesis of previtamin D$_3$ after exposure of a solution of 7-dehydrocholesterol (7-DHC) to sunlight in Boston (42° N) for 1 h (-○-) or 3 h (-●-); in Edmonton, Canada, (52°N) for 1 h (-△-); in Los Angeles (34°N) for 1 h (-▲-), and in Puerto Rico for 1 h (18° N) (-▽-). Measurements were made in the middle of the indicated month on a cloudless day, either from 12 to 1 P.M. (1 h) or from 11 A.M. to 2 P.M. (3 h). Measurements in Los Angeles and Puerto Rico were made only in January. (Adapted from Webb, A. R., Kline, L. and Holick, M. F. [1988] Influence of season and latitude on the cutaneous synthesis of vitamin D$_3$: Exposure to winter sunlight in Boston and Edmonton will not promote vitamin D$_3$ synthesis in human skin. J Clin Endocrinol Metab 67:373–378. © The Endocrine Society.)*

solar UVB radiation that reaches the earth's surface. In winter, vitamin-producing UVB photons pass through the ozone layer at an oblique angle and are absorbed by the ozone in great numbers. More UVB photons are able to penetrate the ozone layer in the spring, summer, and fall months because the sun is directly overhead. At latitude 42° N (Boston), sunlight is incapable of producing vitamin D$_3$ in the skin from November through February. Ten degrees north of Boston (52° N, Edmonton, Canada), this period is extended to include October and March (Fig. 27–2) (Webb et al., 1988).

Because casual exposure to sunlight provides most of our vitamin D requirement, the inability of the sun to produce vitamin D$_3$ in northern and southern latitudes during the winter may require the elderly to take a vitamin D supplement to prevent vitamin D deficiency. For children and young adults, the cutaneous production of vitamin D$_3$ during the spring, summer, and fall is adequate to produce enough for storage in the fat that can be used during the winter months.

Exposure to sunlight at lower latitudes, such as in Los Angeles (24° N), Puerto Rico (18° N), and Buenos Aires (34° S), results in the cutaneous production of vitamin D$_3$ during the entire year. During the summer in Boston, exposure to sunlight from the hours of 7 A.M. to 5 P.M. Eastern Standard Time (EST) results in sufficient UVB photons to produce previtamin D$_3$ in the skin. In the spring and fall months, vitamin D production commences at approximately 9 A.M. and ceases after 3 P.M. EST.

Effect of Aging on the Cutaneous Production of Vitamin D$_3$

Aging affects many different metabolic processes. Therefore, it is not surprising that aging also decreases the capacity of human skin to produce vitamin D$_3$. Aging decreases the concentration of 7-DHC in the epidermis and thereby reduces the capacity of the skin to produce vitamin D$_3$ by approximately 75% by age 70 years compared with younger adults (Fig. 27–3) (Holick et al., 1989).

Effects of Sunscreen Use and Clothing on the Cutaneous Production of Vitamin D$_3$

The public is now very much aware that chronic excessive exposure to sunlight can

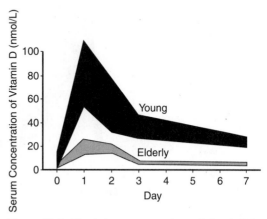

Figure 27–3. *Circulating concentrations of vitamin D in healthy young (20 to 30 years of age) and elderly (62 to 80 years of age) subjects in response to a whole-body exposure (at time zero) to 1 minimal erythemal dose of simulated sunlight. The shaded areas on the graph represent the mean ± 1 SEM for the serum vitamin D concentrations for the two subject groups. (Adapted from Holick, M. F., Matsuoka, L. Y. and Wortsman, J. [1989] Age, vitamin D, and solar ultraviolet. Lancet 2:1104–1105. © The Lancet, 1989.)*

increase the risk of skin cancer and cause photoaging of the skin. This has led to the general recommendation that people of races that sunburn should always wear a sunscreen before going outdoors (Gilchrest, 1993). Commercial sunscreens work by absorbing solar UVB radiation, and some products also absorb some or all of the solar ultraviolet A (320 to 400 nm) radiation. Thus, sunscreens act like melanin and prevent these high-energy photons from having adverse effects on the skin.

Sunscreen use has been proved to decrease the risk of some forms of skin cancer, including squamous cell carcinoma, and to reduce photodamage that causes photoaging of the skin. However, since the solar radiation that is responsible for causing the damaging effects to the skin is the same radiation that causes the cutaneous production of vitamin D_3, it is not surprising that the topical application of a sunscreen can diminish or completely prevent the vitamin D_3 production in the skin. When a young adult exposes the whole body to simulated sunlight that causes a minimal sunburning (1 minimal erythemal dose; MED), the amount of vitamin D_3 that is

produced in the skin and enters the circulation is equivalent to taking between 10,000 and 25,000 IU of vitamin D orally.

When healthy young adult volunteers applied a sunscreen preparation with a sun protection factor of 8 (SPF-8) before being exposed to a whole body dose of 1 MED of simulated sunlight, plasma levels of vitamin D did not rise above the baseline value (Fig. 27–4). To further investigate the impact of sunscreen use on the cutaneous production of vitamin D_3, 10 volunteers who wore typical clothing for a summer day (short-sleeved blouse or shirt and shorts) topically applied a sunscreen with an SPF of 25 only to the face or to unclothed areas with the exception of the face. Twenty-four hours after exposure to 0.9 MED of simulated sunlight, a small increase in the circulating concentration of vitamin D_3, from 3.0 ± 1.0 (mean $\pm$ SEM) to $4.4 + 1.0$ ng/mL of serum, was noted in the volunteers who exposed only their faces. When the face was covered and the arms and legs were exposed, there was a significant increase in the serum vitamin D level: from 1.9 ± 0.3 to 4.4 ± 0.8 ng/mL.

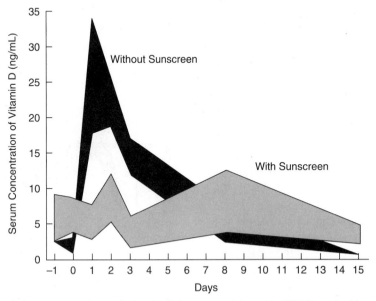

Figure 27–4. Circulating concentrations of vitamin D in young adults with (SPF-8) and without (topical placebo cream) sunscreen after a single exposure (at time zero) to 1 minimal erythemal dose of simulated sunlight. The shaded areas on the graph represent the mean $\pm$ 1 SEM for the serum vitamin D concentrations for the two treatment groups. (Adapted from Matsuoka, L. Y., Ide, L., Wortsman, J., MacLaughlin, J. A. and Holick, M. A. [1987] Sunscreens suppress cutaneous vitamin D_3 synthesis. J Clin Endocrinol Metab 64:1165–1168. © The Endocrine Society.)

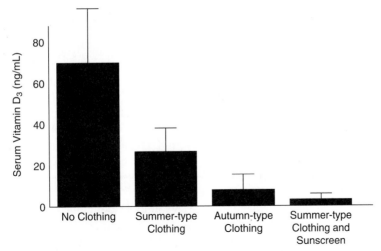

Figure 27–5. *Circulating concentrations of vitamin D in human subjects who wore no clothing, summer-type clothing, or autumn-type clothing, or who wore summer clothing and also used a sunscreen. Serum vitamin D concentration was measured 24 h after whole-body exposure to 1 minimal erythemal dose of ultraviolet B radiation. (Adapted from Matsuoka, L. Y., Wortsman, J., Dannenberg, M. J., Hollis, B. W., Lu, Z. and Holick, M. F. [1992] Clothing prevents ultraviolet-B radiation-dependent photosynthesis of vitamin D. J Clin Endocrinol Metab 75:1099–1103. © The Endocrine Society.)*

Clothing absorbs most ultraviolet radiation; therefore, covering the skin with most types of clothing will prevent the cutaneous production of vitamin D_3 (Matsuoka et al., 1992) (Fig. 27–5). People of cultures such as Bedouins living in the Negev Desert, who are required to have most of the skin surface covered by clothing, are prone to develop vitamin D deficiency (Taha et al., 1984).

It is recommended that children and young adults always wear a sunscreen with an SPF of at least 15 to prevent the consequences of chronic excessive exposure to sunlight. There is no need to be concerned about the effect of sunscreen use on preventing the cutaneous production of vitamin D_3 in this population because it is unlikely that they will always wear a sunscreen or use the proper amount of the agent before going outdoors. However, there is reason for concern with regard to elderly people, who often depend on sunlight for their vitamin D requirement. If they limit their outdoor activities and apply a sunscreen properly before going out, they can substantially reduce or even prevent the production of vitamin D_3 and develop a subclinical vitamin D deficiency (Holick, 1994).

FOOD SOURCES OF VITAMIN D AND THE RECOMMENDED DIETARY ALLOWANCES

Naturally occurring vitamin D is rare in foods. Vitamin D is used to refer to either vitamin D_2 or vitamin D_3, both of which can be converted to active vitamin D metabolites. Vitamin D_2 originates from the yeast and plant sterol ergosterol, whereas vitamin D_3 originates from 7-DHC in animals. The major structural difference between vitamin D_2 and vitamin D_3 is in the side chain. Unlike vitamin D_3, vitamin D_2 has a double bond between carbons 22 and 23 and a methyl group on carbon 24.

The major natural sources of vitamin D are fatty fish like mackerel and salmon and fish oils, including cod and tuna liver oils. The major dietary sources of vitamin D are foods fortified with vitamin D_2 or D_3. Milk has been fortified with vitamin D in the United States since the 1930s. More recently, some cereals and breads have been fortified with vitamin D. Other dairy products, including ice cream, cheeses, and yogurt, are not fortified with vitamin D.

The vitamin D content in milk, however,

is variable. Several recent studies suggest that in the United States and western Canada, up to 80% of samples tested did not contain between 400 and 600 IU/quart (10 and 15 μg/quart) of vitamin D. Almost 50% of the samples did not contain 50% of the vitamin D stated on the label, and approximately 15% of the skim milk samples contained no detectable vitamin D (Holick, 1994). Multivitamin preparations containing vitamin D were found to be a good source of vitamin D and contained between 400 and 600 IU (10 and 15 μg) of vitamin D per tablet; pharmaceutical preparations labeled as 50,000 IU (1250 μg) of vitamin D_2 contained the stated amount ± 10%. Although the 1980 and 1989 RDAs for vitamin D were set at 5 μg/day for adults, there is mounting evidence that in the absence of sunlight the actual requirement for vitamin D in adults may be as much as 15 to 20 μg/day (Dawson-Hughes et al., 1991; Holick, 1994). This is now reflected in the recently released Dietary Reference Intakes for vitamin D (Institute of Medicine, 1997). Although a new RDA was not established, the Adequate Intake (AI) for vitamin D was set at 5 μg/day for individuals 50 years of age and younger, but at 10 μg/day for adults 51 to 70 years of age and at 15 μg/day for adults more than 70 years of age.

VITAMIN D IN BONE HEALTH

Vitamin D plays a critical role in mineralization of the bone, and bone disorders result from inadequate circulating levels of the biologically active metabolite of vitamin D. Vitamin D acts to maintain the plasma calcium and phosphate concentrations so that skeletal mineralization occurs.

Rickets and Osteomalacia

Vitamin D deficiency causes rickets in children (Holick, 1994). Before the epiphyseal plates close, vitamin D deficiency causes a disorganization and hypertrophy of the chondrocytes at the mineralization front as well as a mineralization defect, resulting in short stature and bony deformities that are characteristic of vitamin D deficiency rickets (Fig. 27–6). In adults, the epiphyseal plates are closed, thereby preventing many of the bony deformities seen in rachitic children. Vitamin D deficiency in adults causes osteomalacia. Osteomalacia is a very significant metabolic bone disease, especially in elderly people. Adults with vitamin D deficiency have a mineralization defect in the skeleton that results in poor mineralization of the collagen matrix (osteoid). Although this does not cause bony

---

 Food Sources of Vitamin D

• Fortified milk
• Fatty fish (herring, mackerel, salmon, sardines)
• Fortified cereals

Adequate Intakes (AIs) Across the Life Cycle (1 μg = 40 IU)

	μg vitamin D/day
Infants, birth–1 y	5
Children and adults <51 yr	5
Adults, 51–70 y	10
Adults, 71+ y	15
Pregnant and lactating women	5

Synthesis in the skin as a result of exposure to sunlight is normally the most important source of vitamin D. Vitamin D supplements or intake of vitamin D–fortified foods may benefit individuals with very limited exposure to sunlight or older adults who have a more limited capacity for vitamin D synthesis.

From Institute of Medicine (1997) Dietary Reference Intakes: Calcium, Phosphorus, Magnesium, Vitamin D, and Fluoride. National Academy Press, Washington, D.C.

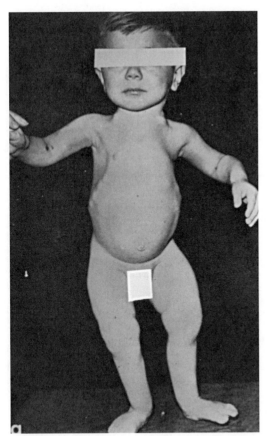

Figure 27–6. *Child with rickets showing the characteristic bony deformities, including bowed legs and rachitic rosary of the rib cage. (From Fraser, D. and Scriver, C. R. [1994] Disorders associated with hereditary or acquired abnormalities of vitamin D function: Hereditary disorders associated with vitamin D resistance or defective phosphate metabolism. In: Endocrinology, [De Groot, L. J., et al., eds.], pp. 797–808. Grune and Stratton, New York.)*

deformities, it can cause severe osteopenia (a decrease in the opacity of the skeleton as seen by x-ray). This mineralization defect can lead to increased risk of skeletal fractures (Aaron et al., 1974). In addition, for unexplained reasons, osteomalacia can also cause localized or generalized, unrelenting deep bone pain.

Consequences of Vitamin D Deficiency

The major function of vitamin D in maintaining a healthy skeleton is to maintain the serum calcium and phosphate concentrations within their physiological ranges to keep the calcium × phosphorus product [e.g., (serum Ca of 10.0 mg/100 mL) × (serum P of 4.0 mg/100 mL) = 40] high enough for skeletal mineralization. (See Chapter 28 for more information on calcium and phosphorus.)

As the body becomes vitamin D deficient, the efficiency of intestinal calcium absorption decreases from the usual 30% to 50% to no more than 15%. This results in a decrease in the ionized calcium concentration in the blood, which signals the calcium sensor in the parathyroid glands to increase the production and secretion of parathyroid hormone (PTH) (Fig. 27–7). PTH, in turn, tries to conserve calcium in the kidney by increasing renal tubular reabsorption of calcium. With vitamin D, PTH helps mobilize monocyte-like stem cells to become active bone calcium

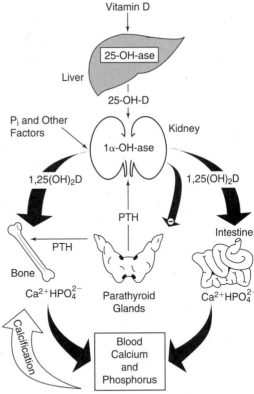

Figure 27–7. *Metabolism of vitamin D and the biological actions of 1,25(OH)$_2$D. 25-OH-ase, vitamin D 25-hydroxylase; 1α-OH-ase, 25-hydroxyvitamin D 1α-hydroxylase. (Reproduced from Holick, M. F., Krane, S. and Potts, J. T. [1994] Calcium, phosphorus, and bone metabolism: Calcium-regulating hormones. In: Harrison's Principles of Internal Medicine [Isselbacher, K. J., Braunwald, E., Wilson, J. D., Martin, J. B., Fauci, A. S. and Kasper, D. L., eds.], 13th ed. pp. 2137–2151. McGraw-Hill, Inc., New York.)*

resorbing multinucleated giant cells known as osteoclasts, which can cause erosion of the skeleton, causing or exacerbating osteoporosis (Fig. 27–7). Although PTH performs an invaluable function in retaining calcium in the kidney, it also induces a leaking of phosphate into the urine, which results in hypophosphatemia. Thus, patients with subclinical vitamin D deficiency often have a normal serum calcium concentration with a low or low-normal serum phosphorus concentration. Patients with long-standing vitamin D deficiency have low serum concentrations of both calcium and phosphorus. This results in a substantial decrease in the calcium × phosphorus product, resulting in a defect in bone matrix mineralization that leads to rickets in children and osteomalacia in adults. The hallmarks for vitamin D insufficiency and deficiency are a low-normal (between 10 and 20 ng/mL) and a low or undetectable (less than 10 ng/mL) serum concentration of 25-hydroxyvitamin D (25-OH-D), respectively.

There is ample clinical evidence that increasing dietary calcium intake to at least 1000 mg/day, along with supplementation of at least 10 to 20 μg of vitamin D daily, will decrease vertebral and nonvertebral fractures and increase bone mineral density (Chapuy et al., 1992). During the winter in New England, when sunlight loses its ability to produce vitamin D_3 in the skin, there is marked loss of bone mineral density of the hip and spine that is related to a decrease in circulating levels of 25-OH-D and an increase in PTH levels (Fig. 27–8) (Rosen et al., 1994).

VITAMIN D METABOLISM AND FUNCTION

In the body, vitamin D undergoes two hydroxylation reactions that convert it to the biologically active form 1,25-dihydroxyvitamin D [1,25(OH)$_2$D]. This active form of vitamin D acts on target tissues, especially intestine and bone. It acts to regulate calcium absorption and bone mineral mobilization in order to maintain calcium homeostasis.

Metabolism

Vitamin D_2 and vitamin D_3 that are used to fortify foods are ingested, mixed with other

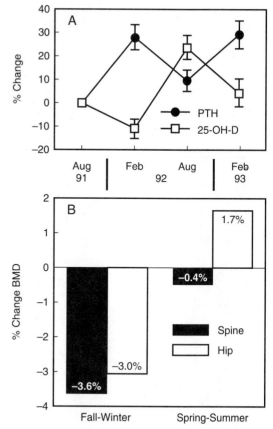

Figure 27–8. (A) Seasonal changes (as percentage of previous measurement) in serum PTH and 25-OH-D. Measurements were made at 6-month intervals over an 18-month period in healthy women with a mean age of 77 years. Results are ± SEM. (B) Percentage change in the bone mineral density (BMD) of the average L_2–L_4 spine and femoral neck of 15 older rural Maine women over a 6-month period consisting of fall and winter or of spring and summer. (Based on data of Rosen, C. J., Morrison, A., Zhou, H., Storm, D., Hunter, S. J., Musgrave, K., Chen, T., Wei, W. and Holick, M. F. [1994] Elderly women in Northern New England exhibit seasonal changes in bone mineral density and calciotropic hormones. Bone Miner 25:83–92.)

lipids, taken up by enterocytes, and incorporated into chylomicrons. Chylomicrons are released by the enterocytes and enter the lymphatic system, which drains into the venous blood stream. Ultimately, this vitamin D (in chylomicron remants) reaches the liver, where it is hydroxylated and again enters the circulation bound to vitamin D–binding protein. Vitamin D_3 that is synthesized in the skin enters the circulation and is bound to the vitamin D–binding protein.

Both vitamin D_2 and vitamin D_3 in the

circulation are taken up by the liver and hydroxylated on carbon 25 to produce 25-OH-D (see Fig. 27–7). 25-OH-D is the major circulating form of vitamin D, and it is present in the circulation bound to the vitamin D–binding protein. It is 25-OH-D that is measured in the blood to determine the vitamin D status of a patient. The hepatic vitamin D 25-hydroxylase is not tightly regulated; therefore, any increase in vitamin D intake or in the cutaneous production of vitamin D_3 leads to an increase in the circulating concentration of 25-OH-D. That is the reason why 25-OH-D is so valuable as a marker for determining the vitamin D status of a patient. Low or undetectable circulating concentrations of 25-OH-D are diagnostic of vitamin D deficiency, and 25-OH-D levels that are two to three times the upper limit of the normal range (normal range, 10 to 55 ng/mL of serum) are diagnostic for vitamin D intoxication (Holick et al., 1994).

Once 25-OH-D is made, it enters the circulation, and most of it is bound to the vitamin D–binding protein. The unbound form of 25-OH-D enters the kidney tubular cells, where it is hydroxylated on carbon 1 to form $1,25(OH)_2D$ (see Fig. 27–7). $1,25(OH)_2D$ is considered to be the biologically active form of vitamin D that is responsible for carrying out most if not all of the biological functions of vitamin D. The major function of $1,25(OH)_2D$ is to increase the efficiency of intestinal calcium absorption, thereby increasing the utilization of dietary calcium (see Fig. 27–7). $1,25(OH)_2D$ can increase the efficiency of intestinal calcium absorption from a basal level of 20% to 30% up to 80%.

Regulation of 25-Hydroxyvitamin D Metabolism

The major factor that regulates the metabolism of 25-OH-D to $1,25(OH)_2D$ is PTH (see Fig. 27–6). The exact mechanism by which PTH stimulates the kidney's production of $1,25(OH)_2D$ is not well characterized. However, there is evidence that the hypophosphatemic effect of PTH on the kidney may be responsible for increasing the renal production of $1,25(OH)_2D$ (Holick et al., 1994). Indeed, hypophosphatemia and hyperphosphatemia are associated with increased and

decreased circulating concentrations of $1,25(OH)_2D$, respectively. A variety of other hormones associated with growth and development of the skeleton or calcium regulation, including growth hormone and prolactin, indirectly increase the renal production of $1,25(OH)_2D$.

It is recognized that elderly people often lose their ability to adapt to a low calcium diet by increasing their efficiency of intestinal calcium absorption (Ireland and Fordtran, 1973). Although the exact mechanism is not fully understood, there is evidence that the ability of the kidney to upregulate the production of $1,25(OH)_2D$ by PTH is no longer operative (Slovik et al., 1981; Riggs et al., 1981).

Extrarenal Production of 1,25-Dihydroxyvitamin D

Although the kidney is the major site for $1,25(OH)_2D$ production, during pregnancy the placenta also has the capacity to make it. This apparently is important during the last trimester of pregnancy, when circulating levels of $1,25(OH)_2D$ are increased to enhance the efficiency of intestinal calcium absorption of the mother to meet the increased need of the fetus for calcium to mineralize its skeleton.

There is mounting scientific evidence that other cells have the capacity to produce $1,25(OH)_2D$. However, it is believed that the local production of $1,25(OH)_2D$ is used in an autocrine or paracrine manner and does not contribute to the circulating concentration of $1,25(OH)_2D$. Although the exact biological function of $1,25(OH)_2D$ in tissues not responsible for calcium metabolism, such as circulating monocytes, skin cells, and bone cells, is not well understood, it is recognized that $1,25(OH)_2D$ is a potent inhibitor of cellular proliferation and a stimulator of differentiation (Holick, 1994).

Biological Functions of 1,25-Dihydroxyvitamin D

The major biological function of vitamin D is to maintain calcium homeostasis in order to maintain cellular metabolic processes and neuromuscular functions. The principal biological function of $1,25(OH)_2D$ is to increase the efficiency of intestinal calcium absorption. $1,25(OH)_2D$ directly affects the entry of calcium through the plasma membrane of the intestinal absorptive cell, thereby enhancing the movement of calcium through the cytosol and across the basolateral membrane of the enterocyte into the circulation. $1,25(OH)_2D$ alters the flux of calcium across the intestinal absorptive cell by increasing the production and activity of several proteins in the small intestine, including calcium-binding protein (calbindin), alkaline phosphatase, low-affinity calcium-dependent ATPase, calmodulin, brush border actin, and brush border proteins with molecular masses of 80 to 90 kDa. Although the exact function of calbindin is not well understood, it is specifically induced by $1,25(OH)_2D$ and is thought to be one of the major proteins responsible for alterations in the flux of calcium across the gastrointestinal mucosa. When $1,25(OH)_2D$ is given as a single intravenous dose to vitamin D–deficient animals, it causes a biphasic response. Within the first 2 hours there is a rapid increase in the flux of calcium across the gastrointestinal mucosa that peaks by 6 hours; another response begins after 12 hours and peaks after 24 hours.

$1,25(OH)_2D$ also increases the efficiency of intestinal phosphorus absorption in the jejunum and ileum of the small intestine. Because dietary phosphate is often plentiful and at least 40% of dietary phosphorus is absorbed passively, the role of $1,25(OH)_2D$ in enhancing phosphorus absorption is less critical.

When dietary sources of calcium are inadequate to maintain calcium homeostasis, $1,25(OH)_2D$ will call upon the bone to mobilize its calcium reserves. $1,25(OH)_2D$ accomplishes this by stimulating monocytic stem cells in the bone marrow to differentiate into bone-resorbing mature osteoclasts. Once the osteoclasts have matured they no longer respond to $1,25(OH)_2D$. It is believed that $1,25(OH)_2D$, through its action on osteoblasts, enhances the production of osteoclast-sensitive cytokines and hormones such as interleukin-6 (IL-6) and interleukin-12 (IL-12), which in turn regulate osteoclastic activity. Therefore, $1,25(OH)_2D$ may indirectly regulate mature osteoclast function by this mechanism.

Mature osteoblasts in the bone possess vitamin D receptors and are responsive to $1,25(OH)_2D$. $1,25(OH)_2D$ increases the expression of alkaline phosphatase, osteopontin, and osteocalcin, as well as a variety of cytokines in the cells. It is likely that $1,25(OH)_2D$ plays an important role in the bone remodeling process. However, $1,25(OH)_2D$ does not directly induce bone to mineralize. Instead, $1,25(OH)_2D$ promotes the mineralization of osteoid laid down by osteoblasts by maintaining extracellular calcium and phosphorus concentrations within the normal supersaturating range, which results in the passive deposition of calcium hydroxyapatite into the bone matrix.

Metabolism of 1,25-Dihydroxyvitamin D

$1,25(OH)_2D$ is metabolized in its target tissues—the intestine, bone, kidney, as well as in the liver. It undergoes several hydroxylations in the side chain, resulting in the cleavage of the side chain between carbons 23 and 24, forming the biologically inert, water-soluble calcitroic acid. Both 25-OH-D and $1,25(OH)_2D$ undergo a 24-hydroxylation to form 24,25-dihydroxyvitamin D and 1,24,25-trihydroxyvitamin D, respectively. These metabolites are considered to be biologically inert and are the first step in the biodegradation of 25-OH-D and $1,25(OH)_2D$. More than 40 different metabolites of vitamin D have been identified to date, but $1,25(OH)_2D$ is believed to be responsible for most, if not all, of the biological actions of vitamin D on calcium and bone metabolism (DeLuca, 1988; Bouillon et al., 1995).

MOLECULAR BIOLOGY OF VITAMIN D

Vitamin D is lipophilic, as is its active form. Therefore, the mechanism of action of $1,25(OH)_2D$ is similar to the action of other small hydrophobic hormones that act via nuclear receptors, such as retinoic acid, thyroid hormone, estrogen, and glucocorticoids. All target tissues for vitamin D contain a nuclear receptor for $1,25(OH)_2D$, known as the vitamin D receptor (VDR). The VDR recognizes $1,25(OH)_2D$ 1000 times better than it recognizes 25-OH-D. It is the unbound (free) $1,25(OH)_2D$ that enters into the target cell

NUTRITION INSIGHT

Cells Involved in Bone Formation and Resorption

The major cells in bone that are concerned with bone formation and resorption are the osteoblasts, the osteocytes, and the osteoclasts. *Osteoblasts* are the bone-forming cells that secrete collagen, forming a matrix around themselves that then calcifies. Osteoblasts have vitamin D receptors and are responsive to changes in circulating concentrations of $1,25(OH)_2D$. Osteoblasts arise from osteoprogenitor cells that are of mesenchymal origin. The osteoblasts seem to form at least a partial membrane that separates bone fluid (the fluid in most immediate contact with hydroxyapatites) from the extracellular fluid of the rest of the body. In this way, the calcium and phosphate concentrations in bone fluid can be carefully regulated.

As osteoblasts become surrounded by new bone (calcified matrix), they become *osteocytes.* Osteocytes remain in contact with one another and with osteoblasts via tight junctions between long protoplasmic processes that run through channels in the bone.

Osteoclasts are multinuclear cells that erode and resorb previously formed bone. Osteoclasts are derived from monocytic stem cells in the bone marrow as a result of stimulation of these cells by $1,25(OH)_2D$ to differentiate into osteoclasts. Osteoclasts appear to phagocytose and break down bone, resulting in a characteristic "chewed-out" edge on the bone surrounding an active osteoclast.

where it is recognized by the VDR. Although the exact mechanism is not completely clarified by which $1,25(OH)_2D$ interacts with its receptor and causes activation of transcription of specific genes, a sequence of events is required before $1,25(OH)_2D$ can carry out its biological functions.

Once $1,25(OH)_2D$ enters the cell, it eventually finds its way to the nucleus, where it is bound to its VDR. The VDR + $1,25(OH)_2D$ complex, in turn, binds a retinoic acid X-receptor (RXR) to form a heterodimeric complex (Pike, 1991; Darwish and DeLuca, 1993). This heterodimeric complex interacts with a specific vitamin D–responsive element (VDRE) within the DNA. The DNA-binding motif for VDR, which is present in the N-terminal part of the molecule, contains two zinc finger motifs that interact with the DNA in the VDRE (Fig. 27–9). The VDRE is composed of two tandemly repeated hexanucleotide sequences separated by three base pairs. This interaction ultimately leads to an increase or a decrease in the transcription of the vitamin D–responsive genes and a change in the rate of synthesis of new mRNAs.

The best-characterized proteins that are induced by $1,25(OH)_2D$ in osteoblasts are osteocalcin, osteopontin, and alkaline phosphatase. The major gene product produced in the small intestine by $1,25(OH)_2D$ is the calcium-binding protein calbindin (Wasserman et al., 1984).

BIOLOGICAL FUNCTIONS OF $1,25(OH)_2D$ IN NONCALCEMIC TISSUES

A wide variety of tissues and cells, including the brain, gonads, breast, skin, mononuclear cells, and activated B and T lymphocytes, possess VDR. The first insight into the biological action of $1,25(OH)_2D$ in noncalcemic tissues was the observation that promyelocytic leukemic cells with a VDR transformed into mature, biochemically functioning macrophages after being treated with $1,25(OH)_2D$ (Tanaka et al., 1982). It is now recognized that $1,25(OH)_2D$ can inhibit the proliferation and induce terminal differentiation of a variety of normal and tumor cells, possibly by directly or indirectly altering transcription of cell growth regulatory genes such as c-myc, c-fos, and c-sis (Fig. 27–9). $1,25(OH)_2D$ has not been found useful for treating a variety of malignant disorders, probably because clones of cells that have a defective receptor become the dominant tu-

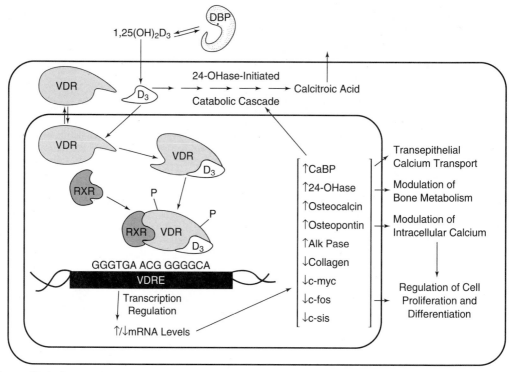

Figure 27–9. *Proposed mechanism of action of 1,25(OH)₂D₃ in target cells resulting in a variety of biological responses. The free form of 1,25(OH)₂D₃ (D₃) enters the target cell and interacts with its nuclear vitamin D receptor (VDR), which is then phosphorylated (P). The 1,25(OH)₂D₃–VDR complex combines with the retinoic acid X-receptor (RXR) to form a heterodimer, which, in turn, interacts with the vitamin D response element (VDRE), causing an enhancement or inhibition of transcription of vitamin D–responsive genes, such as the 25-OH-D-24-hydroxylase (24-OHase). (From Holick, M. F. [1996] Vitamin D: Photobiology, metabolism, mechanism of action, and clinical applications. In: Primer on the Metabolic Bone Diseases and Disorders of Mineral Metabolism [Favus, M. J., ed.], 3rd ed., pp. 74–81. Lippincott-Raven, Philadelphia.)*

mor cell type, resulting in malignant cells that are no longer responsive to the antiproliferative activity of 1,25(OH)₂D (Koeffler et al., 1985). However, there is one clinical application for the antiproliferative activity of 1,25(OH)₂D and its analogs. Because epidermal cells possess a VDR, it was reasoned that patients with the hyperproliferative skin disorder might benefit from either topical or oral 1,25(OH)₂D therapy. A multitude of studies have now demonstrated the therapeutic efficacy of 1,25(OH)₂D and its analogs for treating the hyperproliferative skin disorder (psoriasis) that causes redness, scaling, and raised lesions. This has led to the development of an analog, calcipotriene (Dovonex), which is highly effective when applied topically for the treatment of psoriasis. Unlike other treatments for psoriasis, there is no evidence that the topical application of calcipotriene has any significant undesirable side effects (Kragballe, 1989; Perez et al., 1996).

RECOMMENDATIONS FOR SATISFYING THE VITAMIN D REQUIREMENT FOR MAXIMUM BONE HEALTH

Vitamin D evolved as a calciotropic hormone responsible for maintaining the blood calcium and phosphorus within the normal physiological range. Only when the body's need for calcium to maintain metabolic functions is satisfied is any additional calcium that is absorbed through the intestine deposited into the skeleton.

Vitamin D deficiency is a significant health problem, especially for elderly people. Because most of our vitamin D comes from casual exposure to sunlight, it is important to recognize that adults over the age of 50 years should consider being exposed to suberythemal (not causing sunburn) doses of sunlight to provide their bodies with the vitamin D requirement. In Boston, it has been recommended for middle-aged and older adults that

---

CLINICAL CORRELATION

Vitamin D-dependent Rickets Type II (VDDRII)

The vitamin D receptor (VDR) is a nuclear transcription factor that binds to the vitamin D response element (VDRE) of certain genes to regulate their expression. Vitamin D–dependent rickets type II (VDDRII) is a rare autosomal recessive disease that results from target organ resistance to the action of $1,25(OH)_2D$. Mutations in the gene for VDR result in an inability of VDR to bind $1,25(OH)_2D$ or of the receptor-hormone complex to bind to VDRE in DNA. Affected patients usually present early in childhood with severe rickets, hypocalcemia, and growth retardation. Cultured fibroblasts obtained from these patients fail to respond to $1,25(OH)_2D$ by increasing synthesis of 25-OH-D-24-hydroxylase; this is used as a test for a defect in the $1,25(OH)_2D$ receptor-effector system. In patients with VDDRII, physiological doses of $1,25(OH)_2D$ have no therapeutic effect. In some patients, high-dose calcium therapy or pharmacological doses of vitamin D metabolites have resulted in biochemical and radiological improvement.

Thinking Critically

1. What effect would you expect a defect in the $1,25(OH)_2D$ receptor-effector system to have on calcium absorption? Why?

2. Would high-dose calcium therapy (intravenous or oral) potentially improve bone growth in patients with defects in the $1,25(OH)_2D$ receptor-effector system? Why?

3. For pharmacological doses of $1,25(OH)_2D$ to be effective, would some residual VDR need to be present? Why?

---

exposure of hands, face, and arms two to three times a week to suberythemal doses of sunlight (approximately 5 to 15 minutes a day depending on the skin's sensitivity to sunlight) is adequate to provide sufficient amounts of vitamin D_3.

Vitamin D_3 that is produced in the skin is stored in the body fat; therefore, the vitamin D_3 that is produced in the spring, summer, and fall can be stored and is available during the winter when the sun is incapable of producing vitamin D_3 in the skin. This is the reason why children and most adults do not become vitamin D–deficient during the winter months in far northern and southern latitudes. Because a topical application of a sunscreen can essentially prevent the production of vitamin D_3 in the skin, people who wish to stay outdoors for long periods of time should be exposed only to suberythemal amounts of sunlight for their vitamin D_3 and then apply a sunscreen with a SPF of 15 or greater to prevent the consequences of chronic excessive exposure to sunlight. Children and young adults should always wear a sunscreen before going outdoors to help prevent skin damage

and skin cancer. Because children and young adults will not always wear a sunscreen over all sun-exposed areas, they are still able to produce enough vitamin D from sun exposure to satisfy their body's requirement.

Although milk, some cereals, and bread products may contain vitamin D, this is highly variable and should not be depended on as the only source of the vitamin. A multivitamin tablet that contains 10 μg (400 IU) of vitamin D is an excellent source and will help maintain circulating concentrations of 25-OH-D. However, in the absence of any sunlight, a multivitamin may not be adequate to maintain normal vitamin D status (Holick, 1994). Adults 51 years and older who have little exposure to sunlight likely require at least 10 to 15 μg of vitamin D daily to satisfy the body's requirement. Vitamin D deficiency can be corrected by administering an oral dose of 50,000 IU (1250 μg) vitamin D_2 once a week for 8 weeks. The serum 25-OH-D level can be expected to increase from less than 15 ng/mL to 25 to 40 ng/mL. This treatment will maintain a normal vitamin D status for at least 2 to 4 months. After the 8 weeks, patients can be

LIFE CYCLE CONSIDERATION

Vitamin D Deficiency in Elderly People

Elderly people are more prone to develop a vitamin D deficiency, which may cause osteomalacia, exacerbate osteoporosis, and increase the risk of fractures. A decrease in the capacity of human skin to produce vitamin D occurs with age because of a decrease in the concentration of 7-dehydrocholesterol in the skin. Additionally, production of vitamin D_3 may be restricted in elderly people as a result of limited exposure to sunlight through indoor confinement or use of sun-screen or protective clothing from concern about sun-induced cancer or wrinkles. In a study of sunlight-deprived elderly subjects, a large proportion of homebound elderly persons had below-normal serum 25-OH-D concentrations (Gloth et al., 1995). Vitamin D supplementation or increased exposure to sunlight may improve calcium absorption, suppress PTH levels, and decrease bone loss in elderly people. Calcium intake, hormonal status, exercise, and genetics also may be important factors in the development of osteomalacia and osteoporosis in elderly individuals.

placed on a multivitamin containing 400 IU (10 μg) of vitamin D, which should help maintain their vitamin D status. An adequate source of calcium in combination with vitamin D from sunlight and/or a multivitamin containing vitamin D is essential for guaranteeing a healthy skeleton throughout life.

REFERENCES

Aaron, J. E., Gallagher, J. C., Anderson, J., Stasiak, L., Longton, E., Nordin, B. and Nicholson, M. (1974) Frequency of osteomalacia and osteoporosis in fractures of the proximal femur. Lancet 7851:230–233.

Bouillon, R., Okamura, W. H. and Norman, A. W. (1995) Structure-function relationships in the vitamin D endocrine system. Endocr Rev 16:200–257.

Chapuy, M. C., Arlot, M., Duboeuf, F., Brun, J., Crouzet, B., Arnaud, S., Delmas, P. and Meuner, P. (1992) Vitamin D_3 and calcium to prevent hip fractures in elderly women. N Engl J Med 327:1637–1642.

Clemens, T. L., Henderson, S. L., Adams, J. S. and Holick, M. F. (1982) Increased skin pigment reduces the capacity of skin to synthesize vitamin D_3. Lancet 1:74–76.

Darwish, H. and DeLuca, H. F. (1993) Vitamin D–regulated gene expression. Crit Rev Eukaryot Gene Expr 3:89–116.

Dawson-Hughes, B., Dallal, G. E., Krall, E. A., Harris, S., Sokoll, L. J. and Falconer, G. (1991) Effect of vitamin D supplementation on wintertime and overall bone loss in healthy postmenopausal women. Ann Intern Med 115:505–512.

DeLuca, H. (1988) The vitamin D story: A collaborative effort of basic science and clinical medicine. FASEB J 2:224–236.

Gilchrest, B. A. (1993) Sunscreens—A public health opportunity. N Engl J Med 329:1193–1194.

Gloth, F. M., III, Gundberg, C. M., Hollis, B. W., Haddad, J. G., Jr. and Tobin, J. D. (1995) Vitamin D deficiency in homebound elderly persons. JAMA 274:1683–1686.

Holick, M. F. (1994) Vitamin D: New horizons for the 21st century. Am J Clin Nutr 60:619–630.

Holick, M. F., Matsuoka, L. Y. and Wortsman, J. (1989) Age, vitamin D, and solar ultraviolet. Lancet 2:1104–1105.

Holick, M. F., Krane, S. and Potts, J. T. (1994) Calcium, phosphorus, and bone metabolism: Calcium-regulating hormones. In: Harrison's Principles of Internal Medicine (Isselbacher, K. J., Braunwald, E., Wilson, J. D., Martin, J. B., Fauci, A. S. and Kasper, D. L. eds.), 13th ed., pp. 2137–2151. McGraw-Hill, Inc., New York.

Institute of Medicine (1997) Dietary Reference Intakes: Calcium, Phosphorus, Magnesium, Vitamin D, and Fluoride. National Academy Press, Washington, D.C.

Ireland, P. and Fordtran, J. S. (1973) Effect of dietary calcium and age on jejunal calcium absorption in humans studied by intestinal perfusion. J Clin Invest 52:2672–2681.

Koeffler, H. P., Hirji, K., Itri, L. and The Southern California Leukemia Group (1985) 1,25-Dihydroxyvitamin D_3: In vivo and in vitro effects on human preleukemic and leukemic cells. Cancer Treat Rep 69:1399–1407.

Kragballe, K. (1989) Treatment of psoriasis by the topical application of the novel vitamin D_3 analogue MC 903. Arch Dermatol 125:1647–1652.

Loomis, F. (1967) Skin-pigment regulation of vitamin D biosynthesis in man. Science 157:501–506.

Matsuoka, L. Y., Wortsman, J., Dannenberg, M. J., Hollis, B. W., Lu, Z. and Holick, M. F. (1992) Clothing prevents ultraviolet-B radiation-dependent photosynthesis of vitamin D. J Clin Endocrinol Metab 75:1099–1103.

Perez, A., Chen, T. C., Turner, A., Raab, R., Bhawan, J., Poche, P. and Holick, M.F. (1996) Efficacy and safety of topical calcitriol (1,25-dihydroxyvitamin D_3) for the treatment of psoriasis. Br J Dermatol 134:238–246.

Pike, J. W. (1991). Vitamin D_3 receptors: Structure and function in transcription. Annu Rev Nutr 11:189–216.

Riggs, B. L., Hamstra, A. and DeLuca, H. F. (1981) Assessment of 25-hydroxyvitamin D 1α-hydroxylase reserve in postmenopausal osteoporosis by administration of parathyroid extract. J Clin Endocrinol Metab 53:833–835.

Rosen, C. J., Morrison, A., Zhou, H., Storm, D., Hunter, S. J., Musgrave, K., Chen, T., Wei, W. and Holick, M. F. (1994) Elderly women in northern New England exhibit seasonal changes in bone mineral density and calciotropic hormones. Bone Miner 25:83–92.

Slovik, D. M., Adams, J. S., Neer, R. M., Holick, M. F.

and Potts, J. T. (1981) Deficient production of 1,25-dihydroxyvitamin D in elderly osteoporotic patients. N Engl J Med 305:372–374.

Taha, S. A., Dost, S. M. and Sedrani, S. H. (1984) 25-Hydroxyvitamin D and total calcium: Extraordinarily low plasma concentrations in Saudi mothers and their neonates. Pediatr Res 18:739–741.

Tanaka, H., Abe, E., Miyaura, C., Kuribayashi, T., Konno, K., Nishi, Y. and Suda, T. (1982) 1,25-Dihydroxycholecalciferol and human myeloid leukemia cell line (HL-60): The presence of cytosol receptor and induction of differentiation. Biochem J 204:713–719.

Wasserman, R. H., Fullmer, C. S. and Shimura, F. (1984) Calcium absorption and the molecular effects of vitamin D₃. In: Vitamin D; Basic and Clinical Aspects (Kumar, R., ed.), pp. 233–257. Nijhoff, Boston.

Webb, A. R., Kline, L. and Holick, M. F. (1988) Influence of season and latitude on the cutaneous synthesis of vitamin D₃: Exposure to winter sunlight in Boston and Edmonton will not promote vitamin D₃ synthesis in human skin. J Clin Endocrinol Metab 67:373–378.

Webb, A. R., DeCosta, B. R. and Holick, M. F. (1989) Sunlight regulates the cutaneous production of vitamin D₃ by causing its photodegradation. J Clin Endocrinol Metab 68:882–887.

RECOMMENDED READINGS

Bouillon, R., Okamura, W. H. and Norman, A. W. (1995) Structure-function relationships in the vitamin D endocrine system. Endocr Rev 16:200–257.

Darwish, H. and DeLuca, H. F. (1993) Vitamin D–regulated gene expression. Crit Rev Eukaryot Gene Expr 3:89–116.

Holick, M. F. (1996) Vitamin D: Photobiology, metabolism, mechanism of action, and clinical application. In: Primer on the Metabolic Bone Diseases and Disorders of Mineral Metabolism (Favus, M. J., ed.), 3rd ed. pp. 74–81. Lippincott-Raven, Philadelphia.

Holick, M. F., Chen, M. L., Kong, X. F. and Sanan, D. K. (1996) Clinical uses for calciotropic hormones 1,25-dihydroxyvitamin D₃ and parathyroid hormone–related peptide in dermatology: A new perspective. J Invest Dermatol 1:1–9.

Malabanan, A., Veronikis, I. E. and Holick, M. F. (1998) Redefining vitamin D insufficiency. Lancet 351:805–806.

The Minerals

◆ ◆

From the 90 or so elements that occur naturally in the environment, a limited number (perhaps 22) are essential for human life. The preceding units on carbohydrates, proteins, lipids, and vitamins consider organic compounds or nutrients made up almost entirely of six relatively small elements: hydrogen, carbon, nitrogen, oxygen, phosphorus, and sulfur. In this unit, the biological roles of a number of other essential elements are considered, along with further consideration of phosphorus. Sulfur, as sulfate, is analogous to phosphorus, as phosphate, in many ways, but inorganic sulfur is discussed in Chapter 11 because humans obtain sulfur

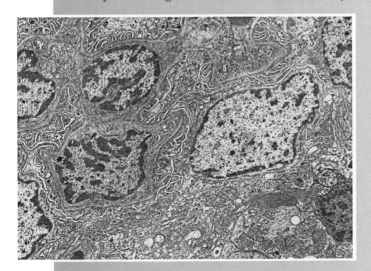

predominantly from their intake of sulfur amino acids. Inorganic phosphate and sulfate are important anions as well as substrates for formation of organic esters. Cobalt also could be considered here but is not because the only requirement humans have for cobalt is as part of preformed vitamin B_{12}, which is discussed in Chapter 21.

Two rather common features of the elements discussed in this unit are that these minerals are required in smaller amounts and for very specialized functions. Additionally, although some of these elements (e.g., phosphorus, selenium, and iodine) are capable of forming covalent bonds, weaker types of bonds are more common. In contrast to the strong covalent bond found in organic molecules, in which each atom donates one electron to form a pair of outer orbital electrons that are shared, the ionic bond (salt bridge) found in salts is formed by a single electron donated by one of the paired atoms. The coordinate covalent bond found in metal chelates (e.g., heme and vitamin B_{12}) possesses properties of both the covalent bond and the ionic bond: two electrons from one atom are donated to form the bond to another atom.

Electron micrograph of kidney; courtesy of Cornell Integrated Microscopy Center, Cornell University, Ithaca, NY.

Minerals or inorganic nutrients are sometimes grouped by the amount of each element that is required by the human body. Essential elements include those classified as macroelements; calcium, phosphorus, magnesium, sodium, potassium, chloride, and sulfur are required at levels of more than 100 mg per day by adults. Because the sulfur requirement is met by intake of sulfur amino acids, sulfur usually is not considered with the macroelements. The microelements may be considered in two groups: trace elements required in amounts ranging between 1 mg and 100 mg per day and ultratrace elements required in amounts in the microgram per day range ($<$ 1 mg per day). Trace elements include iron, zinc, manganese, copper, and fluorine. Ultratrace elements include selenium, molybdenum, iodine, chromium, boron, and cobalt. Some evidence of a benefit of arsenic, nickel, vanadium, and silicon comes from animal studies, but these four ultratrace elements have not been proved to be essential or beneficial for humans.

Minerals serve a diverse range of functions in the body, and many of these functions are discussed in the chapters in this unit. The deposition of calcium and phosphate as hydroxyapatite is essential for bone formation. Calcium is considered to be a second messenger molecule; binding of calcium to various proteins acts as a cellular signaling event. Sodium, potassium, and chloride as well as calcium, magnesium, phosphate, and sulfate are important inorganic electrolytes involved in ionic and osmotic balance and electrical gradients. Many of the trace elements are found in association with enzymes and other proteins in which these metals serve structural, catalytic, or binding roles; examples include the role of zinc in the tertiary structure of various proteins, the catalytic role of copper or zinc at the active site of superoxide dismutase, and the role of iron in oxygen binding by hemoglobin. Some minerals are required solely for the synthesis of specialized organic compounds as demonstrated by the incorporation of iodine into thyroid hormones, of selenium into selenocysteine for synthesis of selenoproteins, and of molybdenum into an organic cofactor required by several mammalian enzymes.

◆ ◆

Martha H. Stipanuk

CHAPTER 28

◆ ◆

Calcium and Phosphorus

Richard J. Wood, Ph.D.

OUTLINE

COMMON ABBREVIATIONS

Gla (γ-carboxyglutamate)
IP$_3$ (inositol 1,4,5-triphosphate)
1,25(OH)$_2$D (1,25-dihydroxyvitamin D)
P$_i$ (inorganic phosphate, mainly HPO$_4^{2-}$ and H$_2$PO$_4^{-}$ at physiological pH)
PIP$_2$ (phosphatidyl inositol 4,5-bisphosphate)
PTH (parathyroid hormone)
PTHrP (parathyroid hormone–related protein)

CHEMICAL PROPERTIES OF CALCIUM AND PHOSPHORUS

A consideration of the chemistry of calcium and phosphorus illustrates the unique biochemical niches filled by these elements. The important roles of these two elements in cell membrane function, cellular homeostasis, and the formation of the inorganic component of the skeleton and the intimate intertwining of the hormonal regulation of calcium and phosphorus homeostasis provide a functional basis for discussing calcium and phosphate in a single chapter.

Calcium

The chemical characteristics of the calcium atom are important in defining the function of this element in living organisms. Calcium belongs to the divalent metals in group IIA of the periodic table. This group of metals has 2 valence electrons that are lost when the metals ionize. Calcium gives up electrons readily and thus forms positive ions (Ca^{2+}) in solution. The double-positive charge on the Ca^{2+} nucleus pulls the outer electronic shells of the calcium ion into a tightly bound configuration. The relatively low ionic radius of calcium produces a high charge density or ionic potential. This electrostatic property of calcium has an important effect on the behavior of the ion in aqueous solution and on its participation in biological processes.

The biological activity of calcium is influenced by the concentration of the ionized or free calcium (Ca^{2+}) in solution; the stability constant of Ca^{2+} with various ligands in solution; and the partition coefficient of Ca^{2+}, which defines the stability of Ca^{2+} binding in a nonaqueous phase such as cell membranes. The rate of movement of Ca^{2+} across cell membranes is limited by the permeability of the membrane to Ca^{2+}, as well as by the effect of Ca^{2+} itself on the membrane. The latter effect is due to an increase in rigidity and electrical resistance of the membrane when Ca^{2+} binds to lipids in the cell membrane. Moreover, binding of Ca^{2+} to the protein components of cell membranes can also change the fluidity of the membrane by influencing the possibilities of cross-linking between proteins. These chemical properties of calcium have particular relevance to the development of specific channels in cell membranes that selectively allow passage of ions; for example, the latter effect is important in determining the permeability of cells to sodium (Na^+) and potassium (K^+) ions. The flow of ions through channels in the membrane creates an electrical circuit that requires energy to drive the flow. The currents generated are a major factor in the control of many cellular functions.

An additional factor that determines the biological activity of Ca^{2+} is related to the notion that the binding constant of Ca^{2+} for some large binding molecules can change under conditions in which the conformation of the binding anion changes. This conformational change can result in the development of a range of binding constants for the interaction of Ca^{2+} with the molecule. This phenomenon has important implications for regulation of cellular activities involving Ca^{2+} binding, because a given response may occur progressively, rather than suddenly, in response to conformational stress at the binding site (Robertson, 1988). For example, calmodulin is a highly conserved, ubiquitous calcium-binding protein in cells, and calmodulin modulates a wide variety of cellular reactions. Calmodulin contains 4 calcium-binding domains that contain a high proportion of glutamyl and aspartyl acid residues. These highly conserved calcium-binding domains are also present in other cellular calcium-binding proteins found in various tissues, such as troponin C in muscle. Other calcium-binding proteins in the body include the Gla proteins that contain high proportions of γ-carboxyglutamyl residues, such as the vitamin K–dependent blood-clotting proteins and some proteins found in bone matrix.

In addition to the aforementioned electrostatic properties of Ca^{2+}, other properties of these ions in aqueous solution also influence their biological activity; these include the high electrical field associated with the Ca^{2+} ion, which causes it to become surrounded with water molecules that shield the charge. This shielding of Ca^{2+} by water molecules increases the effective ionic radius of Ca^{2+} by 5-fold, from about 1 Å to 6 Å. This so-called "water of hydration" depends partly on the charge density of the ion and partly on the coordination number of the element. The latter determines the number of interactions that can occur with other ions in solution. For example, Ca^{2+} has from 6 to 12 possible coordination bonds that may form with other molecules. The net effect of these two properties of calcium ions (charge density and coordination number) determines the effective ionic radius of Ca^{2+}, which in turn influences the solution properties of the Ca^{2+} ion, including its chemical activity, diffusion coefficients, and the ability of Ca^{2+} to traverse semipermeable membranes. Another factor that influences chemical activity of Ca^{2+} is the electrical field produced by other ions in solution. Thus, the effective concentration of Ca^{2+} in solution will differ from its actual chemical concentration by a factor that depends upon the ionic strength of the solution. Moreover, because Ca^{2+} is a divalent cation in solution, it also has the capacity to form soluble ion pairs or complexes with divalent anions based on mutual electrostatic attraction, which effectively reduces the concentration of free Ca^{2+}.

Thus, the selective binding chemistry of Ca^{2+} in biological systems is determined by its charge-to-size ratio and its ability to interact with chelating anions, weak acidic groups such as carboxylates and phosphates, and neutral oxygen donors such as carbonyl and hydroxyl groups. In addition, the high coordination number of Ca^{2+} and its ability to form irregular bond lengths allow it to interact with large molecules that have many possible coordination sites, which facilitates the rapid binding and release processes necessary for Ca^{2+} to act as a signaling messenger for various hormone and growth factor actions. These chemical properties of Ca^{2+} create a need to tightly regulate the free concentration of Ca^{2+} in cells so that it may function properly as a "second messenger" signaling molecule in mediating hormonal action, as a factor involved in motor nerve fiber function, and in its role in mineralization of bone tissue via the formation of calcium phosphate complexes such as hydroxyapatite $[Ca_{10}(OH)_2(PO_4)_6]$ crystals.

Two important energy-requiring membrane pump systems have evolved to help maintain calcium homeostasis in cells by ejecting calcium out of cells. These are the Na^+, Ca^{2+}-exchange system in excitable cells and the magnesium (Mg^{2+})-dependent Ca^{2+}-ATPase enzyme system in nonexcitable cells. In addition, various other strategies are employed by the cell to control intracellular free calcium concentrations, including the binding of Ca^{2+} to various cytosolic Ca^{2+}-binding proteins and small chelating ions, such as citrate, phosphate, ADP, and ATP, and the sequestering of Ca^{2+} within various subcellular compartments.

Phosphate

In biological systems, phosphorus is present as phosphate: free phosphate, phosphate anhydrides, or phosphate esters. The major forms of phosphate in aqueous environments are $H_2PO_4^-$ and HPO_4^{2-}. These two orthophosphates are found at a ratio of 1:4 at a physiological pH of 7.4. Phosphate is an important anion in the body and is involved with a variety of biochemical and physiological functions. Mg^{2+} and other cations, including Ca^{2+}, are found associated with phosphate compounds. In anhydrides and esters, phosphate is always negatively charged, and the terminal phosphate group is always partially protonated.

Examples of anhydrides and esters of phosphate in the body include inositol 1,4,5-trisphosphate (IP_3), an important regulator of calcium release from intracellular stores; ATP, the major energy currency of the body; and phosphatidylcholine, a constituent of cell membranes. DNA and RNA are polymers based on phosphate ester monomers. A variety of enzymatic activities are controlled by alternate phosphorylation and dephosphorylation of proteins by cellular kinases and phosphatases. The metabolism of all major metabolic substrates is dependent on the functioning of phosphate as a cofactor in a variety of enzymes and as the principal reservoir for metabolic energy in the form of ATP, creatine phosphate, and phosphoenolpyruvate.

Another important role of phosphate in the body is based on the fact that neutral molecules are soluble in lipid and will pass through membranes. Because phosphates are ionized at physiological pH, phosphorylation of molecules such as glucose results in the trapping of phosphorylated molecules within cells. The majority of phosphate in the body is found in bone where it combines with calcium to form hydroxyapatite, $Ca_{10}(OH)_2(PO_4)_6$, the principal inorganic compound found in the skeleton. Phosphate is also important in the control of acid-base balance in the body.

PHYSIOLOGICAL OR METABOLIC FUNCTIONS OF CALCIUM AND PHOSPHORUS

Both calcium and phosphate serve numerous roles in the body. These include roles as diverse as their structural role in formation of bone mineral, the regulation of enzyme activity by reversible phosphorylation of specific amino acid residues in the protein, the role of calcium as a second messenger in the cell, and the formation and hydrolysis of energy-rich phosphate bonds in ATP to fuel work.

Calcium as a Second Messenger

Increased Cytosolic Ca^{2+}. Almost all the calcium within cells is bound within organelles such as the endoplasmic reticulum, the nucleus, and other membrane-bound compartments. Consequently, the free calcium in cell cytosol is only about 10^{-7} mol/L, thereby creating a 10,000-fold chemical gradient for Ca^{2+} across cell membranes. A relatively large increase in cytosolic Ca^{2+} concentration can be caused by very small changes in the release of Ca^{2+} from intracellular sites or in its transport across the cell membrane. Changes in intracellular Ca^{2+} concentrations in response to cell surface binding of peptide hormones or growth factors (first message) can act as a "second messenger" to elicit a variety of cellular phenomena, as summarized in Table 28–1.

Ligand binding to cell surface receptor proteins can result in the stimulation of the enzyme phospholipase C and in hydrolysis of phosphatidylinositol to diacylglycerol and IP_3 in the cell membrane. Increased cytosolic IP_3 results in the subsequent release of intracellular Ca^{2+} stores. Depolarization of excitable cells, such as heart muscle and nerve termi-

nals, results in an opening of calcium-selective membrane channels, as well as the release of Ca^{2+} from internal sources, mainly from the endoplasmic reticulum. The subsequent rise in free cytosolic Ca^{2+} concentration triggers muscle contraction or secretion of neurotransmitters.

Calcium-Dependent Trigger Proteins in Cells. Cytosolic Ca^{2+} can bind to cellular Ca^{2+}-binding proteins, including calmodulin, a ubiquitous cytosolic protein that can activate cellular kinases and other enzymes, and troponin C, a muscle protein that is bound to actinomycin contractile fibers. Binding of Ca^{2+} to Ca^{2+}-dependent proteins such as calmodulin results in a conformational change in the protein. This activation of the protein by Ca^{2+} binding results in subsequent activation of calmodulin-dependent enzymes that can then directly or indirectly alter cellular activity, as illustrated in Figure 28–1.

Removal of the Ca^{2+} Stimulus. Cell recovery following stimulation of cellular activity by increased cytosolic concentrations of Ca^{2+} can involve a variety of cellular mechanisms that work to remove the stimulus by lowering Ca^{2+} concentrations. This can be accomplished by buffering free Ca^{2+} via molecular sequestration involving calcium-binding proteins, by physical compartmentalization of Ca^{2+} through uptake into cellular organelles, and by removal of excess Ca^{2+} from the cell through pumping Ca^{2+} out of the cell via energy-dependent Ca^{2+} pumps found on the plasma membrane.

TABLE 28–1
Regulation of Selected Cellular Activities by Intracellular Calcium

Excitation-contraction coupling in muscle
Neurotransmitter release
Microtubule assembly
Membrane permeability to K^+ and Ca^{2+}
Exocrine and endocrine gland secretion of hormones
Cell division and reproduction
Cell-to-cell communication
Certain enzyme activities (e.g., phosphorylase kinase)
Chromosome movement
Initiation of DNA synthesis

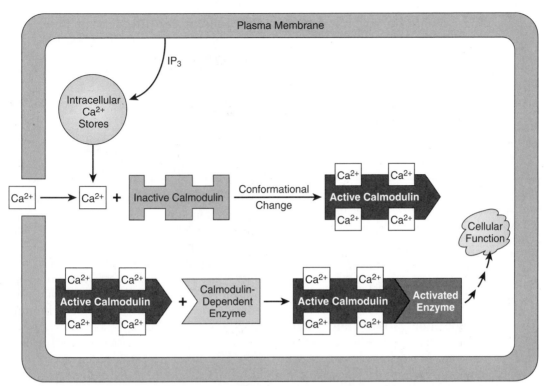

Figure 28–1. *General scheme for activation of Ca²⁺-dependent enzymes by calcium binding to calmodulin. The concentration of free intracellular Ca²⁺ can be increased by inositol triphosphate (IP₃)-dependent release of Ca²⁺ from intracellular stores and/or increased influx of Ca²⁺ across the plasma membrane in response to a signal initiated in the plasma membrane by binding of a hormone or growth factor to its receptor. Calcium ions bind to calmodulin, a ubiquitous cellular calcium-binding protein, resulting in a conformational change in this protein. The Ca²⁺-dependent alteration of calmodulin structure exposes a region of the protein that can now bind to and activate a calmodulin-dependent target enzyme. The activation of the enzyme subsequently results directly or indirectly in a change in cellular function. The Ca²⁺ signal is turned off by lowering the cytosolic Ca²⁺ concentration by sequestering free Ca²⁺ or pumping the Ca²⁺ out of the cell via plasma membrane Ca²⁺-ATPase pumps.*

Role of Calcium in Activation of Other Proteins

Ca^{2+} binding to some proteins can affect cellular activity without first causing a conformational change in the Ca^{2+}-dependent protein. For example, cellular Ca^{2+} concentrations can control biological activity by facilitating the conversion of inactive proenzymes to active enzymes. This process is illustrated by considering some of the enzymes involved in digestion and blood clotting.

Phospholipase A₂. This enzyme has a strong, predetermined fold that generates a rather immobile cavity for Ca^{2+} binding. Thus, the binding of Ca^{2+} to phospholipase A_2 has little effect on the conformation of the protein. In the case of phospholipase A_2, Ca^{2+} is needed to hold the phosphate group of the phospho-

lipid substrate in a suitable location for hydrolysis of the *sn*-2 ester linkage. Arachidonic acid is derived from membrane phospholipids by the action of phospholipase A_2, and this reaction acts as the rate-limiting step in prostaglandin synthesis, as described further in Chapter 15.

Calpain. This Ca^{2+}-dependent neutral proteinase is present as a 110-kDa complex in the soluble fraction of all mammalian cells. The protein complex consists of an 80-kDa catalytic subunit and a 30-kDa regulatory subunit. In the presence of a calpain activator protein, which also is a Ca^{2+}-binding protein, physiological concentrations of Ca^{2+} result in the dissociation and activation of the calpain complex. Progressive binding of Ca^{2+} to the calpain complex is linearly related to the dissociation of the two subunits, which reaches completion when all 8 Ca^{2+}-binding sites of calpain (4 per subunit) are occupied. Moreover, the activity of the 80-kDa catalytic subunit itself also is enhanced in the presence of physiological concentrations of Ca^{2+} (Michetti et al., 1997).

Blood-Clotting Enzymes. In the case of the blood-clotting enzymes, Ca^{2+} has a dual role. Ca^{2+} binds to membrane phospholipids via the negative charge associated with the phospho-moiety of the phospholipid and also plays a role in promoting cross-linking by binding to γ-carboxyglutamyl (Gla) or hydroxyaspartyl residues in pro-blood-clotting enzymes.

Calcium and Phosphorus as Components of Mineralized Tissue

Mineral Composition of Bone and Teeth. The skeleton is an important reservoir for minerals in the body. Approximately 99% of the body's calcium, 80% to 90% of the phosphates, 70% of magnesium, and 40% to 50% of sodium is found in bone (Driessens and Verbeeck, 1990). The mineral component of bone is largely calcium and phosphate. In the body, calcium is found mainly as the calcium phosphate compound hydroxyapatite. Forty-seven percent of skeletal weight is dry, fat-free bone, of which 26% is calcium. The organic matter of compact bone is composed primarily of collagen. The skeleton is made up of two types of bone tissue: cortical bone and trabecular bone. About 80% of the skeleton is composed of dense cortical bone, and the remainder is composed of sponge-like trabecular bone, which is found mostly in the axial skeleton and the ends of long bones. Trabecular bone is a frequent site of osteoporotic bone fracture and is particularly sensitive to calcium deficiency due to its relatively high rate of turnover.

The hard outer layer of teeth is composed of enamel, which is 96% (by weight) inorganic matter, 3% water, and 1% organic matter. The inner dentine layer of the tooth is composed of 70% mineral, 20% organic matter, and 10% water. The major inorganic constituents of teeth are calcium and phosphate. The turnover of calcium in teeth is negligible.

Calcium-Binding Proteins in Bone. The most abundant noncollagenous protein (NCP) produced by bone cells is osteonectin, a phosphorylated glycoprotein, which accounts for about 2% of the total protein in developing bone and which has a high affinity for binding calcium and hydroxyapatite (Termine, 1993). This protein can be found in platelets and nonskeletal tissues that are rapidly proliferating. Its function in bone may be associated with osteoblast proliferation and matrix mineralization. However, the best-studied Ca^{2+}-binding protein in bone is osteocalcin. Osteocalcin is an NCP that requires vitamin K for posttranslational modification of glutamyl residues in the protein to Gla residues. Osteocalcin (also known as bone Gla-protein, BGP) is a 6-kDa, bone-specific, Gla-containing protein in which Ca^{2+} binding occurs via the Gla side chains. Another Gla-protein, matrix-Gla-protein (MGP), is a 9-kDa NCP found in bone and cartilage and also in other tissues in the body. Both osteocalcin and MGP are structurally similar, but the functions of these proteins are unknown. Osteocalcin production in bone is enhanced by 1,25-dihydroxyvitamin D [$1,25(OH)_2D$], and serum osteocalcin is used as a biochemical marker of bone turnover.

Some Important Biological Functions of Phosphate

Oxidative Phosphorylation to Form ATP. ATP serves as a common intermediate between cellular processes that generate free energy, such as glycolysis and respiration, and processes that consume free energy. Important cellular processes that require free energy, such as biosynthesis, contraction and motility, and active transport, depend largely on the energy released from splitting the energy-rich phosphate bond of ATP. Most catabolic pathways appear to be regulated by the energy charge or the phosphorylation potential of the cell. AMP and ADP often serve as stimulatory regulators of catabolic reactions, whereas ATP often acts as an inhibitor of regulatory enzymes controlling the rate of catabolic pathways. Biosynthetic reactions are also regulated by AMP, ADP, and ATP, particularly the pathways leading to fuel storage in the form of glycogen and fat.

HPO_4^{2-} and $H_2PO_4^-$ as an Acid-Base Buffer System.

It is crucial for the body to maintain acid-base balance within narrow limits. One of the major ways in which large changes in H^+ concentration are prevented is by buffering. The body's buffers, which are primarily weak acids, are able to take up or release H^+ so that changes in pH are minimized. Phosphate is an effective buffer in the body. If H^+ ions are added to the extracellular fluid, they will combine with HPO_4^{2-} to form $H_2PO_4^-$ (Rose, 1984). Conversely, if H^+ ions are lost from the extracellular fluid, H^+ will be released from $H_2PO_4^-$.

DNA and RNA.

The hidden plan for an organism's development lies within information-containing elements, called genes, that are carried by chromosomes in the nucleus of a cell. Genetic instructions are coded within the genes by DNA and are transcribed into messenger ribonucleic acid (mRNA) molecules that can be translated in the extranuclear compartment into functional proteins. Both DNA and RNA are linear polymers of nucleotides linked together by covalent phosphodiester linkages that join the 5′-carbon of one nucleotide to the 3′-carbon of the next to form a sugar-phosphate backbone.

Phospholipids.

Phospholipids are small molecules that resemble triacylglycerols because they are composed of fatty acids and glycerol. However, in phospholipids the glycerol is joined to two fatty acids rather than three. The remaining site on glycerol is joined to a phosphate group, which in turn is linked to another small hydrophilic compound such as ethanolamine, choline, or serine. The fatty acid chains provide a hydrophobic tail for the molecule, whereas the phosphate-linked polar head groups of phospholipid molecules provide a hydrophilic head, allowing the molecule to act as a detergent. Phospholipid molecules spread out to form thin films on water, with the hydrophobic tails facing away from the water and the hydrophilic heads in contact with the water. The structural basis of cell membranes is based on two such phospholipid films aligned tail-to-tail in sandwich fashion, creating a lipid bilayer.

Metabolic Trapping of Substrates.

Neutral molecules can pass more readily across cell membranes than charged molecules can. Phosphorylation of substrates can result in the metabolic trapping of the phosphorylated compound within the cell. For example, vitamin B_6 vitamers are released from food during the process of digestion. Nonspecific phosphatases in the intestine hydrolyze the 5′-phosphate of these vitamers, allowing passage of the vitamin into the enterocyte via a nonsaturable, passive absorption process. After absorption, the vitamers can be phosphorylated and thus retained (Leklem, 1996).

Nucleotides, Creatine Phosphate, and Other Phosphoesters.

The principal forms of purine and pyrimidine compounds in cells are nucleotides, which consist of nucleosides (purine or pyrimidine bases attached to β-D-ribose or β-D-2-deoxyribose) that have one or more phosphate groups esterified to the sugar moiety (usually to the 5′-carbon). The most abundant nucleotide in normal cells is ATP. The major purine derivatives in cells are the adenosine and guanosine tri- and diphosphates, certain coenzymes or "activated" compounds that contain adenosine phosphate moieties, nucleotide derivatives such as guanosine diphosphate (GDP)-mannose, and, of course, DNA and RNA, which are polymers synthesized from nucleotide precursors. The major pyrimidine derivatives in cells are the uridine, cytidine, and thymidine tri- and diphosphates, nucleotide derivatives [such as uridine phosphate (UDP)-glucose and cytidine diphosphate (CDP)-choline] that act as substrates for various reactions, DNA (containing deoxycytidine and deoxythymidine residues), and RNA (containing uridine and cytidine residues).

Synthesis of purine and pyrimidine nucleotides is regulated by the concentrations of nucleotides in the cell. For example, the rate-limiting step in de novo purine synthesis is the reaction catalyzed by 5-phosphoribosyl pyrophosphate (PRPP) glutamyl aminotransferase (see Figure 11–14 in Chapter 11), which is strongly regulated by inosine 5′-monophosphate (IMP), guanosine monophosphate (GMP), and AMP.

Nucleotide triphosphates are required for

synthesis of the active forms of a number of substrates and coenzymes for enzymatic reactions. These include synthesis of phosphate-containing "activated" metabolic intermediates such as 3′-phosphoadenosine 5′-phosphosulfate (PAPS) as well as a number of nucleotide diphosphate derivatives such as UDP-glucuronide. Phosphate esters of sugars and their derivatives play major roles as intermediates in metabolism of glucose and other carbohydrates. These phosphate esters are formed mainly by ATP-requiring reactions that transfer a phosphate group from ATP to the sugar and release free ADP.

Coenzymes are molecules that are associated with enzymes and are essential for their catalytic functions. Coenzymes generally participate in reactions as carrier molecules that transfer chemical groups to other molecules. Some coenzymes contain AMP moieties contributed by ATP in the coenzyme synthetic pathway; these include nicotinamide adenine dinucleotide (phosphate) [NAD(P)], flavin adenine dinucleotide (FAD), and coenzyme A. Other coenzymes such as pyridoxal phosphate (PLP), flavin mononucleotide (FMN), and thiamine diphosphate (TPP) are phosphate esters of vitamin precursors. In addition to the adenosine 5′-monophosphate moiety, NADP and coenzyme A contain additional phosphate groups esterified to the 2′- and 3′-positions, respectively, of the adenosine moiety. The negatively charged phosphate groups present in these coenzymes are involved in interactions with their apoenzyme binding sites, and the 2′-phosphate of NADP allows enzymes to discriminate between NAD(H) and NADP(H) (Alberts et al., 1989). Coenzymes are discussed in more detail in Chapters 20–22.

Creatine phosphate is a high-energy phosphate ester that plays a special role in muscle during work. The hydrolysis of ATP provides the energy for driving a large number of biochemical reactions. In addition, both ADP and ATP are powerful effectors of many enzymes. Thus, the concentration and ratios of the adenine nucleotides are tightly controlled, and ATP cannot be increased to provide a reservoir of available energy. As an alternative, the muscle stores large amounts of high-energy phosphate as creatine phosphate. Creatine phosphate is used to replenish ATP levels by transfer of the phosphate group from creatine phosphate to ADP in a reaction catalyzed by creatine kinase. (See Chapter 39 for more detail about the role of creatine phosphate in exercising muscle.)

Signaling Molecules: Cyclic AMP, Cyclic GMP, and Inositol Triphosphate. A more recently recognized function of nucleotides and their derivatives is their role as mediators of key metabolic processes. For example, 3′,5′-cyclic AMP (cAMP) functions as a "second messenger" in hormone-mediated control of glycogenolysis and glycogenesis. Cyclic 3′,5′-GMP (cGMP) also serves as an intracellular messenger by activating a specific protein kinase that phosphorylates target proteins in the cell. In the eye, cGMP acts directly on sodium channels in the plasma membrane of the rod cells. In the absence of a light signal, cGMP is bound to the sodium channel, keeping it open. In the presence of light, a series of reactions occur that lead to an increase in cGMP phosphodiesterase, which hydrolyzes cGMP to 5′-GMP. The drop in cGMP allows the sodium channel to close. In this way, the light signal is converted into an electrical signal.

Inositol triphosphate (IP_3) couples receptor activation at the plasma membrane to Ca^{2+} release from a calcium-sequestering compartment in the cell interior. Phosphatidylinositol (PI) in the cell membrane is converted by a phosphorylation reaction (PI kinase) into the polyphosphatidylinositols: phosphatidylinositol 4-phosphate (PIP) and phosphatidylinositol 4,5-bisphosphate (PIP_2). Activation of a cell surface receptor activates a G-protein in the cell membrane that in turn activates phospholipase C, which cleaves PIP_2 to form IP_3 and diacylglycerol. IP_3 is a water-soluble molecule that releases Ca^{2+} from intracellular stores. Diacylglycerol can be further cleaved to yield arachidonic acid, which can be used to synthesize prostaglandins and other signaling molecules, or it can activate protein kinase C, which is a Ca^{2+}-dependent enzyme. (See Chapters 15 and 16 for more detail about these signaling processes.)

Reversible Covalent Modification of Proteins. Many protein molecules have two or more slightly different conformations available to them, and, by shifting reversibly from one to the other, they can alter their function. A common mechanism employed by the cell to control the shape of certain proteins involves covalent modification by transfer of a phosphate group from ATP to a seryl, threonyl, or tyrosyl residue in the protein, forming a covalent linkage. (See Chapters 9 and 16 for more discussion of the role of phosphorylation in the regulation of enzyme activity.) The alternate phosphorylation and dephosphorylation of proteins via protein kinases and phosphatases is an important cellular control mechanism. In addition, ATP-driven conformational changes in membrane-bound proteins can act as pumps to cause the influx or efflux of ions from a cell. For example, the Na^+,K^+-ATPase in the cell membrane pumps 3 Na^+ into the cell and 2 K^+ out of the cell during each cycle of conformational change driven by ATP-mediated phosphorylation (see Figure 30–2 in Chapter 30).

HORMONAL REGULATION OF CALCIUM AND PHOSPHATE METABOLISM

To maintain homeostasis and supply the mineral needs of the body, calcium and phosphate absorption by the intestine and reabsorption by the kidney and bone mineral turnover are coordinately regulated by the hormones 1,25-dihydroxyvitamin D (1,25$(OH)_2$D, also called calcitriol), parathyroid hormone (PTH), and calcitonin, as summarized in Figure 28–2. A fourth hormone, parathyroid hormone–related protein (PTHrP), which is produced by several different cell types, has been identified recently and shown to cause hypercalcemia in patients with certain cancers. However, the normal physiological function of PTHrP is unknown.

Parathyroid Hormone

PTH is a peptide hormone that is produced in the parathyroid gland and acts on the cell through PTH receptors on the cell surface. The biologically active form of PTH is a single-chain polypeptide of 84 amino acids; however, only the first 31 amino acids of PTH are essential for biological activity. It was discovered recently that the parathyroid gland also contains a protein that acts as a sensor of plasma-ionized calcium levels (Chattopadhyay et al., 1996). A drop in ionized calcium in the blood is detected by the calcium sensor, leading to an increase in PTH secretion. The actions of PTH ultimately lead to an increase in calcium in the extracellular fluid, creating a negative feedback regulatory loop.

Bone and kidney are the primary target organs for PTH. PTH interacts with specific receptors on the plasma membrane of bone cells (osteoblasts) and tubular kidney cells to stimulate the adenylate cyclase system and subsequently cAMP production. Cyclic AMP acts as a second messenger to activate enzymes, such as protein kinases, that result in expression of the biological actions of PTH. Despite the fact that PTH plays an important role in bone resorption, no PTH receptors have been identified on osteoclasts. PTH may produce its bone resorbing effect by changing the shape of osteoblast-like cells that cover bone to make more room for osteoclasts, or through osteoblastic release of an unidentified messenger that enhances osteoclastic activity (Mundy, 1993). Increased plasma PTH concentrations are detected by renal PTH receptors, causing the kidneys to increase the rate of renal calcium reabsorption (which decreases urinary calcium loss) and decrease the rate of phosphate reabsorption (which increases urinary phosphate loss). PTH stimulates the renal conversion of an inactive circulating vitamin D metabolite 25-hydroxyvitamin D (25-OH-D) into the active hormonal form of vitamin D (1,25$(OH)_2$D) by stimulating increased activity of the renal 25-hydroxyvitamin D 1α-hydroxylase. There are no PTH receptors in the intestine, but the PTH-mediated increase in circulating 1,25$(OH)_2$D leads to an increase in intestinal calcium and phosphate absorption. The increased flux of calcium into the plasma compartment from the intestine, kidney, and bone helps restore steady-state calcium levels. Hyperphosphatemia is prevented by the phosphaturic effect of PTH on the kidneys.

1,25-Dihydroxyvitamin D

Vitamin D can enter the circulation after synthesis in the skin or absorption from the diet.

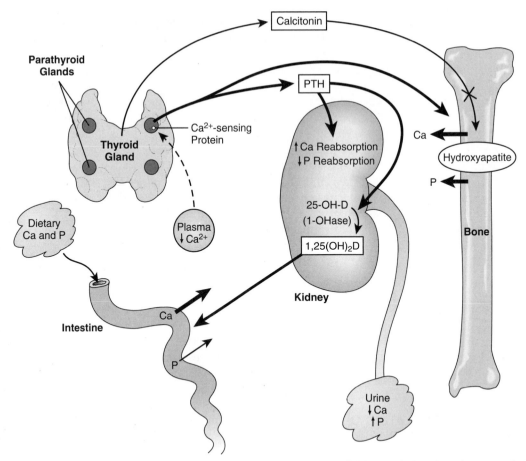

Figure 28–2. *Hormonal control of calcium and phosphate metabolism. Calcium and phosphate homeostasis is maintained by the coordinated actions of three organ systems: intestine, kidney, and bone. A fall in plasma ionic Ca^{2+} is detected by a calcium-sensor protein in the parathyroid glands that subsequently causes an increased secretion of the peptide hormone PTH from the parathyroid glands. Elevated levels of PTH in the plasma activate PTH receptors in the kidneys as well as in bone osteoblasts. The renal effect of PTH is to cause an immediate increase in renal calcium reabsorption and a decrease in renal phosphate reabsorption. PTH also has a delayed effect on calcium and phosphate metabolism by stimulating the activity of the renal 1α-hydroxylase (1-OHase) that converts inactive 25-OH-D to the active vitamin D metabolite $1,25(OH)_2D$. The primary action of $1,25(OH)_2D$ is to significantly increase intestinal calcium absorption and, to a lesser extent, phosphate absorption. In addition, $1,25(OH)_2D$ can also promote bone resorption by stimulating the production of osteoclasts.*
Elevations of plasma ionic Ca^{2+} brought about by these changes in calcium flux serve as a signal to create a negative feedback loop by removing the stimulus to the calcium-sensing protein in the parathyroid gland and promoting a drop in PTH secretion. Hypercalcemia also stimulates the secretion of calcitonin from the thyroid gland. Calcitonin interacts with calcitonin receptors on osteoclasts and inhibits bone resorption. 25-OH-D, 25-hydroxyvitamin D; $1,25(OH)_2D$, 1,25-dihydroxyvitamin D; PTH, parathyroid hormone.

Vitamin D is transported through the body bound to a vitamin D–binding protein. This complex binds to liver cells, allowing vitamin D to enter the hepatocyte. In the liver, the vitamin D molecule is stored or can be hydroxylated at carbon 25. The resulting 25-OH-D leaves the liver and is bound again in the blood by the vitamin D–binding protein. 25-OH-D can then be taken up by the kidney, which can add one additional hydroxyl group

at the carbon 1 position to form $1,25(OH)_2D$, the active hormone form of vitamin D. The renal conversion of 25-OH-D to $1,25(OH)_2D$ is primarily regulated in the renal cell by PTH.

$1,25(OH)_2D$ acts on cells through an intracellular receptor protein called the vitamin D receptor, which is found in many different tissues. In the mammalian intestine, $1,25$-$(OH)_2D$ increases production of calbindin D_{9K}, a 9-kDa intracellular Ca^{2+}-binding protein that facilitates the absorption of calcium. In addition, $1,25(OH)_2D$ also stimulates the synthesis of a Na^+-dependent phosphate pump, that facilitates phosphate absorption in the brush border membrane of the enterocyte (Lee et al., 1981a). Osteoblasts have intracellular receptors for $1,25(OH)_2D$ that when activated by the hormone can interact with specific promoter regions of DNA to increase the transcription of vitamin D–specific genes, such as osteocalcin. However, many of the details of how $1,25(OH)_2D$ affects bone turnover and mineralization at the molecular level remain to be determined. See Chapter 27 for additional information about the hormonal actions of $1,25(OH)_2D$.

Calcitonin

Calcitonin, synthesized by the C cells of the thyroid gland, is a polypeptide containing 32 amino acid residues, almost all of which are needed for biological activity. A rise in plasma Ca^{2+} is the strongest calcitonin secretagogue. When blood Ca^{2+} increases acutely, there is a parallel increase in calcitonin secretion, whereas an acute drop in plasma Ca^{2+} results in a decrease in calcitonin secretion. Osteoclasts have calcitonin receptors on the plasma membrane that respond to the hormone with an increase in cAMP production that in turn mediates the actions of calcitonin, which include inhibition of the movement of the pseudopod-like extensions of osteoclasts. Inactivation of calcitonin occurs primarily in the kidney. Calcitonin acts in opposition to PTH and lowers blood calcium levels by inhibiting osteoclastic bone resorption. However, it should be noted that the role of calcitonin in calcium homeostasis and skeletal metabolism has not been established in humans, and many questions remain unanswered about the physiological significance of the hormone in humans (Deftos, 1993). Nevertheless, the hypocalcemic effect of calcitonin has led to the use of this hormone as a drug to treat diseases associated with high rates of bone resorption and concomitant hypercalcemia, such as Paget's disease, osteoporosis, and hypercalcemia of malignancy.

Parathyroid Hormone–Related Protein

PTHrP is a recently discovered protein that can be produced in an unregulated manner by various types of tumors. This unregulated production of PTHrP in some cancer patients leads to the development of the so-called humoral hypercalcemia of malignancy (Burtis, 1993). PTHrP is normally expressed in small amounts in many tissues in the body, including skin and other epithelia, the central nervous system, many endocrine glands, islet cells, breast, uterus, and urinary bladder. Physiologically, PTHrP is probably acting locally where it is produced as an autocrine or paracrine hormone. However, PTHrP has significant amino acid sequence homology to PTH in the amino-terminal end of the protein and is thereby able to stimulate PTH receptors. When PTHrP is produced in an unregulated fashion by tumors, it acts as a systemic hormone and causes hypercalcemia via its effect on the PTH receptor. A midregion fragment of PTHrP has been shown to stimulate the activity of a placental calcium pump, and the carboxy-terminal region of the molecule may inhibit osteoclastic bone resorption.

Other Hormones Affecting Calcium and Phosphate Metabolism

Although PTH, $1,25(OH)_2D$, and calcitonin are the major calcium and phosphate-regulating hormones, several other hormones, such as glucocorticoids, thyroid hormone, growth hormone, insulin, and estrogen, can also affect bone turnover and mineral metabolism (Favus, 1993).

The main effect of glucocorticoids on bone is an inhibition of osteoblastic activity, although osteoclastic activity is also impaired. There is a reduced incorporation of sulfate into cartilage and of amino acids into collagen. Glucocorticoids also impair both the active and passive transport of calcium through intestinal cells. An excess of glucocorticoids can lead to hypocalcemia and PTH stimulation, which results in a reduction in renal phosphate reabsorption and increased urinary phosphate losses. In Cushing's disease or when cortisol is used to treat arthritis, glucocorticoid excess can lead to bone loss, especially of trabecular bone, and result in osteoporosis. In children, excess glucocorticoid frequently results in delayed growth and skeletal maturation.

Thyroid hormone stimulates bone resorption, and both compact and trabecular bone are lost in hyperthyroidism. Increased urinary phosphate is observed in hyperthyroid patients in association with increased serum phosphate. In hypothyroidism, the bone-mobilizing effect of PTH is impaired, leading to secondary hyperparathyroidism.

Growth hormone can stimulate the growth of cartilage and bone through the trophic action of insulin-like growth factor (IGF). Growth hormone can also stimulate the 1α-hydroxylase enzyme in the kidney, causing increased serum 1,25(OH)$_2$D levels. Growth hormone and IGF levels decline in the aged. In senescent rats, growth hormone administration can increase calcium and phosphate absorption independently of changes in serum 1,25(OH)$_2$D (Fleet et al., 1994).

Insulin, a pancreatic hormone primarily involved with regulating glucose metabolism, also stimulates the osteoblastic production of collagen. In addition, insulin can reduce the renal reabsorption of calcium and sodium and decrease urinary phosphate losses.

Estrogen receptors have been identified in bone, and gonadal hormones are known to play an important role in maintaining bone mass. Estrogen deficiency, which occurs in women after menopause, results in an increased loss of bone mineral and is an important factor in the development of postmenopausal osteoporosis. Estrogen hormone replacement therapy in postmenopausal women reduces the rate of bone loss and the incidence of bone fracture. Hypogonadism in adult men is a risk factor for osteoporosis, which may be related to the effects of testosterone on bone resorption.

CALCIUM AND PHOSPHATE HOMEOSTASIS

Mineral balance represents the equilibrium condition in which the amount of a mineral absorbed from the diet equals the sum of all the daily losses of the mineral from the body.

Because 99% of the calcium in the body is found in the skeleton, changes in calcium balance are reflected in changes in bone mass. During growth, a positive calcium and phosphate balance must be maintained to supply sufficient amounts of these minerals for bone growth. In contrast, during periods of bone loss, as occur with immobilization and commonly during aging, loss of bone calcium results in a negative calcium balance. Coordination of calcium and phosphate fluxes across the intestine, kidney, and bone maintains calcium and phosphate homeostasis in the face of marked changes in daily intakes of these minerals and of longer-term metabolic changes associated with changing calcium and phosphate needs throughout the life cycle.

Intestinal Absorption

The unidirectional absorption of calcium or phosphate from the diet is called "true" absorption. However, there is also some obligatory mineral loss into the gastrointestinal tract, as part of digestive secretions and sloughed intestinal cells, which is referred to as endogenous fecal loss. The difference between true intestinal absorption and endogenous fecal loss is called "net" absorption, which is thus always lower than true absorption. Net absorption of calcium and phosphate is the nutritionally important absorption fraction that is available to build new bone, to maintain steady-state plasma levels of these minerals, and to replace any skeletal and renal losses.

True Intestinal Absorption. The unidirectional rate of intestinal calcium absorption is primarily regulated by the circulating level of 1,25(OH)$_2$D. The efficiency of true calcium absorption varies in response to the dietary calcium intake and throughout the life span as a function of metabolic need. However, it is usually within the range of about 25% to 60%, the latter being observed in infants and the former being typical of young adults (Institute of Medicine, 1997). Aging is associated with a gradual decline in intestinal calcium absorption (Avioli et al., 1965).

Kinetic studies of calcium transport suggest that there are two distinct pathways for calcium absorption in the intestine (Bronner, 1988). One pathway represents an active, energy-dependent, transcellular pathway, with limited capacity, that is under hormonal regulation. The second absorption pathway is a nonsaturable, energy-independent, concentration-dependent, paracellular transport pathway that is not regulated. The active, saturable, transcellular transport pathway is found mainly in the duodenum and proximal jejunum, is regulated primarily by $1,25(OH)_2D$, and involves the vitamin D–dependent cytosolic calcium-binding protein calbindin D. Quantitatively, the most important site of calcium absorption in the intestine is the ileum, due to the relatively long sojourn of calcium in this segment of the intestine. It has been shown in humans that removal of the ileum has a more devastating effect on calcium absorption than does removal of the jejunum. Although calcium can also be absorbed by the colon, in humans this segment of the intestine apparently plays a very minor role in the overall economy of calcium absorption. However, in rats, the cecum has a high rate of vitamin D–dependent calcium absorption, which increases during dietary calcium deficiency (Nellans and Goldsmith, 1983).

The paracellular transport pathway is present throughout the intestine. In humans, calcium intakes above as little as 3 mmol (120 mg) in a meal are mostly absorbed by the diffusion-dependent transport route (Sheikh et al., 1988). Calcium absorption continues to increase with intake of very high amounts of calcium as a result of this diffusion-dependent paracellular route. The total amount of calcium absorbed from the intestine represents the sum of the saturable, carrier-mediated calcium transport process and the nonsaturable concentration-dependent process.

The molecular details of transcellular calcium transport are still not fully understood. A simplified model of the molecular details of calcium transport across the enterocyte is shown in Figure 28–3. Conceptually, the transport of any minerals across the intestinal cell must involve mechanisms that allow the ionic form of the mineral to traverse three formidable cellular barriers: the brush border membrane, the aqueous cell cytosol, and the basolateral membrane (Serfaty-Lacrosniere et al., 1995).

In the case of calcium, two additional important constraints are present, however. First, the final step in the process of transport out of the enterocyte requires that calcium be transported "up-hill" against a 10,000-fold Ca^{2+} concentration gradient because intracellular Ca^{2+} levels are maintained at 10^{-7} mol/L while extracellular Ca^{2+} is 10^{-3} mol/L. This function is performed by an energy-dependent calcium pump (Ca^{2+}-ATPase) on the basolateral membrane of the enterocyte. Second, because intracellular free Ca^{2+} concentration is used by cells as a second messenger to control a large number of intracellular events vital to cell function and survival, Ca^{2+} vectorially transported across the enterocyte must somehow be compartmentalized. This function may be served by the vitamin D–dependent protein calbindin D. In addition, some recent evidence suggests that Ca^{2+} may be physically sequestered inside endosomal and lysosomal vesicles during its absorptive sojourn through the enterocyte (Nemere, 1992).

Studies in isolated brush border membrane vesicle preparations have shown that the rate of calcium transport across the intestinal brush border membrane is greater in vitamin D–replete compared with vitamin D-deplete animals (Fontaine et al., 1981). However, the molecular details of how vitamin D status can alter calcium transport across the brush border membrane are not well understood. The characteristics of calcium movement across the brush border are consistent with the notion of a vitamin D–regulated calcium carrier protein being present in the membrane. This putative brush border membrane calcium carrier has not been isolated, however. A liponomic theory has also been postulated to explain the effects of vitamin D on calcium transport across the brush border membrane (Fontaine et al., 1981). According to this theory, vitamin D–dependent changes in membrane lipid composition and membrane fluidity are responsible for altering the rate of calcium transport across the membrane.

The increased rate of calcium absorption

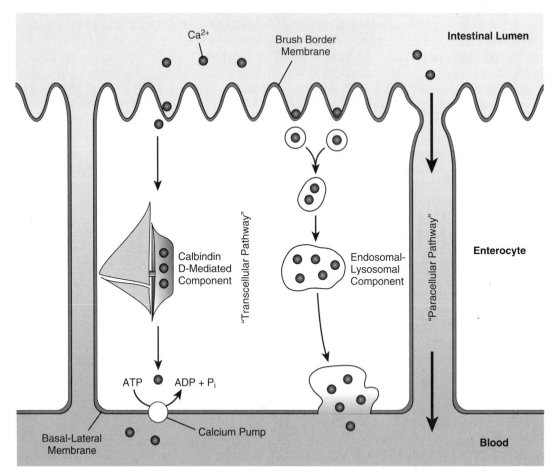

Figure 28–3. *Model of calcium transport pathways across the intestine. Calcium crosses the intestine by two possible routes. One pathway is characterized by a nonsaturable, energy-independent, concentration-dependent, paracellular transport pathway, which probably occurs between the absorptive cells and is not hormonally regulated. The second pathway is characterized by a saturable, energy-dependent, transcellular pathway across the enterocyte, which has a limited transport capacity and is primarily regulated by 1,25(OH)₂D via a genomic mechanism that stimulates the production of calbindin D. Calbindin D is primarily a cytosolic protein that acts as an intracellular "ferry" for calcium across the aqueous cytosolic compartment. This protein may also regulate the activity of Ca²⁺-ATPase pumps on the basolateral cell membrane that extrude Ca²⁺ out of the cell against an electrochemical gradient. Some calcium may also be transported through the cell in endosomal and lysosomal vesicles and exit from the cell via the process of exocytosis.*

observed in response to vitamin D treatment is associated with an increased synthesis of the vitamin D–dependent protein calbindin D. Calbindin is believed to act as an intracellular calcium "ferry" that facilitates the diffusion of calcium across the aqueous cytosol and delivers ionic calcium to the ATP-dependent calcium pumps on the basolateral membrane for extrusion out of the cell. It has been argued, however, based on quantitative estimates of the number and activity of Ca^{2+}-ATPase pumps on the enterocyte, that the basolateral exit step is not the primary rate-limiting step controlling the efficiency of

calcium absorption in the intestine (Bronner et al., 1986). Nevertheless, some evidence suggests that vitamin D status influences the expression of the Ca^{2+}-ATPase mRNA and the number of calcium pumps on the basolateral membrane (Wasserman et al., 1992). Moreover, calbindin D may directly stimulate the activity of the Ca^{2+}-ATPase pumps on the basolateral membrane (Walters, 1989). However, based on quantitative considerations of the relative rates of calcium transport across the brush border and basolateral membranes of intestinal cells, it has been proposed that the rate of passage of calcium across the cytosol is the rate-limiting step in calcium absorption (Bronner et al., 1986).

Recently, it has been suggested that at least part of the transcellular transport of calcium in the intestine may involve trafficking and compartmentalization of calcium by an endosomal-lysosomal pathway (Nemere and Norman, 1988). According to this theory, calcium enters the cell by endocytosis in primary endosomes formed at the cell surface. The calcium in these endosomal vesicles is then passed on to lysosomes from which the calcium can then exit from the cell via the process of exocytosis. However, there is little evidence as yet demonstrating that exocytosis of calcium accounts for the bulk of vectorially transported calcium across the enterocyte. Additional experiments, probably based on modern molecular biology techniques, will be necessary to demonstrate more definitively the important regulatory step(s) in intestinal calcium transport.

About 60% to 70% of phosphate is absorbed from a typical mixed diet. Thus, phosphate absorption is at least twice as efficient as calcium absorption. Phosphate absorption in humans has been shown to be linearly related to phosphate intake over a wide range of phosphate intakes (Lee et al., 1981a). Phosphate absorption is influenced by vitamin D status, although to a less marked degree than calcium absorption is normally affected. Administration of $1,25(OH)_2D$ has been shown to increase phosphate absorption in humans (Ramirez et al., 1986). In rats, $1,25(OH)_2D$ increases phosphate absorption in all segments of the small intestine, but the major effect occurs in the jejunum (Lee et al., 1981b).

Little is known about the molecular details of intestinal phosphate absorption. Transport of phosphate into the intestinal cell is by an active, Na^+-dependent pathway, and the preferred phosphate form transported is HPO_4^{2-} (Lee et al., 1981a). The kinetics of phosphate uptake in vitro by isolated intestinal brush border vesicle preparations is consistent with the suggestion that phosphate is transported across the apical membrane of the enterocyte by a carrier-mediated mechanism. Moreover, a 130-kDa protein has been putatively identified as the brush border, Na^+-sensitive phosphate transporter (Peerce,

1993). Like calcium, phosphate is absorbed by both a saturable and nonsaturable transport pathway.

Endogenous Fecal Loss. Approximately 3.5 mmol/d (140 mg/day) of calcium enters the intestinal lumen in secretions, but about 29% of this is absorbed, so that the minimum endogenous fecal calcium is usually 2.5 mmol/day (100 mg/day) (Heaney and Recker, 1994). Reports of endogenous fecal losses of phosphate have been quite variable but are usually lower than those observed for endogenous fecal calcium losses.

Urinary Excretion

Urinary Calcium. Due to the binding of plasma calcium to albumin, a significant portion of plasma calcium cannot enter the kidneys. However, about 9.7 g of calcium are filtered each day by the kidneys. Urinary calcium excretion is usually only 2.5 to 6 mmol/day (100 to 240 mg/day) among normal individuals, which represents only about 1% to 2.5% of the calcium filtered by the kidney. Renal calcium transport is similar to that in the intestine. Active calcium transport is found in the distal convoluted tubule and possibly the proximal tubule, and it involves a vitamin D–dependent, 28-kDa protein, calbindin D_{28K}. Paracellular calcium transport, by which most renal calcium reabsorption occurs, takes place in the proximal tubule, the thick ascending limb of the loop of Henle, and the connecting and collecting ducts. Approximately 50% of excreted calcium is in the free Ca^{2+} form, and the remainder is complexed with small anions such as sulfate, phosphate, citrate, and oxalate. Patients with renal stones (nephrolithiasis) frequently have hypercalciuria (urinary calcium > 250 mg/day) and kidney stones composed of calcium oxalate crystals.

There are large diurnal fluctuations in the rate of urinary calcium excretion, due mainly to the calciuretic effect of various food components. Dietary calcium intake has a positive, but weak, relationship with urinary calcium excretion. Approximately 8% of the increment in dietary calcium intake over the usual range of dietary calcium intakes of 300 to 1600 mg/

CLINICAL CORRELATION

Dietary Calcium Intake and Renal Calcium Stones

Many patients with calcium kidney stones (nephrolithiasis) have idiopathic hypercalciuria. About 90% of these patients with excess urinary calcium losses are characterized by elevated active intestinal calcium absorption, normal serum calcium and PTH, and elevated serum 1,25(OH)$_2$D. The vitamin D elevation may be the primary defect, and it is associated with a renal phosphate leak (Vosburgh and Peters, 1987). For reasons that are not completely understood, renal stone formers exhibit a lower bone mineral content. Possible explanations are the hypophosphatemia, hypercalciuria, and elevated serum 1,25(OH)$_2$D accompanied by a low calcium intake. Unfortunately, maintenance of stone formers on a low calcium diet may exacerbate bone loss. Epidemiological evidence suggests that low calcium diets are associated with an increased risk of nephrolithiasis, probably due to a greater degree of oxalate absorption from the intestine when diets are low in calcium (Curhan et al., 1993). On the other hand, use of calcium supplements also has been shown to be associated with increased risk of stone formation.

day is lost in the urine (Lemann, 1993). Dietary intake of simple sugars and protein can increase urinary calcium losses. For example, it has been calculated that for each 50-g increment in daily protein intake, an additional 1.5 mmol (60 mg) of calcium is lost in the urine (Kerstetter and Allen, 1990).

The mechanism of protein-induced hypercalciuria involves a reduction of renal calcium reabsorption mediated in part by the sulfur amino acid content of the protein. The metabolism of these amino acids results in the generation of an acid (fixed anion, SO_4^-) load, which can inhibit renal calcium reabsorption. Intake of caffeine and sodium also increases urinary calcium loss. Urinary calcium and urinary sodium losses are frequently found to be positively associated because these two minerals share a common resorption mechanism in the proximal renal tubule.

On the other hand, there is an inverse relationship between dietary phosphate intake and urinary calcium. Elevations in serum phosphate decrease serum ionic calcium and thereby cause an increase in PTH synthesis, which in turn increases calcium reabsorption in the kidney. Phosphate also can affect renal tubular calcium transport independently of PTH (Lau et al., 1982). This anticalciuretic effect of phosphate has practical implications, because the high phosphate content of meat results in a considerable blunting of the usual hypercalciuric effect of consuming a high-protein diet (Spencer et al., 1978).

Urinary Phosphate. The kidneys provide the primary route for phosphate loss from the body and play an important role in the regulation of phosphate homeostasis (Lee et al., 1981a). The great majority of plasma inorganic phosphate is filtered at the renal glomerulus. The fractional excretion of filtered phosphate can be varied by the kidneys from 0.1% to 20%, so the kidney can efficiently regulate plasma phosphate. About 40% of the total phosphate reabsorption in the kidney occurs within the first few convolutions of the proximal tubule, and 60% to 70% has occurred by the time the ultrafiltrate reaches the last segment of the cortical superficial nephrons.

The transport of phosphate in the renal tubules occurs by two processes: one is dependent on sodium and the other is not. In the proximal tubule, phosphate is reabsorbed by an active, Na^+-dependent phosphate transport system. Brush border membranes from proximal tubule cells have a Na^+- and pH-dependent, saturable phosphate transport system, whereas phosphate transport across basolateral membranes (i.e., out of the renal cell) is via a passive transport process only. The primary regulator of the rate of renal phosphate reabsorption is the plasma phosphate concentration. In vitro studies in porcine and monkey renal cell lines have shown that treatment of cells with a low-phosphate medium results in a 2- to 7-fold increase in the rate of phosphate transport (Escoubet et al., 1989). This autoregulatory phenomenon is probably a widespread process that occurs in most, if not all, cell types.

The chief hormonal regulator of renal phosphate reabsorption is PTH. Plasma PTH is positively correlated with urinary excretion of phosphate and affects both the Na^+-dependent and Na^+-independent phosphate transport pathways. In addition, renal phosphate handling is also affected indirectly by PTH inhibition of proximal and distal bicarbonate reabsorption. The full molecular details of PTH action on renal phosphate transport are not precisely understood. Presumably, the steps involve transmembrane transduction of the cell surface signal initiated by PTH binding to its receptor and induction of an intracellular second messenger.

Bone Resorption and Formation

Bone is composed of collagen fibers, noncollagenous proteins, and deposited minerals, primarily hydroxyapatite. Crystals of hydroxyapatite are found in and on the collagen fibers and in the ground substance (glycoproteins and proteoglycans) of bone. Longitudinal bone growth occurs in children until closure of the epiphyses during adolescence. However, bone mineral density continues to increase until about the age of 30 years (Recker et al., 1992), and bone tissue is continually remodeled throughout life. This remodeling process occurs at localized sites in both cortical and trabecular bone. Although the entire bone calcium pool turns over on average every 5 to 6 years, a given local bone surface on trabecular bone may undergo complete remodeling once every 2 years. However, the rate of remodeling varies greatly among specific bones, with the lumbar vertebral bone turning over most rapidly. Two important cell types in bone are the osteoblasts, involved in bone formation, and the osteoclasts, involved in bone resorption.

Bone Formation. The activity of osteoblasts in bone determines the rate of bone matrix (collagen and ground substance) deposition. Osteoblasts originate from a local precursor mesenchymal stem cell that can be stimulated to undergo proliferation and differentiate into preosteoblasts and then into mature osteo-

blasts. Osteoblasts, which have cellular receptors for PTH, estrogen, and $1,25(OH)_2D$, regulate the flux of calcium and phosphate in bone and presumably mediate the deposition of hydroxyapatite in bone tissue. Osteoblasts are usually found in clusters of 100 to 400 cells per bone-forming site along the bone surface (Baron, 1993) lining a layer of uncalcified bone matrix that they are producing. Parenthetically, in vitamin D deficiency there is a defect in mineralization of bone matrix. A cardinal feature of osteomalacia (adult vitamin D deficiency) is an overabundance of unmineralized bone matrix that is evident on histologic staining of bone biopsies. Because the plasma membrane of the osteoblast is rich in the enzyme alkaline phosphatase, biochemical measures of bone-specific serum alkaline phosphatase are used as a convenient marker of bone formation rates. Osteoblasts also synthesize a vitamin D–dependent protein called osteocalcin, which is presumably important to the function of the skeleton. Serum osteocalcin also is used as a biochemical marker of bone formation.

Bone Resorption. The activity of osteoclasts in bone determines the rate of bone breakdown. The osteoclast has a monocytic-phagocytic cell lineage and is characterized histologically as a giant multinucleated cell that is usually found in contact with a calcified bone surface within a lacuna (hole) that is the result of its own resorptive activity (Baron, 1993). Usually only one to five osteoclasts are found associated with one of these resorptive cavities. The contact zone with the bone is characterized by the presence of a ruffled border on the osteoclast. The ruffled border portion of the osteoclast plasma membrane is surrounded by a ring of contractile proteins, which serve to attach the cell to the bone surface and seal off the subosteoclastic bone-resorbing compartment.

The attachment of the cell to the bone matrix is performed by integrin receptors that bind to specific sequences in matrix proteins (Baron, 1993). Lysosomal enzymes are actively secreted via the ruffled border of the osteoclast into the sealed-off extracellular bone-resorbing compartment. The osteoclast also secretes collagenase as well as protons to acidify the bone-resorbing compartment. The acid environment dissolves the hydroxyapatite crystals, and the secreted enzymes break down the bone matrix. The dissolution of bone helps maintain calcium and phosphate concentrations in the plasma. End products of bone matrix breakdown, such as hydroxyproline and amino-terminal collagen peptides, are excreted in the urine and can be used as convenient biochemical measures of bone resorption rates.

The mode of regulation of osteoclast activity is uncertain. Osteoclasts have receptors only for calcitonin, and their activity is decreased by calcitonin. However, osteoclasts also respond to other regulatory signals, such as PTH, $1,25(OH)_2D$, and prostaglandin E_2, presumably via osteoblast mediation.

Bone-Remodeling Cycle: "Coupled" Bone Formation and Bone Resorption. After the osteoclasts have finished removing a certain amount of bone, they are replaced by bone-forming osteoblasts that then proceed to replace the excavated bone material. The total resorptive period at a given bone site takes about 40 days to complete. After about one week of the resorptive phase, the formation activity of osteoblasts begins and continues for about 145 days (Melsen and Mosekilde, 1988). Thus, the remodeling of bone involves a recurring cycle of skeletal events involving the coordinated activities of osteoblasts and osteoclasts. This process of bone remodeling can be divided into four phases: activation, resorption, formation, and a resting phase.

Activation is the process by which osteoclast precursor cells are transformed into osteoclasts. Prostaglandins or lymphokines produced by cells at the bone site probably act to attract osteoclasts to the specific area of bone destined to be resorbed. Bone resorption and formation are mediated by the activity of osteoclasts and osteoblasts. During the process of remodeling, a "coupling" is somehow established between bone resorption and bone formation that ensures the overall integrity of the skeleton despite the ongoing bone-remodeling process. Factors leading to the uncoupling of bone formation and bone resorption are important in the development of osteoporosis.

Because the process of bone remodeling is relatively long, clinical trials evaluating potential therapeutic agents (such as calcium supplementation) on bone mass need to be carried out for at least 2 to 3 years. Otherwise, simple transient effects on bone remodeling caused by the intervention and due to the temporary disruption of the normal remodeling process would not be distinguished from changes that would have a sustained long-term benefit on the skeleton (Heaney, 1994).

DIETARY SOURCES, BIOAVAILABILITY, AND RECOMMENDED INTAKES FOR CALCIUM AND PHOSPHORUS

Dietary Sources of Calcium and Phosphate

The great majority of calcium in American diets is supplied by dairy products. If milk-based products are excluded from the diet or used in limited amounts, then the relatively low calcium content of many foods makes it difficult to achieve recommended amounts of dietary calcium. Other relatively rich vegetarian sources of calcium include calcium-set tofu and certain green vegetables. Recently, calcium-fortified foods, such as orange juice, have appeared on the market in response to recommendations to increase calcium intakes to prevent osteoporosis (National Institutes of Health, 1994).

Phosphate is found widely distributed in foodstuffs. In general, food sources high in protein (meats, milk, eggs, and cereals) are also high in phosphate. Dairy products, meat, fish, poultry, and eggs supply about 70% of typical phosphate intakes in the United States (Life Sciences Research Office, 1989). Phosphate in meat is found mainly as intracellular organic compounds, which are mostly hydrolyzed in the gastrointestinal tract to release inorganic phosphate, which is available for intestinal absorption. Processed meat also contains various polyphosphates and pyrophosphates as additives.

Calcium and Phosphate Bioavailability

Bioavailability refers to the fraction of a nutrient in food that is absorbed and metabolically

Food Sources of Calcium

- Milk, yogurt, and cheese
- Tofu
- Sardines and canned salmon (with bones)
- Corn tortillas processed with lime (calcium hydroxide)
- Various green vegetables

Adequate Intakes Across the Life Cycle

	mg calcium/day
Infants, 0–0.5 y	210
0.5–1 y	270
Children, 1–3 y	500
4–8 y	800
9–18 y	1300
Adults, 19–50 y	1000
>50 y	1200
Pregnant or lactating women	
<19 y	1300
19–50 y	1000

From Institute of Medicine (1997) Dietary Reference Intakes for Calcium, Phosphorus, Magnesium, Vitamin D, and Fluoride. National Academy Press, Washington, D.C.

Food Sources of Phosphorus

- Meats
- Milk
- Eggs
- Cereals

RDAs Across the Life Cycle

	mg phosphorus/day
Infants, 0–0.5 y	100 (AI)
0.5–1.0 y	275 (AI)
Children, 1–3 y	460
4–8 y	500
9–18 y	1250
Adults, 19–50 y	700
>50 y	700
Pregnant or lactating women	
<19 y	1250
19–50 y	700

From Institute of Medicine (1997) Dietary Reference Intakes for Calcium, Phosphorus, Magnesium, Vitamin D, and Fluoride. National Academy Press, Washington, D.C.

available. Ideally, an evaluation of dietary calcium and phosphate adequacy should consider not only the quantitative aspects of consumption but also the relative bioavailability of these minerals from the diet. A variety of dietary factors are known to influence calcium bioavailability (Allen and Wood, 1994). From a practical perspective, the most important dietary factors influencing calcium absorption from food are the levels of dietary fiber, phytate, and oxalate.

Milk has long been considered to be the best dietary source of calcium. However, large segments of the population are lactose-intolerant (see Chapter 5) and may avoid milk or desire to consume only limited quantities. In recent years, investigators have utilized intrinsically incorporated, stable isotopes of calcium to study the bioavailability of calcium from various foodstuffs. Using this approach, the absorbability of calcium from several foods has been shown to be equivalent to or better than that of calcium from milk. However, although some low-oxalate green leafy vegetables have been shown to be sources of highly bioavailable calcium (Heaney and Weaver, 1990), milk is clearly one of the richest sources of highly absorbable dietary calcium on a per serving basis (Fig. 28–4).

Phosphate from meat is well absorbed (>70%) by humans. However, little is known about the bioavailability of phosphate from different plant-based foods. Phosphate in grains is mostly in the form of phytate (myoinositol hexaphosphate), an organophosphate compound used by plants to store phosphate. For example, in wheat, rice, and maize, more than 80% of the total phosphate is found as phytate, whereas as much as 35% of the phosphate in mature potato tubers is in this chemical form.

Recommended Calcium and Phosphorus Intakes

Many people in the United States do not consume recommended levels of dietary calcium (Fig. 28–5), although phosphate intakes appear quite adequate (Fig. 28–6). Recommended calcium and phosphate intakes throughout the life cycle for the American and Canadian populations were updated in 1997 (Institute of Medicine, 1997).

Adequate Intake for Calcium. With the exception of infants, current recommended intakes for calcium are based on the amount of dietary calcium that will result in maximum

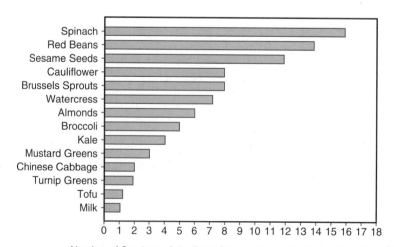

Figure 28–4. *Relative bioavailability of calcium from various food sources. Shown are the estimated number of standard servings of a given food source that would need to be consumed to absorb an equivalent amount of calcium as derived from 1 serving of milk. The numbers of servings of each food are based on the calcium content of the food and the estimated bioavailability of calcium from that food source. Serving sizes are ½ cup, except for milk (1 cup), almonds (1 oz), and sesame seeds (1 oz). The figure was drawn from data derived from Weaver, C. M. and Plawecki, K. L. (1994) Dietary calcium: Adequacy of a vegetarian diet. Am J Clin Nutr 59 (Suppl): 1238S–1241S.*

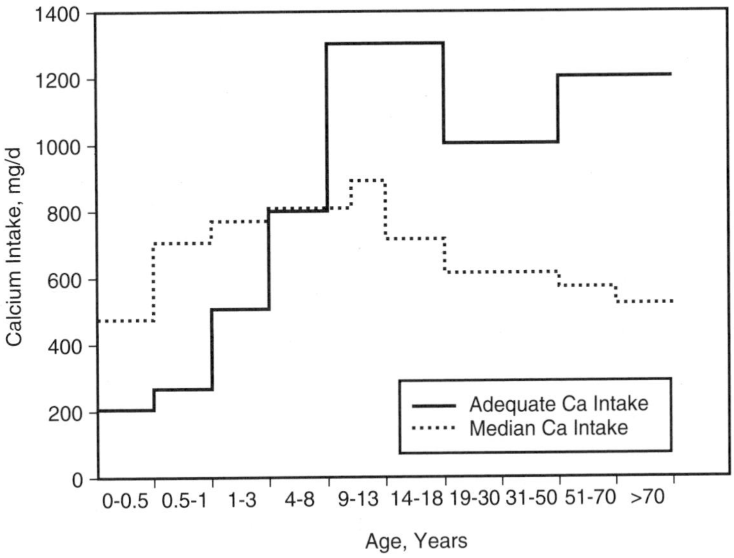

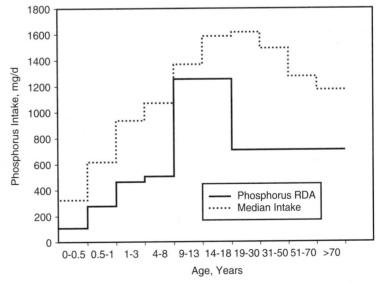

Figure 28–5. Median calcium intakes for girls and women in the United States compared with current recommended intakes for calcium. Shown are median (50th percentile) values for calcium intakes in girls and women of various ages, based on the NFCS Continuing Survey of Food Intake of Individuals (United States Department of Agriculture, 1994), and the current recommended intakes of calcium (Adequate Intakes) for these populations, developed as Dietary Reference Intakes by the Institute of Medicine (1997).

calcium retention, which has been determined from calcium balance studies. However, because of methodological limitations in estimating precisely the dietary calcium intakes needed for maximal calcium retention in all age groups, an Estimated Average Requirement (EAR) for calcium could not be derived with sufficient confidence. Thus, rather than the traditional calcium Recommended Dietary Allowance (RDA), an Adequate Intake (AI) level was estimated for calcium pending the development of a more comprehensive data base (Institute of Medicine, 1997).

The AI levels of calcium for infants are based on the mean intake of calcium in breast-fed infants. The concentration of calcium in breast milk is relatively constant—about 6.6 mmol/L (264 mg of Ca/L) during the first 6 months of lactation and 5.3 mmol/L (210 mg of Ca/L) during the second 6 months of lactation. The average intake of breast milk during the first 6 months of life is 780 mL/day. Thus, the AI was established as

Figure 28–6. Median phosphorus intakes for girls and women in the United States compared with current recommended intakes for phosphorus. Shown are median (50th percentile) values for phosphorus intakes in girls and women of various ages, based on the NFCS Continuing Survey of Food Intake of Individuals (United States Department of Agriculture, 1994) and the current recommended intakes of phosphorus (RDAs) for these populations developed as Dietary Reference Intakes by the Institute of Medicine (1997).

210 mg (5.3 mmol) of Ca per day for up to 6 months. For the second 6 months of infancy, the AI was established based on an estimate of breast milk intake of 600 mL/day, with a calcium concentration in breast milk of 210 mg/L plus an estimate of solid food intake of calcium of 140 mg/day. Thus, the AI for the infant from 6 to 12 months is 270 mg/day.

Special consideration is needed for infants fed infant formulas due to the lower bioavailability of calcium. Intakes of 315 mg Ca/day should be adequate to achieve maximal calcium retention in infants fed infant formulas during the first six months, and intakes of 335 mg Ca/day are adequate for formula-fed infants who are 6 to 12 months of age.

AIs for children aged 1 to 3 years are set at 12.5 mmol/day (500 mg of Ca/day), based on an average calcium absorption efficiency of 20% and the need to achieve a net calcium retention of 100 mg/day. The AI for children 4 to 8 years old is 20 mmol/day (800 mg/day), based on a 20% calcium absorption efficiency and the need to achieve a net calcium retention of about 130 to 174 mg/day. During ages 9 through 18 years, calcium retention increases to a peak and then declines. Peak calcium accretion rates are approximately 212 mg/day in girls and 282 mg/day in boys. The AI during the pubertal growth phase is 1300 mg of Ca/day (32.5 mmol/day), based on the observed maximal calcium retention achieved in balance studies over a wide range of calcium intakes. This peak level of recommended calcium intake is also supported by calcium supplementation trials in which maximum rates of increase in bone mineral content occurred at dietary calcium intakes near 1300 mg/day.

Peak bone mass is achieved during ages 19 to 30 years. Maximal calcium retention based on calcium balance studies in this age group indicates that a plateau in calcium retention occurs at dietary calcium intakes of about 1000 mg of Ca/day (25 mmol/day). Moreover, this level of calcium intake appears to support maximal calcium retention in older middle-aged adults as well. Hence, the AI for men and women aged 19 to 50 years is 1000 mg/day.

Maximal calcium retention values derived from calcium balance studies in older men and women indicate that a plateau value is reached at dietary calcium intakes of about 1200 mg of Ca/day (30 mmol/day). Although a large number of well-controlled calcium intervention studies in which rates of bone loss have been measured have been conducted in older women, only a few have been conducted in older men. Overall, these studies indicate that the effectiveness of dietary calcium to slow bone loss varies depending upon the bone site measured, the time since menopause, and the usual calcium intake of the subjects. In general, women in late menopause tend to be more responsive to calcium supplementation than women in early menopause. The AI for men and women over 50 years of age is 1200 mg/day.

Approximately 25 to 30 g (625 to 750 mmol) of calcium is transferred by the mother to the fetus during pregnancy. Most of this calcium accumulation in the fetus occurs during the third trimester. The increased demand for calcium in pregnancy is compensated for by an increase in calcium absorption efficiency, which may be related to pregnancy-associated increases in circulating 1,25-$(OH)_2D$. Thus, if calcium intake is sufficiently high to maximize calcium retention in the nonpregnant state, then the AI does not have to be increased further during pregnancy.

There is a significant increase in calcium demand during lactation to provide the approximately 210 mg of calcium/day needed for milk production. However, no evidence suggests that the calcium need of lactating women should be increased above that of nonlactating women. The additional calcium needed for milk production is supplied by maternal skeletal stores. The loss of calcium from the skeleton is not prevented by increased dietary calcium. The loss of maternal bone mineral density that occurs during lactation is regained following weaning. Thus, the AI for calcium during lactation is the same as the AI for nonlactating women.

Recommended Dietary Allowance for Phosphorus. In the past, the RDAs for phosphorus were usually set to equal the recommended calcium intakes. However, the most recent RDAs for phosphorus were set indepen-

LIFE CYCLE CONSIDERATION

Calcium Supplementation and Osteoporosis

Osteoporosis is a multifactorial disease that is clinically characterized by low bone mass and bone pain and an increased risk of bone fracture. According to the NHANES III national survey, the prevalence of osteoporosis (defined as a bone mineral density that is more than 2.5 standard deviations below the mean for young adult women) in white, non-Hispanic women over 50 years of age in the United States is between 17% and 20% (Looker et al., 1995). The prevalence of osteoporotic fracture is dramatically increased in elderly people. It has been estimated that osteoporotic bone fracture is found in about 7% of women by age 60 years and in 25% of women by age 80 years (Nordin, 1983). The age-associated increase in the occurrence of osteoporosis has enormous public health significance because it is estimated that one in five of the people in the United States will be elderly in the first quarter of the 21st century. Moreover, the fastest growing segment of our population are those over 85 years old.

Several factors may be involved in the pathogenesis of postmenopausal osteoporosis, including reduced intestinal calcium absorption and increased urinary calcium loss. Some of the bone loss that is seen in elderly people can be ameliorated by calcium supplementation (Dawson-Hughes et al., 1990; Reid et al., 1993; Aloia et al., 1994). However, the role of dietary calcium in the causation and treatment of osteoporosis is still the focus of intense debate. Among the reasons for this debate are the complex nature of osteoporosis and, until recently, the low sensitivity with which bone mineral density could be measured. Certainly the rather abrupt changes in bone and calcium metabolism that accompany menopause in women cannot be attributed solely to an abrupt decrease in calcium intake or absorption. An important question, then, is to what extent high calcium intakes can maximize peak bone mass in younger adults or slow the rate of loss of bone mass with aging.

Despite the fact that a number of investigators have noted a lack of association between current calcium intake and bone mineral density, a significant relationship has been observed between an individual's lifetime history of calcium intake and peak bone mineral density. A higher bone mineral density delays the appearance of symptoms of bone loss but does not change the rate of loss (Matkovic et al., 1979). In designing clinical trials to test the effects of dietary calcium or supplements on bone loss, it is essential to account for potential confounding factors such as age, menopausal status, serum estrogen levels, vitamin D status, smoking, parity, lactation history, history of oral contraceptive use, usual calcium intake, and usual level of physical activity.

---

dently of recommended calcium intakes (Institute of Medicine, 1997). Data from phosphorus balance studies and serum phosphate have been used to estimate phosphorus requirements. In adults, phosphate balance alone is not an adequate criterion to establish an EAR because phosphate balance can be zero at an intake that is inadequate to maintain serum phosphate within a normal range. If serum phosphate is within the normal range, it can be assumed that dietary phosphorus intakes are adequate to meet cellular and skeletal needs. Although phosphorus intake directly affects serum phosphate, the relationship between dietary phosphorus and serum phosphate has been established clearly only in adults.

It is difficult to determine the critical values for phosphorus intakes associated with the normal range of serum phosphate in children. Instead, the requirement for phosphorus during growth has been estimated based on the amount of phosphorus needed to support new tissue growth. Thus the EAR of phosphorus is based on a factorial approach in children and adolescents and on serum phosphate in adults.

Because no functional criteria for phosphate status reflect the response to dietary intake in infants, recommended intakes of phosphorus for infants are AIs based upon the observed mean intakes of infants fed principally with human milk (Institute of Medicine, 1997). The established phosphorus AI is based on an estimated intake of 780 mL of milk/day and an average phosphorus concentration in human milk of 124 mg/L (4 mmol/L). Thus, the AI for infants up to 6 months of age is 100 mg/day (3.2 mmol/day). The AI for infants 6 to 12 months old is based on the average intake of phosphorus from human milk plus that obtained from infant foods and is 275 mg/day (8.9 mmol/day).

An estimate of body accretion of phosphorus was used to establish an EAR for phosphorus for children 1 to 3 years old. These rates of accretion were corrected for predicted absorption efficiency of phosphorus and urinary losses to derive an EAR of 380 mg/day (12.3 mmol/day) based on the factorial approach. The RDA for phosphorus was derived as 460 mg/day (14.8 mmol/day) by assuming a coefficient of variation of 10% associated with the population EAR (Institute of Medicine, 1997). A similar factorial methodology was followed to estimate the EAR of 405 mg/day (13.1 mmol/day) for phosphorus in children aged 4 to 8 years, and the EAR of 1055 mg/day (34 mmol/day) for children 9 to 18 years. Likewise, a coefficient of variation of 10% was used to set the RDAs of 500 mg/day (16.1 mmol/day) for 4- to 8-year-old children and 1250 mg/day (40.3 mmol/day) for individuals between 9 and 18 years of age.

In contrast to the factorial methodology used to derive an EAR for growing children, the EAR for adults was established as 580 mg/day (18.7 mmol/day) on the basis of the amount of ingested phosphorus needed to maintain serum phosphate at the lower limit of the normal range (2.7 mg/100 mL or 0.87 mmol/L) (Institute of Medicine, 1997). The RDA for phosphorus for adults was set as the EAR + 20% or 700 mg/day (22.6 mmol/day).

The phosphorus content of the full-term infant is 17.1 g (552 mol) and must be supplied by the pregnant mother. The lactating woman secretes approximately 90 to 120 mg (2.9 to 3.9 mmol) of phosphorus per day in milk (Institute of Medicine, 1997). Despite this increased need for phosphorus during both pregnancy and lactation, no currently available evidence supports an increase in the phosphorus RDA above the level set for nonpregnant or nonlactating women.

CALCIUM AND PHOSPHORUS DEFICIENCY AND ASSESSMENT OF STATUS

Calcium deficiency is difficult to assess, and many possible indicators of calcium deficiency are also indicators of vitamin D status, bone diseases, and hormonal imbalances. Phosphorus deficiency is rare and seldom is due to a lack of phosphorus in the diet.

Calcium Deficiency and Status Assessment

In experimental animals that are severely restricted in dietary calcium (and that develop hypocalcemia), increased serum levels of PTH and $1,25(OH)_2D$, higher fractional intestinal absorption of calcium and phosphate, and lower calcium but higher phosphate levels in urine are consistently observed. Bone resorption and turnover are also stimulated, and net loss of bone mineral ensues.

In humans, chronic calcium deficiency is difficult to assess. Measurement of serum total and ionic calcium levels are inadequate to judge calcium status because they are tightly controlled. When observed, low total serum calcium levels are usually explainable by low levels of serum albumin, a protein that binds calcium in the plasma, rather than by a calcium deficiency. Moreover, abnormal levels of biochemical measures associated with calcium homeostasis are not necessarily proof of a dietary calcium deficiency, because vitamin D deficiency, bone diseases, and other hormonal imbalances can produce similar symptoms.

Calcium balance data provide useful information on whether the current level of calcium absorption is sufficient to replace calcium lost in urine and sweat and via endogenous intestinal secretions. Because 99% of the body's calcium store is found in bone, it is axiomatic that if an individual is in consistent negative calcium balance, then calcium is being lost from bone. However, balance studies provide no information on the extent to which bone calcium has been lost in the past. During growth, provision of sufficient dietary calcium in humans is necessary to achieve maximal levels of bone mineral density (Bonjour et al., 1997), but a positive calcium balance does not imply optimal bone mineralization.

Precise modern bone densitometry techniques can be used to monitor the response of bone mineral density to dietary intervention. The sensitivity of these techniques has improved dramatically in recent years, and use of these techniques has demonstrated the need for high calcium intakes to maximize bone growth in children and to retard bone loss in the elderly (National Institutes of Health, 1994).

Phosphorus Deficiency and Status Assessment

Dietary phosphorus deficiency is considered to occur very rarely because of the high phosphorus content of the diet, an efficient intestinal absorption of dietary phosphorus, and the ability of the kidneys to elaborate an essentially phosphorus-free urine in response to hypophosphatemia. An exception to this general rule is the premature infant fed human milk. Compared with other animal milks, human milk is relatively low in phosphorus. Despite similar caloric densities, human milk supplies only approximately 150 mg of phosphorus/L in comparison with the 1000 mg/L supplied by cow's milk. Although human milk is a sufficient source of phosphorus for the full-term infant, the phosphorus content of mother's milk is inadequate to meet the phosphorus demand of premature infants, who have a higher rate of phosphorus deposition in the skeleton and soft tissues per unit of body size than do full-term infants. Inadequate phosphorus intake in the preterm infant results in hypophosphatemia and inadequate bone mineralization, and the symptoms of rickets develop despite an adequate vitamin D status.

Phosphorus depletion can also occur in adults from inadequate phosphorus absorption owing to the overingestion of aluminum hydroxide antacids. Phosphate depletion has been induced experimentally in healthy individuals by feeding a very low phosphorus diet accompanied by antacids. Abnormalities of phosphorus homeostasis and phosphorus depletion can also occur in association with various disease states (see later). The symptoms of phosphate depletion include a diminished concentration of intracellular organic phosphoric acid esters, such as 2,3-diphosphoglycerate (in erythrocytes) and ATP (in muscle and other cell types). In the red blood cell, 2,3-diphosphoglycerate interacts with hemoglobin to promote the release of oxygen from oxyhemoglobin. Tissue oxygen levels can be lowered as a consequence of depleted 2,3-diphosphoglycerate levels, because of a shift in the equilibrium for oxyhemoglobin dissociation so that less oxygen is liberated. Additional symptoms of severe phosphorus depletion include hemolysis of red blood cells, diminished phagocytic function of granulocytes, severe muscle weakness, and markedly increased excretion of calcium in the urine.

The most commonly used index of phosphorus status is the serum phosphorus level. However, this measure of status can be an inadequate reflection of body phosphorus stores for a variety of reasons. Only 1% of total body phosphorus is in the extracellular fluid, and plasma phosphorus is under some degree of physiological control. Plasma phosphorus is determined by the tubular reabsorptive capacity of the kidney, which in turn is regulated by the level of PTH, growth hormone, and other factors. The level of phosphorus in the plasma can be artificially elevated due to muscle and bone catabolism or acutely decreased due to rapid shifts of phosphorus into the intracellular compartment. Nevertheless, plasma phosphate is directly related to absorbed phosphorus and was used as a functional criterion to establish the EARs (and RDAs) for phosphorus for the adult population (Institute of Medicine, 1997).

Other approaches to assessing phosphorus status are available. Intracellular phosphorus levels in red blood cells, leukocytes, and platelets have been investigated as possible indicators of phosphorus status and were found to correlate with the circulating phosphorus. Urinary phosphorus levels reflect dietary phosphorus intake under normal conditions. Hypophosphaturia and hypercalciuria occur with phosphate depletion. Likewise, serum alkaline phosphatase and $1,25(OH)_2D$ may be elevated in phosphate deficiency, but these biochemical changes are not specific enough to predict body phosphorus stores accurately. Newer developments in nuclear magnetic resonance (NMR) techniques offer a powerful research tool for assessment in vivo of intracellular phosphorus levels, and whole body neutron activation analysis can be used to measure total body phosphorus in living subjects. However, these expensive and sophisticated methodologies have limited applicability, and additional approaches to the problem of assessing phosphorus status are needed.

CLINICAL DISORDERS INVOLVING ALTERED CALCIUM AND PHOSPHORUS HOMEOSTASIS

Several clinical disorders are associated with altered calcium and phosphorus homeostasis. Changes in calcium and phosphorus stores may be caused by an increase or a decrease in intestinal absorption or renal reabsorption. Also, rapid shifts in serum phosphorus levels occur in response to several conditions that stimulate movement of phosphorus into or out of intracellular compartments.

Intestinal disorders, such as Crohn's disease, celiac disease, and intestinal resection or bypass, result in poor mineral and vitamin D absorption owing to fat malabsorption. In chronic liver disease, poor mineral absorption can occur secondary to vitamin D deficiency caused by impaired hydroxylation of vitamin D. In chronic renal failure, impairment of calcium and phosphate homeostasis is associated with the reduced renal synthesis of $1,25(OH)_2D$ and the development of secondary hyperparathyroidism.

Excessive intestinal absorption of calcium occurs in sarcoidosis, a chronic granulomatous disease, because of enhanced extrarenal $1,25(OH)_2D$ production. Elevated $1,25(OH)_2D$ also explains hyperabsorption of calcium in primary hyperparathyroidism and the hyperabsorption of calcium found in many patients with renal calcium stones (nephrolithiasis).

Hypercalcemia can be found in some cancer patients owing to an excess production by the tumor of PTHrP. This protein is produced by some epithelial cancers and can

act physiologically like PTH to increase renal calcium reabsorption and bone resorption, but its production is not under normal negative feedback control by elevated serum ionized calcium (Stewart, 1993).

Phosphate imbalance can occur in various disease states for a variety of reasons (Berner and Shike, 1988). In starvation, despite underlying phosphorus depletion, normal plasma phosphorus levels may be maintained because of increased muscle catabolism. Excessive amounts of phosphorus can be lost in the urine of uncontrolled diabetics owing to polyuria and the development of metabolic acidosis. However, plasma phosphorus can be normal or slightly elevated in ketotic patients due to the release of large amounts of phosphorus from intracellular sites. Recovering burn patients are at risk of hypophosphatemia due to massive diuresis. Likewise, excessive urinary phosphorus losses are also seen in patients with dysfunctions of the proximal renal tubule, such as seen in Fanconi's syndrome. In alcoholism, phosphate depletion can occur because of low dietary phosphorus, intestinal malabsorption, increased urinary losses, secondary hyperparathyroidism, hypomagnesemia, and hypokalemia.

The clinical sequel of chronic hyperphosphatemia is frequently ectopic calcification (Berner and Shike, 1988). In chronic renal failure, reduced renal function may cause hyperphosphatemia. Chronic hyperphosphatemia can be managed in these patients by limiting dietary phosphorus intake when possible and by administering oral phosphate binders containing aluminum, calcium, or magnesium salts. Hyperphosphatemia can also be seen with severe hemolysis and various endocrine dysfunctions, such as hypoparathyroidism, acromegaly, and severe hyperthyroidism.

REFERENCES

Alberts, B., Bray, D., Lewis, J., Raff, M., Roberts, K. and Watson, J. D. (1989) Molecular Biology of the Cell. Garland Publishing, New York.

Allen, L. H. and Wood, R. J. (1994) Calcium and phosphorus. In: Modern Nutrition in Health and Disease. (Shils, M., Olson, J. and Shike, M., eds.), 8th ed, vol. 1, pp. 144–163. Lea & Febiger, Philadelphia.

Aloia, J. F., Vaswani, A., Yeh, J. K., Ross, P. L., Flaster, E.

and Dilmanian, F. A. (1994) Calcium supplementation with and without hormone replacement therapy to prevent postmenopausal bone loss. Ann Intern Med 120:97–103.

Avioli, L. V., McDonald, J. E. and Lee, S. E. (1965) Influence of aging on the intestinal absorption of ^{47}Ca in women and its relation to ^{47}Ca absorption in postmenopausal osteoporosis. J Clin Invest 44:1960–1967.

Baron, R. (1993) Anatomy and ultrastructure of bone. In: Primer on the Metabolic Bone Diseases and Disorders of Mineral Metabolism (Favus, M., ed.), 2nd ed, pp. 3–9. Raven Press, New York.

Berner, Y. N. and Shike, M. (1988) Consequences of phosphate imbalance. Annu Rev Nutr 8:121–148.

Bonjour, J.-P., Carrie, A.-L., Ferrari, S., Clavien, H., Slosman, D., Theintz, G. and Rizzoli, R. (1997) Calcium-enriched foods and bone mass growth in prepubertal girls: A randomized, double-blind, placebo-controlled trial. J Clin Invest 99:1287–1294.

Bronner, F. (1988) Gastrointestinal absorption of calcium. In: Calcium in Human Biology (Nordin, B., ed.), pp. 93–124. Springer-Verlag, New York.

Bronner, F., Pansu, D. and Stein, W. D. (1986) An analysis of intestinal calcium transport across the rat intestine. Am J Physiol 250:G561–G569.

Burtis, W. J. (1993) Parathyroid hormone–related protein assays. In: Primer on the Metabolic Bone Diseases and Disorders of Mineral Metabolism (Favus, M. J., ed.), pp. 99–102. Raven Press, New York.

Chattopadhyay, N., Mithal, A. and Brown, E. M. (1996) The calcium-sensing receptor: A window into the physiology and pathophysiology of mineral ion metabolism. Endocrinol Rev 17:289–307.

Curhan, G. C., Willett, W. C., Rimm, E. B. and Stampfer, M. J. (1993) A prospective study of dietary calcium and other nutrients and the risk of symptomatic kidney stones. N Engl J Med 328:833–838.

Dawson-Hughes, B., Dallal, G., Krall, E. A., Sadowski, L., Sahyoun, N. and Tannenbaum, S. (1990) A controlled trial of the effect of calcium supplementation on bone density in postmenopausal women. N Engl J Med 323:878–883.

Deftos, L. J. (1993) Calcitonin. In: Primer on the Metabolic Bone Diseases and Disorders of Mineral Metabolism (Favus, M. J., ed.), pp. 70–76. Raven Press, New York.

Driessens, F. C. M. and Verbeeck, R. M. H. (1990) Biominerals. CRC Press, Boca Raton, FL.

Escoubet, B., Djabali, K. and Amiel, C. (1989) Adaptation to P_i deprivation of cell Na-dependent P_i uptake: A widespread process. Am J Physiol 256:C322–C328.

Favus, M. J. (ed.). (1993) Primer on the Metabolic Bone Diseases and Disorders of Mineral Metabolism, 2nd ed. Raven Press, New York.

Fleet, J. C., Bruns, M. E., Hock, J. M. and Wood, R. J. (1994) Growth hormone and parathyroid hormone stimulate intestinal calcium absorption in aged female rats. Endocrinology 134:1755–1760.

Fontaine, O., Matsumoto, T., Goodman, D. B. P. and Rasmussen, H. (1981) Liponomic control of Ca^{2+} transport: Relationship to mechanism of 1,25-dihydroxyvitamin D_3. Proc Natl Acad Sci USA 78:1751–1754.

Heaney, R. P. (1994) The bone-remodeling transient: Implications for the interpretation of clinical studies of bone mass change. J Bone Miner Res 9:1515–1523.

Heaney, R. P. and Weaver, C. M. (1990) Calcium absorption from kale. Am J Clin Nutr 51:656–657.

Heaney, R. P. and Recker, R. R. (1994) Determinants of endogenous fecal calcium in healthy women. J Bone Miner Res 9:1621–1627.

Institute of Medicine (1997) Dietary Reference Intakes for Calcium, Phosphorus, Magnesium, Vitamin D, and Fluoride. National Academy Press, Washington, D.C.

Kerstetter, J. E. and Allen, L. H. (1990) Dietary protein increases urinary calcium. J Nutr 120:134–136.

Lau, K., Goldfarb, S., Goldberg, M. and Agus, Z. S. (1982) Effects of phosphate administration on tubular calcium transport. J Lab Clin Med 99:317–324.

Lee, D., Brautbar, N. and Kleeman, C. (1981a) Disorders of phosphorus metabolism. In: Disorders of Mineral Metabolism, Vol. III, (Bronner, F. and Coburn, J., eds.), pp. 284–423. Academic Press, New York.

Lee, D. B., Walling, M. M., Levine, B. S., Gafter, U., Silis, V., Hodsman, A. and Coburn, J. W. (1981b) Intestinal and metabolic effect of 1,25-dihydroxyvitamin D_3 in normal adult rat. Am J Physiol 240:G90–G96.

Leklem, J. E. (1996) Vitamin B-6. In: Present Knowledge in Nutrition (Zeigler, E. E. and Filer, Jr, L. J., eds.), pp. 174–183. ILSI Press, Washington, D.C.

Lemann, J. (1993) Urinary excretion of calcium, magnesium, and phosphorus. In: Primer on the Metabolic Bone Diseases and Disorders of Mineral Metabolism (Favus, M. J., ed.), pp. 50–54. Raven Press, New York.

Life Sciences Research Office, Federation of American Societies for Experimental Biology (1989) Nutrition Monitoring in the United States—An Update Report on Nutrition Monitoring, DHHS Publication No. [PHS] 89-1255. U.S. Government Printing Office, Washington, D.C.

Looker, A. C., Johnson, Jr., C. C., Wahner, H. W., Dunn, W. L., Calvo, M. S., Harris, T. B., Heyse, S. P. and Lindsay, R. L. (1995) Prevalence of low femoral bone density in older U.S. women from NHANES III. J Bone Miner Res 10:796–802.

Matkovic, V., Kostial, K., Simonovic, I., Buzina, R., Brodarec, A. and Nordin, B. E. (1979) Bone status and fracture rates in two regions of Yugoslavia. Am J Clin Nutr 32:540–549.

Melsen, F. and Mosekilde, L. (1988) Calcified tissues: Cellular dynamics. In: Calcium in Human Biology (Nordin, B., ed.), pp. 187–208. Springer-Verlag, London.

Michetti, M., Salamino, F., Minafra, R., Melloni, E. and Pontremoli, S. (1997) Calcium-binding properties of human erythrocyte calpain. Biochem J 325:721–726.

Mundy, G. R. (1993) Bone resorbing cells. In: Primer on the Metabolic Bone Diseases and Disorders of Mineral Metabolism (Favus, M. J., ed.), pp. 25–32. Raven Press, New York.

National Institutes of Health (1994) Optimal calcium intake. NIH Consensus Development Panel on Optimal Calcium Intake. JAMA 272:1942–1948.

Nellans, H. N. and Goldsmith, R. S. (1983) Mucosal calcium uptake by rat cecum: Identity with transcellular calcium absorption. Am J Physiol 244:G618–G622.

Nemere, I. (1992) Vesicular calcium transport in chick intestine. J Nutr 122:657–661.

Nemere, I. and Norman, A. W. (1988) 1,25-Dihydroxyvitamin D_3-mediated vesicular transport of calcium in intestine: Time course studies. Endocrinology 122:2962–2969.

Nordin, B. E. C. (1983) Osteoporosis with particular reference to the menopause. In: The Osteoporotic Syndrome (Avioli, L. V., ed.), pp. 13–43. Grune and Stratton, New York.

Peerce, B. E., Cedilote, M., Seifert, S., Levine, R., Kiesling, C. and Clarke, R. D. (1993) Reconstitution of intestinal Na(+)-phosphate cotransporter. Am J Physiol 264:G609–G616.

Ramirez, J. A., Emmett, M., White, M. G., Fathi, N., Santa Ana, C. A., Morawski, S. G. and Fordtran, J. S. (1986)

The absorption of dietary phosphorus and calcium in hemodialysis patients. Kidney Int 30:753–759.

Recker, R. R., Davies, K. M., Hinders, S. M., Heaney, R. P., Stegman, M. R. and Kimmel, D. B. (1992) Bone gain in young adult women. JAMA 268:2403–2408.

Reid, I. R., Ames, R. W., Evans, M. C., Gamble, G. D. and Sharpe, S. J. (1993) Effect of calcium supplementation on bone loss in postmenopausal women. N Engl J Med 328:460–464.

Robertson, W. G. (1988) Chemistry and biochemistry of calcium. In: Calcium in Human Biology (Nordin, B. E. C., ed.), pp. 1–26. Springer-Verlag, London.

Rose, D. B. (1984) Clinical Physiology of Acid-base and Electrolyte Disorders. McGraw-Hill Book Co., New York.

Serfaty-Lacrosniere, C., Rosenberg, I. H. and Wood, R. (1995) The process of mineral absorption. In: Handbook of Metal-ligand Interactions in Biological Fluids (Berthon, G., ed.), pp. 322–330. Marcel Dekker, New York.

Sheikh, M. S., Ramirez, A., Emmett, M., Santa Ana, C. and Fordtran, J. S. (1988) Role of vitamin D-dependent and vitamin D-independent mechanisms in absorption of food calcium. J Clin Invest 81:126–132.

Spencer, H., Kramer, L., Osis, D. and Norris, C. (1978) Effect of a high protein (meat) intake on calcium metabolism in man. Am J Clin Nutr 31:2167–2180.

Stewart, A. W. (1993) Humoral hypercalcemia of malignancy. In: Primer on the Metabolic Bone Diseases and Disorders of Mineral Metabolism. (Favus, M. J., ed.), 2nd ed., pp. 169–172. Raven Press, New York.

Termine, J. D. (1993) Bone matrix proteins and the mineralization process. In: Primer on the Metabolic Bone Diseases and Disorders of Mineral Metabolism (Favus, M. J., ed.), pp. 21–24. Raven Press, New York.

United States Department of Agriculture (1994) NFCS Continuing Survey of Food Intakes by Individuals, 1991. U.S. Department of Commerce, National Technical Information Service, Springfield, VA.

Vosburgh, E. and Peters, T. J. (1987) Pathogenesis of idiopathic hypercalciuria: A review. J R Soc Med 80:34–37.

Walters, J. R. F. (1989) Calbindin-D9k stimulates the calcium pump in rat enterocyte basolateral membranes. Am J Physiol 256:G124–G128.

Wasserman, R. H., Smith, C. A., Brindak, M. E., Talamoni, N. D., Fuller, C. S., Penniston, J. T. and Kumar, R. (1992) Vitamin D and mineral deficiencies increase the plasma membrane calcium pump of chicken intestine. Gastroenterology 102:886–894.

Weaver, C. M. and Plawecki, K. L. (1994) Dietary calcium: Adequacy of a vegetarian diet. Am J Clin Nutr 59 (suppl):1238S–1241S.

RECOMMENDED READINGS

Bronner, F., ed. (1990) Intracellular Calcium Regulation. Wiley-Liss, New York.

Bronner, F. and Coburn, J. W., eds. (1981) Disorders of Mineral Metabolism, vols II and III. Academic Press, New York.

Favus, M. J., ed. (1993) Primer on the Metabolic Bone Diseases and Disorders of Mineral Metabolism, 2nd ed. Raven Press, New York.

Nordin, B. E. C., ed. (1988) Calcium in Human Biology. Springer-Verlag, London.

CHAPTER 29

◆ ◆

Magnesium

Robert K. Rude, M.D.

OUTLINE

COMMON ABBREVIATION

PTH (parathyroid hormone)

CHEMISTRY OF MAGNESIUM

Magnesium (Mg^{2+}) is a divalent metal ion with an atomic number of 12 and a molecular weight of 24. It is one of the most abundant elements in the earth's crust and is also prevalent in seawater. In vertebrates, it is the fourth most abundant cation in the body (after calcium, Ca^{2+}; potassium, K^+; and sodium, Na^+) and the second most abundant intracellular cation (after K^+). Throughout evolution it has come to be involved in numerous biological processes, including its role as a component of chlorophyll in plants. Like Ca^{+2}, Mg^{2+} is usually bound to ligands, but unlike Ca^{2+}, Mg^{2+} is strictly octahedral in the symmetry of its complexes and forms relatively stable complexes. Its major role in mammalian biology is to complex highly charged anions, including organic polyphosphates and nucleic acids, by which it can facilitate enzyme-substrate interactions or stabilize conformation of polymers (Frausto da Silva and Williams, 1991).

FOOD SOURCES AND DIETARY INTAKE OF MAGNESIUM

Magnesium is ubiquitous in foods, and moderate to severe magnesium depletion is unusual in the absence of dietary restriction or some disorder causing magnesium loss from the body. The magnesium content of foods does vary substantially, however. Foods such as unpolished grains, nuts, legumes, and green leafy vegetables have high magnesium content, whereas meats, most fruits, and dairy products have intermediate levels. Refined foods generally have the lowest magnesium content. Indeed, with the consumption of more refined foods, dietary intake of magnesium has been estimated to fall below recommended levels in up to 75% of subjects surveyed in the United States (Marier, 1986). Bioavailability of magnesium as well as the effect of other dietary factors also affects dietary magnesium balance.

ABSORPTION AND EXCRETION OF MAGNESIUM

Magnesium homeostasis in the body is obtained by balancing the intestinal absorption of magnesium with renal excretion. Relatively little is understood about the regulation of these processes.

Intestinal Magnesium Absorption

Intestinal magnesium absorption is inversely proportional to the amount ingested. Under normal dietary conditions in healthy individuals, approximately 30% to 50% of ingested magnesium is absorbed (Fine et al., 1991). Magnesium is absorbed along the entire intestinal tract, including the large and small bowel, but the sites of maximal magnesium absorption appear to be the ileum and distal jejunum. There appears to be both a passive and an active transport system for magnesium absorption, which probably accounts for the higher fractional absorption observed at low dietary magnesium intakes (Kayne and Lee, 1993).

Little is known about the regulation of intestinal magnesium transport. Vitamin D, as well as its metabolites 25-hydroxyvitamin D and 1,25-dihydroxyvitamin D, has been found in some studies to enhance intestinal magnesium absorption, but vitamin D affects magnesium absorption to a much lesser extent than it affects calcium absorption (Hardwick et al., 1991).

Bioavailability may be a factor in intestinal magnesium absorption as other nutrients may affect its absorption. High levels of dietary fiber from fruits, vegetables, and grains decrease fractional magnesium absorption (Siener and Hesse, 1995). However, diets high in vegetables are magnesium-rich, and the high magnesium content of these diets offsets decreased fractional absorption associated with the higher fiber intake. Many foods high in fiber also contain phytate, which may decrease intestinal magnesium absorption by binding Mg^{2+} to the phosphate groups on phytic acid (Franz, 1989). The ability of phosphate to bind Mg^{2+} may explain decreases in intestinal magnesium absorption in subjects on high-phosphate diets (Franz, 1989). Although dietary calcium has been reported to both decrease and increase magnesium absorption, recent human studies have shown no effect (Fine et al., 1991). Dietary protein may also influence intestinal magnesium absorp-

Food Sources of Magnesium

- Green leafy vegetables
- Legumes and tofu
- Nuts
- Whole grains

RDAs Across the Life Cycle

	mg magnesium/day
Infants, 0–0.5 y	30 (AI)
0.5–1.0 y	75 (AI)
Children, 1–3 y	80
4–8 y	130
9–13 y	240
Males, 14–18 y	410
19–30 y	400
31+ y	420
Females, 14–18 y	360
19–30 y	310
31+ y	320
Pregnant	+40
Lactating	+ 0

Data from Institute of Medicine (1997) Dietary reference intakes: Calcium, phosphorus, magnesium, vitamin D, and fluoride. National Academy Press, Washington, D.C. Adequate Intakes (AI) are listed for infants for whom RDAs were not set.

tion; magnesium absorption is lower when protein intake is less than 30 g/day (Hunt and Schofield, 1969).

Renal Magnesium Handling

The kidney is the principal organ involved in magnesium homeostasis (Quamme and Dirks, 1986). During dietary magnesium deprivation, the kidney avidly conserves magnesium, and less than 12 to 24 mg is excreted in the urine per day. Conversely, when dietary magnesium is high, excessive amounts are rapidly excreted in the urine. The renal handling of magnesium in humans is a filtration-reabsorption process. About 70% of plasma magnesium is filtered as free Mg^{2+} at the glomerulus, but most of this is reabsorbed.

Micropuncture studies of the nephron in several mammalian species indicate that the proximal tubule and the thick ascending limb of Henle are the major sites of Mg^{2+} reabsorption (Quamme and Dirks, 1986), as shown in Figure 29–1. Approximately 20% to 30% of this filtered magnesium is reabsorbed in the proxi-

mal tubule. Magnesium reabsorption follows changes in sodium and water reabsorption and is also associated with the concentration of magnesium in the filtrate: the higher the tubular luminal magnesium concentration, the greater the amount of magnesium reabsorbed (Quamme and Dirks, 1986). The majority, approximately 50% to 70%, of filtered magnesium is reclaimed in the cortical thick ascending limb of Henle. Recent studies have provided evidence that magnesium transport in this section of the nephron is voltage dependent and essentially passive (de Rouffignac et al., 1993). Micropuncture studies have also demonstrated that hypermagnesemia or hypercalcemia will decrease magnesium reabsorption in the thick ascending limb of the loop of Henle (Quamme and Dirks, 1986).

Micropuncture studies performed during a period in which the concentration of magnesium was gradually increased, in either the tubular lumen or the extracellular fluid, have failed to demonstrate a transport maximum (Tm; maximal rate of transport of a particular solute) for reabsorption of magnesium

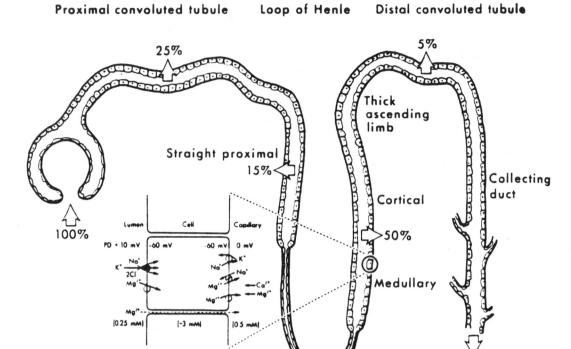

Figure 29–1. Summary of the tubular handling of magnesium. The 100% represents the total filtered load and the other % values represent the fraction of the filtered load absorbed at each tubular site. Inset: schematic illustration of the cellular transport of magnesium within the thick ascending limb of the loop of Henle. (From Quamme, G. A., and Dirks, J. H. [1986] The physiology of renal magnesium handling. Renal Physiol 9:257–269. Reproduced with permission of S. Karger AG, Basel.)

(TmMg) in the proximal tubule (Quamme and Dirks, 1986). Similarly a TmMg was not reached in the loop of Henle during a graduated increase in the luminal filtered magnesium load, although hypermagnesemia did result in a marked depression of fractional magnesium resorption in this segment of the tubule. Studies performed in vivo in animals and humans, however, have demonstrated that a TmMg exists for the renal tubules as a whole; this probably reflects a composite of various tubular reabsorption processes (Rude and Ryzen, 1986).

During magnesium deprivation, magnesium virtually disappears from the urine. Despite the close regulation of magnesium by the kidney, no hormone or factor has been shown to regulate renal magnesium homeostasis. Micropuncture studies have shown that parathyroid hormone (PTH) changes the potential difference in the cortical thick as-cending limb (making the tubular lumen less negative relative to the interior of the proximal tubular cell) and increases magnesium reabsorption (de Rouffignac et al., 1993). When given in large doses in humans or other species, PTH decreases urinary magnesium excretion. However, patients with either excess PTH levels (primary hyperparathyroidism) or PTH deficiency (hypoparathyroidism) usually have normal serum magnesium concentrations and normal tubular Tms for magnesium, suggesting that PTH is not an important physiological regulator of magnesium homeostasis (Rude, 1996). Glucagon, calcitonin, and antidiuretic hormone (ADH) also affect magnesium transport in the loop of Henle; they also change the potential difference, but the physiological relevance of these actions is unknown (de Rouffignac et al., 1993). Little is known about the effect of vitamin D hormone on renal magnesium handling.

Renal magnesium handling is also influenced by dietary factors. High-calcium and high-sodium diets, which increase urinary calcium and sodium excretion, may increase urinary magnesium excretion, presumably by interfering with magnesium transport in the proximal tubule and/or the thick ascending limb of the loop of Henle (Quamme and Dirks, 1986).

BODY MAGNESIUM CONTENT

The normal adult total body magnesium content is approximately 25 g or 1000 mmol, and 50% to 60% of this total resides in bone, as shown in Figure 29–2 (Elin, 1987). One third of skeletal magnesium is on the surface of bone, and this fraction may serve as a reservoir for maintaining a normal extracellular Mg^{2+} concentration (Wallach, 1988).

Extracellular magnesium accounts for only about 1% of total body magnesium, as shown in Figure 29–2. The normal serum magnesium concentration is 0.7 to 1.0 mmol/L. Most of the plasma magnesium, ~60% to 65%, is ionized or free Mg^{2+} (Altura et al., 1992; Elin, 1997). Of the remaining 35% to 40%, 5% to 10% is complexed to anions such as phosphate, citrate, and sulfate, and 30% is bound to proteins (chiefly albumin), as shown in Figure 29–3 (Elin, 1987).

Magnesium is present in higher concentrations inside cells than in the plasma. Soft tissue contains about one half of the total body magnesium, ~470 mmol. The magnesium content of soft tissues varies between 2.5 and 9 mmol/kg wet tissue weight (Elin, 1987). In general, the higher the metabolic activity of the cell, the higher the magnesium content. For example, the magnesium content of liver cells is about four times that of red blood cells.

Within the cell, significant amounts of magnesium are in the nucleus, mitochondria, and endoplasmic (or sarcoplasmic) reticulum as well as in the cytosol (Birch, 1993; Cowan, 1995). Most of the magnesium is bound to proteins and other negatively charged molecules such as nucleoside tri- and diphosphates (e.g., ATP and ADP) and nucleic acids (e.g., RNA and DNA); in the cytoplasm, about 80% of the Mg^{2+} is complexed with ATP (Frausto da Silva and Williams, 1991). One to five percent of the total cellular magnesium is free ionized Mg^{2+} (Romani et al., 1993).

The concentration of free Mg^{2+} in the cytosol of mammalian cells has been reported to range from 0.2 mM to 1.0 mM, but values vary with cell type and means of measurement (Romani et al., 1993). The free Mg^{2+} concentration in the cell cytosol is maintained relatively constant even when the magnesium concentration in the extracellular fluid is experimentally varied above or below the physiological range (Dai and Quamme, 1991). The relative constancy of the free Mg^{2+} concentration in the intracellular milieu is attributed to

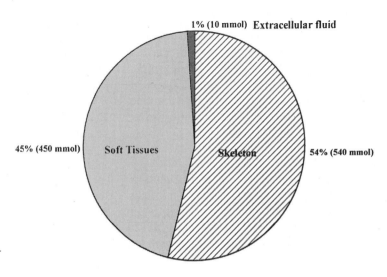

Figure 29–2. Distribution of magnesium in the body.

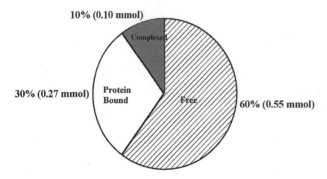

Figure 29–3. Physiochemical states of magnesium in normal plasma.

the limited permeability of the plasma membrane to Mg^{2+} and to the operation of specific Mg^{2+} transport systems that regulate the rates at which Mg^{2+} enters or leaves cells (Romani et al., 1993). Although the concentration differential between the cytosol and the extracellular fluid for free Mg^{2+} is minimal, Mg^{2+} enters cells down an electrochemical gradient owing to the relative electronegativity of the cell interior. Maintenance of the normal intracellular concentrations of free Mg^{2+} requires that Mg^{2+} be actively transported out of the cell.

Tissues vary in the rates at which Mg^{2+} exchange occurs and in the percentage of total magnesium that is readily exchangeable. The rate of Mg^{2+} exchange in heart, liver, and kidney appears to exceed that in skeletal muscle, red blood cells, brain, and testis (Romani et al., 1993). Increased cellular magnesium content has been reported for rapidly proliferating cells, indicating a possible relationship between the metabolic state of a cell and the relative rates of Mg^{2+} transport into and out of cells.

Magnesium transport into or out of cells appears to require the presence of carrier-mediated transport systems (Gunther, 1993). The efflux of Mg^{2+} from the cell appears to be coupled to Na^+ transport, which requires energy (ATP hydrolysis). Magnesium influx also appears to be linked to Na^+ and HCO_3^- transport, but by a different mechanism than for efflux.

Magnesium transport in mammalian cells may be influenced by hormonal and pharmacological factors, including β-agonists, growth factors, and insulin (Romani and Scarpa 1992; Gunther, 1993). It is hypothesized that a regulated Mg^{2+} uptake system controls the free Mg^{2+} concentration in cellular subcytoplasmic compartments. The free Mg^{2+} concentration in these compartments would then serve to regulate the activity of Mg^{2+}-sensitive enzymes. Information is sparse about the free and bound Mg^{2+} concentrations within mitochondria and endoplasmic reticulum (ER), but the free Mg^{2+} concentration of these compartments may not be significantly different than in the cytosol (Birch, 1993).

PHYSIOLOGICAL ROLES OF MAGNESIUM

The main biological role of Mg^{2+} in mammalian cells is involved with anion charge neutralization. Magnesium is particularly found in association with organic polyphosphates such as nucleotide triphosphates and nucleotide diphosphates (e.g., $ATP^{4-} \cdot Mg^{2+}$ and $ADP^{3-} \cdot Mg^{2+}$). Magnesium is also found associated with other highly anionic species, including multisubstituted phosphates of sugars such as inositol triphosphate, nucleic acids (RNA and DNA), and some carboxylates (e.g., isocitrate-Mg^{2+} as substrate for isocitrate lyase; carboxylate groups on proteins) (Frausto da Silva and Williams, 1991; Cowan, 1995).

Magnesium is normally bound between the β- and γ-phosphates of nucleotide triphosphates such as ATP and between the α- and β-phosphates of nucleotide diphosphates such as ADP, as shown in Figure 29–4. This serves to neutralize the negative charge density on the ATP or other nucleotide tri- or diphosphates and to facilitate binding of the nucleotide phosphates to the enzymes that use them as substrates. In most reactions in which Mg^{2+} is involved, it is present as a complex with a

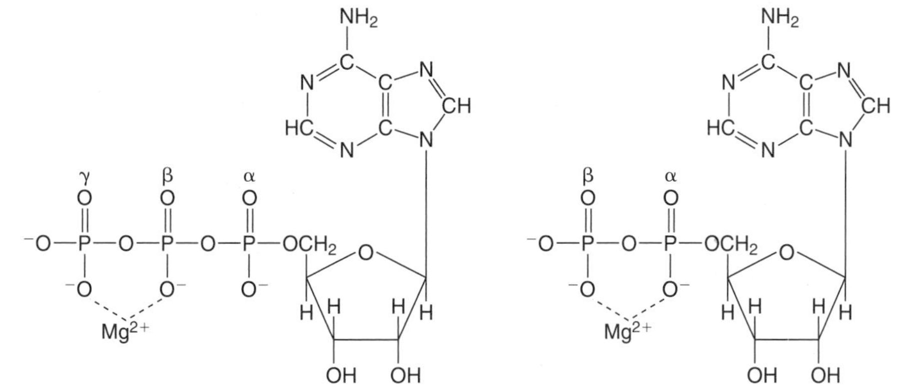

Figure 29–4. *Physiological forms of Mg-ATP and Mg-ADP.*

nucleotide tri- or diphosphate, which serves as substrate. The Mg^{2+} in these complexes does not interact directly with the enzyme in most cases but is linked by the substrate in an enzyme-substrate-metal type of substrate-bridged complex. Hence, Mg^{2+} plays a dominant role in all nucleotide tri- or diphosphate-dependent enzymatic reactions, which are widespread in metabolism. These reactions include those catalyzed by kinases, G-proteins, adenylate cyclase, ATP synthases, ATPases, and reactions coupled to ATP hydrolysis.

Magnesium also is required for binding to some enzymes or other proteins to stabilize them in the active conformation or to induce the formation of a binding site or active site. Some enzymes known to require enzyme-bound Mg^{2+} are enolase and pyruvate kinase; the Mg^{2+} in these enzymes coordinates the binding of substrate to the active site. Magnesium is also bound to the myosin regulatory light chain in the actin-myosin complex and is present in glutamine synthetase. Magnesium also is required for the conformational regulation of the binding of some elongation factors.

Additionally, Mg^{2+} is found in association with nucleic acids, which are negatively charged polymers due to the phosphate groups in the nucleotide chains. Magnesium stabilizes bending of RNA or DNA into particular curved or folded structures. This presumably occurs due to the cross-linking of the oxyanion centers of the phosphate residues by the divalent cation.

Cellular Energy Metabolism

Magnesium is involved in numerous steps in central pathways of carbohydrate, lipid, and protein metabolism and in mitochondrial ATP synthesis. For example, many steps in the glycolytic pathway require Mg^{2+}, either in the form of a complex with the ATP or ADP substrate or as a part of the metalloenzyme itself. The steps catalyzed by hexokinase and phosphofructokinase require Mg-ATP (i.e., $ATP^{4-} \cdot Mg^{2+}$) as substrate, whereas the steps catalyzed by phosphoglycerate kinase and pyruvate kinase require Mg-ADP (i.e., $ADP^{3-} \cdot Mg^{2+}$) as substrate. Both enolase, which interconverts 2-phosphoglycerate and phosphoenolpyruvate, and pyruvate kinase, which converts phosphoenolpyruvate to pyruvate, require enzyme-bound magnesium. Magnesium is bound to these enzymes through several carboxylate groups on the protein and forms an active complex with the enzyme before the substrate is bound. The bound Mg^{2+} in enolase may coordinate the hydroxyl group of 2-phosphoglycerate, making it a better leaving group. Pyruvate kinase requires both K^+ and Mg^{2+}. The K^+ plays a conformational role, while Mg^{2+} coordinates the binding of the substrate phosphoenolpyruvate to the enzyme active site.

Magnesium is required for phosphorylation and dephosphorylation reactions. ADP phosphorylation by mitochondrial ATP synthase (F_1F_0-ATPase) involved in oxidative phosphorylation utilizes Mg-ADP as substrate. In cardiac and skeletal muscle as well as other soft tissues, the creatine-phosphocreatine cycle acts as a reserve for high energy phosphate.

$$\text{Mg-ATP} + \text{creatine} \xleftrightarrow{\text{creatine kinase}} \text{Mg-ADP} + \text{phosphocreatine}$$

Phosphocreatine can be used to convert ADP to ATP when the muscle is subjected to a heavy workload. This occurs via a reversible reaction catalyzed by creatine kinase. As is true for all kinases, Mg^{2+} is an activating ion functioning with ADP and ATP.

Nucleic Acid and Protein Synthesis

The transcription, translation, and replication of nucleic acids (RNA, DNA) require enzymes that catalyze the hydrolysis and formation of phosphodiester bonds. Almost all these enzymes require Mg^{2+} for optimal activity. For example, DNA polymerase I is thought to require Mg^{2+} for stabilization of the conformation required for catalysis. RNA polymerases, which catalyze transcription (the synthesis of RNA using a DNA template) also require Mg^{2+}; the cation again is thought to effect a conformational change in the enzyme to produce a catalytically competent state.

Replicating cells must be able to synthesize new protein, and all cells must continually replace protein that is degraded. Protein synthesis has been reported to be highly sensitive to magnesium depletion. Magnesium is required for virtually every step of protein biosynthesis: the formation of the aminoacyl–transfer RNA species (which requires Mg-ATP) and the maintenance of its conformation (which is required for recognition by messenger RNA), as well as the maintenance of the ribosomes, require Mg^{2+}. Magnesium is also required for structure and activity of elongation factor-guanosine triphosphate (GTP) complexes that allow protein synthesis to begin and for the GTPase activities that occur during elongation and termination of protein biosynthesis.

Second Messenger Systems

Many hormones, neurotransmitters, and other cellular effectors regulate cellular activity via the adenylate cyclase system. The hormone-receptor unit interfaces with adenylate cyclase via a guanine nucleotide-binding protein (G-protein). Activation or inhibition of adenylate cyclase involves the dissociation of a G-protein into α and β-γ subunits; this process requires the presence of GTP and Mg^{2+}. As is the case for other ATP-utilizing enzymes, the actual substrate for adenylate cyclase is Mg-ATP. There is also evidence for a Mg^{2+}-binding site on adenylate cyclase through which Mg^{2+} directly increases enzyme activity. G-proteins, along with GTP and Mg^{2+}, are also required for many other signaling events in cells.

Another group of hormones and neurotransmitters exert their effects by raising the ionized calcium (Ca^{2+}) concentration in the cytosol of their target cells through the activation of the phosphoinositol cycle. One of the principal mechanisms by which this is thought to occur is by receptor-mediated activation of phospholipase C. Phospholipase C hydrolyzes a specific phospholipid present in the plasma membrane, phosphatidylinositol 4,5-bisphosphate (PIP_2), to yield two biologically active products, diacylglycerol and inositol 1,4,5-triphosphate (IP_3). Diacylglycerol activates protein kinase C, and IP_3 triggers calcium release from the ER. The IP_3 is rapidly inactivated by dephosphorylation. It appears that Mg^{2+} is essential for the normal functioning of this phosphoinositol cycle because the kinase that forms the PIP_2, as well as the enzymes that inactivate IP_3, require Mg^{2+} at concentrations that are physiological (Connolly et al., 1985; Volpe et al., 1990). In contrast, higher Mg^{2+} concentrations may decrease intracellular Ca^{2+} by two mechanisms: (1) noncompetitive inhibition of IP_3 binding to its receptor, and (2) inhibition of the release of Ca^{2+} via IP_3-gated channels (Volpe et al., 1990). See Figure 29–5.

Ion Channels

Ion channels constitute a class of proteins that is responsible for generating electrical signals across the cell membrane. These proteins allow passage of ions into or out of cells when the channels are open. Ion channels are classified according to the type of ion they allow to pass, such as Na^+, K^+, or Ca^{2+}

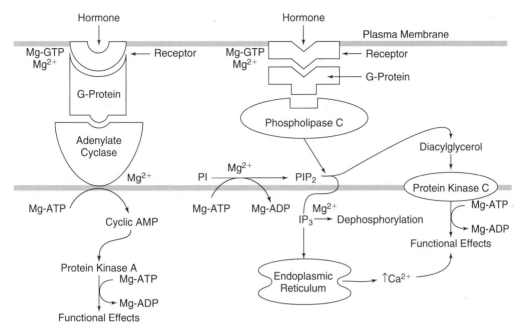

Figure 29–5. *Schematic representation of the role of magnesium in two second messenger systems, adenylate cyclase and phosphatidylinositol. GTP, guanosine triphosphate; G-protein, guanine nucleotide regulatory protein; PI, phosphatidylinositol; PIP₂, phosphatidylinositol 4,5-bisphosphate; IP₃, inositol 1,4,5-triphosphate.*

(Ackerman and Clapham, 1997; O'Rourke, 1993). Mg^{2+} plays an important role in the function of a number of ion channels.

Magnesium deficiency results in cellular potassium depletion. Several mechanisms may contribute to the potassium loss. Magnesium is necessary for the active transport of K^+ out of cells by the Na^+,K^+-ATPase pump. Magnesium-depleted animals and humans have been found to have a reduction in the concentration of Na^+,K^+-ATPase pumps in skeletal muscle, and this reduction in number of transport systems may contribute to the decrease in cellular K^+ (Dorup, 1994). The ATPase activity is also dependent on Mg^{2+}, and therefore Na^+ and K^+ transport may be impaired during magnesium deficiency, as has been reported in heart cells (Ryan, 1991). Another mechanism for the K^+ loss is an increased efflux of K^+ from cells via other Mg^{2+}-sensitive K^+ channels, as has been seen in skeletal muscle (Dorup, 1994). Magnesium is also involved in regulating a number of K^+ channels in heart muscle (Matsuda, 1991; White and Hartzell, 1989). Inwardly rectifying K^+ channels normally allow K^+ to pass more readily inward than outward, and intracellular magnesium appears to block the outward

movement of K^+ through these channels in myocardial cells. In the absence of Mg^{2+}, K^+ is transported equally well in both directions, and a deficiency in Mg^{2+} may lead to a reduced amount of intracellular K^+. As the resting membrane potential of heart muscle cells is determined in part by the intracellular K^+ concentration, a decreased intracellular K^+ concentration will result, by a complex mechanism, in partial depolarization (i.e., a less negative resting membrane potential) of electrical tissues at rest. The arrhythmogenic effect of magnesium deficiency may therefore be related to its effect on maintenance of intracellular K^+, as discussed later.

Magnesium has been called "nature's physiological calcium channel blocker" (Iseri and French, 1984). During magnesium depletion, intracellular calcium rises. This may be due to both uptake from extracellular calcium and release from intracellular calcium stores. Magnesium has been demonstrated to decrease the inward Ca^{2+} flux through slow calcium channels (White and Hartzell, 1989; O'Rourke, 1993). In addition, Mg^{2+} will decrease the transport of Ca^{2+} out of the ER into the cell cytosol. As discussed earlier, the ability of IP_3 to release Ca^{2+} from intracellular stores is inversely related to Mg^{2+} concentrations, and therefore, a fall in Mg^{2+} concentration would allow a greater rise in intracellular Ca^{2+}. Thus, because Ca^{2+} plays an important role in skeletal and smooth muscle contraction, a state of magnesium depletion may result in muscle cramps, hypertension, and coronary and cerebral vasospasm (Altura and Altura, 1995).

MAGNESIUM REQUIREMENTS

The RDA for magnesium was increased in 1997 from 280 to 320 mg per day for adult women and from 350 to 420 mg per day for adult men (Institute of Medicine, 1997). The Institute of Medicine also established an Estimated Average Requirement (EAR) for magnesium, which was 265 mg per day for adult women and 350 mg per day for adult men.

The mean intakes of magnesium by women and men in the United States have been estimated to be 228 mg and 323 mg, respectively. These intakes are close to average requirements but are less than the RDAs recommended to meet the nutrient needs of essentially all individuals within a population (Cleveland et al., 1996). This suggests that magnesium intake is marginal or low for a proportion of the population.

The medical significance of marginal magnesium intakes on human health is not clear. Although low dietary magnesium intakes have not been unequivocally linked to chronic disease, epidemiological studies have suggested an inverse relationship between dietary magnesium intake and blood pressure (Altura and Altura, 1995), atherosclerotic vascular disease and sudden death (Altura and Altura, 1995), and osteoporosis (Freudenheim et al., 1986; Yano et al., 1985).

MAGNESIUM DEPLETION

Magnesium depletion is usually secondary to another disease process or to a therapeutic agent. Some disorders that can be associated with magnesium depletion are summarized in Table 29–1 (Whang et al., 1994; Rude, 1996).

Causes

Magnesium may be lost via the gastrointestinal tract, either by excessive loss of secreted

CLINICAL CORRELATION

Cardiac Arrhythmia in Patients with Diabetes Mellitus

Cardiovascular disease is a common cause of morbidity and mortality in patients with diabetes mellitus. This is in part due to hyperlipidemia and hypertension leading to coronary heart disease. Magnesium deficiency has been linked to hypertension, perhaps by altering Ca^{2+} channels resulting in increased Ca^{2+} in the vascular smooth muscle causing vasospasm. Patients with diabetes mellitus are at risk for magnesium depletion. Renal magnesium loss has been correlated with high blood glucose and high urine glucose excretion. It is thought that the osmotic diuresis due to the glucose causes the kidney to waste magnesium. Dietary magnesium intake in diabetics also tends to fall short of the RDA (Schmidt et al., 1994). Other medications may also contribute to magnesium loss. Patients with high blood pressure and heart disease frequently receive diuretics such as furosemide. Furosemide blocks the reabsorption of magnesium in the thick ascending limb of the loop of Henle, the major site of renal magnesium reabsorption, and this causes marked urinary magnesium loss.

Thinking Critically

1. Does magnesium deficiency contribute to heart arrhythmias? Why?

2. How does magnesium deficiency affect potassium homeostasis?

3. Will potassium therapy alone correct the potassium deficit in magnesium-deficient patients?

TABLE 29–1
Major Causes of Magnesium Deficiency

Gastrointestinal Disorders

Prolonged nasogastric suction/vomiting
Acute and chronic diarrhea
Malabsorption syndromes (e.g., celiac sprue)
Extensive bowel resection
Intestinal and biliary fistulas
Acute hemorrhagic pancreatitis

Renal Loss

Chronic parenteral fluid therapy
Osmotic diuresis (e.g., due to presence of glucose in
 diabetes mellitus)
Hypercalcemia
Drugs
 Diuretics (e.g., furosemide, ethacrynic acid)
 Aminoglycosides
 Amphotericin B
 Pentamidine
 Cisplatin
 Cyclosporine
Alcohol
Metabolic acidosis (e.g., starvation, diabetic
 ketoacidosis, alcoholism)
Renal diseases
 Chronic pyelonephritis, interstitial nephritis, and
  glomerulonephritis
 Diuretic phase of acute tubular necrosis
 Postobstructive nephropathy
 Renal tubular acidosis
 Postrenal transplantation

fluids or impaired absorption of both dietary and endogenous magnesium. The magnesium content of upper intestinal tract fluids is approximately 0.5 mmol/L, and vomiting or nasogastric suction may contribute to magnesium depletion from loss of these fluids. The magnesium content of diarrheal fluids and fistulous drainage is much higher (up to 7.5 mmol/L), and consequently, magnesium depletion is common in patients with acute or chronic diarrhea, regional enteritis, ulcerative colitis, or an intestinal or biliary fistula. Malabsorption syndromes such as celiac sprue may result in magnesium deficiency. Steatorrhea and resection or bypass of the small bowel, particularly the ileum, often result in intestinal magnesium malabsorption and loss from the body. Lastly, acute severe pancreatitis may be associated with hypomagnesemia; this could be due to the clinical problem causing the pancreatitis (e.g., alcoholism) or to magnesium binding to necrotic parapancreatic fat surrounding the pancreas.

Excessive excretion of magnesium into the urine is another cause of magnesium depletion. Renal Mg^{2+} excretion is proportional to tubular fluid flow as well as to Na^+ and Ca^{2+} excretion. Therefore, both chronic intravenous fluid therapy with Na^+-containing fluids and disorders such as primary aldosteronism in which there is extracellular volume expansion may result in magnesium depletion. Hypercalcemia and hypercalciuria have been shown to decrease renal Mg^{2+} reabsorption and are probably the cause of the excessive renal magnesium excretion and the hypomagnesemia observed in many hypercalcemic states. An osmotic diuresis will result in increased renal magnesium excretion due to excessive urinary volume. Osmotic diuresis due to glucosuria can, thus, result in magnesium depletion, and diabetes mellitus is probably the most common clinical disorder associated with magnesium depletion. The degree of magnesium depletion in patients with diabetes mellitus has been related to the amount of glucose excreted into the urine and, hence, with the degree of osmotic diuresis.

A number of drugs can cause renal magnesium wasting and magnesium depletion. These include furosemide, aminoglycosides, amphotericin B, cisplatin, cyclosporine, and pentamidine (Shah and Kirschenbaum, 1991). An elevated blood alcohol level has been associated with hypermagnesuria, and increased urinary excretion of magnesium is one factor contributing to magnesium depletion in chronic alcoholism. Metabolic acidosis may also impair renal conservation of magnesium. Lastly, a number of renal disorders (see Table 29–1) may be associated with magnesium wasting because of impaired renal reabsorption of magnesium.

Manifestations

The biochemical and physiological manifestations of severe magnesium depletion are summarized in Table 29–2.

Hypokalemia. A common feature of magnesium depletion is hypokalemia (Whang et al., 1994). During magnesium depletion there is loss of potassium from the cell with intracellular potassium depletion, which is enhanced

CLINICAL CORRELATION

Magnesium Deficiency in Chronic Alcohol Abuse

Chronic alcoholics are prone to magnesium depletion for several reasons. First of all, as blood alcohol levels rise, the kidney is less efficient at reabsorbing Mg^{2+} from the tubular fluid. Alcoholics also have frequent episodes of diarrhea, which result in loss of large amounts of magnesium. Lastly, these subjects are usually poorly nourished and have a low magnesium intake. Alcohol and refined foods have very low magnesium content. Magnesium is not included in routine blood tests, but other measurements may provide clues that suggest a magnesium deficiency. Low blood calcium is one such clue.

Thinking Critically

1. What is the effect of magnesium deficiency on calcium metabolism?

2. Would high-dose calcium correct the adverse effects of magnesium deficiency on calcium homeostasis? Why?

3. What would be the correct therapy? Why?

---

due to the inability of the kidney to conserve potassium. Attempts to replete the potassium deficit with potassium therapy alone are not successful without simultaneous magnesium therapy. This potassium depletion may be a contributing cause of the electrocardiological findings and cardiac arrhythmias discussed later.

Hypocalcemia. Hypocalcemia is also a com-

mon manifestation of moderate to severe magnesium depletion (Rude, 1994). The hypocalcemia may be a major contributing factor to the increased neuromuscular excitability often present in magnesium-depleted patients. The pathogenesis of hypocalcemia is multifactorial. Impaired PTH secretion appears to be a major factor in hypomagnesemia-induced hypocalcemia. Serum PTH concentrations are usually low in these patients, and magnesium administration will immediately stimulate PTH secretion. Patients with hypocalcemia due to magnesium depletion also exhibit both renal and skeletal resistance to exogenously administered PTH, as manifested by subnormal urinary cyclic AMP (cAMP) and phosphate excretion and a diminished calcemic response. All these effects are reversed following several days of magnesium therapy. The basis for the defect in PTH secretion and PTH end organ resistance is not known. Because cAMP is an important second messenger in PTH secretion and is required for mediating PTH effects in kidney and bone, it has been postulated that there may be a defect in the activity of adenylate cyclase. As previously discussed, Mg^{2+} is both an essential part of the substrate (Mg-ATP) for adenylate cyclase and essential for catalytic activity.

Vitamin D metabolism and action may also be abnormal in hypocalcemic magnesium-deficient patients. Resistance to vitamin

---

TABLE 29–2

Major Manifestations of Magnesium Depletion

Biochemical

Hypokalemia
   Excessive renal potassium excretion
   Decreased intracellular potassium
Hypocalcemia
   Impaired PTH secretion
   Renal and skeletal resistance to PTH
   Resistance to vitamin D

Neuromuscular

Positive Chvostek's and Trousseau's sign
Spontaneous carpal-pedal spasm
Seizures
Vertigo, ataxia, nystagmus, athetoid and chorioform
   movements
Muscular weakness, tremor, fasciculation and wasting
Psychiatric: depression, psychosis

Cardiovascular

Electrocardiographic abnormalities
Cardiac arrhythmias

D therapy has been reported in such cases. This resistance may be due to impaired metabolism of vitamin D because plasma concentrations of 1,25-dihydroxyvitamin D are low. Because PTH is a major stimulator of the synthesis of 1,25-dihydroxyvitamin D production, the decrease in PTH secretion observed in hypomagnesemia/hypocalcemia may also be a cause of the impaired metabolism of vitamin D (Rude, 1994).

Neuromuscular Manifestations. Neuromuscular hyperexcitability may be the presenting complaint of patients with magnesium deficiency. Tetany and muscle cramps may be present. Generalized seizures (convulsions) may also occur. Other neuromuscular signs may include dizziness, disequilibrium, muscular tremor, wasting, and weakness (Whang et al., 1994). Although hypocalcemia often contributes to the neurological signs, hypomagnesemia without hypocalcemia has been reported to result in neuromuscular hyperexcitability.

Cardiovascular Manifestations. Magnesium depletion may also result in electrocardiographic abnormalities as well as in cardiac arrhythmias (Hollifield, 1987). This may be manifested by a rapid heart rate (tachycardia), skipped heart beats (premature beats), or a totally irregular cardiac rhythm (fibrillation). Cardiac arrhythmias are also known to occur during K depletion; therefore, the effect of magnesium deficiency on potassium loss from the body may be the cause of the arrhythmias (Whang et al., 1994; Rude, 1996). Patients with myocardial infarction also commonly have cardiac arrhythmias. Recently, magnesium administration to patients with acute myocardial infarction has been shown to decrease the mortality rate in some (Woods et al., 1992) but not all studies (ISIS-4 Collaborative Group, 1995).

DIAGNOSIS OF MAGNESIUM DEFICIENCY

Although magnesium is a relatively abundant cation in the body, over 99% of it is either intracellular or in the skeleton. The <1% of total magnesium present in the body fluids is the most assessable for clinical testing, and the serum magnesium concentration is the most widely used measure of magnesium status. The total serum magnesium concentration is usually 1.7 to 2.2 mg/100 mL (0.7 to 1.0 mmol/L). A serum concentration of less than 1.7 mg/100 mL usually indicates some degree of magnesium depletion (Rude, 1996), but the measurement of serum magnesium concentration does not necessarily reflect the true total body magnesium content. Low intracellular magnesium has been documented in patients with serum levels above 1.7 mg/100 mL. Intracellular levels of magnesium in muscle, red blood cells, and lymphocytes, as well as in bone, appear to reflect more accurately whole body magnesium status, but these tests have not been developed for clinical use (Rude, 1996). Recently, ion-specific electrodes have become available for determining ionized magnesium (Mg^{2+}) in the plasma. Early results suggest that plasma-ionized magnesium concentration may be a better index of magnesium status than the total serum magnesium concentration, but further evaluation is necessary (Altura et al., 1992).

In patients at risk for magnesium deficiency but with normal serum magnesium levels, magnesium status can be further evaluated by determining the amount of magnesium excreted in the urine following an intravenous infusion of magnesium. Normal subjects excrete at least 80% of an intravenous magnesium load within 24 hours, whereas patients with magnesium deficiency excrete much less. The magnesium load test, however, requires normal renal handling of Mg^{2+}. If excess magnesium is being excreted by the kidneys due to diuresis, the magnesium load test may yield an inappropriate negative result. On the other hand, if renal function is impaired and less blood is being filtered, this test could give a false-positive result.

MAGNESIUM TOXICITY

Magnesium intoxication is not a frequently encountered clinical problem, although mild to moderate elevations in the serum magnesium concentration may be seen in as many as 12% of hospitalized patients (Wong et al.,

1983). Symptomatic hypermagnesemia is virtually always due to excessive intake or administration of magnesium salts (Mordes, 1978). The majority of patients with hypermagnesemia have concomitant renal failure, and hypermagnesemia is usually seen in patients with renal failure who are receiving magnesium as an antacid, enema, or infusion. Magnesium infusions also are sometimes given for pregnancy-induced hypertension and for treatment of magnesium deficiency.

Neuromuscular symptoms are the most common presenting problem of magnesium intoxication. One of the earliest demonstrable effects of hypermagnesemia is the disappearance of the deep tendon reflexes at serum magnesium concentrations of 2 to 3 mmol/L. Depressed respiration and apnea due to paralysis of the voluntary musculature may be seen at serum magnesium concentrations in excess of 4 to 5 mmol/L. Cardiac arrest may occur at concentrations greater than 6 mM. Moderate elevations in the serum magnesium concentration (increases of approximately 1.5 to 2.5 mmol/L) can result in a mild reduction in blood pressure. Other nonspecific manifestations of magnesium intoxication include nausea, vomiting, and cutaneous flushing at serum levels of 1.5 to 4 mmol/L (Mordes, 1978).

REFERENCES

Ackerman, M. J. and Clapham, D. E. (1997) Ion channels—basic science and clinical disease. N Engl J Med 336:1575–1586.

Altura, B. M. and Altura, B. T. (1995) Role of magnesium in the pathogenesis of hypertension updated: Relationship to its actions on cardiac, vascular smooth muscle, and endothelial cells. In: Hypertension: Pathophysiology, Diagnosis, and Management (Laragh, J. H. and Brenner, B. M., eds.), 2nd ed, pp. 1213–1242. Raven Press, New York.

Altura, B. T., Shirey, T. L., Young, C. C., Hiti, J., Dell'Orfano, K., Handwerker, S. M. and Altura, B. M. (1992) A new method for the rapid determination of ionized Mg in whole blood, serum and plasma. Methods Find Exp Clin Pharmacol 14:297–304.

Birch, N. J. (1993) Magnesium and the Cell. Academic Press, New York.

Cleveland, L. E., Goldman, J. D. and Borrud, L. G. (1996) Data tables: Results from USDA's 1994 continuing survey of food intakes by individuals and 1994 diet and health knowledge survey. Agricultural Research Service, U.S. Department of Agriculture, Beltsville, MD.

Connolly, T. M., Bross, T. E. and Majerus, P. W. (1985) Isolation of a phosphomonoesterase from human platelets that specifically hydrolyzes the 5-phosphate of inositol 1,4,5-triphosphate. J Biol Chem 260:7868–7874.

Cowan, J. A. (1995) The Biological Chemistry of Magnesium. VCH Publishers, Inc., New York.

Dai, L. J. and Quamme, G. A. (1991) Intracellular Mg and magnesium depletion in isolated renal thick ascending limb cells. J Clin Invest 88:1255–1264.

de Rouffignac, C., Mandon, B., Wittner, M. and de Stefano, A. (1993) Hormonal control of renal magnesium handling. Miner Electrolyte Metab 19:226–231.

Dorup, I. (1994) Magnesium and potassium deficiency: Its diagnosis, occurrence and treatment in diuretic therapy and its consequences for growth, protein synthesis, and growth factors. Acta Physiol Scand 150:Suppl 618:7–46.

Elin, R. (1987) Assessment of magnesium status. Clin Chem 33:1965–1970.

Elin, R. (1997) Evaluating the role of ionized magnesium in laboratory and clinical practice. In: Advances in Magnesium Research: 1. Magnesium in Cardiology (Smetana, R. ed.), pp. 525–531. John Libbey & Co., London.

Fine, K. D., Santa Ana, C. A., Porter, J. L. and Fordtran, J. S. (1991) Intestinal absorption of magnesium from food and supplements. J Clin Invest 88:396–402.

Franz, K. B. (1989) Influence of phosphorus on intestinal absorption of calcium and magnesium. In: Magnesium in Health and Disease (Itokawa, Y. and Durlach, J., eds.), pp. 71–78. John Libbey & Co., London.

Frausto da Silva, J. J. R. and Williams, R. J. P. (1991) The biological chemistry of magnesium:phosphate metabolism. In: The Biological Chemistry of the Elements, pp. 241–267. Oxford University Press, Oxford.

Freudenheim, J. L., Johnson, N. E. and Smith, E. L. (1986) Relationships between usual nutrient intake and bone-mineral content of women 35–65 years of age: Longitudinal and cross-sectional analysis. Am J Clin Nutr 44:863–876.

Gunther, T. (1993) Mechanisms and regulation of Mg efflux and Mg influx. Miner Electrolyte Metab 19:259–265.

Hardwick, L. L., Jones, M. R., Brautbar, N. and Lee, D. B. (1991) Magnesium absorption: Mechanisms and the influence of vitamin D, calcium, and phosphate. J Nutr 121:13–23.

Hollifield, J. W. (1987) Magnesium depletion, diuretics, and arrythmias. Am J Med 82:(Suppl 3A):30–37.

Hunt, M. S. and Schofield, F. A. (1969) Magnesium balance and protein intake level in adult human females. Am J Clin Nutr 22:367–373.

Institute of Medicine (1997) Dietary reference intakes: Calcium, phosphorus, magnesium, vitamin D, and fluoride. National Academy Press, Washington, D.C.

Iseri, L. T. and French, J. H. (1984) Magnesium: Nature's physiologic calcium blocker. Am Heart J 108:188–193.

ISIS-4 Collaborative Group. Fourth International Study of Infarct Survival (1995) A randomised factorial trial assessing early oral captopril, oral mononitrate, and intravenous magnesium sulphate in 58,050 patients with suspected acute myocardial infarction. Lancet 345:669–685.

Kayne, L. H. and Lee, D. B. N. (1993) Intestinal magnesium absorption. Miner Electrolyte Metab 19:210–217.

Marier, J. R. (1986) Magnesium content of the food supply in the modern-day world. Magnesium 5:1–8.

Matsuda, H. (1991) Magnesium gating of the inwardly rectifying K+ channel. Annu Rev Physiol 53:289–298.

Mordes, J. P. (1978) Excess magnesium. Pharmacol Rev 29:273–300.

O'Rourke, B. (1993) Ion channels as sensors of cellular energy: Mechanism for modulation by magnesium and nucleotides. Biochem Pharmacol 46:1103–1112.

Quamme, G. A. and Dirks, J. H. (1986) The physiology of renal magnesium handling. Renal Physiol 9:257–269.

Romani, A., Marfella, C. and Scarpa, A. (1993) Cell magnesium transport and homeostasis: Role of intracellular compartments. Miner Electrolyte Metab 19:282–289.

Romani, A. and Scarpa, A. (1992) Regulation of cell magnesium. Arch Biochem Biophys 298:1–12.

Rude, R. K. (1994) Magnesium deficiency in parathyroid function. In: The Parathyroids (Bilezikian, J. P., ed.), pp. 829–842. Raven Press, New York.

Rude, R. K. (1996) Magnesium disorders. In: Fluids and Electrolytes (Kokko, J. P. and Tannen, R. L., eds.), 3rd ed., pp. 421–445. W.B. Saunders, Philadelphia.

Rude, R. K. and Ryzen, E. (1986) TmMg and renal Mg threshold in normal man in certain pathophysiologic conditions. Magnesium 5:273–281.

Ryan, M. F. (1991) The role of magnesium in clinical biochemistry: An overview. Ann Clin Biochem 28:19–26.

Schmidt, L. E., Arfken, C. L. and Heins, J. M. (1994) Evaluation of nutrient intake in subjects with non-insulin-dependent diabetes mellitus. J Am Diet Assoc 94:773–774.

Shah, G. M. and Kirschenbaum, M. A. (1991) Renal magnesium wasting associated with therapeutic agents. Miner Electrolyte Metab 17:58–64.

Siener, R. and Hesse, A. (1995) Influence of a mixed and a vegetarian diet on urinary magnesium excretion and concentration. Br J Nutr 73:783–790.

Volpe, P., Alderson-Lang, B. H. and Nickols, G. A. (1990) Regulation of inositol 1,4,5-triphosphate-induced Ca^{2+} release. I. Effect of magnesium ion. Am J Physiol 258:C1077–C1085.

Wallach, S. (1988) Availability of body magnesium during magnesium deficiency. Magnesium 7:262–270.

Whang, R., Hampton, E. M. and Whang, D. D. (1994) Magnesium homeostasis and clinical disorders of magnesium deficiency. Ann Pharmacol 28:220–226.

White, R. E. and Hartzell, H. C. (1989) Magnesium ions in cardiac function: Regulator of ion channels and second messengers. Biochem Pharmacol 38:859–867.

Wong, E. T., Rude, R. K., Singer, F. R. and Shaw, S. T. (1983) A high prevalence of hypomagnesemia and hypermagnesemia in hospitalized patients. Am J Clin Pathol 79:348–352.

Woods, K. L., Fletcher, S., Roffe, C. and Haider, Y. (1992) Intravenous magnesium sulphate in suspected acute myocardial infarction: Result of the second Leicester Intravenous Magnesium Intervention Trial (LIMIT-2). Lancet 339:1553–1558.

Yano, K., Heilbrun, L. K., Wasnich, R. D., Hankin, J. H. and Vogel, J. M. (1985) The relationship between diet and bone mineral content of multiple skeletal sites in elderly women living in Hawaii. Am J Clin Nutr 42:877–888.

RECOMMENDED READINGS

Birch, N. J. (1993) Magnesium and the Cell. Academic Press, New York.

Cowan, J. A. (1995) The Biological Chemistry of Magnesium. VCH Publishers, Inc., New York.

Frausto da Silva, J. J. R. and Williams, R. J. P. (1991) The biological chemistry of magnesium:phosphate metabolism. In: The Biological Chemistry of the Elements, pp. 241–267. Oxford University Press, Oxford.

Rude, R. K. (1996) Magnesium disorders. In: Fluids and Electrolytes (Kokko, J. P. and Tannen, R. L. eds.), 3rd ed., pp. 421–445. W.B. Saunders Co., Philadelphia.

CHAPTER 30

◆ ◆

Sodium, Chloride, and Potassium

Hwai-Ping Sheng, Ph.D.

OUTLINE

COMMON ABBREVIATIONS

ADH (antidiuretic hormone)
ANP (atrial natriuretic peptide)

FUNCTIONS OF SODIUM, CHLORIDE, AND POTASSIUM

Sodium (Na^+), chloride (Cl^-), and potassium (K^+) ions are widely distributed in the body and are the principal electrolytes of body fluids. The concentrations of these ions in body fluids are very tightly controlled. These electrolytes play central roles in electrolytic balances and current, in osmotic control, in the transport of organic metabolites by cells, and in stabilization of polyelectrolytes in cells.

Distribution of Sodium, Chloride, and Potassium in Extracellular and Intracellular Fluids

Sodium, chloride, and potassium exist largely as free hydrated ions that bind only weakly to organic molecules. They function largely in the maintenance of electrolytic and osmotic balances or gradients. The concentration of Na^+ in the extracellular fluid is regulated at approximately 145 mmol/L, whereas its concentration in the intracellular fluid is 12 mmol/L as illustrated in Figure 30–1. The distribution of Cl^- generally follows that of Na^+, and Cl^- is the major anion of the extracellular fluid. The intracellular concentration of Cl^- is low, about 2 mmol/L, whereas its extracellular concentration is about 110 mmol/L. The concentration of K^+ is 150 mmol/L inside the cells and 4 to 5 mmol/L in the extracellular fluid. Thus, Na^+ and Cl^- are present mainly in the extracellular fluid compartment and are responsible for the osmolarity of this compartment, whereas K^+ is the principal cation in the intracellular fluid compartment (Rose, 1989).

The differences in the distribution of electrolytes in fluid compartments are the result of ion pumps, especially the Na^+,K^+-ATPase pump, and of the permeability characteristics of cell membranes. Cells expend a great amount of energy in maintaining these internal/external electrolyte gradients. The Na^+,K^+-ATPase, which actively pumps Na^+ out of the cell in exchange for K^+, is estimated to account for 20% to 40% of the whole-body resting energy expenditure in a typical adult (see Chapter 17). The selective permeability of the cell membrane prevents the movement of proteins, organic and inorganic phosphates, sulfates, and magnesium out of the cells. Because the inside of cells necessarily maintains high concentrations of these organic anions (mainly from phosphate, carboxylate, and sulfate groups of organic molecules such as proteins, phospholipids, nucleic acids, nucleotides, and metabolites), maintenance of high intracellular concentrations of K^+ along with magnesium (Mg^{2+}) serves to neutralize these excess negative charges of the organic cell constituents. Ejection of Na^+ and Cl^- from the cell is necessary to maintain osmotic balance.

Rejection and accumulation of ions by cells require the movement of Na^+, K^+, and Cl^- across membranes. Ion transport can occur by passive diffusion down the concentration gradient through ion channels or by active transport ("pumping") against the concentration gradient coupled to an energy-yielding process, which is usually the hydrolysis of ATP.

The enzyme Na^+,K^+-ATPase, a membrane-bound protein, is closely associated with movements of Na^+ and K^+ across cell membranes (Horisberger et al., 1991). It consists of a heterodimer of an α and a β subunit. Three α and three β subunit isoforms have been described so far. The relative proportion of each subunit isoform varies among tissues. The α subunit spans the membrane, has two large cytoplasmic domains, and contains the catalytic and cation-binding sites. The β subunit is a glycoprotein that also spans the membrane with a large extracellular domain; it modulates the catalytic activity of the Na^+,K^+-ATPase pump. When Na^+ is bound to the inward facing cation-binding sites of the α subunit, the enzyme binds ATP, and the ATPase reacts to phosphorylate, an aspartyl residue on the α subunit. The high-energy aspartyl phosphate intermediate relaxes or changes conformation, resulting in release of Na^+ from the carrier protein into the extracellular fluid, as illustrated in Figure 30–2. The transporter is now in a conformation that allows binding of K^+ to the outward facing cation-binding sites. Binding of K^+ results in dephosphorylation of the α subunit, which then returns to its previous conformation with release of K^+ into the cytosol in the process.

The overall stoichiometry of the Na^+,K^+-ATPase reaction is that three Na^+ ions are

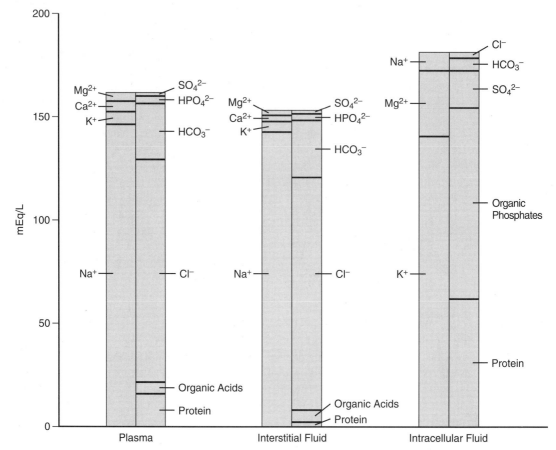

Figure 30–1. *Ionic composition of plasma, interstitial, and intracellular compartments. Concentrations are expressed in milliequivalents (mEq) per liter.*

pumped out of the cell and two K^+ ions are pumped into the cell, with the hydrolysis of 1 molecule of ATP to ADP + inorganic phosphate (P_i). This process creates a high concentration of Na^+ extracellularly and a high concentration of K^+ intracellularly and also creates a negative charge in the cells compared with the outside; the Na^+,K^+-ATPase is, thus, an electrogenic pump. The net extrusion of cations (Na^+) from the cell enables cells to control their osmolarity and, hence, water content; pumping of Na^+ out of the cell also promotes movement of Cl^- out of the cell, as Cl^- tends to move in the same direction as Na^+ to maintain electrical balance. The electrochemical potential gradient across the cell membrane that is maintained by the Na^+,K^+-ATPase is important for the normal functioning of nerves and muscle cells, for secondary active transport of nutrients such as glucose

and amino acids, and for K^+ secretion processes in the kidneys and colon.

Role of the Electrochemical Na^+ Gradient in Nutrient Transport Processes

Sodium is important in many nutrient transport processes (Berry and Rector, 1991). Absorption of Na^+ in the small intestine plays an important role in the absorption of Cl^-, amino acids, glucose, galactose, and water. In the kidney, similar mechanisms are involved in the reabsorption of these nutrients by the renal tubular cells from the plasma filtrate formed by the glomerulus. The driving force for absorption of Na^+ across the brush border membrane of the polar epithelial cells of the small intestinal mucosa or of renal tubules is provided by active transport of Na^+ out of

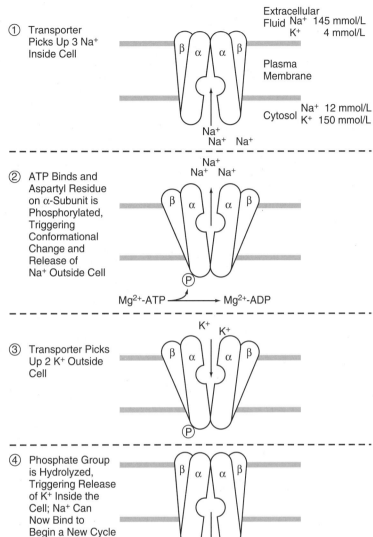

① Transporter Picks Up 3 Na⁺ Inside Cell

Extracellular Fluid Na⁺ 145 mmol/L
K⁺ 4 mmol/L

Plasma Membrane

Cytosol Na⁺ 12 mmol/L
K⁺ 150 mmol/L

② ATP Binds and Aspartyl Residue on α-Subunit is Phosphorylated, Triggering Conformational Change and Release of Na⁺ Outside Cell

Mg²⁺-ATP ⟶ Mg²⁺-ADP

③ Transporter Picks Up 2 K⁺ Outside Cell

④ Phosphate Group is Hydrolyzed, Triggering Release of K⁺ Inside the Cell; Na⁺ Can Now Bind to Begin a New Cycle

Figure 30–2. *Schematic representation of the enzyme Na⁺,K⁺-ATPase, which is responsible for primary active transport of Na⁺ and K⁺ in opposite directions across plasma membranes. The enzyme consists of two types of subunits (α and β) and is thought to have the subunit composition (αβ)₂ and to have one set of cation-binding sites. The α subunit contains the K⁺ and Na⁺ binding sites; it also contains a site for binding ATP and a phosphorylation site in the intracellular portion. Binding of Na⁺ and ATP intracellularly activates the enzyme ATPase, which cleaves 1 molecule of ATP to ADP and phosphorylates an aspartyl residue on a subunit. Phosphorylation causes a conformational change in the carrier protein molecule, thus extruding Na⁺ on the extracellular surface and allowing extracellular K⁺ to bind. K⁺ binding activates intracellular hydrolysis of the bound phosphate group, resulting in a conformational change and release of K⁺ inside the cell. The transporter is now ready to bind Na⁺ for another transport cycle. For each ATP hydrolyzed, 3 Na⁺ ions are moved out of the cell and 2 K⁺ ions are moved into it. This accounts for the low intracellular Na⁺ and high intracellular K⁺ concentrations.*

these same cells across the basolateral membrane into the interstitial space. Large amounts of the Na⁺,K⁺-ATPase are present in the basolateral membranes of these cells. Active extrusion of Na⁺ reduces the concentration of intracellular Na⁺. Sodium moves along its electrochemical gradient from the lumen into the cytosol of the epithelial cells to replace the Na⁺ that is transported out of the cells. The net result is an uptake of Na⁺ from the lumen of the gastrointestinal tract or from the renal tubular fluid into the extracellular fluids of the body.

Entry of Na⁺ across the luminal membrane is through Na⁺ channels or carrier-mediated facilitated diffusion in which other solutes are cotransported or countertransported with it. The absorption of Na⁺ across the epithelial cells creates a slight electronegativity in the lumen and electropositivity on the basal side of the epithelial cells. This provides a driving force for either the absorption of Cl⁻ in the same direction as Na⁺ movement or the secretion of K⁺ or H⁺ in the opposite direction in exchange for Na⁺, as illustrated in Figure 30–3. Absorption of Na⁺ and Cl⁻ across epithelial cells increases their concentrations in the intercellular spaces and provides an osmotic

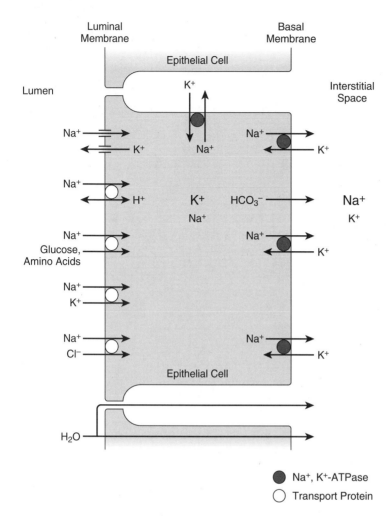

Figure 30–3. Schematic representation of how active extrusion of
Na+ via the enzyme Na+,K+-ATPase
across the basal membrane of an
epithelial cell creates an electrochemical gradient for the entry of
Na+ across the luminal membrane.
Entry of Na+ is by diffusion through
ion channels or carrier-mediated facilitated diffusion, which uses the
electrochemical gradient created
by the Na+,K+-ATPase as a driving
force for cotransport or countertransport of other solutes. Only the
most common types of transport
are shown.

gradient for the absorption of water. A large
proportion of water uptake occurs by a paracellular route through the junctions between
the apical borders of adjacent epithelial cells,
while a small proportion of water flux is
through the cells, involving movement across
the luminal membrane, cytoplasm, and basolateral membrane.

Some of the carrier proteins in the luminal membrane, such as the sodium-glucose
transporter (SGLT1) and a number of the
amino acid transport systems, have receptor
sites for binding both Na+ and an amino acid
or a monosaccharide (Fig. 30–3). Because Na+
is coupled to either an amino acid or a monosaccharide on the carrier protein, entry of Na+
down its electrochemical gradient across the
luminal membrane also brings in an amino
acid or a monosaccharide. Amino acids and

monosaccharides are, therefore, cotransported with Na+ across the luminal membrane; this process frequently is referred to as
secondary active transport. The Na+ gradient
allows cotransport to occur against the concentration gradient for monosaccharides or
amino acids. The increase in concentrations
of amino acids and monosaccharides inside
the epithelial cells allows the diffusion, usually facilitated by another carrier, of these nutrients across the basolateral membrane into
the interstitial fluid.

Membrane Potentials in Nerves and Muscles

Resting Membrane Potential. All cells in
the body have a potential difference across
their membranes under resting conditions,

with the inside of the cell negatively charged with respect to the outside. The resting membrane potential exists because of a small excess of negative ions inside the cell and an excess of positive ions outside. The magnitude of the resting membrane potential is determined by the differences in specific ion concentrations in the intracellular and extracellular fluids and the differences in membrane permeabilities to the different ions. Because Na^+ and K^+ are present in the highest concentrations, they generally play the most important roles in generating the membrane potential.

The higher intracellular K^+ concentration and lower intracellular Na^+ concentration resulting from the activity of the Na^+,K^+-ATPase causes K^+ to diffuse out of the cell and Na^+ into the cell down their concentration gradients through the K^+-Na^+ leak channels. However, passive K^+ efflux is much greater than passive Na^+ influx, because the K^+-Na^+ leak channels are more permeable to K^+ than to Na^+ in the resting state. Because the membrane is impermeable to most of the anions in the cell, the K^+ efflux is not accompanied by an equal efflux of anions, and the membrane is maintained in a polarized state, with the inside negative relative to the outside. The electrical potential developed begins to influence the efflux of K^+ and influx of Na^+ across the membrane. The negativity inside the cells attracts and the positivity outside the cells repulses these cations. For K^+, as long as efflux due to its concentration gradient is greater than influx due to the electrical potential, there will be net efflux. The membrane potential at which efflux of K^+ is equal to its influx is called the equilibrium potential for K^+.

A K^+ equilibrium potential of approximately -95 mV is calculated from its concentrations in the intracellular and extracellular fluids. Similarly, an equilibrium potential of $+60$ mV for Na^+ is calculated from its concentration gradient. Because the membrane is more permeable to K^+ than to Na^+, the resting membrane potential is closer to the K^+ equilibrium potential, about -70 mV for neurons and -90 mV for skeletal muscle fibers. At that resting membrane potential, there is net influx of Na^+ and efflux of K^+ through their channels.

However, the concentrations of intracellular Na^+ and K^+ remain relatively constant due to the activity of the Na^+,K^+-ATPase in the membrane. In the resting state, the number of ions moved by the Na^+,K^+-ATPase equals the number of ions that move in the opposite direction through the membrane channels down their concentration or electrical gradients.

In most cells, because of the absence of an active Cl^- pump, movements of Cl^- across membranes are passive, through Cl^- channels. The negative membrane potential moves Cl^- out, and the concentration gradient moves Cl^- into the cell. Thus, Cl^- concentration gradient across the membrane shifts until the equilibrium potential for Cl^- is equal to the resting membrane potential. Unlike K^+ and Na^+, Cl^- flux responds to the membrane potential and makes no contribution to its magnitude.

Action Potential. Transient activation of nerve and muscle cells depolarizes the cell membrane. A slight decrease in the resting membrane potential (depolarization) leads to increased K^+ efflux, which restores the resting membrane potential. However, membranes of nerve and muscle cells are also capable of producing action potentials in which rapid large depolarization in the membrane potential occurs; the potential may change from -70 mV to $+30$ mV, and then it may repolarize back to its resting membrane potential. In the events of action potential, both the voltage-gated Na^+ channels and voltage-gated K^+ channels play important roles. When the membrane depolarizes by about 20 mV to 40 mV to a value of -50 mV to -30 mV, the voltage-gated Na^+ channels are activated and begin to allow a rapid inflow of Na^+ into the cells. A rapid inflow of Na^+ causes further depolarization and opens more voltage-gated Na^+ channels. This process is a positive feedback cycle, which continues until all the voltage-gated Na^+ channels are opened. As more Na^+ ions enter the cell than K^+ ions leave the cell, the membrane depolarizes. When the firing level is reached, the influx of Na^+ along its inwardly directed concentration gradient is so great that it dominates over the electrical gradient, and the membrane potential moves toward $+60$ mV.

In nerve cells, immediately after the overshoot, the membrane potential returns rapidly to its resting potential. Several events allow for rapid repolarization. The voltage-gated Na^+ channels rapidly enter a closed state, thus preventing further entry of Na^+ ions, and they remain in this state until the membrane potential returns to its original resting level. In the meantime, during the depolarizing phase of the action potential, the voltage-gated K^+ channels also open, but the K^+ channels open more slowly than do the Na^+ channels so that they are mainly open when the Na^+ channels are beginning to close. Therefore, the decrease in Na^+ entry and the simultaneous exit of K^+ cause repolarization of the cell.

At the end of the action potential, the return of the membrane potential to the negative state causes the voltage-gated K^+ channels to close back to their original status, but again after a delay. This slight delay accounts for the slight hyperpolarization of the membrane potential after an action potential. Chloride permeability does not change during the action potential. Chloride distributes passively along its concentration and electrical gradients across the membrane. Thus, depolarization is due to Na^+ influx, whereas repolarization is a manifestation of K^+ efflux. Although Na^+ enters the nerve cell and K^+ leaves it during the action potential, the number of ions involved is minute relative to the total numbers present. In nerve and skeletal muscle cells, the alternation of K^+ steady-state potentials with pulsed sodium potentials due to opening and closing of voltage-gated Na^+ channels gives rise to a traveling wave of depolarization, which is the current message that is conducted along the nerve or muscle fiber.

Cardiac and smooth muscle cells also contain calcium (Ca^{2+})-transporting ATPase, which actively transports Ca^{2+} out of the cells, creating a Ca^{2+} concentration gradient. In addition, voltage-gated Ca^{2+} channels, which are highly permeable to Ca^{2+} but only slightly permeable to Na^+, are also present in cell membranes; these are called Ca^{2+}-Na^+ channels. In contrast to the Na^+ channels, which are fast channels, the Ca^{2+}-Na^+ channels are slow to activate. Opening of these channels during an action potential allows rapid inflow of mostly Ca^{2+} and some Na^+ into the cells.

The increase in intracellular Ca^{2+} concentration plays an essential role in the signal transduction pathway that couples membrane excitability to events within the cells. In some types of smooth muscle cells, the fast Na^+ channels are absent so that the action potentials are caused almost entirely by activation of the slow Ca^{2+}-Na^+ channels.

Importance of Potassium Gradient. The high concentration gradient of K^+ between the intracellular fluid and the plasma is important for maintaining the normal resting membrane potential across cell membranes and for excitability of nerves and muscles. Changes in the concentration of K^+ in the plasma change this gradient and will adversely affect the aforementioned functions (Rodriguez-Soriano, 1995). For instance, in hyperkalemia, when the concentration of K^+ in the plasma exceeds 5.5 mmol/L, the membrane depolarizes, causing muscular weakness, flaccid paralysis, and cardiac arrhythmias. A plasma K^+ concentration of 8 mmol/L can lead to cardiac arrest. In contrast, in hypokalemia, when the concentration of K^+ in the plasma is less than 3.5 mmol/L, the membrane hyperpolarizes, and this can interfere with the normal functioning of nerves and muscles, resulting in muscle weakness and decreased smooth muscle contractility. Severe hypokalemia can lead to paralysis, metabolic alkalosis, and death. Therefore, it is important to regulate the concentration of K^+ in the plasma within narrow limits.

Importance of Extracellular Calcium. The extracellular Ca^{2+} concentration also affects the excitability of nerve and muscle cells by its effect on the voltage-gated Na^+ channels. In low extracellular Ca^{2+} concentration, the voltage-gated Na^+ channels are activated by a very small depolarization of the resting membrane potential, thus increasing the excitability of nerve and muscle cells. An increase in extracellular Ca^{2+} concentration decreases excitability and thereby stabilizes the membrane.

Differences Between Ionic Composition of Interstitial Fluid and Plasma

The ionic composition of the two extracellular fluid compartments, interstitial fluid and plasma, are very similar (see Figure 30–1). The capillary endothelium, which separates them, acts as a semipermeable barrier that allows free movement to solutes of low molecular weight while retaining proteins in the vascular compartment. The small amount of protein that diffuses into the interstitial space is returned to the circulation via the lymphatics. This accounts for the low concentration of protein, less than 10 g/L, in the interstitial fluid, compared with an average of 73 g/L in the plasma. The concentration difference of protein across the capillary endothelium affects the distribution of diffusible ions so that the concentration of any diffusible cation is higher and the concentration of any diffusible anion is lower in the plasma than in the interstitial fluid, in accordance with the Gibbs-Donnan equilibrium (see Chapter 37). This Gibbs-Donnan effect is small at the normal concentration of plasma protein. It causes a difference of about 5% in the concentrations of Na^+, K^+, and Cl^- across the capillary endothelium. For all practical purposes the ionic compositions of plasma and interstitial fluid are considered to be the same.

Sodium, a Major Determinant of Extracellular Fluid Volume

The volume of the extracellular fluid compartment (interstitial fluid and plasma) is determined primarily by the total amount of osmotic particles present. Because Na^+ is the major determinant of osmolarity of extracellular fluid, disturbances in Na^+ balance will change the volume of the extracellular fluid compartment. This can be illustrated simply by the infusion of a hypertonic NaCl solution into the circulation. The added Na^+ distributes rapidly between the vascular and interstitial fluid compartments, causing increases in the Na^+ concentration and hence osmolarity of both of these compartments. Osmoreceptors present in the supraoptic and paraventricular nuclei in the hypothalamus are stimulated by the increase in the osmolarity of fluid bathing them (Baylis and Thompson, 1988). Stimulation of these cells activates the thirst mechanism and also causes the release of antidiuretic hormone (ADH) from the posterior pituitary. Drinking of water in response to

thirst, together with the ADH-induced decrease in water excretion by the kidneys, restores the osmolarity and increases the volume of the extracellular fluid toward normal.

Conversely, a decrease in the osmolarity of the extracellular fluid due to a loss of NaCl in excess of water from the body causes excretion of water by the kidneys. This will restore the osmolarity of the extracellular fluid compartment toward normal and decrease its volume. Thus, alterations in the concentrations of Na^+ and Cl^- in the extracellular fluid result in parallel changes in its volume when the mechanisms for thirst and secretion of ADH function normally.

Other Functions of Electrolytes

Interactions with Macroions. Many macromolecules present in the extracellular and intracellular compartments contain multiple ionizing groups on their surfaces and are classed as macroions. Their behavior in solution depends on their surface charges, which either repel each other so that they remain separated in solution or attract each other so that they associate. Nucleic acids are large polyelectrolytes that carry multiple negative charges, whereas proteins are polyampholytes that contain both acidic and basic groups on their surfaces. Therefore, depending on the pH of the solution, proteins may carry substantial net positive or negative charges. Most plasma and intracellular proteins have net negative charges at plasma pH of 7.4, but a few have net positive charges. Another important macroion is a group of polysaccharides, the glycosaminoglycans, which are of major structural importance and which carry carboxylate and sulfate groups. A major function of the glycosaminoglycans, such as chondroitin sulfates and keratan sulfates of connective tissue and dermatan sulfates of skin, is the formation of a matrix to hold together the protein components of connective tissue and skin. A very highly sulfated glycosaminoglycan is heparin, a natural anticoagulant produced by the mast cells that line the arterial walls. Heparan sulfate, which is less highly sulfated than is heparin, is linked to many cell surface proteins and matrix proteoglycans.

Macroion surfaces are modified by a

counterion atmosphere enriched in oppositely charged small ions, mainly Na^+, K^+, and Cl^-. The counterion atmosphere is greatly affected by the ionic strength of the solution. At low ionic strength, the counterion atmosphere is diffuse, with minimal interference to interactions of macroions, whereas at high ionic strength, the counterion atmosphere is concentrated about the macroions, which then effectively reduces their interactions. This explains the observation that increasing salt concentration of a solution containing protein increases the solubility of the protein.

Activation of Enzymes. Activators of enzyme-catalyzed reactions are frequently metal ions such as Mg^{2+}, zinc (Zn^{2+}), manganese (Mn^{2+}), and Ca^{2+}, whereas only a limited number of enzymes require the presence of Na^+, K^+, or Cl^-. The most common and most widely distributed enzyme in the cell membrane is the Na^+,K^+-ATPase, the activation of which requires the presence of Na^+ and K^+. Enzymes that require the presence of Cl^- for activation include the angiotensin-converting enzyme that catalyzes the conversion of angiotensin I to angiotensin II (Bunning and Riordan, 1987). Although the presence of Mg^{2+} is required for activation of a number of enzymes by K^+ in mammalian tissues, K^+ by itself is important for the activity of pyruvate kinase (Larsen et al., 1994).

SODIUM, CHLORIDE, AND POTASSIUM BALANCE

Total body sodium has been estimated at 100 g, chloride at 95 g, and potassium at 140 g for a 70-kg adult (Forbes, 1987). One mole of Na^+, K^+, or Cl^- is equivalent to 23 g, 39 g, or 35.5 g, respectively. To maintain a stable content of these elements in the plasma and tissues, the amount consumed must equal the amount lost from the body. In the growing child, the amount accreted for tissue formation has to be considered also.

Loss of Sodium, Chloride, and Potassium

Obligatory loss of fluids through skin, feces, and urine invariably causes loss of sodium and chloride (see Chapter 37). Minimum obligatory loss of sodium in the absence of profuse sweating and gastrointestinal and renal diseases has been estimated to be approximately 115 mg/day, with loss of sodium in urine and feces estimated to be about 23 mg/day and dermal losses from 46 to 92 mg/day (National Research Council, 1989). Studies over a 12-day period have shown that sweat and fecal excretion accounted for only 2% to 5% of total sodium excretion in adults consuming an average intake of salt; the remainder of the salt consumed was excreted in the urine (Sanchez-Castillo et al., 1987b). However, loss of sodium can increase greatly under certain circumstances, such as diarrhea, diabetes, and profuse sweating during strenuous physical activity in hot weather. Under most, but not all, circumstances, loss of sodium is accompanied by a similar molar loss of chloride.

As with sodium and chloride, obligatory loss of fluid through feces, sweat, and urine also causes loss of potassium via these routes. In the normal healthy adult, potassium loss via these routes is less than 800 mg/day, with less than 400 mg via fecal loss, 200 to 400 mg via urinary loss, and negligible amounts from sweat (National Research Council, 1989).

Intake of Sodium and Chloride

Dietary Intake. Dietary sodium is consumed mainly as sodium chloride, with small amounts as sodium bicarbonate, sodium glutamate, and sodium citrate. These sodium salts are present in most natural foodstuffs; they are low in vegetables and fresh fruits but high in meat products. Studies in a British population found that only 10% of sodium intake came from natural foods, 15% from table salt added during cooking and at the table, and 75% from salts added during manufacturing and processing (Sanchez-Castillo et al., 1987a). The amount of chloride consumed parallels the amount of sodium, as dietary chloride is consumed almost exclusively as a salt of sodium.

Daily salt consumption has been estimated by assessing salt intake or measuring urinary sodium excretion. Usually consumption far exceeds the needs of an individual, although it varies widely between individuals and cultures. Average Americans consume between 2 and 5 g/day of sodium or between 5 and 13 g/day of sodium chloride (National Research Council, 1989). This wide range of reported intakes is due to the different methods of assessment and to the large variability of discretionary salt intake. Individuals consuming a diet high in processed foods have high salt intakes. In Japan, where consumption of salt-preserved fish and the use of salt for seasoning are customary, salt intake is high, ranging from 14 to 20 g/day (Kono et al., 1983). On the other hand, urinary sodium chloride excretion of the Yanomamo Indians in Brazil averages 87 mg/day (Oliver et al., 1975). These individuals and vegetarians, who consume an average of 760 mg of NaCl per day, do not normally exhibit chronic deficiencies because of the efficiency of the mechanism of salt conservation.

Recommended Intake. Daily minimum requirements of sodium and chloride in the adult can be estimated from the amount needed to replace obligatory losses, which add up to about 115 mg of sodium or 300 mg of sodium chloride. Because of various degrees of physical activities of individuals and environmental conditions, the estimated level of safe minimum intake for a 70-kg adult is 500 mg/day of sodium (National Research Council, 1989). Requirements for chloride parallel those for sodium on a milliequivalent basis, and the estimated minimum requirement for chloride is 750 mg/day for adults. This corresponds to about 1.3 g of sodium chloride for adults, a value considerably less than the average intake in the United States. Although there is no established optimal range of intake of sodium chloride, it is recommended that daily salt intake should not exceed 6 g because of the association of high intake with hypertension (National Research Council, 1989).

The need for sodium chloride is increased in pregnancy and lactation. A normal physiological event during pregnancy is a gradual retention of a total of approximately 20.7 g of sodium, which is associated with increased fetal requirements and expansion of maternal plasma and total extracellular fluid volume (Lowe et al., 1992). This increased need leads to the recommendation of an additional 69 mg/day over the safe minimum intake of 500 mg/day for the duration of pregnancy (National Research Council, 1989). The increased need for the duration of lactation can be estimated from the average milk production and sodium content in milk. Daily milk production averages 0.75 L, and sodium content in milk averages 7.5 mmol/L. Therefore, an additional need of about 135 mg/day is required for the duration of lactation (National Research Council, 1989). These increased needs during pregnancy and lactation can be met by the usual average intake in the United States.

For infants under 1 year of age, during which growth rate is maximal, the sodium requirement per unit of body weight is higher than that of adults in order to support growth. From data derived from daily accretion and losses, the recommended estimated level of minimum daily sodium intake is 120 mg for infants between birth and 5 months of age and 200 mg for infants 6 to 11 months of age (National Research Council, 1989). This criterion is met when either human milk or cow's milk formula supplemented with solid foods is given ad libitum. The estimated minimum requirements of sodium for children range from 225 mg at 1 year of age to 500 mg at 10 to 18 years.

Intake of Potassium

Dietary Intake. Potassium is widely distributed in foods, especially in vegetables and fruits. Intakes of potassium vary widely, depending on dietary habits. An average American adult consumes between 2.5 and 3.5 g/day of potassium (National Research Council, 1989). Individuals consuming large amounts of fruits and vegetables, which are low in sodium and high in potassium, may have a potassium intake of as high as 11 g/day (Eaton and Konner, 1985). Even on this high consumption, a healthy adult can maintain potassium balance because of the large capacity of the kidneys to excrete the excess.

Recommended Intake. To replace the loss of potassium in feces, sweat, and urine, an

Food Sources of Sodium

- Foods and beverages containing NaCl added during food processing
- Table salt
- Other sodium salts (e.g., sodium bicarbonate or monosodium glutamate) used as food additives

Estimated Minimum Requirement Across the Life Cycle

	mg sodium/day
Infants, 0–0.5 y	120
0.5–1.0 y	200
Children, 1 y	225
2–5 y	300
6–9 y	400
10–18 y	500
Adults, >18 y	500

From National Research Council (1989) Recommended Dietary Allowances, 10th ed., pp. 247–261. National Academy Press, Washington, D.C.

adult should consume not less than 800 mg/day. The estimated minimum requirement for potassium as recommended by the National Research Council (1989) is 2 g/day for adults. Because of the growing evidence of the beneficial effects of potassium in hypertension, concern of possible underconsumption of potassium has led to recommendations for increased intake of dietary fruits and vegetables, which would increase the intake to about 3.5 g/day. The need for potassium is increased in pregnancy and lactation. During pregnancy, the increase in maternal supportive tissues and fetal and placental tissues increases the minimum requirement for potassium. The increased need for the duration of lactation has been estimated from the average milk production of 0.75 L/day and potassium content of 13.3 mmol/L and averages 384 mg/day. The estimated minimum requirement for adults and the additional need for potassium for the duration of pregnancy and lactation can be

Food Sources of Chloride

- Foods and beverages containing NaCl added during food processing
- Table salt

Estimated Minimum Requirement Across the Life Cycle

	mg chloride/day
Infants, 0–0.5 y	180
0.5–1.0 y	300
Children, 1 y	350
2–5 y	500
6–9 y	600
10–18 y	750
Adults, >18 y	750

From National Research Council (1989) Recommended Dietary Allowances, 10th ed., pp. 247–261. National Academy Press, Washington, D.C.

met by the usual average intake in the United States of 2.5 to 3.5 g/day.

For infants and children, a higher consumption of potassium per unit body weight is recommended to support growth of new tissues, as well as obligatory losses. The estimated total accretion of potassium averages 5.6 g from birth to 5 months of age and 4.4 g from 6 to 12 months of age, for an average daily accretion rate of 37 mg and 24 mg for the two growth periods (Fomon et al., 1982). To allow for obligatory losses, the estimated minimum requirement is 500 mg/day for infants between birth and 5 months of age and 700 mg for infants 6 to 11 months of age (National Research Council, 1989). This amount is normally met when a diet of either human milk or cow's milk formula, supplemented by solid foods in the second 6 months, is fed to infants. The estimated minimum daily requirements of potassium for children and adolescents range from 1000 mg at 1 year of age to 2000 mg at 10 to 18 years of age.

REGULATION OF SODIUM, CHLORIDE, AND POTASSIUM BALANCE

The kidneys are the main site of regulation of sodium, chloride, and potassium balance; the intestines play a relatively minor role. The kidneys respond to a deficiency of these elements in the diet by decreasing their excretion, and they respond to an excess by increasing their excretion in the urine. Urinary loss of sodium is controlled by varying the rate of sodium reabsorption from the filtrate by tubular cells, whereas urinary loss of potassium is controlled by varying the rate of secretion of potassium.

Renal Excretion of Sodium, Chloride, and Potassium

The rate of renal excretion of Na^+, Cl^-, and K^+ depends on the tubular functions of the kidneys (Berry and Rector, 1991). These electrolytes are filtered freely across the glomerular membrane of the nephrons (functional units of the kidneys) so that their concentrations in the glomerular filtrate are similar to those in the plasma. As the filtrate flows along the renal tubules, reabsorption of Na^+, Cl^-, and K^+ and secretion of K^+ by renal tubular cells alter the final concentrations of Na^+, Cl^-, and K^+ in the urine. Figure 30–4 illustrates the basic renal processing of Na^+, Cl^-, and K^+. Net reabsorption of all three ions occurs in the proximal tubule, the thick ascending limb of the loop of Henle, and the distal convoluted tubule. Normally, 95% to 97.5% of the filtered load of these ions and water is reabsorbed by these segments. Reabsorption of the re-

Food Sources of Potassium

- Fruits (avocado, banana, cantaloupe, orange juice, watermelon)
- Vegetables (lima beans, potatoes, tomatoes, spinach, winter squash)
- Fresh meats

Estimated Minimum Requirement Across the Life Cycle

	mg potassium/day
Infants, 0–0.5 y	500
0.5–1.0 y	700
Children, 1 y	1000
2–5 y	1400
6–9 y	1600
10–18 y	2000
Adults, >18 y	2000

From National Research Council (1989) Recommended Dietary Allowances, 10th ed., pp. 247–261. National Academy Press, Washington, D.C.

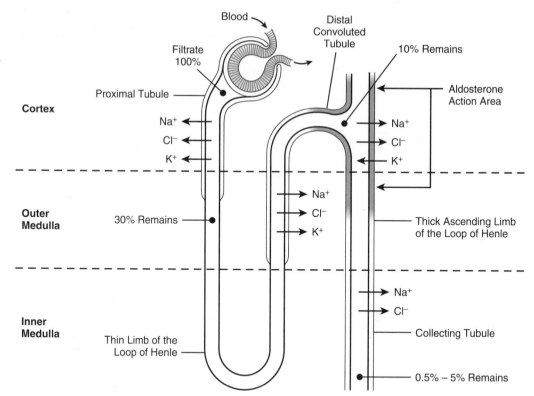

Figure 30–4. *Resorption of Na+, K+, and Cl− and secretion of K+ at different parts of the nephron. The nephron is the functional unit of the kidney; there are ~1,200,000 nephrons in each human kidney.*

maining 2.5% to 5% of the filtrate and secretion of K+ in the cortical collecting tubule are variable and depend greatly on the needs of the individual. Individuals on low-sodium diets have low rates of excretion of Na+. When there is an excess of sodium from high dietary intake, little Na+ is reabsorbed by renal tubular cells, resulting in the excretion of the excess Na+ in the urine. As much as 13 g/day of sodium can be excreted in the urine.

In contrast to Na+, K+ is secreted by the tubular cells of the cortical collecting tubules (Rodriguez-Soriano, 1995). In the absence of disease, changes in K+ excretion are not due to changes in reabsorption of K+ in the proximal tubules but to changes in K+ secretion by the cortical collecting tubules. During potassium depletion, most of the filtered K+ is reabsorbed, and virtually no K+ is secreted. The small amount of K+ excreted comes from the filtered K+ that escaped reabsorption. However, when potassium intake is high, secretion of K+ is increased, thus eliminating the excess potassium. A normal Western diet contains

about 3 g/day of potassium and requires the renal tubular secretion of K+ in order to maintain potassium balance. Reabsorption of Na+, Cl−, and K+ and secretion of K+ are under the control of various homeostatic regulatory mechanisms that effectively maintain a balance of these elements in the body.

Control of Renal Excretion of Sodium and Chloride

Because Na+ is the main determinant of extracellular fluid volume, physiological control mechanisms that control the volume of extracellular fluid effectively maintain a balance for sodium and chloride. Changes in extracellular fluid volume lead to corresponding changes in the effective circulating volume. Any change in this effective circulating volume will affect the "fullness" or "pressure" in the circulation and will cause a change in cardiac filling pressure, cardiac output, and arterial pressure. Located throughout the vascular system are volume or pressure sensors that detect these changes and send either excitatory or inhibitory signals to the central nervous system and/or the endocrine glands to effect appropriate responses by the kidneys.

Renin-Angiotensin-Aldosterone System. The most important regulator of renal excretion of Na$^+$ and Cl$^-$ is the renin-angiotensin-aldosterone system (Laragh, 1985). The baroreceptors located in the afferent arterioles of the glomerulus of each nephron sense changes in perfusion pressure while chemoreceptors located in the macula densa area of the thick ascending limb of the loop of Henle sense changes in the sodium load in the tubular fluid. These sensors respond to changes in renal perfusion and sodium load by influencing the synthesis and secretion of renin by the juxtaglomerular cells located at the afferent arterioles (Levens et al., 1981). Any decrease in effective circulating volume will decrease renal perfusion and sodium load in the tubular fluid. This will then increase the release of renin from the juxtaglomerular cells (Fig. 30–5).

Renin, a proteolytic enzyme, is synthesized and stored in an inactive form called prorenin in the juxtaglomerular cells of the afferent and efferent arterioles in the kidneys (Ballermann et al., 1991). It is released in response to stimuli from the renal sympathetic nerves and by an intrarenal reflex mechanism via the juxtaglomerular apparatus when the effective circulating volume is decreased. In the circulation, renin acts as an enzyme to split off a small polypeptide, angiotensin I (a decapeptide), from angiotensinogen, a protein produced by the liver. Angiotensin I is biologically inactive and undergoes further cleavage to form angiotensin II (an octapeptide), a reaction catalyzed by the angiotensin-converting enzyme present on the luminal surface of the endothelium of blood vessels in the lungs, liver, and kidneys.

Angiotensin II has important physiological functions (Ballermann et al., 1991). First, it conserves body sodium by stimulating Na$^+$ reabsorption by the proximal convoluted tubules and indirectly via secretion of aldoste-

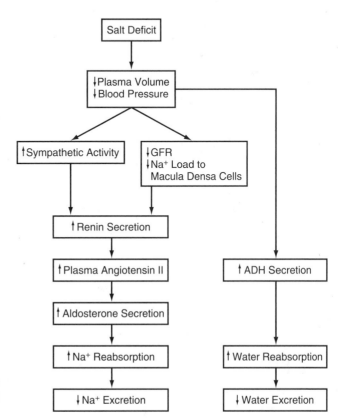

Figure 30–5. *Schematic representation of the control of renal excretion of sodium and water during salt deficit.*

rone. Angiotensin II stimulates the Na^+,K^+-ATPase in the basolateral membrane and the Na^+,H^+-exchanger in the luminal membrane of the tubular cells. The overall effect is an increase in reabsorption of Na^+Cl^- and $Na^+HCO_3^-$. More importantly, angiotensin II is a potent stimulator of aldosterone synthesis and secretion. Angiotensin II also causes arteriolar constriction, thereby raising peripheral resistance and sustaining blood pressure in response to a decrease in blood volume.

Aldosterone is a steroid hormone produced and secreted by the zona glomerulosa cells of the adrenal cortex. Its secretion is stimulated by a low plasma Na^+ concentration, a high plasma K^+ concentration, or angiotensin II. Aldosterone stimulates mainly the cells of the cortical collecting tubules, and to a lesser extent the distal convoluted and medullary collecting tubules, to reabsorb Na^+ and secrete K^+. Aldosterone first binds to cytoplasmic receptors in the tubular cells and then subsequently interacts with specific binding sites on the DNA in the nucleus to regulate the transcription of certain messenger RNAs (mRNAs). This stimulates the translation of specific proteins important in the processes of Na^+ and K^+ transport. The density and activity of Na^+,K^+-ATPase in the basolateral membrane, and the number of electrogenic Na^+ and K^+ channels in the luminal membrane, are increased (O'Neil, 1990). These changes cause an increase in the rate of reabsorption of Na^+ by increasing the active transport of Na^+ out of the cells across the basolateral membrane and the passive influx of Na^+ across the luminal membrane. At the same time, the rate of movement of K^+ into the cells across the basolateral membrane and out of the cells across the luminal membrane into the tubular lumen is increased. The increased reabsorption of Na^+ also increases the potential difference across the tubular epithelial cells (the lumen becomes more negative), so that more K^+ is secreted into the lumen along the electrical gradient.

Vascular Pressure Receptors—Renal Sympathetic and Antidiuretic Hormone Pathways. Essentially two kinds of baroreceptors are present: (1) the vascular low-pressure receptors located in the central venous portion of the circulation, and (2) the vascular high-pressure receptors located in the arterial side of the vascular tree (Moe et al., 1991). The low-pressure receptors respond primarily to distention of the walls of the cardiac atria and the pulmonary vein. These baroreceptors send signals via afferent fibers in the vagus nerve to the hypothalamic and medullary centers of the central nervous system. The high-pressure receptors respond primarily to changes in blood pressure in the walls of the aortic arch and the carotid sinus. The aortic arch and carotid baroreceptors send impulses via the vagus and the glossopharyngeal nerves to the hypothalamic and medullary regions of the central nervous system. Increases in vagal and glossopharyngeal nerve activities from both the low-pressure and high-pressure receptors inhibit secretion of ADH from the posterior pituitary and also inhibit the sympathetic outflow and renal sympathetic activity. In hypervolemia, the activities of the vagal and glossopharyngeal nerves are increased, resulting in a decrease in sympathetic outflow and in secretion of ADH. In hypovolemia, there is a reflex increase in the renal sympathetic activity and in secretion of ADH (Quail et al., 1987).

Under normal arterial pressure, there is minimal sympathetic nerve activity to the kidneys. As part of a reflex response to a fall in systemic arterial pressure, the renal sympathetic nerves are activated to bring about a decrease in renal excretion of Na^+ and Cl^- (Moe et al., 1991). Three mechanisms are involved in sympathetic effects on renal Na^+ and Cl^- transport. First, sympathetic nerve activity stimulates the α_1-adrenergic receptors of the afferent and efferent arterioles of the glomerulus. This increases the overall renal vascular resistance, resulting in a decrease in renal blood flow and the glomerular filtration rate. This in turn leads to an overall reduction in the filtered load of Na^+. Second, sympathetic nerve endings stimulate the α_1-adrenergic receptors on the proximal tubules and loops of Henle, which results in increased reabsorption of Na^+ and Cl^- (Aperia et al., 1996). These two actions decrease renal excretion of Na^+ and Cl^-. Third, in addition to their effects on renal hemodynamics and reabsorption of Na^+, sympathetic nerves also stimulate the juxtaglomerular cells of the afferent and efferent arterioles to release renin. Renin subsequently increases the circulating levels of angiotensin II and aldosterone, which are important in stimulating reabsorption of Na^+. All these adaptive responses restore the effective circulating volume and blood pressure toward their normal values.

ADH primarily increases the permeability of the collecting ducts to water so that water is reabsorbed from the tubular lumen into the hyperosmotic medullary interstitium. It also enhances reabsorption of Na^+ and Cl^- by the thick ascending limb of the loops of Henle and, to a lesser degree, the collecting ducts (Canessa et al., 1994).

This reflex regulation of volume is effective during hypovolemia. When the effective circulating volume is low, the overall effect is a reflex increase in Na^+, Cl^-, and water retention via the activation of renal sympathetic nerves and secretion of ADH. On the other hand, sympathetic nerve activity has much less effect on renal excretion of Na^+ and Cl^- in hypervolemia because the sympathetic nerve activity to the kidneys is minimal in euvolemia and, hence, is not decreased substantially by hypervolemia.

Natriuretic Peptides. A group of peptides found in different organs of the body, such as the atria, brain, and adrenal glands, exhibit potent hypotensive and natriuretic activities. The natriuretic peptides were first found in the myocytes of the cardiac atria, hence they are called atrial natriuretic peptides (ANPs). Volume expansion stretches the atrial myocytes and releases ANP into the circulation. The ANP increases renal Na^+ excretion and also increases the excretion of water by inhibiting the secretion of ADH from the posterior pituitary (Zeidel, 1990).

Demonstration of the presence of natriuretic peptides in the kidneys led to the postulation that these peptides form a renal natriuretic peptide system that regulates renal circulation and local transport of Na^+ and water. ANP acts predominantly in the glomeruli and inner medulla of the kidneys. It causes natriuresis via three different mechanisms. First, ANP causes vasodilation of the afferent and efferent arterioles of the glomerulus, with its actions on the afferent arterioles being predominant. The increase in renal blood flow and glomerular capillary hydrostatic pressure increases the glomerular filtration rate and filtered load of Na^+. Second, ANP also acts directly on the cells in the medullary portion of the collecting duct. It acts through its second messenger, cyclic guanosine monophosphate (cGMP), to inhibit reabsorption of Na^+ and Cl^-. Third, ANP inhibits secretion of aldosterone partly by its direct inhibitory action on the adrenal cortex and partly via its inhibition of the secretion of renin from the juxtaglomerular cells of the kidneys. Taking all these effects together, ANP increases renal excretion of Na^+, Cl^-, and water in hypervolemia. Hypothetically, a decrease in circulating levels of ANP would be expected to decrease renal excretion of Na^+, Cl^-, and water. However, there is no convincing evidence to indicate that circulating levels of ANP play an important role in hypovolemia.

Control of Renal Excretion of Potassium

Over 90% of the potassium in the diet is absorbed by intestinal epithelial cells into the circulation and is distributed throughout the extracellular fluid. In the adult, the volume of extracellular fluid is about 20% of body weight, or 14 L. The rise in the concentration of K^+ in plasma immediately stimulates physiological mechanisms to promote rapid entry of K^+ into cells so that a rapid rise in the plasma concentration is prevented. If the absorbed potassium ingested during a meal (~1.5 g or 40 mmol) were to remain in the extracellular fluid compartment, the concentration of K^+ in the plasma would increase to 6.9 mmol/L, a potentially lethal concentration. Thus, uptake of K^+ by cells is essential in preventing life-threatening hyperkalemia. However, in the long-term, to maintain K^+ balance, the excess K^+ from the diet must be excreted by the kidneys.

Aldosterone. The most important hormone regulating secretion of K^+ is aldosterone, the release of which is triggered by a high concentration of K^+ in plasma, by a low concentration of Na^+ in plasma, or by angiotensin II. These feedback loops regulate K⁺ concentration in the plasma and provide a relatively large tolerance to changes in dietary K⁺. Lack of aldosterone, for example in Addison's disease, causes a marked depletion of body Na⁺ and retention of K⁺ (Nerup, 1974). Conversely, excess aldosterone, for example in Conn's syndrome, is associated with depletion of K⁺ and retention of Na⁺ (Ganguly and Donohue, 1983).

Plasma Concentrations of K^+ and H^+. Other factors that can directly affect secretion of K⁺ by the distal nephrons are plasma concentrations of K⁺ and H⁺ (Rodriguez-Soriano, 1995). These ions act by changing the concentration of intracellular K⁺ in tubular cells. When the concentration of intracellular K⁺ is increased, the concentration gradient for K⁺ across the luminal membrane increases, thus promoting diffusion of K⁺ into the lumen. A decrease in the concentration of intracellular K⁺ decreases the concentration gradient across the luminal membrane, and secretion of K⁺ is reduced. Under normal circumstances, the concentration of intracellular K⁺ in tubular cells reflects that of the plasma. This is because an increase in the concentration of plasma K⁺ directly stimulates the Na⁺,K⁺-ATPase pump at the basolateral membrane of the distal nephrons. In addition, an increase in the concentration of K⁺ in the plasma causes secretion of aldosterone, which further increases uptake of K⁺ by tubular cells and excretion of K⁺ in the urine.

Secretion of K⁺ by the tubular cells in response to changes in acid-base balance is complex. In general, acute acidosis decreases secretion of K⁺, causing retention of potassium, whereas acute alkalosis increases secretion and loss of potassium from the body (Adrogue and Madias, 1981). An increased concentration of H⁺ in plasma probably acts by inhibiting the Na⁺,K⁺-ATPase activity at the basolateral membrane so that the intracellular K⁺ concentration in the tubular cells is decreased, resulting in a decrease in secretion of K⁺ by the tubular cells. However, with chronic acid-base disorders, the response of the kidneys is varied. It depends on the etiology of the disorders and the presence of other factors that may influence secretion of K⁺. Changes in pH alter other processes that influence secretion of K⁺. Metabolic acidosis may be associated with an increase in secretion of K⁺ and mild K⁺ depletion, which may be explained by an acidosis-induced increase in secretion of aldosterone. Metabolic alkalosis is almost always accompanied by depletion of K⁺.

Control of Intestinal Absorption and Excretion of Sodium, Chloride, and Potassium

Under normal circumstances, about 99% of dietary Na⁺, Cl⁻, and K⁺ is absorbed, and the remainder is excreted in the feces. Analogies may be drawn between the excretion of these ions in the kidneys and the intestines. Absorption of Na⁺ and Cl⁻ occurs along the entire length of the intestines; 90% to 95% is absorbed in the small intestine and the rest in the colon. Absorption of K⁺ occurs in the small intestine, but normally there is net secretion of K⁺ in the colon. In the colon, net absorption occurs during K⁺ deficit, and net secretion occurs in K⁺ excess. Intestinal absorption and secretion of Na⁺, K⁺, and Cl⁻ are subject to regulation by the nervous system, hormones, and paracrine agonists released from neurons in the enteric nervous system in the wall of the intestines. The most important of these factors is aldosterone, which stimulates absorption of Na⁺ and secretion of K⁺, mainly by the colon and, to a lesser extent, by the ileum. The mechanism of aldosterone action is similar to that in the renal tubules.

Activation of Salt Appetite

Salt (NaCl) deficiency and hypovolemia have been shown to produce an increase in appetite for salt. Salt deficiency, for example in patients with Addison's disease, may result in taste alterations such that the individual will have a strong desire for salty food (Henkin and Solomon, 1962). A hormonal system involving the brain renin-angiotensin system appears to play a role in the control of salt appetite, especially in hypovolemia. Evidence exists also that peripherally derived angiotensin II stimulates salt appetite in rats by its direct action on the brain (Fitts and Thunhorst, 1996). It has been shown that all components of the renin-angiotensin system (renin, angiotensinogen, angiotensin-converting enzyme, and angiotensin receptors) are present in the neuronal centers in the hypothalamus (Goto et al., 1982). These neuronal centers also are important in the thirst mechanism. Stimulation of this region simultaneously creates a craving for salt and thirst.

Interactions Among Systems in Volume Regulation

The systems of feedback loops with their reinforcing (positive) and modulating (negative) pathways are highly integrated and effective in regulating circulating volume and blood pressure. The integrated pathways of the sympathetic nervous system, renin-angiotensin-aldosterone system, ANP, and ADH, when acting together, provide a multiple backup system that permits the body to regulate the vasomotor tone and excretion of Na^+ and Cl^- in response to changes in volume even when one of the regulatory systems fails. This regulatory feedback mechanism can best be examined by the following examples of changes in dietary NaCl.

To maintain a normal effective circulating volume, termed euvolemia, a precise balance of consumption of sodium and chloride and of their excretion is required. In euvolemic individuals, daily excretion of Na^+ and Cl^- equals the daily consumption. Excretion of Na^+ and Cl^- in the urine can vary over a wide range, from a very low level to as much as 23 g/day, depending on the diet.

In the case of positive salt balance, retention of sodium and chloride increases the volume of extracellular fluid and, hence, body weight. It is mainly this increase in fluid volume that triggers the homeostatic regulatory mechanisms to increase excretion of Na^+ and Cl^-. Expansion of volume causes excretion of Na^+ and Cl^- via the following mechanisms:

1. reflex suppression of the sympathetic nervous discharge to the kidneys, due to stimulation of the low-pressure stretch receptors and high-pressure baroreceptors,
2. suppression of the renin-angiotensin-aldosterone system,

3. stimulation of the secretion of ANP from the cardiac atria, and
4. suppression of the ADH system.

The loss of Na^+, Cl^-, and water from the body returns the volume of extracellular fluid and body weight to their original levels.

The opposite occurs in negative salt balance, in which acute depletion of sodium and chloride decreases the volume of extracellular fluid. The various control systems act together to conserve body sodium and chloride by the following mechanisms:

1. reflex increase in sympathetic nervous discharge to the kidneys,
2. stimulation of the renin-angiotensin-aldosterone system, and
3. stimulation of the ADH system.

These mechanisms act together to conserve sodium and chloride in the body during depletion (see Fig. 30–5).

Factors Affecting Transmembrane Distribution of Potassium

Any change in the concentration of K^+ in the plasma causes either a release of K^+ from the cells or an uptake of K^+ into the cells in order to maintain a relatively constant concentration of K^+ in the plasma. Various factors can affect the uptake and release of K^+ by cells. These are catecholamines, insulin, and plasma pH. Although aldosterone enhances secretion of K^+ by the tubular cells of the distal nephrons, its effects on transmembrane distribution of K^+ are controversial.

Catecholamines. Catecholamines have dual effects on the movement of K^+ across cell membranes because they activate both the α-adrenergic and β-adrenergic receptors on cell membranes (Moratinos and Reverte, 1993). Stimulation of α_1- and α_2-adrenergic receptors induces hyperkalemia by inducing release of K^+ from the liver by activation of hepatic Ca^{2+}-dependent K^+ channels. In contrast, stimulation of β-adrenergic receptors causes hypokalemia by promoting cellular uptake of K^+ in the muscles and myocardium through stimulation of Na^+,K^+-ATPase. Both adrenergic sympathetic activity and circulating catecholamines can influence cellular uptake and release of K^+. The opposing effects of α- and β-adrenergic fibers have important physiological consequences. During exercise, the sympathetic nervous system is activated; epinephrine from the adrenal medulla and norepinephrine from the sympathetic nerve endings are released. The released epinephrine potentially causes an initial hyperkalemia owing to its action on the α-adrenergic receptors in the liver to release K^+, followed by sustained hypokalemia owing to its action on the β-receptors in the muscles to promote cellular K^+ uptake. However, the simultaneous release of norepinephrine from the sympathetic nerve endings during exercise also stimulates release of K^+ from the liver. Thus, the dual effects of the two catecholamines prevent hypokalemia during exercise.

Insulin. During a meal, the high concentrations of glucose, amino acids, gastrointestinal hormones, and K^+ in the plasma cause insulin to be released from the β-cells of the pancreas. Insulin promotes uptake of K^+ by the liver and skeletal muscles, thus attenuating the rapid postprandial rise in plasma K^+ concentration (Hundal et al., 1992). This reflex regulatory feedback mechanism helps maintain the concentration of K^+ in plasma and the concentration gradient between plasma and intracellular fluid. The precise mechanism of insulin-mediated uptake of K^+ by cells is, as yet, not elucidated, but it is certain that insulin's action is independent of its effects on uptake of glucose (Rodriguez-Soriano, 1995). One of the mechanisms may be that insulin stimulates the Na^+,K^+-ATPase activity of the plasma membrane, thereby promoting uptake of K^+.

Plasma pH. The effect of plasma pH on transmembrane distribution of K^+ is complex and depends on the presence of other physiological factors that affect distribution of K^+. In general, acute metabolic acidosis caused by accumulation of nonmetabolizable acids releases intracellular K^+ and increases plasma K^+ concentration. Acute metabolic alkalosis increases cellular uptake of K^+ and decreases the concentration of K^+ in the plasma (Rodriguez-Soriano, 1995).

SODIUM AND CHLORIDE IMBALANCE AND ITS CONSEQUENCES

In general, sodium retention results in proportionate water retention, and sodium loss results in proportionate water loss due to osmoregulation involving ADH. Various situations can cause an isotonic expansion or contraction of the extracellular volume. Physiological regulatory mechanisms for conservation of sodium seem to be better developed in humans than mechanisms for excretion of sodium, possibly because of an evolutionary history during which salt deficit was more common than salt excess. Because of the well-developed capacity for retention of sodium, pathological states characterized by inappropriate retention of sodium are much more common than salt-losing conditions.

Sodium Chloride Retention

Retention of Na^+ occurs when Na^+ intake exceeds renal Na^+ excretory capacity. This situation can occur with rapid ingestion of large amounts of salt (e.g., ingestion of seawater) or during too-rapid saline infusion. Hypernatremia and hypervolemia resulting in acute hypertension usually occur in these situations. The hypervolemia will initiate the Na^+ regulatory mechanisms causing natriuresis. Hypervolemia can occur also in pathological conditions such as congestive heart failure or renal failure and when there is excessive secretion of aldosterone in Conn's syndrome. In congestive heart failure, circulatory insufficiency stimulates the baroreceptors to reflexly increase renal retention of Na^+. This positive Na^+ balance, together with secondary water retention, causes accumulation of fluid in the vascular and interstitial spaces. Accumulation of fluid in the interstitial space is perceived as edema. In renal diseases and hyperaldosteronism, retention of sodium and water by the kidneys also causes hypervolemia and edema. In renal diseases, because retention of fluid is primarily due to failure of the kidneys, the retained fluid is less readily excreted. Therefore, even though there is a sustained release of ANP, hypervolemia persists. Edema and ultimately heart failure are signs of excess Na^+ and Cl^- that exceed the upper limits of tolerance/regulation (Cody et al., 1994).

Sodium Chloride Deficiency

Loss of Na^+ can occur through either renal or nonrenal routes. Hypovolemia and hyponatremia may occur through increased renal loss of Na$^+$ owing to decreased reabsorption (Briggs et al., 1990). Administration of diuretics, which inhibit NaCl reabsorption, or the presence of an osmotic solute in excess of the renal reabsorptive capacity (e.g., in diabetes mellitus) causes diuresis and loss of Na$^+$. Chronic renal diseases that increase the permeability of the glomerular membranes or diseases that cause tubulointerstitial damage, thus decreasing the tubular capacity for reabsorption of Na$^+$, result in Na$^+$ loss. Transient increases in loss of Na$^+$ also occur in tubular necrosis and in certain toxic nephropathies. Deficiency of aldosterone in Addison's disease results in a greatly enhanced excretion of Na$^+$ and retention of K$^+$ (Briggs et al., 1990).

The commonest route for nonrenal loss of Na$^+$ is through the gastrointestinal tract from vomiting and diarrhea (Field et al., 1989). Severe and prolonged diarrhea causes hyponatremia, hypokalemia, and dehydration. Diseases causing diarrhea are among the leading sources of infant mortality and are a major world health problem. In an acute diarrheal episode in which an infant loses 5% of body weight, the infant is at risk for shock. A more gradual depletion of body fluid may not result in shock until the body weight has been reduced by about 10%. Although diarrhea causes losses of K$^+$ and HCO$_3^-$ as well as of Na$^+$, the immediate concern in treating severe diarrhea is to replace Na$^+$ and water to restore the circulatory volume. Dehydration in diarrhea can be reversed by oral or, in emergencies, intravenous rehydration therapy.

Manifestations of hypovolemia are a result of diminished regional tissue perfusion and vary with the degree of volume contraction (Briggs et al., 1990). The loss of Na$^+$ and hypovolemia produce symptoms, including orthostatic hypotension and an increase in pulse rate. Orthostatic hypotension occurs when a person moves suddenly, either from a reclining to an upright position or from a sitting to a standing position. Vasoconstriction and decreased muscle perfusion during hypovolemia may also lead to muscular weakness and cramps. As hypovolemia becomes more severe, dizziness and syncope (fainting) may accompany the orthostatic hypotension. In severe forms of hypovolemia, the circulatory volume can be greatly compromised, and circulatory shock may result. In hypovolemic individuals, mechanisms to conserve sodium are activated. If the loss is not of renal origin, the normal response is an immediate decrease in renal excretion of Na$^+$ to a very low level. In chronic sodium deficiency, the urine is virtually free of Na$^+$.

POTASSIUM IMBALANCE AND ITS CONSEQUENCES

Retention of K$^+$ resulting in hyperkalemia occurs when K$^+$ consumption exceeds the capacity of the kidneys to excrete K$^+$ (Rodriguez-Soriano, 1995). Hyperkalemia is diagnosed when the plasma K$^+$ concentration exceeds 5.0 mmol/L. This rarely happens when the kidneys are functioning normally because their capacity to excrete K$^+$ is substantial. A reduced capacity occurs when there is a defect in the secretory process in the distal nephrons, a lack of aldosterone secretion, or a lack of responsiveness of the renal tubules to aldosterone.

Hyperkalemia can also occur in the absence of retention of K$^+$. A shift of intracellular K$^+$ into the plasma to cause hyperkalemia can occur in metabolic acidosis or from tissue damage as in hemolysis, burns, major trauma, or lysis of tumor cells. In the treatment of hyperkalemia, consumption of K$^+$ is restricted, but most importantly, the underlying causes of hyperkalemia must be treated.

An important clinical manifestation of hyperkalemia is cardiac arrhythmia, which can lead to ventricular fibrillation and asystole (cardiac arrest). Other symptoms include paresthesia, muscle weakness, and, eventually, paralysis.

Hypokalemia is diagnosed when the plasma K$^+$ concentration is less than 3.5 mmol/L. It is usually associated with depletion of body K$^+$ (Rodriguez-Soriano, 1995), and the change in plasma K$^+$ concentration parallels the change in intracellular K$^+$ concentration. However, a low plasma K$^+$ concentration does not necessarily imply a depletion of body potassium or low intracellular concentrations, because other factors may be present that cause a shift of K$^+$ from the extracellular to

CLINICAL CORRELATION

Diarrhea

Each day approximately 8 to 10 L of fluid passes through the gastrointestinal tract. About 2 L of these fluids are from the consumption of liquids and solid foods, and 6 to 8 L are secretions from the various parts of the gastrointestinal tract. The intestines absorb most of these fluids so that only 100 to 200 mL of fluid are lost daily in the stool of an adult. The average electrolyte contents of the stool are 35 to 50 mmol/L for Na^+, 75 to 90 mmol/L for K^+, 16 mmol/L for Cl^-, and 30 to 40 mmol/L for HCO_3^-.

Diarrhea is defined as an increase in stool liquidity and a fecal volume of more than 200 mL/day in adults. Depending on the severity, several liters of fluid can be lost, leading to profound fluid and electrolyte imbalance. Although there are many causes of diarrhea, it can generally be classified pathogenically into (1) osmotic, (2) secretory, (3) structural, and (4) primary motility disorders. Clinically, the most common and important causes of diarrhea are osmotic and secretory.

Osmotic diarrhea can be caused either by ingestion of poorly absorbable solutes such as magnesium sulfate, sorbitol, and lactulose, or by malabsorption or maldigestion of specific solutes because of enzyme deficiencies, as seen in lactase deficiency. The presence of these solutes (and their fermentation products in the large intestine) increases the intestinal luminal osmolarity. This creates an osmotic gradient across the mucosal cells of the intestines, resulting in a diffusion of water from the interstitial fluid compartment into the lumen of the intestines. In addition, the water that would normally be absorbed or reabsorbed along with the solutes remains in the lumen. Osmotic diarrhea ceases once the aggravating factor is passed out of the lumen.

Secretory diarrhea is characterized by either an increased intestinal secretion or failure of distal reabsorption of normal secretions. Viral enteritis and bacterial infections are the most common causes of secretory diarrhea. Bacteria such as *Vibrio cholerae* and *Escherichia coli* release toxins that activate intestinal adenylate cyclase, resulting in increased secretion of sodium chloride and water, whereas enteroinvasive bacteria such as *Shigella* and *Salmonella* invade intestinal mucosa, producing ulceroinflammatory lesions.

The degree of dehydration due to diarrhea can range from mild to severe. This can be assessed clinically by examining the patient for skin turgor, mental status, blood pressure, urine output, and whether the eyeballs are sunken or not. Fluid replacement is of utmost importance to prevent circulatory collapse, especially in cases of severe dehydration such as those seen in cholera. Diarrhea also causes electrolyte and acid-base imbalances, including hypokalemia, hyperchloremia, and metabolic acidosis.

The World Health Organization has recommended the use of oral rehydration therapy for treatment of mild to moderate cases of diarrhea, especially in Third World countries. Due to the high cost of intravenous fluid therapy and the distance of some areas from medical facilities, the program has been very successful in reducing mortality from diarrheal diseases, particularly in infants. Oral rehydration fluid contains 3.5 g of NaCl, 2.5 g of $NaHCO_3$, 1.5 g of KCl, and 20 g of glucose in 1 L of water. An alternative household remedy is to mix 3 "finger pinches" of salt and a "fistful of sugar" with about 1 quart of water to make the solution.

Thinking Critically

Diarrhea is characterized by dehydration, electrolyte imbalance, and acid-base imbalance. Discuss why hypokalemia, hyperchloremia, and metabolic acidosis occur.

the intracellular compartment. This can occur in acute alkalosis or hyperinsulinemia. Depletion of K^+ rarely arises from insufficient consumption of K^+ because the normal amount consumed usually exceeds that required for the replacement of obligatory losses and

maintenance of tissues. Depletion only occurs when intake is inadequate during prolonged fasting or when severe restriction of dietary K^+ occurs.

Depletion of K^+ and hypokalemia can occur through either renal or nonrenal routes.

Renal K^+ loss can occur in endocrine and metabolic disorders such as hyperaldosteronism, metabolic alkalosis, and diuretic therapy. As with Na^+ depletion, the commonest route for nonrenal loss is vomiting and diarrhea; in these situations, the normal reflex response (increased renal and colon K^+ absorption) is prevented because of the hypovolemia that accompanies the vomiting and diarrhea. Hypovolemia initiates regulatory reflex responses to retain Na^+ and water by the kidneys. The enhanced reabsorption of Na^+ from the cortical collecting tubule under the influence of aldosterone further exacerbates the loss of K^+.

Manifestations of K^+ deficiency are due to alterations of cellular metabolism and membrane potentials. Symptoms include depressed neuromuscular functions, such as muscle weakness and cramps, and, in more severe hypokalemia, cardiac arrhythmias, paralysis, and metabolic alkalosis.

NUTRITIONAL CONSIDERATIONS

Habitual high dietary salt intake has been implicated in the development of hypertension (Weinberger, 1996), gastric mucosal damage, and gastric cancer (Correa, 1992). High consumption of potassium, on the other hand, has a protective action against cardiovascular diseases (Young et al., 1995).

Primary hypertension, or abnormally high blood pressure, is a significant risk factor for cardiovascular disease, stroke, and renal failure in industrialized societies. Although there is a genetic predisposition to hypertension, no reliable and specific genetic markers have been identified. This inherited susceptibility is expressed in the presence of other predisposing factors, such as obesity, consumption of alcohol, unbalanced diet, and stress (Folkow, 1982). Both epidemiological and experimental studies implicate a primary role for dietary factors in the control of blood pressure. Consumption of a high-fat, high-sodium (salt), low-potassium, low-calcium, or low-magnesium diet may contribute to the development of hypertension (Reusser and McCarron, 1994).

Association of High-Salt Intake with Hypertension

Although epidemiological and experimental evidence suggest a positive correlation between habitual high-salt consumption and hypertension, controversy remains regarding the importance of sodium salts in the regulation of blood pressure and the mechanisms by which salt influences blood pressure. This is not surprising, because the response of blood pressure depends on an interplay of various dynamic variables, such as genetic susceptibility, body mass, cardiovascular factors, regulatory mechanisms mediated through the neural and hormonal systems, and the kidneys.

Implications of salt intake in hypertension come from observations that the highest incidence of hypertension occurs in northern Japan, where salt intake may be as high as 20 g/day (Kono et al., 1983). In the United States, where salt intake averages between 5 and 13 g/day, hypertension is present in about 15% of the population aged 30 years and above (WHO, 1978). A low incidence of hypertension has been found in societies with low-salt intake (Oliver et al., 1975).

The most comprehensive study on the role of sodium in hypertension was carried out by The Intersalt Cooperative Research Group (Stamler, 1997). This group studied the association between blood pressure and 24-hour excretion of Na^+ and K^+ in the urine in more than 10,000 men and women between 20 and 59 years of age from 52 geographically separate centers in 32 countries. Highly standardized procedures were used in this international collaborative study so that comparisons could be made between centers. Median daily urinary excretion of sodium ranged between 4.6 mg and 5.6 g, but the distribution within this range was uneven. Four centers had mean values below 1.3 g/day, none had values between 1.3 and 2.4 g/day, 4 had values between 2.4 g and 3.2 g/day, and 44 had values between 3.2 g and 5.6 g/day. Therefore, the bulk of the data on the association between blood pressure and excretion of sodium was for the population with mean excretion of 3.2 to 5.6 g/day of sodium.

Cross-center analyses, which involved all 52 centers, showed that median systolic blood pressure, but not diastolic pressure, was significantly related to median values for excretion of sodium, after adjustments for age, sex, body mass index, and consumption of alcohol. However, when the 4 centers with very low median values of sodium excretion were excluded from the analyses, the correlation between systolic blood pressure and excretion of sodium was not significant. The Intersalt study also showed that populations in the 4 centers with median values for sodium excretion that were under 1.3 g/day had low blood pressure, rare or absent hypertension, and no age-related rise in blood pressure, as occurred in populations in other centers. In centers where the subjects' average excretion of sodium was more than 2.4 g/day, median values for excretion of sodium were significantly related to the age-related rise in blood pressure (Rodriguez et al., 1994). Although it was recognized that the association of blood pressure or prevalence of hypertension with median values for excretion of sodium was relatively weak, nonetheless the evidence supports the general contention that habitual intake of salt is an important factor in the occurrence of hypertension.

Genetic Factors. Even though there is evidence suggesting that genetic susceptibility contributes to the relationship between high intake of sodium salts and hypertension, the mode of inheritance has not been determined. Abnormalities in cellular metabolism of Na^+ and Ca^{2+} have been reported in hypertensive patients (Cooper et al., 1995) and in animal models of hypertension (Okada et al., 1993). This may be explained by the altered functions of Na^+,K^+-ATPase, Na^+-K^+ cotransport, or Na^+-H^+ antiport in the arteries of hypertensive patients. An increased intracellular Na^+ concentration may result in an increase in the intracellular Ca^{2+} concentration, which causes an increase of vasomotor tone. It may be possible to identify abnormalities in membrane transport systems that function as markers for genetic susceptibility to hypertension.

Dietary Salt Restriction. Intervention studies of dietary salt restrictions to lower blood pressure have produced mixed results. This may be explained by the fact that not all hypertensive patients are salt-sensitive, and

many cases of hypertension are due to other causes. Nevertheless, a review of various clinical trials indicates some beneficial effects of dietary restriction of sodium on blood pressure (Cutler et al., 1997). Moderate restrictions of salt were found to decrease systolic and diastolic blood pressure over periods of several weeks to a few years in both hypertensive and normotensive patients. The response of blood pressure to salt restriction depended on age, the degree of restriction, and the initial blood pressure (Reusser and McCarron, 1994). Older patients seemed to have a greater response to salt restriction. Patients with the lowest intakes showed the largest decrease in blood pressure. The highest rate of success in reducing hypertension was obtained in non-overweight, mildly hypertensive patients. There was some evidence that salt restriction may also decrease the incidence of stroke and ischemic heart disease.

Protective Action of Dietary Potassium Against Cardiovascular Diseases

The beneficial effect of K^+ on hypertension has been of interest over the past few decades. Evidence supporting high potassium intake in the protection against hypertension and cardiovascular disease comes from epidemiological studies, clinical intervention trials, and animal experiments. Epidemiological studies have demonstrated that populations with diets habitually low in potassium (mainly industrialized cultures) appear to have an increased incidence of cardiovascular disease, whereas those who had higher potassium intakes had a lower incidence of cardiovascular disease (Young et al., 1995). In some studies in which no correlation was found between blood pressure and intake of sodium, an inverse relationship of potassium intake with blood pressure, incidence of stroke, and other cardiovascular diseases was found. Furthermore, there was a direct relationship between blood pressure and the ratio of Na^+ to K^+ excreted in the urine. These results were substantiated by the Intersalt study (Stamler, 1997). Despite evidence supporting the cardiovascular protective action of potassium, its mechanism of action is still unknown. It has been proposed that increased potassium consumption increases plasma K⁺ concentration, which in turn inhibits free radical formation in vascular endothelial cells, vascular smooth muscle cell proliferation, and platelet aggregation such that the rate of formation of atherosclerotic lesions is decreased (Young et al., 1995).

Data on the usefulness of potassium supplementation to reduce blood pressure in hypertensive patients are mixed. As with the restriction of dietary sodium in the treatment of hypertension, the success of supplementation with potassium depends on the presence of other variables associated with hypertension (Krishna, 1994). In some clinical trials, supplementation with potassium or an increase in dietary potassium from natural foods reduced blood pressure and the incidence of stroke mortality (Young et al., 1995). In other trials, the beneficial effects of potassium were short-lived or nonexistent. Animal models of both salt-sensitive and nonsalt-sensitive rats have shown that supplementation with potassium protects against hypertension, stroke, cardiac hypertrophy, and renal glomerular lesions.

Association of High Salt Intake with Gastric Mucosal Damage

The positive association between intake of salt from salted and smoked products and atrophic gastritis and gastric cancer has led to the postulation that sodium salts are an important factor in the development of gastric cancer (Correa, 1992). Both human and animal studies demonstrated that salt alone is not carcinogenic. In rats, a high salt intake increased the absorption of polycyclic aromatic hydrocarbons, which are gastric carcinogens. Most of the salted, smoked meat and fish products contain polycyclic aromatic hydrocarbons and nitrosamines, which induce glandular stomach tumors in rats (Capoferro and Torgersen, 1974). The most probable explanation from current experimental evidence indicates that a diet high in salt may enhance initiation of cancer by damaging the gastric mucosal barrier thereby facilitating the action of any carcinogen present in the diet (Cohen and Roe, 1997).

REFERENCES

Adrogue, H. J. and Madias, N. E. (1981) Changes in plasma potassium concentration during acid-base disturbances. Am J Med 71:456–467.

Aperia, A., Fryckstedt, J., Holtback, U., Belusa, R., Cheng, X. J., Eklof, A. C., Li, D., Wang, Z. M. and Ohtomo, Y. (1996) Cellular mechanisms for bi-directional regulation of tubular sodium reabsorption. Kidney Int 49:1743–1747.

Ballermann, B. J., Zeidel, M. L., Gunning, M. E. and Brenner, B. M. (1991) Vasoactive peptides and the kidney. In: The Kidney (Brenner, B. M. and Rector, F. C., Jr., eds.), 4th ed., pp. 510–583. W.B. Saunders, Philadelphia.

Baylis, P. H. and Thompson, C. J. (1988) Osmoregulation of vasopressin secretion and thirst in health and disease. Clin Endocrinol 29:549–576.

Berry, C. A. and Rector, F. C., Jr. (1991) Renal transport of glucose, amino acids, sodium, chloride, and water. In: The Kidney (Brenner, B. M. and Rector, J. C., Jr., eds.), 4th ed., pp. 245–282. W.B. Saunders, Philadelphia.

Briggs, J. P., Sawaya, B. E. and Schnermann, J. (1990) Disorders of salt balance. In: Fluids and Electrolytes (Kokko, J. P. and Tannen, R. L. eds.), 2nd ed., pp. 70–138. W.B. Saunders, Philadelphia.

Bunning, P. and Riordan, J. F. (1987) Sulfate potentiation of the chloride activation of angiotensin-converting enzyme. Biochemistry 26:3374–3377.

Canessa, C. M., Schild, L., Buell, G., Thorens, B., Gautschi, I., Horisberger, J. D. and Rossier, B. C. (1994) Amiloride-sensitive epithelial Na⁺ channel is made of three homologous subunits. Nature 367:463–467.

Capoferro, R. and Torgersen, O. (1974) The effect of hypertonic saline on the uptake of tritiated 7,12-dimethylbenz[a]anthracene by gastric mucosa. Scand J Gastroenterol 9:343–349.

Cody, R. J., Kubo, S. H. and Pickworth, K. K. (1994) Diuretic treatment for the sodium retention of congestive heart disease. Arch Intern Med 154:1905–1914.

Cohen, A. J. and Roe, F. J. (1997) Evaluation of the aetiological role of dietary salt exposure in gastric and other cancers in humans. Food Chem Toxicol 35:271–293.

Cooper, R. S., Cheng, H. Y. and Rotimi, C. (1995) Basal and stimulated platelet calcium and sodium in hypertensive versus normotensive black people. J Hum Hypertens 9:747–752.

Correa, P. (1992) Human gastric carcinogenesis: A multistep and multifactorial process. First American Cancer Society Award Lecture on Cancer Epidemiology and Prevention. Cancer Res 52:6735–6740.

Cutler, J. A., Follmann, D. and Allender, P. S. (1997) Randomized trials of sodium reduction: An overview. Am J Clin Nutr 65(suppl):643S–651S.

Eaton, S. B. and Konner, M. (1985) Paleolithic nutrition. A consideration of its nature and current implications. N Engl J Med 312:283–289.

Field, M., Rao, M. C. and Chang, E. B. (1989) Intestinal electrolyte transport and diarrheal disease. N Engl J Med 321:800–806.

Fitts, D. A. and Thunhorst, R. L. (1996) Rapid elicitation of salt appetite by an intravenous infusion of angiotensin II in rats. Am J Physiol 270:R1092–1098.

Folkow, B. (1982) Physiological aspects of primary hypertension. Physiol Rev 62:347–504.

Fomon, S. J., Haschke, F., Ziegler, E. E. and Nelson, S. E. (1982) Body composition of reference children from birth to age 10 years. Am J Clin Nutr 35:1169–1175.

Forbes, G. B. (1987) The adult. In: Human Body Composition; Growth, Aging, Nutrition, and Activity, pp. 169–195. Springer-Verlag, New York.

Ganguly, A. and Donohue, J. P. (1983) Primary aldosteronism; Pathophysiology, diagnosis and treatment. J Urol 129:241–247.

Goto, A., Ganguli, M., Tobian, L., Johnson, M. A. and Iwai, J. (1982) Effect of an anteroventral third ventricle lesion on NaCl hypertension in Dahl salt–sensitive rats. Am J Physiol 243:H614–H618.

Henkin, R. I. and Solomon, D. H. (1962) Salt taste threshold in adrenal insufficiency in man. J Clin Endocrinol Metab 22:856–858.

Horisberger, J.-D., Lemas, V., Kraehenbuhl, J.-P. and Rossier, B. C. (1991) Structure-function relationship of Na,K-ATPase. Annu Rev Physiol 53:565–584.

Hundal, H. S., Marette, A., Mitsumoto, Y., Ramlal, T., Blostein, R. and Klip, A. (1992) Insulin induces translocation of α_2 and β_2 subunits of the Na^+/K^+-ATPase from intracellular compartments to the plasma membrane in mammalian skeletal muscle. J Biol Chem 267:5040–5043.

Kono, S., Ikeda, M. and Ogata, M. (1983) Salt and geographical mortality of gastric cancer and stroke in Japan. J Epidemiol Community Health 37:43–46.

Krishna, G. G. (1994) Role of potassium in the pathogenesis of hypertension. Am J Med Sci 307(Suppl 1):S21–S25.

Laragh, J. H. (1985) Atrial natriuretic hormone, the renin-aldosterone axis, and blood pressure–electrolyte homeostasis. N Engl J Med 313:1330–1340.

Larsen, T. M., Laughlin, L. T., Holden, H. M., Rayment, I. and Reed, G. H. (1994) Structure of rabbit muscle pyruvate kinase complexed with Mn^{2+}, K^+, and pyruvate. Biochemistry 33:6301–6309.

Levens, N. R., Peach, M. J. and Carey, R. M. (1981) Role of intrarenal renin-angiotensin system in the control of renal function. Circ Res 48:157–167.

Lowe, S. A., Macdonald, G. J. and Brown, M. A. (1992) Atrial natriuretic peptide in pregnancy: Response to oral sodium supplementation. Clin Exp Pharmacol Physiol 19:607–612.

Moe, G. W., Legault, L. and Skorecki, K. L. (1991) Control of extracellular fluid volume and pathophysiology of edema formation. In: The Kidney (Brenner, B. M. and Rector, J. C., Jr., eds.), 4th ed., pp. 623–676. W. B. Saunders, Philadelphia.

Moratinos, J. and Reverte, M. (1993) Effects of catecholamines on plasma potassium: The role of alpha- and beta-adrenoceptors. Fundam Clin Pharmacol 7:143–153.

National Research Council (1989) Recommended Dietary Allowances, 10th ed., pp. 247–261. National Academy Press, Washington, D.C.

Nerup, J. (1974) Addison's disease—clinical studies: A report of 108 cases. Acta Endocrinol 76:127–141.

Okada, K., Ishikawa, S. and Saito, T. (1993) Enhancement of intracellular sodium by vasopressin in spontaneously hypertensive rats. Hypertension 22:300–305.

Oliver, W. J., Cohen, E. L. and Neel, J. V. (1975) Blood pressure, sodium intake and sodium-related hormones in the Yanomamo Indians, a "no-salt" culture. Circulation 52:146–151.

O'Neil, R. G. (1990) Aldosterone regulation of sodium and potassium transport in the cortical collecting duct. Semin Nephrol 10:365–374.

Quail, A. W., Woods, R. and Korner, P. I. (1987) Cardiac and arterial baroreceptor influences in release of vasopressin and renin during hemorrhage. Am J Physiol 252:H1120–H1126.

Reusser, M. E. and McCarron, D. A. (1994) Micronutrient effects on blood pressure regulation. Nutr Rev 52:367–375.

Rodriguez, B. L., Labarthe, D. R., Huang, B. and Lopez-Gomez, J. (1994) Rise of blood pressure with age. New evidence of population differences. Hypertension 24:779–785.

Rodriguez-Soriano, J. (1995) Potassium homeostasis and its disturbance in children. Pediatr Nephrology 9:364–374.

Rose, B. D. (1989) Physiology of body fluids. In: Clinical Physiology of Acid-base and Electrolyte Disorders, 3rd ed., pp. 3–27. McGraw-Hill Book Company, New York.

Sanchez-Castillo, C. P., Branch, W. J. and James, W. P. (1987a) A test of the validity of the lithium-marker technique for monitoring dietary sources of salt in men. Clin Sci 72:87–94.

Sanchez-Castillo, C. P., Warrender, S., Whitehead, T. P. and James, W. P. (1987b) An assessment of the sources of dietary salt in a British population. Clin Sci 72:95–102.

Stamler, J. (1997) The INTERSALT Study: Background, methods, findings, and implications. Am J Clin Nutr 65(Suppl):626S–642S.

Weinberger, M. H. (1996) Salt sensitivity of blood pressure in humans. Hypertension 27:481–490.

WHO (World Health Organization) (1978) Arterial Hypertension. Report of a WHO Expert Committee. Technical Report Series 628. WHO, Geneva.

Young, D. B., Lin, H. and McCabe, R. D. (1995) Potassium's cardiovascular protective mechanisms. Am J Physiol 268:R825–R837.

Zeidel, M. L. (1990) Renal actions of atrial natriuretic peptide: Regulation of collecting duct sodium and water transport. Annu Rev Physiol 52:747–759.

RECOMMENDED READINGS

Berry, C. A. and Rector, F. C., Jr. (1991) Renal transport of glucose, amino acids, sodium, chloride, and water. In: The Kidney (Brenner, B. M. and Rector, J. C., Jr. eds.), 4th ed., pp. 245–282. W.B. Saunders, Philadelphia.

Briggs, J. P., Sawaya, B. E. and Schnermann, J. (1990) Disorders of salt balance. In: Fluids and Electrolytes (Kokko, J. P. and Tannen, R. L. eds.), 2nd ed., pp. 70–138. W.B. Saunders, Philadelphia.

Cutler, J. A., Follmann, D. and Allender, P. S. (1997) Randomized trials of sodium reduction: An overview. Am J Clin Nutr 65(Suppl):643S–651S.

Moe, G. W., Legault, L. and Skorecki, K. L. (1991) Control of extracellular fluid volume and pathophysiology of edema formation. In: The Kidney (Brenner, B. M. and Rector, J. C., Jr., eds.), 4th ed., pp. 623–676. W.B. Saunders, Philadelphia.

Reusser, M. E. and McCarron, D. A. (1994) Micronutrient effects on blood pressure regulation. Nutr Rev 52:367–375.

Rodriguez-Soriano, J. (1995) Potassium homeostasis and its disturbance in children. Pediatr Nephrol 9:364–374.

Stamler, J. (1997) The INTERSALT Study: Background, methods, findings, and implications. Am J Clin Nutr 65(Suppl):626S–642S.

CHAPTER **31**

◆ ◆

Iron

Roy D. Baynes, M.D., Ph.D., and Martha H. Stipanuk, Ph.D.

OUTLINE

COMMON ABBREVIATIONS

IRE (iron-responsive element)
IRE-BP (iron-responsive element–binding protein)

BIOLOGICAL FUNCTIONS OF IRON

It is doubtful that life on earth would be possible in the absence of iron. Iron is a transition element that is redox active, is a good Lewis acid, and is capable of forming bonds with electronegative elements (oxygen, nitrogen, and sulfur). The common oxidation states of iron are ferrous (Fe^{2+}) and ferric (Fe^{3+}); some higher states occur transiently in certain redox processes.

Iron, as part of various proteins, is particularly involved in the transport and metabolism of oxygen, as can be seen from the partial list of iron-containing proteins shown in Table 31–1. Iron is required for the synthesis and activity of these proteins. These proteins can be grouped by the type of iron structure they contain: heme, iron-sulfur (Fe-S) clusters, single Fe atoms, and oxygen-bridged iron. Often, these are referred to as heme and nonheme proteins, with the nonheme category including proteins with Fe-S clusters, single Fe atoms, and oxygen-bridged iron. Iron tends to be hexacoordinate with octahedral geometry, as is found in heme and in the metalloproteins with single Fe atoms or oxygen-bridged iron atoms. In the Fe-S clusters, however, iron is tetracoordinate and the coordination geometry is tetrahedral (Frausto da Silva and Williams, 1991).

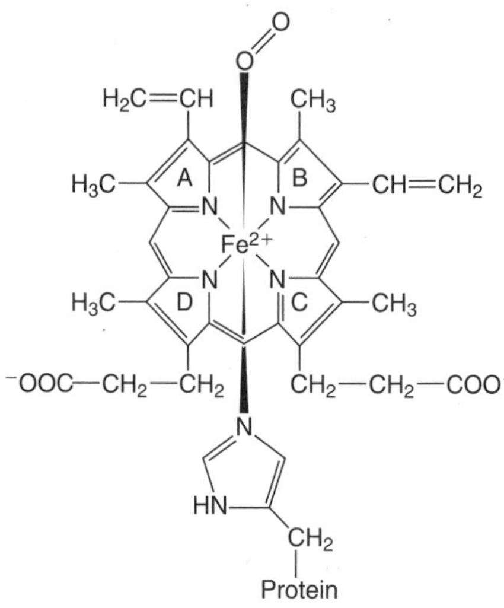

Heme Proteins

Many proteins contain heme prosthetic groups, which are complexes of Fe^{2+} with protoporphyrin IX or a derivative of protoporphyrin IX (Fig. 31–1). These complexes are referred to as hematin when the iron is oxidized to Fe^{3+}. In some heme proteins, some of the tetrapyrrole ring substituents are covalently linked to amino acid residues of the protein. Within the heme group, the heme Fe^{2+} is always coordinated to the four nitrogen atoms of the tetrapyrrole structure. The 5th coordination position is occupied by a histidyl residue of the protein. The 6th coordinate position is the oxygen (O_2)-binding site in proteins that bind O_2, but this 6th coordinate bond is to an amino acid residue of the protein in cytochromes (e.g., cytochrome b) that do not bind O_2. The heme iron of guanylate

Figure 31–1. An example of heme iron. Ferroprotoporphyrin IX is shown with the proximal ligand for the ferrous atom being a histidyl residue on the protein and with the 6th ligand (distal ligand) being to oxygen as it is in oxygenated hemoglobin or myoglobin. In deoxyhemoglobin or deoxymyoglobin, the ferrous atom is 5-coordinated. In contrast, in many of the heme-containing cytochromes, the heme iron is 6-coordinate with no substrate binding site; both the distal and proximal ligands are contributed by side chains from the protein (e.g., imidazole nitrogen of histidine or sulfur of methionine). Protoporphyrin IX has 4 methyl, 2 propionate, and 2 vinyl substituents on the porphyrin structure; other forms of heme are derived from protoporphyrin IX. The b-type cytochromes contain ferroprotoporphyrin IX, as does hemoglobin. In the c-type cytochromes, the vinyl substituents on the A and B pyrrole rings are attached to the protein via thioether linkages. In the a-type cytochromes, the vinyl substituent on the A ring is modified, and a hydrophobic isoprenoid tail is attached to it; additionally, the methyl substituent on the D ring is replaced by a formyl group.

cyclase coordinates with nitric oxide (NO) rather than O_2.

Hemoglobin and myoglobin serve only as O_2 carriers, and the heme iron remains in the Fe^{2+} state. A number of heme-containing enzymes are involved in the activation of O_2 or of peroxides (ROOH) as part of the enzyme's catalytic mechanism. These may be involved in the transfer of $1/2O_2$ or O_2 to the substrate or of electrons to oxygen as an acceptor. Examples of such heme-containing enzymes are listed in Table 31–1 and include monooxygenases (hydroxylases), dioxygenases, oxidases, and peroxidases. The heme substituents of cytochrome a_3 and cytochrome P450 use the 6th coordinate position to bind O_2, like those of many other heme-containing proteins, and

TABLE 31–1

Types and Examples of Iron-Containing Proteins

I. **Heme proteins**
  A. O_2 carriers (globins)
    a. Hemoglobin
    b. Myoglobin
  B. NO binding
    a. Guanylate cyclase
  C. Electron transfer
    Mitochondrial electron transport chain
    a. Cytochrome b_{560} in succinate dehydrogenase/Complex II
    b. Cytochrome b_{562}, b_{566}, and c_1 in the cytochrome c reductase/Complex III
    c. Cytochrome c
    d. Cytochrome a in cytochrome c oxidase/Complex IV
    Mini-electron transport systems
    a. Cytochrome b_{561} in adrenal chromaffin granules
    b. Cytochrome b_5 in fatty acyl CoA desaturases
    c. Cytochrome b_5 in sulfite oxidase
  D. Activation of oxygen (O_2) or peroxides (ROOH)
    Monooxygenases, dioxygenases, and oxidases
    a. Cytochrome P450 systems that are involved in synthesis of steroid hormones, the oxygenation of eicosanoids, heme oxygenase, and the oxidation of a variety of lipophilic xenobiotics
    b. Nitric oxide (NO) synthase
    c. Sulfite oxidase
    d. Tryptophan 2,3-dioxygenase
    e. Cytochrome a_3 of cytochrome c oxidase
    Peroxidases
    a. Catalase
    b. Secretory peroxidases (lactoperoxidase)
    c. Thyroid peroxidase
    d. Peroxidase active site of PGH_2 (prostaglandin H_2) synthase
    e. Chloroperoxidases (myeloperoxidase)

II. **Iron-sulfur cluster proteins**
  A. Electron transfer
    Mitochondrial electron transport chain
    a. NADH dehydrogenase/Complex I: one or more 2Fe-2S clusters; three 4Fe-4S clusters
    b. Succinate dehydrogenase/Complex II: one 2Fe-2S cluster, two 4Fe-4S clusters
    c. Cytochrome c reductase/Complex III: one 2Fe-2S cluster
    d. ETF dehydrogenase: one 4Fe-4S cluster
    Mini-electron transport systems
    a. Adrenodoxin component of cytochrome P450 systems: two 2Fe-2S clusters
    b. Xanthine oxidase: two different Fe-S clusters
    c. Dihydropyrimidine dehydrogenase (uracil and thymine degradation): two 4Fe-4S clusters
  B. Nonredox enzymes containing iron-sulfur clusters
    a. Aconitase (mitochondrial; interconverts citrate and isocitrate): one 4Fe-4S center; the 4Fe-4S center is essential for enzyme activity because one Fe^{2+} of the cluster coordinates the —OH group of citrate so as to facilitate its elimination, followed by rehydration to form isocitrate
    b. Aconitase (cytosolic; iron regulatory protein-1): one 4Fe-4S center that can lose an Fe to become a 3Fe-4S cluster. It is the inactive enzyme (3Fe-4S cluster) that is the active iron regulatory protein, which can bind iron-responsive elements (IREs) on mRNAs.
    c. Ferrochelatase (heme synthesis): one 2Fe-2S center

III. **Single Fe-containing metalloenzymes**
  A. Monooxygenases that contain Fe^{2+} and require tetrahydrobiopterin as a cofactor; hydroxylation of aromatic amino acids
    a. Phenylalanine hydroxylase (tyrosine synthesis)
    b. Tyrosine hydroxylase (DOPA/dopamine synthesis)
    c. Tryptophan hydroxylase (5-hydroxytryptamine/serotonin synthesis)
  B. Dioxygenases that require a keto acid co-substrate (usually α-ketoglutarate), Fe^{2+}, and a reducing agent (ascorbic acid); the substrate is hydroxylated, and the keto acid co-substrate is oxidatively decarboxylated (i.e., α-ketoglutarate is converted to succinate)
    a. Prolyl 3-hydroxylase and prolyl 4-hydroxylase
    b. Lysyl hydroxylase
    c. ε-N-Trimethyllysine hydroxylase and γ-butyrobetaine hydroxylase (carnosine synthesis)
    d. Hydroxyphenylpyruvate dioxygenase (tyrosine metabolism—homogentisate formation; in this example, the keto acid that is oxidatively decarboxylated is the pyruvyl side chain of the same molecule that is hydroxylated)
  C. Dioxygenases that add O_2 to a single substrate and require Fe^{2+}
    a. 5-Lipoxygenase (forms ROOH product)
    b. Cysteine dioxygenase (forms RSO_2^- product)
    c. 3-Hydroxyanthranilate 3,4-dioxygenase (cleaves aromatic ring)

IV. **Enzymes that contain Fe-O-Fe**
  A. Ribonucleotide reductase (Fe-O-Fe may function to stabilize a tyrosyl free radical)

are also redox active. In redox-active cytochromes or enzymes, heme Fe^{3+} must be reduced to Fe^{2+} before O_2 binding can occur.

Most cytochromes (e.g., cytochrome b) do not bind oxygen, and the 6th coordinate position of the Fe^{2+} of the heme in these cytochromes is occupied by a histidyl or methionyl residue of the protein. In contrast to cytochrome a_3 and P450, which both bind oxygen and transfer electrons, most cytochromes only transfer electrons. Cytochromes are capable of only 1-electron reductions. The iron in the heme of these redox-active proteins alternates between Fe^{2+} and Fe^{3+}. Although the cytochromes in electron transport chains all catalyze single electron oxidations/reductions of the heme iron, they may be involved in reactions that require 2 or more electrons. For example, complex IV (cytochrome c oxidase) is able to catalyze the 4-electron reduction of one O_2 molecule (to form two H_2O molecules) because it contains two type a heme groups that alternate between the $3+$ and $2+$ oxidation states and two Cu atoms that alternate between their $2+$ and $1+$ oxidation states.

Proteins with Iron-Sulfur Centers

The most common types of iron-sulfur centers are 2Fe-2S and 4Fe-4S clusters, which consist of equal numbers of iron and sulfide ions; the iron atoms of each cluster are also coordinated to 4 protein cysteinyl sulfhydryl groups, as shown in Figure 31–2. When both the sulfide and cysteinyl residues are considered, one can see that each Fe atom is coordinated by 4 sulfur atoms; these 4 sulfur atoms are tetrahedrally located around the Fe atom. The iron atoms in each center form a conjugated system, and the Fe-S clusters can participate in only 1-electron transfer reactions even though they contain more than one iron atom. For example, one can consider that a 4Fe-4S cluster exists as $2Fe^{2+}2Fe^{3+}•4S$ in the reduced form and $Fe^{2+}3Fe^{3+}•4S$ in the oxidized form.

Fe-S clusters are most commonly found in electron transfer proteins. These include proteins of the mitochondrial electron transport chain as well as various minielectron transport systems, such as the adrenodoxin component of mitochondrial cytochrome P450 systems (Beinert et al., 1997; Sweeney and Rabinowitz, 1980).

A few known examples of Fe-S proteins have one iron somewhat exposed so that it can dissociate and serve as a regulatory mechanism (Rouault et al., 1992). Aconitase contains a 4Fe-4S center, but one of the iron atoms is not liganded to a cysteinyl residue of the protein. This allows this iron atom to coordinate the —OH group of citrate in the mitochondrial reaction by which citrate is converted to isocitrate. In the cytosol, the cytosolic isozyme of aconitase loses this iron atom under conditions of low iron concentration and becomes an active iron regulatory protein that binds to iron-responsive elements (IREs) on certain messenger RNAs (mRNAs). The iron that leaves aconitase when cellular

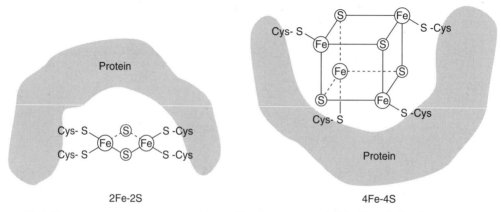

Figure 31–2. *The two most common types of iron-sulfur clusters, namely 2Fe-2S and 4Fe-4S, consisting of equal numbers of iron and sulfide ions coordinated to 4 cysteinyl sulfhydryl groups of the protein.*

iron concentrations are low is able to leave because it is not coordinately linked to a cysteinyl residue; thus, active iron regulatory protein contains a 3Fe-4S cluster.

Single Iron-Containing Metalloenzymes

A number of enzymes contain iron as a single Fe atom, which is coordinately bound to imidazole (histidine) or carboxylate (glutamate and aspartate) ligands on the protein. Generally, the Fe does not form a very stable complex with the protein when in the reduced Fe^{2+} oxidation state, and exchange of iron can occur. These enzymes are involved in reactions that use O_2 as substrate. One subgroup of iron metalloenzymes are those that require a keto acid substrate (usually α-ketoglutarate) and a reducing agent. In these reactions, one of the oxygen atoms from O_2 is transferred to the substrate, which is hydroxylated, and the other oxygen atom is transferred to the keto acid cosubstrate, which is oxidatively decarboxylated. (See Chapter 23, especially Figure 23–7, for examples and an explanation of the role of ascorbic acid in these reactions.) Another subgroup of iron-containing metalloenzymes are aromatic amino acid hydroxylases that require tetrahydrobiopterin as a cofactor. Some other Fe^{2+}-containing enzymes add both oxygen atoms from O_2 to a single substrate; these dioxygenases include the 5-lipoxygenase involved in eicosanoid synthesis (see Chapter 15).

Protein with Oxygen-Bridged Iron

Only one mammalian enzyme has been shown to contain oxygen-bridged iron. This protein is ribonucleotide reductase (nucleotide 5′-diphosphate reductase), and it contains an Fe^{3+}-O^{2-}-Fe^{3+} complex (Fig. 31–3) (Nordlund et al., 1990). Each Fe^{3+} ion is octahedrally coordinated by the O^{2-} ion (the oxo bridge), by 4 carboxylate or imidazole groups on the protein, and by coordination with a H_2O molecule. The cytoplasmic ribonucleotide reductase enzyme system participates in the reduction of the four common ribonucleotides to their corresponding deoxyribonucleotides, which are essential for DNA synthesis. The mechanism by which the iron center

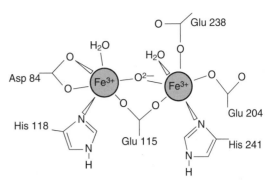

Figure 31–3. *The structure and active site of ribonucleotide reductase. (Adapted from Nordlund, P., Sjoberg, B.-M. and Eklund, H. [1990] Three-dimensional structure of the free radical protein of ribonucleotide reductase. Nature 345:593–598. Reprinted with permission. Copyright 1990 Macmillan Magazines Limited.)*

functions is not clearly understood, but it is thought that the reaction of the apoenzyme with Fe^{2+} and O_2 results in formation of the Fe^{3+}-O^{2-}-Fe^{3+} bridge and of a tyrosyl free radical in the protein, which plays a role in catalysis. It is possible that some other mammalian iron-containing enzymes (e.g., fatty acyl CoA desaturases) also may contain oxo-bridged iron (Shanklin et al., 1994; Thelander and Graslund, 1994).

PROTEINS OF IRON TRANSPORT AND IRON STORAGE

Given the many essential functions of iron in oxygen-requiring processes, electron transport, and deoxyribonucleotide synthesis, it is not surprising that efficient mechanisms have developed for iron assimilation and storage. The properties of iron that are so essential for cellular metabolism also make it possible for iron to participate in the generation of free radicals, which are highly cytotoxic. In the aerobic extracellular environment, ferrous ions are readily oxidized to ferric ions; ferric ions can rapidly form complexes with hydroxide ions or water to form polyhydroxides, which are relatively insoluble. If these polyhydroxides form in body fluids, this results in the iron becoming unavailable for cellular uptake, and precipitation of these iron aggregates in tissues could have pathological consequences. Consequently, the mechanisms of iron exchange, transport, and storage must also serve to maintain an extremely low free iron concentration. A list of proteins involved in iron transport, storage, and recycling is in Table 31–2.

Proteins of Iron Transport

Transferrin. The major plasma protein involved in the transport of iron is transferrin (Aisen, 1989; Baker and Lindley, 1992; Morgan, 1981). Transferrin is a glycoprotein synthesized by the liver. It is composed of a single polypeptide chain that contains approximately 680 amino acid residues and has 2 iron-binding sites; it is encoded on chromosome 3. The carboxyl terminal and amino terminal lobes are each organized into two unlike subdomains; each lobe contains an iron-binding site (Fig. 31–4). The affinity of transferrin for Fe^{3+} is extremely high, but Fe^{2+} is not bound. Four of the six atoms required to coordinate the Fe^{3+} are provided by an aspartyl, a histidyl, and two tyrosyl residues in the protein, and the remaining 2 coordinate bonds are to a carbonate anion (CO_3^{2-}), which is required to stabilize the binding. In the absence of this co-anion, the 4 protein residue ligands are insufficient for strong binding, and release of Fe^{3+} from transferrin would occur. Binding and release of iron by transferrin results in striking conformational

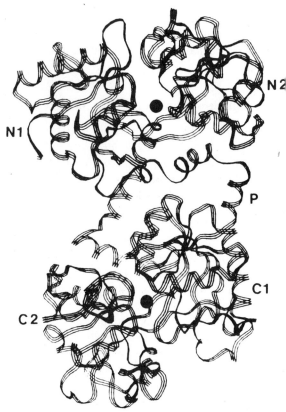

Figure 31–4. *A ribbon diagram showing the characteristic folding of transferrins into 2 lobes (N-lobe above and C-lobe below) and 4 domains (N1, N2, C1, and C2). Iron atoms are shown as filled circles. The interlobe connecting peptide (P) is helical in lactoferrin but irregular in transferrin. (From Baker, E. N. and Lindley, P. F. [1992] New perspectives on the structure and function of transferrins. J Inorg Biochem 47:147–160. Reproduced with permission of Elsevier Science, copyright 1992.)*

TABLE 31–2
Proteins That Bind Iron or Iron-Containing Moieties

Iron-Binding Proteins
Transferrin (Fe^{3+})
Lactoferrin (Fe^{3+})
Ferritin (Fe^{3+})
Hemosiderin (Fe^{3+})

Proteins That Use Iron as a Substrate
Ferroxidase (Fe^{2+}/Fe^{3+})
Ferrochelatase (Fe^{2+})

Heme-Binding Protein
Hemopexin (heme or hematin)

Protein That Uses Heme as a Substrate
Heme oxygenase

Protein That Binds Hemoglobin
Haptoglobins (oxyhemoglobin dimers)

Protein That Binds Transferrin
Transferrin receptor

changes in the two lobes. In the absence of bound Fe^{3+}, the subdomains swing apart and are in the open position. In the presence of bound Fe^{3+}, these subdomains take up the closed position.

The mean normal plasma iron concentration is about 20 μmol/L, and the mean normal plasma transferrin concentration is about 30 μmol/L (with each molecule of transferrin containing 2 iron-binding sites). Consequently, plasma transferrin is normally only about one third saturated with iron, and therefore, the plasma has significant excess iron-binding capacity. Transferrin concentration, reflecting synthesis, is increased in iron deficiency and when estrogen levels are high, such as during pregnancy and in women taking oral contraceptives. Concentrations are reduced in the presence of excess iron, infection, inflammation, neoplasia, and protein catabolic states. Transferrin is distributed throughout most of the extracellular fluid of the body, with a continuous circulation from blood to interstitial fluid. The delivery of transferrin-bound iron to cells is dependent upon the expression of transferrin-binding molecules; these transferrin-binding proteins are known as transferrin receptors.

Transferrin Receptor. Transferrin receptors are involved in the cellular uptake of iron from the circulation, and they have highest affinity for saturated (diferric) transferrin. The transferrin receptor is a transmembrane glycoprotein composed of 2 identical 95-kDa monomers linked by a pair of disulfide bridges. Each monomer consists of 760 amino acid residues organized into an amino terminal cytoplasmic domain of 61 amino acids, a membrane-spanning segment of 28 amino acids, and a large extracellular domain of 671 amino acids. The cytoplasmic domain is required for appropriate intracellular trafficking of the transferrin-receptor complex. The peptide sequence tyrosine-threonine-arginine-phenylalanine in the cytoplasmic domain has been identified as the signal for endocytosis via coated pits, and the seryl residue at position 24 is a phosphorylation site. The transmembrane domain, consisting largely of hydrophobic amino acid residues, functions as a signal peptide for translocation across the endoplasmic reticulum during synthesis and as a membrane anchor for the protein. A cysteinyl residue at position 62 is the major site of posttranslational fatty acid acylation; the significance of this is uncertain, but nonacylated receptors undergo more rapid endocytosis.

Sites of N-linked glycosylation have been identified at amino acid residues 251, 317, and 727 in the extracellular domain, and threonine at amino acid position 104 has been identified as a site of O-linked glycosylation. These glycan chains may play a role in translocation of the receptor to the cell surface and in facilitating the interaction between the receptor and transferrin. The transferrin-binding site is in the extracellular domain, but the details of this site are not yet elucidated. Cysteinyl residues at positions 89 and 98 in the extracellular domain are the sites of disulfide linking that hold the homodimers together. The extracellular domain has serine protease-sensitive sites at arginine 100 and arginine 121. Each receptor dimer can bind 2 transferrin molecules, probably 1 to each subunit. The receptor is fundamental to the cellular binding and uptake of iron-bearing transferrin; the pathway of internal iron exchange is discussed more comprehensively in a subsequent section of this chapter. The transferrin receptor is encoded on chromosome 3 (Testa et al., 1993).

Other Transport Proteins. A number of other proteins present in plasma may play a role in iron transport. This is particularly likely in iron overload, hemolytic anemia, and conditions of ineffective erythropoiesis during which free hemoglobin or heme may be present in the plasma compartment. These transport proteins include haptoglobin, hemopexin, ferritin, lactoferrin, and albumin. The amounts of iron carried by these proteins are uncertain but usually are relatively trivial in comparison with those carried by transferrin.

Haptoglobin binds free oxyhemoglobin dimers. Hemopexin and albumin bind free heme and hematin. All these proteins are synthesized and secreted by the liver, and the bound forms are also taken up by the liver. Hepatocytes have a specific receptor for the haptoglobin-hemoglobin complex, and this complex is internalized by receptor-mediated endocytosis. Both receptor and ligand are degraded. The hemopexin-heme complex is also internalized by the hepatocyte via receptor-mediated endocytosis. The receptor and the hemopexin molecule both appear to be recycled. The mechanism by which heme in association with albumin makes its way into hepatocytes is uncertain.

Haptoglobin is an 85-kDa α-2 glycoprotein encoded on chromosome 16, and hemopexin is a 70-kDa β glycoprotein encoded on chromosome 11. The haptoglobin receptor is as yet incompletely understood, as is the mapping of its gene. The hemopexin receptor is known to be an 85-kDa molecule composed of a 20-kDa and a 65-kDa subunit. The mapping of its gene is as yet undetermined.

The iron storage protein ferritin is primarily an intracellular protein. Minor amounts are present in the circulation in proportion to iron stores. In contrast to cellular ferritin, the plasma ferritin is glycosylated and relatively iron-poor. Consequently, ferritin cannot have a major role in iron transport under normal circumstances. However, in situations of iron overload and tissue injury, the plasma ferritin concentration is raised, with some of the ferritin being nonglycosylated tissue ferritin that has a higher iron content. Ferritin in these circumstances is taken up in the liver both by putative specific ferritin receptors and in the case of tissue ferritin by the asialoglycoprotein receptor. In these circumstances, ferritin may contribute modestly to iron transport.

A more subtle role for ferritin in iron transport has been suggested by observations that macrophages may release ferritin directly, and that this ferritin can be taken up by specific hepatic ferritin receptors. This pathway has been suggested to be of significance in iron transport within the liver. Precise quantitative data, however, are still lacking.

Lactoferrin is an iron-binding protein found predominantly in neutrophils, secretory epithelium, and secretions, including milk. It is structurally similar to transferrin. Amounts on the order of 2 to 3 mg/L (25 to 40 nmol/L) have been reported in human plasma. This concentration is several orders lower than that of transferrin (30 μmol/L). This, together with kinetic data, indicates a doubtful role for lactoferrin in iron transport. Its functional significance in neutrophils and in secretions appears to relate to its antibacterial properties. This antibacterial activity has been thought to be due to lactoferrin's ability to sequester iron, but it may be more a function of the innate bactericidal activity of a portion of the lactoferrin molecule (lactoferricin).

Nontransferrin-Bound Iron. Under normal circumstances, there is virtually no iron in the systemic circulation that is not bound to heme, transferrin, or ferritin: the normal level of nontransferrin-bound iron is less than 1 μmol/L. Much higher levels may be detected in conditions of iron overload (hereditary hemochromatosis) or hemolytic anemia (e.g., thalassemia major). This iron is not dialyzable and can be detected either by the addition of chelators or by the bleomycin assay, which is based on the ability of bleomycin to degrade DNA only in the presence of free iron. The nature of this nondialyzable but available iron is incompletely understood, but candidates for formation of this nontransferrin-bound iron include nonspecific interaction of free iron with other plasma proteins and/or interactions with citrate, ascorbate, histidine, or other amino acids. Regardless of the specific form, this nontransferrin-bound iron is rapidly cleared from the circulation by the liver by a passive carrier-mediated process, and its uptake may contribute significantly to the deposition of iron in parenchymal cells of the liver in conditions of iron overload (Morgan, 1996).

Proteins of Iron Storage

Ferritin. Iron is delivered to the cells of the body by one of the transport mechanisms outlined in the previous section. Certain specialized cells obtain additional iron by other pathways. The cells of the reticuloendothelial system acquire significant amounts of iron from phagocytized and catabolized red blood cells. Mucosal cells of the gastrointestinal tract procure food iron by the process of iron absorption. These aspects of iron exchange are more fully delineated in subsequent sections of this chapter. Most of the iron delivered to or acquired by cells is believed to cross the cell membrane in ferrous form and to enter a poorly characterized intracellular transit pool. This pool reflects the readily available iron within the cell and is believed to be the key regulator of internal and external iron exchange. To prevent the unwanted effects of iron-catalyzed free radical generation or iron oxidation and precipitation, it is imperative that the cell safely store excess iron. Hence, iron storage fulfills a cellular "housekeeping" function in all cells in addition to its role as an iron reservoir in specialized cells (macrophages of the reticuloendothelial system and parenchymal cells of the liver) from which body iron pools can be replenished as iron is utilized or lost.

The ferritin molecule is ideally suited to serve both the housekeeping and repository functions because its structure allows for the housing of vast amounts of iron in a soluble and nontoxic, yet biologically available, form (Harrison et al., 1980). The iron-free or apoferritin molecule has a molecular mass of approximately 480 kDa and is composed of 24 subunits of two biochemically distinct types (Fig. 31–5). The heavier, or H, subunit has a molecular mass of approximately 21 kDa, is encoded by a gene on chromosome 11, and has a more acidic isoelectric point. The lighter, or L, subunit has a molecular mass of approximately 19 kDa, is encoded by a gene on chromosome 19, and has a more basic isoelectric point. Different proportions of H and L subunits may make up the 24-subunit apo-ferritin, leading to distinct isoferritins with various tissue specificities. The L-rich, more basic isoferritins predominate in such tissues as liver and spleen. Iron administration tends to enhance predominantly L subunit synthesis. These observations indicate a predominant storage role for the L ferritin subunit. The H-rich, more acidic isoferritins are found in tissues such as the heart, erythrocytes, and mononuclear leukocytes, which tend not to be major sites of iron storage.

The ferritin subunits are arranged to create an outer shell permeated by a number of channels, each approximately 0.5 nm in diameter. Fe^{2+} moves down these channels, undergoes oxidation to Fe^{3+} by an as yet incompletely understood process that involves the H subunit, and is incorporated into the ferric oxyhydroxide (FeOOH) core of ferritin. The average storage capacity of each ferritin molecule is on the order of 1200 iron atoms. The mechanism of iron release from the ferritin store is incompletely understood. The process does appear to be facilitated by reducing conditions and by more acidic pH, as might be anticipated to pertain in endosomal and lysosomal structures.

Hemosiderins. Hemosiderin is also a storage form of iron. Hemosiderins are observed predominantly in conditions of iron overload, such as hereditary hemochromatosis and transfusion-dependent hemoglobinopathies. The hemosiderins are closely related to the ferritins but are less well characterized. Indeed, in untreated iron overload states the hemosiderin iron core is a ferrihydrite as in

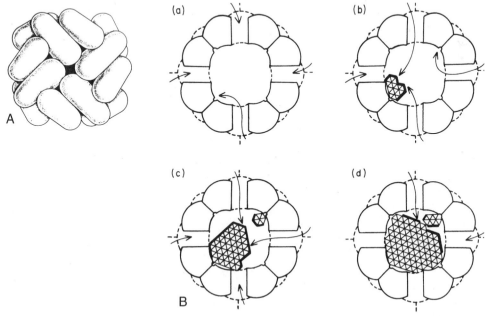

Figure 31–5. A, A molecule of horse spleen apoferritin. The molecule is a symmetrical shell of 24 protein subunits. B, A model for ferritin iron uptake and release. (a) Fe(II) enters the shell through channels and is bound at sites favoring oxidation (arrows). (b) An Fe(III)OOH iron-core nucleus forms on the bound Fe(III). (c, d), The microcrystal builds up by the oxidation of further Fe(II) at its surface (additional nuclei may also form). (From Harrison, P. M., Clegg, G. A. and May, K. [1980] Ferritin structure and function. In: Iron in Biochemistry in Medicine II. [Jacobs, A. and Worwood, M., eds.], pp. 131–171. Academic Press, London.)

ferritin. There is significant amino acid sequence similarity and immunoreactivity between hemosiderins and ferritins. In subjects with transfusion-dependent hemoglobinopathies who are treated with iron chelators, the crystalline nature of the iron core changes character somewhat.

Hemosiderins appear to be the partial degradation products of ferritin packaged into micelles. The iron in these degradation polymers is less available to chelation than is that in ferritin; that in the crystalline goethite form appears even less labile and chelatable than that in the ferrihydrite form.

REGULATION OF CONCENTRATIONS OF PROTEINS OF IRON TRANSPORT AND STORAGE

Given the key role played by iron in cellular metabolism and proliferation, the concentrations of the proteins of iron transport and storage must be highly regulated. Although the mechanisms involved in the regulation of levels of these proteins are incompletely understood, this is an active area of research.

Transcriptional Regulation of Synthesis of Ferritin, Transferrin Receptors, and Transferrin

Tissue differences in the expression of H and L ferritins exist and are in part due to differences in transcriptional activity. Changes in expression of ferritin in response to cellular iron content also differ for the H and L ferritin subunits. Transcriptional control of ferritin expression has been documented in a number of human cells and cell lines. Factors such as cellular differentiation and inflammatory cytokines (such as tumor necrosis factor and interleukin-1) may bring about differential subunit expression (Harrison and Arosio, 1996).

Changes in expression of the transferrin receptor have been observed in response to different phases of the cell cycle, to cellular differentiation, and to cytokines, including α- and γ-interferons. These responses in transferrin receptor expression appear to be predominantly mediated by changes in transcription.

The expression of transferrin also appears to be transcriptionally regulated. Expression of transferrin is predominantly in the liver, and transcription rates are increased in the presence of functional iron deficiency or increased steroid hormone levels (e.g., in pregnancy and in individuals taking exogenous estrogen). Transcription of transferrin is also modulated in relation to inflammatory cytokines; although these cytokines enhance transferrin transcription, catabolism of the molecule is also increased such that the net effect is a reduction in the circulating concentration of transferrin.

The specific mechanisms by which transcription of ferritin, transferrin receptor, and transferrin is altered have not been clearly defined. It has been suggested that the nuclear transcription factor NF-κB may be the modulating factor in the transcriptional regulation of ferritin production. The 5′ promoter region on the transferrin receptor gene has been partially characterized, and it contains sequences that are homologous with the consensus sequence for the Sp1 transcription factor-binding site. Another sequence located −80 to −66 nucleotides 5′ to the transferrin receptor gene may have a PEA1 (plastid envelope ATPase)-like transcription factor–binding site. Several DNA-binding proteins have been identified that interact with the transferrin promoter region.

Posttranscriptional Regulation of Ferritin and Transferrin Receptor Synthesis

Iron-Responsive Elements. It has long been appreciated that ferritin biosynthesis can be regulated in response to changes in cellular iron content even when transcription has been experimentally inhibited. In the last decade it has been established that this regulation involves a sequence of approximately 30 nucleotides in the 5′ untranslated region of the ferritin mRNA. This sequence is highly conserved through all the ferritin genes studied. Biosynthesis of the transferrin receptor is also regulated in the presence of transcriptional inhibition, but in this case the regulation involves nucleotide sequences in the 3′ untranslated portion of the transferrin receptor mRNA. These sequences all show significant homology and have been termed iron-responsive elements or IREs (Klausner et al., 1993; Theil, 1993).

These IREs can be fitted to a consensus motif, as shown in Figure 31–6. They consist of a lower stem of variable length made up of complementary pairs of RNA bases; the lower stems of the IREs in the ferritin H and L subunit mRNAs are guanine-cytosine (GC)-rich, whereas they tend to be adenine-uracil (AU)-rich in the transferrin receptor mRNAs. Above the lower stem is an unpaired cytosine base, which produces a characteristic bulge in the stem structure. Above this is an upper stem that consists of 5 complementary base pairs. A 6-base loop is found on top of the upper stem; 5 of the 6 bases forming this loop are almost always CAGUG.

In the mRNAs for ferritin L and H, there is a single stem-loop IRE in the 5′ untranslated portion. In contrast, transferrin receptor mRNA contains as many as 5 tandem IREs in the 3′ untranslated portion. The binding of the 5′ and 3′ flanking IREs results in different effects on translation, as will be discussed later. In addition to the ferritin H, ferritin L, and transferrin receptor mRNAs, the mRNAs for several other proteins have more recently been found to contain IREs or IRE-resembling sequences. The mRNA for the erythroid form of δ-aminolevulinate synthase (the first enzyme in the heme biosynthetic pathway), the mRNA for the mitochondrial form of aconitase, and the mRNA for transferrin also contain a single IRE in the 5′ untranslated region.

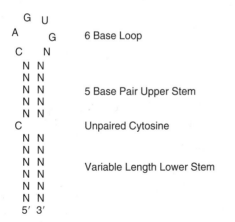

Figure 31–6. *Consensus sequence for iron-responsive elements.*

IRE-Binding Proteins. A cytosolic protein has been identified that directly interacts with the IRE to modulate mRNA translation. This protein has been termed the IRE-binding protein (IRE-BP); it is also sometimes called the iron regulatory factor or protein (IRF or IRP) or the ferritin repressor protein (FRP). The IRE-BP is an iron-sulfur protein with a molecular mass of approximately 90 kDa and is encoded by a gene on chromosome 9. In its iron-saturated state (4Fe-4S), it has aconitase activity and lacks IRE-binding activity. When the cellular iron concentration is low, a labile iron is lost from the 4Fe-4S cluster, and the protein loses aconitase activity but acquires IRE-binding activity.

The specific mechanisms by which IRE/IRE-BP interactions modulate protein biosynthesis are still incompletely understood, but they are clearly different for ferritin than for transferrin receptor synthesis. Interaction of IRE-BP with the 5′ stem-loop of the ferritin mRNA prevents the formation of ferritin-mRNA polysomes. Hence, when the iron supply is low, IRE-BP is active, binds to the IRE on ferritin mRNAs, and acts to block ferritin synthesis. On the other hand, when iron is abundant, the IRE-BP is inactive (iron-saturated), does not bind to the IRE, and does not restrict ferritin synthesis.

When active IRE-BPs bind to the stem-loop structures on the 3′ end of the transferrin receptor mRNA, the transferrin receptor mRNA is stabilized against degradation, and the concentrations of this mRNA increase. It appears that there is a determinant for rapid mRNA turnover within this 3′ untranslated region, and that IRE-BP binding to the stem-loop structure in some way masks the rapid turnover determinant. Thus, when cytoplasmic iron levels are low, transferrin receptor mRNA concentrations increase and more transferrin receptor is synthesized, resulting in higher concentrations of transferrin receptors in cell membranes.

This IRE/IRE-BP regulatory mechanism is one of the first examples of how a single protein can coordinately regulate distinct mRNAs, thereby decreasing the translation of one (ferritin) by inhibiting polysome formation while simultaneously increasing translation of the other (transferrin receptor) by limiting degradation of its mRNA (Binder et al., 1994). Although the major determinant of IRE-BP activity is the cytosolic content of exchangeable iron, recent data indicate that nitric oxide, a metabolite of L-arginine, is able to modulate iron removal from iron-sulfur proteins. Clearly this could also result in modulation of high-affinity IRE-BP and might be one of the factors involved in posttranscriptional regulation of proteins of iron metabolism in situations of inflammation and stimulated cytokine production.

BODY IRON COMPARTMENTS

Understanding the disorders of iron metabolism is greatly facilitated by the consideration of body iron (approximately 40 mg/kg in women and 50 mg/kg in men) as two major compartments, namely functional and storage iron, as summarized in Table 31–3. Functional iron is composed predominantly of the iron in hemoglobin (28 mg/kg in women and 32 mg/kg in men) of red blood cells and erythroid tissues, iron in myoglobin in the muscle (4 mg/kg in women and 5 mg/kg in men), and iron-containing enzymes in all cells of the body (1 to 2 mg/kg). The storage iron compartment is an intrinsically more variable compartment, accounting for between 0 and 20 mg of iron/kg of body weight. This storage iron is held in association with the protein complexes called ferritin and hemosiderin; storage iron is located predominantly in macrophages of the reticuloendothelial system and in parenchymal cells of the liver. These

storage proteins serve as a repository for dietary iron absorbed in excess of that needed to replace losses from the functional compartment; this provides a mechanism to prevent accumulation of free iron ions, which would be toxic, and to provide an emergency reserve supply from which sudden deficits in the functional compartment may be replenished.

A much smaller third compartment can be thought of as the transport system interfacing between the storage and functional compartments. This transport compartment consists of iron bound to transferrin and accounts for approximately 0.04 mg of iron/kg. Although the amount of iron in this compartment at any given time is quantitatively small, flux of iron through this compartment is relatively large on a daily basis (40 mg of Fe/day, or approximately 0.6 mg • kg^{-1} • day^{-1}), and measurements of this transport compartment provide important and clinically useful information for defining the stage of iron deficiency or excess.

INTERNAL IRON EXCHANGE AND IRON DELIVERY TO CELLS

Transferrin is the major iron-transport molecule. Although the total amount of plasma transferrin-bound iron is only about 50 μmol (in 2.5 L of plasma), the rate of plasma iron turnover determined by ferrokinetic evaluation is about 700 μmol/day in an adult. Hence, the plasma iron pool is turned over ten or more times daily. This estimate of iron turnover is much greater than would be predicted from the rate of transferrin synthesis, catabolism, or lymphatic circulation, indicating that transferrin is significantly reutilized, with only limited catabolism during iron delivery (Aisen, 1989; Morgan, 1981).

The Transferrin Cycle

The apotransferrin molecule binds iron released from cells of iron storage (i.e., macrophages of the reticuloendothelial system and parenchymal cells of the liver) and iron procurement (i.e., enterocytes of the intestine). The iron released from cells crosses the plasma membrane in all likelihood as ferrous

TABLE 31–3
Typical Iron Distribution in Adults

	Men	Women
	(mg iron/kg body weight)	
Functional iron		
Hemoglobin	32	28
Myoglobin	5	4
Iron-containing enzymes	1–2	1–2
Storage iron		
Ferritin (and hemosiderin)	≈11	≈6
Transport iron		
Transferrin	0.04	0.04

iron, but during this process or shortly thereafter, the iron is oxidized to the ferric form. The likely oxidase is plasma ceruloplasmin, which has ferroxidase activity (Harris et al., 1995). The ferric iron is rapidly bound by transferrin, which has two Fe^{3+}-binding sites. In plasma, the iron-free (apo) form, the single iron (monoferric) form, and the two-iron (diferric) form are all normally found, with an average overall iron saturation of about one third. The affinity of transferrin for its receptor correlates directly at physiological pH with its degree of iron occupancy; the apo form has negligible affinity, whereas the diferric form has highest affinity.

Because transferrin uptake is mediated by transferrin receptor, transferrin iron is delivered to tissues in proportion to their surface expression of transferrin receptors. In practical terms, fully 80% of the transferrin iron is routinely delivered to erythroid precursors. After binding to the transferrin receptor, the receptor-ligand complexes tend to aggregate over clathrin-coated pits. Thereafter they are internalized by the process of receptor-mediated endocytosis. Within the endocytic vesicles, energy-dependent protonation occurs, and in the more acidic environment that is produced, the transferrin loses its iron-binding avidity and releases its iron. The released iron in all likelihood undergoes a reduction step, and the resulting ferrous iron is transported across the endocytic membrane into the cytosol. The apotransferrin molecule that is generated has an extremely high affinity for the receptor in the more acidic environment of the endosome. By binding to the receptor, apotransferrin largely escapes degradation in the endosome, and the majority of the apotransferrin-receptor complexes are returned to the cell surface after uncoupling of the iron has occurred.

This rapidly recycling endosome passes through the Golgi apparatus prior to fusing with the plasma membrane at the cell surface. After fusion has occurred, the former contents of the endosome are exposed to physiological pH, at which the apotransferrin dissociates from the receptor and is returned to the interstitial fluid. From the interstitial fluid, the apotransferrin returns to the circulation where it is again able to bind iron and participate in further cycles of iron delivery. The cell membrane-bound transferrin receptor is able to participate in further cycles of receptor-mediated endocytosis. This cellular transferrin recycling pathway is extremely rapid; one complete cycle for uptake of the transferrin-transferrin receptor complex, release of the iron, return of the apotransferrin-receptor complex to the plasma membrane, and return of transferrin to the circulation requires only 3 to 10 minutes.

Transferrin Receptor Degradation

A minor portion of the endocytosed transferrin and transferrin receptor is processed via an alternative pathway. In this pathway the endocytic vesicle membrane undergoes internal outpouching. The internal blebs formed are then pinched off in a process that forms a larger vesicle containing numerous small 50-nm-diameter vesicles called exosomes. These exosomes carry the transferrin receptor on their surface with the extracellular domain directed into the cavity of the greater vesicle and the cytoplasmic domain into the interior of the exosome. This whole structure is referred to as the multivesicular endosome or body. By a much slower process, the multivesicular body fuses with the surface membrane to release its contents to the exterior by the process of exocytosis. This process represents a transferrin receptor degradative pathway. Recent evidence suggests that the receptors attached to the exosomes undergo proteolytic cleavage, probably within the multivesicular body, such that a soluble proteolytic product of the intact receptor is released to the circulation (Baynes et al., 1994a). Little, if any, exosomally bound transferrin receptor is detectable in the circulation.

Nontransferrin-Bound Iron

As indicated previously, iron can also be internalized into cells by other pathways that do not involve transferrin. These include the haptoglobin-hemoglobin complex, the hemopexin-heme complex, the iron-albumin complex, ferritin iron, and the nontransferrin-, nonheme-, nonferritin-bound iron. The organ most involved in clearing these forms of iron from the circulation is the liver. In most of these mechanisms the iron is delivered primarily into an endocytic vesicle, as with transferrin. Only in the case of the nonprotein-bound form of iron does it appear that the iron is taken up directly across the plasma membrane.

Postendocytic Transmembrane Iron Transport

After the iron has been freed from its carrier protein by processes within the endocytic vesicle, the iron is still separated from the cytosol by the vesicle membrane. The process of transport across this membrane is poorly understood and somewhat controversial. It appears likely that the iron, either after liberation from its carrier or during the transport process, undergoes reduction, which is possibly mediated by a membrane-associated ferrireductase. Current data suggest that this ferrous iron is transported across the vesicle membrane by a carrier-mediated iron transport system; the putative carrier has not been fully characterized, but it appears to be similar to the ferrous iron carrier in the plasma membrane.

Cytosolic Transport

Once iron has successfully crossed the vesicle membrane into the cytosol, it enters the low molecular weight pool from which it is transported to sites where it is incorporated into heme, ferritin, and nonheme-iron proteins. The nature of the cytosolic transporters is unclear, as is the mechanism by which iron is delivered to such organelles as mitochondria.

The Red Cell Cycle

As shown in Table 31–3, the majority of body iron is present in hemoglobin in red blood cells and erythroid tissues; typically, hemoglobin iron represents about two thirds of the total body iron. Each day in the normal adult approximately 2×10^{11} red blood cells are produced, and this requires more than 2×10^{20} atoms or almost 24 mg of iron. The majority of this (about 17 mg) is incorporated into hemoglobin. Clearly hemoglobin synthesis

and red blood cell turnover dominate the events of iron homeostasis.

Iron is incorporated into red blood cells during their synthesis in the bone marrow. Erythroblasts are synthesized by the bone marrow from stem cells and are nucleated, developing red blood cells. An erythroblast eventually loses its nucleus to become a reticulocyte and ultimately a mature red blood cell, or erythrocyte. Transferrin-bound iron is taken up by erythroblasts and is incorporated into protoporphyrin in the mitochondria to form heme. The incorporation of iron into heme is catalyzed by heme synthetase or by ferrochelatase. The supply of iron to the erythroblast for hemoglobin synthesis is regulated in a feedback manner by heme, which inhibits release of iron from transferrin.

Once released from the bone marrow, mature erythrocytes circulate for approximately 120 days. As erythrocytes circulate in the blood, a number of physicochemical changes occur. These include oxidative damage with modification of membrane lipids and proteins, loss of surface sialic acid and electrostatic charge, the generation of advanced glycation end products, decreases in ion gradients, and metabolic depletion of glycolytic and other enzymes. Which of these changes or combinations is responsible for recognition of senescence is uncertain, but intact senescent cells are removed from the circulation by specialized macrophages of the liver, spleen, and bone marrow. Although quantitatively less significant, some red cells are prematurely cleared on account of failure to reach maturity within the marrow and resultant red cell death in the marrow (ineffective erythropoiesis).

Within the macrophage, hemoglobin iron is liberated under the action of the enzyme heme oxygenase. Heme oxygenase is a substrate-inducible enzyme that catalyzes the cleavage of the α-methene bridge that joins the two pyrrole residues containing the vinyl substituents in the protoporphyrin; action of heme oxygenase releases Fe^{3+} from the tetrapyrrole structure. The liberated iron enters a low molecular weight pool from which it is either incorporated into stores in the form of ferritin or is released into the interstitial fluid and circulation for recycling via transferrin. It is believed that iron crosses the macrophage membrane as ferrous iron and then undergoes oxidation by a ferroxidase (possibly ceruloplasmin) prior to uptake by circulating apo- or monoferric transferrin. Recent data have suggested a possible role for the Nramp1 (natural resistance-associated macrophage protein) gene, whose expression appears to be largely restricted to the reticuloendothelial cells, in regulating iron release from these cells (Fleming et al., 1997). The macrophage system returns an almost equivalent amount of iron (approximately 22 mg Fe/day) to the plasma as it is cleared from the circulation by the transferrin receptor mechanism.

Thus, the iron in hemoglobin is scavenged and returned to the circulation where it exists as transferrin-bound iron. The process of transferrin iron delivery to erythroid bone marrow accounts for at least 80% of transferrin iron turnover. Most of this iron is used for synthesis of hemoglobin for new red blood cells. The other 20% of transferrin iron turnover is accounted for by delivery of iron to other cells, primarily to the liver.

If red blood cells are destroyed in the blood stream and heme or hemoglobin is released into the blood stream, these are bound by haptoglobin (oxyhemoglobin dimers) or hemopexin and albumin (heme and hematin). Normally, little free heme or hemoglobin exists in plasma, and these binding proteins are largely free, but these hemoglobin and heme-binding proteins do serve to remove and recycle any iron present in the plasma as free hemoglobin or heme and may be quantitatively important in conserving iron in hemolytic disease states. Because the protein complexes of heme and hemoglobin are too large to be filtered through the renal glomeruli, heme and hemoglobin are scavenged as long as free haptoglobin or hemopexin is present in the circulation. The haptoglobin-hemoglobin and hemopexin-heme complexes are taken up by the liver by receptor-mediated processes, and the iron is released by action of heme oxygenase.

EXTERNAL IRON EXCHANGE AND IRON ABSORPTION

External iron exchange is concerned with the processes by which iron is either lost from or added to the body. Normally only approximately 0.05% (2 to 2.5 mg) of body iron is lost each day. This iron loss must be replaced by absorption of a similar amount of iron from dietary sources. Net negative balance results when losses exceed absorption. When iron absorption is less than that needed to replace losses and to meet demands for growth, this ultimately results in a depletion of the functional iron compartment. When absorption exceeds losses, positive balance occurs as a result of growth or an increase in iron in the storage compartment. If positive iron balance is sustained in an adult, it may ultimately lead to iron overload.

Iron Losses and Requirements for Absorbed Iron

In the basal state, iron is lost passively in cells that are shed from the skin surface or the epithelial lining of internal organs. Small amounts of red blood cells are also lost via the gastrointestinal tract. The normal amount of iron lost in men is on the order of 14 μg $\cdot$ kg^{-1} $\cdot$ day^{-1}. These losses are distributed between gastrointestinal tract, skin, and urinary tract in a ratio of 6:3:1. In a 70-kg man, this basal loss would average 0.98 mg/day. For a 55 kg-woman, this would be 0.77 mg/day. The variability of these estimates is calculated to be approximately 15%. In iron deficiency these losses may be reduced by 50%, whereas in iron overload these losses are slightly increased. Menstruation increases the amount of iron loss, and absorption of 1.36 mg of iron is required daily to maintain iron balance in 50% of normal menstruating women. To maintain balance in 95% of women, absorption of 2.84 mg/day of iron is required.

The other physiological cause of increased iron loss is pregnancy. Although a pregnant woman should be in positive iron balance during the course of the pregnancy, it is not unusual for the course of pregnancy and parturition to result in a net loss of iron from the mother's body. The iron requirements specific to pregnancy over the 9-month gestational period, for a 55-kg woman, are calculated to be 320 mg for basal losses, 360 mg for the products of conception (fetus, 270 mg; placenta and umbilical cord, 90 mg), and approximately 150 mg as peripartum blood loss. An additional 450 mg of iron is required for expanded maternal red cell mass; however, this iron will not be lost with parturition but will be returned to the mother during postpartum contraction of red cell mass. The greatest increases in total requirements (up to 6 mg of iron/day) are for fetal growth and erythroid expansion during the second and third trimesters, which are only slightly offset by the diminished iron loss as a result of the amenorrhea of pregnancy. Lactation results in a further iron loss of 0.3 to 0.6 mg/day postpartum in the milk, but this additional loss is largely balanced by the accompanying amenorrhea.

Growth markedly increases iron requirements for formation of both erythroid and nonerythroid tissues. Because of more efficient oxygen delivery to tissues, the newborn infant initially experiences a decrease in hemoglobin concentration, with a shift of iron into stores. Growth and erythropoiesis exhaust this supply of iron within 6 months, so that in the first year of life the infant must absorb 0.3 mg of iron/day to maintain iron homeostasis. In the second year of life, growth causes this figure to rise to 0.4 mg/day. Slow growth from this time until puberty results in a gradual increase in requirements to 0.5 to 0.8 mg/day. Puberty and adolescent growth spurts increase iron requirements to 1.6 mg/day in young men and to 2.4 mg/day in young women. The higher requirement in young women reflects concomitant menarche.

Basal iron losses and physiologically enhanced losses as in menstruation, pregnancy, and lactation are normal iron losses. Iron loss may be increased in situations of pathological and nonpathological blood loss. Pathological losses occur in such situations as bleeding from the urinary, genital, and gastrointestinal tracts. The gastrointestinal tract is the most common site of pathological bleeding, secondary to conditions such as esophagitis, gastritis, varices, peptic ulcers, neoplasms, diverticulosis, angiodysplasia, and inflammatory bowel disease. In developing regions of the world, infection with parasites such as hookworm may increase iron loss. Heavy infestation may cause bleeding of sufficient magnitude to increase requirements of iron by as

much as 3 to 5 mg/day. Nonpathological increases in blood loss may be secondary to the effects of aspirin or nonsteroidal antiinflammatory drugs, which may cause gastric bleeding, or to voluntary blood donation.

Stimulated erythropoiesis by administered erythropoietin used to treat various disease states (e.g., renal failure) or by endogenous erythropoietin in hemolytic states related to abnormalities in hemoglobin formation (e.g., thalassemia or sickle cell disease) further increases iron requirements. Endogenous erythropoietin production by the kidney is stimulated when oxygen delivery to the kidney is reduced, as in anemia.

Iron Absorption

Intestinal iron absorption reflects a composite of three determinants: the iron content of the diet, the bioavailability of the dietary iron, and the capacity of the mucosal cells to absorb the iron. In terms of the iron content of the diet, Western diets have remarkably consistent iron contents, averaging 6 mg/1000 kcal. Iron in Western diets tends to be highly bioavailable, with an estimated iron availability in the range of 14% to 17%. Thus, a 2000-kcal diet should provide about 1.8 mg of absorbed iron/day. Clearly, it is difficult for many women with normal activity levels to obtain sufficient iron from the diet alone.

Methods of Assessing Iron Absorption. A number of in vitro and animal models have been evaluated in an attempt to predict iron absorption in humans. In vitro methods generally simulate in vivo digestive processes, including acid hydrolysis, proteolytic digestion, and the addition of bile acids. Released soluble low molecular weight iron is then determined. Such methods give a crude prediction of food iron bioavailability. Although superior to certain animal models, these in vitro techniques are at best indicators of trends in bioavailability rather than indicators of absolute levels of iron absorption.

A variety of experimental animals have been used as models for studying iron absorption. Absorption of radioisotopes of iron has been evaluated in whole animals and in isolated gut loops. The most widely used animal for these studies has been the rat, but significant disparities in nonheme iron absorption have been well documented between rat and humans. Consequently, the rat model is unsuitable as a predictor of human iron absorption (Reddy and Cook, 1993). Other animals have been evaluated only partially as models for studying human iron absorption, but studies of human iron absorption ultimately must be done in humans.

Prior to the ready availability of radioisotopes, iron balance techniques were employed to evaluate human iron bioavailability. Prolonged stool collections make this a cumbersome method, and the small amounts of iron absorbed each day result in this approach being highly inaccurate. Measurements of increases in plasma iron concentration with iron intake also are of marginal value for assessing food iron bioavailability, given variable absorption and the multicompartmental kinetics involved. Changes in plasma iron levels following pharmacological doses of iron, however, are useful as a crude screening test for gastrointestinal malabsorption of iron.

Progress in defining iron bioavailability and iron absorption was facilitated in past decades by the use in humans of radioisotopes. Absorption was estimated from the amount of radioiron (either ^{59}Fe or ^{55}Fe) incorporated into circulating erythrocytes 2 to 3 weeks after ingestion of the radioactive label, or whole body counters were used to assess whole body retention of radioiron. Foods under study could be labeled either intrinsically or by extrinsic tagging. Intrinsic labeling relies on either hydroponic cultivation of vegetable material or biosynthetic labeling of animal material. Extrinsic tagging is a simpler and valid indicator of bioavailability and absorption because the extrinsic iron enters a common pool with intrinsic iron; enhancing and inhibitory influences affect the common pool in aggregate, and neither affect the intrinsic or extrinsic pool selectively.

To facilitate comparison of different iron absorption studies, it is desirable to factor out the effect of variations in body iron status. This has been done by administering a standard reference dose of radiolabeled inorganic iron containing 3 mg of iron as ferrous ascorbate. The ratio of absorption from a given meal to that from the reference dose can be used to measure the relative bioavailability of the nonheme iron in the meal. A more concrete measure may be obtained by standardizing the test measurement to a reference value of 40%, the mean absorption in subjects who are borderline iron-deficient. Clear disadvantages of this method are that additional isotope must be ingested and that day to day variability in individual absorption may affect the results. Serum ferritin concentration, an excellent marker of body iron stores, provides as useful a correction and comparison factor as does the reference iron absorption and may be used instead.

Because of general concern about radioisotopes in human subjects, particularly in children and pregnant women, stable isotopes of iron including ^{54}Fe, ^{56}Fe, ^{57}Fe, and ^{58}Fe have been evaluated as alternative tracers. These techniques are still in their infancy, are extremely costly, and require highly sophisticated laboratory facilities. However, it is very likely that, as the technology is refined, use of stable isotopes will replace the ^{55}Fe and ^{59}Fe methodologies.

Much of what is known of iron bioavailability in the diet and iron absorption is based upon single-meal studies in which the single meal was isotopically labeled. The study protocol, however, is not reflective of the usual conditions pertaining during the absorptive process because the test includes a protracted fast, the meal administration, and a subsequent period of fasting. Significant discrepancies have recently been documented between putative promotory ligands (e.g., ascorbic acid) and inhibitory factors (e.g., soy protein), as documented by single-meal studies when compared with a lack of effect of these factors over the course of longitudinal studies of iron absorption. Recent data comparing results of long-term studies of labeled diets with results of single-meal studies have clearly established that single-meal studies tend to exaggerate enhancing or inhibitory influences grossly (Cook et al., 1991). Although single-meal studies are very useful for evaluation of iron absorption in populations consuming simple diets that consist largely of a single staple, they are relatively unhelpful in the evaluation of more complex diets as consumed in the developed world.

Heme Iron Absorption. Hemoglobin and myoglobin are the major protein sources from which heme iron is derived, and foods derived from animal tissues are the predominant sources of heme iron. Heme iron in meat is an important source of dietary iron not only because of its intrinsic high bioavailability but also because a "meat factor" enhances the bioavailability of the nonheme iron present in the diet. Consequently, in developed regions where heme iron accounts for about 10% to 15% of total dietary iron, heme iron accounts for 35% of the iron actually absorbed. In population studies in developed communities, meat ingestion is the major determinant of iron status.

Heme is released from hemoglobin during digestion in the small intestine. This is a rapid process, with 70% of a specific hemoglobin dose being converted to heme within 30 minutes of ingestion in a dog model. Heme fed by itself is poorly absorbed, possibly due to the formation of relatively nonabsorbable heme polymers, but this is largely only of mechanistic interest because heme is not usually consumed in its free form. The globin moiety and other proteins present in the diet appear, during digestion, to yield residues that inhibit heme polymerization and maintain it in free, absorbable form. The heme appears to bind to a specific receptor on the luminal intestinal surface and to be taken up by enterocytes via endocytosis. The heme moiety is then catabolized within the mucosal cell by heme oxygenase. The release of iron from heme by heme oxygenase appears to be the rate-limiting step in absorption of heme iron. After heme degradation, the liberated iron appears to enter a common iron pool that also includes absorbed nonheme iron; further transport either into mucosal cellular stores or across the basolateral membrane of the enterocyte into the interstitial fluid occurs from this common iron pool.

When physiological amounts of heme iron, ranging from 0.25 mg to 6 mg, are ingested with food, a linear increase in the amount of heme iron absorbed occurs, reflecting a constant percentage absorption of heme iron over this range. Luminal factors other than the presence of proteins to protect against heme polymerization do not appear to influence heme iron absorption. Although heme iron absorption is inversely correlated with body iron status, this relationship is much less pronounced than in the case of nonheme iron. Indeed, the slopes of the regression lines describing the relationship have been calculated to be -0.358 for heme iron as compared with -0.936 for nonheme iron. This has two obvious ramifications. First, iron deficiency is least likely in areas of significant meat consumption. Second, iron overload is most likely in these same areas. The picture is further emphasized by the finding that, although nonheme iron absorption is decreased, heme iron absorption is not decreased in subjects with hereditary hemochromatosis (iron overload). These data all suggest that there is relatively little regulation of heme iron absorption.

Nonheme Iron Absorption. Nonheme iron is the largest component of dietary iron. Its absorption, as determined in single-meal studies, is influenced by the balance between a large number of potentially enhancing and inhibitory influences. These influences, however, appear to be more important in the setting of diets consisting of a single staple or only a few foods, as consumed in certain less-developed regions of the world, than in developed regions where multicomponent mixed diets are the rule.

Nonheme iron compounds are found in foods of both plant and animal origin. Iron in plants is present in three major forms: as metalloproteins, with the predominant example being plant ferritin; as soluble iron in the sap of xylem, phloem, and plant vacuoles; and as nonfunctional iron complexed either to plant structural components or to storage compounds predominantly in the form of phytates (inositol hexa- or pentaphosphates). A large amount of dietary nonheme iron is present as contaminant ferric oxides and hydroxides. Nonheme iron in animal-derived food is found in many forms, including ferritin and hemosiderin in meat products, iron bound to the phosphoprotein phosphovitin in egg yolk, and iron in milk bound to lactoferrin or associated with fat globule membranes and low molecular weight compounds such as citrate. Nonheme iron in the form of ferritin, hemosiderin, contaminating oxides, and hydroxides, as well as certain formulations of iron added in food fortification or enrichment or taken as supplements, enter the common iron pool poorly and may contribute little, if at all, to the overall iron economy.

Once nonheme food iron enters the alimentary canal, it is acted upon by the gastric juices containing pepsin and hydrochloric acid. Because the acid appears to be important in reducing ferric to ferrous iron, the effect of achlorhydria (absence of hydrochloric acid [HCl] from the gastric juice) is most pronounced on absorption of ferric rather than ferrous iron salts. As iron enters the duodenum and pH rises, the ferric iron is rapidly precipitated as ferric oxyhydroxides, whereas the ferrous iron remains relatively soluble as pH rises. Uptake into the mucosal cell occurs rapidly, with the greatest proportion being taken up within the first 5 minutes after the digesta enters the duodenum, and with ferrous salts being better absorbed than ferric salts. The solubility of iron in the duodenum can be greatly modified by the presence of various ligands.

The precise mechanism by which luminal nonheme iron crosses the mucosal cell membrane to enter the enterocyte is poorly understood. In a proposed mechanism, binding is thought to occur via a specific high-affinity acceptor molecule. Several specific surface iron-binding proteins have been putatively identified. A 160-kDa iron-binding protein consisting of three 54-kDa monomeric peptides has been reported to be on the mucosal surface (Teichmann and Stremmel, 1990). More recently, a surface-expressed integrin has been reported to be the mucosal iron-binding moiety. A low-affinity iron-binding mucin is thought to trap the luminal iron and then transfer it to the surface integrin (Conrad et al., 1993). However, recent data obtained by studying mutant *mk* mice suggest that another transporter, the gene product of Nramp2, might be the luminal iron transporter molecule (Fleming et al., 1997). The *mk* mouse has an abnormality of iron metabolism characterized by abnormally reduced iron absorption and hypochromic microcytic anemia. By positional cloning, the defect has been shown to be the consequence of mutation of the Nramp2 gene. These findings, while obviously exciting, do require confirmation and further studies of the protein product of the Nramp2 gene.

Once nonheme iron has undergone surface adsorption, it must then be transported into the enterocyte. Again, this is a poorly defined process with many potential mechanisms, including simple diffusion, facilitated diffusion possibly involving the integrin, entry via a ferrous or ferric ion channel, fluid phase endocytosis, adsorptive pinocytosis, or receptor-mediated endocytosis. The intracellular movement of iron after it enters the enterocyte is also poorly understood. Putative transcellular carrier mechanisms include a newly described protein called mobilferrin (Conrad et al., 1993). The possible role of mobilferrin has not yet been confirmed. The possible role of the Nramp2-related protein also requires further elucidation.

Suffice it to say, once nonheme iron enters the enterocyte, it enters a low molecular weight pool. From this pool, the iron may be rapidly transported across the basolateral membrane into the interstitial fluid from whence it enters the systemic circulation. The mechanism by which iron crosses the basolateral membrane of the intestinal mucosal cells is not known. Alternatively, the iron taken up from the lumen of the gastrointestinal tract can be stored within enterocytes in the iron storage protein ferritin. There appears to be little release of iron from ferritin in the enterocyte once it has been stored; the majority of enterocyte ferritin is apparently destined for excretion via the process of shedding of mucosal cells.

After iron enters the common luminal pool, it is subject to interactions with a number of ligands contained in the food, as well as other food constituents that affect its absorption. Based on a large number of predominantly single-meal studies, foods can be classified as having low, intermediate, and high iron bioavailability, as shown in Table 31–4. These data are based largely on single-meal studies (Bothwell et al., 1989), which in all likelihood exaggerate the effects on iron bio-

TABLE 31–4
Relative Bioavailability of Nonheme Iron in a Number of Foods

Foods	Low	Intermediate	High
Cereals	Maize Oatmeal Rice Sorghum Whole wheat flour	Corn flour White flour	
Fruits	Apple Avocado Banana Grape Peach Pear Plum Rhubarb Strawberry	Cantaloupe Mango Pineapple	Guava Lemon Orange Papaw Tomato
Vegetables	Eggplant Legumes Soy flour Isolated soy protein	Carrot Potato	Beetroot Broccoli Cabbage Cauliflower Pumpkin Turnip
Beverages	Tea Coffee	Red wine	White wine
Nuts	Almond Brazil Coconut Peanut Walnut		
Animal proteins	Cheese Egg Milk		Fish Meat Poultry

availability over those likely to be observed in the setting of a normal mixed diet. The tabulation reflects the net effect of the composite of both enhancing and inhibitory ligands consumed as part of the single meal under test.

The major ligands in food that enhance nonheme iron absorption appear to be the organic acids, including ascorbic, citric, malic, and lactic acids. These organic acids are particularly found in citrus and deciduous fruits. These organic acids, when tested in single-meal studies, all appear to increase nonheme iron absorption, but their significance in mixed diets is less clear. Studies of the effects of chronic ingestion of high doses of vitamin C or multivitamin supplements failed to show any effects of ascorbic acid on long-term iron status in subjects consuming mixed diets. Consequently, the impact of these organic acids on long-term iron balance in subjects consuming a mixed diet appears

modest. It is likely that their effects would be more readily appreciated in populations consuming diets with little variety and consisting of foods with poor iron bioavailability.

A large number of inhibitory ligands are found in ingested foods. These include phytates, polyphenols, calcium, and fiber. Phytates are widely distributed in various grains and vegetable foods and particularly limit iron absorption by the formation of diferric and tetraferric phytate complexes. Polyphenols are also widely distributed in various vegetables and are found in beverages such as tea and coffee. In single-meal studies, polyphenols and phytate are profoundly inhibitory of iron absorption, but their impact on iron nutrition when consumed as part of a mixed diet is not well defined. Calcium may also inhibit nonheme iron absorption. The effect of calcium is most prominent when the basal meal is one of relatively poor iron bioavailability. Finally, certain components of dietary fiber cause a modest reduction in nonheme iron absorption.

Nonheme iron absorption from meals containing significant amounts of vegetable-derived protein, such as soybeans, other legumes, and nuts, tends to be inhibited. Although these foods contain a number of other inhibitory ligands, including phytates and polyphenols, there appears to be a close relationship between the presence of intact vegetable protein and the degree of inhibition of iron absorption. Indeed, the inhibitory effect of soy protein is progressively reduced by increasing the extent of protein hydrolysis (e.g., as produced by fermentation) to the point at which products such as miso and soy sauce actually act as promoters of iron absorption in single-meal studies. Vegetable protein products may also bind to polyphenols and reduce their inhibitory effects on nonheme iron absorption. Consequently, nonheme iron absorption reflects not only iron-ligand interactions but also ligand-ligand interactions.

Animal tissue protein is a rich source of highly absorbable heme iron and also has a marked enhancing effect on nonheme iron absorption. The nature of this "meat factor" that enhances nonheme iron absorption is the subject of much current investigation. Various mechanisms have been suggested, including an interaction of cysteinyl residues or carboxylate groups of the proteins with luminal nonheme iron to maintain iron in a soluble form, enhanced gastric acid production in response to meat ingestion, and interactions between phytates and meat-derived peptides that reduce the inhibitory effects of phytate.

Regulation of Mucosal Iron Absorption. The regulation of nonheme iron absorption appears to be controlled at the luminal brush border membrane absorptive site, whereas the regulation of heme iron absorption appears to reside at the transcellular and basolateral transmembrane transfer sites. Mucosal conditioning appears to occur in the crypts of the intestinal villus, with a brief delay (on the order of 24 to 48 h) before this is reflected in altered absorption in the absorptive villous apical cells. The delay in all likelihood reflects the time for migration of cells from crypt to apex. Regulation at the level of the mucosal cell is reflected in reduced absorption on a high-iron diet. The mucosal cell appears to be conditioned in relation to the amount of iron delivered from food iron, and the mucosal cell is also conditioned in relation to such entities as functional iron deficiency and stimulated erythropoiesis, which appear to be the most significant regulatory influences (Finch, 1994).

The nature of the signal by which erythropoiesis and mucosal iron absorption are coupled remains one of the most important unanswered questions in ferrobiology. Certain data suggest that multifunctional hematopoietic growth factors may have an important role to play in the regulation of iron absorption (Baynes et al., 1995). A quantitatively less impressive but nevertheless significant regulator of iron absorption appears to be body iron stores, with a clear inverse relationship between the iron stores and iron absorption (Finch, 1994). Little is known of the signaling involved by which iron stores influence iron absorption. From single-meal studies it appears that the regulation of nonheme iron absorption may be such that less than 1% up to in excess of 60% of the iron content of the meal in question may be absorbed.

RECOMMENDED DIETARY INTAKES OF IRON

The Recommended Dietary Allowances (RDAs) for iron intake established by the National Research Council (1989) are 10 mg/day for adult men and 15 mg/day for menstruating women. The RDA for women represents a reduction from the 1980 RDA, which was 18 mg/day.

Recommendations for iron intake deserve careful consideration. Iron deficiency severe enough to result in anemia is associated with significant morbidity, whereas uncontrolled iron absorption, as in hemochromatosis, causes multiorgan failure. Preliminary data from the third National Health and Nutrition Examination Survey (NHANES III) demonstrate that the prevalence of iron deficiency anemia in the United States is very low. The implication is that current iron consumption is adequate, because iron deficiency without

Food Sources of Iron

- Meat, poultry, and fish
- Enriched or fortified cereal products
- Vegetables

RDAs Across the Life Cycle

		mg Fe/day
Infants,	0–0.5 y	6
	0.5–1 y	10
Children,	1–10 y	10
Males,	11–18 y	12
	19+ y	10
Females,	11–50 y	15
	51+ y	10
	Pregnant	30
	Lactating	15

From National Research Council (1989) Recommended Dietary Allowances, 10th ed., National Academy Press, Washington, D.C.

anemia is not associated with any proven liability.

The data, however, indicate that, along with a reduction in iron deficiency anemia, a rise has occurred in the iron stores in American men and postmenopausal women. The epidemiological data indicating potential liabilities of such a modest increase in body iron have resulted in the recommended daily iron intake becoming a highly controversial area, with the debate ranging over such areas as whether the recommended intake should factor in positive storage balance, how best to define the iron status of a population, whether a safe upper limit rather than a recommended daily allowance should be the guideline for all groups not at high risk for iron deficiency, and whether the diet is excessively fortified (Lynch and Baynes, 1996). In regions where the diet is less varied and its iron content is less bioavailable, a higher recommended daily iron intake is needed to meet the requirement for absorbed iron.

ASSESSMENT OF IRON STATUS

Much of the confusion relating to prevalence of iron deficiency is a function of the mechanisms used to evaluate iron status of either individuals or populations. To evaluate optimally a population or individual, it is important to define which iron compartment is being assessed and which test is being used to evaluate the compartment in question.

Measurements of Iron Status

The single best measure to assess stores noninvasively is the serum ferritin concentration, because in the range of 20 to 200 ng/mL, it bears a quantitative relationship to iron stores, with 1 ng/mL being indicative of 8 mg of storage iron. Careful phlebotomy studies (in which blood was slowly and systematically removed from a volunteer to deplete the stores without rendering the person anemic) have shown that serum ferritin concentrations decrease until stores are exhausted, which is indicated by a serum ferritin of 12 ng/mL. Beyond this point, the functional compartment becomes depleted. Serum ferritin concentration shows little and somewhat erratic further reduction as the functional compartment becomes depleted. It should be noted, however, that alcohol consumption, infection, inflammation, neoplasia, and hepatic dysfunction may all spuriously raise the serum ferritin concentration relative to stores and therefore result in a misleadingly high serum ferritin concentration. The size of stores also can be assessed invasively by measurements of iron content of bone marrow or liver biopsies or by quantitative phlebotomy as just outlined. These latter methods, however, are unsuitable for routine use. Recent developments in magnetic resonance imaging may allow iron stores to be assessed noninvasively.

At the point when stores are exhausted, the transport compartment begins to become depleted. This is best evaluated by measurements of serum iron, transferrin, and the percentage saturation of transferrin. Once the percent iron saturation of transferrin drops below 16, iron supply becomes limiting for tissue needs and erythropoietic requirements. At this point, functional depletion commences.

To assess functional compartment depletion of iron, the usual measurements of value include the mean red cell volume and the red cell free erythrocyte protoporphyrin. These, however, become abnormal relatively late in the development of functional depletion because red cells survive in the circulation for a relatively long period of time (approximately 120 days). A better measure of functional iron depletion is the soluble form of the transferrin receptor (Baynes et al., 1994b); this soluble form of transferrin receptor is the extracellular domain released by proteolytic cleavage at the surface of the exosome. The cleavage occurs between arginine 100 and leucine 101 and is mediated by a membrane-associated serine protease (Baynes et al., 1994a). The concentration of this cleavage product of transferrin receptor remains relatively constant until stores and the transport compartment are both depleted. Thereafter it shows a highly predictable inverse relationship with functional compartment depletion and, indeed, has been shown to be the single best measure of functional compartment depletion. Ultimately functional depletion can become severe enough and of sufficient duration for anemia to develop. Anemia can be quantified by measuring the hemoglobin concentration in the blood.

These compartment depletions correlate well with the clearly defined stages of storage iron depletion, iron-deficient erythropoiesis, and iron deficiency anemia, as shown in Figure 31–7.

Iron excess is best evaluated noninvasively: an elevated serum ferritin concentration and a percent transferrin saturation in excess of normal both indicate iron excess. When percent saturation exceeds 62, the risk of nonprotein-bound iron being present in the circulation and contributing to parenchymal tissue injury becomes very high. The degree of tissue iron overload can be invasively assessed by quantifying the iron content of a liver biopsy.

Evaluation of Individuals

To evaluate the iron status of an individual, the results of the combination of tests just discussed can accurately define the precise stage of iron nutrition (Baynes, 1996). The importance of defining this in individuals relates to appropriate diagnosis and treatment of iron deficiency in the early stages and to the distinction of anemias due to iron deficiency from those due to other causes. Because of concern about relationships between iron and heart disease and cancer, iron supplements should be used only when there is a definitive iron deficiency. Also, a diagnosis of iron deficiency mandates a search for the underlying cause because serious pathology might be present.

Early diagnosis of iron excess in an individual and early intervention are also important uses of measures of iron status. If iron excess is not diagnosed and treated in its early stages, serious long-term organ damage may occur.

Evaluation of Populations

Accurate determination of the iron nutritional status of a population is crucial for determining national and international nutritional priorities. Once a problematic area is defined and an intervention is initiated, repeat population evaluation is essential to evaluate the response. The initial approach was to use a number of measurements of iron status and to employ an arbitrary threshold value for each to define deficiency; it has been well documented that this approach results in

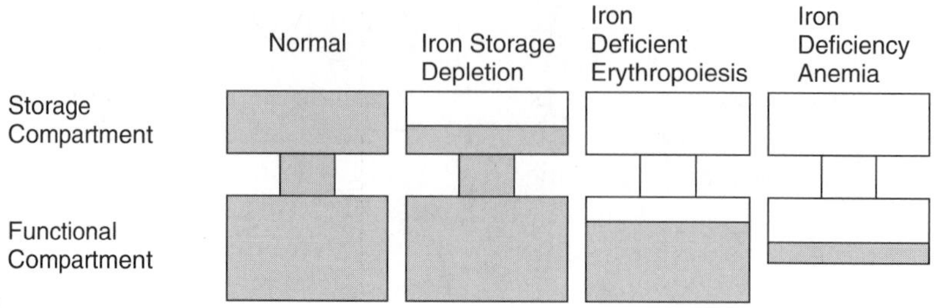

Measurement	Normal	Iron Storage Depletion	Iron Deficient Erythropoiesis	Iron Deficiency Anemia
Marrow Iron[1] (Stainable)	1-3+	0	0	0
Red Cell Distribution Width[2]	<15	<15	>15	>15
Serum Ferritin (μg/L)	>12	<12	<12	<12
Mean Cell Volume (fL)[2]	>80	>80	<80	<80
% Saturation[3]	35±15	>16	<16	<16
Free Erythrocyte Protoporphyrin (μg/100 mL RBC)[2]	<70	<70	>70	>70
Transferrin Receptor (mg/L)[4]	<8.5	<8.5	≥8.5	>>8.5
Hemoglobin Male (g/100 mL) Female	>13 >12	>13 >12	>13 >12	<13 <12

[1] Invasive test; [2] Insensitive and late marker of functional depletion; [3] Lacks sensitivity and specificity; [4] Kansas City Monoclonal ELISA

Figure 31–7. Sequential compartment depletions, stages of iron depletion, and the accompanying changes in iron-related measurements. (Adapted from Bothwell, T. H., Charlton, R. W., Cook, J. D. and Finch, C. A. [1979] Iron Metabolism in Man, p. 45. Blackwell Scientific Publications, Oxford, United Kingdom.)

lower sensitivity for correct assignment of iron deficiency but an increased specificity of that assignment. The other approach is to calculate the iron status of each individual assessed. This employs a formula-driven computation that uses the measurements performed on an individual to define the individual's iron status. This approach markedly increases the sensitivity while preserving excellent specificity. The choice of measurements is to some extent dependent upon whether the highest prevalence is expected to be depleted stores, depleted transport compartment, or functional depletion. The best portrayal of iron status will be provided by combined measurements of serum ferritin (stores), serum transferrin receptor (functional compartment), and hematocrit (degree of anemia) (Cook et al., 1996). Formal evaluation of this combination approach in a large field setting was provided by a study in which pregnant women in the Caribbean were given iron supplements (Simmons et al., 1993).

In the light of increasing concerns over risks of excess iron nutrition, it has become important to assess degrees of iron overload. This is particularly important in regions where the diet is heavily fortified with iron.

IRON DEFICIENCY

Precise data on the prevalence of iron deficiency on a global basis are not readily available. However, much can be inferred from the global prevalence of anemia. Clearly not all anemia is due to iron deficiency, but a crude correction can be arrived at by assuming that anemia in adult men is an estimate of anemia due to causes other than iron deficiency and

LIFE CYCLE CONSIDERATION

Iron Deficiency and Low Iron Stores in Infants, Children, and Women of Child-Bearing Age

Iron deficiency affects a large number of infants, children, and women of child-bearing age in both developed nations and the developing world. Estimates of the prevalence of iron deficiency among women and children in developing countries are as high as 60%. Data from the third National Health and Nutrition Examination Survey (NHANES III), which was conducted during 1988 to 1994, indicated a low rate of iron deficiency in the United States (Centers for Disease Control and Prevention, 1998). About 3% of children aged 12 to 36 months in the United States had iron deficiency anemia, and an additional 6% had low iron stores (based on elevated erythrocyte protoporphyrin concentration, low serum ferritin concentration, and low transferrin saturation). The NHANES III results indicated that 11% of nonpregnant women aged 16 to 49 years in the United States had low iron stores, and 3 to 5% also had iron deficiency anemia. The NHANES III data also indicated that the prevalence of iron deficiency is higher among children and women living at or below the poverty level than among those living above the poverty level.

Iron deficiency is of nutritional concern during infancy and childhood, especially among children less than 24 months of age. The iron stores of full-term infants are estimated to be adequate to meet the infants' iron requirements for 4 to 6 months, whereas those of preterm infants are smaller and may be depleted sooner. A rapid rate of growth, along with frequently inadequate intake of dietary iron, places young children at particular risk. Breast milk provides iron in a highly available form and is sufficient to meet an infant's needs during the first 6 months of life, but other sources of iron are recommended after 6 months. Iron-fortified formula and iron-fortified cereals are important sources of iron for infants in the first year of life. Risk for iron deficiency drops after 24 months of age because of the slower rate of growth and more diversified diet.

Adolescent girls and women of child-bearing age (12 to 49 years) are also at some risk of iron deficiency. Most women in this age group have high iron requirements due to menstrual blood losses and do not meet their needs for iron from dietary intake, partly because of relatively low energy expenditure and food intake. During pregnancy, iron requirement is high due to an increase in blood volume and the growth of fetal and maternal tissues. The iron requirement of 4.5 mg/day during pregnancy is three times higher than during nonpregnancy (1.5 mg/day) and is only partially compensated for by increased iron absorption and decreased menstrual loss throughout pregnancy. Because most women enter pregnancy with low iron stores, routine iron supplementation during pregnancy has been the standard practice in many countries to prevent the development of iron deficiency anemia during the later part of pregnancy.

Consequences of iron deficiency include adverse developmental outcomes and greater risk of lead poisoning in children, reduced work capacity in adults, and possibly an increased risk of poor pregnancy outcomes, such as preterm delivery and higher maternal mortality.

that anemia due to these other causes will occur at similar rates in women. Thus, it can be calculated that roughly 0.5 billion people in the world have iron deficiency anemia. Because anemia reflects the end point of functional iron deficiency, two to three times this number of people must be afflicted by depleted iron stores or lesser degrees of functional compartment depletion. In developed areas of the world, only about 8% of the population are anemic. Conversely, about 36% of the population of underdeveloped and developing regions of the world are anemic. Consequently, the iron nutritional imperatives are clearly different between developed and developing regions. The preliminary data from NHANES III suggest that iron deficiency anemia is currently an unusual finding in the United States (Centers for Disease Control and Prevention, 1998).

Liabilities of Iron Deficiency

The liabilities of iron deficiency correlate with functional iron depletion. Storage iron depletion has not been shown to carry any adverse liabilities. Of the adverse health effects of functional depletion, the demonstration that iron deficiency in infants appears to result in abnormalities of psychomotor development is of major concern. These abnormalities appear to be a consequence of altered dopamine metabolism, and there is some evidence that these abnormalities may be reversible only to a limited extent. Reduced work performance, effort tolerance, and peak effort output are all well documented to result from iron deficiency. Where people depend upon manual labor for their livelihood, these impairments clearly translate into significant economic disadvantage. It now appears clear that iron deficiency contributes to adverse pregnancy outcomes, with higher rates of premature delivery and perinatal mortality in the iron-deficient population. Impaired immune responses, gastrointestinal abnormalities, changes in epidermal appendages, impaired thermogenesis, altered thyroid metabolism, and changes in catecholamine turnover have also been observed in subjects with iron deficiency (Baynes, 1994).

Treatment and Prevention

Treatment of the individual subject with iron deficiency is obviously appropriate, but a search for the cause of the iron deficiency should also be undertaken (Baynes and Cook, 1995). In populations with a low incidence of iron deficiency, identification and treatment of individuals are most appropriate. In most cases, the problem of iron deficiency is correctable with orally administered ferrous iron salts. Side effects of iron supplement ingestion frequently limit compliance, but these side effects may be dramatically reduced by a recently developed formulation of iron that allows for slow release of iron over a number of hours within the stomach. This formulation relies on the use of a matrix that keeps the iron close to the surface of the gastric contents (Simmons et al., 1993).

In populations with a very high prevalence of iron deficiency, the appropriate prevention strategy involves a pilot unscreened therapeutic supplementation trial. If the program is shown to be successful, then it should be rapidly translated into a regional or national program. Recent suggestions have raised the possibility that a weekly supplement may facilitate better compliance and obtain reasonable efficacy compared with daily supplementation; these suggestions are predicated in part on the notion, derived from rat data, that continuous intake is inhibitory to absorption (Fairweather-Tait et al., 1985; Viteri et al., 1995). Recent human absorption data refute this suggestion and confirm the advantage of daily supplementation (Cook and Reddy, 1995).

In regions of intermediate prevalence, one or two intervention strategies appear appropriate. These should take the form of either a pilot fortification trial or a pilot prophylactic unscreened supplementation program. If successful, these should be extended regionally. Surveillance of population iron status should be undertaken to guard against the production of excessive positive iron balance.

In populations in whom the prevalence of iron deficiency is low, a public health initiative aimed at improving overall iron nutrition is inappropriate. The only appropriate activity should be the screening of high-risk groups, such as infants, pregnant women, and trained athletes, and therapeutic supplementation of individuals who are identified as being iron-deficient. Indeed, if it appears that population iron status is increasing above putative normal values, consideration should be given to reducing the levels of iron fortification and supplementation.

IRON EXCESS

There are a number of well-recognized situations of iron overload. The best defined of these is hereditary hemochromatosis. This disorder is autosomally recessively inherited. By positional cloning (Feder et al., 1996), and gene "knock out" experiments (Rothenberg and Voland, 1996; Santos et al., 1996), the putative hemochromatosis gene appears to have been identified. The putative gene is localized on chromosome 6 and encodes a major histocompatibility complex class I-like molecule. Mutations of this gene appear to be found consistently in subjects with this iron-loading condition. Although initially designated HLA-H, this designation had already been used for a previously identified pseudogene, and consequently the hemochromatosis gene has been assigned the name HFE by the nomenclature committee. An antibody raised to a deduced peptide sequence in the HFE protein product has been used to demonstrate by immunohistochemistry that HFE protein is present in mucosal cells of the gastrointestinal tract (Parkkila et al., 1997). The biochemical identification and characterization of the structure and function of the protein product of the HFE gene remain to be accomplished.

In hemochromatosis, iron is absorbed in excess of requirements, leading to transferrin hypersaturation and the accumulation of significant concentrations of nonprotein-bound iron in the circulation. This leads to progressive parenchymal iron loading, resulting in the well-recognized clinical complications of cardiomyopathy, diabetes mellitus, endocrinopathy (other endocrine abnormalities, particularly of pituitary and sex hormones), arthritis, cutaneous pigmentation, liver cirrhosis, and liver cancer. The mechanism by which iron causes organ damage is uncertain, but lipid peroxidation and fibrogenesis appear to be important contributory factors. The frequency of hereditary hemochromatosis in white populations is roughly 3 per 1000, with a high heterozygous carrier rate of about 10% to 15% of the population. The precise metabolic basis of the disease remains to be elucidated, but iron overload is more likely to be manifested in areas of high iron intake and particularly when the dietary iron is highly bioavailable. The disease is in large measure reversible by removal of body iron by phlebotomy therapy (removal of blood over time).

Iron overload with similar organ damage is well recognized in patients suffering from such hemoglobinopathies as β-thalassemia major and who are generally dependent upon frequent blood transfusions. The blood transfusions, along with the increased iron absorption observed in these conditions, lead to a massive increase in body iron content and eventually to saturation of the normal iron carrier proteins and the presence of nontransferrin-bound iron in the circulation, and ultimately to iron loading of tissues and consequent tissue damage. The ravages of iron overload can be ameliorated by iron chelation therapy and significantly reversed by such treatment modalities as allogeneic bone marrow transplantation. In this treatment, the hematopoietic stem cells of the patient are eradicated and replaced with normal stem cells from an HLA-matched donor.

A number of recent publications have suggested that even relatively modest increases in iron status may place subjects at risk for development of occlusive coronary artery disease. In this regard, positive correlations between myocardial infarction and serum ferritin (Salonen et al., 1992) and between myocardial infarction and food iron intake (Ascherio et al., 1994), along with a negative relationship between iron-binding capacity and myocardial infarction (Magnusson et al., 1994), have been documented. It is well known that there is a strong inverse correlation between serum iron-binding capacity and serum ferritin. Although at least 7 epidemiological studies have reported a positive correlation between iron status and ischemic heart disease, 18 studies have failed to confirm the finding (Meyers, 1996).

A recent prospective evaluation of carotid atherosclerosis showed not only that iron status was a significant risk factor but also that in combination with serum LDL it was even more significant (Kiechl et al., 1997). This suggests a possible role for iron in increasing the atherogenic potential of LDL. An association has also been reported between modest increases in body iron status and the occurrence of cancer (Nelson et al., 1994; Stevens et al., 1994). These studies are at this time primarily epidemiological rather than mechanistic. It remains to be conclusively determined whether iron status is an independent risk factor and not merely a surrogate marker of particular dietary patterns. The mechanism by which iron status may relate to these disease states also requires further definition. These reservations, however, do not negate the observations.

Of even greater concern in this regard is the appearance of a progressive increase in the iron nutritional status of the American population as determined by comparisons be-

LIFE CYCLE CONSIDERATION

Iron Overload

Iron overload can result in the impairment of organ structure and function from the excessive deposition of iron in parenchymal cells of the organ. Hereditary hemochromatosis results from homozygosity for a recessive HLA-linked gene on chromosome 6 and is limited largely to people of European origin. Homozygote frequencies are estimated to be between 1 in 100 and 1 in 1000, with about 5% to 20% of the population being heterozygotes for the HLA-linked iron-loading gene. This abnormality leads to absorption of more iron than is required (a greater rate of iron absorption than is appropriate, given the body stores); the amount of iron absorbed in excess of requirements is only a few milligrams per day, but over a number of years, this can result in an increase in iron stores to 20 to 50 times the normal levels, representing the accumulation of 20 to 40 g of surplus iron.

Because of interactions of genetics with iron supply and needs, phenotypic expression of this disorder is rare in populations where iron deficiency is prevalent (due to lack of bioavailable iron in the diet), is encountered about ten times more frequently in men than in women (owing to greater losses by women due to menstruation and pregnancy), and is typically diagnosed after the age of 40 years, with age at onset being younger in men than in women (Bothwell et al., 1995).

The earliest biochemical signs of iron overload are elevations in the plasma iron concentration, a high plasma transferrin saturation, and elevated plasma ferritin concentrations. As iron stores enlarge, hemosiderin deposits become more prominent in the liver; examination of liver biopsy specimens from patients with hereditary hemochromatosis reveals that the hepatocytes (parenchymal cells) are loaded with hemosiderin while the Kupffer cells are relatively free of stored iron. Organ damage occurs only after the concentrations of stored iron are grossly elevated, but this damage is largely irreversible. Early diagnosis and treatment are essential to avoid tissue damage. Repeated venesection (e.g., the removal of 500 mL of blood, which contains 200 to 250 mg of iron, each week over a period of 2 to 3 years) to remove the excess iron, followed by less frequent venesections to prevent reaccumulation, is the usual treatment.

A picture resembling hemochromatosis may also be caused by iron-loading anemias. These iron-loading anemias include thalassemia major and certain other hereditary anemias in which erythropoiesis is ineffective. Thalessemia major occurs in patients who are homozygous for mutations that lead to a decrease in β globin synthesis, which in turn leads to deficient hemoglobin synthesis and the accumulation of α globin chains in the bone marrow. Iron overload occurs in these patients as a consequence of enhanced absorption of iron and of essential treatment of the anemia with multiple blood transfusions. In these chronic hyperplastic anemias, the iron deposition occurs in both reticuloendothelial and parenchymal cells, and organ damage tends to develop as parenchymal loading proceeds. Treatment of iron overload in these patients is by chelation therapy.

Another cause of iron overload is largely of dietary origin and has been observed only in sub-Saharan Africa. This unique type of iron overload is related to the consumption of indigenous beers that are brewed in iron containers and that contain approximately 15 to 40 mg of iron/L. Large quantities of this beer are consumed by many men; it is estimated that an additional 50 to 100 mg of iron in a highly available form are ingested each day. This type of iron overload results in hemosiderin deposits in reticuloendothelial cells throughout the body and, with advanced disease, in the parenchymal cells of the liver. More recent data have suggested that a genetic component also contributes to this form of iron overload (Gordeuk et al., 1992).

Thinking Critically

1. What effect would blood removal or chelation therapy over an extended period of time ($\approx$1 year) have on plasma iron concentration, transferrin saturation, total iron binding capacity, and plasma ferritin levels?

2. Would you expect the prevalence of symptomatic hemochromatosis to increase or decrease with introduction of an iron-fortification program or an increase in the intake of bioavailable iron? Why?

tween HANES II, Hispanic HANES, and HANES III. The increases appear to be greater than can be accounted for by methodological differences among studies, and at this time the prudent course appears to be a very conservative approach to the use of iron fortification and supplementation in developed regions of the world.

REFERENCES

Aisen, P. (1989) Physical biochemistry of the transferrins. In: Iron Carriers and Iron Proteins (Loehr, T. M., Gray, H. B., Lever, H. B. P., eds.). VCH Publishers, Weinheim, Germany.

Ascherio, A., Willet, W. C., Rimm, E. B., Giovannucci, E. L. and Stampfer, M. J. (1994) Dietary iron intake and risk of coronary disease among men. Circulation 89:969–974.

Baker, E. N. and Lindley, P. F. (1992) New perspectives on the structure and function of transferrins. J Inorg Biochem 47:147–160.

Baynes, R. D. (1994) Iron deficiency. In: Iron Metabolism (Brock, J. H., Halliday, J. W., Pippard, M. J. and Powell, L. W., eds.), pp. 190–218. W. B. Saunders, London.

Baynes, R. D. (1996) Assessment of iron status. Clin Biochem 29:209–215.

Baynes, R. D. and Cook, J. D. (1995) Iron deficiency anemia. In: Current Therapy in Hematology-Oncology (Brain, M. C., Carbone, P. O., eds.), 5th ed., pp. 57–61. Mosby Press, Philadelphia.

Baynes, R. D., Cook, J. D. and Keith, J. (1995) Interleukin-II enhances gastrointestinal absorption of iron. Br J Haematol 91:230–233.

Baynes, R. D., Shih, Y. J. and Cook, J. D. (1994a) Mechanism of production of the serum transferrin receptor. Adv Exp Med Biol 356:61–68.

Baynes, R. D., Skikne, B. S. and Cook, J. D. (1994b) Circulating transferrin receptors and assessment of iron status. J Nutr Biochem 5:322–330.

Beinert, H., Holm, R. H. and Munck, E. (1997) Iron-sulfur clusters: Nature's modular, multipurpose structures. Science 277:653–659.

Binder, R., Horowitz, J. A., Basilion, J. P., Koeller, D. M., Klausner, R. D. and Harford, J. B. (1994) Evidence that the pathway of transferrin receptor mRNA degradation involves an endonucleolytic cleavage within the 3' UTR and does not involve poly (A) tail shortening. EMBO J 13:1969–1980.

Bothwell, T. H., Baynes, R. D., MacFarlane, B. J. and MacPhail, A. P. (1989) Nutritional iron requirements and food iron absorption. J Intern Med 226:357–365.

Bothwell, T. H., Charlton, R. W. and Motulsky, A. G. (1995) Hemochromatosis. In: The Metabolic and Molecular Bases of Inherited Disease (Scriver, C. R., Beaudet, A. L., Sly, W. S. and Valle, D., eds.), 7th ed., vol. II, pp. 2237–2269. McGraw-Hill, New York.

Centers for Disease Control and Prevention (1998) Recommendations to Prevent and Control Iron Deficiency in the United States. MMWR 47 (No. RR-3):1–29.

Conrad, M. E., Umbreit, J. N., Peterson, R. D. A., Moore E. G. and Harper, K. P. (1993) Function of integrin in duodenal mucosal uptake of iron. Blood 81:517–521.

Cook, J. D., Dassenko, S. A. and Lynch, S. R. (1991) Assessment of the role of nonheme iron availability in iron balance. Am J Clin Nutr 54:717–722.

Cook, J. D. and Reddy, M. B. (1995) Efficacy of weekly compared with daily iron supplementation. Am J Clin Nutr 62:117–120.

Cook, J. D., Skikne, B. and Baynes, R. (1996) The use of the serum transferrin receptor for the assessment of iron status. In: Iron Nutrition in Health and Disease (Hallberg, L. and Nils-Georg, A., eds.), pp. 49–58. John Libbey, London.

Fairweather-Tait, S. J., Swindell, T. E. and Wright, A. J. (1985) Further studies in rats on the influence of previous iron intake on the estimation of bioavailability of Fe. Br J Nutr 54:79–86.

Feder, J. N., Gnirke, A., Thomas, W., Tsuchihashi, Z., Ruddy, D. A., Basava, A., Dormishian, F., Domingo, R., Ellis, M. C., Fullan, A., Hinton, L. M., Jones, N. L., Kimmel, B. E., Kronmal, G. S., Lauer, P., Lee, V. K., Loeb, D. B., Mapa, F. A., McClelland, E., Meyer, N. C., Mintier, G. A., Moeller, N., Moore, T., Morikang, E. and Wolff, R. K. (1996) A novel MHC class I-like gene is mutated in patients with hereditary hemochromatosis. Nat Genet 13:399–408.

Finch, C. (1994) Regulators of iron balance in humans. Blood 84:1697–1702.

Fleming, M. D., Trenor, C. C., Su, M. A., Foernzler, D., Beier, D. R., Dietrich, W. F. and Andrews, N. C. (1997) Microcytic anemia mice have mutation in Nramp2, a candidate iron transport gene. Nat Genet 16:383–385.

Frausto da Silva, J. J. R. and Williams, R. J. P. (1991) The Biological Chemistry of the Elements. The Inorganic Chemistry of Life. Oxford University Press, Inc., New York.

Gordeuk, V., Mukiibi, J., Hasstedt, S. J., Samowitz, W., Edwards, C. Q., West, G., Ndambire, S., Emmanual, J., Neal, N., Chapanduka, Z., Randall, M., Boone, P., Romano, P., Martell, R. W., Yamashita, T., Effler, P. and Brittenham, G. (1992) Iron overload in Africa. Interaction between a gene and dietary iron content. N Engl J Med 326:95–100.

Harris, Z. L., Takahashi, Y., Miyajima, J., Serizawa, M., MacGillivray, R. T. A. and Gitlin, J. D. (1995) Aceruloplasminemia: Molecular characterization of this disorder of iron metabolism. Proc Natl Acad Sci USA 92:2539–2543.

Harrison, P. M., Clegg, G. A. and May, K. (1980) Ferritin structure and function. In: Iron in Biochemistry in Medicine II (Jacobs, A. and Worwood, M., eds.), pp. 131–171. Academic Press, London.

Harrison, P. M. and Arosio, P. (1996) The ferritins: Molecular properties, iron storage function, and cellular regulation. Biochim Biophys Acta 1275:161–203.

Kiechl, S., Williet, J., Egger, G., Poewe, W. and Oberhollenzer, F. (1997) Body iron stores and the risk of carotid atherosclerosis: Prospective results from the Bruneck study. Circulation 96:3300–3307.

Klausner, R. D., Rouault, T. A. and Harford, J. B. (1993) Regulating the fate of mRNA. Cell 72:19–28.

Lynch, S. R. and Baynes, R. D. (1996) Deliberations and evaluations of the approaches, endpoints, and paradigms for iron dietary recommendations. J Nutr 126(Suppl):2404S–2409S.

Magnusson, M. K., Sigfusson, N., Sigvaldason, H., Johannesson, G. M., Magnusson, S. and Thorgeirsson, G. (1994) Low iron binding capacity as a risk factor for myocardial infarction. Circulation 89:102–108.

Meyers, D. G. (1996) The iron hypothesis—does iron cause atherosclerosis? Clin Cardiol 19:925–929.

Morgan, E. H. (1981) Transferrin, biochemistry, physiology, and clinical significance. Mol Aspects Med 4:3–123.

Morgan, E. H. (1996) Cellular iron processing. J Gastroenterol Hepatol 11:1027–1030.

National Research Council (1989) Recommended Dietary Allowances, 10th ed. National Academy Press, Washington, D.C.

Nelson, R. L., Davis, F. G., Sutter, E., Sobin, L. H., Kikendall, J. W. and Bowen, P. (1994) Body iron stores and risk of colonic neoplasia. J Natl Cancer Inst 86:455–460.

Nordlund, P., Sjoberg, B.-M. and Eklund, H. (1990) Three-dimensional structure of the free radical protein of ribonucleotide reductase. Nature 345:593–598.

Parkkila, S., Waheed, A., Britton, R. S., Feder, J. N., Tsuchihashi, Z., Schatzman, R. C., Bacon, B. R. and Sly, W. S. (1997) Immunohistochemistry of HLA-H, the protein defective in patients with hereditary hemochromatosis, reveals unique pattern of expression in gastrointestinal tract. Proc Natl Acad Sci USA 94:2534–2539.

Reddy, M. B. and Cook, J. D. (1993) Absorption of non-heme iron in ascorbic acid–deficient rats. J Nutr 124:882–887.

Rothenberg, B. E. and Voland, J. R. (1996) Beta-2 knockout mice develop parenchymal iron overload: A putative role for class I genes of the major histocompatibility complex in iron metabolism. Proc Natl Acad Sci USA 93:1529–1534.

Rouault, T. A., Haile, D., Downey, W. E., Philpott, C. C., Tang, C., Samaniego, F., Chin, J., Orloff, D., Harford, J. B. and Klausner, R. D. (1992) Biometals 5:131–140.

Salonen, J. T., Nyyssonen, K., Korpela, H., Tuomilehto, J., Seppanen, R., Salonen, R. (1992) High stored iron levels are associated with excess risk of myocardial infarction in Eastern Finnish men. Circulation 86:803–811.

Santos, M., Schilham, M. W., Rademakers, L. H., Marx, J. J., deSousa, M. and Clevers, H. (1996) Defective iron homeostasis in beta 2-microglobulin knockout mice recapitulates hereditary hemachromatosis in man. J Exp Med 184:1975–1985.

Shanklin, J., Whittle, E. and Fox, B. G. (1994) Eight histidine residues are catalytically essential in a membrane-associated iron enzyme, stearoyl-CoA desaturase, and are conserved in alkane hydroxylase and xylene monooxygenase. Biochemistry 33:12787–12794.

Simmons, W. K., Cook, J. D., Bingham, K. C., Thomas, M., Jackson, J., Jackson, M., Ahluwalia, M., Khan, S. G. and Patterson, A. W. (1993) Evaluation of a gastric delivery system for iron supplementation in pregnancy. Am J Clin Nutr 58:622–626.

Stevens, R. G., Graubard, B. I., Micozzi, M. S., Meriishi, K. and Blumberg, B. S. (1994) Moderate elevation of body iron level and increased risk of cancer occurrence and death. Int J Cancer 56:364–369.

Sweeney, W. V. and Rabinowitz, J. C. (1980) Proteins containing 4Fe-4S clusters: An overview. Annu Rev Biochem 49:139–161.

Teichmann, R. and Stremmel, W. (1990) Iron uptake by human upper small intestine by a membrane iron-binding protein. J Clin Invest 86:2145–2153.

Testa, U., Pelosi, E. and Peschle, C. (1993) The transferrin receptor. Crit Rev Oncogen 4:241–276.

Theil, E. C. (1993) The IRE (iron regulatory element) family: Structures which regulate mRNA translation or stability. Biofactors 4:87–93.

Thelander, L. and Graslund, A. (1994) Ribonucleotide reductase in mammalian systems. In: Metal Ions in Biological Systems (Siegel, H. and Sigel, A., eds.), Vol. 30, pp. 109–129. Marcel Dekker, New York.

Viteri, F. E., Xunian, L., Tolomei, K. and Martin, A. (1995) True absorption and retention of supplemental iron is more efficient when iron is administered every three days rather than daily to iron-normal and iron-deficient rats. J Nutr 125:82–91.

RECOMMENDED READINGS

Bothwell, T. H., Charlton, R. W., Cook, J. D. and Finch, C. A. (1979) Iron Metabolism in Man. Blackwell Scientific Publications, Oxford, United Kingdom.

Brock, J. H., Halliday, J. W., Pippard, M. J. and Powell, L. W. (1994) Iron Metabolism. W. B. Saunders, London.

Jacobs, A. and Worwood, M. (1980) Iron in Biochemistry and Medicine, II. Academic Press, London.

CHAPTER 32

◆ ◆

Zinc, Copper, and Manganese

James C. Fleet, Ph.D.

OUTLINE

THE ROLE OF ZINC, COPPER, AND MANGANESE IN ENZYME SYSTEMS

Copper (Cu), zinc (Zn), and manganese (Mn) are chemically classified as transition elements in the periodic table. Using a broad definition, transition elements are those that have partially filled *d* or *f* subshells in any of their common oxidation states. Because the *d* orbitals of zinc are completely filled, zinc does not fit this common definition of a transition element. However, like copper, manganese, and the other transition elements, zinc has the ability to form complexes in which the metal serves as a central atom (a Lewis acid) that is surrounded by several Lewis bases (usually amino acids in biological systems), as shown in Figure 32–1. As a result, the functions of copper, zinc, and manganese are closely associated with their binding to biological ligands, particularly in enzyme systems. Table 32–1 lists a number of zinc, copper and manganese-dependent enzymes. Because over 200 zinc-containing metalloenzymes with at least 20 distinct biological functions have been identified in various species,

Simplest Terms: Acid + Base – – – – – – – –▶ Complex

Generalized: e⁻ Acceptor + e⁻ Donor – – – –▶ Complex
Lewis Acid   Lewis Base

Specific: Metal Ion + Ligand – – – – – –▶ Metal Ligand
  Zn²⁺   Amino   Complex
       Acid

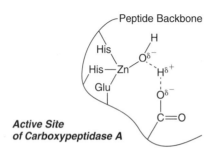

*Active Site
of Carboxypeptidase A*

Figure 32–1. *Metal-ligand complex formation. The biological roles of minerals like copper, zinc, or manganese frequently depend on their interaction with biological ligands such as amino acids in proteins. These interactions are defined by the chemistry of the mineral. This is illustrated in the figure using the general chemical principles of Lewis acid-base theory.*

the metalloenzyme function is particularly associated with zinc. However, the metalloenzyme function is central to our understanding of the biology of copper, zinc, and manganese, and the loss of specific metalloenzyme function may account for the symptoms that we associate with deficiencies of these three metals.

In general, metals can be classified based on four general biological roles: signaling, structural, catalytic, and regulatory. The last three roles relate directly to the functions of metals in proteins and enzyme systems. What makes zinc, copper, and manganese so useful in enzyme systems? Some general guidelines that one can follow to assess the likelihood that a mineral will fit a particular biological role include (1) the charge of the ion (determines the stability and reactivity of the metal in an enzyme), (2) the size of the atom (limits the sites a metal can fit), and (3) the natural abundance of a metal and its natural location within a cell (e.g., cytosolic vs. extracellular localization will define the likelihood of incorporation into specific enzymes) (Glusker, 1991).

When the chemical features of zinc are examined, it becomes apparent why this metal is so prevalent in proteins and enzyme systems. First, with the exception of potassium (K^+) and magnesium (Mg^{2+}), zinc is the most common intracellular metal ion. It is found in the cytosol, in vesicles and organelles, and in the nucleus. Thus, it is in the correct proximity to be incorporated into many cellular enzymes. Next, zinc's flexible coordination geometry makes it ideal for the active site of enzymes. One hypothesis regarding metalloenzymes is that the active site of metalloenzymes is "poised for catalysis," a condition called the entatic state (Vallee and Galdes, 1984).

Researchers have defined the entatic state as the condition in which the geometry of the metal binding site in an enzyme is distorted and asymmetrical (Fig. 32–2). When this strain is released by allowing the metal binding site to return to a less distorted form, the energy released may contribute to lowering the energy of activation of the enzymatic reaction. Theoretically, this permits a faster, more efficient enzymatic reaction. Because

TABLE 32–1
Vertebrate Enzymes Containing or Activated by Copper, Zinc, or Manganese

Enzyme	Function	Role of Metal
Copper		
Lysyl oxidase	Collagen synthesis	Catalytic
Peptidylglycine α-amidating monooxygenase	Neuropeptide synthesis	Catalytic
Superoxide dismutase (cytosolic and extracellular)	O_2^- to H_2O_2	Catalytic
"Ferroxidase"/ceruloplasmin	Release of stored iron	Catalytic
Cytochrome c oxidase	Oxidative phosphorylation	Catalytic
Dopamine β-hydroxylase	Neurotransmitter synthesis	Catalytic
Tyrosine oxidase	Melanin synthesis	Catalytic
Zinc		
Alcohol dehydrogenase	Alcohol metabolism	Catalytic, noncatalytic
Superoxide dismutase (cytosolic)	O_2^- to H_2O_2	Noncatalytic
Superoxide dismutase (extracellular)	O_2^- to H_2O_2	Noncatalytic
Terminal deoxynucleotide transferase	Add dNTPs to 3' end of DNA	?
Alkaline phosphatase	Bone formation	Catalytic, noncatalytic
5'-Nucleotidase	Hydrolysis of 5'-nucleotides	?
Fructose 1,6-bisphosphatase	Glycolysis	Regulatory
Aminopeptidase	Protein digestion	Catalytic, regulatory
Angiotensin-converting enzyme	Angiotensin I to II	Catalytic
Carboxypeptidase A and B	Protein digestion	Catalytic
Neutral protease	Protein digestion	Catalytic
Collagenase	Collagen breakdown	Catalytic
Carbonic anhydrase	$CO_2 \rightarrow HCO_3^-$	Catalytic
δ-Aminolevulinic acid dehydratase	Heme biosynthesis	Catalytic
Manganese		
Arginase	Urea formation	Catalytic
Pyruvate carboxylase	Gluconeogenesis	Catalytic
Superoxide dismutase (mitochondrial)	O_2^- to H_2O_2	Catalytic
Farnesyl pyrophosphate synthetase	Cholesterol synthesis	Catalytic
Glycosyltransferases	Cartilage formation	Regulatory
Phosphoenolpyruvate carboxylase	Gluconeogenesis	Regulatory
Xylosyltransferase	Cartilage formation	Regulatory

zinc has several possible coordination geometries, and because the coordination geometry is easily distorted, zinc can sit in this proposed "entatic" state. Finally, zinc is a strong Lewis acid (only copper is better), and the presence of a strong Lewis acid like zinc at an active site can supply a hydroxyl group (OH^-) that may be important for many enzymatic reactions (see Fig. 32–1). This is accomplished when zinc uses water as a fourth ligand (the other three being amino acids in the enzyme). The hydroxyl group results when the water molecule forms a partial dipole that is loosely associated with zinc and with a negatively charged group in the enzyme (e.g., a carboxyl group from aspartate).

Like zinc, manganese and copper can supply the hard base, OH^-, for enzymatic reactions when they are present in the active sites of enzymes. However, they have the ad-

vantage over zinc when redox reactions are required. Whereas manganese (Mn^{2+}, Mn^{3+}, Mn^{7+}) and copper (Cu^{1+}, Cu^{2+}) have multiple valence states and can cycle between them as part of an enzymatic reaction, zinc has only one common valence state (Zn^{2+}) and cannot function in these situations. For example, Zn^{2+} serves a structural role in cytosolic and extracellular Cu/Zn superoxide dismutase (SOD), whereas the catalytic reaction of SOD in detoxifying superoxide involves a redox reaction that utilizes either copper (cytosolic and extracellular Cu/Zn SODs) or manganese (mitochondrial Mn SOD).

Understanding the central role of zinc, copper, and manganese in association with proteins and enzymes also serves as a framework to explain how researchers have tried to develop functional status assessment tools that can be utilized in defining optimal di-

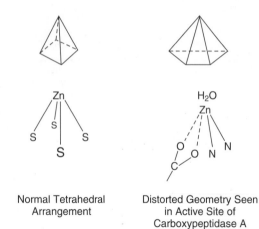

Normal Tetrahedral
Arrangement

Distorted Geometry Seen
in Active Site of
Carboxypeptidase A

Figure 32–2. *Distorted geometry of ligand binding is associated with the entatic state seen in the active site of enzymes. Zinc is shown bound to the enzyme via ligands to the sulfhydryl group of cysteinyl residues (S), the imidazole nitrogen of histidyl residues (N), or the carboxylate group of glutamyl residues (COO⁻).*

etary requirements; this will be discussed further.

REQUIREMENTS AND FOOD SOURCES OF ZINC, COPPER, AND MANGANESE

Recommended Daily Allowance for Zinc

An RDA for zinc has been estimated based upon the amount of dietary zinc needed to replace endogenous zinc losses (National Research Council, 1989). Unfortunately, endogenous zinc losses are not constant and vary with the amount of zinc consumed, so the true requirement of zinc is still uncertain. However, a sufficient number of experiments on human zinc metabolism and balance have been conducted so that these estimates are considered reliable for most people. As with all of the nutrients for which RDAs have been defined, the requirement changes during the stages of life. This is a reflection of changing body size as well as altered needs at different life stages. In the United States, people across the age spectrum have been found to have zinc intakes below the RDA. This is particularly true for elderly people, who have typical intakes of between 7 and 10 mg per day. The average intake for adults in the United States is about 13 mg per day.

Estimated Safe and Adequate Daily Dietary Intakes for Copper and Manganese

At this time insufficient evidence is available to support establishing concrete RDAs for either manganese or copper (National Research Council, 1989). Manganese balance studies suggest that for adults, an intake of between 2 and 5 mg per day is sufficient for health. This is within the estimated range of intake recorded for men in the United States and Canada. The Estimated Safe and Adequate Daily Dietary Intake (ESADDI) for copper is 1.5 to 3 mg. Available evidence suggests that most Western diets do not furnish this amount of copper; a mean intake of about 1 mg per day has been reported.

Food Sources

Zinc. Red meats, organ meats (e.g., liver), and shellfish (e.g., oysters) are generally the best dietary sources for zinc. Whole grain cereals are rich sources of zinc, but refined grain products are poor sources because the zinc is found primarily in the bran and germ. Many breakfast cereals made from refined grain products are supplemented with zinc and other nutrients during production and thus may be good sources of zinc. Nuts and legumes are also relatively good plant sources of zinc. In contrast, fruits and vegetables are generally low in zinc. Excessive intake of phytate-rich foods (e.g., some grains) is known to inhibit zinc bioavailability. Infant formulas are often supplemented with zinc, but this is up to the discretion of the producer.

Copper. As for zinc, shellfish, nuts, legumes, the bran and germ portions of grains, and liver are rich sources of copper (>0.3 mg of copper/100 g). Most meats, mushrooms, tomatoes, dried fruits, bananas, potatoes, and grapes have moderate amounts of copper (0.1 to 0.3 mg of copper/100 g). Poor sources of copper are cow's milk and dairy products, chicken, and many fish, as well as fruits and vegetables other than those just listed.

Manganese. Manganese can be found in unrefined cereals, nuts, tea, and leafy vegetables, but refined grains, meats, seafood, and dairy products are poor sources.

Food Sources of Zinc

- Seafoods, especially oysters
- Meats, especially red and organ
- Whole grain products

RDAs Across the Life Cycle

	mg/day
Infants, 0–1 y	5
Children, 1–10 y	10
Males, >10 y	15
Females, >10 y	12
Pregnant	15
Lactating	16–19

From National Research Council (1989) Recommended Dietary Allowances, 10th ed., National Academy Press, Washington, D.C.

Food Sources of Copper

- Organ meats
- Nuts

Estimated Safe and Adequate Daily Dietary Intake Across the Life Cycle

	mg copper/day
Infants, 0–0.5 y	0.4–0.6
0.5–1 y	0.6–0.7
Children, 1–3 y	0.7–1.0
4–6 y	1.0–1.5
7–10 y	1.0–2.0
11+ y	1.5–2.5
Adults	1.5–3.0

From National Research Council (1989) Recommended Dietary Allowances, 10th ed., National Academy Press, Washington, D.C.

Food Sources of Manganese

- Whole grain products
- Nuts
- Tea

**Estimated Safe and Adequate Daily Dietary Intake
Across the Life Cycle**

	mg/day
Infants, 0–0.5 y	0.3–0.6
0.5–1.0 y	0.6–1.0
Children, 1–3 y	1.0–1.5
4–6 y	1.5–2.0
7–10 y	2.0–3.0
11+ y	2.0–5.0
Adults	2.0–5.0

From National Research Council (1989) Recommended Dietary Allowances, 10th ed., National Academy Press, Washington, D.C.

ABSORPTION, TRANSPORT, STORAGE, AND EXCRETION OF ZINC, COPPER, AND MANGANESE

Humans or animals must effectively obtain and retain zinc, copper, and manganese so that these minerals may be utilized for their primary roles in enzyme systems or in other interactions with proteins and biological ligands. Despite the importance of these minerals in mammalian biology, there are still considerable gaps in our knowledge of their metabolism. Of the three metals, we know more about the metabolism of zinc and copper, whereas very little is known about manganese.

Absorption

Zinc, copper, and manganese are each absorbed throughout the length of the small intestine. Copper may also be absorbed in the stomach. Because of its length and the relatively long period that the digest spends in it, the jejunum is probably where the greatest total amounts of these minerals are absorbed. Absorption is regulated at the intestinal level for copper and zinc; this is probably also true for manganese, although evidence is limited. Absorption can be separated into a saturable, regulated portion and a nonregulated, diffu-

sional component (Fig. 32–3). Because of the existence of both carrier-mediated and nonregulated diffusional absorption of these minerals, the efficiency of absorption falls (lower fractional absorption), although the total amount of mineral entering the body increases, as the dietary level of the mineral increases. Some information is known regard-

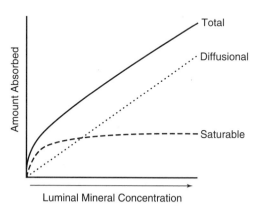

Figure 32–3. A generalized scheme of intestinal mineral absorption kinetics. Regulated intestinal mineral absorption is a combination of both diffusional processes (dotted line) and saturable processes (dashed line). The diffusional component is defined by a linear relationship between the intestinal content of the mineral and the total amount of mineral absorbed. In contrast, the saturable component varies depending upon the mineral content of the intestine. At low mineral content, this component is very effective, and at high mineral content, the saturable component plateaus.

ing the specific mechanisms of zinc and copper absorption and is described here. Little is known about the mechanism of manganese absorption, but there is some evidence that it competes with iron for a common absorption mechanism (see Chapter 31 for a discussion of iron absorption).

Energy-Dependent Zinc Absorption. The general scheme that has been used to describe intestinal transport of minerals is a three-step process including entry into the cell through the brush border membrane, movement through the cell, and extrusion from the basolateral membrane. The proposed model for zinc absorption is shown in Figure 32–4. Zinc uptake across the brush border membrane occurs both through a carrier-mediated system and by simple diffusion. The carrier-mediated mechanism predominates at low zinc content in the diet, and the number of carriers may increase under these conditions. The specific identity of the carrier has not yet been characterized, but molecular studies of patients with the genetic disease acrodermatitis enteropathica (AE) may lead researchers to this answer.

AE is caused by an autosomal recessive mutation and is characterized by symptoms normally associated with severe zinc deficiency. Symptoms include dermatitis, alopecia, poor growth, immune deficiencies, hypogonadism, night blindness, impaired taste, and diarrhea. Studies have shown that a pri-

mary defect in AE patients is reduced intestinal zinc absorption. Other studies have shown that cellular zinc uptake is reduced in intestinal biopsies and in cultured fibroblasts of AE patients (Grider and Young, 1996). This suggests that the genetic defect in AE is a mutated gene for the brush border zinc carrier. An alternative model to explain the reduction of zinc absorption with AE describes the defect as the absence of a low molecular weight zinc-binding factor. This binding factor is proposed to be produced by the pancreas and would bind to zinc and transport it into the enterocyte. Researchers suggest that this factor is present in breast milk, because human breast milk has been known to overcome the low efficiency of zinc absorption and to ameliorate AE. It is not clear at this time whether either of the models will explain the genetic mutation in AE.

The extrusion of zinc from the enterocyte is thought to be by a carrier-dependent ATP-driven mechanism (e.g., a specific Zn^{2+} ATPase). Like the brush border carrier, the identity of the basolateral Zn^{2+} pump has not been established. However, two transporters have recently been cloned that may function in cellular Zn^{2+} transport. The first is a plasma membrane Zn^{2+} transporter called ZnT-1 that is proposed to be responsible for cellular Zn^{2+} extrusion (Palmiter and Findley, 1995; McMahon and Cousins, 1997). (A related transporter, ZnT-2, transports Zn^{2+} into intracellular vesicles and may protect cells from zinc toxic-

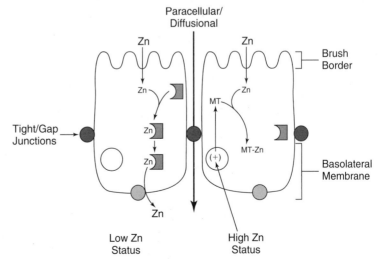

Figure 32–4. A proposed model for intestinal zinc absorption under conditions of high and low zinc status. In this model, the diffusional component of transport is shown as movement of zinc between the cells (paracellular transport), and the regulated, saturable component is shown as the movement through the cells (transcellular transport). The right side of the figure illustrates how zinc absorption may be limited when zinc status is high by induction of metallothionein synthesis and the resulting increased binding of zinc by metallothionein, which results in increased retention of zinc in the enterocyte.

ity by facilitating the movement of zinc into endosomes/lysosomes.) The other transporter is an iron transporter named NRAMP2 or DCT1 that has affinity for Zn^{2+} and other divalent cations and is believed to transport iron (Fe^{2+}) and other divalent metals into cells (Gruenheid et al., 1995; Gunshin et al., 1997). Further study of these transporters, including their location and regulation, is needed to establish their roles in Zn^{2+} transport.

Inhibition of Intestinal Zinc and Copper Absorption by Metallothionein. At low zinc status, transcellular zinc absorption is at its most efficient; at high zinc status, zinc absorption is inhibited. Research suggests that this downregulation of zinc absorption is due to the production of metallothionein, a zinc-binding protein. Metallothionein is a low molecular weight protein (6.1 kDa) found in the cell cytosol, and it is produced in response to high levels of dietary zinc or copper, as well as toxic heavy metals such as cadmium (Cd^{2+}) and mercury (Hg^{2+}) (Cousins, 1985). (See later for potential nonintestinal functions of metallothionein.) It has been proposed that high levels of metallothionein in enterocytes act as a mucosal block by binding zinc and preventing its movement through the cell, thus limiting absorption. The "blocked" metal is later lost from the body as the enterocyte is sloughed off into the intestine. The induced production of metallothionein by copper may also serve to downregulate copper absorption by this same mechanism.

Some studies have shown that high levels of zinc can inhibit intestinal copper absorption; this observation has been used to reduce copper absorption and help minimize the copper toxicity that is characteristic of Wilson's disease. (See later for more details about Wilson's disease.) One possible explanation for this copper-zinc antagonism is that the high zinc diet stimulates the production of metallothionein, which then causes the reduction in copper absorption by serving as a block to transcellular transport. In contrast, high levels of dietary copper, although they induce metallothionein, do not reduce zinc absorption. This may be due to the fact that copper has a higher affinity for metallothionein than does zinc, so that the copper bound

to metallothionein is not displaced by zinc and zinc absorption is not impeded. Another possible explanation for the copper-zinc antagonism is that copper and zinc compete for a common brush border membrane transporter.

The actual proteins that mediate the movement of zinc, copper, and manganese across the cytosol from the brush border membrane to the basolateral membrane have not been discovered. A Zn^{2+}-binding protein, cysteine-rich intestinal protein (CRIP), was proposed as an intracellular zinc ferry [analogous to the intestinal calcium (Ca^{2+})-binding protein calbindin D_{9K}] (Hempe and Cousins, 1992). However, CRIP is found in many tissues other than intestine, is not regulated by zinc status, and appears to be more intimately associated with changes in differentiation than with zinc absorption.

Bioavailability. Just as the biological roles of copper, zinc, and manganese are defined by their chemical interactions with ligands, so are their interactions with dietary components. These interactions can influence how well copper, zinc, or manganese is absorbed from the diet, but the luminal interactions leading to increased or decreased absorption are less well characterized than those for ligand interactions of copper, zinc, and manganese with enzymes (Lonnerdal and Sandstrom, 1995).

Chemical similarities with other nutrients may result in competition for common binding sites between related minerals. This could explain the inhibition of manganese absorption caused by high dietary iron, or the zinc-copper antagonism discussed earlier. Binding of minerals to organic components of the diet in the lumen of the gastrointestinal tract can alter absorption. The classic example of this is the inhibitory effect that the phosphate-rich plant compound phytate (*Myo*-inositol penta- and hexaphosphates) has on the absorption of zinc and many other minerals (e.g., copper and iron) from the diet (Torre et al., 1992). The presence of calcium and phytate together in the same meal enhances the inhibitory effect on mineral absorption due to the stabilization of phytate by calcium. Others have suggested that binding of zinc or copper to low molecular weight ligands such as amino acids (e.g., histidine) may enhance intestinal absorption, but it is not clear how this enhancement would occur. Although ascorbate enhances iron absorption, it inhibits copper absorption. The chemical effects of ascorbate on iron and copper are the same; ascorbate promotes the reduction of both metals (to Fe^{2+} and Cu^{1+}). This suggests that copper is optimally transported in the Cu^{2+} state. Dietary components can also influence other points of copper utilization. For example, high dietary molybdenum has been shown to increase urinary copper losses, and high dietary calcium increases exogenous zinc losses in the intestine.

Transport in Plasma

Once absorbed, both copper and zinc are bound primarily to albumin in the plasma and transported to the liver. After reaching the liver, zinc is repackaged and released into the circulation bound to α_2-macroglobulin. At any given time, the relative distribution of zinc in the circulation is approximately 57% bound to albumin, 40% to α_2-macroglobulin, and 3% to low molecular weight ligands such as amino acids. There is evidence that the uptake of zinc into cells is regulated. Zinc uptake seems to be carrier mediated and energy independent, but the specific mechanistic details are not known.

Once copper reaches the liver, it is incorporated into ceruloplasmin. Then the copper-ceruloplasmin complex is released into the circulation for delivery to peripheral tissues. Scientists have traditionally thought that ceruloplasmin is a critical protein in the metabolism and function of copper (Vulpe and Packman, 1995). It is a large glycoprotein of 132 kDa, which contains 6% to 7% carbohydrate and which can bind 6 atoms of copper; 90% to 95% of serum copper is bound to ceruloplasmin. Ceruloplasmin is produced in the liver, and its synthesis is regulated by copper as well as inflammatory mediators such as interleukin-1 and glucocorticoids. These and other factors associated with the acute-phase response are presumably responsible for the increase in serum copper and ceruloplasmin

that occurs following acute inflammation or infection.

In cell culture studies, the mechanism of copper uptake into cells was through the binding of ceruloplasmin-copper to a cell surface receptor (Percival and Harris, 1990). Whereas the circulating transferrin-iron complex is internalized after it binds to the transferrin receptor on the cell surface, copper is reduced and released from ceruloplasmin, at which point the copper can be taken up by the cell as the free metal. The identity of the cellular copper transport protein is not known. Paradoxically, individuals who have a genetic mutation in the ceruloplasmin gene, leading to a total lack of ceruloplasmin in the serum (i.e., aceruloplasminemia), do not have overt symptoms of copper deficiency as one might predict from the cell culture studies (Harris et al., 1995). Instead, these individuals have altered iron metabolism. This raises questions regarding the biological role of ceruloplasmin in serum copper transport.

Manganese is handled slightly differently than are copper and zinc. Following absorption, it is thought to bind to α_2-macroglobulin for delivery to the liver. Because manganese can be oxidized to the Mn^{3+} state, it can bind to transferrin for subsequent delivery to other tissues. It is not clear, however, whether this system was intended to accommodate manganese or whether the binding is simply opportunistic. Regardless, this suggests that manganese uptake into cells is by the same mechanism as iron uptake, by receptor-mediated endocytosis of the metal-transferrin complex. (See Chapter 31 for details of this process.)

Storage

When animals are fed experimental diets lacking copper, zinc, or manganese, their status rapidly declines. This suggests that there is not a storage pool of these minerals to be used during times of low intake or increased need (i.e., for the production of new metal-containing proteins and enzymes). For example, zinc can be localized in the bones under conditions of high zinc intake, but this zinc cannot be specifically mobilized to serve the needs of the organism under conditions of low zinc intake. When zinc or copper intake is high, metallothionein increases dramatically in liver, kidney, and intestine. Although metallothionein can avidly bind copper and zinc, the functional significance of this is unclear.

Metallothionein. The only serious candidate for a zinc storage protein is metallothionein. Since its discovery in 1960, experiments on the biological role of this protein have been a central feature of zinc research. Metallothionein is a low molecular weight protein of 61 amino acids, of which 20 residues are cysteinyl residues (Cousins, 1985). It is surprising that there are no disulfide bridges in metallothionein; all the thiol groups are involved in metal binding. Seven atoms of zinc or the related transition elements (cadmium, mercury, copper, and silver) have been found to bind to metallothionein in vitro. The metals are normally bound in two clusters, with one cluster binding 4 metal ions and the other binding 3. Under normal physiological conditions, zinc is the primary metal bound to metallothionein. It is unlikely that a significant amount of metal-free metallothionein exists. There are multiple isoforms of metallothionein in mammalian tissues; 4 isoforms have been identified in mice, and at least 12 metallothionein genes have been identified in humans.

Metallothionein is rapidly induced in liver, kidney, pancreas, and intestine by exposure to high levels of heavy metals, particularly zinc, copper, and cadmium. Hepatic levels of metallothionein are also directly induced by glucocorticoids and the cytokine IL-6. This accounts for the redistribution of zinc from the plasma to the liver during the acute-phase response that occurs following bacterial infection or as a result of inflammatory conditions, such as rheumatoid arthritis and intense exercise. Hepatic metallothionein levels are also elevated in the newborn infant and may serve as a short-term depot for zinc during the initial days of life.

The transcription of the metallothionein genes is mediated through regulatory elements in the promoter region of the genes. Studies have only recently elucidated how zinc promotes metallothionein gene transcription (Palmiter, 1994). Under low zinc conditions, metal-response element-binding transcription factor-1(called MTF-1) is normally bound to a zinc-sensitive inhibitor (MTI). MTI dissociates from MTF-1 in the presence of zinc, thus allowing MTF-1 to interact with the metal-response elements in the metallothionein promoter to activate transcription of the metallothionein gene.

Because metallothionein so avidly binds to zinc, researchers have tried to demonstrate a biological role for this protein in normal zinc homeostasis. This goal has been aided by the development of mice lacking or overexpressing the metallothionein genes. Transgenic mice that overexpress metallothionein I (the predominant form of the protein in mice) appear to resist dietary zinc deficiency compared with normal mice, which suggests that metallothionein functions as a repository for zinc (Dalton et al., 1996). In contrast, mice lacking the genes for metallothionein I and II (the forms found in intestine, liver, kidney, and most other cells except the brain) are born healthy and do not show any obvious symptoms of zinc deficiency when their mothers are fed a diet that contains adequate zinc (Kelly et al., 1996). However, kidney abnormalities are seen in newborn pups lacking metallothionein if their mothers are fed zinc-deficient diets while the pups are nursing. This suggests there may be a developmental role for metallothionein as a storage protein that protects the offspring when maternal zinc status is low.

Preliminary studies suggest that animals lacking metallothionein in the intestine do not reduce intestinal zinc absorption in response to high zinc status (Davis et al., 1996). This supports the proposed role of intestinal metallothionein in limiting the amount of zinc that leaves the enterocyte and enters the portal circulation. Finally, metallothionein "knockout" mice are excessively sensitive to cadmium toxicity, which supports the role of metallothionein as a heavy metal detoxification protein. Recent studies have shown that metallothionein is also essential for the redistribution of zinc from the plasma to the liver, which is characteristic of the acute-phase response.

Menkes' Syndrome and Wilson's Disease: Copper Transporting P-type ATPases. Both

Menkes' syndrome and Wilson's disease are genetic disturbances in copper metabolism (Danks, 1995; DiDonato and Sarkar, 1997). Menkes' syndrome is an X-linked recessive disorder that occurs at a rate greater than 1 in 300,000 live births and is usually fatal within 3 years after birth. It is characterized by low serum copper and ceruloplasmin levels and low copper levels in the liver and brain but markedly elevated cellular copper levels in the intestinal mucosa, muscle, spleen, and kidney. Other symptoms include abnormal ("steely") hair and progressive cerebral degeneration.

Wilson's disease has autosomal recessive inheritance and occurs with an incidence greater than 1 in 100,000 live births. The onset of Wilson's disease is much slower than that of Menkes' syndrome, and it is usually diagnosed during or after the third decade of life. As in Menkes' syndrome, serum ceruloplasmin levels are low in patients with Wilson's disease, but, in contrast to Menkes' syndrome, copper accumulates in the liver and brain. Patients with Wilson's disease appear to have a defect in the ability to excrete copper via the bile. Neurological damage and hepatic cirrhosis are end stage effects of uncontrolled Wilson's disease. If diagnosed early, patients can be treated by reducing copper intake, undergoing chelation therapy (with D-penicillamine), and taking oral zinc supplements (which will increase intestinal metallothionein and reduce copper absorption).

It now appears that both these diseases are the result of a genetic mutation in a class of genes encoding copper transporting P-type ATPases (energy-dependent copper transport proteins). Because of the difference in the etiology of the two diseases, it is thought that the ATPases impaired in Wilson's disease and Menkes' syndrome are related but not identical proteins. This has been confirmed by genetic analysis demonstrating that there is 62% amino acid sequence identity between the Menkes' and Wilson's ATPases. Mutations of either of these ATPases result in defective copper export from cells, but the defects are manifested in different tissues. The liver is affected primarily in Wilson's disease, whereas peripheral tissues are the affected sites in Menkes' syndrome. The Menkes' protein has recently been localized to the trans-Golgi network and a vesicular compartment but not to the nucleus or the plasma membrane. The subcellular localization of the Wilson's disease protein is not known. Differences in the severity of Wilson's disease among individuals suggest that the disease is not explained by a single mutation of the ATPase gene; preliminary research has borne out this conclusion. Ongoing research is expected to clarify the function of these two ATPases in copper transport.

Excretion

Under normal circumstances, very little zinc, copper, or manganese is lost through the urine or through cutaneous losses; most of the losses are through the feces. Of the endogenous fecal loss, some is from the sloughing off of intestinal cells into the intestinal lumen and is considered nonspecific. However, when dietary zinc or copper intake is high and metallothionein levels are induced, this loss can be significant. The specific loss of copper and manganese through the gastrointestinal tract is via their secretion in the bile. The incorporation of manganese into bile is thought to be very rapid. When manganese is transported into the liver, it either rapidly enters the mitochondria (where it is incorporated into mitochondrial SOD) or is sequestered into lysosomes. Lysosomal manganese is then actively transported into the bile, and it is concentrated in the gallbladder to a concentration 150-fold greater than that seen in the plasma. Almost all copper excretion is via the bile, and biliary copper appears to be complexed in such a way as to make it unavailable for reabsorption in the intestine.

Zinc excretion in urine will vary with intake but is generally below 10% of total excretion. Ninety percent of zinc excretion is through the feces; the level of actual excretion varies with dietary intake and with the zinc status of the individual. As a result, the fine tuning of zinc balance is through the fecal excretion. Although bile and gastroduodenal secretions contribute to endogenous zinc excretion, pancreatic secretions are the major contributor to endogenous zinc losses. The zinc-containing fraction of pancreatic secretions is made up of zinc-dependent enzymes, including carboxypeptidase A and B. These enzymes can be digested, and most of the zinc from them can be reabsorbed.

SELECTED FUNCTIONS OF ZINC, COPPER, AND MANGANESE

The following sections detail a few of the interesting biological functions of copper, zinc, and manganese for which mechanisms have been proposed.

Zinc-Finger Proteins As Gene Transcription Factors

Since the 1980s, a nonenzymatic role for zinc in proteins has been shown to be important in the regulation of genes. Klug coined the term zinc finger to describe the folding pattern of amino acids around zinc that he observed in the transcription factor TFIIIA (Rhodes and Klug, 1993). In this model, zinc binding to certain transcription factors results in the formation of a loop, or "finger," in the protein that permits the folded region to bind DNA sequences in the promoter region of genes (Fig. 32–5). Thus, without zinc, the tran-

scription factor cannot bind DNA and stimulate transcription of a gene. The zinc-finger motif requires 4 amino acid residues as ligands (2 cysteinyl and 2 histidyl residues) per mole of zinc. Despite the level of acceptance regarding the importance of zinc-finger proteins in biology, there are few proven instances of zinc fingers. Putative zinc-finger motifs have been observed in the primary sequences of various hormone receptors (e.g., the vitamin D receptor and thyroid hormone receptor) and various transcription factors.

Zinc Regulation of Growth

A primary feature of severe zinc deficiency in young animals and in children is slow growth. The classic observation, made over 30 years ago, was that low-zinc, high-phytate, plant-based diets stunted growth of Iranian adolescents (Reinhold, 1971). More recently, researchers have shown that low-income Hispanic children who fall in the lower growth percentiles and infants with a nutritional pattern of failure to thrive respond to zinc supplementation by growing. This suggests that mild zinc deficiency is one of the etiological factors contributing to these conditions.

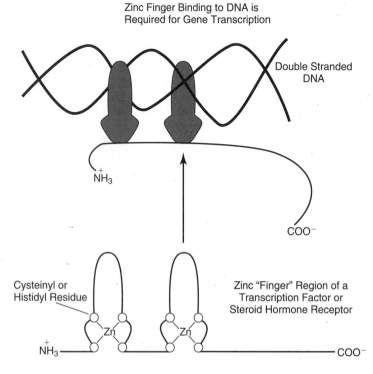

Zinc Finger Binding to DNA is Required for Gene Transcription

Double Stranded DNA

$\overset{+}{N}H_3$

COO⁻

Cysteinyl or Histidyl Residue

Zinc "Finger" Region of a Transcription Factor or Steroid Hormone Receptor

Zn   Zn

$\overset{+}{N}H_3$ ———————————————— COO⁻

Figure 32–5. *Zinc-finger proteins are important for binding of transcription factors to DNA. By binding to histidyl and cysteinyl residues in transcription factors and nuclear hormone receptors, zinc introduces a finger-like secondary structure to the proteins. This structure allows the transcription factors to interact properly with response elements in the promoters of genes.*

Zinc deficiency appears to retard growth by disrupting the function of insulin-like growth factor I (IGF-I), the factor that mediates the cellular effects of growth hormone. Studies have shown that serum IGF-I levels are reduced in zinc-deficient animals (Roth and Kirchgessner, 1994). However, normalizing serum levels of IGF-I by infusing zinc-deficient rats with IGF-I did not increase either food intake or growth, which suggests that additional points of growth regulation are also impaired (MacDonald et al., 1997). One possible mechanism is that zinc deficiency causes a reduction in the cellular levels of the IGF-I receptor (Williamson et al., 1997). Although this observation is preliminary, it is consistent with the observation that the promoter for the IGF-I receptor can be activated by a promoter-specific transcription factor (Sp1) that contains a zinc-finger DNA–binding region.

Immunoregulation by Zinc and Copper

Both zinc and copper deficiency impair immune function. Most of the work in this area has been conducted using mouse models. Studies in humans are more difficult because of the rarity of severe zinc or copper deficiency and the practical difficulties related to the identification of people with marginal zinc or copper deficiency. Nevertheless, in both animals and humans, zinc deficiency appears to reduce immune function because of an overall loss in the total numbers of lymphocytes (B and T cells) of the peripheral immune system (Walsh et al., 1994), whereas copper deficiency results in neutropenia (a lack of circulating neutrophils/granulocytes) (Percival, 1995), as well as lower numbers of T lymphocytes (Failla and Hopkins, 1997).

Preliminary evidence suggests that the loss of lymphocytes and neutrophils results from reduced production of new cells rather than from excessive or early death of existing cells. The effects that zinc deficiency has on the lymphocytes may result partially from atrophy of the thymus, an organ that controls the development of T lymphocytes, and the loss of the zinc-dependent hormone thymulin. In zinc deficiency, the proportion of T lymphocytes and B lymphocytes (and subsets of these cell types) and the functional capacity of the

lymphocytes present in zinc-deficient animals appear to be normal. Addition of copper to cultures of HL-60 cells (a promyelocytic cell line) promotes differentiation of these cells toward the granulocyte/neutrophil phenotype by enhancing the progression of the cells from promyelocytes to myelocytes. Thus, although both copper and zinc are important for optimal development of the immune system, their effects appear to be on different aspects of marrow stem cell differentiation (Fig. 32–6). Exactly how copper or zinc directly influences immune cell differentiation is not known.

Copper deficiency inhibits the proliferation of T cells (particularly the T helper or CD4+ cells) in response to mitogens. More detailed studies show that the T-cell precursors can be activated and become competent during copper deficiency. Interleukin-2 (IL-2) mediates T-cell proliferation in response to mitogens, but copper-deficient cells do not make as much IL-2 as do cells from copper-adequate animals. It is not clear how copper deficiency alters the production of IL-2.

Copper and Iron Metabolism

In addition to its proposed role as a plasma copper transport protein, ceruloplasmin also has an enzymatic function as a ferroxidase, oxidizing Fe^{2+} released from iron stores to Fe^{3+}, which can then bind to transferrin and be delivered to cells for use in processes such as heme synthesis (Fig. 32–7; see also Chapter 31). It also is possible that this ferroxidase function could be important in the plasma to help control the level of free Fe^{3+} and prevent it from initiating free radical damage. Copper is proposed to function in the catalytic site of ceruloplasmin/ferroxidase, where it exchanges electrons with iron. This ferroxidase role of ceruloplasmin was first proposed following observations of anemia in severely copper-deficient animals, which was characterized by normal hepatic iron stores (Owen, 1973). The anemia could be reversed by dietary copper but not iron. Additional data have been generated that are inconsistent with the proposed ferroxidase function of ceruloplasmin. However, researchers recently have identified individuals who lack the ability to produce ceruloplasmin and are thus

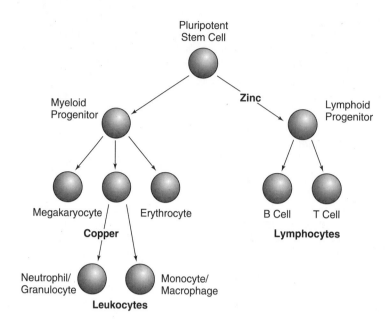

Figure 32–6. The putative sites of action for copper and zinc in immune cell differentiation. Severe copper deficiency results in reduced numbers of neutrophils, whereas severe zinc deficiency results in reduced numbers of T and B lymphocytes. This is partly due to impaired differentiation of these terminally differentiated cells from their precursors. The proposed points of action of copper and zinc on immune cell differentiation are shown in the figure.

aceruloplasminemic. These people also show signs of irregular iron metabolism with tissue deposition of iron and mild anemia, providing additional support for a role for ceruloplasmin in iron metabolism (Harris et al., 1995).

Copper in Bone and Vascular Function

Copper deficiency results in abnormal bone metabolism and skeletal abnormalities in most species. This is not due to abnormal

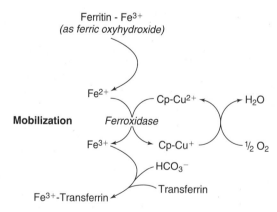

Figure 32–7. The proposed mechanism of the ferroxidase function of ceruloplasmin (Cp) in mobilizing stored iron.

calcium metabolism or mineralization of bone but occurs because the collagen matrix of bone is incompletely formed. The root cause of this defect is reduced activity of the copper-containing enzyme lysyl oxidase (Rucker et al., 1996). Lysyl oxidase is required for the removal of the ε-amino group of lysyl and hydroxylysyl residues and the oxidation of the carbon to an aldehyde, which results in the production of a variety of cross-linkages with amino acid residues in collagen. A loss of lysyl oxidase activity results in lower strength and stability of bone collagen.

The lack of the cross-linking by lysyl oxidase also affects elastin. Elastin is a protein that normally gives the aorta its needed flexibility. During copper deficiency the aorta is weakened and aortic rupture may occur. Additional cardiac abnormalities have been observed in association with copper deficiency; these include cardiac hypertrophy, altered electrocardiograms, abnormal mitochondrial structure, and reduced levels of ATP and phosphocreatine. It is not clear what aspect of copper deficiency causes these latter effects, but they are not thought to be attributable to reduced lysyl oxidase activity.

Superoxide Dismutase and Free Radical Protection

Superoxide dismutases (SODs) are part of the body's natural defense against reactive oxygen

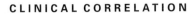

CLINICAL CORRELATION

Role of Ceruloplasmin in Iron Metabolism

Subsequent to the identification of the mutated gene responsible for Wilson's disease, it became possible to screen adult patients with neurological degeneration and low serum ceruloplasmin concentrations for molecular diagnosis of Wilson's disease. Wilson's disease is due to defective coding for a putative copper-transporting ATPase located in hepatic membranes; this transport protein is required for copper trafficking into a common pool for biliary excretion and holoceruloplasmin biosynthesis. Failure to incorporate copper during ceruloplasmin biosynthesis results in unstable ceruloplasmin that lacks oxidase activity.

As patients were referred for molecular diagnosis, it became clear that some of the patients with low or absent ceruloplasmin did not have Wilson's disease. Further molecular genetic analysis of patients with non-Wilson's disease aceruloplasminemia revealed mutations in the ceruloplasmin gene that resulted in truncation of the open reading frame. Harris et al. (1995) described one of two sisters with undetectable ceruloplasmin. This patient was homozygous for a mutation in exon 7 of the ceruloplasmin gene. She had developed degeneration of the retina and basal ganglia during the fifth decade of life. Liver biopsy revealed a normal hepatic copper concentration but elevated iron stores. Indirect evidence for iron deposition in the basal ganglia of the brain was also obtained. The association of defects in ceruloplasmin synthesis with abnormalities in iron metabolism in this and other patients confirms an essential role of ceruloplasmin in human iron metabolism and supports a role of ceruloplasmin as a ferroxidase (Harris and Gitlin, 1996). However, the major problem in patients with aceruloplasminemia seems to be excessive iron deposition or storage, with much milder problems related to iron delivery or utilization. How a plasma protein can be involved in release of iron from tissue ferritin is not yet clear.

Thinking Critically

1. Explain how a lack of ceruloplasmin could result in iron overload in liver and other tissues.

2. A low serum iron concentration and an elevated serum ferritin concentration are found in patients with defects in the ceruloplasmin gene. Anemia is seen in some but not all patients with defects in the ceruloplasmin gene. (a) Explain how each of these clinical/biochemical manifestations could result from a defect in ferroxidase activity. (b) Are these changes in measures of iron status similar to or different from the changes that would occur in iron deficiency anemia? (See Chapter 31 for more information about iron metabolism.)

3. Copper metabolism and transport seem to be relatively normal in patients with defects in ceruloplasmin synthesis. What might this tell us about the role of ceruloplasmin in copper transport in the body?

---

species. Reactive oxygen species are free radicals that, if left uncontrolled, can damage DNA, proteins, and lipids within cells and can alter or inhibit cellular function. (See the review by Halliwell [1994] for an excellent summary of this area of research.) SODs catalyze the reaction by which superoxide is removed: $2O_2^- + 2H^+ \rightarrow H_2O_2 + O_2$. The hydrogen peroxide generated is further metabolized by either catalase (an iron-containing enzyme) or glutathione peroxidase (a selenium-containing enzyme). Cytosolic Cu/Zn SOD is made up of two identical subunits, each of which contains 1 atom of copper and 1 atom of zinc. Extracellular Cu/Zn SOD is a secreted tetrameric glycoprotein that is related, but not identical, to the cytosolic form of Cu/Zn SOD. The manganese-containing SOD catalyzes the same reaction as the Cu/Zn SOD, but Mn SOD is located in the mitochondria as opposed to the cytosol or extracellular fluids. In the active site of the enzymes, copper or manganese is alternately reduced and oxidized by superoxide to produce hydrogen peroxide. Therefore, the enzyme activity is completely inhibited in the absence of these minerals. In contrast, some Cu/Zn SOD activity is retained when zinc is removed or replaced with other chemically similar metals (e.g., cadmium, mercury, or copper). Zinc may serve two functions: it may stabilize the native structure of the enzyme, and a zinc-histidyl-copper triad may act as a proton donor during the oxidation cycle of the enzyme.

The genetic overexpression of cytosolic Cu/Zn SOD or Fe-dependent catalase in the fruit fly, an insect model of aging, prolongs life, presumably due to improved protection from free radical damage (Orr and Sohal, 1994). These types of studies have provided strong support for the free radical theory of aging. Experimental evidence shows that a reduction in cytosolic or extracellular Cu/Zn SOD can also occur in animals fed zinc- or copper-deficient diets. This may have physiological consequences. For example, erythrocytes from copper-deficient animals with low cytosolic Cu/Zn SOD levels are more susceptible to lipid peroxidation and hemolysis in vitro (Rock et al., 1995). In addition, young rats fed a copper-deficient diet have lower Cu/Zn SOD activity in the lung and liver and have lower survival times when exposed to high-oxygen conditions. Collectively, these data suggest that dietary deficiencies of copper and zinc can have functional consequences related to reduced free radical defenses.

The mitochondria are the site of oxidative phosphorylation and are therefore a tremendous source of potentially hazardous reactive oxygen species and free radicals. Thus, deficiency of manganese becomes a condition of superoxide radical poisoning owing to the loss of Mn SOD activity. This can have several identifiable consequences. First, researchers have identified abnormalities in cell function and ultrastructural abnormalities in mitochondria in manganese deficiency. The mitochondrial changes (elongation and reorientation of cristae, presence of vacuoles in the matrix, separation of inner and outer mitochondrial membranes) are likely the result of observed increases in mitochondrial lipid peroxidation. Disruption of mitochondrial integrity may result in disturbed energy metabolism through disruption of oxidative phosphorylation. Man-

ganese deficiency alters carbohydrate metabolism through the destruction of pancreatic β cells. This could account for the decreased glucose utilization, reduced pancreatic insulin, and lower insulin output from perfused pancreas observed in manganese-deficient animals. Although it is not clear how manganese contributes to pancreatic β-cell abnormalities, researchers have proposed that free radical damage resulting from the lack of Mn SOD activity is a factor.

Manganese in Cartilage Formation

As with copper deficiency, skeletal abnormalities that are unrelated to impaired mineralization of bone are a characteristic of manganese deficiency. For example, in growing animals manganese deficiency results in an inhibition of endochondral osteogenesis at the growth plates/epiphyseal cartilages. This is due to a reduction in the synthesis of proteoglycans such as chondroitin sulfate (the proteoglycan affected most by manganese deficiency) (Liu et al., 1994). Proteoglycans (glycosaminoglycan-protein complexes) are essential structural components of cartilage, which explains the sensitivity of the growth plate to manganese deficiency. Chondroitin sulfate synthesis is regulated by manganese at two sites. The polymerase responsible for the polymerization of UDP-*N*-acetylgalactosamine to UDP-glucuronic acid to form the glycosaminoglycan chain requires manganese. Galactotransferase, an enzyme that catalyzes the incorporation of galactose into a galactose-galactose-xylose trisaccharide, which is required for the linkage of the polysaccharide chain to the protein associated with it, is also a manganese-requiring enzyme. Other glycosyltransferases are also activated by manganese.

In the least severe stage of manganese deficiency, animals will give birth to viable offspring, but some of the young will exhibit ataxia and loss of equilibrium. This condition is the result of a structural defect in the development of the inner ear, resulting in impaired vestibular function. As with the bone defects noted earlier, these inner ear structural defects are also the result of impaired cartilage development associated with reduced proteoglycan formation.

ASSESSMENT OF ZINC, COPPER, AND MANGANESE STATUS AND DEFICIENCY SYMPTOMS

Status Assessment

The "Holy Grail" of status assessment is the availability of a functional parameter whose activity changes with the dietary deficiency of a required nutrient. Unfortunately, there are no reliable functional assessment tools for either zinc, copper, or manganese. Researchers have examined a number of metal-dependent enzymes for their ability to serve as sensitive indicators of zinc (e.g., alkaline phosphatase, Cu/Zn SOD, 5′ nucleotidase) and copper (e.g., Cu/Zn SOD) status (Delves, 1985). Although some of these assays show promise, none has to date been proved useful. The remaining option is static assessment tools, such as mineral levels in serum, hair, and red or white blood cells.

In normal, healthy people, the plasma concentration of zinc does not appear to change except under conditions of extreme deficiency. Thus, plasma or serum zinc concentration is an inadequate measure for assessment of more subtle changes in status. The plasma zinc level does fall significantly during pregnancy, but this decrease is associated with a fall in plasma albumin concentration and an expansion of maternal blood volume. These changes may be important to the development of the fetus and the viability of the pregnancy, and it is not clear that this decline in plasma zinc indicates inadequate zinc intake during pregnancy (Swanson and King, 1983). Serum copper and ceruloplasmin have shown some utility as measures of copper status, but these measures (as well as serum zinc) are very sensitive to acute inflammation. During acute inflammation, serum zinc levels fall and serum copper and ceruloplasmin levels increase, giving the false impression that zinc status is low and copper status is high. Hair mineral levels can be a useful crude measure of long-term mineral status, but hair mineral content is sensitive to contamination from the environment (e.g., shampoos and emissions). Recently some researchers have examined erythrocyte or serum metallothionein levels as a measure of zinc status. Although extremes of zinc status can be assessed by this method, there is no indication that metallothionein concentration is useful for assessment of marginal zinc status. Lymphocyte zinc content has been shown to be more sensitive to marginal zinc intake in small, well-controlled studies. However, the association of lymphocyte zinc concentration with zinc intake has not been verified in larger groups, and the difficulty in isolating these white blood cells reduces the utility of this measure for assessing zinc status in the population. Finally, urinary excretion poorly reflects changes in intakes of zinc, copper, and manganese. Clearly, the development of reliable functional assessment tools is essential for establishing the true requirements for zinc, copper, and manganese and for defining the true health risks of inadequate intake of these minerals.

Deficiency Symptoms

Zinc. Zinc deficiency symptoms have been observed in humans in populations consuming diets high in phytate and low in meat (e.g., the classic studies of zinc deficiency in Iranian children), as well as in subjects with acrodermatitis enteropathica (AE). As a result of its occurrence in humans, zinc deficiency has been extensively studied. Many symptoms of zinc deficiency have been characterized (Table 32–2), but the underlying biochemical defects responsible for most of them have not been found. For example, loss of appetite is one of the first signs associated with specific dietary zinc inadequacy. Although this clearly contributes to the growth depression seen in zinc-deficient children, the reason for the loss of appetite is not known. This is also true for the classic symptoms of zinc deficiency, such as loss of normal taste sensation, alopecia, hyperkeratinization of skin, and reproductive abnormalities. Because of the vast array of zinc-dependent enzymes, as well as the proposed importance of the zinc-finger structure in modulating the interaction between transcription factors and DNA, it is unlikely that a single root cause will be determined for many of these conditions.

Copper. Experimental copper deficiency has

TABLE 32–2
Characteristics of Zinc, Copper, and Manganese Deficiency in Animals and Humans

Zinc	Copper	Manganese
Loss of appetite	Anemia	Poor growth
Poor growth	Skeletal defects	Abnormal bone
Alopecia	Cardiac enlargement	Impaired glucose tolerance
Immune dysfunction	Altered pigmentation	Poor reproduction
Hypogonadism	Reproductive failure	Malformations in offspring
Poor wound healing	Lower aortic elasticity	
Impaired taste acuity	Neutropenia	

helped us understand the role of copper in iron metabolism, immune function, and cartilage production. The symptoms listed for copper deficiency in Table 32–2 are all associated with either severe dietary copper deficiency or copper deficiency associated with the genetic condition called Wilson's disease. These conditions are rare in humans. In contrast, researchers have noted several symptoms (e.g., irregular heartbeat and impaired glucose utilization) that occur before the onset of severe deficiency and that may have more general relevance to human health. The degree of copper deficiency or low intake that leads to these milder symptoms is not clearly defined, but epidemiological evidence linking low serum copper levels to an elevated risk of cardiovascular disease suggests that marginal copper status may be of practical concern.

Manganese. Reduced growth is a general feature of manganese deficiency. Although food consumption does fall in manganese-deficient animals, it is not a prominent feature of the deficiency. As discussed earlier, some of the deficiency signs that have been observed for manganese can be linked to the loss of specific enzyme functions. In contrast, the cause of the disrupted reproductive ability (lower conception, increased abortion, stillbirths, lower birth weights, defective ovulation, and testicular degeneration) observed in manganese-deficient animals is unknown. Similarly, although animal studies reveal a greater susceptibility to convulsions and electroencephalogram readings reminiscent of those for epileptics, the underlying basis for these phenomena is not clearly understood.

TOXICITY OF ZINC, COPPER, AND MANGANESE

As a general rule, zinc, copper, and manganese are relatively nontoxic when consumed in the diet. Toxic exposure is most likely to result from accidental exposure or from environmental contamination.

Zinc

Manifestations of overt toxicity will occur with long-term exposure to as little as 100 to 300 mg of zinc per day (6 to 20 times the RDA). The symptoms of zinc toxicity include induced copper deficiency (characterized by anemia and neutropenia), impaired immune function, and reduction of HDL cholesterol levels. Extremely high zinc intake will cause vomiting, epigastric pain, lethargy, and fatigue.

It was recently reported that taking zinc gluconate lozenges within 24 hours of the onset of symptoms can reduce the duration of symptoms of the common cold (Mosssad et al., 1996). Although this is a potentially exciting finding, misuse of this product could result in zinc toxicity. To get the benefit of this product, users must take a lozenge containing 13.3 mg of zinc every 2 waking hours until the symptoms have been eliminated (4 to 7 days). This dose (>150 mg per day) may have toxic effects, particularly if people attempt to use the lozenges prophylactically by consuming them throughout the cold and flu season.

Copper

Under conditions of chronic overconsumption of copper, toxicity occurs only when the capacity of the liver to bind and sequester copper is exceeded. The amount of dietary copper required to cause toxicity is not well established, but gastrointestinal discomfort has been seen with intakes of as little as 5 mg of copper per day. The consequences of copper toxicity are weakness, listlessness, and anorexia in the early stages, which can progress to coma, hepatic necrosis, vascular collapse, and death.

Manganese

Manganese is considered one of the least toxic minerals. Oral toxicity is extremely rare. However, airborne manganese from industrial and automobile emissions can have serious toxic effects if exposure is high enough. Symptoms associated with manganese toxicity include pancreatitis and neurological disorders that are similar to those observed in patients with schizophrenia and Parkinson's disease. Manganese toxicity has been recently observed in children receiving long-term parenteral nutrition. In addition, the recently approved use of methylcyclopentadienyl manganese tricarbonyl as a gasoline additive in the United States has raised concerns that environmental exposure to manganese may increase in the future.

REFERENCES

Cousins, R. J. (1985) Absorption, transport, and hepatic metabolism of copper and zinc: Special reference to metallothionein and ceruloplasmin. Physiol Rev 65:238–309.

Dalton, T., Fu, K., Palmiter, R. D. and Andrews, G. K. (1996) Transgenic mice that overexpress metallothionein-I resist dietary zinc deficiency. J Nutr 126:825–833.

Danks, D. M. (1995) Disorders of copper transport. In: The Metabolic and Molecular Bases of Inherited Disease (Scriver, D. R., Beaudet, A. L., Sly, W. S. and Valle, D., eds.), vol. 2, 7th ed., pp. 2211–2235. McGraw-Hill, New York.

Davis, W., Chowrimootoo, G. F. and Seymour, C. A. (1996) Defective biliary copper excretion in Wilson's disease: The role of caeruloplasmin. Eur J Clin Invest 26:893–901.

Delves, H. T. (1985) Assessment of trace element status. Clin Endocrinol Metab 14:725–760.

DiDonato, M. and Sarkar, B. (1997) Copper transport and its alterations in Menkes and Wilson diseases. Biochim Biophys Acta 1360:3–16.

Failla, M. L. and Hopkins, R. G. (1997) Copper and immunocompetence. In: Trace Elements in Man and Animals—9: Proceedings of the Ninth International Symposium on Trace Elements in Man and Animals (Fischer, R. W. F., L'Abbe, M. R., Cockell, K. A. and Gibson, R. S., eds.), pp. 425–428. NRC Research Press, Ottawa, Canada.

Glusker, J. P. (1991) Structural aspects of metal liganding to functional groups in proteins. Adv Protein Chem 42:1–76.

Grider, A. and Young, E. M. (1996) The acrodermatitis enteropathica mutation transiently affects zinc metabolism in human fibroblasts. J Nutr 126:219–224.

Gruenheid, S., Cellier, M., Vidal, S. and Gros, P. (1995) Identification and characterization of a second mouse Nramp gene. Genomics 25:514–525.

Gunshin, H., Gunshin, Y., Berger, U., Nussberger, S., Mackenzie, B., Gollan, J. L. and Hediger, M. A. (1997) Expression cloning of an iron transporter (lDCT1) in rat duodenum. FASEB J 11:A453.

Halliwell, B. (1994) Free radicals and antioxidants: A personal view. Nutr Rev 52:253–265.

Harris, Z. L. and Gitlin, J. D. (1996) Genetic and molecular basis for copper toxicity. Am J Clin Nutr 63:836S–841S.

Harris, Z. L., Takahashi, Y., Miyajima, H., Serizawa, M., MacGillivray, R. T. and Gitlin, J. D. (1995) Aceruloplasminemia: Molecular characterization of this disorder of iron metabolism. Proc Natl Acad Sci USA 92:2539–2543.

Hempe, J. and Cousins, R. J. (1992) Cysteine-rich intestinal protein and intestinal metallothionein—An inverse relationship as a conceptual model for zinc absorption in rats. J Nutr 122:89–95.

Kelly, E. J., Quaife, C. J., Froelick, G. J. and Palmiter, R. D. (1996) Metallothionein I and II protect against zinc deficiency and zinc toxicity in mice. J Nutr 126:1782–1790.

Liu, A. C., Heinrichs, B. S. and Leach, R. M. (1994) Influence of manganese deficiency on the characteristics of proteoglycans of avian epiphyseal growth plate cartilage. Poult Sci 73:663–669.

Lonnerdal, B. and Sandstrom, B. (1995) Factors influencing the uptake of metal ions from the digestive tract. In: Handbook of Metal-Ligand Interactions in Biological Fluids (Berthon, G., ed.), vol. 1, pp. 331–337. Marcel Dekker, New York.

MacDonald, R. S., Browning, J. D., Williamson, P. S., Thornton, W. H. and O'Dell, B. L. (1997) Food intake by zinc deficient rats is normalized by megestrol acetate (MA) but not by insulin-like growth factor-I (IGF-I). FASEB J 11:A15.

McMahon, R. J. and Cousins, R. J. (1997) Regulation of the zinc transporter ZnT-1 in rat intestine and liver by zinc and lipopolysaccharide. FASEB J 11:A14.

Mossad, S. B., Macknin, M. L., Medendorp, S. V. and Mason, P. (1996) Zinc gluconate lozenges for treating the common cold. A randomized, double-blind, placebo-controlled study. Ann Intern Med 125:81–88.

National Research Council (1989) Recommended Dietary Allowances, 10th ed., National Academy Press, Washington, D. C.

Orr, W. C. and Sohal, R. S. (1994) Extension of life-span by overexpression of superoxide dismutase and catalase in *Drosophila melanogaster.* Science 263:1128–1130.

Owen, C. A. (1973) Effects of iron on copper metabolism and copper on iron metabolism in rats. Am J Physiol 224:514–518.

Palmiter, R. D. (1994) Regulation of metallothionein genes by heavy metals appears to be mediated by a zinc-sensitive inhibitor that interacts with a constitutively active transcription factor, MTF-1. Proc Natl Acad Sci USA 91:1219–1223.

Palmiter, R. D. and Findley, S. D. (1995) Cloning and functional characterization of a mammalian zinc transporter that confers resistance to zinc. EMBO J 14:639–649.

Percival, S. S. (1995) Neutropenia caused by copper deficiency: Possible mechanisms of action. Nutr Rev 53:59–66.

Percival, S. S. and Harris, E. D. (1990) Copper transport from ceruloplasmin: Characterization of the cellular uptake mechanism. Am J Physiol 258:C140–C146.

Reinhold, J. G. (1971) High phytate content of rural Iranian bread: A possible cause of human zinc deficiency. Am J Clin Nutr 24:1204–1206.

Rhodes, D. and Klug, A. (1993) Zinc fingers. Sci Am, February: 56–65.

Rock, E., Gueux, E., Mazur, A., Motta, C. and Rayssiguier, Y. (1995) Anemia in copper-deficient rats: Role of alterations in erythrocyte membrane fluidity and oxidative damage. Am J Physiol 269:C1245–C1249.

Roth, H. P. and Kirchgessner, M. (1994) Influence of alimentary zinc deficiency on the concentration of growth hormone (GH), insulin-like growth factor I (IGF-I) and insulin in the serum of force-fed rats. Horm Metab Res 26:404–408.

Rucker, R. B., Romero-Chapman, N., Wong, T., Lee, J., Steinberg, F. M., McGee, C., Clegg, M. S., Reiser, K., Kosonen, T., Uriu-Hare, J. Y., Murphy, J. and Keen, C. L. (1996) Modulation of lysyl oxidase by dietary copper in rats. J Nutr 126:51–60.

Swanson, C. A. and King, J. C. (1983) Reduced serum zinc concentrations during pregnancy. Obstet Gynecol 62:313–318.

Torre, M., Rodriguez, A. R. and Saura-Calixto, F. (1992) Effects of dietary fiber and phytic acid on mineral availability. Crit Rev Food Sci Nutr 30:1–22.

Vallee, B. L. and Galdes, A. (1984) The metallobiochemistry of zinc enzymes. Adv Enzymol Relat Areas Mol Biol 56:283–430.

Vulpe, C. D. and Packman, S. (1995) Cellular copper transport. Annu Rev Nutr 15:293–322.

Walsh, C. T., Sandstead, H. H., Prasad, A. S., Newbern, P. M. and Fraker, P. J. (1994) Zinc: Health effects and research priorities for the 1990's. Environ Health Perspect 102:5–46.

Williamson, P. S., Brown, E. C., Browning, J. D., Wollard, L. C., Thornton, W. H., O'Dell, B. L. and MacDonald, R. S. (1997) Decreased insulin-like growth factor-I (IGF-I) receptor concentration and IGF-I binding in small intestine of zinc-deficient rats. FASEB J 11:A194.

RECOMMENDED READINGS

Cousins, R. J. (1985) Absorption, transport, and hepatic metabolism of copper and zinc: Special reference to metallothionein and ceruloplasmin. Physiol Rev 65:238–309.

Hill, C. H. and Matrone, G. (1970) Chemical parameters in the study of in vivo and in vitro interactions of transition elements. Fed Proc 29:1474–1481.

Vulpe, C. D. and Packman, S. (1995) Cellular copper transport. Annu Rev Nutr 15:293–322.

Walsh, C. T., Sandstead, H. H., Prasad, A. S., Newbern, P. M. and Fraker, P. J. (1994) Zinc: Health effects and research priorities for the 1990's. Environ Health Perspect 102:5–46.

CHAPTER **33**

◆ ◆

Iodine

Hedley C. Freake, Ph.D.

O U T L I N E

C O M M O N   A B B R E V I A T I O N S

IDD (iodine deficiency disorder)
rT_3 (reverse T_3)
RXR (retinoid X receptor)
T_3 (3,5,3'-triiodothyronine)
T_4 (thyroxine)
TR (thyroid hormone receptor)
TRE (thyroid hormone response element)
TRH (thyrotropin-releasing hormone)
TSH (thyroid-stimulating hormone, thyrotropin)

UNIQUENESS OF IODINE

Iodine is an extremely unusual and interesting nutrient from almost every perspective. For the chemist, it possesses the distinction of being the heaviest element required for human nutrition, with an atomic weight of 127. It is responsible for just a single function in the body, the synthesis of thyroid hormones. However the multiple actions of thyroid hormones mean that it has an impact on a wide range of metabolic and developmental functions. The definition of those functions, and the unraveling of the molecular mechanisms that underlie them, have occupied numerous physiologists, biochemists, and molecular biologists for decades. Deficiency of iodine is common, and the consequences of that deficiency are so profound, particularly in the neonatal period, that it represents one of the largest public health problems in the world today (Micronutrient Deficiency Information System, 1993). The occurrence of iodine in soils is extremely variable, so dietary deficiency depends almost entirely on where food sources are grown, rather than which are selected. Yet eradicating that deficiency is relatively simple and in some parts of the world has resulted in dramatic improvements in human function.

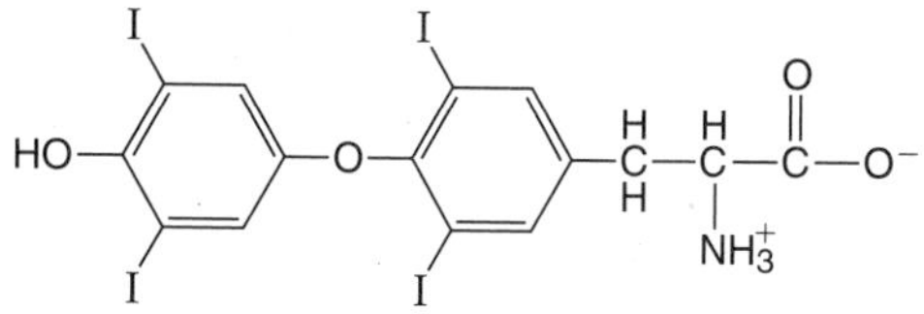

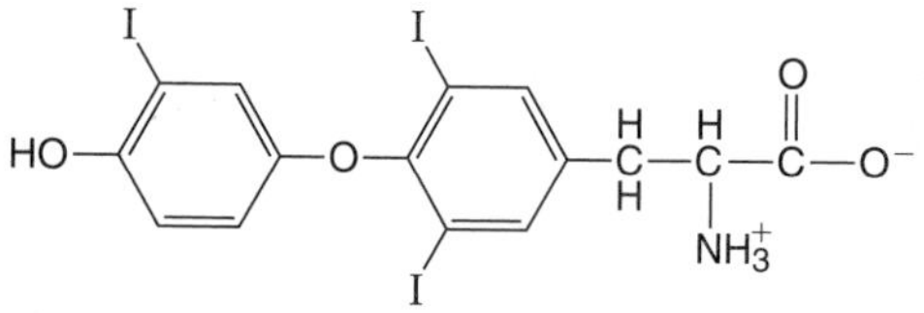

PRODUCTION AND METABOLISM OF THYROID HORMONES

Use of Iodine—Thyroid Hormones

Inorganic iodine occurs predominantly in nature in the form of the anion iodide. The sole function of iodine in humans and other mammals is the synthesis of thyroid hormones. These iodinated derivatives of the amino acid tyrosine, shown in Figure 33–1, are thyroxine, or 3,5,3′,5′-tetraiodothyronine (T_4), and 3,5,3′-triiodothyronine (T_3). Because they are derived from amino acids, thyroid hormones are in the L-form. D-Isomers can be synthesized but have lower biological activity.

Dietary Sources of Iodine

Iodine is a reasonably abundant element, but its solubility leads to wide regional variations

Thyroxine (T_4)

3,5,3′-Triiodothyronine (T_3)

Figure 33–1. *Chemical structures of the thyroid hormones.*

in its availability. The iodine content of soils is diminished by their exposure to rain, snow, and glaciation, which leach out the mineral and deposit it in the oceans. Although iodine is volatilized from the sea and returns to land through rainwater, this does not make up for the long-term loss of iodine from older exposed soils. Iodine-deficient areas include mountainous regions, such as the Himalayas, Andes, and Alps, and also river deltas, such as the Ganges and the Yellow River, where frequent flooding has leached out the mineral (Hetzel and Maberly, 1986).

The iodine content of plants averages 1 mg/kg dry weight, but it may be only 1% of that in plants grown in iodine-deficient areas. Its content in animal foods, including milk, reflects the amount found in the feeds supplied to the animals. Foods arising from the sea, such as fish and seaweed, provide a rich source. In more developed parts of the world, the food available to a particular community is usually drawn from a variety of geographical locations and thus, in aggregate, is less likely to be deficient in iodine. However, supplementation, particularly in the form of iodized salt as has been used in the United States, is the only reliable way to ensure an adequate dietary supply in low-iodine areas. This relatively simple public health program has reaped enormous benefit in many communities. A good example of this is Switzerland, where iodine deficiency, which used to affect the majority of the population, has now

Food Sources of Iodine

- Rich sources
  Seafood (fish, shellfish, seaweed)
- Variable sources
  Vegetables, meats, dairy foods
- Fortified foods
  Salt
- Adventitious sources
  Bread (iodates as dough improvers)
  Milk (iodine-based antiseptics)

RDAs Across the Life Cycle

	μg iodine/day
Infants, 0–0.5 y	40
0.5–1.0 y	50
Children, 1–3 y	70
4–6 y	90
7–10 y	120
Males, 11+ y	150
Females, 11+ y	150
Pregnant	175
Lactating	200

From National Research Council (1989). Recommended Dietary Allowances, 10th ed., National Academy Press, Washington, D.C.

been virtually eradicated. The content of iodine-containing compounds in foods may be increased by the use of iodine-containing products at various points in the production process. For example, iodates are used in bread making, and iodine-containing antiseptics are used in dairy facilities.

Absorption, Storage, and Excretion of Iodine

Iodine (I^-) is the form of the nutrient found in most food sources. It is efficiently absorbed along the length of the gastrointestinal tract. Organic forms of iodine also occur in the diet—for example, the iodates (IO_3^-) added to bread. They too are easily absorbed, although not as completely as iodide itself.

The adult human body contains 15 to 20 mg of iodine, and about three quarters of this is found in the thyroid gland. This gland has a unique and powerful ability to take up iodide actively. Concentrations in the gland are 100-fold those in plasma under normal circumstances and can become higher still in iodine

deficiency. Iodine accumulates to a much lesser extent in other tissues—for example, the salivary glands. The kidneys are the other principal site for iodine uptake, but they are incapable of conserving the mineral, and hence the kidneys represent the main route for excretion. The amount of iodine found in urine is proportional to the plasma concentration and can be used as a convenient index of iodine status. It has been suggested that urinary iodine levels of at least 50 μg/g of creatinine indicate normal iodine status (Querido et al., 1974). Feces and sweat, together with breast milk in lactating women, represent other routes of iodine loss from the body.

Synthesis of Thyroid Hormones

The process of thyroid hormone synthesis is illustrated in Figure 33–2. Iodine is actively transported into the thyroid gland, coupled to the action of Na^+, K^+-ATPase. It traverses the thyroid cells and enters the colloid space. The iodine is then oxidized by thyroid peroxidase,

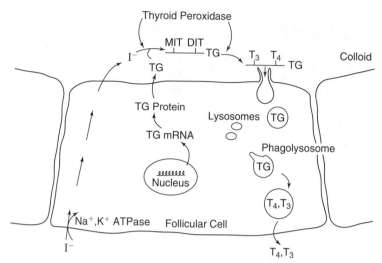

Figure 33–2. Synthesis of thyroid hormones. Iodide is pumped into the follicular cells of the thyroid gland. It diffuses across the cells and enters the colloid space, where it is incorporated into thyroglobulin (TG), leading to the synthesis of MIT and DIT (mono- and di-iodotyrosines), which then condense to form thyroid hormones. The hormones, still within thyroglobulin, are stored in the colloid space. When stimulated by thyroid-stimulating hormone (TSH), the secretion pathway begins with the uptake of a droplet of colloid, which fuses with a lysosome to form a phagolysosome. The lysosomal enzymes degrade the thyroglobulin, leading to release of the thyroid hormones and their secretion from the cell.

using hydrogen peroxide as a co-substrate, and the reactive intermediate is coupled to tyrosyl residues in the protein thyroglobulin. These then become mono- or diiodotyrosyl residues, depending on whether one or two iodine molecules are incorporated. Thyroglobulin is a very large glycoprotein and may constitute up to half the protein in the thyroid gland. Only selected tyrosyl residues in this protein become iodinated. Mono- or diiodotyrosyl residues within thyroglobulin condense with each other to form T_4 or T_3 residues. This reaction is also catalyzed by thyroid peroxidase. When the iodophenolic ring of one iodotyrosyl residue is condensed with another, the rest of the donor residue is left in the thyroglobulin chain in the form of serine. Thyroid hormones are stored in the colloid space, still as a part of thyroglobulin.

For release of thyroid hormones, portions of colloid that contain iodinated thyroglobulin are taken into the follicular cells by pinocytosis. These droplets then fuse with lysosomes within the cells to form phagolysosomes, and the thyroglobulin within them is broken down by proteolytic enzymes. This results in the release of free thyroid hormones, which are able to diffuse out into the circulation. T_4 is the predominant form released, but

a small amount of T_3 is also generated. The proportion of T_3 released appears to be increased under hypothyroid conditions by intrathyroidal deiodination of T_4.

Hypothyroidism can result not only from insufficient dietary iodine but also from the ingestion of goitrogens. These are present in some foods, notably the cruciferous family of vegetables, which includes broccoli and cabbage, and also cassava. The latter may be more important, as it is a dietary staple eaten in large quantities by some populations. Cruciferous vegetables themselves are not likely to be eaten in sufficient quantities to cause concern. Goitrogens work either by competitively inhibiting iodine uptake by the thyroid gland or by blocking its incorporation into the tyrosyl residues of thyroglobulin and their subsequent condensation. Antithyroid drugs, such as propylthiouracil and methimazole, work by the latter mechanism and are used clinically in the treatment of hyperthyroidism.

Circulation

Thyroid hormones are carried in the blood on three proteins: thyroid-binding globulin, thyroid-binding prealbumin, and albumin. The prealbumin is also known as transthyretin and functions with retinol-binding protein in retinol transport. (See Chapter 26.) Over 99% of both T_4 and T_3 circulate bound to these proteins, but T_4 is bound more tightly than T_3. Only the small free fraction is available for tissue uptake, either to exert biological activity or for further metabolism. This tight binding means that thyroid hormones, particularly T_4, have relatively long plasma half-lives and also that there is a large plasma pool of thyroid hormones, which can become available to tissues after dissociation from the binding proteins. The T_4 plasma concentration in normal humans is about 100 nM, which is 50- to 100-fold higher than that for T_3. This reflects the fact that T_4 is the primary product of the thyroid gland and that it has a longer plasma half-life than T_3 does.

Activation

T_4, the predominant circulating thyroid hormone, is really a prohormone that requires deiodination at the 5' position in the outer ring to generate the biologically active T_3. Deiodination serves not only to activate thyroid hormones but also as a deactivation pathway (Fig. 33–3). Removal of iodine from the inner ring of T_4 will result in the production of reverse T_3 (rT_3; 3,3',5'-triiodothyronine), and similar processing of T_3 produces 3,3'-diiodothyronine, both of which are inactive metabolites.

A family of microsomal enzymes is responsible for deiodination (Leonard and Visser, 1986). The type I deiodinase, found in liver, kidney, and thyroid gland, produces most of the T_3 in the body, although it can also convert T_4 to rT_3. Complementary DNA (cDNA) clones encoding this enzyme have recently been isolated (Berry et al., 1991). The cDNA nucleotide sequence revealed that the type I deiodinase contains the unusual amino acid selenocysteine, which is similar in structure to cysteine except that it contains selenium instead of sulfur. At that time, glutathione peroxidase was the only other mammalian enzyme known to contain selenocysteine. Both enzymes require selenium for activity. These findings explained earlier work in the rat that showed that selenium deficiency reduced plasma T_3 levels and thereby impaired thyroid status. It has also given a possible explanation for some of the diversity seen in the spectrum of iodine deficiency disorders, as described later. Selenoenzymes are discussed further in Chapter 34.

Type I deiodinase activity is increased in hyperthyroidism and decreased in the hypothyroid state. This emphasizes its role in the inactivation of T_4. It is also inhibited by propylthiouracil, giving a second site of action for this antithyroid drug.

The type II deiodinase, located in brain, pituitary, and brown adipose tissue, operates solely on the outer ring. It functions to convert T_4 to T_3 for local use within these tissues, rather than to maintain plasma levels of T_3. However, it has been shown that under some circumstances, the brown adipose tissue type II deiodinase makes a significant contribution to circulating levels of T_3. In tissues containing

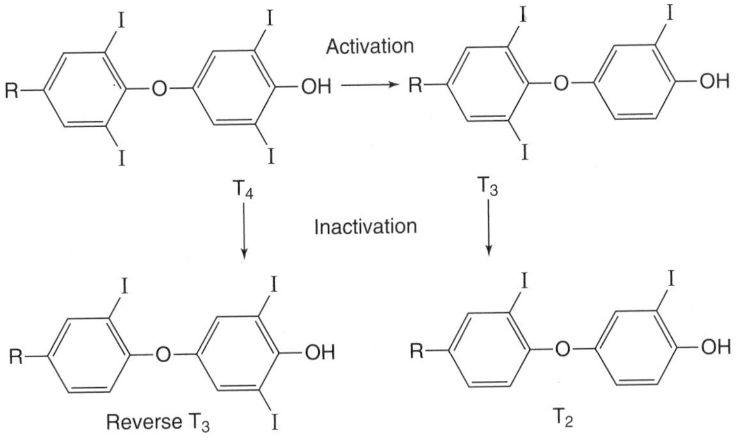

Figure 33–3. Deiodination pathways for thyroid hormones. The parent compound thyroxine (T_4) is activated by monodeiodination of the outer ring to form 3,5,3'-triiodothyronine (T_3). Either one of these may be inactivated by inner ring deiodination to form reverse T_3 or di-iodothyronine (T_2).

the type II enzyme, thyroid hormone status will depend primarily on plasma levels of T_4 rather than T_3. The activity of this enzyme is increased in the hypothyroid state, which means that these tissues may be partially protected from the effects of hypothyroidism by this local production.

Type III deiodinase operates exclusively on the inner ring and therefore inactivates thyroid hormones. It has been found in brain and placenta and appears unresponsive to thyroid status.

Further Metabolism and Excretion

Removal of iodine from the inner ring is an irreversible degradative step. There are additional pathways of thyroid hormone metabolism. The phenolic hydroxyl group of the outer ring can be conjugated with glucuronate or sulfate. This occurs primarily in the liver, with glucuronidation being favored for T_4 and sulfation for T_3. These conjugates are then secreted into the bile and may be lost in the feces. However, a significant amount is likely to be hydrolyzed in the intestine, followed by reabsorption of the free thyroid hormones. Deamination or decarboxylation also occurs, resulting in carboxylate or amine analogs of the thyroid hormones, respectively. Although metabolic activity has been suggested for some of these analogs, this seems unlikely because they are further degraded very quickly.

Any iodine produced by the peripheral metabolism of thyroid hormones will be either taken up by the thyroid gland and used for further synthesis or lost in the urine.

Regulation of Thyroid Hormone Status

From the preceding discussion, it is apparent that thyroid hormone status can be modified at a number of different levels. The primary site may be output from the thyroid gland, but the rate of conversion of the prohormone to active T_3 is also important.

Under normal circumstances, circulating thyroid hormone levels are well maintained, because of a negative feedback loop on their production (Fig. 33–4). Thyrotroph cells in the anterior pituitary produce thyrotropin, or thy-

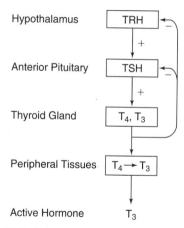

Figure 33–4. *Feedback regulation of thyroid hormone status. TRH, thyrotropin-releasing hormone; TSH, thyroid-stimulating hormone; T_4, thyroxine; T_3, 3,5,3′-triiodothyronine.*

roid-stimulating hormone (TSH), a glycoprotein that is a heterodimer of two subunits, which are encoded by separate genes. The α subunit is similar to those of the gonadotropic pituitary hormones, luteinizing hormone, and follicle-stimulating hormone, whereas the β subunit is unique. TSH acts on the thyroid gland, primarily by a cyclic AMP-mediated mechanism, to stimulate iodine uptake and organification and also the release of thyroid hormones. T_4 travels back to the pituitary, where it is deiodinated by the type II enzyme. The T_3 produced operates at a transcriptional level to inhibit the production of both subunits of TSH, thereby completing the cycle. TSH is also under the control of the hypothalamic tripeptide thyrotropin-releasing hormone (TRH), which is responsible for basal production of TSH by the pituitary. It provides a mechanism by which thyroid status can be modulated either positively (e.g., in response to cold) or negatively (e.g., in response to stress or illness) at a central level. T_3 has also been shown to inhibit transcription of the TRH gene, showing that the negative feedback loop extends up to the hypothalamus.

This hypothalamic/pituitary/thyroid axis is responsible for producing the appropriate amounts of thyroid hormones, but thyroid status can also be regulated by altering the rate of T_4 to T_3 conversion. The deiodinase enzymes can be differentially regulated. This allows the possibility that tissues may differ in thyroid status, according to whether they depend on the type I or type II deiodinase for supply of T_3. For example, plasma T_3 is reduced by fasting and increased by carbohydrate feeding in humans, and these effects are achieved by altering the activity of the type I deiodinase. This response to decreased food availability helps conserve fuel by reducing metabolic rate. In particular, protein catabolism is minimized by a reduction in its T_3-stimulated turnover rate. However, because the type II enzyme is not affected by fasting, generation of T_3 in the brain and pituitary, and therefore T_3-dependent functions in those tissues, is maintained.

Although T_3 is the active thyroid hormone, thyroid status is usually better determined by measuring plasma T_4. This provides a more sensitive indicator of hypothyroidism, such as that resulting from iodine deficiency, than does plasma T_3. Circulating levels of T_3 may be maintained, even in the face of inadequate thyroid hormone production, both by increasing the proportion of T_3 produced by the thyroid gland and by stimulating peripheral conversion. Thus plasma T_3 values may be within the normal range, despite reduced levels of T_4. This compensation may occur at the expense of the brain, because brain derives T_3 from plasma T_4 by the type II deiodinase-catalyzed reaction. The body uses T_4 as its own indicator of thyroid status; as mentioned, TSH production in the pituitary is downregulated by T_3 that is locally produced from T_4. Measurement of plasma TSH is also widely used clinically as a sensitive indicator of thyroid status, because elevated levels indicate hypothyroidism. Plasma TSH level is used to confirm normal thyroid status in newborn infants.

MECHANISM OF ACTION OF THYROID HORMONES

In recent years it has come to be accepted that most and perhaps all actions of thyroid hormones are mediated by effects within the nucleus. This mechanism is outlined in Figure 33–5. Following dissociation from plasma proteins, T_4 and T_3 enter the cell. The T_4 is deiodinated and T_3 enters the nucleus. There it is bound by specific nuclear receptor proteins, which in turn bind to and alter the rate of transcription of target genes. The changed amount of messenger RNA is translated to a corresponding amount of protein, and therefore the physiological state is altered.

Nuclear Receptors

Attempts to understand thyroid hormone action on a molecular level received an enormous boost in 1986 with the unintentional cloning of thyroid hormone receptors (TRs). The glucocorticoid and estrogen receptors had previously been cloned, leading to the realization that not only were they very similar to each other in amino acid and nucleotide sequence but also to the viral oncogene *v-erb A*. Oncogenes are DNA or RNA sequences found within viruses, which derive their name from their ability to produce unregulated proliferation of the cells they infect. The oncogene *v-erb A* is found in some retroviruses (i.e., viruses in which the infection is transmitted by a particle containing RNA rather than DNA). The oncogenes within retroviruses are derived from chromosomal material and thus each has its own cellular counterpart, the proto-oncogene, in this case *c-erb A*. Usually the proto-oncogene encodes a protein that plays an important role in the control of cellular growth, explaining the effects of its unregulated expression following viral infection. Complementary DNAs (cDNAs) derived from the *c-erb A* gene were isolated from chick and human sources in two independent laboratories (Sap et al., 1986; Weinberger et al., 1986), with the expectation that they might encode another hormone receptor. This supposition proved accurate, and binding studies using proteins derived from the cloned cDNAs demonstrated that ligand was T_3. This adventitious and relatively straightforward cloning of the receptors was ironic in that it followed many years of essentially unsuccessful attempts to purify receptor proteins by conventional means.

Functional Regions of Receptors. The realization that TRs are part of a class of nuclear acting proteins has facilitated progress in understanding their mechanism of action, be-

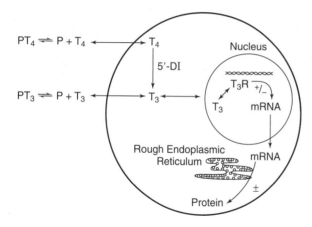

Figure 33–5. *Outline of thyroid hormone action. Thyroid hormones circulate bound to plasma proteins (P), from which they must dissociate to enter the cell. Tissues containing the deiodinase enzyme (5'DI) convert T_4 to T_3. T_3 travels to the nucleus, where it is bound by specific receptor proteins (R). Together they interact with target genes, resulting in a change of their transcriptional rate. This results in altered mRNA levels, leading to different rates of protein synthesis and therefore different amounts of the protein products of the target genes, which ultimately produce the biological effect.*

cause analogies can be drawn with other members of the class. This includes receptors not only for steroid hormones but also for retinoic acid, 1,25-$(OH)_2$ vitamin D, and a host of other less well-known or uncharacterized ligands (Evans, 1988). These receptors have a modular structure (Fig. 33–6). They all have a carboxy-terminal region that binds to hormone and therefore provides each receptor with its ligand specificity. The area that is most highly conserved across the family is the DNA-binding region, through which the receptors recognize and bind to their target genes. Regions that appear to be required for nuclear localization of the protein and others that facilitate dimerization between receptors have also been described.

The DNA-binding region contains multiple cysteinyl residues, which do not vary in their relative location between different members of the receptor class. By analogy to other nuclear DNA-binding proteins, it was suggested that these receptors would use 8 of

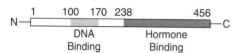

Figure 33–6. *The modular structure of thyroid hormone receptors (TRs). In common with other members of the nuclear receptor family, the TRs have defined regions for DNA and hormone binding, separated by a hinge region. Sequences required for dimer formation have been described within both the DNA- and hormone-binding domains. The amino-terminal region does not appear to be required for function of TRs although in other nuclear receptors this region has been assigned a role in transcriptional activation. The numbers shown represent amino acids in the human TRβ1 sequence.*

these cysteinyl residues to chelate 2 atoms of zinc and that the mineral would then stabilize a receptor conformation appropriate for DNA binding. Much evidence in favor of this hypothesis has accumulated for various members of the receptor class, and it is generally accepted that they are zinc proteins (Vallee et al., 1991). The significance of this fact remains to be determined; for example, does zinc deficiency ever cause levels of zinc within the nucleus to drop to an extent that would cause its dissociation from receptor proteins and therefore interrupt their function? The role of zinc as a component of nuclear proteins involved in the transcriptional process is discussed in Chapter 32.

Multiple Thyroid Hormone Receptors. The cloning of TRs has also served to complicate our understanding of their mechanism of action. It had been assumed previously that a single receptor was responsible for mediating T_3 action. The two receptors cloned in 1986, although they were derived from different species, also appeared to be generated from independent genes. The existence of two human TR genes (α on chromosome 17 and β on chromosome 3) has subsequently been confirmed. In addition, these two genes result in multiple protein products. There are two thyroid hormone β receptors: β1 that has a broad tissue distribution and β2 that appears to be restricted to the pituitary and certain areas of the brain. Multiple products derived from the α gene have also been described, though only one of them, α1, retains an intact hormone-binding region and therefore appears capable of performing a receptor function. Other forms may play important roles, however, and it has been suggested that they may antagonize T_3 action. In particular, the nonhormone-binding variant α2 is expressed at high levels in the brain and in the testis, and it has been suggested that this could explain the metabolic nonresponsiveness of these tissues to T_3 in the adult (Lazar, 1993).

Hereditary disorders, termed thyroid hormone resistance, have been described in which individuals appear hypothyroid despite normal or elevated circulating thyroid hormone levels (Refetoff and Weiss, 1993). Families with this condition are located very rarely, but they provide a useful opportunity to learn more of the mechanism of action of T_3. When the genetic loci of thyroid hormone resistance in these families have been determined, they have all been found in the carboxy-terminal, ligand-binding portion of the TRβ gene. These mutations result in a diminished ability of the receptors to bind T_3 and also in a decreased ability of the TRβ to mediate a transcriptional response to T_3 in various systems in vitro. The disorder is almost always heterozygous, i.e., the affected individuals also possess a normal β-receptor gene. This means that the mutant receptors must have a dominant negative activity and can inhibit the transcriptional activation that would operate through the normal wild-type receptors. This might be predicted, because mutations in the ligand-binding region leave the DNA-binding region of the TRβ unaffected, and therefore the mutant receptors may block the access of biologically active receptors to TR-binding sites on their target genes.

Response Elements in Target Genes. The TR must be capable of selecting the genes whose transcription it regulates from among the background of the entire genome. This specificity is achieved by DNA sequences in the control regions of target genes, known as thyroid hormone response elements, or TREs. A TRE consists of a hexanucleotide with the sequence AGGTCA, although some substitutions within that sequence are permissible. The TREs are usually found in pairs, although sometimes three or even more copies of this sequence are present. The same recognition motif is used by some other members of the nuclear receptor family, notably receptors for retinoic acid and vitamin D, which indicates that not only the recognition sequences but also their arrangement within the promoter are important for determining target gene specificity. It has therefore been suggested that a TRE consists of two repeats of the sequence AGGTCA with a four-nucleotide separation. Although such a sequence certainly is able to respond to the thyroid hormone–receptor complex, the sequences actually found within target genes frequently deviate from this. Thus the exact requirements for a DNA sequence to confer responsiveness to thyroid hormone remain to be established.

Heterodimerization of Receptors. The fact that recognition motifs for TRs, as well as for other members of the nuclear receptor family, are found in pairs suggests that the receptors might bind to the response elements as dimers. This has proved to be the case, though for thyroid hormone, hetero- rather than homodimers appear to be the favored form. Retinoic acid has a naturally occurring isomer, 9-*cis*-retinoic acid, which has its own nuclear receptor, termed the RXR or retinoid X receptor. This is distinct from the receptor for all-*trans*-retinoic acid, the RAR. These retinoid receptors are discussed in detail in Chapter 26. Studies in vitro have shown that, in the presence of T_3, heterodimers between TRs and RXRs bind more tightly to TREs and confer a more robust transcriptional response than do homodimers of TRs (Yen and Chin, 1994). RXRs heterodimerize in a similarly effective way with both RARs and vitamin D receptors. Three distinct RXR genes have been discovered, and each of these generates multiple isoforms of the receptor. Given the multiplicity of TRs, it appears reasonable to suppose that the combination of different receptor isoforms as heterodimerization partners would give a host of possibilities for achieving gene- and tissue-specific responses to thyroid hormone. The fact that a range of receptor heterodimers is available may also help explain why variations are observed in the response elements of target genes. The particular organization of a response element may favor a specific pair of TR/RXR isoforms.

Effects on Transcription

The occupation of TRs by T_3 leads to a change in the transcription rate of the target genes, although the precise way in which this occurs is not well understood. A depiction of the current model is shown in Figure 33–7. Studies in vitro have indicated that the TRs are bound to the TREs in both the presence and absence of hormone. Thus the hormone does not cause binding of the receptor to the target gene. Rather, T_3 binding to TR alters the interaction between this ligand-activated transcription factor and the proteins that constitute the basal transcriptional apparatus. Additional proteins called coactivators (Lee et al., 1995) and corepressors (Horlein et al., 1995), which are required for receptor function and appear to mediate this linkage between the receptors and the basic transcriptional machinery, have recently been described. In the absence of ligand, the TR:RXR heterodimer, bound to the response element, is associated with a corepressor protein, which mediates an inhibitory interaction with the proteins of the basal transcriptional apparatus. Addition of hormone leads to dissociation of the corepressor and recruitment of the coactivator, which then switches on transcription. In this model, absence of hormone is not just a lack of stimulation of transcription but actually an inhibition.

Transcription can be either stimulated or inhibited by T_3, depending on the target gene. Although the majority of the actions described are stimulatory, the autoregulation of thyroid status is an example of negative transcriptional control. T_3 acts at the transcriptional level in the anterior pituitary gland to limit the production of TSH, which results in decreased production of thyroid hormones.

S14—A Model Thyroid Hormone–Responsive Gene

Several target genes for T_3 have been identified and proved useful for understanding the physiology of thyroid hormone action, as well as the molecular events occurring within the nucleus that initiate the biological effects. A partial listing of target genes is given in Table 33–1. The physiology of thyroid hormone action is described next. Here, one example of a thyroid hormone–responsive gene will be taken to illustrate the regulatory mechanisms.

A key metabolic target for T_3 is the liver. In 1981, Oppenheimer, Towle, and coworkers sought to identify hepatic gene products

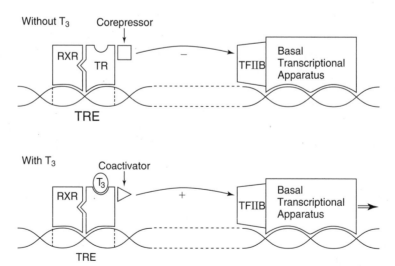

Figure 33–7. *Thyroid hormone action in the nucleus. The efficient regulator of transcription that binds to the thyroid hormone response element (TRE) of target genes appears to be a heterodimer between a thyroid hormone receptor (TR) and a retinoid X receptor (RXR). In the absence of T_3, this dimer is associated with a third protein, the corepressor. This complex interacts with the basal transcriptional apparatus through one of its associated proteins, transcription factor IIB (TFIIB), and inhibits transcription. In the presence of T_3, the corepressor is replaced by a coactivator, resulting in initiation of transcription. A break is shown between the two portions of the DNA to indicate that TREs are often far upstream of the transcriptional start site, requiring folding of the DNA to bring the two regions together.*

TABLE 33–1
Selected Target Genes for Thyroid Hormones

Metabolic
  Fatty acid synthase
  Malic enzyme
  Pyruvate kinase
  Spot 14
  Phosphoenolpyruvate carboxykinase
Cardiac
  Myosin heavy chain
  Calcium ATPase
Endocrine
  Growth hormone
  TSH
  TR (α and β)
Mitochondrial
  Cytochrome c
Ion Transport
  Na$^+$, K$^+$-ATPase

whose abundance was altered in response to thyroid status (Seelig et al., 1981). Nineteen such products were identified, some of which increased and some of which decreased with T_3 treatment. Attention was particularly focused on one product, called spot 14 or S14, and a cDNA clone coding for this product was isolated. The identify of the S14 protein was and still is unknown, but T_3 treatment results in a rapid and large induction in the expression of the mRNA. This stimulation occurs at the level of transcription and can be detected as soon as 10 minutes after intravenous T_3 injection into a hypothyroid rat. The S14 gene clearly represents a direct target for T_3 action, and subsequent effort has been directed toward elucidating the steps involved in its transcriptional regulation.

The regions of DNA that contain the TRE and mediate the response to T_3 have been identified and are noteworthy because they are relatively far (about 2700 base pairs) from the transcriptional start site (Zilz et al., 1990). Other sites in the S14 gene promoter that mediate a positive transcriptional response to carbohydrate feeding or a negative response to polyunsaturated fatty acids have been found. The carbohydrate response is particularly relevant here because it is synergistic with that to T_3. Use of a specific antibody has demonstrated that the S14 protein is located within the nuclear compartment of the cell (Kinlaw

et al., 1992). This suggests a role for S14 in nuclear functions, perhaps in coordinating the regulation of a subset of genes involved in lipid metabolism. Supporting this idea is the recent demonstration that specifically blocking the production of S14 protein within cultured hepatocytes also removed the ability of the cells to increase lipogenesis in response to T_3 (Kinlaw et al., 1995).

Most studies regarding the regulation of S14 have been limited to liver. The gene is expressed in several other tissues, in particular adipose tissue, and this distribution has supported a role for the protein in lipid metabolism. However, the responsiveness of S14 gene expression to T_3 is quite tissue-specific. For example, tissues like lung and brain, which actively synthesize fatty acids, do not alter either S14 expression or lipogenesis in response to T_3 (Blennemann et al., 1995). Identifying the elements of the S14 promoter and the nuclear proteins that interact with them to dictate this cell-specific regulation of expression is an important area of research for both S14 and other T_3-regulated genes.

Non-nuclear Pathways

The nuclear pathway for thyroid hormone action is now well established. Non-nuclear mechanisms have also been suggested, but evidence in their favor is much less complete and sometimes contradictory. The stimulatory effects of thyroid hormones on oxygen consumption are well known, and this knowledge led to the suggestion that they might act directly on mitochondria. Mitochondrial receptors for T_3 have been described, but such descriptions have been inconsistent. Although T_3 clearly affects mitochondrial structure and function, it appears likely that such actions are mediated by the nuclear transcriptional pathway described earlier. Binding proteins that recognize thyroid hormones have also been identified in the plasma membrane and the cytoplasm. These may serve transport functions governing the delivery of T_3 to the nucleus, rather than initiating biological functions independently of nuclear receptors. The means whereby T_3, which is not very soluble and binds easily to proteins, enters the cell and reaches the nucleus are not clear.

PHYSIOLOGICAL FUNCTIONS OF THYROID HORMONES

The physiological actions of T_3 can be divided into two components, metabolic and developmental. These actions are best known in terms of the regulation of basal metabolic rate (BMR) on the one hand and the thyroid hormone requirement for normal brain development on the other. It is interesting to note that, although these actions of thyroid hormone have been known for decades and although the molecular mechanism of T_3 action within the nucleus has been increasingly well delineated, large gaps remain in our physiological understanding of how thyroid hormone regulates these processes.

Regulation of Basal Metabolic Rate

Thyroid hormone increases oxygen consumption in all warm-blooded animals. The effect is seen in the basal portion of metabolic rate (i.e., that measured in the postabsorptive, resting state). Basal or resting oxygen consumption is reduced about 30% in hypothyroid individuals and is increased 50% in hyperthyroidism (Freake and Oppenheimer, 1995). Thus, overall, basal metabolism can be doubled by alterations in thyroid state. It is generally assumed that most tissues, with the exception of brain, spleen, and testis, respond to thyroid hormone by increasing oxygen consumption. However, this is based on measuring oxygen consumption in vitro in tissue preparations taken from animals of different thyroid state. The extent to which this faithfully represents their metabolic activity in vivo is clearly open to question.

There is a considerable lag time following administration of thyroid hormone before an increase in oxygen consumption can be detected. This delay is approximately 1 day and is consistent with the nuclear pathway for thyroid hormone action. Appearance of the physiological effects requires the transcription of mRNAs and the translation and accumulation of the relevant proteins, a process that is likely to take hours.

Efficiency of Energy Production. An early and attractive explanation for the stimulation of metabolic rate observed with thyroid hormone treatment was that the hormone acted directly on mitochondria to uncouple electron transport from ATP synthesis. Indeed, such effects could be demonstrated in vitro. However, this required very high concentrations of thyroid hormone and could not be reproduced at physiological levels. Thus this concept was discarded. More recently, it has been revived, although in a very different form. Treatment with thyroid hormone produces numerous effects on mitochondria (Freake and Oppenheimer, 1995). These include induction of several components of the electron transport chain, increased activity of the ADP translocator protein, which is responsible for the import of ADP into mitochondria and therefore a prerequisite for oxidative phosphorylation, increases in mitochondrial membrane surface area, and changes in membrane lipid composition. Some investigators believe that a considerable portion of resting oxygen consumption can be attributed to the passive leak of protons back into mitochondria (Harper et al., 1993). The operation of the electron transport chain is coupled to the extrusion of protons from the inner mitochondrial space. The mitochondrial membrane contains proton ports, which allow their return coupled to the synthesis of ATP. However, in addition to these ports, it has been shown that the mitochondrial membrane itself is not completely impermeable to protons. Moreover, such thyroid-induced effects as increased membrane surface area or changed membrane lipid composition may enhance this permeability; this would result in increased oxygen consumption without altering ATP production, and thus enhance basal metabolic rate.

Even the proponents of these ideas calculate that these effects on energy production can account for only a part of the thyroid hormone–dependent increase in metabolic rate. In addition, treatment with T_3 not only results in increased amounts of respiratory chain components but also in a greater state of reduction of these components. This implies an enhanced delivery of reducing equivalents to the chain, which is equivalent to increased energy consumption. It has also been shown that T_3 increases the production of ATP, which must then be utilized at a faster rate. Otherwise respiration will be limited by a lack of ADP. Numerous ATP-consuming processes are enhanced by thyroid hormone and collectively account for the increased load on mitochondria.

Effects on Energy-Consuming Processes. A well-known effect of hyperthyroidism is increased heart rate (Klein, 1990). Cardiac size, stroke volume, and output are all increased. These changes may be partially attributed to direct transcriptional effects on cardiac genes, but the increased load on the heart also plays an important role. Increased oxygen consumption overall results in an enhanced requirement for oxygen supply and therefore blood flow.

A second target of thyroid hormone is the cell membrane Na^+,K^+-ATPase. This protein utilizes ATP to pump sodium out and potassium into cells, both against a considerable concentration gradient. The expression of the gene encoding Na^+,K^+-ATPase is stimulated by thyroid hormone treatment, and earlier experiments suggested this could account for the major portion of increased oxygen consumption in some tissues. However, these experiments, which involved measurement of oxygen consumption in tissue preparations in vitro, have been criticized as nonphysiological. Subsequent studies in more intact systems have suggested a much more limited role for this protein, perhaps accounting for 5% to 10% of the enhanced oxygen consumption (Clausen et al., 1991).

Changes in heart rate and ion pumping provide only a partial explanation for the thyroid hormone–dependent increase in ATP consumption. T_3 stimulation of fat, carbohydrate, and protein metabolism also increases requirements for ATP, and these effects are discussed in the next section.

Regulation of Macronutrient Metabolism

The nutritional significance of iodine and the thyroid hormones is magnified by the fact that T_3 regulates the metabolism of all the macronutrients. An unusual characteristic of this regulation is that it operates on both the anabolic and catabolic arms of these pathways. Although construction and destruction of macromolecules may appear to be wasteful, it is completely consistent with the central role of thyroid hormones to generate heat for the maintenance of body temperature.

Lipids. Thyroid hormone stimulates fatty acid synthesis by enhancing expression of the genes involved in this process. The principal target is liver, but smaller inductions also occur in other tissues. The target genes, which respond in a coordinated fashion, include acetyl CoA carboxylase and fatty acid synthase, which are directly responsible for assembling the carbon skeleton, as well as enzymes of the hexose monophosphate shunt and malic enzyme, which generate the reducing equivalents as NADPH. The esterification of fatty acids into triacylglycerols and phospholipids is also increased by T_3. (See Chapter 13 for details of lipid metabolism.)

This induction of lipid synthesis might surprise a clinician who would be more familiar with the reduced triacylglycerol stores associated with hyperthyroidism. Thyroid hormone also enhances lipolysis, probably by increasing the sensitivity of adipose cells to circulating catecholamines. The fatty acids released are also oxidized at an enhanced rate. This is because thyroid hormone also stimulates the expression of carnitine palmitoyltransferase, the protein that governs the entry of fatty acids into mitochondria for β-oxidation. Many of these pathways of lipid metabolism are counter-regulated. For example, the activity of carnitine palmitoyltransferase is inhibited by malonyl CoA, the product of acetyl CoA carboxylase, which catalyzes the first step of fatty acid synthesis. Similarly, long-chain fatty acids, which are elevated in catabolic states, inhibit the activity of acetyl CoA carboxylase and therefore limit fatty acid synthesis. This counterregulation is overcome by thyroid hormone by increasing the expression of the genes encoding these enzymes. The increased enzyme mass then allows greater flux through both pathways, in spite of the mutual inhibition.

A negative relationship between thyroid status and plasma cholesterol levels is another feature of thyroid disease well known to clinicians. Regulation of cholesterol metabolism is also an example of the double actions of thyroid hormone. T_3 treatment increases the levels of mRNA encoding the hydroxymethyl-glutaryl CoA reductase enzyme, thereby increasing cholesterol synthesis. However, it also stimulates the biliary clearance of cholesterol; this effect predominates and results in the lower levels observed in the circulation. Attempts have been made to produce a thyroid hormone agonist that would be active in liver and therefore reduce circulating cholesterol levels but leave heart rate unaffected. Such a drug might be extremely useful for treating hypercholesterolemia.

Carbohydrates. Hyperthyroidism increases and hypothyroidism decreases substrate cycling through multiple pathways of glucose metabolism. Glycolysis is accelerated as well as gluconeogenesis. Glycogen stores are depleted in the hyperthyroid state, which further emphasizes the importance of lipid stores to meet the energy demands under this condition. It seems reasonable to suppose that these effects are mediated by transcriptional regulation of the enzymes involved. Perhaps the best-investigated step in this context is phosphoenolpyruvate carboxykinase, which plays a key regulatory role in gluconeogenesis.

Treatment with thyroid hormone stimulates transcription of this gene, at least in the rat, and a TRE has been identified in its promoter.

Proteins. Protein turnover is also sensitive to thyroid state. Less is known about T_3 regulation of these pathways in comparison with those involving the other macronutrients. Hyperthyroidism leads to a generalized increase in RNA synthesis in both cardiac and skeletal muscle, which in turn accelerates protein synthesis. However, muscle mass has been shown to be decreased in the thyrotoxic state, so that, as with lipid and carbohydrate metabolism, the overall effect of high T_3 is catabolic.

The pathways underlying the thermogenic effects of thyroid hormone are summarized in Figure 33–8. Many specifics, including the relative contributions of these various components and of different organ systems to the overall effect, remain to be determined. (Additional information on regulation of energy metabolism can be found in Chapters 17 through 19.)

Regulation of Growth and Development

It is quite clear in the rat that T_3 stimulates transcription of the growth hormone gene,

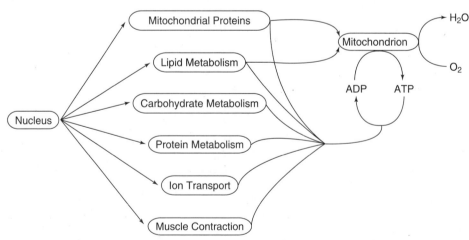

Figure 33–8. *Mechanisms underlying the stimulation of oxygen consumption by thyroid hormone. T_3, acting via its nuclear receptors, regulates the levels of proteins required for the synthesis and breakdown of macronutrients, for ion transport, and for muscle contraction. Both the synthesis and operation of these proteins consume ATP and therefore stimulate respiration. Thyroid state also affects mitochondrial function by changing the membrane lipid composition and by altering the level of mitochondrial proteins encoded by both the mitochondrial and nuclear genomes. (Adapted from Freake, H.C. and Oppenheimer, J.H. [1995] Thermogenesis and thyroid function. Reproduced, with permission, from the Annual Review of Nutrition, Volume 15, pp. 263–291. © 1995 by Annual Reviews Inc.)*

and indeed this system has been widely used as a model for the regulation of gene expression by thyroid hormone (Samuels et al., 1988). The situation is less clear in humans and attempts to demonstrate responsiveness of the human growth hormone gene to T_3 using various preparations in vitro have met with mixed results. However, it appears that growth hormone secretion is impaired in hypothyroid individuals, as is signaling through the insulin-like growth factor 1 pathway. Thus T_3 does appear to be necessary for normal growth hormone activity in humans. The effects of thyroid hormone on growth and development, at the level of a particular tissue or organ system, are the aggregate of direct T_3 effects and of those produced by growth hormone as well as by other secondary signals influenced by thyroid state.

Brain Development. The brain has traditionally represented a fascinating conundrum to investigators of thyroid hormone action. On the one hand, the devastating effects of a lack of thyroid hormones are all too apparent in the syndrome of cretinism (discussed in the next section). On the other hand, the brain is one of the few organs that does not appear to respond to thyroid hormone in terms of alterations in metabolic rate. The mystery has been solved only partially. One key to the solution is the realization that brain growth and development are completed relatively early in the life span of the organism. In humans, it appears to be complete in the third year of life (Porterfield and Hendrich, 1993).

Much of the work looking at thyroid hormones and brain development has utilized rodents. This is appropriate as long as it is appreciated that the chronology of brain development in these animals differs from that in humans. Although of course the human time line is much longer than the rat's, brain development in the rat occurs relatively late, so that more neurogenesis occurs postnatally. In humans, most neuronal cell division is complete at birth. However, the development of these neurons, including axonal outgrowth and synaptogenesis, continues into the first 2 years of life, as does the production of glial cells and the process of myelinogenesis. These processes (i.e., the development of appropriate brain architecture and organization) are thyroid hormone-dependent. The effects are presumed to be mediated by the nuclear pathway at the transcriptional level. Some gene targets have been identified, including those encoding myelin basic protein, cytoskeletal components, and various growth factors (Porterfield and Hendrich, 1993).

In humans, the fetal thyroid begins to function in the 3rd month of gestation. Prior to that time, requirements for thyroid hormone are met by placental transport of maternally synthesized hormones (Porterfield and Hendrich, 1993). During the 2nd and 3rd trimesters, fetal requirements are met by a combination of fetal and maternal sources. Iodine deficiency compromises both maternal and fetal thyroid hormone synthesis. The significance of the maternal supply is indicated by comparing the consequences of iodine deficiency with those of congenital hypothyroidism. In the latter condition, the maternal iodine supply is intact and the neurological symptoms in the newborn infant are distinctly milder.

Receptors for thyroid hormone are present in fetal brain by the 10th week of gestation. It appears likely that thyroid hormone plays a role in brain development from this early point through the first 2 years of life. The consequences of deficiency at any particular time may not be reversible by later supplementation. The extent of the reversibility will depend on the timing and the severity of the deficiency. Although in some cases cretinism may not be prevented by supplementation as early as the second trimester, the effects of congenital hypothyroidism are at least partially alleviated by treatment postnatally. The routine screening of the thyroid status of neonates in the United States is useful because postnatal treatment with thyroid hormones can improve the status of these infants, even though as a group they still have learning difficulties.

Although it is clear that thyroid hormone is required for normal brain development, it is less certain whether it plays a role in the functioning of the mature brain.

Developmental Effects on Other Tissues. Hypothyroidism leads to reduced muscle mass and delayed skeletal maturation (Brown et al., 1981). Lung maturation in the fetus has also been reported to be dependent on thyroid hormone. The effects of thyroid state on the heart have already been mentioned, in terms of their contribution to energy expenditure. A part of these effects is mediated by differential effects of T_3 on the expression of the myosin heavy chain genes (Izumo et al., 1986). There are two myosin heavy chain genes, α and β, and T_3 stimulates transcription of the α form. Growth hormone also has important influences on these tissues, and thus at least some of the consequences of hypothyroidism are likely to be mediated by lack of this trophic hormone.

IODINE DEFICIENCY

Scope of the Problem

Iodine deficiency is classically recognized by the enlargement of the thyroid gland, known as goiter. An insufficient supply of iodine results in reduced accumulation of the mineral in the thyroid gland and diminished production of thyroid hormones. Lower plasma levels of T_4 lead to an increased production of TSH by the anterior pituitary gland. This stimulates many aspects of thyroid gland function, including the hyperplasia that leads to the goiter. This chronic stimulation of the thyroid gland also causes more efficient iodine uptake. This uptake can be measured clinically using a radioactive isotope of iodine, and radioactive iodine uptake has been used to assess iodine status.

Goiter is only one of many symptoms resulting from lack of iodide, and the broader term iodine deficiency disorders (IDD) is now preferred. The World Health Organization considers iodine deficiency to be the "greatest single cause of preventable brain damage and mental retardation" in the world today (Micronutrient Deficiency Information System, 1993). This statement is based on the assumption that all people living in areas where the prevalence of goiter among school-age children is greater than 5% are at risk. It also assumes that the effects of limited iodine on brain development fall on a spectrum, ranging from severe neurological cretinism to mar-

ginal effects on intellectual performance. Although the assumptions behind these estimates are arguable, it is indisputable that iodine deficiency is an enormous public health problem.

Estimates made in 1997 suggest that 14.4% of the world's population, or 845 million people, had a goiter (Table 33–2). Those afflicted were found in all regions of the world. In many parts of Europe, IDD is still widespread. For example, in Italy, although iodized salt is available it accounts for only 2% of domestic consumption. Thus, in 1993, the WHO estimated a goiter prevalence of 20% of schoolchildren in Italy (Micronutrient Deficiency Information System, 1993). In contrast, in Switzerland, which historically has had very high goiter rates, the condition has now been eliminated. In Switzerland, 92% of domestically consumed salt is iodized. Estimates of those at risk from iodine deficiency disorders worldwide amount to 1.6 billion people, approaching 30% of the total population.

Cretinism

Although goiter may be the most obvious form of IDD, the effects on neurological development are the most important. The extent of the neurological impairment depends on the timing and severity of the iodine deficiency. One critical period is in the 1st trimester of pregnancy, when a lack of maternally supplied thyroid hormones at a time of very active fetal brain development has irreversible consequences. Severe effects of iodine lack are called cretinism and have classically been divided into two types, neurological and myxedematous. In the former, the neurological symptoms are severe and include mental retardation, deaf mutism, and spastic diplegia (paralysis) of the legs. Myxedematous or hypothyroid cretinism has less severe neurological symptoms, but those affected are more clinically hypothyroid and growth retarded. It has been suggested that concurrent selenium deficiency may at least in part explain some of these symptomatic differences.

Other Consequences

In addition to the long-term consequence of cretinism, an insufficient supply of iodine dur-

TABLE 33–2
Prevalence of Iodine Deficiency Disorders

Groupings	Total Goiter Rate	
	Prevalence (%)	*Population Affected (millions)*
Global		
Male	13.0	380.1
Female	15.8	464.6
Both sexes	14.4	844.7
Age Groups		
School age 6–12 y	17.6	159.3
General population	14.4	844.7
WHO Regions		
Africa	21.9	135.7
Americas	5.7	45.6
Eastern Mediterranean	29.0	138.9
Europe	9.0	78.3
Southeast Africa	14.3	210.5
Western Pacific	14.4	235.7
Level of Development		
(1) Developed market-economy countries	2.8	23.1
(2) Developing countries (excluding least developed)	14.9	602.7
(3) Developing countries (least developed)	29.7	185.1
(4) Economies in transition	8.6	33.8

The population at risk for IDD is approximately twice the goiter-affected population. Tabulated values are taken from WHO Global Database on Prevalence of IDD (1997 update). Used with permission of the World Health Organization.

ing pregnancy is also associated with an increased occurrence of spontaneous abortions, stillbirths, and congenital abnormalities, as well as perinatal and infant mortality (Hetzel, and Maberly, 1986). It is quite clear that profound iodine lack results in cretinism and that this damage is irreversible by later treatment with thyroid hormones. What is less apparent is the extent to which mild iodine deficiency causes much smaller decrements in neurological function and whether or not these may be reversible. In areas of iodine deficiency, supplementation with iodine of mothers prior to conception results in children with improved cognitive performance relative to those given a placebo (Pharoah et al., 1971). Also, comparison of children in communities that are similar other than in the amount of iodine available suggests that iodine deficiency may lead to developmental delays (Pharoah, and Connolly, 1995). However these effects may all be due to fetal iodine deficiency.

Iodine deficiency after birth can result in hypothyroidism and goiter. Whether it also leads to impaired neurological function and, if so, whether these effects can be reversed by iodine supplementation is an open question. It used to be said that the adult brain was

refractory to thyroid hormone treatment. This was based on animal studies showing that brain was one of the few tissues in the body that did not increase oxygen consumption in response to thyroid hormone treatment. In addition, a number of morphological and biochemical parameters that were sensitive to thyroid hormone in the neonatal period, but not at later times, were identified. However, in the last few years some biochemical responses to thyroid hormone in adult brain have been identified, at least in the rat (Alvarez-Dolado et al., 1994). This allows the possibility that milder consequences of thyroid insufficiency, if they exist, can be remedied at later ages.

Other Thyroid Abnormalities

Deficiencies of iodine are entirely manifested through abnormalities in thyroid hormone metabolism and function. Situations are often seen clinically in which the latter are disordered in the face of normal iodine supply. Hypothyroidism can result from a primary defect in the thyroid gland itself, from a pituitary or hypothalamic dysfunction leading to insufficient stimulation of the gland by TSH, or

---

CLINICAL CORRELATION

Interaction of Iodine and Selenium Status in the Development of Cretinism

Nutrient deficiencies are likely to occur in combination. The symptoms caused by the lack of one nutrient may be modified by the concurrent shortage of a second. It has been suggested that the division of cretinism into the neurological and myxedematous types may be explained by selenium status (Corvilain et al., 1993). An interesting conjunction of molecular, animal, and population data has come together in support of this hypothesis. The type I deiodinase contains the amino acid selenocysteine, and thus its synthesis is inhibited by selenium deficiency (Berry et al., 1991). This molecular prediction has been validated by animal studies that have shown impaired enzyme activity and reduced conversion of T_4 to T_3 (Beckett et al., 1992). Iodine deficiency will limit T_4 production, but concurrent selenium deficiency, by limiting peripheral conversion to T_3, will help preserve circulating T_4 levels. This will then be available to the brain, where the selenium-independent type II deiodinase will catalyze local production of T_3. Thus the selenium deficiency may help preserve neurological function.

However, selenium lack will also impair another selenium-dependent enzyme, glutathione peroxidase. The production of thyroid hormones by thyroid peroxidase requires an oxidative environment, and glutathione peroxidase protects against damaging effects of that environment. An impaired antioxidant defense system will result in irreversible damage to the thyroid gland, particularly when the gland is stimulated in an attempt to make up for insufficient iodine (Corvilain et al., 1993). Thus the brain may be protected, but the thyroid gland is damaged and the myxedematous type of cretinism results. When selenium is sufficient, the thyroid gland will be protected, but the T_4 it produces will be more quickly metabolized to T_3, leaving less available for the brain. At early stages of life this leads to irreversible damage and neurological cretinism.

This is an interesting hypothesis, which has yet to be fully supported. One consequence would be that care needs to be taken that the iodine supply is adequate when treating selenium deficiency. Otherwise, selenium supplementation would restore conversion of T_4 to T_3 by the type I deiodinase, lessen the supply of T_4 for the brain, and therefore potentially increase neurological damage.

Thinking Critically

What additional studies would you propose to confirm the hypothesis that impaired selenium status is responsible for the development of myxedematous as opposed to neurological cretinism?

---

from a peripheral resistance to thyroid hormone. The latter has usually been attributed to a defect in the receptor signaling pathway. The resulting clinical symptoms are fairly generalized, and most organ systems are affected. The symptoms include fatigue, cold intolerance, mental slowness, reduced cardiac function, and increased serum cholesterol. Increased serum TSH is a biochemical characteristic, and patients are treated with sufficient T_4 to return TSH levels to the normal range.

Hyperthyroidism is most often caused by Graves' disease, which results in a continuous stimulation of the thyroid gland and overproduction of thyroid hormones. This is an autoimmune disease, more often seen in women, caused by antibodies directed against the TSH receptor. Hyperthyroidism can also result from thyroid adenomas or thyroiditis. The symptoms include weight loss, increased heat production, tachycardia, muscular tremor, irritability, and nervousness, as well as exophthalmos (protrusion of the eyes) and enlargement of the thyroid. Treatment is by antithyroid drugs, radioactive iodine to cause necrosis of the thyroid cells, or surgical thyroidectomy. The latter two treatments can result in hypothyroidism, which may require thyroid hormone replacement.

Prevention

Iodine deficiencies can be combated by programs directed at the whole population or targeted at those particularly at risk. Iodization of salt represents a simple, inexpensive, and effective measure to supply iodine to a population, and there are several examples of it being used to eliminate IDD. Either potassium iodide or potassium iodate (which is more stable) can be used. However, the high prevalence of IDD in the face of the decades-old knowledge of how to prevent the condition shows that reality is more complex. The amount of iodized salt required is enormous, and its distribution to many of the communities at risk is very difficult. Most if not all populations in the world use salt and so have developed their own local means to produce it. The introduction of iodized salt, therefore, either means replacing the local product with potentially unacceptable, centrally produced iodized salt, or putting the technology in place to allow fortification on a local basis. Ensuring a stable and reliable supply of iodized salt may be very difficult or impossible using the latter approach. Fortification of other foods has been attempted, often with success, but it is unlikely that fortification of other foods would have as widespread applicability as a salt supplementation program. Water represents another fortification vehicle

that has been used to deliver iodine to a population.

Apart from iodized salt, the most common vehicle used for delivery of iodine is iodized oil (Hetzel et al., 1987). The fatty acids of the oil are chemically modified by iodination, and, once inside the body, the iodine is slowly released over a period of months to years. Injection of the oil is the usual route of administration; oral preparations, which are cheaper but less effective, are also available. These treatments are most often used in remote areas, where interactions with health services are rare and introduction of iodized salt is problematic. They permit the supply of iodine to those segments of the population who are particularly at risk (i.e., women of child-bearing age and infants and children).

Supplementation to individuals who have had lifelong iodine deficiency can lead to thyrotoxicosis. The long-term stimulation of the thyroid gland can lead to its autonomous functioning; in other words, it continues to take up iodine and synthesize and secrete thyroid hormones even when adequate iodine is supplied and the stimulus of high TSH is removed. This complication is easily treated with antithyroid drugs.

NUTRITION INSIGHT

"Please Pass the Iodine"

Large areas of the northern United States have soil with low iodine, presumably because of mineral losses during the glaciation of the Ice Age. Thus IDD and goiter were endemic at the beginning of this century. The magnitude of this problem was noted at the time of World War I, when conscripts were turned away because they had goiters. Treatment with sodium iodide was shown to be effective. Thus both the cause and cure for the problem were apparent. The question was what was to be done or, more specifically, how could the iodine intake of large numbers of people be increased?

Many solutions were considered and rejected, including use of iodine-containing fertilizers, supplementing cows to increase the iodine content of milk, and iodination of public water supplies. Table salt, a product that is commonly eaten and that can be supplemented easily and cheaply, was selected as the vehicle for fortification. Iodization of salt began in 1924. The program was and is voluntary. Thus consumers had to be persuaded to buy the new fortified product. "Please Pass the Iodine" was a story that ran in the Saturday Evening Post at that time. In Michigan, where 40% of the population had goiters, a state-run education campaign was assisted by manufacturers and grocers and only iodized salt was sold. Four years later, the incidence of goiter had dropped to 10%, and it then declined further until 1951 when only 1.4% of schoolchildren in Michigan had goiters (Brush and Atland, 1952).

Acknowledgment is made to contributions of Linda Daube, M.S., in the preparation of this material.

IODINE REQUIREMENTS

The 1989 edition of the Recommended Dietary Allowances (National Research Council, 1989) set the iodine requirement at 150 μg for both male and female adults. This allowance is set at about twice that needed to maintain urinary iodine levels greater than 50 μg/g of creatinine, the level that has been determined to indicate normal function. This safety margin allows for the presence of dietary goitrogens. The allowances for infants and children have been set at lower levels in proportion to energy requirements "in the absence of a better basis." Additional allowances of 25 μg/day for pregnancy and 50 μg/day for lactation have been set. Intakes in the United States are usually well in excess of these levels, due to the use of iodized salt, which contains 76 μg of iodine/g, and also to the use of iodates in bread production.

REFERENCES

Alvarez-Dolado, M., Iglesias, T., Rodriguez-Pena, A., Bernal, J. and Munoz, A. (1994) Expression of neurotropins and the trk family of neurotropin receptors in normal and hypothyroid rat brain. Mol Brain Res 27:249–257.

Beckett, G. J., Russell, A., Nicol, F., Sahu, P., Wolf, C. R. and Arthur, J. R. (1992) Effect of selenium deficiency on hepatic type I 5-iodothyronine deiodinase activity and hepatic thyroid hormone levels in the rat. Biochem J 282:483–486.

Berry, M. J., Banu, L. and Larsen, P. R. (1991) Type I iodothyronine deiodinase is a selenocysteine-containing enzyme. Nature 349:438–440.

Blennemann, B., Leahy, P., Kim, T.-S. and Freake, H. C. (1995) Tissue-specific regulation of lipogenic mRNAs by thyroid hormone. Mol Cell Endocrinol 110:1–8.

Brown, J. G., Bates, P. C., Holliday, M. A. and Millward, D. J. (1981) Thyroid hormones and muscle protein turnover. Biochem J 194:771–782.

Brush, B. E. and Altland, J. K. (1952) Goiter prevention with iodized salt: Results of a thirty-year study. J Clin Endocrinol Metab 12:1380–1388.

Clausen, T., Van Hardeveld, C. and Everts, M. E. (1991) Significance of cation transport in control of energy metabolism and thermogenesis. Physiol Rev 71:733–774.

Corvilain, B., Contempre, B., Longombe, A. O., Goyens, P., Gervy-Decoster, C., Lamy, F., Vanderpas, J. B. and Dumont, J. E. (1993) Selenium and the thyroid: How the relationship was established. Am J Clin Nutr 57(Suppl):244S–248S.

Evans, R. M. (1988) The steroid and thyroid hormone receptor superfamily. Science 240:889–895.

Freake, H. C. and Oppenheimer, J. H. (1995) Thermogenesis and thyroid function. Annu Rev Nutr 15:263–291.

Harper, M. E., Ballantyne, J. S., Leach, M. and Brand, M. D. (1993) Effects of thyroid hormone on oxidative phosphorylation. Biochem Soc Trans 21:785–792.

Hetzel, B. S., Dunn, J. T. and Stanbury, J. B., eds. (1987) The Prevention and Control of Iodine Deficiency Disorders. Elsevier, Amsterdam.

Hetzel, B. S. and Maberly, G. F. (1986) Iodine. In: Trace Elements in Human and Animal Nutrition (Mertz, W. ed.), pp. 139–208. Academic Press, New York.

Horlein, A. J., Naar, M., Heinzel, T., Torchia, J., Gloss, B., Kurokawa, R., Ryan, A., Kamei, Y., Soderstrom, M., Glass, C. K. and Rosenfeld, M. G. (1995) Ligand-independent repression by the thyroid hormone receptor mediated by nuclear receptor corepressor. Nature 377:397–404.

Izumo, S., Nadal-Ginard, B. and Mahdavi, V. (1986) All members of the MHC multigene family respond to thyroid hormone in a highly tissue-specific manner. Nature 231:557–560.

Kinlaw, W. B., Church, J. L., Harmon, J. and Mariash, C. N. (1995) Direct evidence for a role of the "spot 14" protein in the regulation of lipid synthesis. J Biol Chem 270:16615–16618.

Kinlaw, W. B., Tron, P. and Friedmann, A. S. (1992) Nuclear localization and hepatic zonation of rat "spot 14" protein: Immunochemical investigation employing anti-fusion protein antibodies. Endocrinology 131:3120–3122.

Klein, I. (1990) Thyroid hormone and the cardiovascular system. Am J Med 88:631–637.

Lazar, M. A. (1993) Thyroid hormone receptors: Multiple forms, multiple possibilities. Endocrinol Rev 14:184–193.

Lee, J. W., Ryan, F., Swaffield, J. C., Johnston, S. A. and Moore, D. D. (1995) Interaction of thyroid-hormone receptor with a conserved transcriptional mediator. Nature 374:91–94.

Leonard, J. L. and Visser, T. J. (1986) Biochemistry of deiodination. In: Thyroid Hormone Metabolism (Hennemann, G., ed.), pp. 189–229. Marcel Dekker, New York.

Micronutrient Deficiency Information System (1993) Global Prevalence of Iodine Deficiency Disorders, World Health Organization, Geneva.

National Research Council (1989) Recommended Dietary Allowances, 10th ed. National Academy Press, Washington, D. C.

Pharoah, P. O. D., Buttfield, I. H. and Hetzel, B. S. (1971) Neurological damage to the fetus resulting from severe iodine deficiency during pregnancy. Lancet 1:398–410.

Pharoah, P. O. D. and Connolly, K. J. (1995) Iodine and brain development. Dev Med Child Neurol 38:464–469.

Porterfield, S. P. and Hendrich, C. E. (1993) The role of thyroid hormones in prenatal and neonatal neurological development—current perspectives. Endocrinol Rev 14:94–106.

Querido, A., Delange, F., Dunn, J. T., Fierro-Benitez, R., Ibbertson, H. K., Koutras, D. A. and Perinetti, H. (1974) Definitions of endemic goiter and cretinism, classification of goiter size and severity of endemics, and survey techniques. In: Endemic Goiter and Cretinism: Continuing Threats to World Health (Dunn, J. T. and Medeiros-Neto, G. A., eds.). Scientific Publ. No. 292, pp. 267–272. Pan American Health Organization, Washington, D. C.

Refetoff, S. and Weiss, R. E. (1993) The syndromes of resistance to thyroid hormones. Endocrinol Rev 14:348–399.

Samuels, H., Forman, B., Horowitz, Z. and Ye, Z.-S. (1988) Regulation of gene expression by thyroid hormones. J Clin Invest 81:957–967.

Sap, J., Munoz, A., Damm, K., Goldberg, Y., Ghsydael, J., Leutz, A., Beug, H. and Vennstrom, B. (1986) The c-erb-A protein is a high affinity receptor for thyroid hormone. Nature 324:635–640.

Seelig, S., Liaw, C., Towle, H. C. and Oppenheimer, J. H. (1981) Thyroid hormone attenuates and augments hepatic gene expression at a pretranslational level. Proc Natl Acad Sci USA 78:4733–4737.

Vallee, B. L., Coleman, J. E. and Auld, D. S. (1991) Zinc fingers, zinc clusters, and zinc twists in DNA-binding protein domains. Proc Natl Acad Sci USA 88:999–1003.

Weinberger, C., Thompson, C. C., Ong, E. S., Lebo, R., Gruol, D. J. and Evans, R. M. (1986) The c-erb-A gene encodes a thyroid hormone receptor. Nature 324:641–646.

Yen, P. M. and Chin, W. W. (1994) New advances in understanding the molecular mechanisms of thyroid hormone action. Trends Endocrinol Metab 5:65–72.

Zilz, N. D., Murray, M. B. and Towle, H. C. (1990) Identification of multiple thyroid hormone response elements located far upstream from the rat S14 promoter. J Biol Chem 265:8136–8143.

RECOMMENDED READINGS

Brent, G. A., Moore, D. D. and Larsen, P. R. (1991) Thyroid hormone regulation of gene expression. Annu Rev Physiol 53:17–35.

Freake, H. C. and Oppenheimer, J. H. (1995) Thermogenesis and thyroid function. Annu Rev Nutr 15:263–291.

Hetzel, B. S. and Maberly, G. F. (1986) Iodine. In: Trace Elements in Human and Animal Nutrition (Mertz, W., ed.), pp. 139–208. Academic Press, New York.

McNabb, F. M. A. (1992) Thyroid Hormones. Prentice-Hall, Englewood Cliffs, N.J.

CHAPTER **34**

◆◆◆◆◆◆◆◆◆◆◆◆◆◆◆◆◆◆◆◆◆◆◆◆◆◆◆◆◆◆◆◆◆◆◆◆◆◆

Selenium

Roger A. Sunde, Ph.D.

OUTLINE

COMMON ABBREVIATIONS

Sec (selenocysteine)
SECIS (selenocysteine insertion sequence)
SEL-A (selenocysteine synthetase)
SEL-B (selenocysteine-specific elongation factor)
Sel-C (tRNA$^{Ser \rightarrow Sec}_{UCA}$)
SEL-D (selenophosphate synthetase)
U (1-letter symbol for Sec)

CHEMISTRY OF SELENIUM

Selenium (Se) was discovered in 1817 by the Swedish chemist Berzelius in the flue dust of iron pyrite burners, and this new element was named after the Greek *selene* (moon). The remainder of the 19th century saw limited use of selenium as CdSe in the ruby red coloring of glass. Selenium's notoriety as a toxic element emerged in the 1930s with its identification as the causative agent of several forms of "loco diseases" in horses and cattle caused by the ingestion of high selenium-containing plants. In 1943, a 5 mg/kg selenium diet was reported to cause the development of neoplasms in rat liver, thus marking selenium as a carcinogenic agent. It was therefore surprising when Schwarz and Foltz (1957) reported that liver necrosis in rats could be prevented by inorganic selenium, leading to the demonstration that selenium was a nutritionally essential trace element. In the 1960s and 1970s, epidemiological data and animal research began to demonstrate that selenium also possesses anticarcinogenic activity. Since the discovery that glutathione peroxidase-1 (GPX1; discussed in the section on Mammalian Selenoproteins) is a selenoenzyme, at least ten additional selenoenzymes have been identified in higher animals (Burk, 1994; Stadtman, 1996; Sunde, 1994, 1997; Xia, 1997).

Selenium lies below oxygen and sulfur in the group VIa elements in the periodic table. Thus selenium has both metallic and nonmetallic properties, resulting in its unique chemistry and biochemistry. Its 34 electrons are distributed with 18 in the argon shell, 10 3d electrons, and 6 electrons in the 4s and 4p orbitals. The 4s and 4p electrons, when lost, give rise to the common $+6$ and $+4$ oxidation states, whereas the addition of 2 electrons to the 4p orbitals completes the octet to yield the -2 oxidation state. The atomic weight of the naturally abundant isotope of selenium is 78.96, and 6 naturally occurring stable isotopes of selenium have potential for use as tracers.

Selenium's chemical properties (Cotton and Wilkinson, 1972) have a strong impact on selenium biology. First, the empty $d\pi$ orbitals of selenium can be filled by $p\pi$ electrons of oxygen, resulting in multiple "$d\pi$-$p\pi$ bonds" similar to those of sulfur, thus permitting the formation of more than 4 σ bonds to other atoms, as might occur during selenium-catalyzed enzyme reactions (see Fig. 34–1 for common structures). These $d\pi$-$p\pi$ orbitals also confer the unique electronic properties taken advantage of by enzymes. Second, selenium and sulfur have similar radii, so that covalent sulfur and selenium compounds (C—S—X or C—Se—X) are not readily distinguished by enzymes based upon bond length. Third, selenium and sulfur also have similar chemical reactivity.

Two aspects of selenium and sulfur chemistry are significantly different, however, permitting ready separation of selenium and sulfur under physiological conditions. First, hydrogen selenide (H_2Se) is a much stronger acid than is hydrogen sulfide (H_2S). At physiological pH, the amino acid selenocysteine (Sec) has a selenol pK_2 of 5.24 and is predominantly deprotonated, whereas the cysteine thiol with a pK_2 of 8.25 is largely protonated. Second, the reduction potentials of selenious and selenic acid are much greater than those of the analogous sulfur acids, so biological metabolism directs selenium toward reduction and sulfur toward oxidation.

SELENIUM DEFICIENCY AND ESSENTIALITY

The use of purified and semipurified diets led to the identification of selenium as a nutritionally essential mineral element. A water-soluble factor present in American brewer's yeast was found to prevent liver necrosis in rats fed a diet based on torula yeast as the protein source. Supplementation of this diet with cystine, vitamin E, or this water-soluble "factor 3" would prevent liver necrosis in rats. This degenerative liver disease was distinct from fatty liver and liver cirrhosis and, if untreated, resulted in death in 21 to 28 days. In 1957, Schwarz and Foltz discovered that factor 3 isolated from pig kidney contained selenium, and that a variety of inorganic as well as organic forms of selenium would prevent liver necrosis in rats. Selenium alone was later shown to be unconditionally essential for rats

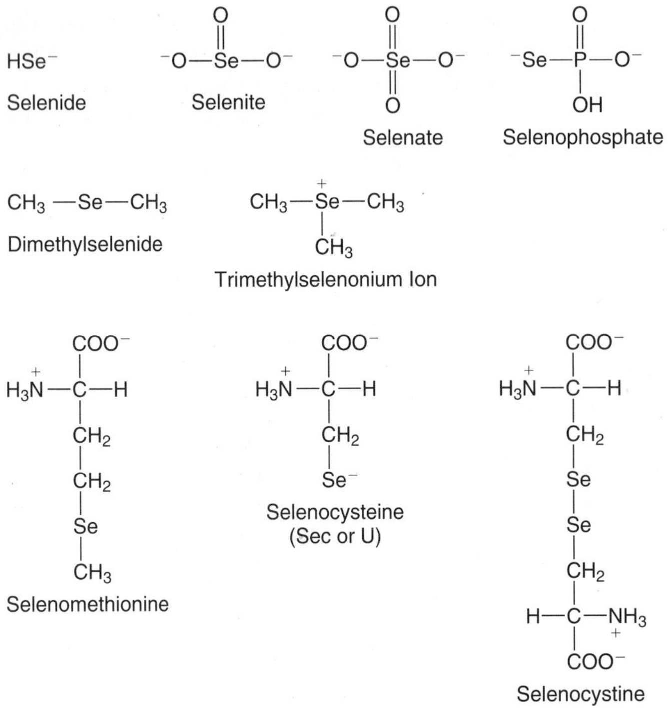

HSe⁻

Selenide

$$^-O—\overset{\overset{\displaystyle O}{\|}}{Se}—O^-$$

Selenite

$$^-O—\overset{\overset{\displaystyle O}{\|}}{\underset{\underset{\displaystyle O}{\|}}{Se}}—O^-$$

Selenate

$$^-Se—\overset{\overset{\displaystyle O}{\|}}{\underset{\underset{\displaystyle OH}{|}}{P}}—O^-$$

Selenophosphate

$CH_3—Se—CH_3$

Dimethylselenide

$$CH_3—\overset{+}{\underset{\underset{\displaystyle CH_3}{|}}{Se}}—CH_3$$

Trimethylselenonium Ion

Selenomethionine

$$\overset{\displaystyle COO^-}{H_3\overset{+}{N}—\overset{|}{C}—H}$$
$$\overset{|}{CH_2}$$
$$\overset{|}{CH_2}$$
$$\overset{|}{Se}$$
$$\overset{|}{CH_3}$$

Selenocysteine
(Sec or U)

$$\overset{\displaystyle COO^-}{H_3\overset{+}{N}—\overset{|}{C}—H}$$
$$\overset{|}{CH_2}$$
$$\overset{|}{Se^-}$$

Selenocystine

$$\overset{\displaystyle COO^-}{H_3\overset{+}{N}—\overset{|}{C}—H}$$
$$\overset{|}{CH_2}$$
$$\overset{|}{Se}$$
$$\overset{|}{Se}$$
$$\overset{|}{CH_2}$$
$$H—\overset{|}{C}—\overset{+}{NH_3}$$
$$\overset{|}{COO^-}$$

Figure 34–1. Structures of common selenium metabolites at physiological pH.

and chickens in diets containing adequate levels of vitamin E and sulfur amino acids.

Clear-cut evidence for the essentiality of selenium in humans was not reported until 2 decades later. Human selenium deficiency in a New Zealand patient undergoing total parenteral nutrition (TPN) was first reported in 1979. The patient lived in a rural area with low-selenium soils; endemic white muscle disease in sheep was controlled by selenium

NUTRITION INSIGHT

Selenium Geochemistry Influences Nutrition and Disease

Selenium is present in soils at both toxic and deficient levels. The origin of high-selenium soils is principally volcanic. Soil selenium in the Dakotas has been estimated to average as high as 0.1 g of Se/cm³ and to reach down to a thickness of 800 m. Rainfalls of less than 20 in/y do not leach soil sufficiently, resulting in retention of the high soil concentrations of selenium. The hard wheat grown in these areas of the Great Plains gives rise to bread that is a good source of dietary selenium. These high-selenium areas also harbor plants that accumulate toxic levels of selenium, which caused the "loco diseases" (alkali disease, blind staggers) and other equine problems (loss of hair and hooves) that were reported in 1860 around Fort Randall in the Dakota Territory (Rosenfeld and Beath, 1964).

Toxic buildup of selenium in the Kesterson Reservoir of California is due to irrigation of Se-rich soils in the San Joaquin Valley. This reservoir, or wetland, was developed in the late 1970s to collect subsurface drainage from the tile drainage systems used to irrigate the agricultural land of the San Joaquin Valley. The problem of selenium buildup was identified when fish and wildlife in the reservoir began dying in the early 1980s.

In contrast to areas with selenium-rich soils, lack of recent volcanic activity and low annual rainfall in some other regions of the country, such as Ohio and New York, have left some areas with soils so deficient in selenium that livestock were formerly commonly afflicted by diseases that are now known to be due to selenium deficiency and are prevented by selenium supplementation.

dosing. Following surgery, she was given TPN. After 20 days, she had dry, flaky skin, and after 30 days she developed bilateral muscular discomfort and muscle pain. Plasma selenium had dropped to 9 ng/mL of Se versus 25 ng/mL immediately before the start of TPN. The muscle pain was sufficient to aggravate walking, and a generalized muscular wasting occurred. The patient was then infused intravenously with 100 μg/day of Se; within the next week, muscle pain disappeared and she returned to full mobility. TPN-associated selenium deficiency in humans is not restricted solely to countries with low-selenium content in the soil. A similar TPN-induced case of muscle pain and cardiomyopathy leading to death has been reported in the United States. These cases are associated with very low levels of selenium in plasma and red blood cells, with low erythrocyte GPX1 activity, with elevated plasma marker enzymes indicative of tissue damage, and often with white nail beds.

Selenium deficiency is not just a clinical curiosity. Just as with animal species consuming feed produced locally, humans linked solely to regional food production are potentially susceptible to nutrient deficiency disease. An endemic Se-responsive disease, Keshan disease, formerly affecting peasant populations in Se-deficient areas of China, has now been completely eradicated by an aggressive Se-supplementation program. A regional disease of unknown origin, called Kashin-Beck disease, which continues to affect 8 million individuals in regions of northern China eating corn-based diets, also has been hypothesized to have selenium deficiency as a contributing factor.

SELENIUM ABSORPTION, DISTRIBUTION, AND EXCRETION

Selenium metabolism in the body is incompletely understood. Absorption is highly efficient, and selenium is lost from the body primarily in the urine. Most of the selenium present in body tissues is present as Sec in selenoproteins.

Selenium in Foods

The majority of selenium in most plants is selenomethionine. In "selenium-accumulator" plants, however, selenium is accumulated as selenium analogs of intermediates in sulfur amino acid metabolism, such as selenocystathionine and methylselenocysteine. The majority of selenium in products from animals fed usual levels of dietary selenium is present as selenoproteins and thus mostly Sec. Only elemental selenium, dimethylselenide, and the mercury-selenium complex in tuna are forms of selenium that are basically not available for conversion to biologically active selenium forms. In large part, most of the concern about the particular dietary form of selenium is a moot academic point, because selenium absorption from most sources is very high; homeostasis at the organism level does not occur via regulation of absorption.

Inorganic selenium is commonly used to supplement animal feeds and to provide inexpensive selenium in vitamin-mineral supplements. The most common inorganic form of selenium used in animal supplements is sodium selenite (Na_2SeO_3); sodium selenate (Na_2SeO_4) is increasingly used because, without the free electron pair, selenate is far less likely than selenite to oxidize other components of the diet.

Intake of selenium varies widely depending on the selenium content of the soil in which foods are grown as well as on supplement use. Typical intakes from food are 20 μg/day in China, 35 μg/day in Finland and New Zealand, and 50 to 200 μg/day in North America.

Selenium Absorption

In humans, both selenite and selenomethionine are highly available. In kinetic modeling experiments (Patterson et al., 1989), absorption from relatively large doses providing 200 μg of Se (~three times the recommended intake) was 84% for selenium provided as selenite and 98% for selenium provided as selenomethionine; these studies illustrate that a high absorption rate is not a microtracer phenomenon. Thus under physiological conditions, selenium homeostasis is clearly not regulated by absorption, but rather urinary excretion is likely to be important for homeostasis (Burk, 1976). The enzymes/transporters responsible for absorption or movement of selenium

CLINICAL CORRELATION

Keshan Disease

The dramatic impact of selenium deficiency in humans is revealed in the descriptions of Keshan disease, an endemic cardiomyopathy that occurred until the 1980s in China. Keshan disease affected primarily children under 15 years of age and women of child-bearing age. Prevalence rates prior to the start of selenium supplementation were on the order of 6.5 to 13.5 per thousand, and the disease was primarily localized in the peasant populations in certain hilly and mountainous regions with low soil selenium. Urban inhabitants and families of managerial classes living in the same areas were unaffected owing to an improved diet with more animal products and with products from a more diverse geographical range.

The main pathological feature of Keshan disease is a multiple focal myocardial necrosis scattered throughout the heart muscle. Criteria for diagnosis include acute or chronic heart function insufficiency, heart enlargement, gallop rhythm or arrhythmia, ECG changes, and pulmonary edema. Subacute cases may also have facial edema.

The demonstration that selenium was essential for laboratory animals and livestock in the 1960s, and the observations that the cardiomyopathy associated with Keshan disease was similar to that observed in Se-deficient mice and swine suggested trials with selenium. Encouraging preliminary results indicated selenium might be preventive. All affected areas were found to be invariably poor in selenium, and a large-scale study was begun in 1974 with all children in 119 production teams in three communes (Chen et al., 1980). Half the children were given weekly sodium selenite tablets orally and the other half were given a placebo. Children 1 to 5 years old received 0.5 mg and children 6 to 9 years old received 1 mg of sodium selenite (0.23 and 0.46 mg of Se/week, respectively). A total of 46,033 children were in this study. In the first 2 years, there were 5.6 deaths per thousand in the control group versus 0.08 per thousand in the treatment group. Because of the effectiveness of selenium supplementation, the control group was omitted for the last 2 years of the study. Total cases in the selenium-treatment group were not immediately eliminated but progressively declined over the 4-year study period, suggesting that more than restoration of selenium status may be involved in the disease.

The average hair selenium in nonaffected sites was above 0.2 μg of Se/g versus an average below 0.12 μg of Se/g for all affected sites. GPX1 activity in the blood of peasant children was two thirds of that observed in staff children. The average daily selenium intake for women in these affected areas was estimated to be 12 μg of Se/day, which is considerably lower than the New Zealand estimate of 20 μg of Se/day necessary for maintenance of normal human health (Chen et al., 1980; Robinson and Thomson, 1983).

The disease has now been virtually eliminated by selenium supplementation, but troubling questions remain about the etiology. The ineffectiveness of selenium to eradicate the disease completely in one season following selenium supplementation and a seasonal prevalence of the disease both suggest that other factors are involved. A cardiotoxic virus has been isolated from the hearts of individuals who died from Keshan disease, suggesting that a viral infection may be the underlying cause.

across membranes are mostly unknown. Selenomethionine is actively transported by the same system that transports methionine.

Selenium Excretion

Urinary methaneselenol, urinary trimethylselenonium ion, and expired dimethylselenide are the excretory forms of selenium. Both the size of the dose as well as the selenium status of an animal influences the form and amount of urinary selenium excretion. Methaneselenol is the usual major form of urinary selenium, and trimethylselenonium constitutes only a small fraction of urinary selenium in rats with low selenium status. However, trimethylselenonium is the major urinary selenium form in animals ingesting supernutritional levels of selenium. When pharmacological doses of selenium are injected into rats, selenium is expired in the breath as dimethylselenide; 50% of the Se from selenite and

35% of that from selenomethionine are expired as dimethylselenide in the first 24 hours after rats are injected with 5 mg of Se/kg of body weight.

In humans, methaneselenol is the major urinary form of selenium under deficient and adequate conditions; between 7% and 17% of urinary selenium is present as trimethylselenonium ion. Following administration of 200 μg of selenium to selenium-adequate adult humans, 17% of tracer selenite and 11% of tracer selenomethionine appeared in the urine over the following 12 days (Patterson et al., 1989). Trace amounts of dimethylselenide, which has a garlic-like odor, may be detected in the breath of people ingesting high levels of selenium.

Models of Selenium Metabolism

Elegant studies using the radioactive tracer ^{75}Se or stable isotopes have been conducted in rats and humans to monitor selenium flux. Figure 34–2 shows a whole-body model of human selenium metabolism from selenite, based on recent stable isotope kinetic modeling in humans as well as information from other studies with humans and rats. The diagram illustrates the fate of 70 μg of Se as selenite over a 12-day period in a Se-adequate subject. The diagram consists of intestine, the major site of selenium absorption, and compartments for blood, liver/pancreas, kidney, and muscle. Muscle represents muscle plus other tissues. An important aspect of this model is that plasma selenium is shown to consist of three distinctly different compartments: selenoprotein P (SEL-P), plasma glutathione peroxidase (GPX3; see section on Mammalian Selenoproteins), and a low molecular weight compartment of mainly hydrogen selenide (HSe$^-$).

Selenium absorption is 84%, or 59 μg of Se, with 16% released in the feces. Biliary recycling returns an additional 32 μg to the intestine, and 12 μg (17%) of the dose is released in the urine over the first 12 days. The remaining absorbed selenium is incorporated into tissue selenoproteins as part of normal protein turnover, thus displacing the original selenium, which mixes with the low molecular weight pool and is excreted, keeping the subject in selenium balance.

Intestinal selenite is most likely reduced to selenide during absorption, and red blood cells and other tissues also readily reduce selenite to selenide; thus selenide in the low molecular weight pool in plasma peaks about 2 h after ingestion and disappears with a half life of 20 min. The majority of this selenium is taken up by liver, incorporated into SEL-P, and secreted into the circulation. Plasma SEL-P concentration peaks at 10 h, with a half life of 3 h. Kidney is the major source of GPX3 in humans, and GPX3 levels in plasma peak at 13 h, with a half life of 12 h. To date, specific uptake of neither secreted SEL-P nor GPX3 has been demonstrated for any tissue, so the fates of these species are unknown. Thus the diagram shows distribution of SEL-P and GPX3 selenium directly to reticulocytes, muscle, and other tissues, although turnover of these species may occur in liver or kidney, with passage of this selenium through the plasma selenide pool before uptake by these other tissues.

Tissue Distribution of Selenium

Estimates of total selenium content of humans, determined from cadavers, range between 13.0 and 20.3 mg (Schroeder et al., 1970). Metabolic stable isotope methodology models predict that total body selenium asymptomatically approaches 30 mg, but these studies are based on subjects dosed with 200 μg of Se as the tracer (Patterson et al., 1989). Individuals living in New Zealand or China with considerably lower selenium intakes would be presumed to have a much lower total body burden of Se. Muscle, liver, blood, and kidneys contain 61% of the estimated total body selenium in humans; if skeleton is included, this increases to 91.5%.

METABOLIC PATHWAYS OF SELENIUM

The intracellular metabolism of selenium is complex not only because this trace "metal" bonds covalently to carbon, but also because unique metabolic pathways are necessary to convert simple dietary forms of selenium into the form found in selenium-containing en-

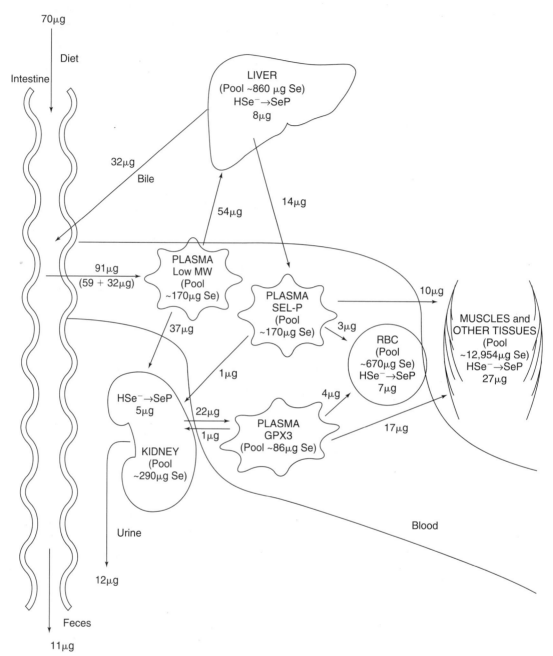

Figure 34–2. *Whole body model of human selenium metabolism. This model shows the following compartments: intestine, liver (plus pancreas), kidney, muscle plus other tissues, and blood, including a low molecular weight pool of selenium (HSe⁻) and the SEL-P, GPX3, and red blood cell (RBC) pools. Pool values within compartments indicate the estimated pool sizes (in micrograms of Se). Values adjacent to arrows show the estimated flux between pools (in micrograms of Se) arising from ingestion of 70 μg of Se as selenite, as followed over the subsequent 12 days in a selenium-adequate human. Fluxes were estimated from the observed percentage absorption and excretion values and from fractional fluxes associated with plasma pools, as reported by Patterson et al. (1989) and as described by Sunde (1997). Within liver, kidney, RBC, and muscle, HSe⁻ → SeP indicates the estimated incorporation of the ingested Se (in micrograms of Se) into tissue selenoproteins (SeP).*

zymes. These pathways include inorganic selenium metabolism, pathways of metabolism for low molecular weight organic selenium compounds, and the main as well as several alternative pathways that result in selenium-containing proteins or enzymes.

Inorganic Selenium Metabolism

Conversion of dietary selenate to selenite, shown in path 1 of Figure 34–3, is thought to involve adenosine phosphoselenate (APSe) or phosphoadenosine phosphoselenate (PAPSe) intermediates. Selenite is reduced nonenzymatically (path 2) by glutathione to a formal zero-oxidation state in selenodiglutathione (GS-Se-SG), which in the absence of oxygen is further reduced by glutathione reductase

(path 3) to selenide. This reduction usually occurs in intestinal cells or in red blood cells but also readily occurs in other cells. Selenide and ATP are the substrates for selenophosphate synthetase (path 4), which produces selenophosphate, the activated selenium compound used for the transfer RNA (tRNA)-mediated synthesis of selenoproteins (paths 5, 6, 7). In addition, selenide can bind nonenzymatically to proteins (path 16), which is likely to account for the acute toxicity of selenium.

Catabolism of Organic Selenium

Selenomethionine, like methionine, is not synthesized by higher animals. Selenomethionine is the common form of selenium in most plant-derived foods and is metabolized by the

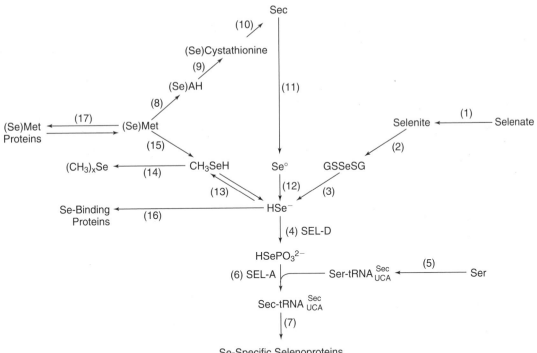

Figure 34–3. *Metabolic pathways of selenium. Path (1), selenate reduction to selenite via adenosine phosphoselenate (APSe) or phosphoadenosine phosphoselenate (PAPSe); path (2), glutathione (GSH)-dependent nonenzymatic reduction of selenite; path (3), glutathione reductase-catalyzed reduction; path (4), selenophosphate synthase, or SEL-D; path (5), seryl-tRNA synthase; path (6), selenocysteine synthase, or SEL-A; path (7), translational selenocysteine insertion, mediated by tRNA^{Sec} and SEL-B at the position specified by the UGA codon; path (8), formation of adenosylselenomethionine and transmethylation resulting in formation of adenosylselenohomocysteine (SeAH); path (9), cystathionine β-synthase; path (10), cystathionine γ-lyase; path (11), selenocysteine lyase; path (12), nonenzymatic reduction via GSH; path (13), S-methyltransferase; path (14), thioether S-methyltransferase; path (15), transamination pathway resulting in methaneselenol; path (16), selenide binding to proteins; path (17), selenomethionine acylation of tRNA^{Met} followed by incorporation at positions specified by an AUG codon. (From Sunde, R. A. [1997] Selenium. In: Handbook of Nutritionally Essential Mineral Elements [O'Dell, B. L. and Sunde, R. A., eds.], pp. 493–556. Marcel Dekker, New York. Redrawn by courtesy of Marcel Dekker, Inc.)*

same enzymes responsible for methionine catabolism. Thus selenomethionine is activated to form adenosylselenomethionine (SeAM). SeAM, like adenosylmethionine, is an excellent methyl donor in mammalian systems and thus is converted to adenosylseleno-homocysteine (SeAH) (path 8 in Fig. 34–3). SeAH in turn is a substrate for cystathionine β-synthase and cystathionine γ-lyase (paths 9 and 10 in Fig. 34–3) and thus is converted to Sec in mammalian tissues. Here the sulfur and selenium paths diverge.

Sec is degraded by a selenium-specific enzyme, Sec lyase (path 11 of Fig. 34–3), which directly releases elemental selenium. The elemental selenium is reduced nonenzymatically to selenide (path 12) by glutathione or other thiols. Selenide can be methylated (path 13) using S-adenosylmethionine by either microsomal or cytosolic methyltransferases in liver to form methaneselenol, the usual major urinary form of selenium. Under high dietary intakes of selenium, further methylation steps (path 14) result in dimethylselenide or trimethylselenonium ion. Methaneselenol is also produced more directly from methionine via the enzymatic transamination and decarboxylation reactions (path 15) of the methionine transamination pathway.

SELENIUM INCORPORATION INTO SELENOPROTEINS

Selenium incorporation into selenoproteins occurs cotranslationally during protein synthesis, proceeds through several unusual intermediates, and requires four unique gene products (SEL-A, SEL-B, and SEL-D, which are proteins, and Sel-C, which is a unique tRNA) and two unique messenger RNA (mRNA) elements (the UGA [uracil-guanine-adenine] codon and the SECIS [selenocysteine insertion sequence] element) in the mRNA for the selenoprotein itself. Selenium is incorporated as the amino acid, Sec. This process illustrates the importance of biochemistry and molecular biology in understanding the nutrition of a trace element. This area has recently been reviewed by Stadtman (1996).

The Selenocysteine Moiety

Experiments with GPX1 conducted just after it was shown to contain selenium revealed that this metalloenzyme was different from many other metalloproteins. Dialysis would not remove the trace element nor would dialysis with inorganic selenium restore GPX1 activity when selenium-deficient hemolysates were incubated with selenite alone or with components of the selenite-reduction pathway. Pioneering studies on bacterial selenoproteins led to the identification of Sec as the chemical form of the selenium moiety in mammalian selenoproteins. Furthermore, this Sec is incorporated into the peptide backbone. The presence of Sec in both prokaryotes and eukaryotes indicates that this amino acid is of ancient origin. Because Sec is specifically incorporated into proteins during translation, it is considered the 21st amino acid required for protein synthesis. Sec is the 3-letter code commonly used for selenocysteine, and U is increasingly used as the 1-letter code in protein sequences. The codon for Sec is TGA (thymine-guanine-adenine) in DNA and UGA in mRNA, as shown in Figure 34–4 for GPX1. Intact Sec from the diet or from selenomethionine catabolism is not used for synthesis of selenoproteins. Instead, inorganic selenium is activated: serine provides the carbon skeleton for Sec, and the reaction proceeds while the serine is esterified to a tRNA, as shown in Figure 34–5.

Selenophosphate Synthetase

Selenophosphate synthetase (SEL-D) catalyzes formation of the active selenium donor species from selenide and ATP, as shown in Figure 34–5. Human SEL-D has been cloned, has an apparent molecular weight of 45 kDa, and contains a conserved ATP/GTP-binding consensus sequence. The reaction begins with ATP binding, formation of an enzyme-pyrophosphate intermediate, and liberation of AMP. Subsequent addition of selenide forms selenophosphate ($HSePO_3^{2+}$) containing the γ-phosphate of ATP, and liberates orthophosphate arising from the β-phosphate of ATP. Selenophosphate is labile.

SEL-D is the product of expression of at

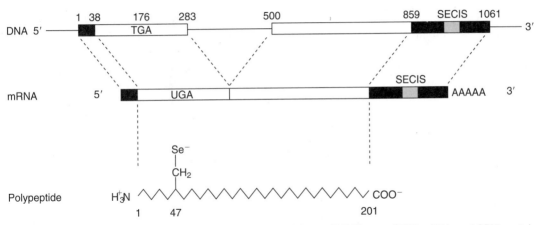

Figure 34–4. Diagrammatic alignment of the glutathione peroxidase-1 (GPX1) gene, GPX1 mRNA, and GPX1 protein. Solid bars indicate UTRs (untranslated regions), gray bars the SECIS (selenocysteine insertion sequence) element, and open bars indicate exons. Numbers indicate the position of the nucleotide base and amino acid residues in the genomic, message, and polypeptide sequences, respectively.

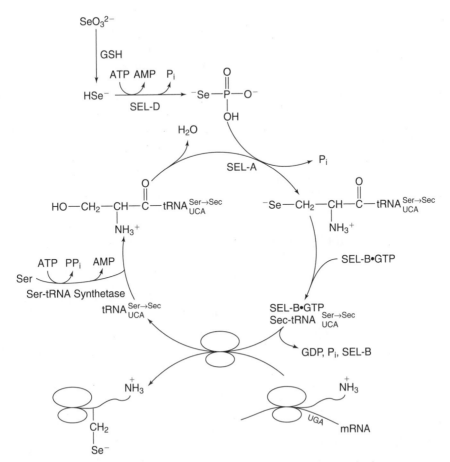

Figure 34–5. Diagram of cotranslational selenocysteine synthesis.

least two distinct Sel-D genes. The more typical Sel-D gene contains cysteine, but a second Sel-D gene has a UGA-encoded Sec located at the corresponding position. This gene offers the possibility of downregulating selenophosphate synthesis under selenium-deficient conditions.

Selenocysteine tRNA$_{UCA}^{Sec}$

Synthesis of selenoproteins requires a unique RNA gene product—the tRNA$_{UCA}^{Sec}$ (Sel-C) (Fig. 34–6). The mammalian tRNA$_{UCA}^{Sec}$ has a UCA (uracil-cytosine-adenine) anticodon and has 90 nucleotides, compared with 76 nucleotides for all common tRNAs. The extra base pairs are in the acceptor stem of the tRNA (8 to 9 versus the usual 7 base pairs) and in a longer d-loop (with approximately 16 bases and 5 base pairs, compared with the usual 5 bases and no base pairs). These tRNAs comprise about 1% to 3% of the total seryl tRNAs in mammalian tissues. Mammalian tRNA$_{UCA}^{Sec}$ can have methylcarboxy-methylated uridine at the

5′ position of the UCA anticodon, as well as partial ribosylation on the same residue.

Serine, from the same cellular pool used for protein synthesis, is esterified to the 3′ terminal adenosine (A) of the tRNA$_{UCA}^{Sec}$ to form the corresponding seryl-tRNA, as shown in Figure 34–5; thus this tRNA is more completely designated tRNA$_{UCA}^{Ser\rightarrow Sec}$. This reaction is catalyzed by cellular seryl-tRNA synthases, which apparently do not differentiate between the 76-nucleotide tRNA^{Sec} and the 90-nucleotide tRNA$_{UCA}^{Ser\rightarrow Sec}$.

Selenocysteine Synthase

Sec is synthesized enzymatically from serine in a novel mechanism catalyzed by selenocysteine synthase (SEL-A). The reaction is specific for seryl-tRNA^{Sec}. The enzyme catalyzes the dehydration of L-serine while attached to the tRNA to form aminoacrylyl-tRNA^{Sec}, followed by a C2-C3 addition of selenium as selenophosphate, to form the Sec moiety still esterified to the tRNA^{Sec}, as shown in Figure 34–5. The mammalian gene and enzyme have yet to be identified but are likely to be similar to *Escherichia coli* SEL–A, which has a subunit molecular weight of 51 kDa and a native weight of approximately 600 kDa and which contains pyridoxal phosphate. SEL-A and SEL-D, thus, along with Sel-C, are involved in synthesis of the direct precursor or Sec donor—Sec-tRNA$_{UCA}^{Sec}$—used in the translational incorporation of selenium into selenoproteins. An additional unique protein, SEL-B, and two *cis*-acting mRNA elements are necessary for the actual synthesis of mammalian selenoproteins.

The UGA Codon in Selenoprotein mRNA

The GPX1 gene was the first selenoprotein gene to be cloned and sequenced (see Fig. 34–4). The gene, consisting of two exons, encodes a 201-amino acid polypeptide. Most significantly, a TGA codon in the middle of the open reading frame of the first exon specifies the position of Sec. All characterized mammalian selenoproteins to date also contain Sec that is encoded by TGA. This is also true for all Sec-containing bacterial selenoproteins.

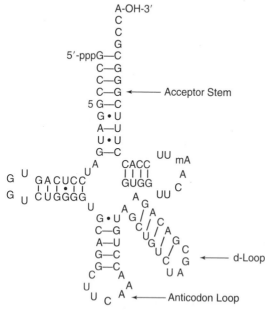

Figure 34–6. *Eukaryotic tRNA$_{UCA}^{Ser\rightarrow Sec}$ consisting of 90 nucleotides. (From Amberg, R., Urban, C., Reuner, B., Scharff, P., Pomerantz, S. C., McCloskey, J. A. and Gross, H. J. [1993] Editing does not exist for mammalian selenocysteine tRNAs. Nucleic Acids Res 21:5583–5588. Redrawn and used with the permission of Oxford University Press.)*

Because UGA in the mRNA unambiguously serves as a termination codon for many mammalian proteins, it is obvious that a UGA alone is not sufficient to specify Sec incorporation into the small number of selenoproteins.

The Selenocysteine Insertion Sequence Element in Selenoprotein mRNA

Studies on expression of cloned selenoproteins revealed that the 3′UTR (3′ untranslated region) of the mRNA was necessary for UGA-encoded Sec incorporation. Berry et al. (1991) fused the coding region of 5′-deiodinase (DI1) and the 3′UTR of GPX1 and used this chimeric to identify a consensus 87-base stem-loop element in rat DI1 or GPX1 3′UTR that catalyzes the insertion of selenium into DI1. This element is called a eukaryotic SECIS element. A single SECIS is also present in the 3′UTR of GPX4, GPX3, GPX2, and selenoprotein W (SEL-W), and two SECIS elements are present in the 3′UTR of plasma SEL-P.

A model SECIS element is shown in Figure 34–7. The consensus SECIS element is a stem-loop structure with a variable loop consisting of 7 to 10 unpaired bases, including a consensus AAA (adenine-adenine-adenine) sequence. A consensus AUG (adenine-uracil-guanine) sequence is 5′ to the loop, and a consensus UGR (uracil-guanine-purine base) sequence is located 3′ to the loop. The second and third As in the AAA sequence appear to be especially important, as do the AUG and UGR sequences, but base pair changes in the intervening stem do not affect efficacy for mediating selenium incorporation (Berry et al., 1993). The model SECIS element has two helical regions separated by an internal loop. The top helix ends in the consensus AUG and UGR sequences and forms a quartet motif of non-Watson and Crick base pairs, which results in a greater than 90-degree kink in the stem-loop (Walczak et al., 1996). The specific secondary structure of the SECIS elements found in different selenoproteins may affect the rate of Sec insertion. The role of the two SECIS elements in SEL-P is unknown.

In bacteria, recognition of UGA as a Sec codon rather than a stop codon also requires a prokaryotic SECIS (or pSECIS) element. This pSECIS, however, is a 38-nucleotide stem-loop element in the open-reading frame of the pro-

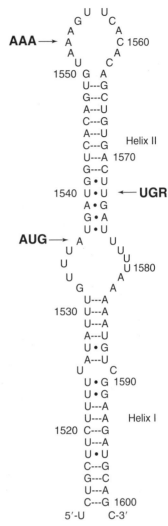

Figure 34–7. *Selenocysteine insertion sequence (SECIS) elements. Eukaryotic SECIS element that resides in the 3′UTR of rat DI1. (From Walczak, R., Westhof, E., Carbon, P. and Krol, A. [1996] A novel RNA structural motif in the selenocysteine insertion element of eukaryotic selenoprotein mRNAs. RNA 2:367–379. Redrawn and used with the permission of Cambridge University Press.)*

karyotic selenoprotein mRNA that immediately follows the UGA. The constraints of maintaining this secondary structure and varying the amino acid sequence defined by the primary structure must limit the ability of bacterial genes to place Sec at the active site of enzymes.

Selenocysteine-Specific Elongation Factor

A Sec-specific elongation factor (SEL-B) is also necessary for incorporation of UGA-encoded Sec. In bacteria, this factor is the 68-kDa Sel-B gene product, SEL-B, that is similar to elongation factor EF-Tu, the prokaryotic equivalent of the eukaryotic elongation factor eEF-1α. Native EF-Tu has a molecular mass of 43 kDa. The SEL-B protein is very specific for Sec-tRNA^{Sec} and for the SECIS element on the mRNA. This mechanism thus serves to increase the concentration of the Sec-tRNA on the mRNAs. The eukaryotic SEL-B has not yet been identified unequivocally, but several candidate proteins have been reported. This factor must exist to facilitate recognition and assembly of the Sec insertion complex.

The selenoprotein mRNA, SEL-B, and Sel-C, along with guanosine triphosphate (GTP), assemble in a quaternary complex on the ribosome for cotranslational Sec incorporation, as illustrated in Figure 34–8. The quaternary SEL-B–GTP–Sec-tRNA^{Sec}–mRNA complex is hypothesized to orient the Sec at just the correct position to facilitate the specificity of Sec insertion. On eukaryotic ribosomes, the SECIS element can be visualized as located on its flexible 3'UTR tether, which permits interaction of the SEL-B–GTP–Sec-tRNA^{Sec} with the ribosome in a favorable position for the

anti-codon on the tRNA to interact with the approaching acceptor site (also called the aminoacyl site, or A-site) on the ribosome. Peptide bond formation is then catalyzed by peptidyltransferase, resulting in the formation of a peptide bond between Sec and the nascent polypeptide.

MAMMALIAN SELENOPROTEINS

Currently, 11 distinct mammalian selenoenzymes or selenoproteins have been cloned and identified. These proteins are listed in Table 34–1. These species all contain selenium as Sec encoded by a UGA codon.

Glutathione Peroxidase-1

Virtually all cells and animal plasma seem to contain glutathione peroxidase (GPX) activity. GPX activities decrease in plasma and cells in selenium deficiency, and selenium supplementation restores these activities to normal. Although it was initially assumed that a single gene was responsible for GPX activities, careful biochemical studies have established dis-

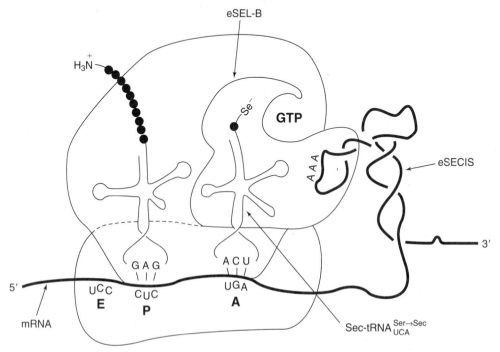

Figure 34–8. Model for the ribosomal mRNA–SEL-B–Sec-tRNA$^{Ser \rightarrow Sec}_{UCA}$ complex. See text for explanation. (From Sunde, R. A. [1997] Selenium. In: Handbook of Nutritionally Essential Mineral Elements [O'Dell, B. L. and Sunde, R. A., eds.], pp. 493–556. Marcel Dekker, New York. Redrawn by courtesy of Marcel Dekker, Inc.)

TABLE 34–1
Mammalian Selenoenzymes, Selenoproteins, and Related Proteins

Abbreviation	Name	Se Moiety
DI1	Iodothyronine 5′-deiodinase-1 (Type I DI)	Sec
DI2	Iodothyronine 5′-deiodinase-2 (Type II DI)	Sec
DI3	Iodothyronine 5′-deiodinase-3 (Type III DI)	Sec
GPX1	Classical glutathione peroxidase (classical GSH-Px)	Sec
GPX2	Gastrointestinal glutathione peroxidase (GPX-GI)	Sec
GPX3	Plasma glutathione peroxidase (plasma GPX)	Sec
GPX4	Phospholipid hydroperoxide GPX (PHGPX)	Sec
GPX5	Androgen-regulated epididymal secretory protein	(Cys)
GPX6	Odorant metabolizing protein	(Cys)
SEL-P	Plasma selenoprotein P	ten Sec
SEL-W	Muscle selenoprotein W (formerly selenoprotein G)	Sec
SEL-D	Selenophosphate synthetase (SPS1)	(Cys)
SEL-D2	Selenophosphate synthetase-2 (SPS2)	Sec
TRR	Thioredoxin reductase	Sec

tinct differences in the nature of the GPXs. We now know that there are at least six distinct members of the GPX family in higher animals (see Table 34–1).

Glutathione peroxidase (glutathione: H_2O_2 oxidoreductase) was discovered by Mills (1957) in a search for factors that protect erythrocytes against oxidative hemolysis. GPX1 is unique with respect to many other peroxidases because it is not inhibited by azide or cyanide, and hydroperoxides as well as H_2O_2 are substrates for the enzyme. The enzyme catalyzes the following reaction:

$$2\,GSH + ROOH \rightarrow GSSG + ROH + H_2O$$

GPX1 is very specific for glutathione (GSH) as the donor substrate, and no other substrate results in more than 30% of the activity obtained with GSH as substrate. However, GPX1 is not specific at all for the acceptor substrate and thus destroys many organic hydroperoxides (ROOH) at rates very similar to those for H_2O_2. Only cholesterol 25-hydroperoxide, cholesterol-7α hydroperoxide, and phospholipid hydroperoxides such as phosphatidyl choline hydroperoxide are poor substrates for GPX1. The enzyme reaction is a ter-uni ping-pong mechanism as shown in the following equation. The intermediates, beginning with the deprotonated selenium Se⁻ in the Sec residue of the enzyme (E), are also indicated.

ROOH ROH	GSH HOH	GSH GSSG
↓ ↑	↓ ↑	↓ ↑
E-Se⁻ E-Se-OH	E-Se-SG	E-Se⁻

GPX1 is a tetrameric protein with 4 identical subunits, each with a molecular mass of approximately 23 kDa and each containing 1 Se atom. The bovine erythrocyte GPX1 has been crystallized, and it consists of 4 spherical subunits, each with a diameter of 3.8 nm, arranged in an almost flat, square planar configuration ($9 \times 11 \times 6$ nm). Selenium atoms located in slight depressions are no closer than 2 nm, strongly suggesting that each Se atom functions independently. The Sec moiety is located at the end of an α-helix associated with two parallel β-sheets in a βαβ structure. Charged amino acids within the active site apparently confer specificity for glutathione. Recombinant analogs of murine GPX1, with cysteine or serine replacing the Sec moiety, have been prepared; the analog with serine in place of Sec is completely without activity, whereas the cysteine mutant has 1/1000 the activity of the wild type of enzyme, clearly demonstrating the biochemical essentiality of selenium.

Glutathione Peroxidase-2 in Intestine

GPX2 has 66% amino acid sequence identity to GPX1. GPX2 is also called GPX-GI because the species is expressed in gastrointestinal cells as well as epithelial cells and some cultured cells. The mRNA for GPX2 is detected in human liver and colon, but not in kidney, heart, lung, placenta, or uterus. More than 70% of the total GPX activity in the rat small bowel is due to GPX2. The discovery of this second GPX might at first glance suggest that various GPX activities are redundant, but it appears that individual GPXs have somewhat unique niches.

Glutathione Peroxidase-3 in Plasma

Almost immediately after the discovery that GPX1 was a selenium-dependent enzyme, researchers observed that plasma GPX activity responded more quickly than GPX1 to selenium deficiency and to selenium resupplementation. We now know that plasma GPX is a distinct enzyme. The specific activity of the purified plasma enzyme, however, is only 10% of GPX1 specific activity. Plasma GPX is called GPX3 because the cloning of human plasma GPX in 1990 from a human placenta cDNA library (collection of complementary DNAs synthesized using mRNA as the template) was the third protein for this family. The sequence encodes a 226-amino acid polypeptide with a molecular weight of 25,389 and with 44% homology with human GPX1, including a Sec residue encoded by a UGA at residue 73. Screening of tissues for GPX3 mRNA suggests that the kidney is the major source of circulating GPX3. Human patients undergoing chronic dialysis due to renal failure have low levels of plasma GPX3 in spite of normal plasma selenium content. After renal transplantation, plasma GPX3 increases up to 200% of normal. GPX3 is a secreted enzyme, and thus it is not surprising in hindsight that 90% of human milk GPX activity is precipitated by anti-GPX3 antibodies, demonstrating the genetic origin of milk GPX activity. The expression of GPX3 in milk may have evolved specifically to maintain milk selenium levels rather than to protect milk from peroxidation in the (short) trip from breast to infant stomach.

Phospholipid Hydroperoxide Glutathione Peroxidase

Phospholipid hydroperoxide glutathione peroxidase, or GPX4, is an intracellular selenoperoxidase, and it is active as a monomer. Its peroxide substrate specificity is broader than for the other glutathione peroxidases; the enzyme will reduce phospholipid hydroperoxides as well as cholesterol hydroperoxides, which are not substrates for GPX1 (Maiorino et al., 1990). GPX4 is a 170-amino acid polypeptide with a calculated molecular weight of 19.5 kDa, and the Sec residue is located 46 amino acids from the N-terminal end. The full-length nucleotide and amino acid sequences have 39% identity with rat GPX1. The enzyme uses a ter-uni ping-pong mechanism, the same as that of GPX1. Addition of detergents stimulates the activity of this enzyme, suggesting that GPX4 may work the interface between the membrane and the aqueous phase of the cell. GPX4 may "roll along" membrane surfaces in the cytosol and in the mitochondrial intermembrane space and may protect membrane components by detoxifying hydroperoxides that would otherwise damage or impair membrane function.

Other Glutathione Peroxidases

In addition to the four Sec-containing GPXs, two cysteine-containing members of the glutathione peroxidase family have been identified in mammals. GPX5 is an androgen-regulated epididymal secretory protein with about 67% identity to GPX1. GPX6 is an odorant-metabolizing protein, with about 40% amino acid sequence identity to GPX1, which appears to be expressed only in Bowman's gland of the olfactory system. The existence of intracellular and secreted GPX-like proteins strongly suggests that enzymatic removal of peroxides is an important means by which organisms cope with an oxidant-filled environment.

A nonselenium-dependent GPX activity found in the liver of selenium-deficient humans and animals is due to activity of several of the glutathione S-transferases. (See Chapter 40 for more about glutathione S-transferases.) Levels of glutathione S-transferases increase two-fold in selenium-deficient liver only after liver glutathione peroxidase is fully depleted. This delayed response to selenium deficiency indicated that more than just loss of GPX is occurring, and this observation helped point the way to the discovery of additional mammalian selenoenzymes.

Iodothyronine 5′-Deiodinase-1

Iodothyronine 5′-deiodinase-1, often referred to in the literature as type I 5′-deiodinase

(DI1), is the major enzyme that converts thyroxine (T_4) to triiodothyronine (T_3). Liver DI1 is responsible for the majority of the circulating plasma T_3 levels, but two additional deiodinase isozymes are also found in more specialized tissues. In the early 1990s, three research groups independently discovered that the deiodinases were selenoenzymes (see review by Sunde, 1997). John Arthur in Scotland observed elevated T_4 and reduced T_3 in Se deficiency and focused in on a new selenoprotein. Concurrently, Dietrick Behne in Germany used ^{75}Se-labeling to discover a 28-kDa selenoprotein at high concentrations in thyroid, liver, and kidney. And in 1991, Marla Berry and Reid Larsen in Boston used expression cloning to isolate and sequence DI1. These three approaches revealed that DI1 is a 257-amino acid (27 kDa) polypeptide that contains a Sec at residue 126. DI1 appears to function as a homodimer, with a molecular mass of approximately 55 kDa.

DI1 is localized in the membrane and co-purifies with microsomal (endoplasmic reticulum) markers from liver and with the basolateral membrane of kidney proximal convoluted tubule cells. A single transmembrane segment of the protein is located at the N-terminus of the protein and orients the catalytic portion toward the cytoplasm.

DI1 catalyzes both outer and inner ring deiodination of thyroxine, but the preferred reaction is removal of the outer ring 5′ iodine from either T_4 or reverse T_3 (rT_3) leading to T_3 or T_2, respectively. Formation of T_3 is thought to be the most important physiological role for DI1, but production of T_2 from rT_3 may also be of biological importance in the elimination of excess thyroid hormone from the circulation. The catalyzed reaction is analogous to the GPX1 reaction:

$$T_4 + 2\ GSH \rightarrow T_3 + GSSG + I^- + H^+$$

Reduced GSH is the likely physiological substrate, and thus the mechanism is best described as a ter-uni ping-pong mechanism similar to that for GPX1, which proceeds via formation of an enzyme-Se-I intermediate.

Deiodinase-2 and Deiodinase-3

Although more than 90% of plasma T_3 is produced by DI1 in liver, kidney, and muscle, two additional deiodinases, deiodinase-2 (DI2) and deiodinase-3 (DI3), also contain selenium as Sec and arise from distinct genes. DI2 catalyzes the 5′-deiodination of the outer ring of T_4 and is found in brain, pituitary, brown adipose tissue, placenta, and skin. Its principal physiological role is for local, intracellular production of T_3.

DI3 catalyzes the 5′-deiodination of the inner ring of T_4, and DI3 activity levels are highest in adult brain, skin, and placenta and in fetal liver, muscle, brain, and central nervous system. The role of DI3 has been proposed as protecting fetal tissue from high levels of T_3 and T_4 during development by converting them to the inactive rT_3 and T_2, respectively.

This array of three deiodinases may confer additional regulation on iodine metabolism. In iodine deficiency, downregulation of DI1 conserves precious iodine by limiting DI1's conversion of T_4 to circulating T_3, thus making the limited T_4 available for intracellular conversion by DI2 in important endocrine organs. Combined selenium and iodine deficiency may contribute to the etiology of endemic myxedematous cretinism in populations in Zaire; administration of selenium alone appears to aggravate this disease by restoring DI1 activity, leading to increased utilization of T_4 (and I) for production of plasma T_3, which in turn further reduces the concentration of T_4 substrate for DI2 in critical endocrine tissues. (See Chapter 33 for more discussion of the relation of selenium and iodine.)

Thioredoxin Reductase

Thioredoxin reductase (TRR) is an important enzyme—it regulates the intracellular redox state, reduces small intracellular molecules, and may be important in cell cycling. This NADPH-dependent flavoenzyme, found in animals, plants, and bacteria, transfers reducing equivalents from NADPH through a tightly bound flavin adenine dinucleotide (FAD) to a disulfide in the enzyme, and then to thioredoxin (Trx):

$$NADPH + H^+ + Trx\text{-}S_2 \rightarrow NADP^+ + Trx\text{-}(SH)_2$$

TRR is a 497-amino acid (57 kDa) selenoprotein that contains Sec as the penultimate amino acid. Selenium deficiency studies in rats indicate that TRR activity in liver and other tissues is less affected by selenium deficiency than is GPX1 activity but is more affected than are plasma SEL-P levels. Loss of TRR activity may be important in the development of the signs and symptoms of selenium deficiency. Recent exciting research indicates that TRR will reduce dehydroascorbic acid and that ascorbate levels are decreased in Se-deficient rat liver. This offers a new potential antioxidant role for selenium.

Plasma Selenoprotein P

SEL-P is a plasma selenoprotein that can be labeled rapidly with ^{75}Se within 3 to 4 h after rats are injected with ^{75}Se. Mature human SEL-P is a 362-amino acid protein with five or six glycosylation sites. The native molecular mass is approximately 57 kDa. As expected for a secreted protein, the cDNA sequence contains an N-terminal 15-amino acid secretion signal. The concentration of SEL-P mRNA is highest in liver, with smaller amounts in kidney, heart, testis, and some in lung, suggesting that liver is the major source of SEL-P (Burk and Hill, 1994). SEL-P contains about 40% of the plasma selenium in normal individuals, and the level of SEL-P decreases in patients with liver disease.

Analysis of purified SEL-P revealed that it contains 7.5 ± 1 Se atoms/molecule, whereas the cDNA sequence has 10 TGA codons in the open-reading frames. When selenium is limiting, early termination at the second or a later UGA in the mRNA would reduce the selenium content of SEL-P and result in smaller circulating proteins.

SEL-P concentrations in plasma of selenium-deficient Chinese are 10% to 20% of American levels, showing that this protein reflects Se intake in human populations and may be associated with the onset of selenium deficiency disease. Immunohistochemical localization studies indicate that SEL-P coats both the luminal and the interstitial surfaces of the vascular system except in brain where the blood-brain barrier apparently restricts access to brain interstitium. Burk and colleagues (1994) have shown that injecting selenium-deficient rats with 50 μg of selenium rapidly

protects against toxicity of the herbicide diquat and raises SEL-P levels with virtually no change in GPX1 activity 10 h after injection, suggesting that SEL-P may function as an antioxidant protein in the interstitial space. There are preliminary reports that SEL-P may have peroxidase activity.

Other hypotheses suggest that SEL-P might be a selenium transport protein. Alternative hypotheses include a role for SEL-P in disulfide exchange, based solely on the high cysteine plus Sec content, and a role for SEL-P associated with regions rich in histidyl residues, which may potentiate interaction with membranes or serve as a metal-binding motif.

Muscle Selenoprotein W

The search for a mammalian selenoprotein to explain white muscle disease in selenium-deficient sheep and cattle pointed in 1972 to a small selenoprotein that was lacking in lambs suffering from white muscle disease. This protein has now been purified and named selenoprotein W (SEL-W); it is a single polypeptide of 9.8 kDa containing 1 atom of Se/molecule. It is interesting that purified SEL-W is often isolated with 1 tightly bound GSH. Human, monkey, sheep, rat, and mouse SEL-W have been cloned. Cloned SEL-W encodes an 87- or 88-amino acid polypeptide that includes a UGA-encoded Sec at residue 13. SEL-W mRNA abundance in muscle of rats fed adequate levels of selenium (0.1 μg of Se/g diet) increases four-fold above the abundance in selenium-deficient rats (Vendeland et al., 1995). The role of this low molecular weight protein in protecting muscle against white muscle disease is unknown.

Additional Selenoproteins in Higher Animals

In the 1970s and early 1980s, a number of groups used column chromatography to examine ^{75}Se labeling of selenoproteins in various mammalian tissues. Behne et al. (1988) used sodium dodecyl sulfate–polyacrylamide electrophoresis to separate 13 selenium-containing polypeptides with molecular masses of 12.1, 15.6, 18.0, 19.7, 22.2, 23.7, 27.8, 33.3, 55.5, 59.9, 64.9, 70.1, and 75.4 kDa from tissue homogenates. At that time only the 23.7 kDa protein was positively identified as a GPX1 subunit. It is now clear that the 19.7 kDa protein is GPX4, the 27.8 kDa protein found in thyroid is DI1, and the 55.5 and 59.9 KDa proteins are likely to be SEL-P and TRR. It is important to note that pretreatment with cycloheximide (an inhibitor of protein synthesis) completely eliminated ^{75}Se labeling of these selenoproteins, demonstrating that protein synthesis is required for selenium incorporation and strongly suggesting that the selenium is present in all these proteins as Sec and is encoded by a UGA in the mRNA. The other important concept to emerge from these studies is that in selenium deficiency, selenoproteins other than GPX1, especially in brain, endocrine, and reproductive organs, appear to have priority for the selenium. Subsequent estimates for the number of selenium-containing proteins in higher animals range from 30 to 50 selenoproteins. The nature of these additional potential selenoproteins awaits characterization.

Selenium-Binding Proteins

Several additional apparent "selenium-binding proteins," identified as ^{75}Se-labeled proteins, have been reported for proteins with known cDNA sequences that do not contain an in-frame UGA or a SECIS element in the 3′UTR of the mRNA. Many of these reports now appear to be due to co-purification of the identified protein with trace levels of a contaminating selenoprotein of the same size. Nevertheless, selenide binding to proteins (path 16 of Figure 34–3), such as the 130-kDa Cd-Se-binding protein found in plasma or the eukaryotic initiation factor 2α (eIF-2α) involved in initiation of translation, clearly indicates that the full nutritional impact of selenium is likely to be mediated by more than just the UGA-encoded selenoproteins.

Selenomethionine-Containing Proteins

Selenomethionine from dietary sources can be incorporated nonspecifically into proteins because selenomethionine is an excellent analog for methionine in protein synthesis. Selenomethionine can be esterified to methionyl-tRNA at rates only slightly less favorable than that for methionine itself (K_m of 11 μmol/L for selenomethionine versus 7 μmol/L for methionine), and thus dietary selenomethionine in higher animals is readily incorporated into protein (path 17 of Figure 34–3). Hemoglobin and plasma proteins can be major pools of blood selenium in human populations, such as those in rural China, who obtain their selenium primarily from plant-derived foods, which are rich in selenomethionine.

Prokaryotic Selenoenzymes

A number of selenoenzymes have been identified in microorganisms (Stadtman, 1996; Sunde, 1997; Xia, 1997). The study of these selenoenzymes has led to the discovery of many unique aspects of selenium biochemistry. These enzymes are also likely to serve as models for additional new roles for selenium in higher organisms; examples include enzymes using selenocysteine as a ligand for nickel and enzymes containing molybdenum-selenium cofactors that do not involve Sec.

SELENIUM REQUIREMENTS

A number of direct as well as indirect measures could be used to determine selenium requirements. Death and development of overt disease are obviously the most stringent as well as clear-cut. Growth and reproductive success are other practical measures. Tissue selenium concentrations or levels of specific selenoenzymes or selenoproteins are biochemical assays that offer potential convenience and precision if they can be shown to be relevant. Just as a series of parameters are often necessary fully to describe a curve, a series of measures or parameters are needed fully to describe the nutritional status of an individual with regard to a specific nutrient. This is readily apparent in the case of selenium if one considers that some biochemical pools turn over rapidly (e.g., SEL-P) and thus reflect recent Se intakes, other pools average Se status over the life span of the molecules in the pool (e.g., erythrocytes), and some pools most strongly reflect past Se status (perhaps Se in bone). For this discussion, parameter is defined as a measured concentration, rate, or level whose value can vary with the nutrient status of the subject. The parameters that are most useful as markers for assessment of selenium status or requirement remain to be identified (Levander, 1983; National Research Council, 1983, 1989; Sunde, 1994, 1997).

Studies of Selenium Requirements and Status in Experimental Animals

Studies with experimental animals, especially the rat, have provided the basis for understanding the nutritional biochemistry of selenium as well as the nutritional requirement for selenium. Although Schwarz and Foltz (1957) first estimated the selenium requirement for prevention of overt disease (prevention of weanling rats from dying from liver necrosis within 30 days) at 0.05 to 0.1 mg of Se/kg diet, these studies were conducted with rats that were selenium-deficient at the beginning of the experiment and that also were fed diets deficient in vitamin E and sulfur amino acids. It has since been established that less than 0.002 mg of Se/kg diet is necessary to prevent overt disease in rats fed diets with adequate levels of vitamin E and other nutrients. Rats purchased commercially in 1971 and fed the Se-deficient diet of Schwarz, but with adequate sulfur amino acids and vitamin E, grew at 85% of the rate of animals supplemented with 0.1 mg of Se/kg diet. Supplementation with 0.05 mg of Se/kg diet or higher raised growth to that of animals supplemented with 0.1 mg of Se/kg diet. Experiments conducted with commercially available weanling rats in the 1990s, however, did not show any effect on growth from feeding similar selenium-deficient diets, nor any impact on growth or disease from feeding crystalline amino acid diets containing 0.002 to 0.003 mg of Se/kg diet for 28 days (Lei et al., 1995; Sunde, 1997). Pups from selenium-deficient dams, however, grew at markedly lower rates when fed a selenium-deficient diet than when fed a diet with 0.1 mg of Se/kg, demonstrating that severe selenium deficiency does impair growth. These studies illustrate the value of body stores of a nutrient in maintenance of function during prolonged deficiency.

A number of efforts have been focused on identification of a biochemical parameter that would be a useful measure of selenium status. Effects of selenium intake on erythrocyte GPX1 activity, plasma GPX3 activity, liver GPX1 activity, liver GPX4 activity, plasma SEL-P level, liver DI1 activity, and liver TRR activity have indicated that liver GPX1 decreases to the greatest extent in Se-deficient rats. As shown in Figure 34–9, hepatic GPX1 activity fell to undetectable levels when weanling (21-day-old) rats were fed a selenium-deficient diet for 21 days, whereas hepatic GPX4 decreased only to 41% of the level in selenium-adequate animals (Lei et al., 1995). The other selenoproteins that have been assessed also decreased with selenium deficiency, usually to levels in the range of 5% to 20% of the levels in selenium-adequate animals. The dietary level of selenium required to reach maximal or plateau levels of various selenoproteins also ranges; liver GPX1 reaches a maximal level at about 0.1 mg of Se/kg diet whereas liver GPX4 activity reaches a plateau by 0.05 mg of Se/kg diet (Lei et al., 1995). It is important to note that plasma GPX3 activity reaches a plateau at 0.07 mg of Se/kg diet (Weiss et al., 1996) and thus reflects a level of dietary Se that provides sufficient Se for maximal GPX4 synthesis but not for maximal GPX1 synthesis. A level of 0.1 mg of Se/kg diet is sufficient to obtain maximal concentrations of most selenoproteins; an exception is erythrocyte GPX1 activity, which continues to increase with addition of Se beyond the level of 0.1 mg of Se/kg diet.

Tissue selenium levels are another possible measure of selenium nutritional status. Increases in dietary selenium levels increase erythrocyte selenium concentration in the rat between 0 and 0.1 μg of Se/g, but the erythrocyte selenium concentration continues to increase at higher levels of dietary selenium, following a pattern similar to that observed for erythrocyte GPX1 activity. Although blood or erythrocyte Se levels or GPX1 activity is a convenient measure of Se status, they are not very useful as markers for the purpose of setting Se requirements because they do not become saturated at levels of intake that otherwise are clearly adequate or even in excess. Liver and kidney Se concentrations generally

NUTRITION INSIGHT

Selenium and Viral Resistance

Exciting studies by Beck et al. (1994b) have demonstrated that a virulent Coxsackie virus B3 (CVB3/20) that induces myocardial lesions in the hearts of mice is more virulent in Se-deficient than in Se-supplemented mice. Subsequent to viral infection, lesions occur more quickly and more severely, and a higher virus titer is detected in heart and liver of selenium-deficient mice versus selenium-adequate mice. In addition, infection of mice with a cloned and sequenced benign amyocarditic Coxsackie virus B3 (CVB3/0), which causes no pathology in the hearts of selenium-adequate mice, induces extensive cardiac pathology in selenium-deficient mice. However, CVB3/0 virus recovered from the hearts of selenium-deficient mice and inoculated into selenium-adequate mice did induce significant heart damage, suggesting that the mutation of the virus to a virulent genotype was predisposed by culturing in the selenium-deficient mice (Beck et al., 1994a). Coxsackie virus has been isolated from patients who died from Keshan disease, suggesting a possible antiviral component to selenium's role in preventing human disease.

Taylor et al. (1994) have suggested a novel hypothesis that selenium deficiency may potentiate mutation of viruses, including human immunodeficiency virus (HIV) and other retroviruses. The foundation of the hypothesis is the presence of highly conserved alternative reading frames in viral genomes, which are accessed by formation of a thermodynamically stable "pseudo knot" secondary structure in the mRNA. In viruses, Taylor has found that putative alternative reading frames often contain UGA codons and eSECIS elements so that selenocysteine might be inserted in a Se-adequate host, thus sustaining survival pressure to retain the native viral genome sequence. As the hypothesis goes, in selenium deficiency these alternative frame shift proteins would not be made, thus promoting and selecting for mutations of the virus that do not require selenium. The hypothesis is intriguing but remains untested. An alternative hypothesis is simply that in selenium deficiency there may be increased reactive oxygen species, resulting in altered immune response and allowing the virus a chance to achieve higher titers or persist longer (Beck et al., 1994a).

Shisler and colleagues (1998) have recently reported that a human skin poxvirus, molluscum contagiosum, has acquired in its genome a cDNA sequence for mammalian GPX1. The discoverers propose that the poxvirus expresses the captured mammalian GPX1 as a countermeasure to the host antivirus mechanisms, which include peroxidative stimulation of programmed cell death.

follow the same relative pattern as liver GPX1 activity, but after 0.1 mg of Se/kg diet, tissue Se concentration can further increase in a manner similar to that of erythrocyte Se, making tissue Se concentrations difficult to interpret. The presence of selenomethionine-containing proteins further complicates the use of tissue selenium concentration as a marker for functional selenium status.

The amount of dietary selenium required to produce maximal levels is different for the various parameters that have been studied. Responses for most occur within the range of 0.002 to 0.1 mg of Se/kg diet, but a few continue to increase with Se levels above 0.1 mg/kg. The selenium requirement for maximal response varies in the following order, from lowest to highest, for the different possible outcome parameters; growth < overt disease < GPX4 activity < GPX3 activity < GPX1 activity, liver Se, and erythrocyte Se. The choice of the appropriate parameter to use as the biochemical marker is clearly difficult at this point, but characterization of the molecular mechanisms that underlie these biochemical parameters should enable more precise determination of selenium requirements in the future.

Selenium requirements have been established for a wide variety of animals, and most current estimates of requirements are based on liver or erythrocyte GPX1 activity. Unlike the requirements for almost all the other trace elements, the selenium requirement is virtually the same for all species, ranging from humans to laboratory animals to domestic an-

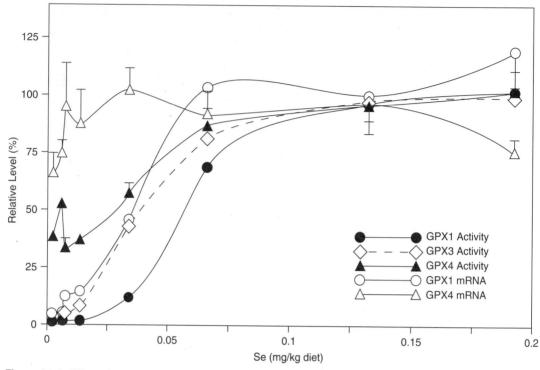

Figure 34–9. *Effect of dietary selenium concentration on liver GPX1 and GPX4 activity and mRNA in male rats. Male weanling rats were fed graded levels of dietary Se from 0 to 0.19 mg/kg for 28 days, following which liver GPX1 activity, GPX1 mRNA level, GPX4 activity, GPX4 mRNA level, and plasma GPX3 activity were determined. (Based on data of Lei, X. G., Evenson, J. K., Thompson, K. M. and Sunde, R. A. [1995] Glutathione peroxidase and phospholipid hydroperoxide glutathione peroxidase are differentially regulated in rats by dietary selenium. J Nutr 125:1438–1446.)*

imals to most poultry and even fish. The minimal selenium requirement for most species is 0.1 mg of Se/kg diet when based on dietary selenium levels necessary for maximal tissue levels of GPX1 activity. Specific molecular mechanisms must be maintaining the dietary requirement across this range of species. Some published recommendations for Se levels in the diets of various species, however, are higher than 0.1 mg of Se/kg diet because these recommendations include margins of safety or have been expanded to include unique situations in which additional dietary selenium seems to be protective.

Human Selenium Requirements

The current Recommended Dietary Allowance (RDA) for selenium is the sole human dietary requirement for a mineral element that is based on a biochemical parameter (as opposed to dietary assessment or balance stud-

ies). This shows the fortuitousness of the discovery of GPX1, as balanced approaches to determine selenium requirements were of little help because of homeostatic mechanisms regulating selenium balance.

The 1989 RDA was set at 70 and 55 μg/day for North American men and women, respectively (National Research Council, 1989). This value is equivalent to 0.13 mg of Se/kg diet based on the recommended energy, protein, and fat intakes. Selenium repletion studies in China suggested that 40 μg of Se/day was an adequate intake to maintain plasma GPX3 activity in adult Chinese men. This estimate, along with adjustments for body weight and addition of a 30% safety factor, yields the values of 70 and 55 μg of Se/day, respectively, for men and women. Deletion of the safety factor results in the value of 0.1 mg of Se/kg diet. To date, use of DI1 activity or SEL-P level to set selenium requirements has not shown advantage over use of GPX1 activity.

Food Sources of Selenium

- Meat and seafood
- Bread and other hard-wheat products
- Brazil nuts

RDAs Across the Life Cycle

	µg Se/day
Infants, 0–0.5 y	10
0.5–1 y	15
Children, 1–6 y	20
7–10 y	30
Males, 11–14 y	40
15–18 y	50
19+ y	70
Females, 11–14 y	45
15–18 y	50
19+ y	55
Pregnant	65
Lactating	75

From National Research Council (1989) Recommended Dietary Allowances. 10th ed. National Academy Press, Washington, D.C.

The RDA for selenium, however, may be high. Comparison of dietary selenium intakes in adult Chinese people living in areas susceptible to Keshan disease with those of Chinese people living in areas seemingly protected from Keshan disease suggests a protective level of 21 µg of Se/day for 65-kg men and 16 µg/day for 55-kg women. Estimates of daily selenium intakes that are not associated with any selenium deficiency symptoms in the New Zealand population suggest that 33 and 23 µg/day for men and women, respectively, are adequate. These and other studies demonstrate that daily selenium intakes below the RDA are typical for much of the world's population and that selenium intakes that are half or less than half the RDA are not associated with any apparent adverse impact on health.

The more recent assessment of trace elements in human nutrition conducted by the World Health Organization (1996) resulted in a new approach for setting Se requirements that was not based on attainment of maximal glutathione peroxidase activity. WHO established a basal requirement of 21 and 16 µg of Se/day for men and women, respectively, based on the selenium intake of Chinese populations that were protected from Keshan disease, as the intake necessary to prevent pathological and clinical signs of selenium deficiency. They also defined a normative requirement that would maintain a desirable level of selenium storage and reserves; this was calculated by estimating the dietary intake needed to achieve two thirds of the maximal attainable activity of plasma GPX3 and was set at 26 µg of Se/day for a 65-kg man. Further adjustment for a hypothetical 16% interindividual variation results in calculated estimates of 40 µg of Se/day for adult men and 30 µg of Se/day for adult women as lower limits of the safe range of population mean intakes. Extrapolation, used to derive requirements for other age and sex groups using basal metabolic rates as justification for these calculations, yielded requirements of 20, 24 and 25 µg of Se/day for children aged 1 to 3 years, 3 to 6 years, and 6 to 10 years, respectively. Requirements of 39 µg of Se/day for pregnant women and 42 to 52 µg of Se/day were estimated for lactating women due to increased needs. These 1996 WHO requirements are thus considerably below the 1989

RDA recommendations but far more in line with typical Se consumption world-wide.

The basis for selenium requirements is clearly more solid than for many of the other nutrients, but a better understanding of the underlying biochemistry and molecular biology is necessary to ensure that the calculations and extrapolations are indeed reasonable so that we can reliably and safely make nutrient recommendations to an entire nation. Does a dietary selenium requirement sufficient to maintain GPX3 activity at 67% of its maximum have a biological foundation? What processes do cells and organisms use to regulate the level of a biochemical parameter such as GPX3 or GPX1?

MECHANISM AND FUNCTION OF REGULATION OF GPX1 EXPRESSION BY SELENIUM

It makes sense that GPX1 activity declines when selenium is lacking, because selenium is the integral cofactor necessary for activity, but what about the GPX1 protein and mRNA? When weanling rats are fed a selenium-deficient diet, GPX1 mRNA levels in liver fall to approximately one tenth of those found in selenium-adequate animals. In progressive selenium deficiency there is a coordinated dramatic exponential drop in GPX1 mRNA ($t\frac{1}{2}$ = 3.2 days), as well as GPX1 activity ($t\frac{1}{2}$ = 3.3 days) and GPX1 protein ($t\frac{1}{2}$ = 5.0 days), suggesting that GPX1 is regulated at the level of mRNA (Sunde et al., 1989; Sunde, 1990).

As illustrated in Figure 34–9, in a study with male weanling rats, both liver GPX1 activity and mRNA levels responded sigmoidally to increasing dietary selenium concentration. Liver GPX1 mRNA levels in rapidly growing young rats fed Se-deficient diets were as low as 5% to 10% of levels in rats fed diets with 0.05 mg of Se/kg diet. In contrast, liver GPX4 mRNA decreased nonsignificantly in Se deficiency, and maximal levels of GPX4 mRNA in male rat liver (and other tissues) were obtained with a 0.015 mg of Se/kg diet. Note that plasma GPX3 activity rises with the GPX1 mRNA level but reaches the plateau levels at 0.07 mg of Se/kg, which is after GPX1 mRNA but before GPX1 activity plateaus. It is im-

portant to note that further increases in selenium intake above 0.1 mg of Se/kg diet had no additional effect on either liver GPX1 mRNA or GPX1 activity. In female rats, which have more than 2.5 times the levels of liver GPX1 mRNA and activity found in male rats, the relationships of dietary selenium level to liver GPX1 activity and GPX1 mRNA (expressed as a percentage of the maximal level) are virtually identical to those in male rats, in spite of the increased need for Se incorporation into GPX1 (Weiss et al., 1996).

Other studies on the impact of selenium deficiency on levels of mRNAs for various selenoproteins show a hierarchy of impact such that GPX4 mRNA is little affected, SEL-W and SEL-P mRNAs are less affected than DI1 mRNA, and DI1 mRNA is less affected than GPX1 mRNA. In selenium-deficient liver, for instance, GPX1 mRNA levels fall by an order of magnitude or more, whereas mRNA levels for GPX4, DI1, and SEL-P typically do not change or decrease only to 30% to 50%. The result is that GPX4, GPX3, SEL-W, SEL-P, and DI1 proteins all are protected from selenium deficiency relative to liver GPX1. This suggests that GPX1 may have a unique physiological role.

All the GPXs can function as antioxidants, and this has long been assumed to be the role of GPX1. Sunde (1994) suggested that selenium regulation of GPX1 expression is an important component of the function of GPX1 and that GPX1 has a second important function as a "biological selenium buffer." This hypothesis suggests that an important role of GPX1 in the liver, and perhaps other tissues, is to be part of the homeostatic mechanism. Upregulation of GPX1 expression when cellular selenium concentrations rise facilitates Se incorporation into GPX1 and thus keeps the concentration of free selenium at a rather fixed, low, and nontoxic level. The effect of this homeostatic regulation of GPX1 is to expand the range of dietary selenium intakes that do not cause a rise in intracellular free selenium, just as a buffer expands the capacity of a solution to absorb protons without a major change in pH. In turn, downregulation of GPX1 in times of selenium deficiency makes selenium available for other functions. This dynamic and homeostatic ability of GPX1 to regulate selenium metabolism is why Sunde (1994) described GPX1 as a biological selenium buffer, rather than as a "selenium store" or "selenium sink." The recent demonstration that GPX1 knockout mice, completely lacking GPX1, grow and reproduce normally (Spector et al., 1996) provides solid proof that this enzyme is not essential when mice are fed diets that contain a moderate level of selenium!

The mechanism for the regulation of GPX1 mRNA level in response to selenium status has been established. Transcription of GPX1 mRNA is not affected by Se deficiency nor is translocation of GPX1 mRNA from the nucleus. Thus, this regulation must occur post-transcriptionally. The most logical mechanism is that the intracellular concentration of one particular selenium species (e.g., selenite, selenophosphate, or selenocysteinyl-tRNA) specifically regulates GPX1 mRNA stability in a manner analogous to iron regulation of transferrin receptor mRNA stability (see Chapter 31). Recent research has shown that the location of the UGA within the first exon of GPX1 is important for the regulation of GPX1 mRNA stability by selenium status (Weiss and Sunde, 1998). This promises to be an exciting area for future research. The key nutrition concepts arising from this hypothesis are that there is a molecular regulatory mechanism that controls GPX1 mRNA level and GPX1 activity, that this process, like a "selenium thermostat," monitors selenium status, and thus that changes in selenium parameters associated with this regulation can be used to determine selenium status and selenium requirements.

These concepts can be used to analyze the underlying assumptions used by the World Health Organization to set the normative Se requirements. The rat model shows that setting requirements based on a second, noninvasive parameter, such as plasma GPX3 activity, could have sound scientific basis if it accurately reflects the cellular Se status (Fig. 34-9). In the experiment summarized in Figure 34-9, a dietary level of 0.05 mg of Se/kg diet resulted in plasma GPX3 activity levels that were 67% of maximum (Lei et al., 1995). As discussed earlier, 0.05 mg of Se/kg provides selenium at a rate sufficient to meet cellular needs for synthesis of selenoproteins such as GPX4, TRR, SEL-P, and SEL-W. At this level of dietary Se, liver GPX1 (the selenium buffer) will be at about 40% of maximum. If the dietary supply of selenium is increased and exceeds needs, the excess will promote GPX1 mRNA stability and then be incorporated into GPX1. If selenium intake is decreased, selenium from GPX1 turnover will be used for synthesis of other selenoproteins, and GPX1 levels will decrease.

SELENIUM AND VITAMIN E

Vitamin E and selenium have been inexorably linked since the discovery that selenium would prevent liver necrosis. Early studies showed that combined selenium and vitamin E deficiency results in elevated levels of tissue malondialdehyde, which arises from the free radical attack on polyunsaturated fatty acids. A more specific indicator of peroxidation, ethane and pentane evolution in the breath, is due to the peroxidative breakdown of $\omega 3$ or $\omega 6$ unsaturated fatty acids, respectively. Ethane and pentane evolution is minimized by vitamin E alone, and it is partially reduced to 40% of the rate in doubly deficient rats by a 0.2 mg of Se/kg diet.

F_2-Isoprostanes are an exciting new marker of in vivo peroxidation. These prostaglandin F_2-like compounds result from the free radical–catalyzed peroxidation of arachidonic acid in vivo. They are found esterified to phospholipids in tissues and are also found as free F_2-isoprostanes in plasma. Plasma F_2-isoprostanes in rats fed a diet deficient in vitamin E are two times control levels, whereas plasma F_2-isoprostanes in rats fed a diet deficient in both vitamin E and selenium are five times the level in animals fed an adequate control diet (Awad et al., 1994). Selenium deficiency alone is not associated with any excess production of F_2-isoprostanes. F_2-Isoprostanes present in phospholipids in various tissues also show similar results, with selenium deficiency exacerbating vitamin E deficiency in most tissues but with selenium deficiency alone being without effect.

These studies suggest that vitamin E is the primary antioxidant molecule that intercepts and detoxifies damaging prooxidants before these species cause detectable damage. In general, selenium-dependent protective mechanisms appear to be an important "second arm" of the overall protective mechanism, although it is possible that selenium may play a more critical role than does vitamin E under certain conditions. The specific physiological roles of all the selenoproteins are still unknown, but it appears that GPX1 selenium-dependent functions are not an essential component of the protective functions of selenium. The minimal role of GPX1 could be due to overlapping functions of the various GPXs or to no role for GPX1 in antioxidant function under normal conditions; GPX1 activity can fall to near-zero levels in selenium deficiency or in GPX1 knockout mice without appreciable tissue damage, whereas substantial activities of other selenium-dependent enzymes are maintained. Circulating GPX3 or SEL-P in the plasma, GPX4 rolling along membranes of the endoplasmic reticulum or in the mitochondrial intermembrane space, TRR in cells, SEL-W in muscle, or another as yet undiscovered selenoprotein could be the major selenium-dependent antioxidant agent. Alternatively, a number of selenium-dependent antioxidant agents with somewhat overlapping functions may serve to defend the body against prooxidant species.

SELENIUM TOXICITY

The range of dietary selenium concentrations that is adequate and yet not toxic is very narrow. In rats, the minimum dietary requirement is 0.1 mg of Se/kg diet, and dietary levels above 2 mg of Se/kg diet are chronically toxic, resulting in a factor of 20 between the dietary selenium requirement and the onset of selenium toxicity. In rats, hydrogen selenide is the most toxic form of selenium, and exposure to 0.02 mg of H_2Se per liter of air for 60 min results in death in 25 days. The relative toxicity of various low molecular weight selenium compounds is illustrated by the following LD_{50} or LD_{75} values (the lethal dose resulting in death of 50% to 75% of the animals) in rats given intraperitoneal injections (in mg of Se/kg body weight):

>sodium selenite, 3.25 to 3.5;
>DL-selenocysteine, 4;
>DL-selenomethionine, 4.3;

>sodium selenate, 5.5 to 5.8;
>diselenodipropionic acid, 25 to 30;
>trimethylselenonium chloride, 49;
>dimethylselenide, 1600.

Long-term intake of dietary selenium at levels of 4 to 5 mg of Se/kg diet are sufficient to cause growth inhibition and result in tissue damage as shown by elevated levels of marker enzymes released into the plasma from damaged tissues. Liver toxicity and hyperplastic hepatocytes have been reported in rats receiving 0.5 to 2 mg of Se/kg diet for 30 months, and higher concentrations of between 4 and 16 mg of Se/kg diet cause edema and poor hair quality, as well as shortened life spans. The biochemical mechanism underlying selenium toxicity is unknown.

Selenium toxicity in humans is initially associated with nausea, weakness, and diarrhea. With continuous intakes of excess selenium, these symptoms lead to loss of hair, changes in nail structure, lesions of the skin and nervous system, and mottling of the teeth. These toxicity symptoms are present with selenium intakes ranging from 3200 to 6700 μg of Se/day. Milder symptoms of selenium toxicity include morphological changes in the fingernails of individuals consuming an average of 1260 μg of Se/day. Mildly prolonged prothrombin times and reduced glutathione concentrations were observed in 400 Chinese subjects, and regression analysis evaluating blood selenium levels relative to selenium intoxication indicated "no observed adverse effect level," or safe upper level, of intake of 853 μg of Se/day, which was associated with typical blood selenium levels of ≤1 mg of Se/L (Abernathy et al., 1993).

Similarly, there was no evidence of selenium poisoning in a study of 142 subjects in seleniferous areas of South Dakota and Wyoming who were consuming as much as 724 μg of Se/day. The danger of selenium toxicity in the United States, however, is not just a question for Great Plains residents and academic researchers. Increasing interest in anticancer nutriceuticals and in self-medication makes an improved biochemical marker of selenium toxicity an important research goal.

SELENIUM AND CANCER

The selenium and cancer story began in 1943 with the report that rats fed 10 mg of Se/kg diet for up to 24 months developed liver cell adenoma or low-grade carcinoma without metastasis (National Research Council, 1982). A repeat of this study 24 years later was not able to confirm these findings, but the stigma of selenium being a carcinogen has remained. Epidemiological studies conducted in the late 1960s and 1970s provided solid evidence of an inverse relationship between selenium intake and cancer mortality, as well as the incidence of leukemia and cancers of the colon, rectum, pancreas, breast, ovaries, prostate, bladder, lung, and skin. Thus it is clear that selenium is anticarcinogenic under at least some conditions.

In a number of systems, selenium supplementation at levels that are chronically toxic (2 to 5 mg of Se/kg diet) will decrease the tumor incidence in animals treated with chemical carcinogens such as 7,12-dimethylbenz[a]anthracene, in animals infected with virally transmitted spontaneous mammary tumors, or in animals given intraperitoneally injected ascites tumor cells. Selenium must be provided both during the initiation and promotional stages of tumor formation for maximal effectiveness. Near-maximal inhibition is obtained when selenium is provided 1 to 2 weeks after administration of the carcinogen, indicating that the major role of selenium may be to inhibit proliferation of tumors.

Excitement about selenium's anticarcinogenic role arose in the 1980s as a result of a retrospective study using prediagnostic serum selenium concentrations, which found that subjects in the lowest quintile of serum selenium concentration had a risk for breast and several other cancers that was twice as high as for those in the highest quintile. This excitement, however, has been reduced because a number of case control and prospective studies looking at tissue selenium concentrations and risk of breast cancer found no evidence of a protective effect of selenium. Recently, a randomized trial with 1312 patients who had histories of basal cell or squamous cell carcinomas of the skin, who were given either an oral supplement of 200 μg of Se/day or a placebo, did not demonstrate any significant effect of selenium supplementation on the incidence of new basal or squamous cell carcinoma of the skin. Selenium treatment however, was associated with a statistically significant reduction in several secondary end points that were not the primary focus of the study; these included total mortality and lung cancer mortality, total cancer incidence, colon and rectal cancer incidence, and prostate cancer incidence. Total cancer incidence was 42% lower in the selenium group (Combs et al., 1997). In two randomized nutrition intervention trials conducted in a rural county in north central China, involving nearly 30,000 participants over 5 years, there was a small but significant reduction in total mortality in subjects receiving a combination of 15 mg of β-carotene, 50 μg of Se as selenized yeast, and 30 mg of α-tocopherol, whereas no appreciable effects were found for other supplements, including retinol, zinc, riboflavin, niacin, ascorbate, and molybdenum. Although the story about selenium and cancer is not yet clear, studies such as these continue to stimulate interest in the role of selenium in human health (Hunter and Willett, 1994; National Research Council, 1982).

REFERENCES

Abernathy, C. O., Cantilli, R., Du, J. T. and Levander, O. A. (1993) Essentiality versus toxicity: Some considerations in the risk assessment of essential trace elements. In: Hazard Assessment of Chemicals (Saxena, J., ed.), pp. 81–113. Taylor and Francis, Washington, D.C.

Awad, J. A., Morrow, J. D., Hill, K. E., Roberts, L. J. and Burk, R. F. (1994) Detection and localization of lipid peroxidation in selenium- and vitamin E–deficient rats using F_2-isoprostanes. J Nutr 124:810–816.

Beck, M. A., Kolbeck, P. C., Rohr, L. H., Shi, Q., Morris, V. C. and Levander, O. A. (1994a) Benign human enterovirus becomes virulent in selenium-deficient mice. J Med Virol 43:166–170.

Beck, M. A., Kolbeck, P. C., Shi, Q., Rohr, L. H., Morris, V. C. and Levander, O. A. (1994b) Increased virulence of a human enterovirus (Coxsackievirus B3) in selenium-deficient mice. J Infect Dis 170:351–357.

Behne, D., Hilmert, H., Scheid, S., Gessner, H. and Elger, W. (1988) Evidence for specific selenium target tissues and new biologically important selenoproteins. Biochim Biophys Acta 966:12–21.

Berry, M. J., Banu, L., Chen, Y., Mandel, S. J., Kieffer, J. D., Harney, J. W. and Larsen, P. R. (1991) Recognition of a UGA as a selenocysteine codon in Type I deiodinase requires sequences in the 3′ untranslated region. Nature (Lond) 353:273–276.

Berry, M. J., Banu, L., Harney, J. W. and Larsen, P. R. (1993) Functional characterization of the eukaryotic SECIS elements which direct selenocysteine insertion at UGA codons. EMBO J 12:3315–3322.

Burk, R. F. (1976) Selenium in man. In: Trace Elements in Human Health and Disease (Prasad, A.S., ed.), pp. 105–133. Academic Press, New York.

Burk, R. F. (1994) Selenium in Biology and Human Health; pp. 1–221. Springer-Verlag, New York.

Burk, R. F. and Hill, K. E. (1994) Selenoprotein P. A selenium-rich extracellular glycoprotein. J Nutr 124:1891–1897.

Chen, X., Yang, G., Chen, J., Wen, Z. and Ge, K. (1980) Studies on the relations of selenium and Keshan disease. Biol Trace Elem Res 2:91–107.

Combs, G. F., Jr, Clark, L. C. and Turnbull, B. W. (1997) Reduction of cancer risk with an oral supplement of selenium. Biomed Environ Sci 10:227–234.

Cotton, F. A. and Wilkinson, G. (1972) Advanced Inorganic Chemistry, pp. 421–457. John Wiley & Sons, New York.

Helzlsouer, K., Jacobs, R. and Morris, S. (1985) Acute selenium intoxication in the United States. Fed Proc 44:1670 (abs.).

Hunter, D. J. and Willett, W. C. (1994) Diet, body build, and breast cancer. Annu Rev Nutr 14:393–418.

Lei, X. G., Evenson, J. K., Thompson, K. M. and Sunde, R. A. (1995) Glutathione peroxidase and phospholipid hydroperoxide glutathione peroxidase are differentially regulated in rats by dietary selenium. J Nutr 125:1438–1446.

Levander, O. A. (1983) Considerations in the design of selenium bioavailability studies. Fed Proc 42:1721–1725.

Maiorino, M., Gregolin, C. and Ursini, F. (1990) Phospholipid hydroperoxide glutathione peroxidase. Methods Enzymol 186:448–457.

Mills, G. C. (1957) Hemoglobin catabolism. I. Glutathione peroxidase, an erythrocyte enzyme which protects hemoglobin from oxidative breakdown. J Biol Chem 229:189–197.

National Research Council (1982) Diet, Nutrition, and Cancer, pp. 163–169. National Academy Press, Washington, D.C.

National Research Council (1983) Selenium in Nutrition. National Academy Press, Washington, D.C.

National Research Council (1989) Recommended Dietary Allowances. 10th ed. National Academy Press, Washington, D.C.

Patterson, B. H., Levander, O. A., Helzlsouer, K., McAdam, P. A., Lewis, S. A., Taylor, P. R., Veillon, C. and Zech, L. A. (1989) Human selenite metabolism: A kinetic model. Am J Physiol 257:R556–R567.

Robinson, M. F. and Thomson, C. D. (1983) The role of selenium in the diet. Nutr Abst Rev 53:3–26.

Rosenfeld, I. and Beath, O. A. (1964) Selenium: Geobotany, Biochemistry, Toxicity and Nutrition. Academic Press, New York.

Schroeder, H. A., Frost, D. V. and Balassa, J. J. (1970) Essential trace metals in man: Selenium. J Chron Dis 23:227–243.

Schwarz, K. and Foltz, C. M. (1957) Selenium as an integral part of factor 3 against dietary necrotic liver degeneration. J Am Chem Soc 79:3292–3293.

Shisler, J. L., Senkevich, T. G., Berry, M. J. and Moss, B. (1998) Ultraviolet-induced cell death blocked by a selenoprotein from a human dermatotropic poxvirus. Science 279:102–105.

Spector, A., Yang, Y., Ho, Y.-S., Magnenat, J.-L., Wang, R.-R., Ma, W. and Li, W.-C. (1996) Variation in cellular glutathione peroxidase activity in lens epithelial cells, transgenics, and knockouts does not significantly change the response to H_2O_2 stress. Exp Eye Res 62:521–540.

Stadtman, T. C. (1996) Selenocysteine. Annu Rev Biochem 65:83–100.

Sunde, R. A. (1990) Molecular biology of selenoproteins. Annu Rev Nutr 10:451–474.

Sunde, R. A. (1994) Intracellular glutathione peroxidases—structure, regulation and function. In: Selenium in Biology and Human Health (Burk, R. F., ed.), pp. 45–77. Springer-Verlag, New York.

Sunde, R. A. (1997) Selenium. In: Handbook of Nutritionally Essential Mineral Elements (O'Dell, B. L. and Sunde, R. A., eds.), pp. 493–556. Marcel Dekker, New York.

Sunde, R. A., Saedi, M. S., Knight, S. A. B., Smith, C. G. and Evenson, J. K. (1989) Regulation of expression of glutathione peroxidase by selenium. In: Selenium in Biology and Medicine (Wendel, A., ed.), pp. 8–13. Springer-Verlag, Heidelberg, Germany.

Taylor, E. W., Ramanathan, C. S., Jalluri, R. K. and Nadimpalli, R. G. (1994) A basis for new approaches to the chemotherapy of AIDS: Novel genes in HIV-1 potentially encode selenoproteins expressed by ribosomal frameshifting and termination suppression. J Med Chem 37:2637–2654.

Vendeland, S. C., Beilstein, M. A., Yeh, J. Y., Ream, W. and Whanger, P. D. (1995) Rat skeletal muscle selenoprotein

W: cDNA clone and mRNA modulation by dietary selenium. Proc Natl Acad Sci USA 92:8749–8753.

Walczak, R., Westhof, E., Carbon, P. and Krol, A. (1996) A novel RNA structural motif in the selenocysteine insertion element of eukaryotic selenoprotein mRNAs. RNA 2:367–379.

Weiss, S. L., Evenson, J. K., Thompson, K. M. and Sunde, R. A. (1996) The selenium requirement for glutathione peroxidase mRNA level is half of the selenium requirement for glutathione peroxidase activity in female rats. J Nutr 126:2260–2267.

Weiss, S. L. and Sunde, R. A. (1998) Cis-acting elements are required for selenium regulation of glutathione peroxidase-1 mRNA levels. RNA 4:801–812.

World Health Organization (1996) Selenium. In: Trace Elements in Human Nutrition and Health, pp. 105–122. World Health Organization, Geneva.

Xia, Y. M. (1997) Proceedings of the 6th International Symposium on Selenium in Biology and Medicine. Biomed Environ Sci 10:113–368.

RECOMMENDED READINGS

Burk, R. F. (1994) Selenium in Biology and Human Health, pp. 1–221. Springer-Verlag, New York.

Chen, J.-S. (1997) Proceedings of the 6th International Symposium on Selenium in Biology and Medicine. Biomed Environ Sci 10:113–368.

Sunde, R. A. (1997) Selenium. In: Handbook of Nutritionally Essential Mineral Elements (O'Dell, B. L. and Sunde, R. A., eds.), pp. 493–556. Marcel Dekker, New York.

CHAPTER 35

◆ ◆

Fluoride

Gary M. Whitford, Ph.D., D.M.D.

OUTLINE

OVERVIEW OF FLUORIDE

Fluoride (F^-), the ionic form of the element fluorine, is the 13th most abundant element in the crust of the earth and, as such, it has been found in all animate and inanimate materials ever analyzed. Due to its high affinity for di- and trivalent cations, fluoride exists in the earth mainly in combination with calcium, magnesium, aluminum, and other metals. Similarly, the bulk of fluoride in the human body (about 99%) is associated with the skeleton and teeth.

The results from some early studies with rodents suggested adverse effects on growth, reproduction, and hematopoiesis when the diet contained only traces of fluoride. Based on such findings, fluoride was classified as an essential element by the National Research Council in 1974. Subsequent studies, however, were unable to confirm these effects. Although no longer considered essential, fluoride is regarded as beneficial owing to its ability to prevent dental decay.

The behavior and effects of fluoride in biological systems differ in several important ways from those of other halogens. The ability of fluoride to bond with hydrogen to form a weak acid, HF (pKa = 3.4), is unique among the halogens and accounts for several aspects of its physiology. Whereas other halogens are largely excluded from the intracellular fluids of soft tissues, the tissue-to-plasma concentration ratios of fluoride range from 0.5 to 0.9 except in adipose tissue and brain, in which the ratios are lower, and kidney, in which the ratio is higher. The rate at which fluoride is removed from the body by the kidneys is many times higher than the rates for excretion of the other halogens. Fluoride is concentrated in calcified tissues. As a general rule, about 50% of the fluoride absorbed by adults each day is deposited in calcified tissues, and the rest is excreted in the urine. Unlike iodide, fluoride does not accumulate in the thyroid gland. Fluoride has the ability to inhibit the activity of a wide variety of enzymes, and its potential to cause acute toxicity is relatively high. The ability of fluoride to stimulate new bone formation is unique among osteoactive agents. Its ability to inhibit the initiation and even reverse the progression of dental caries

is also unique. The remainder of this chapter will develop some of these characteristics and actions in greater detail.

DENTAL FLUOROSIS AND DENTAL CARIES

Early in the 20th century, Dr. Frederick McKay and other investigators drew attention to several regions in the southwestern United States where opacities and discoloration of the teeth were endemic. The identification of fluoride as the etiologic factor involved the efforts of chemists, biologists, and epidemiologists during the following 3 decades. The condition, previously known by several descriptive names such as "Colorado brown stain," is now called dental fluorosis.

Characteristics of Dental Fluorosis

Dental fluorosis is a developmental disorder of the enamel that occurs only pre-eruptively (Fejerskov et al., 1977). After enamel mineralization is complete, no amount of fluoride intake (or of topically applied fluoride) can cause dental fluorosis. Dental fluorosis is classified as mild, moderate, or severe, with the degree of involvement being dependent on the amount of fluoride intake during tooth development. In the milder forms, the enamel has whitish, horizontal striations that may be localized to certain regions of the teeth, frequently the incisal thirds (biting edges) of the anterior teeth and cusps of the posterior teeth ("snow-capping"). Mild fluorosis is not easily noticed by the casual observer and requires some experience to recognize. The moderate and severe forms are characterized by graded degrees of brownish discoloration, sometimes with pitting of the enamel. Histologically, the enamel is more porous, i.e., less dense than normal enamel. The discoloration, which is due to diffusion of sulfur, iron, and other dietary pigments into the porous enamel, occurs slowly over time after the teeth have erupted. Chemically, the enamel has a relatively high protein content, which accounts for the porosity. Dental fluorosis is generally regarded as an aesthetic problem, not an adverse health effect.

Fluoride Intake and the Prevalence of Dental Fluorosis

An average daily fluoride intake of 0.05 mg/kg body weight (range: 0.03 to 0.09 mg/kg) by children with developing teeth is associated with the milder forms of fluorosis in approximately 10% of the population. These levels of fluoride intake (average and range) are those found when the water fluoride concentration is optimal (about 1.0 ppm, or 1.0 mg/L) and the water is the main source of fluoride intake. An average daily intake of 0.10 mg/kg is associated with a prevalence of mild fluorosis of about 50% in a population, with about 5% of the population exhibiting moderate fluorosis.

Water Fluoridation and Dental Caries

The investigators who documented the relationship between fluoride concentrations in drinking water and dental fluorosis in the 1930s also recorded a striking effect on dental caries (Fig. 35–1). It was concluded that the consumption of water containing 1.0 ppm of fluoride was associated with near-maximum protection against dental caries and an acceptably low prevalence of the milder forms of dental fluorosis. This is how 1.0 ppm was

established as the "optimum" concentration in drinking water. The optimal range is from 0.7 to 1.2 ppm, depending on the average regional temperature. The lower concentrations are recommended for warmer climates, where water intake tends to be higher.

The first study of controlled water fluoridation began on January 25, 1945, in Grand Rapids, Michigan. After 6.5 years, the caries experience among 4- to 6-year-old children in Grand Rapids was approximately 50% lower than in the control city of Muskegon, Michigan. Many subsequent studies confirmed this effect, with caries reductions ranging from 20% to 80% and averaging approximately 50%. At present, community water supply systems with controlled fluoride concentrations serve over 60% of the American population. Another 4% of the population lives in some 3340 communities with natural water fluoridation. Some of these water systems are equipped with defluoridating units because the natural concentrations are too high.

The difference in the prevalence of dental decay between American communities with and without water fluoridation is lower today than it was prior to 1970. A national survey conducted in 1979–1980 found a 33%

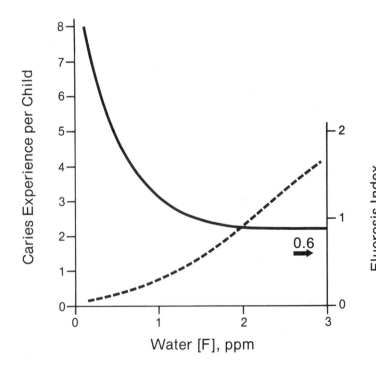

Figure 35–1. The relationships of caries experience (—) and the community dental fluorosis index (- - -) with the fluoride concentration in drinking water as reported by Dean (1942). A total of 7257 12- to 14-year-old children were examined. A fluorosis index value of 0.6, which occurred when the water fluoride concentration approached 2.0 ppm, was judged to represent the threshold for a problem of public health significance. (From Whitford, G.M. [1983] Fluorides: Metabolism, mechanisms of action, and safety. Dent Hyg 57(5):16–29. © 1983 by the American Dental Hygienists' Association.)

lower prevalence among 5- to 17-year-old children who had always been exposed to fluoridated water compared with those who had never been exposed; a 1986–1987 survey found a 25% lower prevalence (Brunelle and Carlos, 1990). The widespread use of topical fluoride products and the "halo" effect, which is discussed later, appear largely to account for the smaller differences.

Topical Fluoride Products

Several kinds of products designed for the topical application of fluoride to the teeth have become available since the mid-1960s. These include gels and solutions with high fluoride concentrations, which are applied in the dental office, and toothpastes and mouth rinses used at home. The fluoride concentrations in these products range from 230 ppm in the over-the-counter mouth rinses to 12,300 ppm in the professionally applied gels. Most toothpastes sold in the United States have a fluoride concentration in the 900 to 1100 ppm (mg/kg) range; one (Extra Strength Aim) contains 1500 ppm. Clinical studies with toothpastes have resulted in caries reductions that ranged from 18% to 28%, with an average reduction close to 25%. When water fluoridation and fluoridated toothpastes are used together, the reductions in dental caries are roughly additive.

Three national epidemiological surveys conducted in 1971 to 1973 (National Center for Health Statistics), 1979–1980 and 1986–1987 (National Institute of Dental Research) revealed a progressive decline in tooth decay. Compared with the 1971 to 1973 data, there were 53% fewer affected tooth surfaces in the 1986–1987 survey. In 1979–1980, 36.6% of the 5- to 17-year-old children surveyed had no dental decay; in 1986–1987, the percentage had increased to 49.9%. It is generally agreed that the combination of water fluoridation and increased use of topical fluoride products has been responsible for these findings.

How Fluoride Prevents Dental Caries

The main minerals of tooth enamel and dentin are various calcium phosphate salts, principally hydroxy- and hydroxyfluorapatite [$Ca_{10}(PO_4)_6(OH)_{2-n}F_n$; $n = 0, 1,$ or 2]. Fluoride-containing apatite is less soluble in acid than is hydroxyapatite that contains no fluoride. Dental caries are caused by the action of acid produced several times each day during the metabolism of carbohydrates by bacteria in dental plaque. The mechanisms by which fluoride prevents dental caries include (1) increased resistance of enamel to acid attack; (2) promotion of remineralization of incipient enamel lesions, which are initiated at the ultrastructural level several times daily according to the frequency of eating or drinking foods containing carbohydrates (Ten Cate, 1990); (3) increasing the deposition of minerals in plaque, which, especially under acidic conditions, provides mineral ions (calcium, phosphate, and fluoride) that retard demineralization and promote remineralization (Tatevossian, 1990); and (4) a reduction in the amount of acid produced through inhibition of bacterial enzymes (especially enolase) and glucose uptake (Hamilton, 1990). These various mechanisms require frequent exposure to fluoride throughout life in order to maintain adequate concentrations of the ion in the dental plaque and enamel. The plaque and enamel receive fluoride from the blood via the saliva (saliva is a continuous source of fluoride except during sleep) and from water, food, and dental products (Whitford, 1996).

FLUORIDE INTAKE

The major sources of ingested fluoride are the diet, especially water and beverages made with fluoridated water, and dental products. The ingestion of fluoride from dental products may be intentional, as with dietary supplements, or unintentional, which occurs to varying degrees when toothpastes or mouth rinses are used.

Fluoride Concentrations in Foods

The fluoride concentrations of most unprepared foods are less than 0.5 ppm (0.5 mg/kg). The concentrations occurring naturally in American drinking waters range from 0.05 to 6 ppm; the great majority are considerably less than 1.0 ppm. The higher concentrations are mainly found in the southwestern United States. The concentrations in foods may increase or decrease depending on the fluoride concentration of the water used for cooking. Tea and marine fish (without bones) have higher concentrations that typically range from 1 to 6 ppm (1 to 6 mg/L or mg/kg).

Table 35–1 shows the average and range of concentrations of fluoride in ready-to-eat foods fed to adult hospital patients in Rochester, New York (Taves, 1983). When preparation required the use of water (e.g., some beverages, juices, and boiled vegetables), the local water was used (1.0 ppm). It was estimated that the average daily intake of fluoride from this hospital diet was 1.8 mg, which is midway between the extreme average values of 1.2 and 2.4 mg/day determined in seven other studies of fluoride intake conducted from 1958 to 1985 (Burt, 1992).

Fluoride Intake by Infants and Young Children

Human breast milk, like cow's milk, has a low fluoride concentration (about 0.01 ppm). Thus, a liter of milk provides not more than 0.01 mg of fluoride, an intake level that has been shown to result in a negative fluoride balance (total excretion > total intake) in infants, which indicates a net loss from calcifying tissues of fluoride that was acquired in utero (Ekstrand et al., 1984).

Prior to 1980, many American manufacturers of ready-to-feed infant formulas prepared their products using fluoridated water, which resulted in concentrations ranging from 0.6 to 1.2 ppm. Since the mid-1980s, a number of reports showing an increase in the prevalence of dental fluorosis have been published. At a meeting sponsored by the American Dental Association, investigators discussed the possible relationship between infant formulas and fluorosis with the manufacturers, who then agreed to prepare their products with low-fluoride water. Today ready-to-feed formulas manufactured in the United States have fluoride concentrations that range from 0.09 to 0.20 ppm. These provide 0.20 mg or less of fluoride with each liter consumed. The fluoride concentrations of prepared liquid concentrates and powdered formulas span a wide range (0.1 to 1.2 ppm), depending mainly on the water used in the home to reconstitute these products.

Of particular interest is fluoride intake by young children at risk of dental fluorosis. When drinking water containing 1.0 ppm of fluoride is the major source of the ion, the average daily intake by young children is approximately 0.05 mg/kg. Table 35–2 shows the results of six studies of dietary fluoride intake by children up to 2 years of age (Burt, 1992). Data were obtained for diets prepared with or without fluoridated water. In 1979, daily fluoride intake by 2- to 6-month-old infants living in areas with fluoridated water ranged from 0.09 to 0.13 mg/kg. These levels of intake were well above the optimum range and due partly to high-fluoride formulas. The more recent studies found lower daily intakes that were remarkably similar and close to 0.05 mg/kg. Table 35–2 also shows lower intakes in areas with low water fluoride concentrations. Average daily dietary fluoride intakes by older children and adults are somewhat less than 0.05 mg/kg because intake does not keep up with body weight (Burt, 1992).

TABLE 35–1

Fluoride Concentrations in 12 Ready-to-Eat Food Classes Served to Hospital Patients in Rochester, NY, in 1982–1983

Food	Fluoride Concentration, mg/kg	
	Average	Range
Fruits	0.06	0.02–0.08
Meat, fish, poultry	0.22	0.04–0.31
Dairy products	0.25	0.02–0.82
Oils and fats	0.25	0.02–0.44
Leafy vegetables	0.27	0.08–0.70
Sugar and adjunct	0.28	0.02–0.78
Root vegetables	0.38	0.27–0.48
Grain and cereal products	0.42	0.08–2.01
Potatoes	0.49	0.21–0.84
Leguminous vegetables	0.53	0.49–0.57
Nonclassifiable	0.59	0.29–0.87
Beverages	0.76	0.02–2.74

Nonclassifiable foods included certain soups, puddings, and so on. Data from Taves, D. R. (1983) Dietary intake of fluoride: Ashed (total fluoride) v. unashed (inorganic fluoride) analysis of individual foods. Br J Nutr 49:295–301. 1.0 mg/kg = 1.0 ppm = 0.052 mmol/kg.

TABLE 35–2

Average Dietary Fluoride Intake by U.S. Children as Reported in 5 Studies Conducted from 1979 to 1988

Year	Age	mg F/day		mg F • kg body weight^{-1} • day^{-1}	
		F	*No F*	*F*	*No F*
1979	2 mo	0.63	0.05	0.13	0.01
	4 mo	0.68	0.10	0.10	0.02
	6 mo	0.76	0.15	0.09	0.02
1980	6 mo	0.21	0.35	0.03	0.04
1980	2 y	0.61	0.32	0.05	0.03
1985	6 mo	0.42	0.23	0.05	0.03
	2 y	0.62	0.21	0.05	0.02
1988	6 mo	0.4	0.2	0.05	0.03

F, foods processed and mixed with fluoridated water (> 0.7 ppm). No F, foods not processed and mixed with fluoridated water (< 0.4 ppm). Data from Burt, B. A. (1992) The changing patterns of systemic fluoride intake. J Dent Res 71(Spec. Issue):723–727.

Fluoride Intake from Dental Products

Unlike the situation that existed 30 or more years ago, when the diet was the only important source of fluoride intake, fluoridated dental products now contribute significantly to intake by both children and adults. An important observation that drew attention to this fact was the increase in the prevalence of dental fluorosis in the United States (Leverett, 1982). The products that are used most frequently and contribute most to fluoride intake are toothpastes, mouth rinses, and dietary fluoride supplements.

When the toothbrush bristles are covered with toothpaste, a weight of approximately 1.0 g is used, which, in the case of a standard 1000-ppm fluoridated product, contains 1.0 mg of fluoride. Studies have shown that from 10% to nearly 100% of the amount used by individual children is swallowed. Among children who are less than 6 years of age, the amount ingested is inversely related to age because of inadequate control of the swallowing reflex. The overall average is close to 30%, so that about 0.3 mg of fluoride is ingested with each brushing. This is equal to or more than the average total daily intake with the diet in nonfluoridated areas and at least 50% of the daily intake where the water is optimally fluoridated (Table 35–2). Similar amounts of unintended fluoride intake have been documented when over-the-counter mouth rinses are used as recommended by the manufacturers.

Several recent studies have shown that the use of fluoridated toothpaste at an early age increases the risk of dental fluorosis (mostly the milder forms) by factors ranging from 3 to 11 (Burt, 1992). As a result of such findings, several workshops conducted since 1985 have produced several precautionary recommendations for children with developing teeth, including (1) parental supervision of brushing, (2) the use of pea-sized portions of toothpaste, (3) teaching how to rinse and empty the mouth at an early age, and (4) the production of products with lower concentrations of fluoride. Some American manufacturers now market toothpastes for children, but so far the changes have been limited to flavors, appearance (e.g., sparkles) and colorful packaging. Several European countries, however, market toothpastes with 250 ppm of fluoride for use by children.

Recommended Fluoride Intake

The Food and Nutrition Board of the Institute of Medicine (1997) has recently published its recommendations for the Adequate Intakes (AIs) of fluoride across the life cycle. The AIs are based on estimated intakes that have been shown to reduce significantly the occurrence of dental caries in a population without causing unwanted side effects, including moderate dental fluorosis. Except for infants up to the age of 6 months, for whom intake from breast milk is regarded as adequate, the AI values

Sources of Fluoride

- Fluoride in the water supply
- Fluoride in dental products

Adequate Intake Across the Life Cycle

	mg fluoride/day
Infants, <0.5 y	0.01
0.5–1.0 y	0.5
Children, 1–4 y	0.7
4–8 y	1.1
8–14 y	2.0
Males, 14–19 y	3.2
19+ y	3.8
Females, 14–19 y	2.9
19+ y	3.1

From Institute of Medicine (1997) Dietary Reference Intakes: Calcium, Phosphorus, Magnesium, Vitamin D, and Fluoride. National Academy Press, Washington, D.C.

are based on an average daily intake of 0.05 mg/kg body weight.

Dietary Fluoride Supplements

Dietary fluoride supplements intended for use by children whose drinking water contains low fluoride concentrations became available in the United States in the 1960s. When taken as recommended, they have been shown to be nearly as effective as water fluoridation in the control of dental decay. The major disadvantages of fluoride supplements are their relatively high cost and frequent lack of compliance with the dosage schedule.

Supplements have also been identified as a risk factor for dental fluorosis (Leverett, 1982; Pendrys and Morse, 1995). Because of this risk, a new dosage schedule was approved by the American Academy of Pediatrics and American Dental Association in 1994 (Table 35–3). The new schedule contains four changes: (1) the drinking water fluoride concentration above which supplements are not recommended was reduced from 0.7 ppm to 0.6 ppm; (2) supplementation should begin at 6 months rather than at birth; (3) the dose for children between the ages of 2 and 6 years was reduced by 50%; and (4) the upper age limit was increased from 13 to 16 years. The second change was based on clinical studies that failed to demonstrate clearly the efficacy of supplementation prior to 6 months of age. The third and probably most important change was based on clinical and laboratory studies showing that the permanent anterior teeth are most susceptible to fluorosis during the 2nd and 3rd years of life. Evaluation of the effects of these recent changes on the prevalence of dental fluorosis and decay must await future studies.

Total Fluoride Intake: Complicating Factors

As shown in Table 35–2, dietary fluoride intake by young children since 1980 has re-

TABLE 35–3

Supplemental Fluoride Dosage Schedule Recommended by the American Dental Association and the American Academy of Pediatrics

Age	Drinking Water Fluoride Concentration, ppm		
	< 0.3	*0.3–0.6*	*> 0.6*
6 mo–3 y	0.25	0	0
3–6 y	0.50	0.25	0
6+ (up to 16 y)	1.00	0.50	0

Values are given in milligrams of fluoride per day (2.2 mg NaF = 1.0 mg F).

Data from American Dental Association, Council on Dental Therapeutics (1994) New fluoride guidelines proposed. J Am Dent Assoc 125:366.

mained relatively constant in areas both with and without water fluoridation. The literature indicates that intake with the diet has also been relatively constant among adults. Prior to the mid-1960s, the diet accounted for nearly all fluoride intake so that total intake could be estimated rather easily. Today, however, the situation is considerably different. The variable intake associated with the use of dental products was discussed earlier. Other factors of current importance include (1) increased sales of bottled water, (2) the use of home water purification systems, and (3) the "halo" or "diffusion" effect.

Most bottled waters contain small amounts of fluoride (<0.2 ppm), but some, such as Vichy water from France, contain 5 ppm or more. Filtration purification systems remove little or no fluoride from water, but fluoride is effectively removed by distillation or reverse osmosis systems. The halo effect refers to the distribution of foods and beverages prepared with fluoridated water to other communities where the water is not fluoridated. Dietary fluoride supplements are recommended for children in communities where the water supplies are low in fluoride, but, because of the halo effect, some children in these communities may already have sufficient fluoride intake. The ingestion of dietary supplements by such children increases their risk of dental fluorosis. Considering all these variables, it is clear that some persons living in

communities without water fluoridation can ingest as much or more fluoride as some persons in fluoridated communities.

FLUORIDE PHYSIOLOGY

Figure 35–2 shows the main features of fluoride metabolism, a subject covered in detail by Whitford (1996). The overall process is relatively uncomplicated because fluoride is not known to undergo biotransformation to form complex chemical compounds, each of which might have its own special metabolic characteristics.

Fluoride Absorption

In the absence of high concentrations of calcium and certain other cations with which fluoride forms insoluble compounds that are poorly absorbed, 80% to 90% of ingested fluoride is absorbed. When taken with milk or other foods high in calcium, absorption is reduced to 50% to 70%. The average half-time for absorption is 30 minutes. Although the stomach is not structurally or functionally designed for absorption, as much as 40% of ingested fluoride can cross the gastric mucosa. The rate and extent of gastric absorption are directly related to the acidity of the stomach contents. This is due to the formation of the highly permeating weak acid hydrogen fluo-

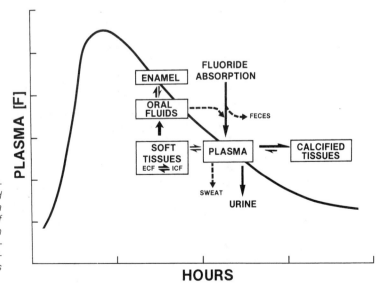

Figure 35–2. *The major characteristics of fluoride metabolism and a typical curve showing plasma concentrations after ingestion of a small amount of fluoride. (From Whitford, G.M. [1990] The physiological and toxicological characteristics of fluoride. J Dent Res 69[Spec. Issue]: 539–549.)*

ride (HF, pKa 3.4). Most of the fluoride that leaves the stomach will be absorbed from the upper intestine, where the pH of the contents appears to have little effect on fluoride absorption. Regardless of the site, there is no evidence for any absorptive mechanism other than diffusion.

Fluoride in Calcified Tissues

Fluoride concentrations in plasma and most soft tissues are low and typically between 0.01 and 0.05 ppm. Approximately 99% of the fluoride in the body is contained in the skeleton and teeth, where it exists mainly as hydroxyfluorapatite. Fluoride concentrations in calcified tissues usually range from 600 to 1500 ppm and depend on past intake and the age of the individual. Higher soft and hard tissue concentrations may occur in people who work in or live near certain industries, such as phosphate fertilizer and aluminum factories, or who live in areas with unusually high fluoride concentrations in drinking water.

As indicated by the double arrows in Figure 35–2, fluoride is strongly, but not irreversibly, bound in calcified tissues. The skeleton has both rapidly exchangeable and slowly exchangeable fluoride pools. Fluoride in the latter pool is found firmly bound within the mineral latticework of mature calcified tissues. Fluoride is mobilized from this pool during the slow but continuous process of bone resorption by osteoclasts.

The rapidly exchangeable pool is located in the hydration shells on the surface of bone crystallites to which fluoride is attracted electrostatically. There appears to be a fixed ratio for the fluoride concentrations in the hydration shell and the surrounding extracellular fluid. Thus, when the plasma concentration increases, as after a meal, there is net uptake

LIFE CYCLE CONSIDERATION

Prenatal Fluoride Supplementation Followed by Breast Feeding

Research on the benefits of prenatal fluoride supplementation for the deciduous teeth of the offspring has yielded conflicting results. A large and well-designed study (randomized and double-blind; Leverett et al., 1997) was unable to detect a statistically significant difference in dental caries between two groups of 5-year-old children whose mothers did or did not take fluoride supplements during pregnancy. Although no longer recommended by professional pediatric or dental organizations, some physicians and dentists still recommend that women take additional fluoride during pregnancy in the belief that it will make the child's deciduous teeth more resistant to dental caries. Much of the fluoride acquired by the fetal calcified tissues, however, could be lost if the infant is breast-fed.

Strong evidence for the mobilization of fluoride from the rapidly exchangeable pool came from a Swedish study (Ekstrand et al., 1984). Two groups of infants born to mothers residing in the same community were studied for several weeks. One group was fed human milk, which has a low fluoride concentration (about 0.01 ppm). The other group was fed a formula reconstituted with the local drinking water that had a fluoride concentration of 1 ppm. The average daily fluoride intakes by the two groups were 10.6 and 861 μg, respectively. The average daily excretions (urinary plus fecal) were 32 and 383 μg. Thus, the breast-fed infants were in a negative balance, while the formula-fed infants were in a strongly positive balance. These findings indicated that the higher fluoride intake was sufficient to maintain or increase the plasma concentrations established in utero and to promote accumulation in calcifying tissues. The lower intake by the breast-fed infants, which would have resulted in gradually declining plasma concentrations, caused mobilization from the rapidly exchangeable pool.

Thus, if it is assumed that prenatal fluoride supplementation of the mother has some beneficial effect on the child's deciduous teeth, it appears that the practice is rational only if the neonate's fluoride intake is substantially greater than that provided by breast milk.

into the rapidly exchangeable pool. After approximately 30 minutes, when the plasma concentrations are falling, net migration of most of the fluoride back into the extracellular fluid occurs. A small fraction of it, however, becomes associated with newly forming bone crystallites so that skeletal concentrations usually increase gradually throughout life. In the postabsorptive state when plasma concentrations are steady, there is little or no net fluoride uptake. The movement of fluoride into and out of calcified tissues has implications for fluoride intake during infancy.

Excretion of Fluoride

The excretion of fluoride occurs mainly via the kidneys. The fecal excretion of fluoride usually accounts for only 10% to 20% of daily intake. Even under extreme conditions of heat or exercise, only minor amounts of fluoride are excreted in sweat, which has a low fluoride concentration close to that of plasma (about 0.02 ppm). Thus, a liter of sweat contains only about 0.02 mg of fluoride.

The renal handling of fluoride is charac-terized by free filtration through the glomerular capillaries, followed by a variable degree of tubular reabsorption. The renal clearance of fluoride, i.e., the volume of plasma from which it is completely removed per unit of time, is approximately 35 mL/min in healthy adults. Various studies found averages ranging from 27 to 42 mL/min but a much wider range among individuals (12 to 71 mL/min). The clearances in children are lower, but, when factored for body weight, they are practically the same as for adults. The efficiency with which the kidneys clear fluoride from the body is due to the relatively large hydrated radius of the ion that restricts its migration (reabsorption) from the renal tubular fluid back into the blood.

Urinary pH and the Balance of Fluoride

Like absorption from the stomach, the reabsorption of fluoride from the renal tubular fluid is strongly dependent on pH and the diffusion of HF (Fig. 35–3). The fraction of fluoride that exists in the form of HF is directly related to the acidity of the renal tubular fluid.

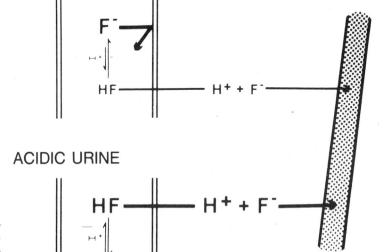

Figure 35–3. The mechanism for the reabsorption of fluoride from the kidney tubule. The tubular epithelium is virtually impermeable to ionic fluoride (F⁻); it is easily permeated by the undissociated acid, HF, which lacks a charge. (From Whitford, G.M. [1990] The physiological and toxicological characteristics of fluoride. J Dent Res 69[Spec. Issue]:539–549.)

When the pH is high, say 7.4, only 0.01% of the fluoride is in the form of HF and available for reabsorption. This results in a high clearance rate. When the pH is close to the physiologically possible lower limit (~ 4.0), nearly 20% exists as HF. Under this condition, reabsorption is rapid and the clearance rate is low.

The dependence of the renal clearance on urinary pH is a major factor in determining the metabolic balance (intake minus excretion) of fluoride. Urinary pH may be affected significantly by several conditions or factors, including (1) certain diseases such as diabetes mellitus, renal tubular acidosis, the chronic obstructive pulmonary diseases, and some hormonal disorders, (2) acidifying or alkalinizing drugs, (3) the altitude of residence, and (4) the composition of the diet. The latter factor is probably the most important in that it affects the urinary pH of all people.

Skeletal Development and the Balance of Fluoride

About 50% of the fluoride absorbed by adults each day is deposited in calcified tissues and the rest is excreted in the urine. This is only a rough generalization, however, as is indicated by the variability among individuals in the renal excretion of fluoride, as discussed in the preceding section.

Another factor important in determining fluoride balance is the stage of skeletal development. The uptake of fluoride by calcified tissues is directly related to the total surface area of the crystallites. Developing crystallites are small in size, large in number, loosely organized, and heavily hydrated, and they have a large surface-to-volume ratio. Thus, the fraction of absorbed fluoride that is retained in the body is inversely related to age during growth. A longitudinal study with growing dogs determined the retention (percent of dose not excreted in the urine) of intravenously administered fluoride for nearly 20 months (Whitford, 1990). The results are shown in Figure 35–4. Shortly after the pups were weaned, only about 10% of the dose was excreted so that retention was close to 90%. Retention declined throughout the study and reached a final value close to 50%, which is the average for adult dogs several years of age. These findings are similar to those from studies with human infants and adults (Ekstrand et al., 1994). Although there are no data with which to judge, it is likely that in the later years of life, when bone resorption begins to exceed accretion, retention of fluoride falls to even lower levels.

NUTRITION INSIGHT

Urinary pH and the Balance of Fluoride

Many infants are fed either breast milk, which has a low acid load, or a cow's milk–based formula, which has a much higher acid load. The urinary pH of breast-fed infants ranges from the middle 6s to the lower 7s, whereas that of infants fed a cow's milk formula ranges from the lower 5s to the lower 6s (Moore et al., 1977). A diet consisting largely of vegetables and fruits (excluding cranberries, plums, and prunes) produces urinary pH values in the upper 6s and middle 7s, whereas a diet of meats and dairy products causes distinctly acidic pH values ranging from the upper 4s to the upper 5s.

Although data showing the effects of feeding infants human milk (breast feeding) or cow's milk formulas are not available, it is likely that fluoride excretion is higher and balance is lower in the former group. Research with young adults eating a vegetarian diet showed that the renal clearance of fluoride was significantly higher than when they were restricted to a meat and dairy product diet (Whitford and Weatherred, 1996). Compared with laboratory rats kept at sea level, rats residing at simulated high altitude (hypobaric hypoxia) have a more acidic urine and significantly higher fluoride concentrations in plasma and calcified tissues. Thus, several environmental and physiological variables can influence the renal handling of fluoride sufficiently to alter its retention and potentially affect its actions in the body.

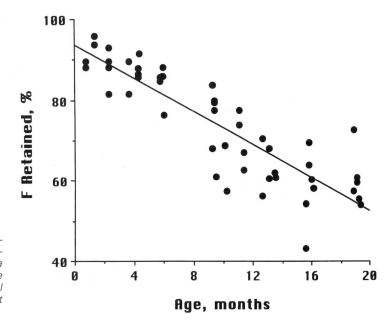

Figure 35–4. The inverse relationship between age and fluoride retention in growing dogs. (Data
from Whitford, G. M. [1990] The
physiological and toxicological
characteristics of fluoride. J Dent
Res 69(Spec. Issue):539–549.)

ACUTE FLUORIDE TOXICITY

Life-threatening or fatal cases of acute fluoride
toxicity are now extremely rare. Substantial
amounts of fluoride in toothpastes, mouth
rinses, or dietary supplements, however, are
found in most American homes. Because of
the suspected or actual overingestion of these
products, especially by young children, several thousand calls to poison control centers
are made each year.

Signs, Symptoms, and Treatment

Acute fluoride toxicity can develop with
alarming rapidity. Nausea and vomiting almost
always occur immediately after swallowing a
large amount of fluoride and should be
treated as initial signs of a potentially serious
sequence of events. A variety of nonspecific
signs and symptoms, including excessive sali-
vation and tearing, sweating, headache, diarrhea, and generalized weakness, may follow
within minutes. Spasm of the extremities, tetany, and/or convulsions may develop if a potentially fatal dose has been swallowed. These
effects will be accompanied by hypotension
and possibly cardiac arrhythmias, all of which
are consequences of hyperkalemia and severe
hypocalcemia. As renal function and respiration become depressed, a mixed metabolic

and respiratory acidosis develops progressively and may end in coma.

Treatment on site and in the hospital is
aimed at reducing absorption, promoting excretion, and supporting the vital signs. It
should begin immediately. The oral administration of 1% calcium gluconate or calcium
chloride reduces absorption. If calcium solutions are not available, milk may slow absorption. While these actions are taken, the hospital should be advised that a case of acute
fluoride poisoning is in progress so that preparations for appropriate treatment can be made
before arrival.

Doses Producing Serious Systemic Toxicity

The "probably toxic dose" (PTD) is defined as
the "minimum dose that could cause serious
or life-threatening systemic signs and symptoms and that should trigger immediate therapeutic intervention and hospitalization"
(Whitford, 1996). Based on reasonably well-
documented case reports, the PTD has been
estimated at 5 mg of fluoride/kg. One 3-year-
old child died in an emergency room 3 hours
after swallowing a fluoride solution in a dental
office. The estimated dose was between 24
and 35 mg/kg. Another 3-year-old died in a
hospital after swallowing about 200 1.0-mg

fluoride tablets. In this case the dose was approximately 16 mg/kg. A third 27-month-old child died 5 days after swallowing an unknown number, but less than 100, of 0.5-mg fluoride tablets. The dose in this case was estimated to be slightly under 5 mg/kg. In each of these cases, the child vomited almost immediately so that the absorbed dose was less than the ingested dose. The survival times after the doses were inversely related to the size of the doses. Based on these reports, it has been concluded that a fluoride dose of 15 mg/kg will probably cause death and that a dose of 5 mg/kg may be fatal. It should be noted that acute toxicity stemming from the ingestion of optimally fluoridated water (1 mg/L) is not possible because 5 L/kg of body weight would be required to reach the PTD.

Dental Products as Sources of High Fluoride Doses

During the first half of this century, sodium fluoride was a popular pesticide. Large amounts of it were stored in the kitchens of some homes and institutions. Being a finely divided white powder easily mistaken for powdered milk, flour, sodium bicarbonate, and similar products, there were numerous individual and several mass poisonings (Hodge and Smith, 1965). In 1941, for example, about 17 pounds of sodium fluoride was mistaken for powdered milk and used to prepare scrambled eggs at the Oregon State Hospital. There were 263 cases of poisoning, 47 of which were fatal. More than 600 deaths were due to fluoride ingestion in the United States between 1933 and 1965, which accounted for nearly 1% of all fatal poisoning during that period.

Other compounds have replaced sodium fluoride as a pesticide, and fluoride-related fatalities are now rare. Owing to the presence of vitamins, dietary supplement tablets, and dental products containing fluoride in most American homes, however, the number of nonfatal cases has increased sharply. The American Association of Poison Control Centers reported that about 11,000 fluoride-related reports were made to American poison control centers annually from 1989 to 1995. Among these, approximately 7% of the cases were treated in a health facility each year.

Toothpastes and mouthwashes were involved in 25% to 34% of the total number of reports each year. More than 90% of the cases involved young children. The "medical outcome" classification of the great majority of cases was "none" (transient and minor signs and symptoms), but 19 to 51 cases each year were classified in the more serious categories, including 3 "major" cases (long-term sequelae) and 2 deaths.

The PTD for a 1-year-old child of average weight (10 kg) is 50 mg of fluoride. Each gram of a conventional, 1000-ppm toothpaste contains 1.0 mg of fluoride, so that ingestion of 50 g (1.6 oz.) could cause serious toxicity. For an average 5- to 6-year-old (20 kg), the PTD is contained in 100 g of toothpaste. Most of the over-the-counter mouth rinses have a fluoride concentration of 230 ppm, or 0.23 mg/mL. Thus, the PTD for a 10-kg child is contained in 217 mL (7.3 oz.) of mouth rinse. These products should be stored out of the reach of small children, and their use should be supervised by an adult.

CHRONIC FLUORIDE TOXICITY

Perhaps because of its early use as a pesticide, fears and claims of harm surrounding the fluoridation of water, including a variety of allergic reactions, cancer, birth defects, and genetic disorders, were heard from the beginning. None of these claims has stood the test of controlled scientific research, as indicated most recently in reviews by Kaminsky et al. (1990), the U.S. Public Health Service (1991), and the National Research Council (1993). It was noted, however, that further epidemiological studies are required to determine whether an association exists between levels of fluoride in the drinking water and bone fractures. This latter subject is currently receiving considerable research attention.

Effects on the Skeleton

Chronic, Low-Level Intake. The results of epidemiological studies investigating the possible relationship between the concentration of fluoride in drinking water and bone fractures have produced a murky picture (National Research Council, 1993). Most of the studies were "ecological" in design—i.e., they compared population-based data without information concerning previous fluoride intake or bone fluoride concentrations for individuals with or without fractures. The studies compared populations living in different areas and having different water fluoride concentrations (geographic studies) or the same population before and after fluoridation of the water supply (time-trend studies). Time-trend studies are less likely to be confounded by uncontrolled variables. Four of the geographic studies found weakly positive correlations between water fluoridation and bone fractures. A fifth geographic study found no relationship. Of the two time-trend studies, one found no relationship, whereas the other found a weak, inverse relationship—i.e., the risk of fracture was slightly lower in the community after the water had been fluoridated.

The 1993 report by the National Research Council concluded that the current database is limited and confusing. It recommended that ". . . additional studies of hip and other fractures be conducted in geographic areas with high and low concentrations in the drinking water, and that studies should use information from individuals rather than population groups." The recommendation specified risk factors for individuals that should be evaluated in such studies, including ". . . fluoride intake from drinking water and from all other sources, reproductive history, past and current hormonal status, intake of dietary and supplemental calcium and other cations, bone density, and other factors that might influence risk of fracture."

Chronic, High-Level Intake: Skeletal Fluorosis. Skeletal fluorosis is a condition characterized by several stages of severity. The changes progress from the asymptomatic preclinical stage in which there is a slight increase in bone mass detectable by X-ray, through stage II in which there is further osteosclerosis, some stiffness and pain in the joints, and slight calcification of ligaments, and ultimately to crippling skeletal fluorosis, which is characterized by irregular, bony outgrowths (exostoses) on previously smooth bone surfaces and marked calcification of lig-

aments, which limits joint mobility. Among adults with lifelong exposure to optimally fluoridated water, bone ash fluoride concentrations are usually less than 1500 ppm. Bone ash concentrations range from 3500 to 5500 ppm in the preclinical stage to over 9000 ppm in the crippling stage of skeletal fluorosis. The latter condition may develop when approximately 20 mg of fluoride are ingested daily for 10 years or more. Only 5 cases of crippling fluorosis in the United States have been documented in the last 30 years. The U.S. Environmental Protection Agency has set the MCL (maximum contaminant level) for fluoride in drinking water at 4 ppm to protect against the first signs of this disorder.

Treatment of Osteoporosis. Based on its ability to increase bone mass, fluoride is used as an experimental drug in the treatment of osteoporosis (10 to 30 mg/day, usually for 3 to 5 years). Fluoride stimulates bone-forming cells (osteoblasts) to increase the production of several proteins, collectively called osteoid, which undergo rapid mineralization to form new bone. Although the literature contains conflicting reports concerning the effects of this treatment on bone strength, recent studies with a slow-release fluoride formulation have shown positive results (Pak et al., 1997).

REFERENCES

American Dental Association, Council on Dental Therapeutics (1994) New fluoride guidelines proposed. J Am Dent Assoc 125:366.

Brunelle, J. A. and Carlos, J. P. (1990) Recent trends in dental caries in U.S. children and the effect of water fluoridation. J Dent Res 69(Spec. Issue):723–727.

Burt, B. A. (1992) The changing patterns of systemic fluoride intake. J Dent Res 71(Spec. Issue):1228–1237.

Dean, H. T. (1942) The investigation of physiologic effects by the epidemiologic method. In: Fluorine and Dental Health (Moulton, F. R., ed.), pp. 23–31. American Association for the Advancement of Science, Washington, D.C.

Ekstrand, J., Hardell, L. I. and Spak, C. J. (1984) Fluoride balance studies on infants in a 1-ppm-water-fluoride area. Caries Res 18:87–92.

Ekstrand, J., Ziegler, E. E., Nelson, S. E. and Fomon, S. J. (1994) Absorption and retention of dietary and supplemental fluoride by infants. Adv Dent Res 8:175–180.

Fejerskov, O., Thylstrup, A. and Larsen, M. J. (1977) Clinical and structural features and possible pathogenic mechanisms of dental fluorosis. Scand J Dent Res 85:510–534.

Hamilton, I. R. (1990) Biochemical effects of fluoride on oral bacteria. J Dent Res 69(Spec. Issue):660–667.

Hodge, H. C. and Smith, F. A. (1965) Biological properties

of inorganic fluorides. In: Fluorine Chemistry (Simons, J. H., ed.), vol. 4, pp. 1–42. Academic Press, New York.

Institute of Medicine (1997) Dietary Reference Intakes: Calcium, Phosphorus, Magnesium, Vitamin D, and Fluoride. National Academy Press, Washington, D.C.

Kaminsky, L. S., Mahoney, M. C., Leach, J., Melius, J. and Miller, M. J. (1990) Fluoride: Benefits and risks of exposure. Crit Rev Oral Biol Med 1:261–281.

Leverett, D. H. (1982) Fluoride and the changing prevalence of dental caries. Science 217:26–30.

Leverett, D. H., Adair, S. M., Vaughan, R., Proskin, H. M. and Moss, M. E. (1997) Randomized clinical trial of the effect of prenatal fluoride supplements in preventing dental caries. Caries Res 31:174–179.

Moore, A., Ansell, C. and Barrie, H. (1977) Metabolic acidosis and infant feeding. Br Med J 1:129–131.

National Research Council (1993) Health Effects of Ingested Fluoride, pp. 1–181. National Academy Press, Washington, D.C.

Pak, C. Y., Sakhaee, K., Rubin, C. D. and Zerwekh, M. (1997) Sustained release of sodium fluoride in the management of established postmenopausal osteoporosis. Am J Med Sci 313:23–32.

Pendrys, D. G. and Morse, D. E. (1995) Fluoride supplement use by children in fluoridated communities. J Public Health Dent 55:160–164.

Tatevossian, A. (1990) Fluoride in dental plaque and its effects. J Dent Res 69(Spec. Issue):645–652.

Taves, D. R. (1983) Dietary intake of fluoride: ashed (total fluoride) v. unashed (inorganic fluoride) analysis of individual foods. Br J Nutr 49:295–301.

Ten Cate, J. M. (1990) In vitro studies on the effects of fluoride on de- and remineralization. J Dent Res 69(Spec. Issue):614–619.

U.S. Public Health Service (1991) Review of Fluoride: Benefits and Risks, pp. 1–134. U.S. Public Health Service Department of Health and Human Services, Bethesda, MD.

Whitford, G. M. (1990) The physiological and toxicological characteristics of fluoride. J Dent Res 69(Spec. Issue):539–549.

Whitford, G. M. (1996) The Metabolism and Toxicity of Fluoride, 2nd ed., pp. 1–156. Monographs in Oral Science, No. 16. S. Karger, New York.

Whitford, G. M. and Weatherred, T. W. (1996) Fluoride pharmacokinetics: Effects of urinary pH changes induced by the diet. J Dent Res 75(Spec. Issue):354 (abs. 2695).

RECOMMENDED READINGS

Proceedings, Joint IADR/ORCA International Symposium on Fluorides (1990) Mechanisms of Action and Recommendations for Use. J Dent Res 69(Spec. Issue):505–835.

Burt, B. A. (1992) The changing pattern of systemic fluoride intake. J Dent Res 71:1228–1237.

CHAPTER **36**

◆ ◆

The Ultratrace Elements

Forrest H. Nielsen, Ph.D.

O U T L I N E

C O M M O N   A B B R E V I A T I O N S

ESADDI (estimated safe and adequate daily dietary intake)
GTF (glucose tolerance factor)

CHARACTERISTICS OF ULTRATRACE ELEMENTS

Trace minerals essential for health are those elements of the periodic table that occur in the body in microgram per gram of tissue amounts and are usually required by humans in amounts of milligrams per day. In 1980, the term ultratrace element began to appear in the nutritional literature; the definition for this term was an element that was required by animals in amounts of 50 ng or less per gram of diet. For humans, the term has been used recently to indicate elements with established, estimated, or suspected requirements quantified by micrograms per day.

The quality of the experimental evidence for nutritional essentiality varies widely for the ultratrace elements. The evidence for the essentiality of three ultratrace elements, iodine, molybdenum, and selenium, is substantial and noncontroversial; specific biochemical functions have been defined for these elements. Iodine and selenium are recognized as elements of major nutritional importance and receive their deserved attention in Chapters 33 and 34. Very little nutritional attention, however, is given to molybdenum, because a deficiency has not been unequivocally identified in humans other than a few individuals nourished by total parenteral nutrition or with genetic defects that cause metabolic disturbances involving the functional roles of this element. Thus, molybdenum will be discussed here.

Two additional elements, cobalt and manganese, perhaps should be listed with iodine, molybdenum, and selenium as established essential ultratrace elements. However, although cobalt is required in ultratrace amounts, it has to be in the form of vitamin B_{12}; thus, it is usually discussed as a component of this vitamin and is covered in Chapter 21. Although manganese has an estimated safe and adequate daily dietary intake (ESADDI) of 2.5 to 5.0 mg/day for adults, recent studies with humans suggest that the actual requirement is less than this, about 1 mg/day or less and may be more correctly classified as an ultratrace element. Nevertheless, manganese is discussed as a trace element in Chapter 32.

Two other elements, boron and chromium, should be considered ultratrace elements, even though biochemical functions have not been firmly established for them, because they have been shown to have at least beneficial, if not essential, actions in humans. Only circumstantial evidence from animal studies suggests that there are other ultratrace elements of nutritional significance. The evidence for some of these elements is briefly summarized at the end of this chapter.

People involved in professions providing nutritional guidance should be aware of the possible importance of the ultratrace elements in nutrition; this may include those that lack a defined biochemical function, which hinders their acceptance as nutritionally essential. The public is continuously exposed to health claims that appear in the popular media, pamphlets, and advertisements for these elements. Knowledge of the bases for these claims will help give informed guidance to those inquiring about usefulness of some ultratrace element in maintaining health and well-being. An uninformed "It is not needed or important" without giving some scientific support to the statement often is not well accepted by the inquirer, who usually has read some convincing statements that have been expertly prepared, as often is done by persons interested in selling supplements. Additionally, because some of the ultratrace elements have beneficial, if not essential, effects in humans, promoting diets that provide luxuriant amounts of these elements is a justifiable action to ensure health and well-being.

BORON

Nutritional and Physiological Significance

Findings involving boron deprivation in humans have come mainly from two studies (Nielsen, 1994a) in which men over the age of 45 years, postmenopausal women, and postmenopausal women on estrogen were fed a diet low in boron—about 0.25 mg/2000 kcal for 63 days, and then were fed the same diet supplemented with 3 mg of boron/day for 49 days. These dietary intakes were near the low and high values in the range of dietary boron intakes (0.5 to 3.1 mg/day) that have been found in a limited number of surveys. The only major differences in these two experiments were the intakes of copper and magnesium, which apparently affected the response to the changes in dietary boron, as shown in Table 36–1. In one experiment, copper was marginal and magnesium was inadequate; in the other experiment, both elements were adequate. Some of the effects of boron supplementation, after 63 days of boron depletion, that were found in these experiments are listed in Table 36–1. Boron supplementation after depletion also enhanced the elevation in serum 17 β-estradiol and plasma copper

TABLE 36–1
Responses of Boron-Deprived Subjects to a 3-mg B/Day Supplement for 49 Days*

Metabolism Affected	Evidence for Effect
Macromineral and electrolyte	Increased serum 25-hydroxy-vitamin D Decreased serum calcitonin†
Energy	Decreased serum glucose† Increased serum triacylglycerols‡
Nitrogen	Decreased blood urea nitrogen Decreased serum creatinine Increased urinary hydroxyproline excretion
Oxidative	Increased erythrocyte superoxide dismutase Increased serum ceruloplasmin
Erythropoiesis/hematopoiesis	Increased blood hemoglobin‡ Increased mean corpuscular hemoglobin content‡ Decreased hematocrit‡ Decreased platelet number‡ Decreased red cell number‡

*Deprivation consisted of 0.25 mg/2000 kcal of boron for 63 days. Subjects included men over the age of 45 years, postmenopausal women not on hormone replacement therapy, and postmenopausal women on estrogen therapy.
†Found when dietary copper was marginal and magnesium was inadequate.
‡Found when dietary copper and magnesium were adequate.
From Nielsen, F. H. (1994a) Biochemical and physiologic consequences of boron deprivation in humans. Environ Health Perspect 102(Suppl):59–63.

caused by estrogen ingestion (Nielsen, 1994a), altered encephalograms such that they suggested improved behavioral activation (e.g., less drowsiness) and mental alertness, improved psychomotor skills, and elicited improvements in the cognitive processes of attention and memory (Penland, 1994).

Changes similar to several of these found in humans also have been found in animal models (Hunt, 1994). For example, many findings indicate that boron deprivation impairs calcium and energy metabolism. These findings include the alleviation by boron of vitamin D deficiency-induced changes in bone, impaired energy substrate utilization, and impaired growth. Boron deprivation also was found to influence brain electrical activity systematically, as assessed by an electrocorticogram in mature rats; the principal effect was on the frequency distribution of electrical activity (Penland, 1994). Another finding suggesting that boron affects macromineral metabolism is that the apparent absorption and balance of calcium, magnesium, and phosphorus were found to be higher in boron-supplemented (2.72 μg/g diet) than in boron-deprived (0.158 μg/g diet) rats fed a vitamin D-deficient diet.

Biochemical Forms and Actions Involved or Implicated in Physiological Actions

Boron exists in biological material mainly bound to oxygen. Thus, boron biochemistry is essentially that of boric acid. Boron has three L-shell electrons available for bonding as in boric acid, but there is a tendency for boron to acquire an additional electron pair to fill the fourth orbital. Thus, boric acid acts as a Lewis acid and accepts an electron pair from a base (H_2O) to form tetracovalent boron compounds such as $B(OH)_4^-$. Thus, the reaction

$$B(OH)_3 + H_2O \rightarrow B(OH)_4^- + H^+$$

at the pH of blood (7.4) results in dilute aqueous boric acid solutions being composed of $B(OH)_3$ and $B(OH)_4^-$. Because the pKa of boric acid is 9.2, the abundance of these two species in blood should be 98.4% and 1.6%, respectively.

Boric acid forms ester complexes with hydroxyl groups of organic compounds; this preferably occurs when the hydroxyl groups are adjacent and *cis*. Among the hydroxylated substances of biological interest with which boron complexes are adenosine 5'-phosphate, pyridoxine, riboflavin, dehydroascorbic acid, and pyridine nucleotides. Formation of these complexes may be biologically important because in vitro formation of these complexes results in the competitive inhibition of some enzymes, including oxidoreductases, that require the *cis*-hydroxyl-containing pyridine of flavin nucleotides as cofactor. The added stabilization of hydrogen bonding between hydroxyl bound to boron and hydrogen of imidazole or amino groups allows complexes to be formed between boric acid and compounds containing single hydroxyl groups. Through formation of this type of complex, borate ($B_4O_7^{2-}$) and boronic acid derivatives [$RB(OH)_2$] can form transition state analogs that inhibit the activity of some enzymes. For example, serine proteases are inhibited when a tetrahedral complex is formed between the serine hydroxyl group and borate, with hydrogen bonding to an imidazole ring of an adjacent histidine adding stabilization.

Five naturally occurring organoboron compounds have been identified; they contain boron bound to four oxygen groups. Among these compounds are aplasmomycin, an antibiotic isolated from strain SS-20 of *Streptomyces griseus,* and boromycin, an antibiotic synthesized by *Streptomyces antibioticus.* Boromycin has the ability to encapsulate alkali metal cations and increase the permeability of the cytoplasmic membrane to potassium ions.

Boron recently has been found to be required for normal development and reproduction of the frog (Fort et al., 1998) and the zebrafish (Eckhert and Rowe, 1999). However, a biochemical function to explain the requirement has not been elucidated.

Two hypotheses recently have been advanced for the biochemical function of boron in higher animals. These hypotheses accommodate a large and varied response to boron deprivation and the known biochemistry of boron. One hypothesis is that boron has a role in cell membrane function or stability such that it influences the response to hormone action, transmembrane signaling or transmembrane movement of regulatory cations or anions (Nielsen, 1994a). This hypothesis is supported by the recent findings that boron influences the transport of extracellular calcium and the release of intracellular calcium in rat platelets activated by thrombin, and that boron deprivation signs in zebrafish include membrane blebbing with cytoplasmic extrusion during the zygote and cleavage periods of embryogenesis and eye cone dystrophy in the adult, changes occurring in cells that produce prodigious quantities of membranes (Eckhert and Rowe, 1999). The other hypothesis is based upon the knowledge that two classes of enzymes are competitively inhibited in vitro by borate or its derivatives and upon findings showing that dietary boron can alter the activity in vivo of a number of these enzymes. Thus, it has been hypothesized that boron is a metabolic regulator; that is, boron controls a number of metabolic pathways by competitively inhibiting some key enzyme reactions (Hunt, 1994). It is emphasized that these are speculated, not confirmed, functions of boron.

Dietary Considerations

In the human studies just described, the subjects responded to a boron supplement after consuming a diet supplying only about 0.25 mg of B/2000 kcal for 63 days. Thus, humans apparently receive benefit from, or have a dietary boron requirement above, this amount. Based on animal studies, an intake of 1 mg of B/day should be considered beneficial.

CHROMIUM

Nutritional and Physiological Significance

A large amount of circumstantial evidence supports the view that chromium is an essential nutrient (Nielsen, 1994b). The evidence includes the finding that humans on long-term

Food Sources of Boron

- Fruits
- Leafy and cruciferous vegetables
- Nuts
- Legumes and pulses
- Wine, cider, beer

total parenteral nutrition containing a low amount of chromium developed impaired glucose tolerance, or high blood sugar with glucose spilling into the urine, and a resistance to insulin action; these abnormalities were reversed by chromium supplementation. Additionally, a number of reports from numerous research groups have described beneficial effects of chromium supplementation of subjects with varying degrees of glucose intolerance, ranging from hypoglycemia (low blood sugar) to insulin-dependent diabetes (Anderson, 1993). Beneficial effects of chromium supplementation on blood lipid profiles also have been reported.

Even with this evidence, chromium is not unequivocally accepted as being essential by all scientists; there are two major reasons for this. First, it has been difficult to induce signs of chromium deficiency in experimental animals. Nutritional, metabolic, physiological, or hormonal stressors generally have to be employed to induce experimental animals to respond to chromium deprivation; in most cases, the responses have not been remarkable. Second, as indicated earlier, a specific biochemical role has not been firmly established for chromium.

Biochemical Forms and Actions Involved or Implicated in Physiological Actions

In spite of the shortcomings in the evidence, chromium most likely is an essential nutrient for higher animals, including humans. Even the skeptics usually accept the fact that chromium can at least be a beneficial element because of the desirable effects it has on glucose and lipid metabolism in some individuals.

Cr^{3+} is the most stable oxidation state of chromium and most likely is the valence state of importance in biological systems. In aqueous solutions, Cr^{3+} complexes are characterized by relative kinetic inertness such that ligand-displacement reactions have half-times in the range of several hours. Thus, chromium is unlikely to be involved as the metal catalyst at the active site of enzymes where the rate of exchange needs to be rapid. Such relatively inert chromium complexes, however, may function as structural components; for example, they may bind ligands in the proper orientation for enzymatic catalysis to occur, or be necessary for the tertiary structures of proteins and/or nucleic acids.

A biochemical role recently has been reported for chromium. A naturally occurring, biologically active form of chromium called low-molecular-weight chromium-binding substance (LMWCr) has been identified that apparently has a role in carbohydrate and lipid metabolism as part of a novel insulin-amplification mechanism (Davis and Vincent, 1997). LMWCr is a mammalian oligopeptide of about 1.5 kDa that binds four chromic ions and potentiates the ability of insulin to stimulate the conversion of glucose into lipids and carbon dioxide by isolated rat adipocytes. A biological role for LMWCr in the stimulation of insulin receptor protein kinase activity after the receptor is activated by insulin has been proposed. Chromium has been determined to be specifically needed by the oligopeptide for activity because ApoLMWCr was inactive in stimulating receptor kinase activity, but titration with chromic ions completely restored activity while other transition metals known to be essential failed to restore activity.

It has been found that RNA synthesis directed by free DNA in vitro is enhanced by the binding of chromium to the template. Furthermore, chromium is concentrated in he-

NUTRITION INSIGHT

Use of Chromium Picolinate Supplements for Weight Reduction and Muscle Building

The general media and health-food or supplement industry, frequently with help from the scientific community, have reported on various nutrients in such a way that the American public is misguided, bewildered, or uncertain as to what to believe. Quite often, a nutrient bursts onto the scene and is touted everywhere as an aid to improving health or body image; shortly thereafter, findings are reported that dispute these claims. Promotion of chromium, especially as chromium picolinate, as an ergogenic aid or weight-loss inducer fits into this category.

The most compelling evidence that chromium picolinate can help build muscles has come from the laboratory of the scientist who patented the method to make this compound. Several studies reported subsequently have not confirmed that the use of chromium supplements, including the picolinate form, will bring forth the overzealously touted propitious effects on muscle accretion, strength gain, or athletic performance.

A number of studies indicate little or no effect of chromium picolinate supplements, and also the studies used as a basis for the claims for chromium picolinate as an aid for weight reduction and muscle building do not themselves offer much support. For example, weight reduction claims are based on the conjecture that insulin action is affected by chromium so that glucose is less likely to be converted into fat and will suppress appetite; a few studies using chromium picolinate found very small reductions in body weight. In one study, the average fat loss was 4.2 pounds, with an average 1.4-pound increase in fat-free mass over a 72-day period of chromium supplementation; this translates to a loss of only 2.8 pounds after 10 weeks of treatment. This amount of weight loss does not conform to the usual claims for chromium supplements. In another study, the weight loss program was not limited to chromium supplementation; it included moderate caloric restriction and other dietary modifications. Thus, although a respectable average weight loss of 15 pounds was achieved in 8 weeks in this study, the loss could not be attributed solely to the chromium picolinate supplement. These studies, coupled with a small fat loss with a weight-training program reported by the holder of the chromium picolinate patent and with hearsay and testimonial evidence, are the basis for the weight loss claims for chromium. In contrast to weight-loss claims, most studies of participants in weight-training programs involving chromium picolinate supplementation gained weight. In other words, there are no data from well-controlled studies to support the astonishing weight-loss claims made for the use of chromium picolinate supplements.

Thinking Critically

1. One advertisement claims that a supplement containing chromium picolinate can "blast off" 49 pounds in only 29 days without exercising and with no problem in eating up to six times a day. Does this claim seem possible given what you know about energy metabolism? (See Chapters 17 and 18.)

2. It has been found that a supplement of 1000 μg of chromium per day as chromium picolinate can reduce some of the abnormalities of diabetes. Should this intake of chromium be considered nutritional?

patic nuclei 48 hours after intraperitoneal injection of $CrCl_3$. The chromium is preferentially bound to DNA in chromatin and increases the number of initiation sites, which enhances RNA synthesis. Perhaps chromium, or a biologically active form of chromium, has a role in regulating gene expression of a critical substance in glucose metabolism. Some

support for this suggestion is the finding that insulin-potentiating substances are often found in materials high in chromium (e.g., brewer's yeast), although one cannot assume that the chromium in these materials is part of the molecules that potentiate insulin action. Further support is the finding of a 4-hour lag period between the administration of chromium and its optimal effect on insulin action in vivo.

Dietary Considerations

Although the Estimated Safe and Adequate Daily Dietary Intake (ESADDI) for chromium is 50 to 200 μg/day, contrary to what some reports lead people to believe, consuming less than 50 μg/day does not mean that one would eventually become chromium-deficient. Balance studies have demonstrated that healthy elderly people maintain metabolic chromium balance despite consuming diets low in chromium (Offenbacher, 1992). Additionally, the average daily intake of chromium apparently is well below 50 μg and may be closer to 25 μg, yet widespread apparent cases of chromium deficiency have not been documented. That is, supplemental chromium fed to many individuals apparently consuming chromium at these low amounts did not result in any improvement in glucose tolerance or in plasma insulin, cholesterol, or triacylglycerol concentrations. Thus, for many people, a daily intake of 25 to 35 μg of chromium may be adequate. However, some data suggest that an intake of less than 20 μg/day is inadequate.

Based on dietary surveys, apparently a significant number of people are consuming less than 20 μg of chromium/day. As a result,

it is not surprising that a large number of studies have found individuals who respond to chromium supplementation.

Regardless of the uncertainties about chromium, substantial evidence exists to suggest that a significant number of individuals would benefit from an increased intake of chromium (Anderson, 1993). The best and most enjoyable way of doing this is by eating a varied diet incorporating foods and beverages that are good sources of chromium.

MOLYBDENUM

Nutritional and Physiological Significance

Although molybdenum is an established essential element, it apparently is not of practical concern in human nutrition. Reports describing molybdenum deficiency signs in humans are very few (Rajagopalan, 1988), and the signs were not very marked for the one study in which a somewhat normal diet was consumed. In this study, 4 young men were fed a low-molybdenum diet (22 μg/day) for 102 days; no clinical symptoms of molybdenum deficiency were observed (Turnlund et al., 1995). However, the low molybdenum resulted in decreased urinary excretion of uric acid and an increased urinary xanthine excre-

---

Food Sources of Chromium

• Processed and organ meats
• Whole grain products, including some ready-to-eat bran cereals
• Nuts

Estimated Safe and Adequate Daily Dietary Intake
Across the Life Cycle

	μg chromium/day
Infants, Birth–0.5 y	10–40
0.5–1.0 y	20–60
Children, 1–3 y	20–80
4–6 y	30–120
7+ y	50–200
Adolescents and adults, 11+ y	50–200

From National Research Council (1989) Recommended Dietary Allowances, 10th ed. National Academy Press, Washington, D. C.

tion after the administration of a load of adenosine monophosphate (AMP); the findings indicate that xanthine oxidase activity was decreased by the low-molybdenum regimen. The most convincing case of molybdenum deprivation was found in a patient receiving prolonged parenteral nutrition therapy. Signs and symptoms exhibited by this patient, which were exacerbated by methionine administration, included high methionine and low uric acid levels in blood, high oxypurines and low uric acid in urine, and very low urinary sulfate excretion. The patient suffered mental disturbances that progressed to coma. Supplementation of the patient with ammonium molybdate improved the clinical condition, reversed the sulfur-handling defect, and normalized uric acid production. A human genetic disorder caused by the lack of functioning molybdenum as part of the enzyme sulfite oxidase has been identified. This genetic deficiency is characterized by severe brain damage, mental retardation, and dislocation of ocular lenses and results in increased urinary output of sulfite, S-sulfocysteine, and thiosulfate and a marked decrease in sulfate output.

Molybdenum deficiency signs also are difficult to induce in animals (Mills and Davis, 1987). In rats and chicks, excessive dietary tungsten was used to restrict molybdenum absorption and thus induce molybdenum deficiency signs of depressed molybdoenzymes, disturbed uric acid metabolism, and increased susceptibility to sulfite toxicity. Under field conditions, a molybdenum-responsive syndrome was found in hatching chicks. This syndrome was characterized by a high incidence of late embryonic mortality, mandibular distortion, and defects in leg bone development and feathering. Skeletal lesions, subsequently detected in older birds, included separation of the proximal epiphyses of the femur, osteolytic changes in the femoral shaft, and lesions in the overlying skin that were ultimately attributed to intense irritation in those areas. The incidence of this syndrome was particularly high in commercial flocks reared on diets containing high concentrations of copper (a molybdenum antagonist) as a growth stimulant. These apparently dissimilar pathological changes were suggested to be caused by a defect in sulfur metabolism.

Biochemical Forms and Actions Involved or Implicated in Physiological Actions

Molybdenum is a transition element that readily changes its oxidation state and can thus act as an electron transfer agent in oxidation-reduction reactions in which it cycles from Mo^{6+} to reduced states. This explains why molybdenum functions as an enzyme cofactor. Molybdenum as $MoOS^{2+}$ is present at the active site of all molybdoenzymes in a small nonprotein cofactor containing a pterin nucleus (Rajagopalan, 1988). More than 40% of molybdenum not attached to an enzyme in the liver exists as this cofactor bound to the mitochondrial outer membrane. This form can be transferred to an apomolybdoenzyme, which transforms it into an active (holo) enzyme molecule. The enzymes in mammalian systems also contain Fe-S centers and flavin cofactors. Molybdoenzymes catalyze the hydroxylation of various substrates using oxygen atoms from water. Aldehyde oxidase oxidizes and detoxifies various pyrimidines, purines, pteridines, and related compounds. Xanthine oxidase/dehydrogenase catalyzes the transformation of hypoxanthine to xanthine and of xanthine to uric acid. Sulfite oxidase catalyzes the transformation of sulfite to sulfate.

These enzymatic functions provide biochemical bases for the signs and symptoms of molybdenum deficiency. For example, with the molybdenum-deficient patient on total parenteral nutrition, the symptoms were indicative of a defect in sulfur amino acid metabolism at the level of sulfite oxidation to sulfate (sulfite oxidase deficiency) and a defect in uric acid production at the level of xanthine and hypoxanthine transformation to uric acid (xanthine oxidase deficiency).

Molybdate might also be involved in stabilizing the steroid-binding ability of the unoccupied glucocorticoid receptor. During isolation procedures, molybdate protects steroid hormone receptors, particularly the glucocorticosteroid receptor, against inactivation. It is hypothesized, however, that molybdate affects the glucocorticoid receptor because it mimics an endogenous compound called "modulator" (Bodine and Litwack, 1988).

Dietary Considerations

Although molybdenum apparently is normally of minor nutritional concern, it should not be ignored. There may be unrecognized situations in which molybdenum nutriture is of importance. For example, the molybdenum hydroxylases apparently are as important as the microsomal monooxygenase systems in the metabolism of drugs and foreign compounds (Beedham, 1985); perhaps a low molybdenum hydroxylase activity caused by molybdenum deficiency would have undesirable consequences when a person is stressed by high intakes of xenobiotics.

Data to support the current molybdenum ESADDIs are scant. These values, including 75 to 250 µg for adults, apparently were set using questionable balance data and through the reasoning that usual dietary intakes are within this range and do not result in signs of deficiency or toxicity. A recent study of molybdenum absorption, excretion, and balance using stable isotopes resulted in an estimation that the minimum dietary molybdenum requirement is about 25 µg/day (Turnlund et al., 1995), which suggests that the lower end of the ESADDI for adults could be decreased.

Recent surveys indicate that the daily intake of molybdenum is 50 to 350 µg. Thus, most diets apparently meet the need for molybdenum.

PROSPECTIVE ULTRATRACE ELEMENTS—NICKEL, VANADIUM, SILICON, ARSENIC, AND FLUORINE

The circumstantial evidence for some of the remaining ultratrace elements has been strengthened by findings other than dietary deprivation effects (Nielsen, 1994c; Table 36–2). That is, they exhibit actions in biological systems, are components of naturally occurring, biologically important molecules, and have biological roles in lower forms of life, which indicate that they may function similarly to known essential mineral elements in higher forms of life, including humans. Thus, some of these characteristics for these ultratrace elements will be described here.

Nickel

Since 1975, nickel has been found to be an essential component of numerous enzymes in lower forms of life (Ankel-Fuchs and Thauer, 1988). Nickel apparently is a universal component of ureases (urea amidohydrolases).

Text continued on page 838

Food Sources of Molybdenum

- Milk and milk products
- Pulses or dried legumes
- Organ meats (liver and kidney)
- Cereals

Estimated Safe and Adequate Daily Dietary Intake

	µg molybdenum/day
Infants, birth–0.5 y	15–30
0.5–1.0 y	20–40
Children, 1–3 y	25–50
4–6 y	30–75
7–10 y	50–150
Adolescents and adults, 11+ y	75–250

From National Research Council (1989) Recommended Dietary Allowances, 10th ed. National Academy Press, Washington, D. C.

TABLE 36–2

Ultratrace Elements of Possible Human Nutritional Significance Based upon Animal Experimentation*†

Element	Reported Deficiency Signs	Apparent Deficient Dietary Intake	Other Apparent Beneficial or Physiological Actions	Dietary Sources for Humans
Aluminum (Al)	Goat: Increased spontaneous abortions, depressed growth, incoordination and weakness in hind legs, and decreased life expectancy Chick: Depressed growth	Goat: 162 µg/kg Chick: not given	Activates adenylate cyclase; enhances calmodulin activity; stimulates DNA synthesis in cell cultures; stimulates osteoblasts to form bone through activating a putative G-protein-coupled cation sensing system	Baked goods prepared with chemical leavening agents (e.g., baking powder), processed cheese, grains, vegetables, herbs, tea, antacids, buffered analgesics
Arsenic (As)	Goat: Depressed growth, abnormal reproduction characterized by impaired fertility and elevated perinatal mortality, depressed serum triacylglycerols, death during lactation, myocardial damage Rat: Depressed growth, decreased liver concentrations of S-adenosylmethionine and activity of glutathione S-transferase, increased kidney calcium in females, and liver concentrations of S-adenosylhomocysteine Pig: Depressed growth Hamster: Depressed plasma taurine	Goat: 10 µg/kg Rat: 10 µg/kg Pig: less than 50 µg/kg Hamster: 10 µg/kg	As arsenocholine, is antiperotic and growth-promoting in fowl; activates some enzymes by acting as an alternate substrate in place of phosphate; induces heat shock or stress proteins; enhances DNA synthesis in human lymphocytes and in lymphocytes stimulated by phytohemagglutinin	Fish, grain, and cereal products
Bromine (Br)	Goat: Depressed growth, fertility, milk-fat production, hematocrit, hemoglobin, and life expectancy; increased spontaneous abortions	Goat: 0.8 mg/kg	Alleviates growth retardation caused by hyperthyroidism in mice and chicks; substitutes for part of chloride requirement for chicks; insomnia exhibited by many hemodialysis patients associated with bromide deficit	Grains, nuts, fish

Element	Signs of deficiency	Amount	Possible functions	Food sources
Cadmium (Cd)	Rat: Depressed growth Goat: Depressed growth	Rat: <4 µg/kg Goat: 20 µg/kg	Has transforming growth factor activity or stimulates growth of cells in soft agar	Shellfish, grains—especially those grown on high-cadmium soils, leafy vegetables
Fluorine (F)	Rat: Depressed growth and incisor pigmentation Goat: Depressed growth and lifespan, histological changes in kidney and endocrine organs	Rat: 0.04–0.46 mg/kg Goat: <0.3 mg/kg	High dietary fluoride improves fertility, hematopoiesis and growth in iron-low mice and rats; is anticarcinogenic; can be antiosteoporotic; prevents phosphorus-induced nephrocalcinosis	Fish, tea, fluoridated water
Germanium (Ge)	Rat: Altered bone and liver mineral composition, and decreased tibial DNA	Rat: 0.7 mg/kg	Reverses changes in rats caused by silicon deprivation; some organic germanium compounds have antitumor activity	Wheat bran, vegetables, leguminous seeds
Lead (Pb)	Rat: Depressed growth; anemia; disturbed iron metabolism; decreased liver glucose, triacylglycerols, LDL cholesterol, phospholipids, aspartate aminotransferase activity and pyruvate aminotransferase activity; increased liver cholesterol and alkaline phosphatase activity; increased serum ceruloplasmin and decreased blood catalase Pig: Depressed growth, and elevated serum cholesterol, phospholipids and bile acids	Rat: 200 µg/kg Rat: 18–45 µg/kg Pig: 30–32 µg/kg	Alleviates iron deficiency signs in young rats	Seafood, plant foodstuffs grown under high-lead conditions
Lithium (Li)	Goat: Depressed fertility, birth weight, lifespan, liver monoamine oxidase activity; depressed serum isocitrate dehydrogenase, malate dehydrogenase, aldolase, and glutamate dehydrogenase activities, and increased serum creatine kinase activity Rat: Depressed fertility, birth weight, litter size, and weaning weight	Goat: <1.5 mg/kg Rat: 0.6–15 µg/kg	Stimulates growth of some cultured cells; exhibits insulinomimetic action; incidence of violent crimes higher in areas with low-lithium drinking water; hair lithium low in violent criminals, learning-disabled subjects, and heart disease patients	Eggs, meat, processed meat, fish, milk, milk products, potatoes, vegetables (content varies with geographical origin)

Table continued on following page

TABLE 36-2

Ultratrace Elements of Possible Human Nutritional Significance Based upon Animal Experimentation*† Continued

Element	Reported Deficiency Signs	Apparent Deficient Dietary Intake	Other Apparent Beneficial or Physiological Actions	Dietary Sources for Humans
Nickel (Ni)	Goat: Depressed growth and reproductive performance Pig: Changed distribution and proper functioning of calcium and zinc Rat: Depressed growth and plasma glucose, changed distribution and proper functioning of iron, manganese, and vitamin B_{12} Sheep: Depressed erythrocyte count, ruminal urease activity, hepatic total lipids, cholesterol, and copper Chicks: Depressed hematocrit and ultrastructural abnormalities in liver Cow: (fed low protein) Depressed growth, ruminal urease, serum urea, and serum nitrogen	Goat: 137 µg/kg Pig: 100–160 µg/kg Rat: 15–25 µg/kg Sheep: 30 µg/kg Chicks: 25–50 µg/kg Cow: 310–400 µg/kg	Activates numerous enzymes in vitro, including arginase and calcineurin; alleviates some signs of copper and iron deficiencies in animals; can replace Mg^{2+} in the formation of the two C3 convertases of the complement system	Chocolate, nuts, dried beans and peas, grains
Rubidium (Rb)	Goat: Depressed food intake, growth, and life expectancy; increased spontaneous abortions	Goat: 180 µg/kg	Rubidium may be factor R, which prevents hind leg paralysis, swelling of abdomen, and death	Coffee, black tea, fruits, vegetables (especially asparagus), poultry, fish
Silicon (Si)	Chick: Long bone structural abnormalities characterized by small, poorly formed joints and defective endochondral bone growth: depressed articular cartilage, water, hexosamine, and collagen Rat: Skull structural abnormalities; increased humerus hexose; decreased humerus hydroxyproline and femur alkaline and acid phosphatase	Chick: 1–2 mg/kg Rat: 1–2 mg/kg	Incorporated in drugs, such as methylsilanetriol, used for the treatment of circulatory ischemias and osteoporosis; required for maximal propyl hydroxylase activity in frontal bones from chick embryo incubated in culture media	Unrefined grains of high-fiber content, cereal products, beer

Element	Signs of deprivation	Apparent requirement	Possible biochemical function	Food sources
Tin (Sn)	Rat: Depressed growth, response to sound, feed efficiency; heart zinc and copper, tibial copper and manganese, muscle iron and manganese, spleen iron, kidney iron, and lung magnesium; increased lung calcium; alopecia	Rat: 17 µg/kg	Influences heme oxygenase activity; associated with thymus immune and homeostatic function	Canned foods
Vanadium (V)	Goat: Increased spontaneous abortions; increased death during the first 56 days after birth; decreased life span; skeletal deformation in forelegs with forefoot tarsal joints thickened Rats: Increased thyroid weight/body weight ratio, altered response to stressors of thyroid metabolism	Goat: 10 µg/kg	Stimulates mineralization of bones and teeth; required for optimal growth of fibroblasts in tissue culture; stimulates bone cell proliferation and collagen synthesis in vitro; exhibits numerous pharmacological actions, including mimicking the actions of insulin in preventing signs of diabetes associated with streptozotocin administration to rats; mimics growth factors such as epidermal growth factor and fibroblast growth factor	Shellfish, mushrooms, parsley, dill seed, black pepper, some prepared foods

*Table does not include cobalt, iodine, manganese, molybdenum, and selenium, which have defined biochemical functions, nor boron and chromium, which human studies have shown to have beneficial, if not essential, actions in humans.

†References for the material presented are given in a review by Nielsen (1996).

Nickel has been found in ureases from bacteria, mycoplasmata, fungi, yeasts, algae, higher plants, and invertebrates. Highly purified urease contains two Ni^{2+} ions per 96.6-kDa subunit. An elegant model has been proposed for the urease mechanism of action, which involves the polarization of the urea carbonyl by one nickel ion to allow nucleophilic attack by an activated hydroxyl anion associated with the second nickel ion.

The hydrogenases are an extremely heterogeneous group of enzymes that catalyze the simplest oxidation-reduction process of $H_2 \leftrightarrow 2H^+ + 2e^-$. Hydrogenases that contain nickel have been identified for over 35 species of bacteria, including methanogenic, hydrogen-oxidizing, sulfate-reducing, phototrophic, and aerobic N_2-fixing bacteria. Nickel may be a common constituent of hydrogenases that function physiologically to oxidize rather than to evolve H_2. Nickel is redox active in hydrogenases and interacts with the substrate H_2.

In addition to its redox role, nickel apparently also has a regulatory role in the production of hydrogenase (Kim et al., 1991). Evidence has been presented that nickel is required for the synthesis of the hydrogenase messenger RNA in *Bradyrhizobium japonicum*. For the hydrogenase gene to be expressed, O_2 and H_2 diffuse into the cell and affect the redox state of the nickel bound to a nickel-containing, DNA-binding protein, which in turn leads to transcriptional upregulation of expression of the hydrogenase gene.

Carbon monoxide dehydrogenase, which oxidizes CO to CO_2, is a nickel enzyme that has been found in acetogenic, methanogenic, phototrophic, and sulfate-reducing anaerobic bacteria. In addition to oxidizing CO to CO_2, carbon monoxide dehydrogenase in acetogenic bacteria catalyzes the reduction of CO_2 to CO and the synthesis and degradation of acetyl CoA, and thus can also be designated as an acetyl CoA synthase.

Methyl-*S*-coenzyme M reductase is the terminal enzyme in the conversion of CO_2 to methane in methanogenic bacteria. The enzyme catalyzes the reductive cleavage of methyl-*S*-coenzyme to methane and coenzyme M. The enzyme contains a nickel tetrapyrrole known as factor F_{430}, which is thought to be the site of substrate reduction. Factor F_{430} has been called a tetrahydrocorphin because of its hybrid relationship to corrin and porphyrin structures; nickel-corphin has been suggested to be a "missing link" between iron porphyrin and cobalt corrin systems.

The preceding shows that nickel has been found to participate in hydrolysis and redox reactions, to regulate gene expression, and, possibly, to stabilize certain structures. In these roles, nickel forms ligands with sulfur, nitrogen, and oxygen, and exists in oxidation states of $3+$, $2+$, $1+$, and perhaps 0 and $4+$. Because nickel is so dynamic in lower forms of life, it most likely has an essential functional role in higher forms of life, including humans. Supporting this supposition is the response of experimental animals when they are deprived of dietary nickel (see Table 36–2).

Vanadium

Numerous biochemical and physiological functions for vanadium have been suggested, based upon its in vitro and pharmacological actions. These include insulin-mimetic properties, numerous stimulatory effects on cell proliferation and differentiation, effects on cell phosphorylation/dephosphorylation, inhibitory effects on the motility of sperm, cilia, and chromosomes, effects on glucose and ion transport across the plasma membrane, interfering effects on intracellular ionized calcium movement, and effects on oxidation-reduction processes (Willsky, 1990). In studies done in vitro with cell-free systems, vanadium inhibits numerous ATPases, phosphatases, and phosphoryl transfer enzymes. The pharmacological action of vanadium receiving the most attention is its ability to mimic insulin.

Recently functional roles for vanadium (Wever and Krenn, 1990; Eady, 1990) have been defined for some algae, lichens, fungi, and bacteria. These roles, along with results of animal deprivation studies (see Table 36–2), may provide clues to the possible biochemical role of vanadium in humans.

In 1984, vanadium was found essential to enzymatic activity of a bromoperoxidase from the brown algae *Ascophyllum nodosum*. Since then vanadium-dependent bromoperoxidases have been found in a number of marine brown algae, marine red algae, and a terrestrial lichen. Vanadium-dependent iodoperoxidases have been detected in brown seaweeds, and a vanadium-dependent chloroperoxidase has been identified in the fungus *Curvularia inaequalis.*

Haloperoxidases catalyze the oxidation of halide ions by hydrogen peroxide, thus facilitating the formation of a carbon-halogen bond. The mechanism of action of vanadium in the haloperoxidases has not been firmly established. However, findings to date do not favor a mechanism in which V^{5+} is reduced to V^{4+} or V^{3+} and reoxidized to V^{5+} by H_2O_2. Rather, as indicated by studies of the bromoperoxidases, H_2O_2 reacts with vanadium as V^{5+} to form a dioxygen species that reacts with the halide to yield an oxidized halide species, which is the intermediate that forms the carbon-halogen bond.

Conversion of atmospheric nitrogen to ammonia by nitrogen-fixing microorganisms is catalyzed by the enzyme nitrogenase. Some nitrogenases are vanadium-dependent. The reduction of dinitrogen by nitrogenase involves the sequential MgATP-dependent transfer of electrons from an iron-protein to a vanadium-iron-cofactor center at the substrate-binding site in nitrogenase.

Silicon

In addition to the animal findings shown in Table 36–2, the finding that silicon is essential for lower forms of life (Carlisle, 1984) provides support for the nutritional essentiality of silicon. Silicon has a structural role in diatoms, radiolarians, and some sponges. It may be needed by some higher plants, including rice. Diatoms, which are unicellular microscopic plants, have an absolute requirement for silicon as monomeric silicic acid for normal cell growth. Moreover, silicon affects gene expression in diatoms, which suggests that a similar role could exist in higher animals.

Arsenic

In addition to the animal findings listed in Table 36–2, some correlation-type findings suggest that arsenic is nutritionally important (Nielsen, 1991; Nielsen, 1996). Decreased serum arsenic concentrations in people under-going hemodialysis treatment were correlated to injuries of the central nervous system, vascular diseases, and cancer. Also, it has been observed that the incidence of skin cancer is higher in areas where no arsenic is detected in drinking water than in areas where detectable amounts of arsenic are found in the water.

Humans have enzymes that are used specifically to methylate inorganic arsenic. Methylation of arsenate takes place in the liver, following glutathione-dependent reduction of arsenate to arsenite, and is catalyzed by an arsenite methyltransferase that utilizes *S*-adenosylmethionine as the methyl donor. The monomethylarsonate precursor formed from arsenite can be methylated again to form dimethylarsinate. In animals, the methylation of arsenic can be modified by changing glutathione, methionine, or choline status.

Arsenite can induce the production of certain proteins known as heat shock or stress proteins in isolated cells. The control of production of these proteins in response to arsenite apparently is at the transcriptional level and has been suggested to involve changes in the methylation of core histones. Because some forms of cancer have been associated with DNA hypomethylation, it is possible that arsenic can influence the susceptibility to some cancers, as indicated by epidemiological studies, by affecting DNA methylation.

Fluorine

To date, most of the findings that often are accepted as evidence for fluoride essentiality reflect a pharmacological, not a physiological, action of fluoride. That is, high amounts of orally administered fluoride alleviate a disorder caused by something other than a fluoride deficiency. In the late 1930s, fluoride was found to be useful for preventing human dental caries. Subsequently, epidemiological findings suggested that fluoride is beneficial for the maintenance of a normal skeleton in adults. However, if tooth mottling is evidence of toxicity, near-toxic amounts of fluoride are needed to prevent the tooth decay caused by bacterial plaque. Also, near-toxic levels of fluoride are needed for preventive or therapeutic action against osteoporosis, which is a disorder of calcium-phosphorus metabolism.

Pharmacological actions do not establish essentiality; only limited animal findings shown in Table 36–2 support the concept that fluoride is an essential element. Still fluoride must be recognized as a trace element with beneficial properties. Based upon amounts considered protective against dental caries and perhaps osteoporosis, adequate dietary intakes have been established for fluoride. The recommendations and the benefits of fluoride in prevention of dental disease are covered in Chapter 35.

ABSTRUSE ULTRATRACE ELEMENTS

The evidence for essentiality, and thus nutritional importance of the other ultratrace elements not specifically described in this chapter, is quite limited and is effectively summarized in Table 36–2. The evidence is generally limited to a few gross observations in one or two species by one or two research groups. Moreover, some of the changes described as evidence for essentiality were not very marked, were not necessarily indicative of a suboptimal biological function, or were obtained under less than satisfactory experimental conditions. Thus, because they are not usually considered essential nutrients, discussion of their nutritional or biochemical significance is judged to be premature at this time.

REFERENCES

Anderson, R. A. (1993) Recent advances in the clinical and biochemical effects of chromium deficiency. In: Essential and Toxic Trace Elements in Human Health and Disease: An Update (Prasad, A. S., ed.), pp. 221–234. Wiley-Liss, New York.

Ankel-Fuchs, D. and Thauer, R. K. (1988) Nickel in biology: Nickel as an essential trace element. In: The Bioinorganic Chemistry of Nickel (Lancaster, J. R., Jr., ed.), pp. 93–110. VCH Publishers, New York.

Beedham, C. (1985) Molybdenum hydroxylases as drug-metabolizing enzymes. Drug Metab Rev 16:119–156.

Bodine, P. V. and Litwack G. (1988) Evidence that the modulator of the glucocorticoid-receptor complex is the endogenous molybdate factor. Proc Natl Acad Sci USA 85:1462–1466.

Carlisle, E. M. (1984) Silicon. In: Biochemistry of the Essential Ultratrace Elements (Friedien, E., ed.), pp. 257–291. Plenum Press, New York.

Davis, C. M. and Vincent, J.B. (1997) Chromium oligopeptide activates insulin receptor tyrosine kinase activity. Biochemistry 36:4382–4385.

Eady, R. R. (1990) Vanadium nitrogenases. In: Vanadium in Biological Systems (Chasteen, N. D., ed.), pp. 99–127. Kluwer Academic, Dordrecht, The Netherlands.

Eckhert, C. D. and Rowe, R. I. (1999) Embryonic dysplasia and adult retinal dystrophy in boron deficient zebrafish. J Trace Elem Exp Med 12:213–219.

Fort, D. J., Propst, T. L., Stover, E. L., Strong, P. L. and Murray, F. J. (1998) Adverse reproductive and developmental effects in *Xenopus* from insufficient boron. Biol Trace Elem Res 66:237–259.

Hunt, C. D. (1994) The biochemical effects of physiologic amounts of dietary boron in animal nutrition models. Environ Health Perspect 102 (Suppl):35–43.

Kim, H., Yu, C. and Maier, R. J. (1991) Common *cis*-acting region responsible for transcriptional regulation of *Bradyrhizobium japonicum* hydrogenase by nickel, oxygen, and hydrogen. J Bacteriol 173:3993–3999.

Mills, C. F. and Davis, G. K. (1987) Molybdenum. In: Trace Elements in Human and Animal Nutrition (Mertz, W., ed.), vol. 1, pp. 429–463. Academic Press, San Diego.

Nielsen, F. H. (1991) Nutritional requirements for boron, silicon, vanadium, nickel, and arsenic: Current knowledge and speculation. FASEB J. 5:2661–2667.

Nielsen, F. H. (1994a) Biochemical and physiologic consequences of boron deprivation in humans. Environ Health Perspect 102 (Suppl):59–63.

Nielsen, F. H. (1994b) Chromium. In: Modern Nutrition in Health and Disease (Shils, M. E., Olson, J. A. and Shike, M., eds.), 8th ed., vol. 1, pp. 264–268. Lea and Febiger, Philadelphia.

Nielsen, F. H. (1994c) Ultratrace minerals. In: Modern Nutrition in Health and Disease (Shils, M. E., Olson, J. A. and Shike, M., eds.), 8th ed., vol. 1, pp. 268–286. Lea and Febiger, Philadelphia.

Nielsen, F. H. (1996) Other trace elements. In: Present Knowledge of Nutrition (Ziegler, E. and Filer, J., eds.), 7th ed., pp. 353–377. ILSI Press, Washington, D.C.

Offenbacher, E. G. (1992) Chromium in the elderly. Biol Trace Elem Res 32:123–131.

Penland, J. G. (1994) Dietary boron, brain function, and cognitive performance. Environ Health Perspect 102 (Suppl):65–72.

Rajagopalan, K. V. (1988) Molybdenum: An essential trace element in human nutrition. Annu Rev Nutr 8:401–427.

Turnlund, J. R., Keyes, W. R., Peiffer, G. L. and Chiang, G. (1995) Molybdenum absorption, excretion, and retention studied with stable isotopes in young men during depletion and repletion. Am J Clin Nutr 61:1102–1109.

Wever, R. and Krenn, B. E. (1990) Vanadium haloperoxidases. In: Vanadium in Biological Systems (Chasteen, N. D., ed.), pp. 81–97. Kluwer Academic, Dordrecht, The Netherlands.

Willsky, G. R. (1990) Vanadium in the biosphere. In: Vanadium in Biological Systems (Chasteen, N. D., ed.), pp. 1–24. Kluwer Academic, Dordrecht, The Netherlands.

RECOMMENDED READINGS

Mertz, W. (1993) Essential trace metals: New definitions based on new paradigms. Nutr Rev 51:287–295.

Nielsen, F. H. (1986) Other trace elements: Sb, Ba, B, Br, Cs, Ge, Rb, Ag, Sr, Sn, Ti, Zr, Be, Bi, Ga, Au, In, Nb, Sc, Te, Tl, W. In: Trace Elements in Human and Animal Nutrition (Mertz, W., ed.), vol 2, pp. 415–463. Academic Press, Orlando, Florida.

Nielsen, F. H. (1996) Other trace elements. In: Present Knowledge of Nutrition (Ziegler, E. and Filer, J., eds.), 7th ed, pp. 353–377. ILSI Press, Washington, D.C.

Nutrition, Diet, and Health

◆ ◆

During the first half of the 20th century, the major emphasis of nutrition research was the identification and prevention of nutrient deficiency diseases and the determination of nutrient requirements. Much more attention was given during the latter decades of the 20th century to the role of nutrition in the maintenance or enhancement of health and in the reduction of the risk of certain chronic diseases, such as heart disease and cancer. This latter focus will likely continue during the 21st century as much remains to be understood about the relationships of nutrition, diet, and health. How we put the knowledge of the biochemistry and physiology of nutrition into practice is another book in itself, but knowledge of the biochemistry and physiological bases of human nutrition is of only academic interest unless it is applied to improvement of the health and well-being of individuals and populations.

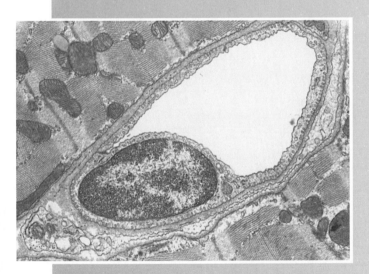

Chapters on a wide number of topics potentially could be included in this unit, but only six were chosen. Because water is also an essential component of the diet, body fluids and water balance are discussed in Chapter 37; this chapter should be considered in conjunction with Chapter 30 because of the close association of electrolytes with fluid balance. The role of diet in oral disease is discussed in Chapter 38; this chapter relates to Unit II because the interactions of food with bacteria and tissues in the oral cavity occur prior to nutrient absorption from the gut. In Chapter 39, the specific fuel needs of muscle during exercise are discussed; this chapter is closely related to discussions of fuel utilization in Units III and IV. The role of diet and nutrition in the body's antioxidation and detoxification systems is discussed in Chapter 40; many of the details of these systems are considered in earlier chapters,

Electron micrograph of rat heart; courtesy of Cornell Integrated Microscopy Center, Cornell University, Ithaca, NY.

but this topic deserves the emphasis and integration provided by a separate chapter.

The role of diet in the etiology of cardiovascular disease has been a major focus of study and treatment during the past several decades, and the vast amount of information on this topic seemed to justify devoting Chapter 41 specifically to this particular chronic disease. Chapter 41 connects to the discussions of lipid metabolism in Unit III. Obesity is another major health concern that is appropriate to this unit, but it is discussed in Chapter 19 of Unit IV along with other aspects of energy nutrition. Finally, Chapter 42 is an overview of how nutrient requirements and nutritional recommendations translate into dietary recommendations that can be implemented in our food choices.

◆ ◆

Martha H. Stipanuk, Ph.D.

CHAPTER **37**

◆ ◆

Body Fluids and Water Balance

Hwai-Ping Sheng, Ph.D.

COMMON ABBREVIATIONS

ADH (antidiuretic hormone)
C_{osm} (osmolar clearance)
C_{water} (free-water clearance)

BODY WATER COMPARTMENTS

Water is an essential nutrient vital to the existence of both animals and plants. In the body, water performs several functions that are essential to life: it is the principal fluid medium in which nutrients, gases, and enzymes are dissolved; the extracellular water bathing the cells serves as a medium for the transport of nutrients and oxygen to the cells and for removing wastes from the cells; and intracellular water establishes the physicochemical medium that allows various metabolic processes to take place. Furthermore, the volume of the intracellular fluid provides turgor to the tissues, which is important for the tissue or organ form and, ultimately, the body form. Another important physiological function of water is its role in the regulation of body temperature. This is achieved by removing excess heat from the body by evaporative water loss from the skin.

Body Water Content

Water makes up the largest component of the body; its content in the body varies with age, sex, and adiposity of the individual. In the neonate, body water makes up about 75% of body weight, decreasing progressively to about 60% in the young adult, and continuing to decline to about 50% at around 50 years of age. The higher proportion of body weight as water in the neonate is, for the most part, the result of a larger fraction of body mass as extracellular fluid space in the infant. The proportion of body mass as extracellular fluid space decreases gradually with an increase in age. This decrease is the consequence of a combination of factors, including an increase in the amount of cellular tissues, such as muscle, at the expense of extracellular space, and an increase in the proportion of body mass made up of adipose tissues and the supporting structures of skeleton, cartilage, and connective tissues, all of which contain a relatively low water content.

Adult women have a lower water content when compared with men of comparable age, and obese individuals have a lower water content than their leaner counterparts. These variations can be attributed to differences in the proportion of adipose tissue relative to lean tissue in the body. Fat cells have a relatively low content of water, about 10%, whereas other cellular tissues such as muscles contain an average of 70% water. Therefore, water content in the body varies inversely with the relative proportion of adipose tissue. The lower water content in both obese individuals and in women is explained by their larger relative proportion of adipose tissue and smaller relative proportion of lean body mass. However, when body water is calculated on a lean body weight basis, it constitutes a higher and relatively constant proportion, 73.2% of lean body mass for adults and 82% for neonates.

Distribution of Body Water

Water in the body is distributed throughout the various body fluid compartments. As shown in Figure 37–1, the simplest subdivision is into an intracellular and an extracellular compartment, with the two compartments separated by the cell membrane. In adults, the intracellular fluid compartment makes up about 40% of body weight whereas the extracellular fluid compartment makes up about 20%; of the 42 L of body water in a 70-kg adult, about two thirds (28 L) is in the intracellular compartment and about one third (14 L) is in the extracellular compartment. The extracellular fluid is made up of the following subdivisions: interstitial fluid, plasma, lymph, and specialized fluids commonly referred to as transcellular fluids. Interstitial fluid and plasma are the two largest components of the extracellular fluid compartment, with the interstitial fluid constituting about three fourths of the extracellular fluid (10 L, or 15% of body weight), and plasma making up about one fourth of the extracellular fluid (3 L, or 5% of body weight) (Rose, 1994).

Plasma circulates throughout the body and provides the medium for transporting solutes, gases, and water from one part of the body to another. Through fenestrations (20- to 100-nm-diameter pores that permit passage of relatively large molecules) of the capillary endothelium, plasma communicates with the interstitial fluid bathing the cells. These fenestrations are highly permeable to almost all solutes in plasma except proteins, so that in-

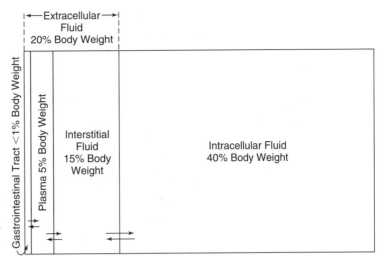

Figure 37–1. *Major body fluid compartments of an adult. Arrows denote direction of water movement along an osmotic gradient.*

terstitial fluid and plasma have a similar composition except for proteins, which are at a higher concentration in the plasma. Forces across the capillary endothelium cause an ultrafiltration of plasma to form interstitial fluid near the arterial ends of capillaries and cause entry of interstitial fluid into the venous ends of capillaries. Thus, interstitial fluid is continuously delivered to tissues by ultrafiltration near the arterial ends and returned to the circulation near the venous ends. In this way, the absorbed solutes and water from the gastrointestinal tract and dissolved oxygen from the lungs are carried to the tissues by plasma and by interstitial fluid to the cells. Similarly, metabolic waste products, including dissolved carbon dioxide, are carried by the same route, but in the opposite direction, from the tissues to the kidneys and lungs to be eliminated. Therefore, the interstitial fluid constitutes the immediate environment of the body cells; it was first described by Claude Bernard (1813–1879) as the *milieu intérieur* (Walser, 1992).

The interstitial fluid protects the cells in the body from direct contact with the external environment and acts as a buffer for the cells from sudden changes in the solutes and water contents in the body caused by ingestion or loss from the body. The body possesses various physiological control systems that regulate the elimination of solutes and water from the body, so that the composition and volume of the plasma and, indirectly, the composition and volume of the interstitial fluid and intra-

cellular fluid, are maintained relatively constant.

A small fraction of interstitial fluid is continuously drained away through lymphatic channels. This fluid, called lymph, drains into the thoracic duct, which returns the fluid to the circulation via the right subclavian vein. The total volume of lymph fluid is small, about 1 to 2 L. Transcellular, or cavity, fluids are generally considered to be specialized secretory fluids produced by active transport processes occurring across epithelial cells. These fluids differ from interstitial fluid in that they are not simple ultrafiltrates of plasma; their compositions differ markedly from that of plasma and are adapted specifically to the function of particular organs. Examples of transcellular fluids are fluids in the lumen of the gastrointestinal tract, cerebrospinal fluid, and fluids in the intraocular, pleural, peritoneal, and synovial spaces. Of these, intraluminal gastrointestinal water constitutes the largest fraction. The total volume occupied by these fluids is small, about 1 to 2 L.

Water Movement Across Cell Membranes

The distribution of water in the various compartments determines the size of the compartments and is governed by solute particles and physical forces that maintain an equilibrium across membranes separating these compartments. To understand the distribution and direction of water movement between the cells and interstitium, it is important to understand the concepts of osmosis, osmolality, and osmotic pressure.

Osmosis. The concept of osmosis can be explained simply by Figure 37–2. A membrane that is impermeable to solutes but permeable to water separates the two compartments A and B, which contain the same volume of fluid but different numbers of solute particles. Water diffuses across the membrane in both directions, but more water molecules diffuse from compartment A, a region of higher water concentration (lower solute concentration), to compartment B, a region of lower water concentration (higher solute concentration). This net movement of water from compartment A to compartment B results in the expansion of compartment B at the expense of compartment A. When the solute concentration in compartment B equals that in compartment A, no further net diffusion of water occurs. The process of net movement of water caused by a concentration difference of water or solutes is called osmosis (Rose, 1994).

The process of osmosis also explains the movement of water across cell membranes. Cell membranes are relatively impermeable to most solutes but highly permeable to water. In the steady state, the volume of water that diffuses across the membrane in either direction is balanced precisely so that no net diffusion of water occurs and the volume of the cell remains unchanged. However, under certain conditions, when a concentration difference for water develops across the cell membrane, water diffuses across the membrane along its concentration gradient. When this happens, either net influx or net efflux occurs, causing the cell to expand or to contract.

Osmolality and Osmotic Pressure. As noted, a difference in the solute concentrations of two fluids separated by a semipermeable membrane causes osmotic movement of water. Therefore, it is useful to have a concentration term that refers to the total concentration of solute particles that cause osmotic movement of water. Because it is the number, and not the size or type, of solute particles that causes water movement, the term osmole

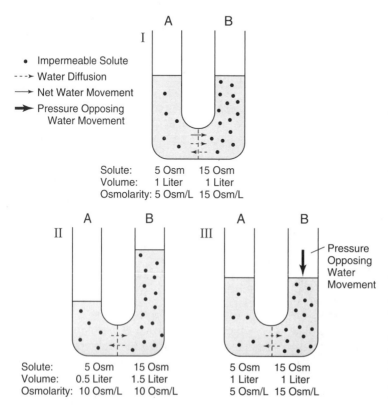

- Impermeable Solute
- - - ► Water Diffusion
— ► Net Water Movement
➡ Pressure Opposing Water Movement

I

	A	B
Solute:	5 Osm	15 Osm
Volume:	1 Liter	1 Liter
Osmolarity:	5 Osm/L	15 Osm/L

II

	A	B
Solute:	5 Osm	15 Osm
Volume:	0.5 Liter	1.5 Liter
Osmolarity:	10 Osm/L	10 Osm/L

III

Pressure Opposing Water Movement

	A	B
	5 Osm	15 Osm
	1 Liter	1 Liter
	5 Osm/L	15 Osm/L

Figure 37–2. Osmosis and osmotic pressure can be illustrated by two compartments separated by a semipermeable membrane, permeable to water but not to solutes (circles). In diagram I, compartments A and B are shown filled with equal volumes of solution, but the solution added to compartment A is hypo-osmotic with reference to the solution added to compartment B. Water will move from A to B until the solutions in the two compartments are iso-osmotic, as shown in diagram II. The movement of water across the semipermeable membrane leads to a change in the initial volumes at equilibrium. In this example, the volume of compartment B increased, while the volume of compartment A decreased. Because the volume of compartment B increased, there were no significant changes in hydrostatic pressure in the compartments. As shown in diagram III, application of a pressure can prevent osmotic movement of water across the semipermeable membrane.

(Osm) is used to describe the number of solute particles, regardless of their mass (Rose, 1994). One Osm is the number of particles (Avogadro's number or 6.02×10^{23}) in 1 mole (mol) or 1 gram molecular weight of an undissociated solute. A solution containing either 1 mol of glucose (180 g) or 1 mol of albumin (70,000 g) in 1 kg of water has a concentration of 1 Osm/kg of water because neither glucose nor albumin dissociates in solution. If the solute in solution dissociates into 2 ions, then 1 mol of the dissociated solute will contain 2 Osm. For example, 1 mol of sodium chloride (NaCl) dissociates to yield 1 mol each of sodium and chloride ions; thus 1 mol of NaCl in 1 kg of water will have an osmolal concentration of 2 Osm/kg of water. Likewise, a solution that contains 1 mol of a solute that dissociates into 3 ions (for example, $CaCl_2$) has an osmolal concentration of 3 Osm/kg.

Strictly speaking, ions in solutions exert interionic attraction to, or repulsion from, each other and can, therefore, cause a decrease or an increase in the actual number of osmotically active particles in the solution. Any deviations can be corrected for if the osmotic coefficient for the molecule is known. For example, the osmotic coefficient for NaCl is 0.93. Therefore, 1 mol of NaCl in 1 kg of water has an osmolal concentration of 1.86 instead of 2 mOsm/kg. In practice, the osmotic coefficients of different solutes are often disregarded when determining the osmolal concentrations of physiological solutions.

The osmolal concentration of a solution can be expressed as Osm/kg of water (osmolality) and osmolar concentration as Osm/L of solution (osmolarity). Therefore, osmolarity, but not osmolality, is affected by the volume of solutes in the solution. The normal osmolarity of plasma is about 290 mOsm/L. Solutes, mainly proteins, occupy about 5% of plasma volume. Therefore, the osmolality of plasma is about 305 mOsm/kg of water. Because body fluids are dilute solutions, differences between osmolality and osmolarity are small so that the two terms are used synonymously. In practice, it is easier to express solute concentrations of plasma in mOsm/L than in mOsm/kg.

Osmosis of water across cell membranes can be opposed by applying a pressure in the direction opposite to that of the diffusion (see Fig. 37–2). The amount of pressure to be applied in order to prevent the diffusion of water through the membrane is called the osmotic pressure (Rose, 1994). The osmotic pressure of a solution, therefore, reflects the concentration of osmotically active particles in that solution. Whenever a difference in the osmolar concentrations occurs between the intracellular and interstitial fluid compartments, osmotic forces will develop across the cell membrane, and water will move rapidly between these two compartments until an osmotic equilibrium is achieved. Therefore, at equilibrium, the osmolarity of the intracellular and interstitial fluid compartments is similar, at about 290 mOsm/L.

Iso-osmotic, Hypo-osmotic, and Hyperosmotic Solutions. These terms are used to describe the osmolar concentrations between different solutions. When two solutions are of equal osmolarity, they are iso-osmotic. A solution is hypo-osmotic when its osmolarity is lower, and hyperosmotic when its osmolarity is higher than that of the reference solution (Rose, 1994). When cells are suspended in a hypo-osmotic solution, water enters the cells, causing them to expand. Conversely, when cells are suspended in a hyperosmotic solution, water diffuses out of the cells, causing them to contract. When cells are suspended in an iso-osmotic solution, no net movement of water occurs, and cell size remains the same. However, this is not the case if cells are suspended in an iso-osmotic solution containing a highly permeant solute, for example urea. Urea diffuses into cells along its concentration gradient, causing an osmotic flow of water into cells, and the cells expand (Fig. 37–3). Therefore, tonicity is used to describe the physiological osmolar concentration of a solution.

Isotonic, Hypotonic, and Hypertonic Solutions. The term tonicity refers to the osmolarity of a solution relative to plasma and refers to whether the solution will affect cell volume. An isotonic solution has an osmolarity of 290 mOsm/L, and when cells are placed in this solution, no net diffusion of water occurs. Solutions in which suspended cells shrink are

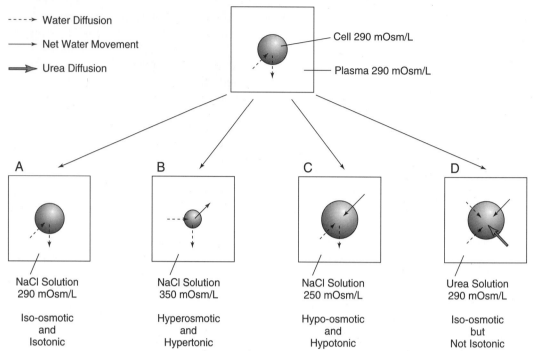

Figure 37–3. *The concepts of osmolarity and tonicity can be illustrated by a red blood cell suspended in various media. In the body, red blood cells are suspended in plasma; because plasma is iso-osmotic and isotonic, the rate of water diffusion out of the cell is equal to that into the cell. No net movement of water occurs, and the cell volume remains the same. (A) When a red blood cell is suspended in a 290-mOsm/L NaCl solution, no net movement of water occurs. The solution is iso-osmotic and isotonic. (B) When a red blood cell is suspended in a 350-mOsm/L NaCl solution, there is a net movement of water out of the cell along an osmotic gradient. The cell will shrink. The solution is hyperosmotic and hypertonic. (C) When a red blood cell is suspended in a 250-mOsm/L NaCl solution, there is a net movement of water into the cell, causing cell expansion and hemolysis. The solution is hypo-osmotic and hypotonic. (D) When a red blood cell is suspended in a 290-mOsm/L urea solution, urea diffuses into the cell along its concentration gradient and water follows, resulting in net entry of water, which causes the cell to hemolyze. (The increased volume of water and solute in the cell causes the cell membrane to rupture.) The solution is iso-osmotic but not isotonic.*

called hypertonic, and solutions in which suspended cells expand are called hypotonic (Rose, 1994). Sodium chloride solution at a concentration of 290 mOsm/L is an isotonic solution because sodium is kept out of cells by active transport processes. On the other hand, a solution of urea or dextrose at a concentration of 290 mOsm/L is iso-osmotic to plasma but not isotonic. Red blood cells suspended in an iso-osmotic solution of urea or dextrose will hemolyze. Urea diffuses readily into cells along its concentration gradient, causing an osmotic flow of water into the cells (Fig. 37–3). Glucose, on the other hand, is taken up and metabolized by red blood cells, causing a progressive decrease in the osmolarity of the suspension fluid and causing water to move into the cells to maintain iso-osmolarity. It is important, therefore, to understand the difference between osmolarity and tonicity, especially in intravenous fluid therapy. A solution containing 0.9% NaCl (290 mOsm/L) is isotonic with plasma. This isotonic saline solution is commonly used as replacement fluid during the postoperative period.

Osmolarity and Volume of Intracellular and Extracellular Fluid Compartments. In contrast to movement of water across cell membranes, movement of solutes is more variable and depends on the presence of specific membrane transporters. Not only are cell membranes relatively impermeable to proteins and organic phosphates, but also they selectively extrude sodium out of the cell in exchange for potassium. Therefore, sodium and its accompanying anions, mainly chloride, are the major solutes in the extracellular fluid. Inside the cells, the major cations are potassium, calcium, and magnesium, and the major anions are proteins and organic phosphates. Water will distribute passively between the intracellular and extracellular compartments according to the osmolar concentrations, which are determined by the quantity of diffusible and nondiffusible solutes present in each of these compartments. Therefore, the volume of each of these compartments depends on the amount of solutes present and the total volume of body water. Whenever an inequality of osmolar concentration occurs across the cell membrane, water diffuses rapidly from the compartment of lower osmolarity to one of higher osmolarity so that any differences in osmolarity are corrected within a few minutes. Thus, in the steady state, the osmolarity of intracellular and extracellular fluids is equal.

Water Movement Across Capillary Endothelium

The major difference in the ionic composition between plasma and interstitial fluid is the higher concentration of protein in the plasma, because the capillary endothelium is essentially impermeable to plasma proteins. On average, the concentration of proteins in the interstitial fluid is less than 10 g/L, compared with 73 g/L in the plasma. This differential concentration of protein affects the distributions of diffusible ions and osmotic pressures across the capillary endothelium.

Gibbs-Donnan Equilibrium. When two fluid compartments, A and B, are separated by a semipermeable membrane, the concentrations of any diffusible cation or anion are equal across the membrane so that no differences in concentration exist for any of the ions. On the basis of thermodynamic principles, Gibbs and Donnan showed that, at equilibrium, the product of the concentrations of diffusible cations and anions in the two compartments are equal, and electrical neutrality is maintained:

$$[Cation]_A \times [Anion]_A = [Cation]_B \times [Anion]_B$$

When a nondiffusible cation or anion is added to one of the compartments, the diffus-

ible ions will redistribute themselves so that the concentration of each of the ions will no longer be equal across the cell membrane.

At normal plasma pH of 7.4, the majority of plasma proteins behave as negatively charged particles. Because proteins are confined to the vascular compartment, electrical neutrality in the plasma can be maintained only by an unequal distribution of the smaller diffusible ions, resulting in lower concentrations of each of the diffusible anions and higher concentrations of the diffusible cations. At a normal concentration of plasma protein (73 g/L), this effect is small, with the concentration of monovalent anions (for example, chloride) about 5% lower and that of monovalent cations (for example, sodium) about 5% higher in the plasma than in the interstitial fluid. For all practical purposes, the concentrations of ions in the plasma and interstitial fluid can be considered to be about equal.

Colloid Osmotic Pressure. The concentration difference of proteins across capillary endothelium not only affects the distribution of diffusible ions, it also causes an osmotic gradient across the capillary endothelium. This osmotic gradient exerts a pressure that is called the colloid osmotic pressure, or oncotic pressure. Colloid osmotic pressure is of physiological importance in determining net water movement across the capillary endothelium.

Starling's Law. Starling first proposed the concept that two opposing forces govern water movement across the capillary endothelium; these two forces are created by the difference in hydrostatic pressure and the difference in colloid osmotic pressure between the plasma and interstitial fluid. Thus, the movement of fluid depends on four variables: hydrostatic pressures in the plasma and interstitial fluid and protein concentrations in the plasma and interstitial fluid. The following equations describe the forces responsible for net water movement across an idealized capillary endothelium:

$$\text{Net driving pressure} = (P_c - P_{if}) - (\pi_c - \pi_{if})$$
$$\text{Net volume of water flow} = K_f[(P_c - P_{if}) - (\pi_c - \pi_{if})]$$

where K_f is the product of water permeability and filtration surface area of the capillary endothelium, P_c is the capillary hydrostatic pressure, P_{if} is the interstitial fluid hydrostatic pressure, π_c is the capillary colloid osmotic pressure, and π_{if} is the interstitial fluid colloid osmotic pressure.

Under normal circumstances, the balance of these forces results in a net pressure gradient favoring the movement of a small amount of fluid from the arterial end of the capillary into the interstitium. Because of a fall in capillary hydrostatic pressure along the length of the capillary, much of the fluid reenters the capillary at the venous end (Fig. 37–4). The small amount of fluid that remains in the interstitium is returned to the circulation by the lymphatic vessels, which empty into the subclavian vein via the thoracic duct (Taylor, 1981).

An imbalance in any of these forces affects net movement of water across the capillary endothelium and ultimately will affect distribution of fluid between the plasma and interstitial compartments. For example, a decrease in plasma protein concentration in disease states, such as liver and kidney diseases, results in an accumulation of fluid in the interstitial spaces, causing edema (discussed later).

Other factors that may affect the distribution of fluid across capillary endothelium include the integrity of the capillary endothelium and the lymphatic drainage system. An increase in capillary permeability allows plasma albumin to enter the interstitium to an abnormal extent, thus reducing the difference in $(\pi_c - \pi_{if})$ in Starling's equation. This increase in permeability occurs in sepsis, venom shock, drug overdose, and anaphylactic reactions, and it can cause large volumes of fluids to leak from the vascular to the interstitial space. The lymphatic system can reduce the volume of edema fluid by returning the fluid to the intravascular system via the thoracic duct. Blockage of lymphatic drainage causes accumulation of fluid in the interstitial fluid compartment.

WATER BALANCE

For an individual to maintain water balance, the amount of water consumed must equal the amount lost from the body. This is illustrated in Table 37–1 for a 65-kg man in a normal environment and consuming a balanced diet that provides adequately for his energy requirements. Even with the excretion of a maximally concentrated urine, water nor-

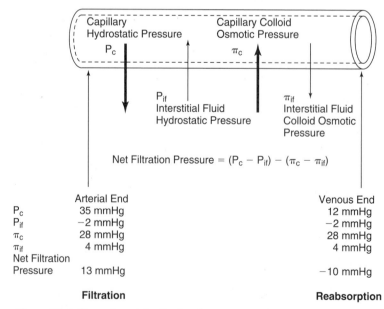

Figure 37–4. Illustration of the Starling forces across the capillary endothelium.

TABLE 37–1

Daily Water Balance in a 65-Kg Man Calculated to Illustrate Minimal Required Drinking Water Intake

Water Intake		Water Loss	
Source	*Liters*	*Route*	*Liters*
Preformed water	0.85	Insensible—lungs	0.30
Metabolic water	0.37	Insensible—skin	0.40
Drinking—minimum	0.22	Feces	0.10
		Urine	0.64
TOTAL	1.44	TOTAL	1.44

mally contained in the food (preformed water) and water produced by oxidation of food (metabolic water, or water of oxidation) are inadequate to provide for losses of water from the respiratory tract, skin, gastrointestinal tract, and kidneys. Therefore, an individual requires ingestion of free water to maintain water balance. The body possesses several homeostatic regulatory mechanisms capable of maintaining balance of water over a wide range of water intake so that health remains unimpaired. An inequality between intake and loss of water ultimately alters the composition and osmolarity of body fluids (Robertson and Berl, 1991).

Loss of Water

Water is lost from the body by essentially four different routes: respiratory tract, skin, gastrointestinal tract, and kidneys. Of the four routes, water loss from kidneys is the most important because renal water excretion is regulated to maintain a constant osmolarity of the body fluids.

Insensible Water Loss. Water is lost continuously from the body by two routes: evaporation from the upper respiratory tract during respiration and passive evaporation from the skin. These passive evaporative losses from the respiratory tract and skin are termed "insensible losses" or "insensible perspiration" because they occur continuously and without our awareness. Evaporative water loss from the respiratory tract occurs during respiration because expired air is saturated with moisture

to a vapor pressure of about 47 mm Hg, whereas the vapor pressure of inspired air is usually less than 47 mm Hg. The insensible water loss from the lungs increases in cold, dry climates when the atmospheric vapor pressure decreases. Evaporative water loss from the respiratory tract averages between 0.14 and 0.47 L daily and depends on body size, the degree of physical activity, and environmental temperature and humidity (Geigy Scientific Tables, 1981).

Insensible water loss from the skin, which occurs independently of sweating, averages between 0.3 and 0.5 L daily for an individual living in a temperate environment and doing minimal physical activity. Therefore, this individual will lose a total of 0.4 to 0.9 L of water daily from insensible loss through both the respiratory tract and skin. This insensible water loss increases in fever and in obese individuals, who usually have an increased evaporative water loss owing to a greater total heat output compared with normal individuals (Irsigler et al., 1979). Therefore, water intake needs to be higher in these individuals.

Water loss occurs also through sweating, during which excess heat is dissipated from the skin. The volume of water lost as sweat is highly variable, depending on the environment and the physical activity of the individual. Evaporation of sweat from the skin is an effective means of removing excess heat from the body. For every gram of water that evaporates from the skin, 0.58 kcal of heat is lost from the body. Water loss as sweat is substantially less in an environment of moderate temperature and humidity than in a warm, humid environment where loss through perspiration can be considerable.

Normally, the volume of sweat in a 65-kg adult doing light work at an ambient temperature of 29°C (84.2°F) amounts to about 2 to 3 L daily, but it can increase to a maximum of about 2 to 4 L per hour for a short time in an unacclimatized individual who is performing heavy physical activity in a hot, humid environment. This levels off to about 0.5 L per hour over a 24-hour period as the duration of perspiration increases (Geigy Scientific Tables, 1981). Even at maximal sweating, the rate of heat loss may not be rapid enough to dissipate the heat from the body. When the body temperature rises to a critical level, above 40.5°C (105°F), the individual is likely to develop heatstroke. However, after acclimatization to hot weather for a few weeks, an individual will have greater tolerance of the hot, humid environment, with as much as a two-fold increase in sweat production. Evaporation of this large volume of sweat effectively removes the excess heat from the body. Acclimatization also involves a decrease in the concentration of sodium chloride in the sweat, allowing for better conservation of sodium chloride. The loss of several liters of sweat a day in a hot climate results in serious losses of both sodium chloride and water, which need to be replaced.

Water Loss by the Gastrointestinal Tract. The volume of water loss in feces is small, about 0.1 L a day, and does not cause problems with water balance unless excessive loss occurs during diarrhea. The volume of fluid ingested varies among individuals but averages about 1.7 L daily. Added to this ingested volume are salivary, gastric, biliary, pancreatic, and intestinal secretions, which amount to 7 L a day. Normally, the small intestine absorbs most of these fluids, approximately 8.3 L, and the colon another 0.3 L, resulting in the excretion of only about 0.1 L of water in the feces. Absorption of water in the intestine is passive, along an osmotic gradient created by the absorption of nutrients from the lumen of the intestine into the plasma. In diseases of the gastrointestinal tract, large volumes of water can be lost in the feces, causing diarrhea. This occurs in gastroenteritis due to bacterial or viral infection or in any situation where absorption of nutrients is compromised. Certain bacterial toxins, such as cholera toxin, can increase the secretion of sodium chloride from the crypt cells of the small intestinal mucosa into the lumen of the small intestine.

CLINICAL CORRELATION

Heat Acclimatization

Acclimatization is an adaptive process in which an individual's ability to withstand a certain environmental stress is enhanced after prolonged exposure to that stress. When persons are first exposed to an environment of high temperature, their capacity to work is hampered by their inability to tolerate the heat. In a couple of days, their bodies adjust to the heat through increased sweating in order to dissipate body heat and prevent a rise in body temperature. Not only does sweating become more profuse, it also begins sooner at a lower body temperature. The concentration of sodium chloride in the sweat is also reduced; this is achieved by increased reabsorption of sodium chloride back into the blood as it passes through the sweat gland ducts.

In some individuals, an inability to dissipate body heat in a hot climate can lead to heat stroke. Individuals with heat stroke may die within a few hours unless immediate treatment is instituted. Prompt transfer to a cooler environment with adequate ventilation to accelerate body heat dissipation, as well as vigorous hydration, is essential.

During prolonged strenuous physical activity in hot weather, a person can develop heat cramps or heat exhaustion. Heat cramps are an acute disorder of skeletal muscle characterized by brief, intermittent, and excruciating muscle cramps. Heat cramps often occur in people who are well acclimatized to work in hot climates and who consume a large amount of water to replace water losses without salt replacement. Although acclimatization is associated with diminished sodium concentration in the sweat, the sodium concentration in sweat still rises sharply as the rate of sweat secretion increases. This condition can be prevented by adequate salt intake together with water replacement.

Heat exhaustion is caused by profuse sweating in a hot environment, when the volume of water loss is not replaced by voluntary drinking and the plasma volume becomes depleted. In an attempt to dissipate body heat, there is an extreme dilation of blood vessels in the skin, thus decreasing peripheral resistance to blood flow. The depletion of plasma volume and the decreased peripheral resistance cause hypotension, culminating in weakness and fainting. Prevention consists of wearing light clothing in hot weather and adequate water ingestion to replace body water losses.

The lumen becomes hyperosmotic, and diffusion of water occurs from the plasma into the lumen, causing diarrhea. Several liters of fluid, up to 10 to 20 L, can be lost, resulting in dehydration (Geigy Scientific Tables, 1981).

Water Loss by the Kidneys. As shown in Table 37–1, the minimal urine volume that an adult must produce, assuming a normal renal function, is about 0.64 L a day. Metabolism of 70 g dietary protein results in the production of about 21 g of urea, which cannot be utilized by the body and has to be excreted in the urine. This 21 g of urea contributes 350 mOsm to the total osmotic load of substances presented to the kidneys. If the sodium chloride intake is 320 mmol and potassium salt intake is 100 mmol, this will add a further 420 mOsm to the total osmotic load. The total load of osmotically active substances requiring excretion by the kidneys is 770 mOsm a day. Because the human kidneys can maximally concentrate urine to an osmolar concentration of 1200 mOsm/L, the minimal volume of urine at maximal attainable osmolarity for this individual is 0.64 L a day.

Intake of Water

The minimal amount of water required daily to replace obligatory water losses from the respiratory tract, skin, feces, and urine is about 1.44 L. Water consumed by an individual comes from beverages, preformed water in food, and water produced by oxidation of food. If the composition of the ingested food is known, the yield of metabolic water can be calculated. Oxidation of 1 g each of carbohydrate, fat, and protein will yield approximately 0.6 g, 1.0 g, and 0.4 g of water, respectively. Assuming that the 65-kg man used as an example in Table 37–1 consumes 400 g of carbohydrate, 100 g of fat, and 70 g of protein, the total yield of metabolic water from the food he eats amounts to 370 g. Preformed water in food can be calculated from the difference between wet and dry weights of food; however, usually it is assumed that water makes up 60% of the wet weight. Therefore, the weight of preformed water in the sample diet is about 850 g, and the total volume of water (preformed plus metabolic) derived from ingested food is about 1.22 L a day (1.22 kg/day). To remain in water balance, the individual has to drink a minimum of 0.22 L of additional water. The ingested volume of water and other beverages varies greatly among individuals depending on habit, custom, physical activity, and environment. On average, humans habitually drink between 1 and 2 L or more of water and beverages a day. The excess water is excreted by the kidneys.

A reasonable allowance for water intake based on recommended energy intake is 1 mL/kcal for adults and 1.5 mL/kcal for infants (National Research Council, 1989); or 35 mL/kg body weight in adults and 150 mL/kg in infants. Infants require more water on a body weight basis because of their relatively larger body surface area and metabolic rate, resulting in higher obligatory losses, and the relatively limited capacity of their kidneys to handle the renal solute load. This is especially important for infants on formula, as most formula has a higher solute load than does human milk. Water loss can be increased greatly in individuals doing heavy work or in athletes undergoing severe training in a hot climate, and in individuals with fever, vomiting, diabetes, or diarrhea. Under these circumstances, water need is increased.

RENAL EXCRETION OF WATER

As discussed in Chapter 30, the kidneys contribute significantly to homeostasis by stabilizing the volume and osmolarity of the body fluids. In their regulatory function, the kidneys process blood by removing substances that are in excess and conserving substances that are in deficit as these substances pass through the kidneys. In water excess, caused by drinking large volumes of fluid, a large volume of dilute (hypo-osmotic with respect to plasma) urine is excreted. Conversely, in water deficit, when there is a need to conserve body water, a smaller volume of concentrated (hyperosmotic) urine is excreted. Excretion of a dilute urine involves the reabsorption of filtered solutes in excess of water, whereas the excretion of a concentrated urine entails the reabsorption of water in excess of solutes (Knepper and Rector, 1991).

To understand how the kidneys produce either a dilute or a concentrated urine, the following has to be considered: (1) the transport and permeability properties of the various segments of the nephron, (2) the countercurrent multiplier system of the loops of Henle, (3) the countercurrent exchanger system of the vasa recta, and (4) the change of the collecting tubules from a diuretic to an antidiuretic state.

Transport and Permeability Characteristics of Various Segments of the Nephron

There are approximately 1 million nephrons in each kidney. Each nephron consists of an initial filtering component, called the renal corpuscle, and a tubular component responsible for transporting solutes and water. The renal corpuscle is made up of the glomerular capillaries, which protrude into the Bowman's capsule. Plasma is filtered across the glomerular membrane into the Bowman's capsule of the nephrons. The ultrafiltrate formed is protein-free, and its ionic composition is similar to that of plasma except for the 5% difference due to the Gibbs-Donnan effect. As the filtrate flows along the nephrons, its volume and composition are altered so that normally only 1% of the filtered load is excreted as urine, the composition of which differs markedly from that of the initial filtrate. The proximal tubules reabsorb 65% of the filtrate, and the loops of Henle reabsorb another 25%. The final reabsorption of solutes (especially sodium chloride and urea) and water in the distal nephron (distal convoluted and collecting tubules) is highly variable; it depends on the needs of the body and is under the influence of hormones (Berry and Rector, 1991). The alterations in the composition and volume of the filtrate are made possible by (1) the various transport processes that occur across the tubular cells of the nephrons, and (2) the permeability characteristics of the various nephron segments. As discussed later, solutes are transported across tubular cells, resulting in the establishment of a concentration gradient in the medullary region of the kidneys. The establishment of a concentration

gradient allows the kidneys to excrete either a concentrated or a dilute urine.

Proximal Tubule. In the proximal tubule, active reabsorption of sodium ions results in cotransport of other solutes, the passive reabsorption of chloride ions, or the secretion of hydrogen ions. Water is reabsorbed passively along the osmotic gradient created. The rates of reabsorption of solutes and water are equal in the proximal tubule so that the osmolarity of the tubular fluid leaving the proximal tubule is similar to that of plasma, at 290 mOsm/L. This iso-osmotic reabsorption applies regardless of whether a dilute or a concentrated urine is produced. Therefore, segments distal to the proximal tubule must be responsible for the production of either a dilute or a concentrated urine.

Distal Tubule. The ability of the kidneys to produce either a dilute or a concentrated urine is due to the different transport and permeability characteristics of sodium chloride, urea, and water of the various segments distal to the proximal tubule.

With the exception of the ascending and descending thin limbs of the loops of Henle, active transport processes occur along the distal tubules to transport sodium chloride out of the tubular fluid. The ascending and descending thin limbs are relatively permeable to sodium chloride, and sodium chloride can diffuse passively along its concentration gradient between the tubular and interstitial fluids.

Urea diffuses passively along its concentration gradient in most segments of the nephron but not the ascending thick limbs, distal convoluted tubules, and cortical and outer medullary collecting tubules.

The permeability to water differs in different segments. The descending thin limb is highly permeable to water, whereas the ascending thin limb, ascending thick limb, and first part of the distal convoluted tubule are relatively impermeable to water. The latter part of the distal convoluted tubule and the cortical and medullary collecting tubules are impermeable to water in the absence of antidiuretic hormone (ADH), but in the presence of ADH, their permeability to water is increased.

Countercurrent Multiplier System of the Loop of Henle

The loop of Henle consists of two parallel limbs of small diameter, with the tubular fluid flowing in opposite directions (countercurrent flow) and in close proximity. The hairpin conformation of the loop of Henle is such that fluid flows from the corticomedullary region to the inner medullary region in the descending thin limb and in the opposite direction in the ascending thin and thick limbs. Because of the flow and permeability characteristics of these segments, the loops of Henle operate as a countercurrent multiplier system and establish and maintain an osmotic gradient between the fluids in the corticomedullary region and the inner medullary region (Knepper and Rector, 1991). This osmotic gradient is made up of concentration gradients of mainly sodium chloride and urea and is essential for formation of a concentrated urine in the collecting ducts. As illustrated in Figure 37–5,

the osmolarity of the interstitial fluid increases steadily from 290 mOsm/L in the corticomedullary region to about 1200 mOsm/L in the inner medullary region.

Active transport of sodium chloride out of the ascending thick limb of the loop of Henle is fundamental to the development of the osmotic gradient between the cortex and inner medulla. However, the passive movement of urea down its concentration gradient from the tubular fluid into the interstitium also plays an important role, especially when the kidney is maximally concentrating urine. The mechanisms that contribute to the buildup of solutes, especially sodium chloride and urea in the medullary region are as follows:

The ascending thick limb actively transports sodium chloride out of the tubular fluid to the interstitium. Because the ascending thin and thick limbs are impermeable to water, active movement of sodium chloride into the interstitium dilutes the fluid in the lumen and produces a hypo-osmotic tubular fluid but a

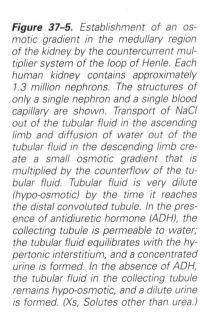

Figure 37–5. Establishment of an osmotic gradient in the medullary region of the kidney by the countercurrent multiplier system of the loop of Henle. Each human kidney contains approximately 1.3 million nephrons. The structures of only a single nephron and a single blood capillary are shown. Transport of NaCl out of the tubular fluid in the ascending limb and diffusion of water out of the tubular fluid in the descending limb create a small osmotic gradient that is multiplied by the counterflow of the tubular fluid. Tubular fluid is very dilute (hypo-osmotic) by the time it reaches the distal convoluted tubule. In the presence of antidiuretic hormone (ADH), the collecting tubule is permeable to water; the tubular fluid equilibrates with the hypertonic interstitium, and a concentrated urine is formed. In the absence of ADH, the tubular fluid in the collecting tubule remains hypo-osmotic, and a dilute urine is formed. (Xs, Solutes other than urea.)

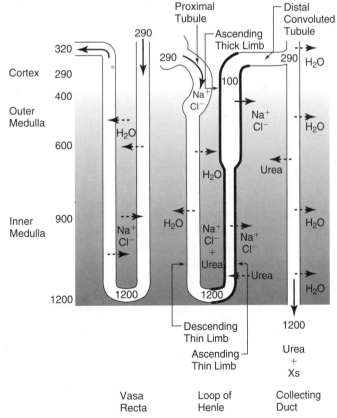

hyperosmotic interstitial fluid. In antidiuresis, under the influence of ADH, water is removed from the late distal convoluted and the cortical and outer medullary portions of the collecting tubules, thus concentrating urea in the tubular fluid. In the inner medullary portion of the collecting duct, urea moves from concentrated tubular fluid down its concentration gradient into the interstitium, thus increasing the osmolarity in the inner medullary region. Some of the urea in the interstitium diffuses passively into the lumen of both the descending and ascending thin limbs along its concentration gradient. Because the descending thin limb is very permeable to water but less so to sodium chloride and urea, water moves out of the tubule so that the osmolarity of the fluid flowing into this segment equilibrates with the surrounding hyperosmotic interstitial fluid. The fluid that enters the ascending limb has a high concentration of sodium chloride because of the removal of water from the descending thin limb. Sodium chloride then moves passively from the tubular fluid in the ascending thin limb down its concentration gradient into the interstitium and adds further to the hyperosmolarity of the inner medullary region. There is more passive efflux of sodium chloride than passive influx of urea because the ascending thin limb is more permeable to sodium than urea, so that there is a net efflux of osmotically active solutes. Because of low water permeability, luminal fluid in the ascending limb is hypo-osmotic relative to its surrounding interstitium. Thus, both passive and active transport of sodium chloride out of the tubular fluid of the ascending limbs results in the formation of tubular fluid that is hypo-osmotic, with reference to plasma, when it enters the distal convoluted tubule.

The continuous countercurrent flow of fluid, together with the movement of sodium chloride out of the ascending limb and water out of the descending limb, multiplies the small osmotic gradient created with each pass of a volume of tubular fluid from the proximal tubule through the loop of Henle. This maintains the osmotic gradient between the interstitial fluids in the corticomedullary region and the inner medullary region.

The collecting tubules run parallel, and in close vicinity, to the loops of Henle through the area of high osmolarity to drain into the ureter (see Fig. 37–5). The fluid entering the collecting tubules is hypo-osmotic. In the absence of ADH, the collecting tubules are relatively impermeable to water and the tubular fluid remains hypo-osmotic; a dilute urine is excreted. Under the influence of ADH, the collecting tubules are permeable to water, the tubular fluid in the collecting tubules equilibrates with the hyperosmotic interstitial fluid, and a concentrated urine is excreted. Thus the countercurrent multiplier of the loop of Henle provides the mechanism for excretion of either a dilute or concentrated urine. The high osmolarity of the interstitial fluid provides the driving force for the absorption of water from the descending thin limb of the loop of Henle and from the inner and outer medullary portions of the collecting tubule.

As discussed earlier, urea contributes substantially to the establishment of the osmotic gradient in the renal medulla, and hence, to the ability to form a concentrated urine. In the presence of ADH, the permeability of the inner medullary collecting tubules to water is increased. Further absorption of water by this segment results in an even higher concentration of urea to diffuse passively out of the tubule into the interstitium. The movement of urea and water out of the inner medullary collecting tubule maintains a high concentration of urea in the tubular fluid and the interstitium in this region. The contribution of urea to the osmotic gradient varies with the amount of urea filtered and hence with the dietary intake of protein. Normally, sodium chloride and urea each contribute about 600 mOsm/L to the osmolarity of the inner medullary region.

The countercurrent multiplier system in the kidneys is an energy-efficient process. By its operation a considerable osmotic gradient ($\sim$900 mOsm/L) is generated between the plasma (290 mOsm/L) and the tubular fluids in the inner medullary region (1200 mOsm/L). The energy cost associated with the establishment of this large osmotic gradient of 900 mOsm/L represents only the energy expended in generating small osmotic gradients between adjacent segments of the descending and ascending limbs of the loops of Henle.

Countercurrent Exchanger of the Vasa Recta

It is essential that the osmotic gradient that is established by the countercurrent multiplier system in the medullary interstitium is maintained and not dissipated by the blood supply. This goal is achieved by the specialized anatomical arrangement of the medullary blood vessels, the vasa recta. The vasa recta are arranged in the form of hairpin loops parallel to the loops of Henle. They represent a passive countercurrent exchange system that perfuses the medullary area while maintaining the medullary interstitial osmotic gradient.

Because of the permeability of the capillary endothelium to both solutes and water, the osmolarity of the plasma in the vasa recta equilibrates with that of the medullary interstitial fluid at each level. The osmolarity of plasma in the descending vasa recta is 290 mOsm/L, similar to that of the systemic plasma. As the plasma flows deeper into the medulla, it equilibrates with the surrounding hyperosmotic interstitial fluid by gaining solutes and losing water, so that by the time the plasma reaches the inner medullary region, its osmolar concentration is that of the surrounding interstitium (that is, 1200 mOsm/L). The opposite process happens in the ascending vasa recta. As plasma flows from a region of higher to lower osmolarity, it becomes less and less hyperosmotic by passive loss of solutes and passive uptake of water. As a result, the osmolarity of the plasma in the ascending vasa recta leaving the medulla is only slightly higher than that of systemic plasma. By this arrangement, the vasa recta remove the excess solutes and water that are added to the interstitial fluid by the various nephron segments in the medulla while at the same time preserving the hyperosmotic medullary interstitium.

Excretion of Dilute and Concentrated Urine

Human kidneys can dilute urine to one sixth the osmolarity of plasma or concentrate it up to four times that of plasma; that is, humans can excrete urine of between 50 and 1200 mOsm/L. A dilute urine is produced when the circulating level of plasma ADH is low. Under this condition the permeability to water in the more distal portion of the distal convoluted tubule and in the collecting tubule is low. As seen in Figure 37–5, tubular fluid leaving the ascending thick limb of the loop of Henle is hypo-osmotic, about 100 mOsm/L. In the production of this dilute fluid, the ascending thick limb of the loop of Henle plays an important role because of its large reabsorptive capacity. Because it is the major site of dilution of tubular fluid, the ascending thick limb is often referred to as the diluting segment of the kidney. Further reabsorption of solutes, especially sodium chloride, by the tubular cells of the distal nephron dilutes the tubular fluid to an osmolarity of 50 mOsm/L.

The production of a concentrated urine occurs when the permeability to water is increased in the more distal portions of the distal convoluted tubules and collecting tubules by the action of circulating ADH. As the collecting tubule passes through the inner medullary region, the tubular fluid equilibrates with the hyperosmotic interstitial fluid, water is removed, and a concentrated urine of an osmolarity as high as 1200 mOsm/L is excreted. Because a hyperosmotic medullary interstitium is essential for the concentration of urine, any process that reduces this hyperosmolarity will impair the ability of the kidneys to concentrate urine maximally.

Concept of Free-Water Clearance

The fundamental process in the dilution and concentration of urine is the separation of solutes and water by both the ascending thin and thick limbs of the loop of Henle, which may be thought of as the generation of a volume of water that is free of solutes. When plasma osmolarity is low due to an excess of water in the body, the circulating level of ADH is low and the permeability of the collecting tubule to water is low, resulting in the excretion of solute-free water from the body. The clearance of this solute-free water by the kidney is called free-water clearance (C_{water}). Free-water clearance is sometimes calculated because it can provide a means to quantify the loss or gain of water from the kidneys by the excretion of a dilute or concentrated urine;

this will reflect the ability of the kidneys to maintain osmolarity of the body fluids (Rose, 1994).

Free-water clearance is calculated as the difference between the rate of urine flow and the clearance of total solutes from the plasma in osmoles. The clearance of total solutes from the plasma by the kidneys is called osmolar clearance (C_{osm}) and can be defined as the volume of water necessary for the excretion of the osmotic load in the urine so that urine is iso-osmotic with plasma. The osmolar clearance, C_{osm}, can be calculated and has the unit of volume/unit time, or liters/day (L/day):

$$C_{osm} = (U_{osm} \times V)/P_{osm}$$

where U_{osm} = osmolarity of urine (mOsm/L), V = rate of urine flow (L/day), and P_{osm} = plasma osmolarity (mOsm/L).

$$C_{water} = V - C_{osm}$$

Therefore, when the rate of urine flow is greater than C_{osm} (i.e., when C_{water} is positive) relatively more water than solute is excreted in the urine; dilute or hypo-osmotic urine is excreted. Conversely, when the rate of urine flow is smaller than C_{osm} (i.e., when C_{water} is negative) relatively more solute is excreted in the urine and urine is hyperosmotic.

The minimal urine volume (excretion of hyperosmotic urine) possible for an adult was calculated for Table 37–1 based on excretion in the urine of about 770 mOsm of solutes per day. Excretion of the solute load can be accomplished by producing urine that is either iso-osmotic (U_{osm}/P_{osm} = 1), hyperosmotic (U_{osm}/P_{osm} > 1), or hypo-osmotic (U_{osm}/P_{osm} < 1) with respect to plasma. In the example used in Table 37–1, the urinary flow rate of the individual was 0.64 L/day and the osmolarity was 1200 mOsm/L. C_{osm} can be calculated as C_{osm} = (1200 mOsm/L × 0.64 L/day)/300 mOsm/L = 2.6 L/day. Because the urinary flow rate (0.64 L/day) is less than C_{osm} (2.6 L/day), a negative C_{water} is obtained. This negative C_{water} expresses the renal conservation of water in which solute-free water is reabsorbed by the kidneys and a concentrated urine is excreted. To excrete an iso-osmotic urine, the 770 mOsm of solutes would need to be ex-

creted in 2.6 L/day of urine, or about four times the minimum obligatory urine volume. In this case of iso-osmotic urine excretion, C_{osm} equals urinary flow rate, C_{water} is equal to zero, and no excretion of solute-free water occurs. The production of a dilute urine requires a flow rate of more than 2.6 L/day; in this case, solute-free water is excreted by the kidneys and C_{water} is positive.

The determination of C_{water} provides important information on the functions of the segments of the nephron involved in the production of dilute and concentrated urine. In the absence of ADH, the renal tubular structures (ascending thin and thick limbs of the loop of Henle, the distal convoluted tubule, and the collecting tubule) are involved in the dilution of luminal fluid by separating solutes from water in the lumen; quantitatively, the ascending thick limb is the most important in reabsorbing solutes. For the kidneys to excrete a maximal volume of solute-free water, ADH must be absent so that water reabsorption by the collecting tubules does not occur. On the other hand, for the kidneys to excrete a concentrated urine, solute-free water must be reabsorbed by the collecting tubules, and this occurs only in the presence of ADH secretion.

REGULATION OF WATER BALANCE

Disturbances of water balance lead to a change in plasma osmolarity, whereas disturbances of sodium balance result in a change in the volumes of body fluids. For an individual to maintain a constant osmolarity of the body fluids at 290 mOsm/L, the ratio of sodium chloride to total body water has to be regulated within narrow limits. Water excess or water deficit will invariably affect the ratio of sodium chloride to water, thus changing the plasma osmolarity. To maintain water balance, physiological feedback mechanisms are present to modify either water loss or water intake (Thompson et al., 1986). Changes in blood volume and blood pressure will also affect thirst and renal excretion of water via feedback mechanisms (Robertson, 1983) (Fig. 37–6).

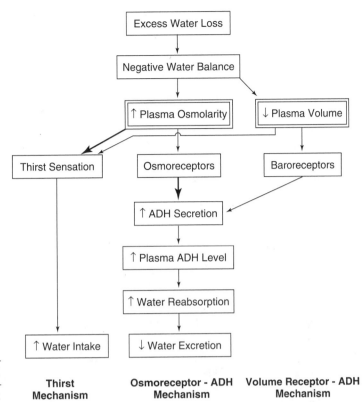

Figure 37–6. Integration of the osmoreceptor-ADH, baroreceptor-ADH, and thirst mechanisms in the regulation of water balance in water deficit.

Renal Excretion of Water

Water excess results in the excretion of a dilute urine, whereas water deficit results in the excretion of a concentrated urine. This ability to excrete either a concentrated or a dilute urine depends on the circulating level of plasma ADH.

Synthesis of ADH. ADH, or arginine vasopressin, is a small peptide, 9 amino acids in length. It is synthesized by the magnocellular neurons located within the supraoptic and paraventricular nuclei of the hypothalamus; synthesis in the supraoptic nuclei is more important quantitatively (Baylis and Thompson, 1988). The synthesized hormone is packaged as granules in vesicles; transported in combination with a carrier protein, neurophysin, down the axons of these neurons; and stored as secretory granules in the nerve endings located in the posterior pituitary gland (neurohypophysis) until released. When the supraoptic and paraventricular nuclei are stimulated, nerve impulses are transmitted along the hypothalamic-hypophysial tract to the

nerve endings at the neurohypophysis to release the secretory granules by exocytosis. After release, the neurophysin and ADH separate, and the ADH enters the circulation to act on the tubular cells of the collecting tubule.

Release of ADH. The two primary physiological factors regulating ADH secretion are changes in plasma osmolarity and effective circulating volume (Menninger, 1985) (see Fig. 37–6). Secretion of ADH can be changed by other stimuli to the central nervous system as well as by various hormones and drugs. For example, nausea-producing agents such as morphine and nicotine stimulate secretion (Verbalis et al., 1987), and ethanol inhibits secretion (Carney et al., 1995).

Effects of ADH in the Kidney. In antidiuresis, when there is a need to conserve water, the circulating level of ADH is high. ADH increases the permeability to water in the collecting tubule, resulting in the reabsorption of water, and a concentrated urine is excreted. In water diuresis, the circulating level of ADH is low and the collecting tubule is impermeable to water, resulting in the excretion of large volumes of solute-free water.

The actual mechanism of ADH in eliciting an increase in water permeability of the luminal membrane of the collecting tubule has been elucidated recently. Large numbers of transporter proteins, called aquaporin-2, that function as water channels are present in intracellular vesicles beneath the luminal membrane of the collecting tubules. It is proposed that when ADH binds to receptors located on the basolateral membrane of the tubular cell, adenylate cyclase is activated, and the intracellular level of cyclic AMP increases. This activates one or more protein kinases that then cause aquaporin-2 water channels to "shuttle" from intracellular vesicles to the luminal membrane, thus providing areas of high water permeability in the membrane (Fig. 37–7) (Knepper et al., 1996). The time course for these reactions to occur is rapid, within 40 seconds. This process temporarily provides channels that allow free diffusion of water from the tubular fluid into the cells. When ADH is removed, these aquaporin-2 water channels are reinternalized into the cell, and the luminal membrane becomes impermeable to water. Again, this process occurs within minutes. The insertion and removal of membrane vesicles containing water channels provides a rapid mechanism for controlling the permeability of the luminal membrane to water.

Once water enters the cell, it exits across the highly permeable basolateral membrane to the interstitium. The water permeability of the basolateral membrane of the collecting tubule is due to the presence of large numbers of aquaporin-3 and aquaporin-4 channels. Aquaporin-3 water channels are located mainly in the lateral membrane, whereas aquaporin-4 water channels are located in both the basal and lateral membranes and allow water taken up across the luminal brush border membrane (aquaporin-2 channels) to pass through the other side of the tubular cell into the interstitial fluid. These aquaporin water channels in the basolateral membrane are not affected by ADH (Knepper et al., 1996).

Osmoreceptor-ADH System in the Regulation of Osmolarity. A change in plasma osmolarity is the most potent stimulus in control-

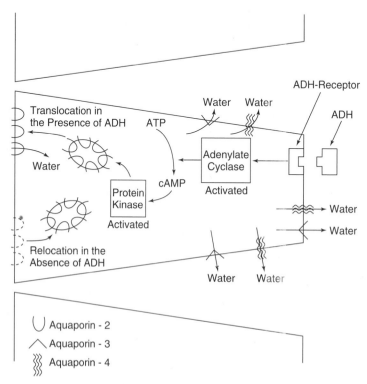

Figure 37–7. Proposed mechanism for the action of antidiuretic hormone (ADH) to increase water permeability of the collecting tubule.

ling the secretion of ADH (see Fig. 37–6). When a hypertonic sodium chloride solution is injected into the artery supplying the hypothalamus, the neurons in the supraoptic and paraventricular nuclei immediately send nerve impulses to the nerve endings in the neurohypophysis to release ADH into the circulation. Conversely, injection of a hypotonic sodium chloride solution into the same artery inhibits the secretion of ADH (Zerbe and Robertson, 1983).

The precise mechanism by which a change in plasma osmolarity affects the secretion of ADH is unclear. In the vicinity of the neuroendocrine cells that synthesize ADH are cells that are sensitive to changes in osmolarity of body fluids. These cells are thought to be located either in the hypothalamus or in the organum vasculosum located in the anteroventral wall of the third ventricle (Zimmerman et al., 1987). Regardless of their location, these cells respond to changes in osmolarity of the extracellular fluid and send appropriate signals either to increase or inhibit the secretion of ADH. When the extracellular fluid bathing these cells is hypertonic, water diffuses out of the cells along an osmotic gradient and causes the cells to decrease in size. Transmission of nerve impulses to the neurohypophysis increases, and the secretion of ADH is increased. Conversely, a hypotonic extracellular fluid causes water to move into these cells, transmission of nerve signals to the neurohypophysis decreases, and the secretion of ADH is inhibited. Therefore, these cells behave essentially as osmometers and are called osmoreceptors. Normally, the plasma osmolarity is set at 290 mOsm/L. An increase in plasma osmolarity above this set point by as little as 0.5% is sufficient to stimulate ADH secretion (Thompson et al., 1986). Because the half-life of the released ADH is short, less than 20 minutes, the concentration of ADH in the circulation can decrease or increase rapidly within minutes in response to changes in the osmolarity of the plasma.

Volume Receptor-ADH System in the Regulation of Osmolarity.
A decrease in effective circulating volume stimulates secretion of large amounts of ADH from the neurohypophysis (see Fig. 37–6). However, the sensitivity

of this system is less than that of the osmoreceptors (Menninger, 1985). An increase in plasma osmolarity of only 0.5% is sufficient to increase ADH secretion, whereas a decrease of about 5% to 10% in blood pressure or blood volume is required before ADH secretion is stimulated.

Volume receptors or sensors are located in the central venous portion of the circulation (right atrium and pulmonary vein) and in the arterial side of the vascular system. These receptors respond primarily to stretch and are termed baroreceptors. In hypervolemia, excitation of the baroreceptors sends signals to the hypothalamus via the afferent fibers in the vagus nerve to inhibit ADH secretion. In hypovolemia, these baroreceptors are not stimulated, and the secretion of ADH is increased.

Thirst Mechanism in Control of Water Intake

In addition to the increase in secretion of ADH during water deficit to minimize water loss by the kidneys, fluid intake is necessary to counterbalance fluid loss through insensible perspiration, sweating, and the gastrointestinal tract (see Table 37–1). Fluid intake is regulated by the thirst mechanism, which, together with the osmoreceptor-ADH feedback mechanism, maintains a relatively constant plasma osmolarity.

Thirst Center. The neural centers for thirst have not been defined completely. It appears that two areas are involved in the perception of thirst. Osmoreceptors similar to, but distinct from, those involved in ADH release are present in the area along the anteroventral wall of the third ventricle and respond to changes in plasma osmolarity. Another small area that promotes drinking is located anterolaterally in the preoptic nucleus (Zimmerman et al., 1987). Very little is known about the pathways involved in the response of thirst to decreased blood volume or pressure, but both the renin-angiotensin system and baroreceptors are believed to be involved.

Stimuli for Thirst. Many stimuli alter the perception of thirst, but the most important ones are changes in plasma osmolarity and changes in effective circulating volume or blood pressure (Andersson, 1978). When plasma osmolarity is increased or when the blood volume or pressure is reduced, the individual perceives thirst. As for ADH secretion, the most potent of these stimuli is hypertonicity; an increase of only 0.5% in plasma osmolarity stimulates the sensation of thirst, whereas a decrease of about 5% to 10% in blood pressure or blood volume is required before a similar thirst response is produced (Thompson et al., 1986, Zimmerman et al., 1987). Another factor that influences drinking is dryness of the mucosa of the mouth and esophagus.

The person finds relief from thirst by the act of drinking even before water is absorbed from the gastrointestinal tract to have an effect on the plasma osmolarity. Receptors in the pharynx, esophagus, and stomach probably are involved in this response (Thrasher et al., 1981). However, these mechanisms provide relief only temporarily. The increase in plasma osmolarity has to be corrected before the desire to drink is satisfied.

Integration of Osmoreceptor-ADH, Volume Receptor-ADH, and Thirst Mechanisms

The preceding systems work in concert to regulate the osmolarity of body fluids and maintain water balance. In water deficit, plasma osmolarity increases and blood volume contracts. This will stimulate the release of ADH to increase water reabsorption from the kidneys. However, the volume of water reabsorbed may be insufficient to correct fully for the water deficit. Stimulation of the thirst sensation to promote drinking returns the plasma osmolarity and blood volume back to normal. Conversely, when the plasma osmolarity is decreased and blood volume is increased in water excess, thirst sensation is suppressed, ADH is not secreted, and solute-free water excretion is enhanced in the absence of ADH to restore the plasma osmolarity and blood volume.

ABNORMAL STATES OF OSMOLARITIES AND VOLUMES

Disturbances of water balance consist of either depletion or excess of water and are manifested by alterations in the body fluid osmolarity. Because the major determinant of plasma osmolarity is sodium ions, these disorders alter the plasma concentration of sodium ions. To understand the disturbances in volume, osmolarity, and distribution of body fluids, two fundamental physiological facts must be kept in mind:

(1) Fluid compartments are in osmotic equilibrium because water permeates the cell membrane and diffuses freely between the extracellular and intracellular fluid compartments, and

(2) When the extracellular fluid becomes hypertonic, water diffuses out of cells until the osmolarities of the extracellular and intracellular fluids are equal, whereas the reverse is true when extracellular fluid becomes hypotonic.

Changes in the osmolarity of the extracellular compartment will invariably affect the volume of the intracellular compartment.

Water deficit is usually associated with hypernatremia (high plasma sodium concentration) and water excess with hyponatremia (low plasma sodium concentration). Under normal circumstances, if the disturbances are not of renal origin, the kidneys compensate for the deficit or excess by appropriately adjusting urine volume and composition, thereby ensuring that the osmolarity of the body fluids is stabilized within narrow limits.

Hyponatremia in Positive Water Balance

Ingestion of an excessive amount of water will dilute all the body fluid compartments; the volumes of both the intracellular and extracellular compartments increase and their osmolarities decrease (hyponatremia and hypervolemia). The excess water will distribute throughout the body in proportion to the initial volumes of the intracellular and extracellular compartments. Under normal circumstances, secretion of ADH is inhibited and the excess water excreted. However, in conditions in which the low plasma osmolarity fails to inhibit secretion of ADH, such as in severe low-output congestive heart failure (Uretsky et

CLINICAL CORRELATION

Edema Formation

Edema is the accumulation of an excessively large amount of fluid in the interstitial space. The amount depends upon the capillary fluid pressure, the interstitial fluid pressure, the interstitial oncotic pressure, the plasma oncotic pressure, the extracellular fluid volume, and the lymph flow. Normally, efflux of fluid exceeds influx across the capillary wall; the extra fluid drains back into the blood stream through the lymphatics. Edema signals the presence of a pathological process that affects the balance of forces regulating the movement of fluid between the intravascular and the interstitial compartments.

Edema can be localized or generalized. Localized edemas are restricted to a discrete vascular area, such as the swelling that accompanies inflammation. Generalized edema exists when an abnormally large amount of fluid accumulates in the interstitial spaces throughout the body. Some common causes of generalized edema are congestive heart failure, nephrotic syndrome, and nutritional or "hunger" edema.

In congestive heart failure, impaired cardiac emptying results in a rise in ventricular end diastolic pressure, which causes an increase in venous pressure that in turn promotes transudation of fluids out of the vascular channel into the interstitial spaces. The loss of fluid from the vascular tree diminishes effective blood volume, and the kidneys respond by retaining salt and water in an effort to increase intravascular fluid volume. However, because the cardiac output remains low, this leads to a vicious cycle that is self-perpetuating unless treatment to increase cardiac output is instituted. Treatment consists of reducing sodium and fluid retention through use of diuretics, improving cardiac output with inotropic agents such as digitalis, and reducing vascular resistance through use of vasodilating drugs. The edema due to congestive heart failure is usually most prominent in the lower extremities when the patient is standing or sitting. When the patient is lying down, edema shifts to the sacral area. Because gravity influences the distribution of the edema, it is termed "dependent edema."

Some kidney diseases such as membranous glomerulonephritis and focal segmental glomerulosclerosis cause nephrotic syndrome owing to increased permeability in the glomerular capillary wall. Nephrotic syndrome is characterized by massive proteinuria, hypoalbuminemia, generalized edema, hyperlipidemia, and lipiduria. Although very little protein is lost in the urine of normal subjects, massive quantities of proteins are filtered and passed out through the urine of patients with nephrotic syndrome because of the increase in glomerular capillary wall permeability. The edema of nephrotic syndrome is largely due to decreased plasma oncotic pressure as a consequence of loss of plasma protein and the resultant hypoalbuminemia. Compensatory secretion of aldosterone and a reduction of glomerular filtration rate as a consequence of the drop in plasma volume further aggravate the condition. Therapies consist of treatment of the underlying cause, sodium restriction, and judicious use of diuretics. Edema due to renal dysfunction tends to be massive and more equally distributed than is edema of cardiac origin. Generalized massive edema is termed anasarca. When finger pressure is applied to the edematous area, temporary displacement of fluid leaves a pitted depression, hence the term "pitting edema."

Another cause of edema is impaired lymphatic drainage. In filariasis, a parasitic worm infestation of the lymphatic system, lymphatic flow is obstructed. Obstruction to lymphatic flow is also seen following radical surgery for breast cancer in which axillary lymph nodes are removed. This edema is usually located distal to the point of obstruction.

Thinking Critically

Children with kwashiorkor, a form of protein-energy malnutrition, often present with signs of inanition and edema. Kwashiorkor is usually characterized by a diet poor in protein and relatively more adequate in total energy.

1. Why does edema develop in these children?

2. Discuss the occurrence of edema with regard to the Starling forces that determine fluid movement in and out of the vascular and interstitial spaces.

al., 1985), cell expansion, hypervolemia, and hyponatremia occur. Acute water intoxication caused by too rapid parenteral fluid replacement will cause expansion of brain cells, leading to symptoms of headache, nausea, vomiting, muscle twitching, convulsion, and finally death (Sterns and Spital, 1990).

Hypernatremia in Negative Water Balance

In general, water is never lost without ions, nor ions without water, although the relative proportions of ions and water lost vary in different circumstances. When loss of water exceeds loss of ions, the osmolarity of the extracellular fluid increases. Water diffuses out of the cells until the osmolarities across the cell membrane are equal. The volumes of both compartments will decrease and their osmolarities will increase. Secretion of ADH is stimulated, the kidneys conserve water, and a concentrated urine is excreted. Excessive sweating during heavy physical exertion in a hot and humid climate causes loss of both electrolytes and water, but water loss exceeds that of electrolytes, leading to hypernatremia and hypovolemia (Randall, 1976). Although the kidney will conserve both electrolytes and water during dehydration by excreting a concentrated urine low in sodium, fluid loss ultimately has to be replaced by fluid intake. Inadequate replacement of water loss leads to pronounced thirst, fatigue, decreased urine output, and fever.

Accumulation of Excess Fluid in Tissues: Edema

In edema, there is an accumulation of excess fluid in body tissues. Edema occurs when there is an imbalance of forces governing the diffusion of water across either the cell membrane or the capillary endothelium or when the permeability of these membranes is increased. The most common edema occurs in the interstitial fluid compartment, but intracellular edema may occur also.

Intracellular edema occurs when the permeability of the cell membrane to solutes is increased, when the concentration of a permeable solute in the plasma is increased, or

in hyponatremia. Both the increase in membrane permeability and the increase in plasma concentration of a permeable solute cause an influx of solutes into the cells. Water diffuses passively along the osmotic gradient into the cells, and the cells expand. In tissue inflammation, permeability of the cell membrane increases, and this causes an influx of sodium and other ions and, subsequently, water into the cells. In hyponatremia, water enters the cells along the osmotic gradient, causing the cells to expand.

Edema commonly involves expansion of the interstitial space. Edema formation may be a result of an increase in filtration of plasma into the interstitial space or a failure of the lymphatics to return the filtered fluid to the circulation. An increase in filtration of plasma can result from an imbalance in any of the factors that affect net movement of water across the capillary endothelium. Examples include an increase in capillary endothelium permeability that results from endothelial cell contraction elicited by chemical mediators of inflammation, such as histamine and bradykinin, and the decrease in plasma oncotic pressure that results from a decrease in plasma protein concentration in individuals with liver cirrhosis, kidney diseases, or protein malnutrition. An increase in filtration pressure due to venous congestion secondary to congestive heart failure is another common cause of edema (Kumar et al., 1992).

REFERENCES

Andersson, B. (1978) Regulation of water intake. Physiol Rev 58:582–603.

Baylis, P. H. and Thompson, C. J. (1988) Osmoregulation of vasopressin secretion and thirst in health and disease. Clin Endocrinol 29:549–576.

Berry, C. A. and Rector, F. C., Jr. (1991) Renal transport of glucose, amino acids, sodium, chloride, and water. In: The Kidney (Brenner, B. M. and Rector, F. C., Jr., eds.), 4th ed., vol. 1, pp. 245–282. W.B. Saunders, Philadelphia.

Carney, S. L., Gillies, A. H. and Ray, C. D. (1995) Acute effect of ethanol on renal electrolyte transport in the rat. Clin Exp Pharmacol Physiol 22:629–634.

Geigy Scientific Tables (1981) (Lintner, C., ed.), 8th ed., vol. 1, p. 108. Ciba-Geigy Limited, Basel, Switzerland.

Irsigler, K., Veitl, V., Sigmund, A., Tschegg, E. and Kunz, K. (1979) Calorimetric results in man: Energy output in normal and overweight subjects. Metabolism 28:1127–1132.

Knepper, M. A. and Rector, F. C., Jr. (1991) Urinary concentration and dilution. In: The Kidney (Brenner, B. M.

and Rector, F. C., Jr., eds.), 4th ed., vol. 1, pp. 445–482. W.B. Saunders, Philadelphia.

Knepper, M. A., Wade, J. B., Terris, J., Ecelbarger, C. A., Marples, D., Mandon, B., Chou, C.-L., Kishore, B. K. and Nielsen, S. (1996) Renal aquaporins. Kidney Int 49:1712–1717.

Kumar, V., Cotran, R. S. and Robbins, S. L. (1992) Disorders of vascular flow and shock. In: Basic Pathology, 5th ed., pp. 61–81. W. B. Saunders, Philadelphia.

Menninger, R. P. (1985) Current concepts of volume receptor regulation of vasopressin release. Fed Proc 44:55–58.

National Research Council (1989) Recommended Dietary Allowances, 10th ed., National Academy Press, Washington, D.C.

Randall, H. T. (1976) Fluid, electrolyte, and acid-balance. Surg Clin North Am 56:1019–1058.

Robertson, G. L. (1983) Thirst and vasopressin function in normal and disordered states of water balance. J Lab Clin Med 101:351–371.

Robertson, G. L. and Berl, T. (1991) Pathophysiology of water metabolism. In: The Kidney (Brenner, B. M. and Rector, F. C., Jr., eds.), 4th ed., pp. 677–736. W.B. Saunders, Philadelphia.

Rose, D. R. (1994) Physiology of body fluids. In: Clinical Physiology of Acid-Base and Electrolyte Disorders, pp. 3–42. McGraw-Hill, New York.

Sterns, R. H. and Spital, A. (1990) Disorders of water balance. In: Fluids and Electrolytes (Kokko, J. P. and Tannen, R. L., eds.), 2nd ed., pp. 139–194. W.B. Saunders, Philadelphia.

Taylor, A. E. (1981) Capillary fluid filtration; Starling forces and lymph flow. Circ Res 49:557–575.

Thompson, C. J., Bland, J., Burd, J. and Baylis, P. H. (1986) The osmotic thresholds for thirst and vasopressin release are similar in healthy man. Clin Sci 71:651–656.

Thrasher, T. N., Nistal-Herrera, J. F., Keil, L. C. and Ramsay, D. J. (1981) Satiety and inhibition of vasopressin secretion after drinking in dehydrated dogs. Am J Physiol 240:E394–E401.

Uretsky, B. F., Verbalis, J. G., Generalovich, T., Valdes, A. and Reddy, P. S. (1985) Plasma vasopressin response to osmotic and hemodynamic stimuli in heart failure. Am J Physiol 248:H395–H402.

Verbalis, J. G., Richardson, D. W. and Stricker, E. M. (1987) Vasopressin release in response to nausea-producing agents and cholecystokinin in monkeys. Am J Physiol 252:R1138–R1142.

Walser, M. (1992) Phenomenological analysis of electrolyte homeostasis. In: The Kidney; Physiology and Pathophysiology (Seldin, D.W. and Giebisch, G., eds.), 2nd ed., vol. 1, pp. 31–44. Raven Press, New York

Zerbe, R. L. and Robertson, G. L. (1983) Osmoregulation of thirst and vasopressin secretion in human subjects: Effect of various solutes. Am J Physiol 244:E607–E614.

Zimmerman, E. A., Ma, L. Y., and Nilaver, G. (1987) Anatomical basis of thirst and vasopressin secretion. Kidney Int 32:S14–S19.

RECOMMENDED READINGS

Baylis, P. H. (1987) Osmoregulation and control of vasopressin secretion in healthy humans. Am J Physiol 253:R671–R678.

Jamison, R. J. (1987) The renal concentrating mechanism. Kidney Int 32(suppl 21):S43–S50.

Menninger, R. P. (1985) Current concepts of volume regulation of vasopressin release. Fed Proc 4:55–58.

Rose, D. R. (1994) Physiology of body fluids. In: Clinical Physiology of Acid-base and Electrolyte Disorders, pp. 3–42. McGraw-Hill, New York.

Sterns, R. H. and Spital, A. (1990) Disorders of water balance. In: Fluids and Electrolytes (Kokko, J. P. and Tannen, R. L. eds.), 2nd ed., pp. 139–194. W.B. Saunders, Philadelphia.

CHAPTER **38**

◆◆◆◆◆◆◆◆◆◆◆◆◆◆◆◆◆◆◆◆◆◆◆◆◆◆◆◆◆◆◆◆◆◆◆◆◆◆

Diet and Oral Disease

Dominick P. DePaola, D.D.S., Ph.D., and
Charles F. Schachtele, Ph.D.

OUTLINE

PERSPECTIVES ON THE ROLE OF CARBOHYDRATES IN ORAL DISEASE

Virtually all human diseases have a genetic component, yet the expression of disease is modulated by the environment. In particular, the environmental variables of diet and nutrition have an influential role in the development and maturation of human tissues and organs, as well as their ability to withstand untoward challenges. Indeed, the contemporary paradigm for human disease centers on the notion that human diseases and disorders are a consequence of complex interactions among genes, environment, and behavior.

The oral tissues offer one of the best examples of how disease processes and disorders, seemingly isolated to teeth and their surrounding hard and soft tissues, are, in reality, linked to general physiological and biological processes and thus to systemic health and disease. For example, dental caries and periodontal disease, both infectious diseases, were thought to be expressions of local accumulation of dental plaque, linked to poor oral hygiene, poor diet, and other human behavioral characteristics. Now, however, there is compelling evidence that periodontal disease in pregnant women is linked to low birth weight infants and that periodontal disease is also a risk factor in cardiovascular disease, stroke, and pulmonary disease. At the same time, cleft lip and/or palate, one of the most prevalent birth defects in the world, has both genetic and environmental components, and the expression of clefting can be a result of inadequate maternal folate status as can neural tube defects.

The oral tissues are also an expressive site of osteoporosis, a variety of essential dietary deficiency diseases, musculoskeletal disorders, taste and neurosensory disorders, neoplastic disease, acquired immunodeficiency syndrome (AIDS), human immunodeficiency virus (HIV), and other infectious diseases, as well as a host of other physiological perturbations. Poor oral health can result in pain, changes in dentate status, inability to chew food properly, and alterations in food selection behaviors. The net result can be compromised nutritional status with consequent effects on general health. Thus, in viewing the role of diet in oral disease, it is important not to lose sight of effects of proteins, fats, vitamins, minerals, water, calories, and other nutrient sources on oral tissues. Without question, the oral cavity is a mirror of the human physiological condition, and, in the words of former Surgeon General Dr. C. Everett Koop, ". . . without oral health you are not healthy."

Historical Perspectives

The literature is replete with observations regarding the establishment of dental caries in the teeth of individuals who lived hundreds of years ago. The prevalence of dental caries has continued into this century. Even though it may have peaked in certain Western populations, it remains one of the most prevalent infectious diseases in the world. There is an unequivocal link of frequency of fermentable carbohydrate consumption, increased sugar consumption in developing populations, and the retention of fermentable carbohydrates in the oral cavity with dental caries prevalence. In early studies, tube-fed rodents that were given a high-carbohydrate diet did not develop dental caries, demonstrating the necessity for food to be in contact with the tooth surface for caries to occur. Similarly, when germ-free animals were fed a high-sucrose diet, no caries developed, further illustrating the necessity of sugar and plaque bacteria to be in intimate contact with the tooth surface. Three frequently cited studies with humans propelled our understanding of this linkage in the human population.

From 1946 to 1951, a study was conducted in a mental institution in Sweden where residents were provided a number of dietary regimes that contained variable amounts of fermentable carbohydrates that were eaten either with or between meals at various frequencies. They were given specific foods that had varying degrees of "stickiness" (Gustafsson et al., 1954). The Vipeholm Study, named after the institution where it was conducted, offered some startling observations and conclusions. Residents who ingested up to ten times as much sugar as the control group did not have an appreciable increase in dental caries over the control when the sugars were ingested at meals. However, as the frequency of sugar intake increased between meals, dental caries increased dramatically, and the caries process was exacerbated when the source of the dietary sugar was a sticky toffee. The inescapable conclusions were that (1) the frequency of sugar ingestion is directly related to caries formation, and (2) the more retentive the sugar, the greater its participation in the dental caries process. Thus, form and frequency of fermentable carbohydrate ingestion emerged as critical determinants of the caries process.

An equally important study took place in an Australian home for boys, the Hopewood House (Harris, 1963). The children who were residents of the House were placed on a dietary regimen that contained few refined sugars and an abundance of complex carbohydrates. The Hopewood children had low caries increments, adding more evidence to the observation that fermentable carbohydrate ingestion and caries prevalence are linked.

A 2-year clinical trial in Finland, known as the Turku Study, demonstrated that young adults ingesting foods sweetened solely with the sugar alcohol xylitol did not develop new caries, compared with the caries increment experienced in those groups that consumed foods sweetened with the monosaccharide fructose or the disaccharide sucrose (Scheinin et al., 1975). In a comparison study, subjects chewed four sticks of xylitol-containing gum per day with a normal dietary regimen (Scheinin et al., 1975). After 1 year, the experimental group who chewed the xylitol gum had a very low level of caries surfaces compared with a control group. The control group chewed the same amount of gum as the experimental group and ate the same relative diet, but the control gum contained sucrose instead of xylitol.

In addition to these important human studies, epidemiological surveys, extensive animal experiments, and other controlled human studies have linked carbohydrates to the development of dental caries. A particularly noteworthy example relates to the rare metabolic disorder hereditary fructose intolerance, which requires patients to subsist on a diet that is essentially sugar-free for their life span. Patients with hereditary fructose intolerance

demonstrate an exceedingly low caries rate, but some caries are found among the patients who do consume a relatively small amount of sucrose (Newbrun et al., 1980).

The minimal concentration of a fermentable carbohydrate in a food that will cause caries in humans is still unknown. However, foods that contain 15% sugars by weight are considered high-sugar foods. It is clear that any food that contains fermentable carbohydrate can, if ingested frequently, potentially contribute to the caries process, given the presence of a susceptible host, plaque on the teeth, substrate, and time for the fermentation process to occur. Figure 38–1 is an illustration of the relationship of fermentable carbohydrate and nutritive and non-nutritive sweeteners to the caries process.

Modern Approaches Relating Carbohydrates to Oral Disease

At one time, sucrose was considered the "arch enemy" of dental caries because of its direct relationship to the caries process and because of its unique biochemical properties (Newbrun, 1969). Indeed, there is biochemical evidence that sucrose is more cariogenic than other fermentable carbohydrates due to its role in the production of extracellular polysaccharides, which are involved in the adherence of plaque to the teeth. Yet other evidence suggests that fructose and glucose are not dissimilar to sucrose in terms of their acidogenicity. Even sorbitol and mannitol, which are hexose sugar alcohols, are fermentable and could contribute to the caries process, however, they are metabolized slowly by plaque bacteria and, therefore, permit the buffering capacity of saliva to mitigate harmful acid production. Utilizing plaque pH telemetry testing (described later), it is clear that all fermentable carbohydrates, whether added to a food or naturally occurring, can contribute to the caries process. In addition, when potentially cariogenic foods are ingested with meals, the ability of the food to participate in the caries process can be somewhat mitigated. At the same time, the order in which foods are eaten during a meal can affect their cariogenic potential; for example, the inges-

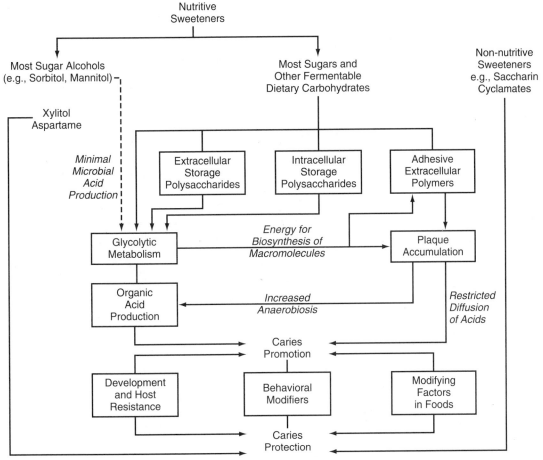

Figure 38–1. *The relationship of nutritive and non-nutritive sweeteners to oral microbial metabolism and dental caries. (Adapted from Alfano, M. C. [1980] Nutrition, sweeteners, and dental caries. Food Technol 34:70–74. Redrawn for DePaola, D. P., Faine, M. P. and Vogel, R. I. [1994] Nutrition in relation to dental medicine. In: Modern Nutrition in Health and Disease [Shils, M. E., Olsen, J. and Shike, M., eds.], 8th ed., vol. 2, pp. 1007–1028. Lea and Febiger, Philadelphia.)*

tion of sugar-rich foods has a low cariogenic potential when followed by eating aged cheeses. In the modern era, it is not appropriate to single out specific foods as cariogenic or to rank foods according to their potential acidogenicity, because the manner in which foods are ingested, the form in which they are ingested, the frequency of their ingestion, and the sequence in which they are eaten all can either potentiate or impede the caries process. Thus, fermentable carbohydrates need to be viewed in terms of the individual's total dietary intake, and the individual's risk for disease must be considered. High-risk caries patients (e.g., individuals with limited access to health care or with salivary dysfunctions) must be assessed in a different manner from the general population.

BIOLOGICAL BASIS FOR THE ROLE OF CARBOHYDRATES IN ORAL DISEASE

To appreciate the role that carbohydrates play in dental caries formation, it is necessary to understand the nature and activities of dental plaque, the specific bacterial etiology of the disease, and the hard mineralized tooth tissue that is destroyed during the disease process. The well-known contributions of dietary carbohydrate, cariogenic bacteria, and tooth enamel must be placed within the time course of disease development. Some of the interactions, such as the production of acid from carbohydrates by cariogenic bacteria, are very rapid. Demineralization of the teeth is a much slower process, requiring repeated cycles of loss of tooth mineral due to acidic dissolution and remineralization when there is less acid in the environment. Key issues are the presence of dental plaque and specific sucrose-metabolizing cariogenic bacteria on the teeth, the fermentation of dietary carbohydrate to acidic end products by these bacteria, and, finally, dissolution of the tooth enamel to yield carious lesions.

Dental Plaque and Cariogenic Bacteria

The ingestion of food containing carbohydrates causes dramatic biochemical changes in the oral cavity because of the high concentrations of bacteria that live in this environment. Over 200 different species of bacteria have been isolated from the human mouth, the surfaces of which contain distinct microcosms, each with a characteristic collection of bacteria. The largest masses of bacteria are found on the surface of teeth where dental plaque accumulates. Ingestion of food is not required for maintenance of the oral bacterial populations; high concentrations are found in humans fed by intubation. Adequate nutrition for the bacteria can be supplied from saliva, gingival crevicular fluid from between the teeth and gums, and from the epithelial cells of the various oral tissues.

Dental plaque can be described as a dense mat of bacteria that covers the teeth and that is not removed by rinsing with water. Plaque formation and metabolism have been extensively studied, and it is clear that this material places a large amount of metabolic potential on the tooth surface where interactions with dietary components can occur. In the anaerobic environment of plaque, the fermentative capacity of the bacteria is not only localized but also appears to be very efficient in converting dietary carbohydrates to acidic metabolic end products. Although the exact stoichiometry of substrate conversion to products within such a concentrated and complex mixture of bacteria would be impossible to describe, it is very clear that plaque has the capacity to rapidly metabolize carbohydrates to acids.

Human dental caries are caused by one or more members of a group of bacteria called the mutans streptococci (Loesche, 1986). *Streptococcus mutans, Streptococcus so-brinus, Streptococcus cricetus, Streptococcus ferus,* and *Streptococcus rattus* make up this complex group of bacteria. *S. mutans* and *S. sobrinus* are the species normally found on human teeth. Important characteristics of these unique bacteria are that they normally live only on the surfaces of teeth, they produce extracellular polymers of glucose from sucrose, they are capable of producing large quantities of acid (they are highly acidogenic), and they can survive and grow at very low pH values (they are very aciduric). These features provide a selective survival advantage for these bacteria, especially in sites on the teeth that are sheltered from the buffering activities of saliva and where food residues can be retained. Consequently, most decay develops between the teeth and in the pits and fissures on the biting surfaces of the molar teeth.

Carbohydrate Metabolism by Cariogenic Bacteria

Because the focus of carbohydrate metabolism by oral bacteria has been on *S. mutans,* this bacterium will be used as a paradigm for the overall fermentation processes that can lead to high concentrations of plaque acids. As shown in Figure 38–1, there are three main pathways by which dietary carbohydrate is metabolized by plaque. *S. mutans* uses these pathways to produce extracellular polymers involved in the bacteria's retention on the teeth, to produce extracellular and intracellular storage polysaccharides, and for production of acid via glycolysis.

The extracellular glucosyltransferases (GTFs), which are extracellular enzymes capable of producing both water-soluble and water-insoluble glucans from sucrose, are a critical virulence factor for *S. mutans.* Strains of bacteria that lack these enzymes do not produce caries in animal model systems. Production of the water-insoluble glucans is essential for caries development because the glucans foster bacterial colonization and retention on the teeth. The production of glucans from sucrose explains the critical role that this dietary sugar plays in the development of dental caries. The GTFs are being studied extensively as possible antigens for development of a vaccine to control *S. mutans* and prevent dental caries.

Both extracellular and intracellular storage polysaccharides play a role in plaque metabolism and caries production. The fructosyl moiety of sucrose can be converted into extracellular polymers by fructosyltransferases produced by *S. mutans*, and these polymers can be degraded and fermented to acidic end products when fermentable carbohydrate from the diet is no longer available. In addition, the mutans streptococci can produce glycogen-like intracellular polysaccharides, which can be degraded to produce acid when fermentable carbohydrate is not available. Thus, the mutans streptococci have adapted to an environment that has marked fluctuations in carbohydrate and can store fructose and glucose for subsequent utilization at times of low availability from their environment.

S. mutans utilize the major sugars found in the human diet and can produce various acidic end products. Transport mechanisms have been demonstrated for the uptake of sucrose, glucose, fructose, mannitol, sorbitol, lactose, mannose, maltose, trehalose, raffinose, stachyose, melibiose, isomaltosaccharides, and palatinose, with subsequent intracellular fermentation. Oral bacteria do not all metabolize dietary sugars to the same end products because they utilize divergent metabolic pathways. For example, pyruvate, an intermediate produced by glycolysis, may be metabolized via several paths. Pyruvate may be reduced to lactic acid by the enzyme lactic acid dehydrogenase or split into formic acid and acetyl CoA by the enzyme pyruvate formate lyase. The acetyl moiety is then converted to acetic acid or ethanol. The proportion of lactic or other organic acids formed by plaques may be markedly affected by the oral environment and by the bacterial types present. When the concentrations of cariogenic bacteria and sugars in plaque are high, the pathway leading to lactic acid formation is dominant. On the other hand, when carbohydrate is limited, more diverse end products are produced.

Relationship of Caries to the Changes in Enamel Structure

After sleep, the pH of human dental plaque is at its highest level due to the production of ammonia, amines, and other basic components by bacterial metabolism of proteins, peptides, urea, and other nitrogen-containing compounds. Some acid-neutralizing activity in plaque may also come from metabolic conversion of lactic acid to weaker organic acids by plaque bacteria such as *Veillonella*. If carbohydrate is not ingested, the pH of the plaque will remain close to 7.0 or neutral. However, after carbohydrate ingestion the metabolism of sugars by plaque bacteria causes the pH to drop dramatically (Fig. 38–2). A drop in pH from 7 to 4 represents a 1000-fold increase in plaque H^+ concentration. With time, the pH will rise back toward neutrality as the acids diffuse from the plaque or are neutralized by the buffers entering plaque from saliva. This plaque pH response, or "Stephan curve," has been proposed by dental scientists to reflect the acidic challenge to the teeth imposed by ingestion of a foodstuff containing fermentable carbohydrate (Stephan, 1940).

The loss of tooth mineral during caries formation is caused by the lowering of plaque pH to the point where the hydroxyapatite mineral of enamel dissolves. The concept of a critical pH has evolved to indicate the pH at which saliva or the fluid phase of plaque or both are no longer saturated with respect to calcium and phosphate ions, thereby permitting hydroxyapatite to dissolve. Both saliva and plaque fluid cease to be saturated at pH values in the range of 5 to 6, with an average of 5.5. The critical pH will vary in different plaques depending on the concentrations of calcium and phosphate ions, and it is also influenced by the buffering power and ionic strength of the environment. However, it is unlikely that demineralization would occur above pH 5.7, and a pH of 5.7 or above has often been accepted as being "safe for the teeth."

The frequency of ingestion of food plays an important role in the caries process. Theoretically, if food is ingested at three times during the day, the plaque acid attack on the teeth will be limited to the three time periods when the pH remains below the critical level. However, increased frequency of ingestion of carbohydrate-containing food would lead to more numerous attacks on the dentition and

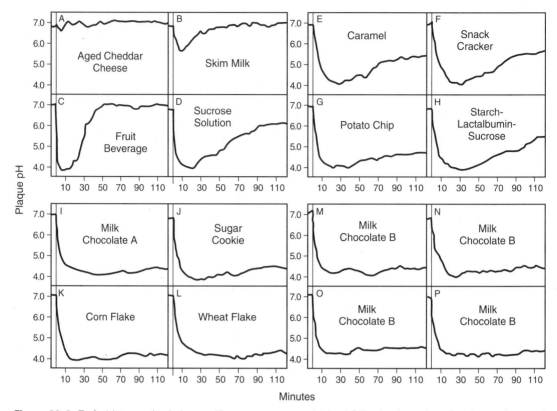

Figure 38–2. *Typical interproximal plaque pH response curves obtained following ingestion of various substrates/ foods by human volunteers. The pH at the beginning of the telemetry runs was close to neutral (pH 7) because the subjects had not ingested food since the previous evening.*

greater exposure to harmful acids. This simple explanation of the caries process emphasizes the important and deleterious effects of snacking with carbohydrate-containing foods and serves to provide some explanation for the results obtained in the Vipeholm study.

Caries development is not a process in which the teeth are simply dissolved by plaque acids when they are present. The dissolution of enamel and lesion formation is a complex process, and several key activities must be appreciated to understand fully the role of diet in the development of lesions. The first detectable sign of dental caries is the appearance of translucent areas on the teeth called white spots. Clinically, no cavitation is evident, although the surface may be rougher than normal. At this early stage of caries development, the incipient lesion may be arrested or even reversed by a process of remineralization. The plaque bacteria ferment dietary carbohydrate into various organic acids, which diffuse into the enamel. As diffu-

sion proceeds, the undissociated acid molecules continuously dissociate, providing H+ ions. These ions interact with the enamel to release calcium and phosphate, which can diffuse out of the lesion. This process continues as long as sufficient acid is available.

Because calcium and phosphate diffuse outward and remineralization is more likely closer to the surface, the enamel surface layer appears intact with a higher mineral content than in the lesion. This remineralization phenomenon, which allows the maintenance of the surface layer of the tooth enamel, is important, and the balance between demineralization and remineralization is critical for maintenance of the tooth structure. Under repeated acid attacks, subsurface dissolution continues, and if remineralization cannot keep pace with mineral loss, the lesion eventually gets to the stage of open cavitation.

As discussed later, the presence of various calcium- and phosphate-containing compounds in the diet may provide anticaries effects by supplying ions to be used in the remineralization process. In addition, it is known that one of the important anticariogenic effects of fluoride is enhancement of the remineralization process.

HUMAN DATA LINKING CARBOHYDRATES TO ORAL DISEASE

Although the caries process is well understood, the specific role of carbohydrates in the caries process in the human population has been difficult to characterize. Beyond the classical Hopewood and Vipeholm studies discussed previously, there are few data on the cariogenicity of foods in humans. For both ethical and practical reasons it is impossible to perform properly controlled human clinical trials on the numerous products continuously being developed by the food processing industry. Consequently, dental scientists have used food analysis and various model test systems to gain an understanding of the cariogenic components in food.

Chemical and Physical Properties of Foods

It seems reasonable that foods could be screened for their cariogenic potential based on their chemical composition. However, although the relationship between fermentable carbohydrates and caries is clear, it has been difficult to relate the carbohydrate content of a particular product with its cariogenic potential. This is due to observations of numerous food components that can alter the cariogenic potential of a food. In addition to the total fermentable carbohydrate content, one needs to consider the concentrations and types of mono-, di-, oligo-, and polysaccharides, proteins, and lipids. The presence of fluoride, calcium, phosphate, and other minerals also influences cariogenic potential. Other compounding factors are the total buffering capacity of the food and saliva and the presence of sialogogues, which stimulate the flow of saliva. Saliva that is rapidly flowing is more alkaline and more supersaturated with calcium and phosphate than resting saliva and, thus, may be more caries-inhibitory.

Some dietary items are highly acidic and therefore affect the pH in plaque and saliva, usually in a transient manner. Distinction should be made between destruction of teeth by a carious process and dissolution of enamel by chemical erosion. In the former process, the production of acids by bacteria acting on a substrate is essential; in the latter, enamel is dissolved by excessive and frequent contact with ingested fluids of low pH (usually below 4). Natural foods, such as lemons, apples, fruit juices, and carbonated beverages, are sufficiently acidic to cause demineralization of enamel. Under normal dietary use, such products are of no consequence in the caries process. However, frequent and excessive use of these foods and beverages may cause etching of enamel and cavitation. Reports of excessive frequency of consumption of carbonated beverages, which have low pH, and continuous chewing or habitual sucking of lemons as causes of dental erosion are well documented.

From a dental standpoint, the physical properties of food may have significance by affecting food retention, food clearance, solubility, and oral hygiene. The incorporation of dyes into toffee has demonstrated the tenacious retention of candy on enamel surfaces. Adhesive properties of food have been measured and correlated with their retention in the mouth. In addition, the physical texture of food is known to affect salivary flow rates, which could affect the cariogenic potential of the food. Indeed, the addition of water to an experimental animal diet or modification of particle size of a diet is known to induce significant effects on caries.

Key Research Findings

Techniques for evaluating the cariogenic potential of foods in the laboratory have been developed to simulate the oral environment. The simulated tests include mixing food with saliva containing viable bacteria and, after incubation, measuring acid production; quantification of release of minerals from enamel; enamel decalcification (demineralization/remineralization studies); and plaque pH studies.

Data from these simulated tests indicate

that only a few foods do not contribute to human plaque acid production. Dental scientists have used various types of pH microelectrodes to demonstrate in studies with human volunteers that most commonly ingested foods (Table 38–1) contain sufficient fermentable carbohydrate to cause the production of plaque acids. All the foods in Table 38–1 cause the pH at interproximal sites (areas between adjoining teeth) in the dentition to fall to close to pH 4 (also see Fig. 38–2). These findings reflect the high sensitivity of the electrodes, the presence of some fermentable carbohydrate in most foods, and the capacity of plaque for rigid metabolism of low concentrations of a wide range of dietary carbohydrates. Table 38–2 lists foods that are hypoacidogenic, nonacidogenic, or minimally acidogenic when tested by interproximal plaque pH telemetry. This limited range of "safe for the teeth" products illustrates the problems involved in attempting to make dietary recommendations for oral health. The wide range of highly acidogenic products (Table 38–1) emphasizes the amazing breadth of the cariogenic challenge presented by the human diet.

TABLE 38–2

Food Products That are Hypoacidogenic, Nonacidogenic, or Minimally Acidogenic as Determined by Interproximal Plaque pH Telemetry

Almonds	Edam cheese	Pepperoni
Beef jerky	Flounder fish	Popcorn (plain)
Beef steak	Gouda cheese	Port du salut
Bologna	Green pepper	cheese
Brie cheese	Ham	Red snapper fish
Broccoli	Hazelnuts	Sugarless candy
Carrots, raw	Monterey jack	Sugarless gum
Cauliflower	cheese	Swiss cheese
Celery	Muenster cheese	Tilsit cheese
Cheddar cheese	Peanuts, plain	Trout fish
(aged)	Pecans	Walleye fish
Cucumber		

The attack on the human teeth from plaque acids may be far greater than previously envisioned. Plaque pH studies using biotelemetry have clearly demonstrated that up to 1000-fold increases in plaque acid concentrations can occur at caries-prone sites between the teeth, and that the resulting low pH can be maintained at these sites for 2 or more hours. Such prolonged intervals at low pH may explain the capacity of dental plaque to demineralize a tissue as hard as enamel and cause development of carious lesions.

Stimulation of the flow of saliva can aid in clearance of food particles from the mouth and can have a dramatic effect on the level of plaque acids. Human saliva has a high buffering capacity owing to the presence of carbonic acid–bicarbonate, phosphate, proteins, ammonia, and urea. Salivary flow can be stimulated physically by the mechanics of chewing or chemically by the presence of sialogogues, such as citric acid, in a food. Consequently, when the pH at interdental sites has decreased through the ingestion of carbohydrate-containing food, the pH can be dramatically elevated toward neutrality by the chewing of paraffin wax or gum. Stimulation of salivary flow brings into the mouth various components capable of enhancing the repair of enamel that has been damaged by plaque acids. Saliva is known to contain high concentrations of calcium and phosphate essential for the natural tooth repair process of remineralization. Enhanced remineralization of dam-

---

TABLE 38–1

Selected List of Acidogenic Foods as Determined by Interproximal Plaque pH Telemetry

Apples, dried	Corn starch	Oats, rolled
Apples, fresh	Crackers, rye	Orange juice
Apple drink	Crackers, soda	Oranges
Apricots, dried	Crackers, wheat	Peaches
Bananas	Dates	Peanut butter
Beans, baked	Doughnuts, jelly	Pears, fresh
Beans, green,	Doughnuts,	Pears, dried
canned	plain	Peas, canned
Bread, white	Fruit bars	Potato, amylose
Bread, whole wheat	Gelatin,	Potato, boiled
Bread, high fiber	sweetened	Potato, French
Cake, chocolate	Graham crackers	fries
Caramel	Granola bar	Potato chips
Carrots, cooked	Granola cereal	Raisins
Cereals,	Grapes	Rice, instant,
nonpresweetened	Gumdrops	cooked
Chocolate, milk	Milk, whole	Soft drinks,
Cola beverage	Milk, 2%	sugarless
Cookies, cream-	Milk, chocolate	Sponge cake,
filled	Nut, fruit mix	filled
Cookies, sugar	Oatmeal, cooked	Tomato, fresh
Cookies, vanilla,		Wheat, flakes
sugar		

aged tooth enamel may occur because of elevated levels of the appropriate ions during and following ingestion of nonacidogenic snacks.

Fluoride, Carbohydrates, and Dental Caries

Fluorides have been shown to play a critical role in the prevention of human dental caries. The metabolism, toxicology, and effectiveness of fluoride and its mechanism of action have been thoroughly studied.

It has been fully documented that the presence of fluoride in enamel crystals improves crystallinity, decreases solubility, and catalyzes a stable apatitic phase, all of which contribute to a reduction of caries formation. The presence of fluoride in plaque has been shown to promote remineralization of the tooth surface. In addition to these activities, it has been suggested that fluoride in plaque may decrease the production of acid from fermentable carbohydrate. It is known that plaque concentrates fluoride, yielding levels thousands of times greater than in saliva. Studies performed in vitro indicate that fluoride may inhibit the enolase in plaque bacteria and thus reduce the active transport of sugars by the phosphoenolpyruvate-dependent bacterial phosphotransferase systems. Enolase is sensitive to 0.5 to 1.0 ppm of fluoride, and such concentrations can easily be found in plaque. Other effects of fluoride in plaque could relate to inhibition of bacterial phosphatases involved in the degradation of sugar phosphates and interference with potassium transport, which is associated with carbohydrate metabolism. It is difficult to evaluate the relative importance of these potential anticaries mechanisms, although clearly the effects on enamel are likely to be the most significant. See Chapters 35 and 36 for more discussion of fluoride.

THE ROLE OF CARBOHYDRATES AND FOODS IN ORAL DISEASE PREVENTION

Studies in various model systems, including caries formation in rats, have failed to demonstrate a linear relationship between the carbohydrate content of a food and its cariogenic potential. It has been shown that many factors in foods can alter the complex interactions involved in disease development (Bowen, 1994; Forward, 1994).

Caries Protective Factors in Foods

Minerals. The effects of mineral constituents of food on caries development have been well documented, with phosphorus-containing compounds being the most numerous. Phosphates have been found to be anticariogenic in animal diets when applied directly to the teeth. These agents include simple inorganic salts ranging from sodium and potassium to more complex polyphosphates, such as trimetaphosphate and pyrophosphate. Organic phosphates such as α-glycerophosphate and phytate have also shown cariostatic activity in animal studies. The presence of phytate has been proposed as the reason for the cariostatic activity of diet additives such as oat or rice seed husks. Phosphates have also been used in human clinical studies as diet additives in bread, flour, sugar, and chewing gum. Positive results have been reported for calcium phosphates in various food products; both trimetaphosphate in chewing gums and sucrose phosphate in the diet reduced caries incidence.

Trace Elements Other than Fluoride. Epidemiological studies in which correlations have been sought between trace elements in drinking water and the prevalence of caries have provided equivocal findings. Both epidemiological data and results from animal studies have demonstrated that ingestion of selenium is associated with an increased prevalence of caries, possibly due to disruption of the formation of the enamel matrix and mineralization of the teeth. Copper appears to decrease acid production in dental plaque and caries formation in rodents. Inclusion of low levels of copper in sugar during the manufacturing process makes the sugar virtually noncariogenic.

Lipids. Various studies indicate that diets high in fat have decreased cariogenic potential. There is minimal information on the role of lipids, although it has been demonstrated that several fatty acids in low concentrations inhibit the growth of the mutans streptococci. The monoglyceride of lauric acid (lauricidin) is inhibitory to gram-positive organisms and has been shown to have modest cariostatic effects. Various cheeses have been shown to have anticariogenic effects; this may be due to their content of inorganic calcium and phosphates, but also it may reflect their lipid content.

Proteins. Reactions involving dietary proteins can effectively raise the pH of plaque. Arginine released from proteins can be metabolized by mutans streptococci to produce ammonia, with the potential to raise the pH of plaque. It is also possible that plaque acids can be removed via the Stickland reaction by which lactate donates two protons to proline, resulting in the production of δ-aminovaleric acid. δ-Aminovaleric acid has been shown to exist in relatively high concentrations in dental plaque.

Food Preservatives. Foods containing preservatives in the form of borate, benzoate, salicylate, and propionate all have the potential to demonstrate anticariogenic activity. These weak acids may diffuse into plaque, stay there for extended intervals, and express antimicrobial activity at low pH.

Human Epidemiological Data and Caries Prevalence/Prevention

Despite voluminous research in the area of caries etiology, many questions persist regarding the exact relationship among caries, the total amount of sugar intake, the frequency of sugar intake, and the sequence in which food items are eaten. Drawing firm conclusions about the relationship between caries and sugars in the human diet is made difficult for several reasons:

1. Sugars are consumed in a variety of physical forms that affect their rate of clearance from the oral cavity.
2. Data concerning sugar consumption at best only approximate the actual sugar consumption.
3. Sugar consumption data are given for

a particular year, but a carious lesion may take years to develop.
4. Other etiological factors such as hygiene, fluoride, and education have important effects on caries prevalence.

Many epidemiological observations have linked increased caries prevalence in developing societies that have adopted westernized dietary patterns and lifestyles, including increased sugar consumption. Perhaps the best example of this type of study was done in the remote Tristan da Cunha islands in the South Atlantic. Historically, the islanders subsisted on a fish-rich diet and showed little evidence of dental caries (Holloway et al., 1963). As the islanders' contacts with "outsiders" increased, dental caries increased dramatically. The compelling feature of the Tristan da Cunha data is the continuity of the caries prevalence data from 1932 through the early 1960s. Sreebny (1982) reviewed the voluminous literature that related sucrose consumption to dental caries; he concluded that groups or communities that had high sugar diets developed high levels of dental caries, whereas others who had low intakes of sugar demonstrated lower levels of dental caries.

On the other hand, Woodward and Walker (1994) conducted an exhaustive statistical analysis of sugar consumption and dental caries among 12-year-old children in 90 countries. For the entire dataset, total dental caries scores rose with total sugar consumption. However, when data from the 29 industrialized nations were analyzed separately, there was no statistically significant sugar-caries relationship. The investigators found their data to be in agreement with the growing body of evidence indicating that the relationship between total sugar consumption and caries incidence in Western countries is not as strong as once believed. Konig and Navia (1995) recently reviewed the role of sugars in oral health and concluded that other factors, such as good oral hygiene and exposure to fluoride, have important effects on caries occurrence and that sugar exposure, per se, does not exert the same strong causative effect on caries activity it once did in the pre-oral hygiene era. Indeed, more recent studies and reviews of epidemiological evidence aimed at assessing the specific relation among human sugar intake, dietary and nutritional patterns, and dental caries demonstrate that sugar consumption alone does not adequately explain the caries incidence or prevalence.

For example, in a study conducted on 405 English children, a high daily consumption of sugar was significantly correlated with increased incidence of caries (Hackett et al., 1984). However, daily sugar intake explained only 4% of the variance in caries increment; 96% of the variance was thus attributable to other factors. Another study was performed in Canada on 232 11-year-old children (LaChapelle et al., 1990). This study showed no relationship between frequency of sugar intake and caries incidence. A third study examined the caries incidence of 499 children aged 11 to 15 years in a nonfluoridated community in Michigan (Burt and Szpunar, 1994). This 3-year study found that caries incidence was poorly related to sugar intake whether measured as total daily consumption, between meal intake, a proportion of total energy intake, or frequency of consumption. These studies suggest that, although sugar continues to be a major etiological factor in dental caries, it is not a sole determinant of the caries experience and is clearly modulated by overall dietary and nutritional intake patterns as well as by fluoride consumption and oral hygiene behaviors. Therefore, caries prevention programs are more likely to benefit from attention paid to a variety of factors that have an impact on the caries process, rather than sugar intake alone. Those other factors, as outlined by Konig and Navia (1995) include

- Oral hygiene
- Fluoride from all sources (including foods, water, tea)
- Plaque bacteria
- Quantity of food residues retained in the oral cavity
- Salivary flow and consumption
- History of and access to oral health care
- Immunological response of the individual
- Nutritional and dietary practices, including dietary intake during tooth and salivary gland development, posteruption food intake patterns, the order and frequency with which foods are eaten, and overall nutritional intake

It is particularly important to note that one of the confounding variables that can affect caries studies data in the human population is the dietary and nutritional intake patterns during tooth and salivary gland development. Cross-sectional surveys demonstrate an apparent inverse correlation between caries prevalence rates in deciduous (baby) teeth and permanent teeth. However, longitudinal data show exactly the opposite correlation. Alvarez and Navia (1989) demonstrated that caries development is delayed as a consequence of delayed tooth eruption due to malnutrition during tooth development. The result is the apparent negative association between caries in deciduous and permanent teeth. However, once the delayed tooth eruption is taken into account, the contribution of malnutrition to increased caries susceptibility is observed.

A growing body of research has been directed at examining the effects of food intake patterns on the oral environment. Food intake patterns involve several factors:

1. Choice of food items
2. Combination of food items eaten together
3. Sequence of consumption of those food items
4. Time lapse between consumption of each item

Human plaque pH measurements have been utilized to assess effects of these variables and have provided important information on food interactions and cariogenic potential.

Geddes (1994) reviewed three such studies that investigated the oral effects associated with different eating patterns. The first and most complete study tested the intraoral acidity of subjects following a meal consisting of a "meat course," a sugary course, sugared coffee, and cheese. Each item was consumed during a predetermined time span, and the order of food item consumption was altered throughout the experiment. Sugar-containing items consistently caused a fall in pH. The cheese always significantly raised the plaque pH, thus protecting against enamel demineralization. The meat source did not alter the plaque pH and did not influence the pH change caused by the other items. If the cheese was consumed immediately following the sugary item, the pH increase counteracted the pH-lowering effect of the sugary item. If the sugary item and the sugared coffee were taken in succession, the pH decrease was greater than if just one of the items had been eaten. Furthermore, an additional test was conducted in which the sugary item was eaten and then the cheese was eaten after a delay of 10 minutes. In this case, the pH had already reached a minimum before the cheese could exert its pH-raising effect. Thus, the interval between consumption of different food items is of great importance. The acidogenic challenge to the teeth by sugared coffee was markedly altered by the timing of drinking during the meal. A similar experiment with a soft-boiled egg, bread and butter, and sugared coffee showed that the plaque pH decrease was kept to a minimum if the coffee was taken before or between the other food items.

The final study reviewed by Geddes (1994) examined whether a noncariogenic snack counters the pH decrease caused by a sugar-containing item (Geddes et al., 1977). In one test, a sugar lump was eaten, followed by an apple eaten for 1 minute. The second test was a sugar lump followed by salted peanuts, eaten for 1 minute. The peanuts had the greatest pH-increasing effect. The pH-raising effect of apples was modest. These studies show that a food item containing sugar will be quickly metabolized and fermented by plaque bacteria, causing a fall in pH. Also, the last item eaten seems to have the greatest effect on the final plaque pH.

In another study, Papas and colleagues (1995) demonstrated that a high intake of cheese was negatively associated with root caries in an elderly population. This added further supportive human evidence for the potential protective effects of cheese on caries, this time on root surfaces. It is clear that the challenge to the teeth can be reduced by the timing and sequence of ingestion of foods without carbohydrate, and the last food ingested may be the most important. The practice of ending a meal with a carbohydrate-containing product (dessert) is not consistent with the health of the teeth.

The concept that dietary patterns that lead to enhanced salivary flow and consequent buffering of plaque acids will have an anticaries effect has led to emphasis on the use of chewing gums after snacks or meals that contain fermentable carbohydrate. A positive effect of the chewing of gum, with no specific anticaries agent, has been demonstrated by plaque pH measurements, but few human caries studies (such as the Turku chewing gum study) have been performed to support this suggestion. Food items that promote salivary stimulation and that promote release of calcium, phosphate, or fluoride are likely to enhance remineralization of enamel damaged by plaque acids. For example, the eating of cheese not only stimulates the flow of saliva but releases calcium from plaque to the tooth surface. Foods that do not contain rapidly fermentable carbohydrate but that do stimulate saliva should not harm and may protect the teeth when taken at the end of a meal or as snacks.

Carbohydrate Substitutes and Dental Caries

The dietary needs of diabetic patients and problems with obesity have driven the search for carbohydrate substitutes or non-nutritive sweetening agents that can be used in food. The relationship between dietary carbohydrate and caries formation has encouraged dental scientists to explore the effects of these substitutes on disease development (Newbrun, 1991). Theoretically, replacement of fermentable carbohydrate in between-meal snacks with sweeteners that cannot be converted to acid by plaque bacteria should reduce the overall cariogenic challenge to the teeth. The evaluation of carbohydrate substitutes has included tests performed in vitro with cariogenic bacteria, animal model studies in which decay can be measured, plaque pH and enamel dissolution tests performed in vivo, and clinical trials in humans. Although the ideal substitute has not been discovered, the potential to make noncariogenic or slightly cariogenic food products has been achieved (Table 38-3).

Sorbitol (D-glucitol) is found in various fruits and berries, seaweeds, and algae and

TABLE 38–3
Cariogenic Potential of Caloric and Noncaloric Sweeteners

Mono- and Disaccharides		Sugar Alcohols		Noncaloric Intense Sweeteners	
Sweetener	*Caries*	*Sweetener*	*Caries*	*Sweetener*	*Caries*
Sucrose	Very high	Xylitol	Nil	Na saccharin	Slight
Glucose	High	Sorbitol	Nil	Acesulfame K	—
Fructose	High	Mannitol	Nil	Aspartame	Nil
High fructose corn syrup	High			Sucralose	Nil
Lactose	Slight to moderate				
Maltose	Probably high				

Adapted from Tanzer, J. M. (1993) Sweeteners and caries: Some emerging issues. In Cariology for the Nineties (Bowen, W. H., Tabak, L. A., eds.), p. 388. University of Rochester Press, Rochester, N. Y.

can be chemically prepared inexpensively from glucose. It is about half as sweet as sucrose and is used in chewing gum, cookies, and soft drinks. Consumption of high concentrations of it can result in laxative effects. It is interesting that although most oral bacteria will not ferment sorbitol, many strains of the cariogenic mutans streptococci will ferment the compound. However, plaque pH measurements have demonstrated minimal acid production from sorbitol. Human clinical studies have shown that chewing sorbitol-containing gum does not promote the development of dental caries.

Xylitol is a pentose alcohol found in fruits and vegetables. It is obtained commercially from birch trees, cottonseed hulls, and coconut shells. Its sweetness is equal to that of sucrose. Like sorbitol, it is only slowly absorbed from the gastrointestinal tract and, therefore, draws water into the bowel by osmotic effects; it causes diarrhea if ingested in excessive amounts. Plaque pH studies have demonstrated that xylitol rinses do not cause plaque acid production (Birkhed, 1994). The Turku study clearly demonstrated that xylitol is noncariogenic in humans. The mechanism for xylitol-induced reductions in caries incidence is not clear. Proposed mechanisms include stimulation of salivary flow, reduction in the level of *S. mutans,* and enhancement of remineralization. Xylitol is approved for use in foods, cosmetics, and pharmaceuticals in about 40 countries. In the United States, xylitol has been approved for special dietary use since 1963. It is used as a sweetener in non-

cariogenic confectionery, in dietetic foods for diabetics, in pharmaceutical products, and in some dentifrices. A deterrent to the use of xylitol as a sweetener is its cost, compared with sucrose.

Other carbohydrate substitutes that have been evaluated, although on a limited basis relative to dental caries, include lactitol (β-D-galactopyranosyl-1,4-sorbitol), maltitol (α-D-glucopyranosyl-1,4-sorbitol), starch hydrolysates, glycosylsucrose, and L-sorbose. A variety of artificial sweeteners or non-nutritive sweeteners are also used in food products. These include aspartame, acesulfame potassium, and saccharin, which are widely used in the United States, as well as sucralose, cyclamate, and alitame, which are not presently approved for use in this country.

THE ROLE OF CARBOHYDRATES IN OTHER ORAL DISEASES

Although the role of carbohydrates in dental caries is well characterized, its roles in the myriad of other oral diseases, such as craniofacial anomalies, osteoporosis, cancer, and infection, have not been extensively studied. Periodontal disease is a collection of a variety of multifactorial infectious diseases of the soft tissues (gingiva) surrounding the teeth and their supporting structures, including alveolar bone. Many studies have concluded that, although periodontal disease is initiated by plaque microorganisms, nutrition can modulate the initiation and progression of the dis-

NUTRITION INSIGHT

Artificial Sweeteners

Aspartame, acesulfame potassium, and saccharin are approved for use as artificial sweeteners in the United States. Because these compounds are not substrates for fermentation by oral bacteria, as well as because of their intense sweeteners or non-nutritive value, they have been used widely in products such as gums, sweeteners for coffee and tea, and various desserts.

Aspartame (L-aspartyl-L-phenylalanyl methyl ester) is a dipeptide that is approximately 200 times as sweet as sucrose. The Food and Drug Administration (FDA) has approved its use as a table-top sugar substitute, as a tablet, or as an additive in cereals, drink mixes, carbonated beverages, instant coffee and tea, chewing gums, gelatins, puddings, fillings, dairy products, and toppings. More recently, approval has been extended for its use in noncarbonated fruit juices, fruit drinks, frozen stick-type confections, breath mints, and as a sweetening agent in drug products. Encapsulated forms are available for commercial baking. The relative cost of sweetening with aspartame is nearly six times that of sucrose. Aspartame is not metabolized to acid by oral bacteria, may reduce plaque formation, and is considered noncariogenic. Products that contain aspartame carry a warning label because individuals with phenylketonuria (PKU), an inborn error of metabolism, must limit their intake of phenylalanine. Although aspartame is a nutritive sweetener because it is digested and its amino acid components are metabolized, its intense sweetness makes it essentially noncaloric.

Acesulfame K (3,4-dihydro-6-methyl-1,2,3 oxathiazine-4-one-2,2-dioxide potassium salt) is approximately 200 times as sweet as sucrose. Unlike aspartame, which loses it sweetness when heated, acesulfame K retains its sweetness when heated and is suitable for cooking and baking. This sweetener has been approved by the FDA for use in dry food products, such as chewing gums, dry mixes for beverages, instant coffee, instant tea, gelatins, puddings, and nondairy creamers and for use as a table-top sweetener. It has also been approved for use in hard and soft candies, baked goods and mixes, yogurt, frozen and refrigerated desserts, sweet sauces, toppings, and syrups. It compares well with sucrose for cost, is stable in many food products, may decrease the growth of mutans streptococci, and is considered noncariogenic. Acesulfame K is noncaloric.

Saccharin is a noncaloric sweetener that is about 300 times as sweet as sucrose. It has a slightly bitter aftertaste. It is currently used in soft drinks, table-top sweeteners, chewing gums, other beverages and foods, and pharmaceuticals. Since 1977, when studies showed that high doses of saccharin caused bladder cancer in rodents and hence it was labeled as a potential carcinogen, the FDA has required that products that contain saccharin carry a warning label indicating that saccharin has been determined to cause cancer in laboratory animals. The issue of whether saccharin belongs on the list of cancer-causing chemicals remains controversial.

ease. Some animal studies have suggested that sugars can influence periodontal health by contributing to the volume of plaque, resulting in the establishment of a more "virulent" or "altered" subgingival microflora. Although the relationship between general nutrition and cellular and molecular immune response is clear, there appears to be few supportive data linking carbohydrates to the etiology and progression of periodontal disease. One relationship of note that has important implications is that diabetes mellitus, a metabolic dysfunction affecting glucose me-

tabolism, is an important risk factor in the initiation and progression of periodontitis.

PREVENTION OF ORAL DISEASE

Perhaps the most fundamental advance in recent years related to food intake patterns and dental caries is the recognition that oral health preventive programs must transcend the previous sole focus on sugar intake. Rather than making blanket recommendations for the general public to reduce intake of sugar or other potentially cariogenic foods, attention must be directed to those populations, groups, and individuals who are at high risk for dental caries. These populations include individuals from lower socioeconomic backgrounds, recent immigrants from developing or "non-Western" cultures, individuals with salivary gland dysfunctions, individuals who are on medications that restrict salivary flow, patients receiving chemotherapy or radiation for head and neck cancers, populations with limited access to fluoride, and individuals with chewing dysfunctions.

When diet is improved, particularly as sugar intake is decreased, all aspects of the individual's health will be affected in a positive manner, including the ability to withstand bacterial and antigenic infectious challenges. Additionally, when the dietary and nutritional assessments are extended to prospective parents, pregnant women, and infants, one can be assured of tissues and organs that have optimal likelihood of reaching their genetic potential. Rational and judicious use of dietary and nutritional information, targeted when necessary to high-risk populations, groups, or individuals, will provide an acceptable and effective basis for prevention of dental caries while improving systemic health and preventing disease.

REFERENCES

Alvarez, J. O. and Navia, J. M. (1989) Nutritional status, tooth eruption, and dental caries: A review. Am J Clin Nutr 49:417–426.

Birkhed, D. (1994) Cariologic aspects of xylitol and its uses in chewing gum: A review. Acta Odontol Scand 52:116–127.

Bowen, W. H. (1994) Food components and caries. Adv Dent Res 8:215–220.

Burt, B. A. and Szpunar, S. M. (1994) The Michigan Study: The relationship between sugar intake and dental caries over three years. Int Dent J 44:230–240.

Forward, G. C. (1994) Non-fluoride anticaries agents. Adv Dent Res 8:208–214.

Geddes, D. A. M. (1994) Diet patterns and caries. Adv Dent Res 8:221–224.

Geddes, D. A. M., Edgar, W. M., Jenkins, G. N. and Rugg-Gunn, A. J. (1977) Apples, salted peanuts, and plaque pH. Br Dent J 140:317–319.

Gustafsson, B. E., Quensel, C. E., Lanke, L. S., Lundqvist, C., Grahnen, H., Bonow, B. E. and Krasse, B. (1954) The Vipeholm Dental Caries Study: The effect of different carbohydrate intake on caries activity in 436 individuals observed for five years. Acta Odontol Scand 11:232–264.

Hackett, A. F., Rugg-Gunn, A. J., Appleton, D. R., Allinson, M. and Eastoe, J. E. (1984) Sugar-eating habits of 405 11- to 14-year-old English children. Br J Nutr 51:347–356.

Harris, R. (1963) Biology of the children of Hopewood House, Bowral, Australia. 4. Observations on dental caries experience extending over five years (1957–1961). J Dent Res 42:1387–1399.

Holloway, P. J., James, P. M. C. and Slack, G. C. (1963) Dental diseases in Tristan Da Cunha. Br Dent J 115:19–25.

Konig, K. and Navia, J. M. (1995) Nutritional role of sugars in oral health. Am J Clin Nutr 62(suppl):275S–283S.

LaChapelle, D., Couture, C., Brodeur, J. M. and Servigny, J. (1990) The effects of nutritional quality and frequency of consumption of sugary foods on dental caries increment. Can J Public Health 81:370–375.

Loesche, W. J. (1986) Role of *Streptococcus mutans* in human dental decay. Microbiol Rev 50:353–380.

Newbrun, E. (1969) Sucrose: The arch enemy of dental caries. J Dent Child 36:239–248.

Newbrun, E. (1991) Dental effects of sugars and sweeteners. In: Sugars and Sweeteners (Kretchmer, N. and Hollenbeck, C. B., eds.), pp. 175–202. CRC Press, Ann Arbor, MI.

Newbrun, E., Hoover, C., Mettraux, G. and Graf, H. (1980) Comparison of dietary habits and dental health of subjects with hereditary fructose intolerance and control subjects. J Am Dent Assoc 109:619–626.

Papas, A. S., Joshi, A., Belanger, A., Kent, R., Palmer, C. and DePaola, P. F. (1995) Dietary models for root caries. Am Clin Nutr 61(suppl):417S–422S.

Scheinin, A., Makinen, K. K. and Ylitalo, K. (1975) Turku sugar studies. 1. An intermediate report on the effect of sucrose, fructose and xylitol diets on the caries incidence in man. Acta Odontol Scand 70:5–34.

Sreebny, L. M. (1982) Sugar and human dental caries. World Rev Nutr Diet 40:19–65.

Stephan, R. M. (1940) Changes in hydrogen-ion concentration on tooth surfaces and in carious lesions. J Am Dent Assoc 27:718–723.

Woodward, M. and Walker, A. R. (1994) Sugar consumption and dental caries: Evidence from 90 countries. Br Dent J 176:297–302.

RECOMMENDED READINGS

Bowen, W. H. and Tabak, L. (1993) Cariology for the Nineties. University of Rochester Press, Rochester, N.Y.

Navia, J. M. (1994) Carbohydrates and dental health. Am J Clin Nutr 59(suppl):719S–727S.

Rugg-Gunn, A. J. (ed.) (1994) Sugarless—Towards the Year 2000. The Royal Society of Chemistry, Special Publication No. 144, Cambridge, U.K.

Tougher-Decker, R. (1996) Nutrition in dental health. In: Food, Nutrition, and Diet Therapy, (Mahan, L. K. and Escott-Stump, S., eds.), 9th ed., pp. 581–593. W. B. Saunders, Philadelphia.

CHAPTER 39

Fuel Utilization by Skeletal Muscle During Rest and During Exercise

Anton J. M. Wagenmakers, Ph.D.

OUTLINE

COMMON ABBREVIATIONS

RQ (respiratory quotient, defined as moles CO_2 produced/moles O_2 consumed; also
  known as respiratory exchange ratio, RER)

VO_{2max} (maximum aerobic capacity; measure of maximum volume of O_2 consumption)

SKELETAL MUSCLE FUEL UTILIZATION DURING REST

Skeletal muscle is the largest body compartment in humans, accounting for 40% to 50% of body mass in an ordinary lean subject. As such, skeletal muscle can have major effects on human metabolism, whole-body energy expenditure, and nutritional requirements.

Skeletal Muscle Fuel Needs During Rest

During rest, energy expenditure is low, and resting skeletal muscle needs less energy for maintenance than intra-abdominal tissues such as liver, gut, or kidney. The latter tissues not only have to take care of their own maintenance but also serve many essential functions in whole-body metabolism (e.g., digestion, absorption, fluid retention, urea synthesis, fatty acid synthesis, lipoprotein synthesis) and as the sites of synthesis of many export proteins (e.g., albumin, fibrinogen, apolipoproteins, digestive enzymes). Apart from a few muscles that continuously are active in the maintenance of posture, skeletal muscle in resting conditions has a low energy expenditure. At rest, energy in the form of ATP, the universal energy donor, as in all other cells is required only

> to maintain electrolyte and calcium gradients via ATP-dependent ion pumps
> to maintain amino acid gradients (much higher intracellular than extracellular concentrations)
> to replace fuel stores lost via oxidation (glycogen and intramuscular triacylglycerols)
> to keep substrate cycles going (e.g., the fructose-6-phosphate/fructose 1,6-bisphosphate cycle and the triacylglycerol-free fatty acid cycle)
> and to maintain the continuous synthesis and breakdown of proteins (protein turnover).

Even from the point of view of protein turnover, skeletal muscle needs less energy than intra-abdominal tissues because the mean turnover rate of skeletal muscle protein (0.05% per h) is lower than that of most other proteins of the human body and much lower than that of the intracellular and export proteins of liver and gut (e.g., apolipoprotein B-100, which is synthesized in the liver, with a turnover rate of 16% per h). The need, therefore, for ATP synthesis during rest is easily met by aerobic metabolism (oxidation). For these reasons, skeletal muscle oxygen consumption constitutes only 25% of whole body oxygen consumption during resting conditions, despite the fact that the skeletal muscle compartment constitutes 40% to 50% of body mass.

Skeletal muscle oxidizes a mixture of carbohydrate and fat during rest. Although the impact of skeletal muscle gas exchange on the whole-body (systemic) respiratory quotient (RQ) is small, measurements of the arteriovenous difference for oxygen and carbon dioxide across skeletal muscle have demonstrated the relative importance of fats and carbohydrates as fuels for the resting muscle. The RQ is defined as moles CO_2 produced/moles O_2 consumed, and it is usually measured as volume of CO_2 produced/volume of O_2 consumed. In 1927, Himwich and Rose, using such techniques in dogs, observed that the RQ of skeletal muscle in fed dogs was about 0.92, and that in starved dogs the value decreased to 0.80 and lower. As an RQ of 1.00 indicates 100% carbohydrate oxidation and a value of 0.70 indicates 100% fat oxidation, it is clear that skeletal muscle at rest always oxidizes a mixture of carbohydrate and fat. This finding has been confirmed in humans on many occasions, using the same techniques.

Use of Plasma Glucose and of Fatty Acids Obtained from Plasma Free Fatty Acids and Lipoproteins During the Resting State

The next question is which carbohydrate sources and which fat sources are oxidized by skeletal muscle. In both cases there is a choice between intramuscular and extracellular sources. For carbohydrates the sources are the glycogen stores in skeletal muscle and blood glucose. Blood glucose originates from the diet in the first hours after a meal (i.e., during the postprandial period) and originates from the liver in the postabsorptive and fasted state. In the fed state, the liver contains about 70 to 80 g of glycogen. The breakdown of liver glycogen to glucose is the major source of hepatic glucose output in the first 16 h of fasting, whereas gluconeogenesis from glycerol and amino acids becomes the primary source of hepatic glucose output after 16 to 24 h of fasting. Blood glucose is the major source of carbohydrate for oxidation in skeletal muscle at rest, and breakdown rates of muscle glycogen are insignificant both in the fed and in the postabsorptive state. Skeletal muscle of an adult contains about 350 to 800 g of glycogen when the intramuscular stores are full.

Fatty acids may be obtained for oxidation by muscle from three potential sources. The first source consists of the free fatty acids circulating in the blood bound to albumin. Free fatty acids originate either from the diet (the plasma concentration is about 0.3 mmol/L after ingestion of a mixed diet) or, in the postabsorptive state and during fasting, from mobilization from the large triacylglycerol stores in adipose tissue (leading to plasma concentrations of 1.0 to 1.5 mmol/L after a few days of fasting). A 70-kg individual of normal body composition contains some 16 kg of adipose tissue (composed of 12.5 kg of lipid, 3.1 kg of water, and 0.5 kg of protein).

The second potential source of fatty acids lies in the triacylglycerols circulating in the blood as lipoproteins. The endothelial wall of the capillary bed in skeletal muscle (as in many other tissues) contains the enzyme called lipoprotein lipase, which liberates fatty acids from chylomicrons and very low density lipoproteins (VLDL). Most of the fatty acids thus liberated are directly taken up by muscle, although some escape and enter the circulation as free fatty acids.

A third potential source of fatty acids lies in the intramuscular triacylglycerols. These are present in the muscle fibers as small lipid droplets and are also in the adipocytes present between fibers. Skeletal muscle contains hormone-sensitive lipase, which can liberate fatty acids from the intramuscular triacylglycerol stores. Although blood free fatty acids traditionally have been seen as the main source of fatty acids for oxidation in muscle, especially during fasting, the possibility that direct mobilization of fatty acids from chylomicrons and VLDL, and maybe also from intramuscular triacylglycerols, contributes significant amounts of fatty acids for oxidation in muscle should be considered. The relative proportion of these sources that are used by muscle, either during rest or during exercise, is not known because of lack of suitable methods for making these determinations.

The Transition from Carbohydrate Utilization in the Postprandial State to Fat Utilization in the Fasted State

RQ measurements across the leg have shown that carbohydrates are the main fuel for skeletal muscle in the fed situation, whereas fat oxidation accounts for 80% to 90% or more of oxygen consumption in the postabsorptive and fasted situation. The transition from the fed to the fasted state is carefully controlled, as described in Chapters 9, 13, and 16. In the postprandial situation, high plasma insulin concentrations lead to a rapid uptake of blood glucose by skeletal muscle. The insulin-stimulated translocation of glucose transporter-4 (GLUT4) from membranes of the endoplasmic reticulum into the plasma membrane plays an important role in the insulin-stimulated glucose uptake into skeletal muscle (Brozinick et al., 1994). From a quantitative point of view, skeletal muscle is the most important tissue for the removal of glucose that enters the blood after oral ingestion of carbohydrates. Glucose uptake by skeletal muscle, therefore, is extremely important for glucose homeostasis and prevents large peaks in blood glucose concentration following meals. The glucose is used both for glycogen synthesis (especially in individuals who are regularly involved in exercise and who, therefore, regularly deplete their muscle glycogen stores) and for fuel.

Simultaneously, the high insulin concentrations, via inhibition of hormone-sensitive lipase, restrict lipolysis in adipose tissue and skeletal muscle so that no mobilization of fatty acid from these triacylglycerol stores occurs. Malonyl CoA concentrations in muscle, furthermore, are high in the fed state and keep the rate of fatty acid oxidation low by inhibiting carnitine palmitoyltransferase I (Sugden and Holness, 1994). The fatty acids present in

NUTRITION INSIGHT

Nutritional Ergogenic Aids

Athletes have long been searching for means that will give them an additional advantage over their competitors. Even small positive effects are considered to be important as the time difference separating number one and two in competition in most cases is minimal, whereas the social and material/financial consequences will be vastly different (beyond proportion when compared with other disciplines/professions). The battery of means in use to improve performance are generally known as ergogenic aids. The term ergogenic means "work-generating" and is derived from the Greek word *ergo,* meaning work. Ergogenic aids can be classified into different categories (Williams, 1992)—i.e., mechanical aids (e.g., lighter sports equipment and improved aerodynamics); psychological aids (e.g., stress and anxiety control), pharmacological aids (e.g., caffeine, anabolic steroids, erythropoietin, clenbuterol), physiological aids (e.g., sodium bicarbonate, blood infusion), and nutritional aids (e.g., carbohydrate loading and the use of dietary supplements like vitamins, carnitine, creatine, special amino acids, and special fatty acids).

Most pharmacological and physiological aids, when taken in abnormal quantities, meet the definition of doping and, therefore, are included in the list of substances banned by the International Olympic Committee. The reason for banning is that the use of many of these compounds also presents considerable health risks to the users, either in the acute period of usage or in the long-term. For example, erythropoietin, a hormone that leads to an increase in the number of circulating red blood cells, may increase the viscosity of the blood so far that fatal circulatory problems could occur either during high-intensity exercise or during periods of low cardiac output, e.g., in the overnight resting state. The long-term use of clenbuterol, a drug with β-agonist action and a proven ability to reduce fat mass and increase muscle mass in meat-producing farm animals, could lead to a further increase in size of the already enlarged heart in a top athlete and increase the risk for development of cardiovascular complications.

In contrast to the use of pharmacological aids, the use of nutritional supplements that are expected to have performance-enhancing effects is generally accepted and has become very popular. Some of the most common nutritional supplements are creatine, carnitine, branched-chain amino acids, and medium-chain fatty acids. Despite their widespread use, there is little metabolic basis or evidence from controlled studies to support the beneficial claims made for most of these supplements (Wagenmakers, 1999).

the diet appear in the circulation mainly as triacylglycerols in chylomicrons. They are primarily directed to the adipose tissue stores, because the activity of lipoprotein lipase in adipose tissue is much higher than the activity of lipoprotein lipase in skeletal muscle in animals in the fed state (Sugden et al., 1993). All these mechanisms limit fat utilization and make carbohydrates the main skeletal muscle fuel in the fed state.

In the transition to the fasted state, the insulin concentrations gradually fall, leading to a return of GLUT4 from the plasma membrane to the endoplasmic reticulum, and to a reduction of glucose uptake by the muscle. This is paralleled by a decrease of the malonyl CoA concentration in muscle and relief of inhibition of carnitine palmitoyltransferase I, allowing fatty acids to enter the mitochondria

for β-oxidation. Simultaneously, free fatty acid mobilization from adipose tissue is accelerated owing to the removal of the inhibitory effect of insulin on hormone-sensitive lipase and via an increase of the direct nervous activity to the fat tissue. As a result, the plasma concentrations of free fatty acids rise, making more free fatty acids available for oxidation in muscle. The increased oxidation of free fatty acids in skeletal muscle suppresses glucose oxidation and uptake via the glucose–fatty acid (Randle) cycle.

The Randle cycle originally was discovered in rat heart in vitro, but it also operates under resting conditions in human skeletal muscle in vivo (Nuutila et al., 1992). The Randle or glucose–fatty acid cycle refers to the inhibition of glucose utilization when fatty acids are available as an alternative fuel. The

Randle cycle also helps suppress glucose oxidation in muscle in the postabsorptive and fasted situation, thus saving glucose for tissues that depend more heavily on glucose as a fuel (e.g., the brain).

Skeletal muscle lipoprotein lipase activities have been reported to increase dramatically between 9 and 12 h of fasting in rats, whereas adipose tissue lipoprotein lipase activities declined by 50% after 6 h of fasting and continued to fall when fasting was continued for 24 h (Sugden et al., 1993). During the first hours of refeeding, following 12 h of fasting, skeletal muscle lipoprotein lipase remained high (in comparison with values in rats fed ad libitum). A programmed shift in the expression of lipoprotein lipase in different tissues in response to the dietary intake, therefore, seems to direct fatty acids from chylomicrons and very low density lipoproteins (VLDL) into adipose tissue for storage in the fed state, and fatty acids from VLDL into muscle for oxidation in the postabsorptive and fasted state. Some of the fatty acids from chylomicrons also seem to be directed into the muscle during the refeeding period, potentially to refill the part of the intramuscular triacylglycerol store that was lost during overnight fasting (Sugden et al., 1993).

THE ENERGY COST OF MOVEMENT

Muscle shortening and movement are brought about by repeated formation of cross-bridges between the thin (actin) and thick (myosin) filaments of the myofibrils. This process costs energy and requires hydrolysis of ATP by the myofibrillar ATPase. The contraction cycles are under nervous control. Whenever a minimal number of nerve impulses during a limited time period arrive at the muscle fiber, the following sequence is set into action: (1) The plasma membrane is depolarized by a short-term loss of potassium ions and uptake of sodium ions in the muscle; (2) the formed action potential is propagated along the sarcolemma into the transverse (T) tubules, where (3) the signal is transmitted to the sarcoplasmic reticulum; this then leads to (4) a rapid release of calcium ions (Ca^{2+}) from the sarcoplasmic reticulum and a 1000-fold increase in the cytosolic Ca^{2+} concentration. This in-

crease in cytosolic Ca^{2+} leads to (5) cross-bridge formation and (6) activation of the myofibrillar ATPase and ATP hydrolysis to break the formed cross-bridges again. The cytosolic Ca^{2+} concentration simultaneously is reduced again by the action of the calcium ATPase in the sarcoplasmic reticulum, and the muscle is ready for the next contraction.

The myofibrillar ATPase, the Na^+, K^+-ATPase (needed to restore the membrane potential following a depolarization), and the Ca^{2+}-ATPase all are much more active during exercise than at rest, and, therefore, greater amounts of ATP are needed during exercise. A muscle can in seconds increase its aerobic ATP turnover rate more than 100-fold (see calculation made later). The higher the exercise intensity, the more contraction cycles are needed per unit of time, the more ATP needs to be synthesized, and the more fuels need to be oxidized. Energy expenditure of skeletal muscle, therefore, is greatly influenced by the increased contractile activity needed to walk, work, or run.

At rest, whole-body energy expenditure of humans is about 80 watts or 68 kcal/h (comparable to that of a light bulb), with about 25% (20 watts or 17 kcal/h) being expended in the skeletal muscles. Energy expenditure during a marathon run covering 42 km in a little over 2 hours is about 20 times resting energy expenditure (1600 watts or 1377 kcal/h). As more than 90% of the increase in energy expenditure originates from fuel oxidation in the active muscle (part is needed for the cardiovascular response), and assuming that maximally about half of skeletal muscle mass is actively used in running a marathon, the energy expenditure of the active muscle can be estimated to go up more than 130-fold (from 10 watts to 1368 watts), as shown in Figure 39–1. Skeletal muscle, therefore, must have powerful mechanisms to increase the rates of ATP synthesis and fuel oxidation. In an individual running a marathon, most of the required ATP is produced by aerobic oxidation of carbohydrate and fat.

A top-class sprinter during a 100-m sprint can achieve a power output of around 3600 watts—that is, about 45 times resting energy expenditure at whole-body level. As over 95% of the increase in energy expenditure origi-

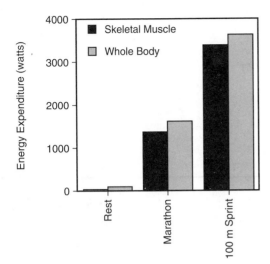

Figure 39–1. Whole-body and muscle energy expenditure at rest, during marathon running, and during a 100-meter sprint. One watt is equivalent to 1 J/s or 2.39 × 10⁻⁴ kcal/s. One thousand watts, thus, is equivalent to an energy expenditure of 0.239 kcal/s or 14 kcal/min or 860 kcal/h.

nates from increased fuel metabolism in the active muscle during a sprint, the energy expenditure of the active muscle is estimated to go up more than 300-fold. Most of the ATP for a 100-m sprint is produced anaerobically by net breakdown of muscle creatine phosphate and by conversion of glycogen to lactate.

FUELS FOR SPRINTING

As the energy requirement of a 100-m sprint is extremely high and the sprint lasts only 10 s, only the fuels present in muscle can be used for ATP synthesis. Moreover, oxygen cannot be transported quickly enough to the active skeletal muscle mass. Even a top-class athlete does not consume more than 0.5 L of oxygen during the 100-m sprint. This implies that more than 95% of the phenomenal need for ATP synthesis (24 g/s) must be derived from anaerobic metabolism. This leaves only two energy sources as main contributors to the ATP production during the 100-m sprint: muscle creatine phosphate and muscle glycogen stores. The use of these fuels over the duration of a 10-s sprint is illustrated in Figure 39–2.

Use of Creatine Phosphate for Maintenance of ATP Levels During the First Few Seconds of Sprinting

In the first seconds after leaving the starting block, ATP is not yet synthesized by glycolysis at the required rate. At the same time, only about 20% of the ATP content of the muscle is lost. Greater losses probably would lead locally to ATP concentrations that are too low to allow the myofibrillar ATPase and ion pumps to function at maximal velocity during exercise. Creatine phosphate plays a critical role in maintenance of ATP levels under these conditions. During the first seconds of the sprint, ATP lost during contraction is almost instantaneously regenerated from creatine phosphate. The concentration of creatine phosphate in human muscle is 80 to 85 μmol per g of dry muscle—that is, some four to five times higher than the ATP concentration. During the first 4 to 5 s of sprinting, about 80% of the creatine phosphate pool is lost and used to regenerate ATP. The transfer of the phosphate group from creatine phosphate to ADP generated during contraction is catalyzed by the enzyme creatine kinase in the following reaction:

$$\text{Creatine phosphate} + \text{ADP} + \text{H}^+ \leftrightarrow \text{Creatine} + \text{ATP}$$

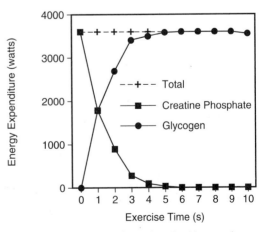

Figure 39–2. Utilization of creatine phosphate and muscle glycogen as fuels over the course of a 100-meter sprint.

NUTRITION INSIGHT

Use of Creatine as an Ergogenic Aid

The main sources of creatine for humans are dietary intake (1 to 2 g per day, mostly from meat products) and endogenous biosynthesis in liver and kidney (1 to 2 g per day). Creatine absorbed from the diet and endogenously synthesized is transported via the blood to the muscle and taken up by muscle by an active transport mechanism against a concentration gradient. In a 70-kg man, the total body creatine pool is approximately 120 g, 95% of which is found in muscle.

In muscle, creatine can be converted to creatine phosphate by creatine kinase. Creatine phosphate is present in resting muscle in a 25- to 30-μmol/g concentration, which is three to four times the concentration of ATP. During high-intensity exercise, regeneration of ATP, split by muscle contraction to ADP, is important if fatigue is to be delayed. An important function of creatine phosphate in muscle is to provide the high-energy phosphate group for ATP regeneration during the first seconds of high-intensity exercise, thus allowing time for glycogen breakdown and glycolysis to speed up to the required rate. Increased generation of ATP by the creatine kinase reaction reduces the necessity to accelerate glycolysis and, therefore, could lead to a reduced lactate production and better maintenance of the intramuscular pH. Decreases of the ATP concentration and of the intramuscular pH play important roles in the mechanisms leading to fatigue during intense maximal exercise. The creatine kinase reaction also has a buffering action in muscle as it uses a hydrogen ion during the regeneration of ATP from creatine phosphate and ADP.

The creatine phosphate store in muscle is finite and can fall to almost zero within 4 to 5 seconds of maximal sprinting. Therefore, nutritional means that lead to an increase of the creatine phosphate content ought to lead to a more prolonged maintenance of the ATP concentration and of the intramuscular pH and would, therefore, from a theoretical point of view, improve performance during intense maximal exercise (e.g., sprinting). This advantage also is expected to be present during sport activities involving intermittent high-intensity exercise, allowing sufficient time for recovery of the creatine phosphate pool or part of it between subsequent sprints (tennis, football, soccer, etc.). Such a theoretical advantage is not to be expected during prolonged aerobic endurance exercise, as creatine phosphate breakdown is minimal in that case.

Oral ingestion of creatine (about 20 g/day for 5 to 6 days) increases the muscle total creatine content in men by about 20% (30% to 40% of this increase is creatine phosphate). A subsequent daily dose of 2 to 3 g is enough for maintenance of this increased concentration and is likely to be safe during long-term use as it hardly exceeds the normal dietary intake. When the creatine is ingested in carbohydrate-containing solutions, then the increase in muscle total creatine has been suggested to be about 30% (Greenhaff, 1997).

Continued

Use of Glycogenolysis and Glycolysis (Lactate Production) to Provide Energy for Sprinting

The 20% decrease in the ATP content during the first seconds of sprinting is also extremely important in muscle fuel utilization during anaerobic metabolism, because it leads to a rapid increase in the concentration of free AMP and free ADP. (Note that most of the AMP and ADP in muscle is bound to myosin and actin; "free" refers to the portion of these nucleoside phosphates that is not bound to proteins and hence is available for metabolic regulation.) Free AMP and free ADP are important allosteric regulators of the key enzymes in the glycolytic pathway (glycogen phosphorylase and phosphofructokinase), and increases in their concentrations in combination with the contraction-induced rise in cytosolic calcium (and changes in the concentrations of several other allosteric effectors) lead to a massive increase in the rate of glycogenolysis and glycolysis (lactate production) during the first seconds of sprinting.

The rise in free ADP during the first me-

NUTRITION INSIGHT

Use of Creatine as an Ergogenic Aid *(Continued)*

Creatine loading (20 g for 5 to 6 days) in agreement with the theory significantly increased the amount of work performed during repeated bouts of short-lasting high intensity exercise (both dynamic and isokinetic) in many studies published so far although not all (Greenhaff, 1997). Only a few studies have shown an ergogenic effect during single bouts of competition-type maximal exercise in highly trained athletes. No studies have shown an ergogenic effect on endurance performance. The increase in body weight (1 to 2 kg) that is observed in many consumers could be disadvantageous for marathon runners or in sports in which part of the energy output is required to counteract gravitational forces (long jump, high jump, cycling, and running on hills or mountains). It is still not clear whether this increase in body weight is the consequence of water retention or whether it reflects an increase in lean body or muscle mass.

Only a few studies have investigated the combined effects of long-term (>4 weeks) creatine ingestion and strength training (for references, see Wagenmakers, 1999). These studies report larger improvements of the maximal strength and maximal intermittent exercise capacity of the muscle groups trained in subjects combining a strength-training program with creatine ingestion. It is also suggested that muscle mass and fat-free mass increase more in the subjects ingesting creatine. This apparent enhancing effect on the effectiveness of strength training may be explained both by the possibility that the higher creatine content enables the athletes to do more repetitions during training at a higher speed or workload and by the possibility that creatine exerts a direct anabolic effect in the muscle. Further research is needed to clarify this point. The effect of long-term creatine ingestion in subjects involved in endurance training programs has yet to be investigated.

In summary, short-term creatine loading (20 g/day for 5 to 6 days) leads to an increase in the muscle content of creatine and creatine phosphate. There is a sound metabolic basis to expect a performance effect of creatine loading on performance during brief intense and maximal exercise and repetitive intense exercise with an anaerobic component. Creatine loading has been shown to enhance performance during repeated bouts of high-intensity exercise (dynamic and isokinetic) in the laboratory. Therefore, creatine loading could be of use to enhance performance in sports practice, particularly in track sprinting events (100 to 800 m), during short-distance swimming, and in team sports with an intermittent high exercise intensity (football, soccer, tennis, hockey, basketball, and so on). The long-term ingestion of creatine in combination with strength training appears to enhance muscular strength and potentially may increase muscle mass. Long-term creatine ingestion, therefore, could be useful in body builders and weight lifters and those in other sports with strength components. For safety reasons, creatine loading (20 g for 5 to 6 days) should be followed by a much lower maintenance dose (2 to 3 g/day) if the creatine ingestion is prolonged for many weeks.

ters of sprinting, coupled with the decrease in cytosolic pH (as a consequence of ATP hydrolysis and lactate production), also forces the creatine kinase equilibrium to rapid ATP production. The contribution of this reaction to ATP synthesis is greatest in the first second of sprinting and then gradually falls to zero in the next 4 s, during which glycolysis (lactate production) is coming up to full speed.

Breakdown of the glycogen stores and subsequent glycolysis with formation of lactate is quantitatively the most important process for ATP production during sprinting. In about 4 to 5 s from the start of a sprint, the rate of glycolysis goes up 1000-fold or more. This increase in rate implies that the rate at which the muscle glycogen stores are broken down is very high during sprinting at top speed. Theoretically, there is enough glycogen in the muscle for about 800 to 1500 m of sprinting at maximal speed. However, even world-class athletes begin to slow down after 80 to 100 m and cannot maintain full speed. The reason for this is that fatigue processes come into operation and start to reduce the force-generating capacity of the muscle. The exact mechanism of fatigue during sprinting is not known, but the rapid increase in the concentration of inorganic phosphate, the decrease of the muscle pH (due to lactate accumulation), and disturbed ion balances (K^+ and Ca^{2+}) have all been implicated in these mechanisms. (For a review of fatigue mechanisms, see Fitts, 1994.) Most of the energy demand of the 100-m sprint is covered by anaerobic metabolism of muscle glycogen. During a 400-m sprint, athletes deliberately have to reduce maximal power output, so that fatigue develops less rapidly and a reasonable pace can be maintained. Part of the ATP production is covered, in that case, by aerobic oxidation of glycogen by glycolysis, pyruvate dehydrogenase, and the citric acid cycle, coupled with the electron transport chain and oxidative phosphorylation; the contribution of aerobic oxidation rapidly increases between the start and finish of a 400-m sprint.

Role of Type II or Fast-Twitch Muscle Fibers in Sprinting

A distinction can be made between different muscle fiber types at the microscopic level. In human muscle, the main fiber types are I, II A, and II B. Because of their electrophysiological properties, type I fibers are also known as slow-twitch fibers and type II as fast-twitch fibers. Type I fibers have a high oxidative capacity (high activities of enzymes of the citric acid cycle, of fatty acid oxidation, and of the electron transport chain), a high content of triacylglycerols, and moderate glycolytic capacity. Type II A fibers have a moderate oxidative and a high glycolytic capacity. Type II B fibers have a lower oxidative capacity and an even higher glycolytic capacity than do type II A fibers. It traditionally is assumed that type II A fibers are specialized to perform sprinting exercise, whereas type I fibers are more suited to perform endurance exercise. In agreement with this, the better sprinters tend to have a high percentage of type II fibers, although some world-class sprinters have a 50% type I–50% type II distribution. Sprint or high-intensity training leads to only small increases in the activity of the glycolytic enzymes, with the small increases being seen in both type I and type II fibers. Sprint or high-intensity training

leads to hypertrophy of type II fibers, which have a high glycolytic capacity, and thus high-intensity training leads to increases in the maximal power output of the muscles involved in sprinting.

FUELS FOR THE MARATHON

The marathon distance is 42.195 km (26 miles, 385 yards) and is completed by elite runners in a little over 2 h. The total energy expenditure during a marathon is about 12,000 kJ (12 MJ or 2868 kcal) independent of running speed. This is equivalent to burning about 750 g of carbohydrate or 330 g of fat. These figures immediately illustrate that it is unlikely that a marathon is run solely on carbohydrate, because the human body in the fed state has only about 400 to 900 g of carbohydrate on board (about 80 g in liver and the remainder in the combined skeletal muscles) and as only half of the muscle mass is involved in marathon running.

Carbohydrate and Fat Mixture

Recreational runners run a marathon at 70% to 80% of maximal aerobic power (VO_{2max} or maximal rate of oxygen uptake) and at an oxygen consumption of 1500 mL/min up to 4000 mL/min, depending on how well trained they are. The slowest runners tend to slow down more than the better trained ones do during the latter part of the race. Both a reduction in running efficiency and a gradual reduction in exercise intensity (as a percentage of VO_{2max}) may contribute to the reduction in running speed. Whole-body RQ can be measured in the laboratory while simulating a marathon run using a treadmill, and the RQ can be used to estimate muscle fuel utilization. Such experiments reveal that the RQ in recreational runners falls from values of 0.90 to 1.00 in the first 30 min to about 0.80 to 0.85 after 2 h of running. These observations indicate that carbohydrates are the most important fuel in the first hour of the marathon and that fat gradually increases in importance.

Elite runners are able to maintain a relatively constant pace during the marathon and run at a higher intensity (85% to 90% of VO_{2max}

or 4000 to 5000 mL of O_2/min). The gradual reduction in running efficiency is smaller in their case, and it also is assumed that they are able to maintain a more constant fuel mixture, with less pronounced switching from carbohydrate as the major fuel in the beginning to fat as the major fuel in the last part of the race. Studies in the laboratory investigating the effect of exercise intensity on RQ have shown that RQ becomes elevated with increasing work intensity in a given individual, indicating that the fractional contribution of fat to total energy expenditure is suppressed at high exercise intensities (Fig. 39–3). Trained subjects, however, have a higher capacity to oxidize fat than do untrained subjects when comparisons are made at high absolute work rates. This increased capacity for fat oxidation leads to glycogen sparing and enables the trained subjects to use their glycogen stores more economically.

Muscle Glycogen, Blood Glucose, Plasma Free Fatty Acids, and Intramuscular and VLDL Triacylglycerols as Fuels

From the RQs measured in the laboratory, we now know that carbohydrate and fat are both

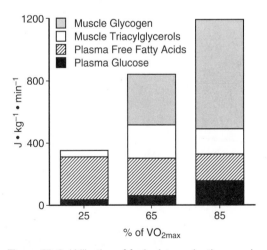

Figure 39–3. *Utilization of fuel mixtures by the exercising muscle at different exercise intensities. (Modified from Romijn, J. A., Coyle, E. F., Sidossis, L. S., Gastaldelli, A., Horowitz, J. F., Endert, E. and Wolfe, R. R. [1993] Regulation of endogenous fat and carbohydrate metabolism in relation to exercise intensity and duration. Am J Physiol 265:E380–E391.)*

oxidized during a marathon. The next question is which fuel stores are oxidized: muscle stores or exogenous sources. Two techniques are available to investigate this question under laboratory conditions. The combination of percutaneous muscle biopsies with arteriovenous difference measurements of blood metabolites across the exercising leg muscles (e.g., Kiens et al., 1993) theoretically may provide all the required information. The limitation of this approach is that blood flow to the exercising muscle is increased ten-fold or more when going from rest to exercise, which sometimes leads to very small arteriovenous differences (smaller than the analytical precision of the assays) of the metabolites of interest so that the differences may not be detectable. Another approach is the use of stable isotopes as metabolic tracers (e.g., Romijn et al., 1993) to measure oxidation rates of blood glucose and fatty acids and to measure the rates of exchange of these metabolites between the muscle and plasma pools.

The use of such techniques opens new possibilities to further our understanding of human physiology, but care is required because many potential pitfalls exist that may lead to incorrect interpretation of the data. Both techniques indicate that both muscle glycogen and blood glucose are used as sources of carbohydrates, as illustrated in Figure 39–4. The blood glucose must originate from glycogen breakdown in the liver, and possibly to a small extent from gluconeogenesis in the liver, especially during the last part of the marathon. Elite runners also ingest carbohydrate drinks during a marathon, which further increases the availability of blood glucose. The absolute rate of both muscle glycogen oxidation and blood glucose oxidation increases with exercise intensity, with muscle glycogen accounting for over 50% of energy expenditure at 85% of maximal aerobic capacity. The contraction-induced translocation of GLUT4 to the plasma membrane plays an important role in the gradual increase of blood glucose uptake and oxidation during prolonged exercise (Brozinick et al., 1994).

Sources of fatty acids for oxidation by skeletal muscle during prolonged exercise are summarized in Figure 39–5. Plasma free fatty acids mobilized from adipose tissue stores are

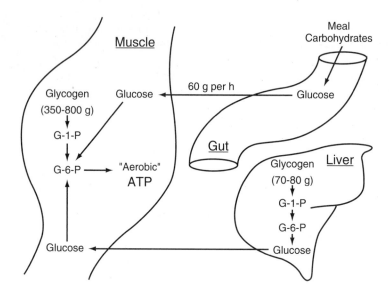

Figure 39–4. Sources of glucose available for oxidation by skeletal muscle during prolonged exercise.

a source of fatty acids for oxidation, and this source gradually increases in importance during prolonged exercise. As noted earlier, the typical basal free fatty acid concentration after ingestion of a mixed diet is 0.3 mmol/L. This concentration drops to half the pre-exercise level early after the onset of exercise, but during prolonged exercise this concentration can increase to reach 1.5 to 2.0 mmol/L. Plasma free fatty acids are oxidized at all exercise intensities, but the rate of lipolysis in the fat pads is reduced at very high work intensities ($>85\%$ of VO_{2max}), leading to a lower supply of plasma free fatty acids and a decrease of the absolute and relative contribution of plasma free fatty acids and total fat to energy expenditure. The muscle triacylglycerols and plasma VLDL also contribute fatty acids for oxidation in muscle (Kiens et al., 1993; Romijn et al., 1993). At intensities of 60% of VO_{2max} and higher, about 50% of the muscle fat oxidation originates from these sources. The liter-

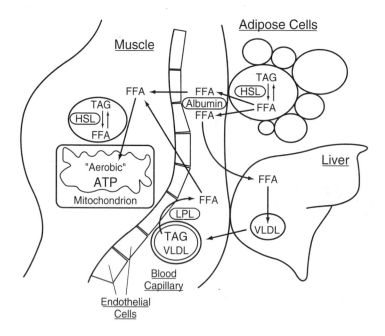

Figure 39–5. Sources of fatty acids for oxidation by skeletal muscle during prolonged exercise. FFA, free fatty acid; HSL, hormone-sensitive lipase; LPL, lipoprotein lipase; TAG, triacylglycerol; VLDL, very low density lipoproteins.

ature, however, is equivocal on the relative contribution of intramuscular and VLDL triacylglycerols (Saltin and Åstrand, 1993).

Anaerobic Versus Aerobic Oxidation of Muscle Glycogen and Blood Glucose

The next question is: How are the carbohydrate sources metabolized? Is carbohydrate oxidized completely (aerobically) or only to lactate (anaerobically)? In recreational runners, high blood lactate concentrations are often observed during the first hour of exercise at 70% to 80% of maximal aerobic power, after which lactate falls to very low levels until the finish has been reached. Measurement of the arteriovenous lactate concentration difference during one-leg exercise in the laboratory also showed a substantial lactate release by the leg (Kiens et al., 1993). This indicates that part of the ATP production in the early period originates from lactate production via glycolysis. The oxygen tension in skeletal muscle is never decreased during submaximal exercise, so it is unlikely that this lactate production is driven by lack of oxygen.

It seems possible that there is some kind of limitation at the level of the mitochondria, leading to a limited rate of pyruvate uptake (pyruvate translocase in the mitochondrial membrane) or oxidation (pyruvate dehydrogenase) or to an inadequate rate of acetyl CoA oxidation via the citric acid cycle. An imbalance between energy delivery and energy need is the consequence of such a limitation, and this leads to increases in the free AMP and free ADP concentrations in muscle, which in turn lead to a temporary increase in the rate of glycolysis and increased pyruvate and lactate production.

It also has been suggested that type II fibers are increasingly recruited in sedentary or moderately trained subjects during the first 30 min of exercise. These fibers start to produce lactate because of their low oxidative capacity. This release of lactate is reduced by training (Kiens et al., 1993). Elite marathon runners appear to metabolize muscle glycogen and blood glucose almost entirely aerobically from the first minute of a marathon until the last despite the fact that they run at a very

high percentage (up to 90%) of aerobic power.

SKELETAL MUSCLE ADAPTATIONS IN RESPONSE TO TRAINING AND THE CONSEQUENCES FOR FUEL UTILIZATION AND PERFORMANCE

Sedentary individuals can markedly increase their endurance by means of regularly performed exercise. After a few weeks of endurance training, individuals can exercise comfortably for prolonged periods at exercise intensities that they could maintain for only a few minutes prior to training. For a long time it was thought that the improved endurance was exclusively the result of the cardiovascular adaptations to endurance training (increased cardiac output, increased gas exchange in the lungs, increased capillary density in skeletal muscle). However, from the perspective of improved endurance, the most important training-induced adaptation is the increase in the number of mitochondria per unit mass of skeletal muscle.

Increase in Mitochondrial Content of Skeletal Muscle as a Result of Training

Training can lead to a five-fold increase in the mitochondrial content of skeletal muscle of sedentary human subjects. Also, in elite athletes the mitochondrial content may vary through the year as a function of training intensity. Cyclists in the Tour de France, which covers a distance of 3000 km over a period of 3 weeks, have only about half the mitochondrial content in the winter season (reduced frequency and intensity of training) that they have in the middle of summer when they are competing daily in cycling races covering 200 to 300 km and often including the ascent of several mountain passes. Their VO_{2max} is only 2% to 5% lower in winter than in summer because it takes much longer for the cardiovascular system to adapt. Their endurance performance, however, is much better in summer due to the higher mitochondrial content of skeletal muscle.

Advantages of an Increased Mitochondrial Content

The major advantage of the increased number of mitochondria in muscle of trained subjects is that the disturbance of the energy status of the muscle is smaller at a given absolute and relative (percentage of VO_{2max}) intensity. Decreases in the muscle ATP and creatine phosphate content, and increases in free ADP, free AMP, and inorganic phosphate, are smaller in trained muscles with a high mitochondrial content (Dudley et al., 1987). Because increases in free AMP, inorganic phosphate, and other allosteric regulators activate glycolysis (see Fig. 9–7 of Chapter 9), the untrained muscle will produce more lactate than the trained muscle. Therefore, elite runners with very high mitochondrial contents are able to run at very high exercise intensities without lactate production, whereas recreational runners and sedentary subjects start to produce lactate at much lower exercise intensities. Because aerobic oxidation of glycogen delivers much more energy than glycolysis alone (~38 versus 3 ATPs per glucose molecule), elite runners also are able to run a much greater distance using the same amount of muscle glycogen.

A second advantage of the higher mitochondrial content is that more fat can be oxidized at moderate to high exercise intensities. The exact biochemical mechanism of this increase in fat oxidation in the trained muscle is not known, but it has been clearly shown that trained muscles extract a greater percentage of the plasma free fatty acids delivered to the muscle than do untrained muscles (Kiens et al., 1993). For this reason, elite marathon runners (in contrast to recreational runners) are still able to oxidize fat at considerable rates when working at 80% to 90% of maximal aerobic power. The major metabolic consequences of the high mitochondrial content in elite marathon runners are a slower utilization of muscle glycogen and blood glucose, a greater reliance on fat oxidation, and less lactate production during exercise of moderate to high intensity. For all these reasons, elite marathoners can run at a speed of 20 km/h for over 2 h, whereas most recreational runners are exhausted within minutes at such a speed.

Role of Training in Reduction of Exercise Stress

Increases in the muscle concentrations of inorganic phosphate, hydrogen ions (H+), and lactate during exercise stimulate group III and group IV afferent nerve fibers in skeletal muscle, which signal to the brain that the muscle is approaching a critical energy deficit leading to contraction failure (Kaufman and Forster, 1996). This activates the muscle-heart reflex and leads to further increases of the heart rate, the ventilation rate, and the blood concentration of catecholamines, which are all experienced as an increase in exercise stress. In trained muscles with a high mitochondrial content, the increases in the muscle concentrations of inorganic phosphate, H+, and lactate are lower at the same absolute exercise intensity, and, therefore, less exercise stress will be experienced. For these reasons, elite runners can run at a higher pace than untrained individuals yet experience only a similar or even lower amount of exercise stress.

FUELS FOR OTHER SPORTING EVENTS

Sports like soccer, football, baseball, basketball, rugby, squash, tennis, and many others can be qualified as intermittent high-intensity exercise. Speed of running or intensity of work varies widely during a game in these sports. Soccer will be used here as an example of an intermittent high-intensity sport, but similar considerations apply to all of them.

A game of soccer lasts 90 min in total with a 10-min break after 45 min. The total distance covered by soccer players depends on the position of the player, but the mean distance covered is 10 km. The speed of running varies from zero to maximal, with a major part of the distance covered at a walking or dribbling pace. Soccer players, however, make many short sprints of 10 to 60 m at full speed throughout the game. The total distance run at full speed is between 800 and 1500 m; this is the distance that theoretically could be covered while consuming muscle glycogen at the rate required to meet the energy demand of sprinting. Part of the energy demand for these sprints is covered by creatine phosphate breakdown, with creatine phosphate resynthesis occurring between sprints. Muscle glycogen breakdown and subsequent lactate production is the other main energy source. Each sprint empties part of the glycogen stores, until the glycogen stores are depleted and the sprints cannot be run at full speed anymore.

The mean heart rate during a game in the highest-class professional league is 85% of maximum; the average oxygen consumption is 80% of maximum; and the mean blood lactate is 8 to 10 mmol/L with peaks up to 12 mmol/L. The lactate produced during sprinting is used as a fuel by the heart and in the intervals at lower intensity also by skeletal muscle. Some lactate also may be converted to glucose by the liver (Cori cycle; see Chapters 9 and 16). Professional soccer players run about the same distance in the first and second half and also run about the same distance in both halves at full speed. Recreational players tend to cover less distance in the second half, run less distance at full speed, and slow down during sprinting in the second half. Muscle biopsy studies have shown that recreational players who start with low muscle glycogen concentrations will have emptied most of their muscle glycogen by half-time.

It is as important for soccer players as for marathon runners to be endurance trained. The better-trained players have a higher aerobic power and therefore depend on anaerobic glycolysis with lactate production less frequently during a game. Thus they are able to spare muscle glycogen during submaximal exercise. During the intervals at lower intensity, they probably also can oxidize more fat, and in this way also save glycogen for a few more sprints (and scoring chances) at the end of the game. Soccer players also should train at high intensity in order to increase speed and maximal anaerobic power, so that they can outrun their opponents during the short sprints.

The body carbohydrate stores are too small to meet the energy cost of ultramarathons, triathlons, and cycling races. Distances covered in athletic events in recent years have tended to become greater, and the selected tracks have tended to become more difficult, often including many steep slopes in moun-

tainous areas. Ultramarathons can be as long as 200 km. In the Tour de France, a professional cycling race, a distance of 3000 km is covered in 3 weeks, and the daily energy expenditure ranges from 27 MJ (6453 kcal) on a flat course to 38 MJ (9082 kcal) when cycling over mountain passes. The latter represents more than three times the daily energy expenditure of a sedentary man. Extremely popular also is the triathlon. In Ironman triathlons, athletes first swim 3800 m, then cycle 180 km, and finally run a full marathon (42 km, 195 m). Although the pace is slower than during a marathon run, elite athletes still are able to exercise at 70% to 80% of maximal aerobic power for continuous periods of 7 to 10 h. At these high intensities, carbohydrates remain an important energy source, but the need for carbohydrates by far exceeds the size of the glycogen stores of the body. During these types of events, therefore, it is extremely important to ensure that the carbohydrate stores at the start of the race are as large as possible and that carbohydrates are ingested before and during the competition if possible.

HOW NUTRITION MAY HELP IMPROVE PERFORMANCE

Resting glycogen concentrations in human skeletal muscle range from about 10 to 23 g per kg of wet muscle. Between 350 and 800 g of glycogen are present in the combined skeletal muscles if one assumes that a lean, 70-kg subject has a skeletal muscle mass of about 35 kg. In highly trained athletes, the reported resting muscle glycogen concentrations tend to be higher than in sedentary subjects, suggesting that glucose deposition and glycogen resynthesis are increased by exercise training.

Interventions to Increase Muscle Glycogen: Carbohydrate Loading

Several nutritional interventions on the days prior to exercise have been shown to increase the resting glycogen concentration at the start of exercise. The first thing for endurance athletes to do is to increase the carbohydrate content of their regular daily diets to 50% to 55% or more of total caloric intake.

Scandinavian researchers have proposed the "supercompensation diet" as best preparation for a marathon. One week before the marathon, a demanding exercise bout is performed to exhaustion to empty the muscle glycogen stores. For the next 3 days, a high-fat diet (<20% of total energy as carbohydrate) is consumed, and for the last 3 days a high-carbohydrate diet (<20% of total energy as fat) is used. No exercise training is performed in the 6 days before competition. This combined diet-training intervention was shown to lead to a 160% to 200% increase of the resting muscle glycogen concentration. However, in practice, this protocol has several disadvantages. It is far from easy to prepare tasteful meals containing less than 20% of calories from carbohydrate or less than 20% of calories from fat. Furthermore, athletes feel weak on the days of the high-fat diet and lose self-confidence when they do not train for 6 days prior to competition.

Therefore, in practice, another diet-training intervention, the so-called "tapering" protocol, has become much more popular. As illustrated in Figure 39–6, the tapering protocol starts 1 week before competition with a demanding exercise session leading to exhaustion in order to empty the muscle glycogen stores. During the next 6 days, the carbohydrate content of the diet is increased from the usual 50 to 55% up to 70 to 75% of total calories. The training volume is gradually decreased in the same period from 100% (until exhaustion) 7 days before competition to 10%

the day before competition. In the last 2 days before competition, the carbohydrate intake should be about 600 to 700 g per day, which is an amount equal to optimal muscle glycogen stores. This carbohydrate-loading protocol also results in a significant increase in the muscle glycogen stores and is more acceptable to athletes and their families. The high-carbohydrate diet used in this intervention can be realized with normal food products (pastas, rice, potatoes, and so on). Alternatively, a basic diet providing 50% of energy from carbohydrates can be supplemented with drinks for athletes, energy bars, or carbohydrate powders to achieve the higher carbohydrate intakes.

Usefulness of Carbohydrate Loading and Ingestion for Endurance Events

Muscle glycogen is the main fuel during marathon running, for both elite and recreational marathoners. Both, therefore, have to ensure that they have enough carbohydrate on board to reach the finish while oxidizing aerobically a fuel mixture consisting of both carbohydrate and fat. If muscle glycogen is emptied a few kilometers before they reach the finish, then fatigue will occur (i.e., they "hit the wall"), and they have to reduce the pace. Carbohydrate loading on the days before the race is, therefore, of utmost importance for optimal performance. Recreational runners cannot use the glycogen stores as efficiently as elite runners can. Carbohydrate loading leading to

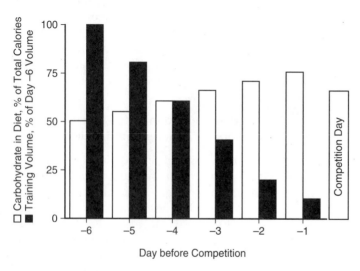

Figure 39–6. Most popular combined diet-training intervention used by elite athletes to obtain maximal muscle glycogen stores on the day of an endurance competition. Beginning 1 week before competition, the "tapering protocol" involves depletion of the muscle glycogen stores by exercise to exhaustion followed by 5 days of gradually increasing the carbohydrate content of the diet (percentage of total calories) and gradually decreasing the daily training "volume" from 100% (exercise to point of exhaustion) to 10% volume the day before competition.

high glycogen content at the start, nevertheless, does help them maintain the pace chosen in the beginning of the race as long as possible.

Ingestion of a carbohydrate-rich meal 2 to 4 hours prior to competition also improves performance as it helps replenish the liver glycogen stores that have been emptied during overnight fasting. In competitions of less than 2 h duration, these carbohydrates preferably should be taken as easily digestible food products or sports drinks. In more prolonged competitions, athletes often prefer solid products, such as bread, bananas, and energy bars. The percentage of protein and fat always should be low in the pre-exercise meal to prevent a reduction of the rate of gastric emptying and the occurrence of gastrointestinal disturbances during exercise. In very few subjects hypoglycemia may occur during the first minutes of exercise when the pre-exercise meal is taken less than 1 h before exercise. Therefore, it is advised to build up experience with pre-exercise meals during training sessions.

Ingestion of carbohydrate drinks during cycling or running exercise of long duration (>2 h) and moderate to high intensity (50% to 90% VO_{2max}) has been shown to improve performance in both elite and recreational athletes. Thus it is advised to refuel carbohydrates during competition. Carbohydrate ingestion maintains both blood glucose concentration and the glucose oxidation rate at higher values during prolonged exercise. The rate of muscle glycogen breakdown is not reduced by carbohydrate ingestion, but the supply of blood glucose to the exercising muscle is increased. Carbohydrates ingested during exercise are oxidized at a maximal rate of about 60 g/h even when much larger amounts are ingested. This suggests that the maximal rate of intestinal absorption or gastric emptying is about 60 g/h during exercise; therefore, ingestion of 60 g of carbohydrate per hour of exercise is advised. The ideal athletic drink also should supply water to compensate for the sweat losses during exercise. Dehydration due to excessive sweating is a well-known cause of a gradual reduction in performance during exercise in the heat. Large volumes of a low-carbohydrate drink should be ingested

in the heat, whereas smaller volumes of a drink with a higher carbohydrate content are advised in cold weather conditions. Sodium chloride should be added to increase intestinal glucose absorption.

The ideal sports drink to be used during exercise has a carbohydrate content of between 40 and 80 g/L, is hypo- to isotonic, and has a sodium chloride content of 400 to 1200 mg/L. To fill the stomach, 6 to 8 mL of this drink per kilogram of body weight should be ingested 5 min prior to exercise, followed by repeated boluses of 2 to 3 mL/kg of body weight each 15 to 20 min during exercise. During exercise in the heat, the volumes taken should be as large as tolerated because sweat losses (>2 L/h) always exceed fluid tolerance under these conditions. Again, it is advised that athletes build up personal experience with fluid losses (or needs) and fluid tolerance in training sessions under different weather conditions.

During ultra-endurance events, a high starting glycogen concentration also helps postpone the point in time when the muscle glycogen stores are empty and the pace has to be reduced. As these events last for many hours, carbohydrates also should be ingested during exercise for the aforementioned reasons. During events like the Tour de France that requires a massively high energy expenditure continuously for 3 weeks, carbohydrates are ingested the whole day prior to, during, and after competition, as both carbohydrate-containing drinks and solid food. Easily digestible carbohydrates should be ingested at a high rate (100 g/h or more) immediately after competition to start glycogen resynthesis as early as possible. Failure to have fully replenished glycogen stores by the start of exercise on the next day (e.g., due to insufficient carbohydrate intake or digestive problems) in most cases leads to the inability to follow the speed of the main group, and the cyclists will either give up voluntarily or be disqualified for finishing too late.

Usefulness of Carbohydrate Loading and Ingestion for Intermittent High-Intensity Events

In intermittent high-intensity sports involving many repeated short distance sprints, the size of the glycogen stores in the muscle determines the total distance that can be covered at full speed. Carbohydrate loading, therefore, is very important. In those sports in which regular drinking is allowed (e.g., tennis) it is advisable to ingest carbohydrate-containing drinks so that orally ingested carbohydrates may contribute at least part of the carbohydrate oxidized during lower intensity exercise, saving some of the muscle glycogen stores for a few more full speed sprints at the end of the game. During sports with a break at halftime, the break can be used to refuel carbohydrate.

PROTEIN AND AMINO ACID METABOLISM IN SKELETAL MUSCLE DURING REST AND DURING EXERCISE

In the middle of the 19th century, the renowned German physiologist von Liebig assumed that the protein of skeletal muscle was consumed during muscular work as a fuel and that large quantities of meat and protein should be eaten by industrial workers to replenish the protein losses during physical exercise. Although this was shown to be incorrect in the late 19th century when careful nitrogen balance studies failed to show increased nitrogen losses during periods of increased physical activity, today—more than a century later—a large percentage of athletes and coaches still believe that vast amounts of protein should be eaten during periods of heavy exercise and training to replace the oxidized protein.

Measurements of the activities of enzymes involved in branched-chain amino acid oxidation in muscle, estimates of leucine incorporation into skeletal muscle protein that can be made with stable isotope techniques, and measurement of urea production rates at various exercise intensities all fail to show net breakdown and increased oxidation of muscle and whole-body protein, especially when the exercise is performed in the fed state as athletes do in practice during competition (for references see Rennie, 1996). Modest increases in plasma urea concentration and urinary urea excretion have been observed only during ultramarathons and during exercise in

the laboratory after overnight or more prolonged fasting.

Therefore, the protein needs of athletes are at most only slightly higher than those of sedentary individuals, especially when the energy balance is adequate. A diet that provides 12% of total energy from protein should easily meet the protein requirement of athletes, especially when, due to the daily exercise and training sessions, they have an increased energy expenditure and, therefore, an increased energy and protein intake per kilogram of body weight.

SKELETAL MUSCLE ADAPTATIONS IN RESPONSE TO DISUSE AND DISEASE AND THE CONSEQUENCES FOR FUEL UTILIZATION AND WELL-BEING DURING NORMAL DAILY LIFE

Although the main part of this chapter focuses on fuel utilization in healthy people during sports events requiring high energy expenditures, a reduced use of skeletal muscle also has consequences for fuel utilization, exercise tolerance, and feelings of fitness, fatigue, and well-being in the daily life of inactive people. Not only training but also disuse (a reduction of muscular activity for a prolonged period of time) leads to a remarkable adaptation in skeletal muscle. Patients with very low energy outputs in habitual activities may have mitochondrial contents that are as little as 10% of those of sedentary individuals (Wagenmakers et al., 1987, 1988).

The ranges of the rates of palmitate oxidation and cytochrome c oxidase activity (both of which are mitochondrial oxidative processes and a reflection of mitochondrial content) in muscle homogenates of individuals with a wide range of habitual physical activities are shown in Figure 39–7. The lowest activities ever reported have been observed in young children with Duchenne muscular dystrophy and with hypotonia due to spinal muscular atrophy type I. Their muscle contained as little as 3% to 4% of the mitochondrial activities observed in the muscle of elite marathoners. Low mitochondrial contents also are seen in the muscle of patients who are bedridden for a long time due to an acquired dis-

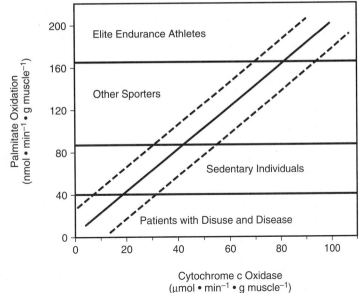

Figure 39–7. Ranges of the activities of two mitochondrial enzymes in populations with high, intermediate, and low habitual activities. (Based on data of Wagenmakers, A. J. M., Kaur, N., Coakley, J. A., Griffiths, R. D. and Edwards, R. H. T. [1987] Mitochondrial metabolism in myopathy and myalgia. In: Advances in Myochemistry: 1 [Benzi, G., ed.], pp. 219–230. John Libbey [Eurotext Ltd., London].)

ease; of subjects who are very inactive due to psychic problems; of those who prefer to avoid exercise-induced pains originating from metabolic defects or from unknown causes; of astronouts traveling through space in a weightless condition for several months; and of subjects deliberately subjected to hypokinesia for 90 days as part of a space research program (for references see Wagenmakers et al., 1988). An 80% to 90% decrease within a period of days is also seen in the mitochondrial contents of skeletal muscle of patients entering intensive care units with severe trauma, sepsis, or septic shock (Helliwell et al., 1990).

Subjects with such low mitochondrial contents have maximal aerobic powers of 60 to 120 watts or 50 to 100 kcal/h (Wagenmakers et al., 1988), and during incremental cycle exercise they start to produce significant amounts of lactate at energy expenditure rates of 30 to 80 watts or 25 to 70 kcal/h. This implies that they quite often experience the stress of severe exercise while performing normal daily activities and that they walk around in their home or at work with high heart and ventilation rates and high blood concentrations of catecholamines. They may empty their muscle glycogen stores while traveling to work or walking to and from the shops. In such a condition it is not unusual for subjects

who entered this situation without a clear causal disease to respond by trying to avoid exercise and then to spiral down in a vicious cycle of further inactivity leading to a further decrease of the mitochondrial contents of their muscle cells. Professional help and physiotherapy programs may be indicated to break this cycle.

The adaptation to disuse is similar to adaptation to training, but in the reverse direction. For optimal health, to reduce the severity of effort syndrome symptoms, and for a good quality of life, patients with disuse and disease should regularly take part in exercise programs. Effort syndrome symptoms include palpitations, dizziness, disturbances of consciousness/vision, breathlessness, chest pain, epigastric pain, dysphagia, aerophagy, muscular pains especially in the neck and shoulder area, tremor, excessive sweating, fatigue, weakness, headache tension, and anxiety. These symptoms often reduce the quality of life and are experienced by all subjects with low mitochondrial contents independent of the reason leading to their physical inactivity. Therapeutic exercise programs may be useful to speed up recovery and improve fitness and the quality of life of patients recovering from prolonged acquired diseases or from an acute critical illness. Subjective muscle weakness and rapid fatigue often prevent these patients from taking up their professional life for periods of 6 to 12 months after discharge from the hospital. Therapeutic exercise programs also may slow down the gradual loss of muscle function and greatly improve the quality of life and well-being of patients who are disabled due to progressive inherited neuromuscular diseases.

REFERENCES

Brozinick, J. T., Etgen, G. J., Yaspelkis, B. B. and Ivy, J. L. (1994) The effects of muscle contraction and insulin on glucose-transporter translocation in rat skeletal muscle. Biochem J 297:539–545.

Dudley, G. A., Tullson, P. C. and Terjung, R. L. (1987) Influence of the mitochondrial content on the sensitivity of respiratory control. J Biol Chem 262:9109–9114.

Fitts, R. H. (1994) Cellular mechanisms of muscle fatigue. Physiol Rev 74:49–94.

Greenhaff, P. L. (1997) The nutritional biochemistry of creatine. Nutr Biochem 11:610–618.

Helliwell, T. R., Griffiths, R. D., Coakley, J. H., Wagenmakers, A. J. M., McClelland, P., Campbell, I. T. and Bone, J. M. (1990) Muscle pathology and biochemistry in critically-ill patients. J Neurol Sci 98:329.

Himwich, H. E. and Rose, M. I. (1927) The respiratory quotient of exercising muscle. Am J Physiol 81:485–486.

Kaufman, M. P. and Forster, H. V. (1996) Reflexes controlling circulatory, ventilatory and airway responses to exercise. In: Handbook of Physiology; Section 12, Exercise: Regulation and Integration of Multiple Systems (Rowell, L. B. and Shepherd, J. T., eds.), pp. 381–447. Oxford University Press, New York.

Kiens, B., Éssen-Gustavsson, B., Christensen, N. J. and Saltin, B. (1993) Skeletal muscle substrate utilization during submaximal exercise in man: Effect of endurance training. J Physiol 469:459–478.

Nuutila, P., Koivisto, V. A., Knuuti, J., Ruotsalainen, U., Teräs, M., Haaparanta, M., Bergman, J., Solin, O., Voipio-Pulkki, L.-M., Wegelius. U. and Yki-Jarvinen, H. (1992) Glucose-free fatty acid cycle operates in human heart and skeletal muscle in vivo. J Clin Invest 89:1767–1774.

Rennie, M. J. (1996) Influence of exercise on protein and amino acid metabolism. In: Handbook of Physiology; Section 12, Exercise: Regulation and Integration of Multiple Systems (Rowell, L. B. and Shepherd, J. T., eds.), pp. 995–1035. Oxford University Press, New York.

Romijn, J. A., Coyle, E. F., Sidossis, L. S., Gastaldelli, A., Horowitz, J. F., Endert, E. and Wolfe, R. R. (1993) Regulation of endogenous fat and carbohydrate metabolism in relation to exercise intensity and duration. Am J Physiol 265:E380–E391.

Saltin, B. and Åstrand, P.-O. (1993) Free fatty acids and exercise. Am J Clin Nutr 57:752S–757S.

Sugden, M. C. and Holness, M. J. (1994) Interactive regulation of the pyruvate dehydrogenase complex and the carnitine palmitoyltransferase system. FASEB J 8:54–61.

Sugden, M. C., Holness, M. J. and Howard, R. M. (1993) Changes in lipoprotein lipase activities in adipose tissue, heart and skeletal muscle during continuous or interrupted feeding. Biochem J 292:113–119.

Wagenmakers, A. J. M. (1999) Nutritional supplements: Effects on exercise performance and metabolism. In: Perspectives in Exercise Science and Sports Medicine; Vol. 12: The Metabolic Basis of Performance in Sport and Exercise (Lamb, D. R. and Murray, R., eds.). Cooper Publishing Group, Carmel, Indiana, in press.

Wagenmakers, A. J. M., Coakley, J. H. and Edwards, R. H. T. (1988) The metabolic consequences of reduced habitual activities in patients with muscle pain and disease. Ergonomics 31:1519–1527.

Wagenmakers, A. J. M., Kaur, N., Coakley, J. H., Griffiths, R. D. and Edwards, R. H. T. (1987) Mitochondrial metabolism in myopathy and myalgia. In: Advances in Myochemistry: 1 (Benzi, G., ed.), pp. 219–230. John Libbey Eurotext Ltd., London.

Williams, M. H. (1992) Ergogenic and ergolytic substances. Med Sci Sports Ex 24:S344–S348.

RECOMMENDED READING

Rowell, L. B. and Shepherd, J. T., eds. (1996) Handbook of Physiology; Section 12, Exercise: Regulation and Integration of Multiple Systems. Oxford University Press, New York.

◆ ◆

CHAPTER 40

Detoxification and Protective Functions of Nutrients

Dean P. Jones, Ph.D., and Mary J. DeLong, Ph.D.

O U T L I N E

C O M M O N   A B B R E V I A T I O N S

ARE (antioxidant response element)
GST (glutathione *S*-transferase)
GSH (glutathione)
PAPS (3′-phosphoadenosine-5′-phosphosulfate)
ROS (reactive oxygen species; also called ROI for reactive oxygen intermediate)
XRE (xenobiotic response element)

DEFENSE SYSTEMS

Humans are constantly exposed to an array of compounds termed xenobiotics (from Greek: *xenos,* foreign; *bios,* life), which include toxic, mutagenic, and carcinogenic chemicals. Many of these chemicals are found in the human diet. These chemicals can react with cellular macromolecules, such as proteins and DNA, or directly with cell structures to cause cell damage. In addition, some nonreactive chemicals can be biologically transformed to reactive molecules within our cells. Formation of reactive oxygen species (ROS) and other free radicals occurs in the processes of various electron transport systems (e.g., mitochondrial electron transport chain, cytochrome P450) involving oxygen as an electron acceptor. In addition to diet and normal metabolism, many environmental factors, such as cigarette smoke, polluted air (ozone), chlorinated hydrocarbons, and heavy metals or extensive exposure to ultraviolet light or x-rays, can induce formation of free radicals and cell damage. To counteract these challenges, the human body has developed two primary defense systems: detoxification enzymes that may be controlled by the level of the xenobiotic and antioxidant systems that reduce free radical species and maintain the redox state of the cell.

OXIDATIVE PROCESSES

Protective functions and oxidative processes are involved in nutrition (Halliwell et al., 1995). Oxidative processes are frequently addressed in nutrition because oxidation of fats affects palatability of foods, and oxidation products of lipid peroxidation are toxic. In addition, several nutrients, including vitamins C and E, as well as selenium, affect susceptibility to oxidative injury. Although many of these specific antioxidant functions are considered in other chapters (e.g., see Chapters 23, 25, 32, and 34) in association with the individual nutrients, it is worthwhile to consider how the various nutrients interact to provide efficient detoxification of oxidants and protection against oxidative stress.

Oxidative Stress

Oxidative stress is a term used to describe any challenge in which pro-oxidants predominate over antioxidants. Pro-oxidants are compounds that interfere with normal metabolism by oxidizing (removing electrons from) normal cellular macromolecules. If the normal macromolecule is DNA, the result can be a mutation. If the normal macromolecule is an enzyme, the result can be loss of that enzyme activity. Any type of macromolecule can be affected, so the process of oxidative stress can result in a range of deleterious consequences determined by the tissue and type of oxidant present.

A large fraction, perhaps as many as half, of all enzyme-catalyzed reactions involve electron transfers. These include most enzymes that contain Fe^{2+}/Fe^{3+} and enzymes utilizing flavocoenzymes, pyridine nucleotides, glutathione, or ascorbic acid as electron donors or acceptors. In most of these oxidative reactions, an even number of electrons are transferred so that free radicals are not formed. However, some aspects of metabolism require that reactive (free radical-producing) species be formed in the process of producing or eliminating specific compounds. For example, hydrogen peroxide (H_2O_2) is normally considered a reactive oxygen species (ROS) that is deleterious, but hydrogen peroxide is required for the synthesis of the thyroid hormone thyroxin and also for the generation of bacteriocidal hypochlorous acid by myeloperoxidase in neutrophils. Generation of reactive oxidants, such as H_2O_2 and hypochlorous acid (HOCl), is a carefully controlled process; these reactions are adequately compartmentalized so that other cells and tissues are not exposed and/or are adequately protected by detoxification enzymes that minimize the risk of exposure of the cell to oxidative stress.

Although generation of ROS is a normal component of oxidative metabolism and effective defenses are present, the electron transfer machinery of the cell is not 100% efficient. Mitochondria, for instance, are responsible for most of the body's oxygen consumption in a process that yields water as the product. A small fraction of the oxygen, however, is reduced to ROS as a byproduct of this mechanism. Chemicals, infectious agents, and genetic defects that disrupt normal mitochondrial function can greatly increase the fraction that is converted to ROS. Moreover, the fraction that is reduced to ROS may also increase as a consequence of normal aging processes by which mitochondria lose efficiency because of age-dependent changes in the mitochondria. Other enzymes, such as cytochrome P450 systems, can similarly contribute to ROS generation, especially in the presence of ethanol, drugs, and environmental toxicants. Differences in age, health, and environmental exposures thus create a nutritional challenge for meeting specific antioxidant needs.

Reactive Oxygen Species

A broad spectrum of reactive species can cause oxidative damage to critical macromolecules in cells. Among the most common are the ROS (Fig. 40–1). The ROS are various forms of oxygen that are much more reactive and damaging to biological systems than the normal molecular oxygen we breathe. Superoxide anion (O_2^-) is a free radical anion that is formed from O_2 by transfer of 1 electron. It is normally produced by an enzyme in neutrophils (white blood cells) when these cells are activated to kill microorganisms. However, it

---

Reactive Oxygen Species

O_2^-	Superoxide Anion
H_2O_2	Hydrogen Peroxide
$^\bullet OH$	Hydroxyl Radical
$^1\Delta_g O_2$	Singlet Oxygen
O_3	Ozone

Possible Reactions Involved

Haber-Weiss Reaction

$$O_2^- + H_2O_2 \rightarrow {}^\bullet OH + {}^- OH + O_2$$

Fenton Reaction (Iron-catalyzed Haber-Weiss Reaction)

$$O_2^- + Fe^{3+} \rightarrow O_2 + Fe^{2+}$$

$$Fe^{2+} + H_2O_2 \rightarrow {}^\bullet OH + {}^- OH + Fe^{3+}$$

Figure 40–1. *Reactive oxygen species (ROS) and their reactions.*

---

is also produced by many other enzymes and by certain toxic reactions. Superoxide is normally eliminated by enzymes termed superoxide dismutases, which convert 2 molecules of superoxide to 1 molecule each of H_2O_2 and O_2. One type of superoxide dismutase, found in the cytosol of cells and in blood plasma, contains copper and zinc. The other type, found in mitochondria, contains manganese. Nutritional deficiencies affecting these enzymes are rare, if they occur at all.

The product of the superoxide dismutase reaction, H_2O_2, is another ROS that is also produced directly by some 2-electron transfer reactions. H_2O_2 is detoxified by glutathione peroxidases and by catalase. Glutathione peroxidases are the most important enzymes for eliminating H_2O_2 under most conditions in the cytosol and mitochondria of cells and in blood plasma. The major forms of glutathione peroxidase require selenium, and geographical regions with low selenium in the soil can have significant populations at risk of selenium deficiency and associated decreased activity of glutathione peroxidases, as discussed in detail in Chapter 34. Catalase is another enzyme that decomposes H_2O_2, but it is mostly found in membrane-bound organelles (peroxisomes) and requires a much higher concentration of H_2O_2 for its catalytic function than does glutathione peroxidase. Although catalase is an iron-containing enzyme, a decrease in catalase activity is usually not of primary concern during iron deficiency because the glutathione peroxidases carry out detoxification of peroxides at the low H_2O_2 concentrations present.

Although O_2^- and H_2O_2 are toxic, their greatest toxicity occurs when both are present and they react to form the more toxic ROS, the hydroxyl radical (·OH). This occurs very rapidly when transition metals such as Fe^{2+} and Cu^{1+} are present (Fig. 40–1). Consequently, in addition to the presence of the enzymes needed to detoxify superoxide and H_2O_2, avid metal ion-binding proteins, such as transferrin, ferritin, and metallothionein, function to protect against oxidative damage by lowering free metal ion concentrations.

Other ROS include ozone and singlet oxygen. Ozone (O_3) is largely derived from photochemical processes in the atmosphere, and mammals have no specific system for its detoxification. However, singlet oxygen can be formed in tissues and is effectively detoxified by reaction with carotenoids. Singlet oxygen is an electronic form of O_2 that differs from the usual ground state form, triplet oxygen, only by suborbital spin pairing of electrons. In other words, triplet oxygen has 2 unpaired electrons, whereas these electrons are paired in singlet oxygen. Singlet molecules react more readily with other singlet molecules, and triplet molecules similarly react more readily with triplet molecules. Because most biomolecules are singlet, this means that most molecules are more susceptible to oxidation by singlet oxygen. Unfortunately, singlet oxygen is very difficult to study in biological systems, and much of what is known is derived from model systems; the specific role of singlet oxygen in oxidative damage in vitro and the protection provided against this by carotenoids can only be inferred.

Trafficking of Redox-Active Nutrients

Although often overlooked, there is a critical interaction of nutrient transport systems and compartmentation of oxidative processes. For instance, energy-yielding oxidative processes are largely confined to mitochondria, which contain iron, copper, and flavocoenzymes tightly bound to proteins that minimize their ability to generate ROS. Maintenance of very low concentrations of free iron and copper is of extreme importance because these ions can catalyze free radical reactions. One well-characterized reaction is the iron-catalyzed Haber-Weiss reaction, also termed Fenton's reaction, in which iron catalyzes the reaction of superoxide anion (O_2^-) with H_2O_2 to yield the potent oxidant, the hydroxyl radical ($\cdot OH$):

$$O_2^- + Fe^{3+} \rightarrow O_2 + Fe^{2+}$$

$$Fe^{2+} H_2O_2 \rightarrow Fe^{3+} + OH^- + \cdot OH$$

The hydroxyl radical is such a powerful oxidant that it can initiate lipid peroxidation, cause destruction of DNA, inactivate proteins, and degrade polysaccharides. Maintenance of low concentrations of H_2O_2 and superoxide in different subcellular compartments requires distribution of catalase, glutathione peroxidase, and superoxide dismutases into these different compartments. Maintenance of very low concentrations of free iron and copper further ensure that these ROS do not cause oxidative damage. However, this requires a complex array of binding and transport proteins as essential mechanisms to protect against oxidative stress. Excess nutritional iron or disruption of these carrier mechanisms by genetic mutation or competition by other metal ions can result in pathological consequences as a result of oxidative damage.

Antioxidant Systems

Antioxidant systems have interacting and complementary functions (Buettner, 1993; Sies and Stahl, 1995; Thomas et al., 1995). To protect effectively against the array of reactive oxidants, multiple mechanisms of protection with broad specificities for potentially damaging agents are required. This interactive and complementary function is illustrated by the enzymes superoxide dismutase and glutathione peroxidase described earlier. Together, they function to keep O_2^- and H_2O_2 concentrations very low so that the hydroxyl radical will not be formed. To understand further the interactive roles of the antioxidant system, it is helpful to consider a simplified scheme of lipid peroxidation. Lipid peroxidation can be initiated by ROS and other mechanisms that result in abstraction of an electron from a polyunsaturated fatty acid, as shown in Figure 40–2.

The resulting carbon-centered radical undergoes rearrangement and, in the presence of O_2, addition of O_2 to form a peroxyl radical (ROO·). Propagation of the free radical reaction can occur by reaction of the peroxyl radical with another polyunsaturated fatty acid, generating the corresponding fatty acid hydroperoxide (ROOH) and another carbon-centered radical. The fatty acid hydroperoxide can result in an amplification of the free radical process by reacting with a transition metal ion such as Fe^{2+} to generate an oxygen-centered radical RO·, which can initiate a new cycle of lipid peroxidation.

Vitamin E reacts with lipid radicals generated in cell membranes to protect against fur-

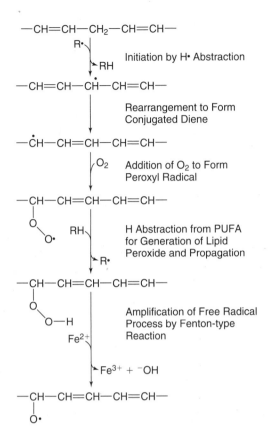

Figure 40–2. *Generalized scheme for peroxidation of polyunsaturated fatty acids (PUFA).*

ther lipid peroxidation, as shown in Figure 40–3. Because this reaction if nonenzymatic, vitamin E can protect against a broad range of radicals. Extensive studies of the rate constants of different reactions indicate that vitamin E is most effective against carbon-centered radicals and peroxyl radicals (ROO·). Both of these types of radicals are important in propagation of lipid peroxidation in cell membranes, and vitamin E thus functions as a chain-breaking antioxidant or free radical scavenger.

Vitamin C (ascorbic acid) also has an important role in protection against lipid peroxidation because it has a high reactivity with oxygen-centered radicals (RO·). Although vitamin C is present in the aqueous phase, the oxidized RO· has sufficient polarity to be accessible to vitamin C. When vitamin E reacts with a radical, it is converted to a radical form, which can be recycled to vitamin E by reaction with vitamin C. Thus, depletion of

vitamin E due to oxidation does not readily occur unless vitamin C is also depleted. Vitamin C is oxidized to a radical form, semidehydroascorbic acid, in its reaction with the radical form of vitamin E or in reaction with RO·. Semidehydroascorbic acid is a relatively stable radical that is probably always present in cells. Its concentration does not normally accumulate to high amounts because 2 molecules of semidehydroascorbic acid rapidly react to form ascorbate and dehydroascorbic acid. Dehydroascorbic acid is reduced back to ascorbate by glutathione (γ-glutamylcysteinylglycine), which is also a very important antioxidant in cells. Because of this reaction, the antioxidant functions of vitamins E and C are largely preserved until there is a significant oxidation of glutathione.

Glutathione has an additional role in protection against lipid peroxidation. Although catalase decomposes H_2O_2 it has no activity toward lipid hydroperoxides. These latter compounds, which are generated during lipid peroxidation and by certain lipoxygenases, are reduced to their corresponding alcohols by the selenium-containing glutathione peroxidases.

Glutathione peroxidase activity depends upon the availability of glutathione (GSH) and results in its oxidation to glutathione disulfide (GSSG). Glutathione disulfide is reduced back to glutathione via a flavoprotein, GSSG reductase. This enzyme requires NADPH as a source of reducing equivalents and FAD as a coenzyme. Blood levels of this enzyme are often used as an early indicator of riboflavin deficiency. Because of the requirement of selenium for glutathione peroxidase, selenium deficiency makes red cells sensitive to oxidant-induced hemolytic anemia. Similarly, individuals who are deficient in glucose 6-phosphate dehydrogenase activity (which catalyzes the first step of the pentose phosphate pathway of glucose metabolism) have an inadequate NADPH supply to protect against oxidative stress. Consequently, they too are sensitive to hemolytic anemia when treated with oxidative therapeutic drugs such as antimalarials.

As can be seen from this brief overview of lipid peroxidation and the function of some critical antioxidant systems, each component has multiple functions and interacts with

Vitamin E as a Chain-breaking Antioxidant:

$R\cdot + E \rightarrow RH + E\cdot$

$ROO\cdot + E \rightarrow ROOH + E\cdot$

Ascorbate as a Radical Scavenger and a Reductant of the Vitamin E Radical:

$RO\cdot + ASC \rightarrow ROH + SDA\cdot$

$E\cdot + ASC \rightarrow E + SDA\cdot$

Glutathione as a Reductant of Dehydroascorbic Acid and Lipid Hydroperoxides:

$2\ SDA\cdot \rightarrow ASC + DHA$

$DHA + 2\ GSH \rightarrow ASC + GSSG$

$ROOH + 2\ GSH \rightarrow ROH + GSSG + H_2O$

GSSG is Reduced Back to GSH by the Flavoprotein GSSG Reductase:

$GSSG + NADPH + H^+ \rightarrow 2\ GSH + NADP^+$

Figure 40–3. Reactions of vitamin E (E), ascorbate (ASC), and glutathione (GSH) in protection against lipid peroxidation. SDA, semidehydroascorbic acid; DHA, dehydroascorbic acid; ROOH, lipid hydroperoxide.

other antioxidants. Failure of antioxidant protection cannot be attributed to any single component because all are affected by an oxidative challenge. This is further complicated by the existence of other antioxidants. For instance, carotenoids function to protect against singlet oxygen and also can function as an antioxidant in protection against lipid peroxidation. Uric acid has been found to have free radical scavenging activity similar to that of ascorbate, and coenzyme Q has been found to have activities similar to those of vitamin E. Thus, one must view the protective mechanisms against oxidative stress as a network of antioxidants, for which the optimal composition has yet to be defined.

Role of Oxidative Mechanisms in the Detoxification of Xenobiotics

Nonpolar organic compounds are not readily excreted by the kidneys because they are permeable to cell membranes and cannot be concentrated in the urine. Consequently, these compounds must be made polar to allow effective elimination. Introduction of polarity into these relatively nonreactive compounds occurs principally by the family of enzymes known as cytochrome P450 monooxygenase systems. The reactions catalyzed by cytochrome P450 require NADPH and molecular oxygen. The overall reaction is shown here:

$$XH + O_2 + NADPH + H^+ \rightarrow$$
$$XOH + H_2O + NADP^+$$

where XH is the substrate. These enzymes contain iron as part of a heme group; this iron interacts with the sulfur of a cysteine residue to create a reactive center that can catalyze diverse oxidation reactions. These reactions are partially determined by the specific isoform of the cytochrome P450, by the nature of the hydrophobic binding site for the substrate, and by the reactivity of the substrate. The electrons are transferred to the cytochrome by a flavoprotein, NADPH cytochrome P450 reductase.

Of particular importance with regard to nutrition is that cytochrome P450 systems are differentially induced by dietary components and are responsible for bioactivating dietary compounds to reactive electrophiles and oxidants. Ethanol is a potent inducer of one form of cytochrome P450. Polycyclic aromatic hydrocarbons, such as the benzo(a)pyrene found in charbroiled foods and cigarette smoke, are inducers of other forms of cytochrome P450. Consequently, dietary components can have a great impact on bioactivation by the cytochrome P450 systems. Because products of these reactions are oxidants, diets high in inducers and substrates of these enzymes are likely to increase the need for antioxidants. Unfortunately, however, the complexities of the human diet and polymorphic variations in P450 in humans make this a difficult hypothesis to test.

Oxidative Stress Associated with Occupational and Therapeutic Exposure to Chemicals

Halogenated hydrocarbons can be reductively activated by cytochrome P450 to generate free radicals. For instance, carbon tetrachloride (CCl_4), a solvent that was previously used as a dry-cleaning agent, is metabolized by cytochrome P450 to a free radical that causes extensive liver injury. An inhalation anesthetic, halothane, similarly can cause extensive liver injury by a similar mechanism. Although these agents are ones that have been studied extensively because of life-threatening toxic reactions, a variety of similar compounds that have been less thoroughly investigated are used in industrial and medical applications. The extent of injury from these agents is dramatically dependent upon both the induction of cytochrome P450 and on the adequacy of antioxidant systems.

Among the most often used oxidative molecules in a medical setting are cancer chemotherapeutic agents, such as doxorubicin (Adriamycin), which are designed to preferentially kill rapidly dividing tumor cells. Adequate nutritional support remains an issue during the course of cancer treatment because the tumor cells compete for the same antioxidants as do normal cells. Similarly, individuals who have excessive exposure to sunlight or who have hyperreactive immune systems are chronically exposed to an increased oxidant burden and may therefore have increased nutritional demands for antioxidants. Unfortunately, carefully controlled intervention trials are costly, and little information is available concerning the utility of supplementation with antioxidants for chronic inflammation, chronic exposure to sunlight, or occupational exposures to various chemicals.

Oxidative Mechanisms Involved in Pathological Processes

Of particular importance to human health are the findings that many pathological processes are associated with an accumulation of oxidant damage. For instance, large deletions in the mitochondrial genome have been found in association with oxidative myocardial injury. Fluorescent lipofuscin pigments, characteristic of lipid peroxidation in the presence of proteins, accumulate in aging and neurodegenerative diseases. Cataracts and macular degeneration can be experimentally induced by chemical- and light-induced oxidative injury. These are just a few of many age-related disease processes that appear to be enhanced, if not entirely caused, by oxidative mechanisms.

Evidence is now accumulating that antioxidant systems that would normally protect against oxidant mechanisms decline with aging. For instance, blood levels of vitamin E, carotenoids, and selenium decline with aging. In addition, antioxidant enzymes such as glutathione peroxidase and superoxide dismutase decrease in activity. Although it remains unclear whether these changes are a cause or a consequence of age-related disease, it appears likely that such changes make tissues more vulnerable to various types of toxicity. This would be especially true for elderly populations whose use of therapeutic agents dramatically increases with time. Whether antioxidant nutritional supplementation can prevent age-related pathological processes continues to be investigated.

Issues Related to Establishment of Recommended Levels of Antioxidant Intake

Because antioxidants overlap in their protective functions, any specific antioxidant cannot be considered to be truly "required." This problem is further complicated because, unlike most vitamins, antioxidants appear to primarily function chemically rather than catalytically as a coenzyme associated with an enzyme activity. This means that the antioxidant function does not clearly obtain a saturation level. Based upon this, one might argue that the efficacy of antioxidants should increase infinitely with dose. However, such a conclusion is unreasonable for several reasons.

First, pharmacokinetics of absorption and elimination have been well studied for some antioxidants, and these studies indicate that there is a maximum attainable body concentration because of absorption limitations and the efficiency of excretory mechanisms. For instance, the efficiency of absorption of ascorbate decreases with increasing dose, and renal clearance increases with increasing plasma concentration, so that very little increase in total body ascorbate occurs at doses above 500 mg.

A second critical issue concerning high doses of antioxidants is that most also have the potential to be pro-oxidants under certain conditions. The major distinguishing feature between antioxidants and pro-oxidants is that antioxidants tend to terminate free radical processes and eliminate highly oxidizing chemicals. They typically do this by becoming oxidized themselves, usually to relatively stable, oxidized forms. However, this also means that antioxidant compounds can readily donate electrons to other species, and at high concentrations in the presence of transition metal ions, antioxidants actually can initiate oxidative stress.

A third issue that is of particular concern for carotenoids is that many different chemicals with very similar structures compete for the same transport mechanisms (Krinsky, 1993). For example, β-carotene competes with lutein for intestinal absorption. Thus excessive supplementation with β-carotene is likely to impair absorption of lutein. Although it remains unclear whether lutein has beneficial functions that are not replaceable by β-carotene, lutein is specifically accumulated in the retina; therefore, supplementation with β-carotene at levels that impair lutein absorption potentially could interfere with any function dependent upon lutein.

Although these arguments are based upon a limited number of examples, they illustrate the complexity of establishing recommendations concerning antioxidant supplementation. In the absence of proof that antioxidant supplements are beneficial, many nutritionists maintain that a balanced diet rich in fresh fruits and vegetables provides an optimal balance of antioxidants and should not be supplemented. Others feel that few can maintain such an ideal diet and believe that some supplementation with well-character-

ized antioxidants, including vitamins C and E, and with selenium is appropriate. Still others maintain that oxidative stress is a common component of disease processes affecting a majority of our aging population. They advocate more aggressive antioxidant therapies. All these approaches have a rational basis. Which is the best remains for future researchers to answer.

DETOXIFICATION OF XENOBIOTIC COMPOUNDS

To facilitate elimination of toxic xenobiotics by formation of reactive intermediates, Phase I activating enzymes are employed. Then Phase II detoxification enzymes further protect against a large array of reactive intermediates and nonactivated xenobiotics.

Sources of Xenobiotics and Chemoprotectors

Dietary sources of toxic, mutagenic, and carcinogenic substances include compounds produced in the cooking of fat, meat, or protein, and naturally occurring carcinogens associated with plant food substances, such as mold byproducts or alkaloids. The best-studied and most relevant carcinogens produced by cooking are the polycyclic aromatic hydrocarbons benzo(a)pyrene and heterocyclic aromatic amines generated by pyrolyzed meat protein (Lin et al., 1994). 2-Amino-1-methyl-6-phenylimidazol[4,5-b]pyridine is the most abundant of the heterocyclic aromatic amines in cooked food and is found at levels from 0.5 to 70 ng/g in cooked meat, depending on the temperature and method of meat preparation, with greatest levels in well-done charbroiled beef. People also ingest xenobiotics that are environmental or industrial contaminants (e.g., particulate matter of diesel exhaust, contaminating pesticides in food and water supplies, and many prescribed and over-the-counter medicinals that can be injurious to health depending on dosage).

On the other hand, many dietary microconstituents from plant sources (e.g., isothiocyanates, dithiolthiones, allyl sulfides, coumarins, and lactones) are associated with protection against cancer and toxicity (Steinmetz and Potter, 1991). These substances are termed chemoprotectors and all possess several common characteristics. They protect against both the initiation and promotion phases of neoplasia, protect against a broad range of procarcinogens and toxicants, protect in a variety of tissues, and induce endogenous xenobiotic detoxification enzymes that inactivate carcinogens and toxicants.

Not all the effects of chemoprotectors have been examined critically. However, the possibility that protection arises from alterations in the metabolism of the carcinogen or toxicant and its subsequent detoxification has received the most attention. Mounting evidence suggests that the enhancement of detoxification enzyme activity by chemoprotective compounds is an important aspect of the anticarcinogenic process (Wattenberg, 1985, 1992). The intervention of chemoprotective compounds at various stages in the carcinogenic process is shown in Figure 40–4.

Activation and Detoxification of Xenobiotics and Endogenous Compounds

As mentioned earlier, most xenobiotics are hydrophobic in nature and require metabo-lism to more hydrophilic forms to be readily eliminated from the body. This often involves insertion or addition of oxygen and transfer of an electron to the xenobiotic to create a reactive compound or an unstable compound that rearranges to form a reactive compound. The reactive intermediate is often an electrophile, an electron-seeking compound that readily reacts with nucleophilic (electron-donating) centers in DNA and cellular proteins. Because formation of a reactive intermediate is essential for elimination of some compounds, biological systems have evolved a balance between the rates of formation and elimination of these reactive intermediates. Imbalance in the rates of formation and detoxification of intermediates results in excessive covalent binding of xenobiotics to cellular macromolecules and causes cellular toxicity, cell injury, or carcinogenesis.

The enzymes that activate xenobiotics are termed Phase I activation enzymes and are represented by the multigene cytochrome P450 family, aldehyde oxidase, xanthine oxidases, and peroxidases. The majority of oxidation reactions that xenobiotics undergo are catalyzed by one family of enzyme systems, the cytochrome P450 monooxygenase systems. Treatment of cells with dietary toxic compounds, such as benzo(a)pyrene or 2-amino-1-methyl-6-phenylimidazol[4,5-b]pyri-

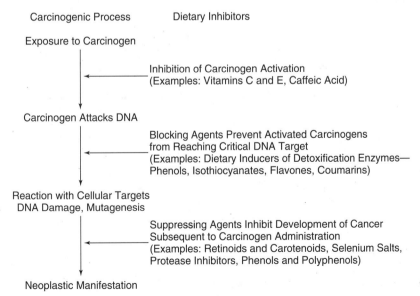

Figure 40–4. *Nutritional chemoprevention of cancer. (Based on Wattenberg, L. W. [1985] Chemoprevention of cancer. Cancer Res 45:1–8.)*

dine, or therapeutic drugs, such as phenobarbital, leads to an increase in the synthesis of one or more isoenzymes of cytochrome P450, leading to an increase in overall activity with respect to a particular substrate.

Endogenous detoxification (Phase II) enzymes eliminate xenobiotics biotransformed by the activation (Phase I) enzymes, as illustrated in Figure 40–5. Phase II detoxification enzymes conjugate the reactive intermediate or reduce an oxidative intermediate. Phase II enzymes include several enzymes or families of enzymes: the sulfotransferases, UDP glucuronosyltransferase, glutathione S-transferases, epoxide hydrolase, NAD(P)H:quinone reductase, and amine oxidases.

Phase II Detoxification Enzymes

Although the Phase II detoxification enzymes protect against a large number and variety of xenobiotics, they all possess several common properties. They usually catalyze the formation of a single type of functional group, have catalytic rates dependent on the enzyme protein and substrate concentrations (and are not regulated by allosteric effectors), are readily inducible by external signals such as dietary microconstituents, and are at highest concentration in the liver. The location of these enzymes in the liver provides efficient clearance of the compounds absorbed into the portal circulation and protects the rest of the body against exposure to compounds entering the body via the gastrointestinal tract and portal circulation. However, these enzymes also occur in most barrier epithelia and can be induced to very high levels in extrahepatic tissues by dietary inducers. Thus, these enzymes can protect against incoming harmful exposure to xenobiotics that produce damaging electrophiles in the lining of the gastrointestinal tract, lung, and skin. This is especially important in that 95% of all cancers are of epithelial cell origin, indicating the importance of environmental exposure of these cells to carcinogens and the significance of their endogenous complement and level of inducibility of the detoxification enzymes.

The Multigene Family of Glutathione S-transferases. The glutathione sulfur-transferases, which are often designated as the GSTs, catalyze the conjugation of xenobiotics with glutathione. The GSTs are a family of versatile isoenzymes that promote the conjugation of many electrophilic and usually lipophilic compounds with glutathione (Daniel, 1993; Jones et al., 1995). The reactions represent the initial steps in the formation of mercapturic acids, which are the ultimate excretory forms of many xenobiotics. The GSTs are present in many tissues in substantial quantities, and conjugation with glutathione is regarded as one of the most important mecha-

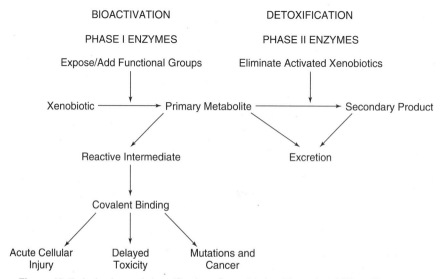

Figure 40–5. Activation and detoxification of xenobiotics: Phase I and Phase II reactions.

nisms for protection of tissues against the damaging effects of electrophiles. The protective function of these enzymes extends beyond their catalytic function, because these proteins also bind (and store) a wide range of compounds, and under some circumstances, may even scavenge electrophiles by undergoing covalent interactions with them. Glutathione conjugates are themselves excreted in the bile and are also converted to mercapturic acid metabolites, which are excreted in urine. (See Chapter 11 for more discussion of GSH synthesis and GSH conjugation reactions.)

The cytosolic GSTs are divided into four broad classes: alpha, mu, pi, and theta, which were originally distinguished by their basic, neutral, and acidic isoelectric points or by their relative substrate specificities. The four classes are each made up of different subunits (currently 12 subunits are known to be present in the rat), which form both homo- and heterodimers. Organ- and cell-specific expression of different GSTs with differing specificities for various electrophilic substrates allows tissues to detoxify a specific toxicant or carcinogen effectively.

The activities of GSTs are often limited by the availability of glutathione (GSH), a tripeptide synthesized from glutamate, cysteine, and glycine. With sulfur amino acid deficiency, GSH levels fall dramatically, and susceptibility to chemically induced injury is increased. The small intestine, which is the primary barrier to reactive electrophiles and lipid peroxides, has a relatively poor capacity to synthesize GSH. However, this epithelium can utilize GSH from food and from the bile to support its detoxification reactions. In addition, the rate-limiting enzyme for synthesis of GSH, γ-glutamylcysteine synthetase, is induced by chemical inducers found in the diet.

The importance of GST levels and their control is reflected in the elevated risk of lung cancer in populations of various ethnic origins who are deficient in the GST M1 gene. Odds ratio analysis indicates that smokers with this polymorphic variant have a higher risk of also developing larynx and bladder cancer.

UDP-Glucuronosyltransferases. These maximize biliary secretion and urinary excretion of xenobiotics. The formation of glucuronides represents a major mechanism of detoxification for many xenobiotics and metabolites of endogenous origin in higher organisms, because this process prepares these substances for excretion via the urine or the bile. Of all the conjugation reactions of the detoxification enzymes, glucuronidation has the highest capacity. Conjugation with glutathione and formation of sulfate esters (sulfo-conjugates) generally are quantitatively less significant for xenobiotic elimination. The formation of glucuronides depends on the generation and availability of the universal glucuronyl donor (UDP-glucuronic acid) in the cell cytosol (see Chapter 9) and the activation of the acceptor molecule by a series of microsomal glucuronosyl transferases of restricted specificities. Glucuronide conjugates are readily excreted in bile and urine, dependent on their molecular weight.

Sulfotransferases. These provide an alternative mechanism to glucuronidation to enhance excretion of compounds containing hydroxyl groups. Phenolic compounds present in the diet, as well as endogenously generated catecholamines, hydroxysteroids, and numerous therapeutic agents, are converted to charged compounds that are readily excreted by conjugation with a sulfate group. The sulfate group is transferred via one of four classes of sulfotransferases, which utilize 3'-phosphoadenosine-5'-phosphosulfate (PAPS) as the active sulfate donor.

The four classes of sulfotransferases recognize different types of hydroxylated compounds. Enzymes of the arylsulfotransferase class conjugate a wide range of dietary phenols and catechols. The other classes of sulfotransferases conjugate hydroxysteroids, phenolic steroids (e.g., estrogens), and bile acids. The capacity for conjugation by sulfotransferases is typically less than for conjugation by glucuronidation so that glucuronidation predominates at very high exposure to phenolic compounds. However, the sulfotransferases typically have a higher affinity for xenobiotics and thus play a greater proportionate role when the concentration of the substrate is low. Thus, at low concentrations of xenobiotics that are metabolized by both sulfation and glucuronidation, sulfation is often the predominant route of metabolism.

NUTRITION INSIGHT

Detoxification of Acetaminophen

Acetaminophen is widely used as an analgesic and antipyretic drug and has been marketed in the United States as an over-the-counter preparation since 1960. Acetaminophen is largely metabolized by Phase II enzyme systems, undergoing conjugation with glucuronate and sulfate in the liver. These nontoxic conjugates are excreted by the kidney. Most of an acetaminophen dose can be recovered in the urine within 24 h as glucuronide conjugates (~50% to 65%) and sulfate conjugates (~30% to 45%). Only about 1% of the dose is excreted in the urine as free acetaminophen. The extent of metabolism to glucuronide versus sulfate conjugates, but not total conjugation, has been shown to be influenced by diet, with a high-carbohydrate, low-protein diet favoring glucuronidation and a high-protein, low-carbohydrate diet favoring sulfation (Pantuck et al. 1991).

A smaller fraction of an acetaminophen dose is metabolized by a Phase I enzyme system to a hepatotoxic reactive intermediate. If this reactive intermediate is not detoxified by conjugation with glutathione, it can covalently bind to cellular macromolecules or cause other injurious effects (oxidative stress), which lead to hepatocellular necrosis. Glutathione conjugates are further metabolized to form cysteine conjugates and N-acetylcysteine conjugates (mercapturic acids), which account for 2% to 3% of the acetaminophen excreted in the urine. A small amount of glutathione-derived conjugates may also be excreted in the bile. A study of acetaminophen disposition in subjects with Gilbert's syndrome, which is an inherited deficiency of UDP-glucuronosyltransferase, demonstrated an inverse relationship between glucuronidation and bioactivation (De Morais et al., 1992). This observation suggests that a decrease in a major pathway of elimination (Phase II system) can shunt more drug through the toxifying route (Phase I system).

Although acetaminophen is generally considered to be safe at doses of less than 6 g/day, it is a potential hepatotoxin. The upper recommended dose is 4 g/day. Overdoses (usually single doses of more than 15 g) can be fatal. The toxicity of acetaminophen is enhanced by alcohol intake, which decreases Phase II and increases Phase I metabolism. There have been a number of reports of liver damage related to therapeutic use of acetaminophen (in some cases, at reported acetaminophen doses less than 4 g/day) by alcoholics or regular alcohol consumers. The effect of ethanol on acetaminophen hepatotoxicity is thought to result primarily from the induction of cytochrome P450(2E1) by ethanol, which allows greater conversion of acetaminophen to its active metabolite. Depletion of hepatic glutathione and malnutrition may also play a role. Zimmerman and Maddrey (1995), based on analysis of 161 cases of hepatic injury in alcohol consumers who took acetaminophen with therapeutic intent, have recommended that individuals who take more than 60 g of ethanol/day should take no more than 2 g/day of acetaminophen. (Approximately 60 g of ethanol is contained in 5 fluid ounces of 80-proof liquor, such as whiskey, gin, or vodka, 15 to 20 fluid ounces of wine, or 50 fluid ounces of beer.)

Epoxide Hydrolase. This protects against oxidative stress–producing epoxides. Epoxide hydrolase (microsomal and cytosolic) promotes the hydrolytic cleavage of a broad range of alkyl and cycloalkyl epoxides and arene oxides to the corresponding *trans*-dihydrodiols. Epoxides and arene oxides are important ultimate forms of many mutagens and carcinogens and are also the toxic metabolites of certain xenobiotics. Like the P450 mixed-function oxidases, epoxide hydrolase appears to serve both metabolic activation and detoxification functions. Thus, epoxide hydrolase is an essential participant in the formation and elimination of the short-lived ultimate carcinogenic species, such as diol-epoxides, formed during benzo(a)pyrene metabolism. There is considerable evidence for the role of this enzyme system in restraining the action of carcinogens, mutagenicity, and other forms of toxicity.

NAD(P)H:Quinone Reductase. This enzyme eliminates the redox cycling of activated xenobiotics and reactive oxygen radical production (Pius et al., 1994; Rushmore and Pickett, 1993). This enzyme, officially named NAD(P)H:quinone acceptor oxidoreductase (QR), was first termed vitamin K reductase, and it subsequently has been known as DT diaphorase and NAD(P)H dehydrogenase. QR is a cytosolic flavoprotein that is distinguished by a mandatory 2-electron reduction of quinones and similar compounds, thus eliminating generation of radical oxygen species that would cause cellular oxidant damage and stress. Like the other detoxification enzymes, it is distributed in all tissues and is readily induced in all tissues. It is unique in its ability to use NADH or NADPH as the electron donor. The function of this enzyme is particularly important because many plant foods contain quinones that are reactive electrophiles. This enzyme reduces quinones to phenolic compounds, which can be conjugated to less reactive glucuronides and sulfate esters and excreted. Many cruciferous vegetables and other plant foods that contain phenolic-type compounds induce QR, providing an effective method for their elimination and the prevention of toxicity and possibly carcinogenesis.

QR has been demonstrated to be preventive against formation of DNA-adducts of benzo(a)pyrene-quinone (Joseph and Jaiswal, 1994). It is clinically important in the bioreduction of antineoplastics such as mitomycin C.

Enhancement of Expression of Detoxification Enzymes in Response to Dietary Microconstituents

Dietary microconstituents can enhance genic transcription of detoxification enzymes. Many of the Phase II enzymes are coordinately and readily induced by dietary constituents present in fruits and vegetables (e.g., isothiocyanates and coumarins) and by food preservative antioxidants (e.g., butylated hydroxyanisole). This mechanism of induction by dietary factors is most understood for the enzymes glutathione *S*-transferase and QR (Pius et al., 1994; Rushmore and Pickett, 1993). Coordinate induction of GSTs and QR by minor dietary constituents occurs because of the common expression of a control sequence in the 5′ flanking region of their genes, as illustrated

in Figure 40–6. This region is termed the antioxidant response element (ARE) and is present in the promoter regions. The mechanism of enzyme elevation by nutritional factors is modulated through a chemically initiated redox signal activating c-Jun and possibly other transcription factors. It is postulated that this redox signal is mediated through the production of an intracellular oxidant state by exposure of cells to the dietary microconstituents, resulting in a decrease in glutathione levels. The oxidant state increases binding of c-Jun to the AP1 sites (activator protein-1 binding sites) in the ARE region of the promoter and results in an increased level of transcription of QR and GSTs.

The dietary inducers of GST and QR are divided into two major classes: (1) monofunctional inducers (e.g., isothiocyanates, coumarins, fumarates, and antioxidants), which act through the ARE region and elevate only detoxification enzymes, and (2) bifunctional inducers (e.g., planar compounds such as benzo(a)pyrene, dioxin, phenobarbital), which act through the xenobiotic response element (XRE) and which elevate both Phase I cytochrome P450 enzymes and Phase II detoxification enzymes. The xenobiotics that act through the XRE are compounds that are first metabolized to electrophilic oxidant signal metabolites by the cytochrome enzymes they induce; these metabolites subsequently act on the ARE region of the GST or QR gene to induce transcription of the detoxification enzymes.

Role of Dietary Intake and Genetics in Modification of Detoxification Enzyme Levels

Although there is a paucity of detailed mechanistic information in this area, it is clear that dietary deficiencies can affect the metabolism of foreign compounds by altering enzymes involved. For example, a low-protein diet will generally decrease the activity of monooxygenases and decrease the content of cytochrome P450. Rats fed a low-protein (5%) diet show 50% of the in vitro microsomal cytochrome P450 enzyme activity of rats fed a normal diet (20% protein diet). A decrease in

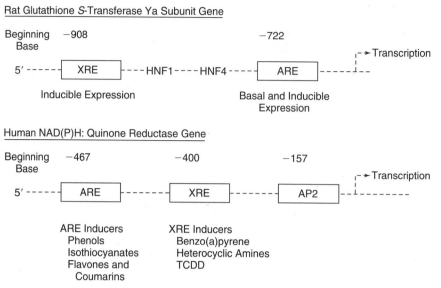

Figure 40–6. *Control of genic expression of detoxification enzymes by dietary compounds. Genic sites in the 5'-flanking region of glutathione S-transferase (GST) and NAD(P)H:quinone reductase are sensitive to dietary components, resulting in elevated enzyme levels. The AREs of both the GST Ya and the NAD(P)H:quinone reductase genes contain AP1 or AP1-like elements. ARE, antioxidant response element; XRE, xenobiotic response element; AP, activator protein; HNF, hepatic nuclear factors (liver-specific enhancer elements). (Based on data from Pius, J., Xie, T., Yuehang, X., and Jaiswal, A. K. [1994] NAD(P)H:quinone oxidoreductase [DT-diaphorase]: Expression, regulation, and role in cancer. Oncology Res 6:525–532; and Rushmore, T. H. and Pickett, C. B. [1993] Glutathione S-transferases; Structure, regulation, and therapeutic implications. J Biol Chem 268:11475–11478.)*

activity is apparent within 24 h, and the enzyme activity reaches the new lower steady state level by 4 days. This decrease of microsomal enzyme activity due to a low-protein diet may result in either reduced or enhanced toxicity. For example, carbon tetrachloride (CCl_4) hepatotoxicity is less in protein-deficient rats than in rats fed a control diet. However, acetaminophen is more hepatotoxic in protein-deficient animals, possibly owing to decreased glutathione levels. As with protein deficiency, a dietary deficiency of essential fatty acids such as linoleic acid also tends to decrease levels of cytochrome P450.

Changes in carbohydrate intake have fewer effects on drug metabolism, although an increase in glucose intake seems to decrease hepatic cytochrome P450 and inhibit barbiturate metabolism. The effects of starvation seem to be variable, with some microsomal enzyme activities being increased and others decreased. Deficiencies in vitamins in general also reduce the activity of the monooxygenases, although there are exceptions to this rule (e.g., thiamin deficiency results in an elevation of cytochrome P450). Several studies

have shown that ascorbate deficiency in guinea pigs is associated with decreased cytochrome P450 activity and with increased glucuronidation activity.

Variation in enzyme expression is an important underlying factor in the effect of nutrients on detoxification and cancer prevention. In addition to mutations that result in loss of expression of specific enzymes, differences exist in tissue expression, and polymorphisms exist for most of the detoxification enzymes. An important example for Phase I enzymes is the difference in cytochrome P450(1A2) expression. This enzyme is involved in the bioactivation of benzo(a)pyrene, a common environmental and dietary component, to a DNA-binding and mutagenic metabolite. This bioactivation is dramatically increased by prior exposure to cigarette smoke, charbroiled foods, cruciferous vegetables, and polybrominated biphenyls because these contain agents that increase the expression of cytochrome P450.

Variable susceptibility to carcinogenic aryl and heterocyclic amines has been related to differences in basal or induced expression of cytochrome P450(1A2). Genetic studies suggest that individuals who have high activities of a specific form of cytochrome P450 in the liver and the enzyme *N*-acetyltransferase 2 in the colon have an increased risk of colon cancer. Deficiency of human GST mu isoenzymes, which detoxify polyaromatic hydrocarbon oxides, diol-oxides, and *trans*-stilbene oxide substrates, is correlated with increased susceptibility to cancers of the lung, stomach, and colon.

Polymorphisms for carcinogen metabolism in humans are receiving increasing attention. As indicated, there are wide variations in carcinogen and toxicant metabolism and detoxification among humans, and these may serve as determinants of individual susceptibility. Polymorphisms can exist in the exons that encode expressed mRNAs that are translated into protein and also in the control regions that determine the conditions and extent of that expression. The former has been extensively studied in terms of multiple alleles, or copies of a single gene, which are inheritable and can differ in terms of expressed enzymatic activity. Genetic differences can result in different abilities to detoxify or bioactivate carcinogens or other toxicants and thereby alter susceptibility to cancer or toxicity. Although less studied and not discussed here, inheritable differences in control regions (e.g., ARE) also exist, and these can affect the expression of a gene as a consequence of environmental exposures.

Diet and Protective Functions

Current dietary recommendations to reduce risk of toxicity and chronic disease such as cancer are largely based upon epidemiological data. Dietary recommendations for daily intake of five servings of fruits and vegetables, especially cruciferous vegetables, are based on their content of fiber, vitamins, non-nutritive phytochemicals, and other minor constituents that act as inducers of endogenous detoxification enzymes as well as epidemiological studies. Increased intake of fruits and vegetables increases detoxification enzyme levels, and less intake of meats and fats lowers levels of reactive carcinogenic and toxic substances.

Several avenues of research are critical to a better understanding of the nutritional control of endogenous detoxification enzymes. These include

(1) differences in human tissue and cellular distribution of the detoxification enzymes and the effect of these differences on target-specific toxicity and carcinogenesis,

(2) the importance of epithelial cellular differentiation on the levels of detoxification enzymes, especially as differentiation relates to normal cell turnover and xenobiotic exposure,

(3) differences in genetic susceptibility to toxicity and carcinogenesis based on detoxification enzyme profiles at a genotypic and phenotypic level,

(4) the ability to elevate levels of these enzymes in humans in specific organs by nutritional intervention only.

Perhaps the least understood and most needed area for further study is the interaction during simultaneous administration of multiple dietary factors known to affect detoxification enzyme levels. Normal diets are composed of many types of foods, each containing microconstituents that affect the detoxification enzyme levels. Studies of such interactions in normal diets ultimately will provide us with a clearer understanding of the best balance of food constituents to reduce the risk of chronic diseases and improve general good health.

REFERENCES

Buettner, G. R. (1993) The pecking order of free radicals and antioxidants: Lipid peroxidation, alpha-tocopherol, and ascorbate. Arch Biochem Biophys 300:535–543.
Daniel, V. (1993) Glutathione S-transferases: Gene structure and regulation of expression. Clin Rev Biochem Mol Biol 28:173–207.
De Morais, S. M. F., Uetrecht, J. P. and Wells, P. G. (1992) Decreased glucuronidation and increased bioactivation of acetaminophen in Gilbert's syndrome. Gastroenterology 102:577–586.
Halliwell, B., Murcia, M. A., Chirico, S. and Aruoma, O. I. (1995) Free radicals and antioxidants in food and in vivo: What they do and how they work. Crit Rev Food Sci Nutr 35:7–20.
Jones, D. P., Brown, L. A. and Sternberg, P. (1995) Variability in glutathione-dependent detoxification in vivo and its relevance to detoxification of chemical mixtures. Toxicology 105:267–274.
Joseph, P. and Jaiswal, A. K. (1994) NAD(P)H:quinone

reductase (DT diaphorase) specifically prevents the formation of benzo(a)pyrene quinone-DNA adducts generated by cytochrome P4501A1 and P450 reductase. Proc Natl Acad Sci USA 91:8413–8417.

Krinsky, N. I. (1993) Actions of carotenoids in biological systems. Annu Rev Nutr 13:561–587.

Lin, D., Meyer, D. J., Ketterer, B., Lang, N. P. and Kadlubar, F. F. (1994) Effects of human and rat glutathione S-transferases on the covalent DNA binding of the N-acetoxyderivatives of heterocyclic amine carcinogens in vitro: A possible mechanism of organ specificity in their carcinogenesis. Cancer Res 54:4920–4926.

Pantuck, E. J., Pantuck, C. B., Kappas, A., Conney, A. H. and Anderson, K. E. (1991) Effects of protein and carbohydrate content of diet on drug conjugation. Clin Pharmacol Ther 50:254–258.

Pius, J., Xie, T., Yuehang, X. and Jaiswal, A. K. (1994) NAD(P)H:quinone oxidoreductase (DT-diaphorase): Expression, regulation, and role in cancer. Oncology Res 6:525–532.

Rushmore, T. H. and Pickett, C. B. (1993) Glutathione S-transferases; Structure, regulation, and therapeutic implications. J Biol Chem 268:11475–11478.

Sies, H. and Stahl, W. (1995) Vitamins E and C, beta-carotene, and other carotenoids as antioxidants. Am J Clin Nutr 62:1315S–1321S.

Steinmetz, K. A. and Potter, J. D. (1991) Vegetables, fruit, and cancer. II. Mechanisms. Cancer Causes Control 2:427–442.

Thomas, S. R., Neuzil, J., Mohr, D., and Stocker, R. (1995) Coantioxidants make alpha-tocopherol an efficient antioxidant for low density lipoprotein. Am J Clin Nutr 62:1357S–1364S.

Wattenberg, L. W. (1985) Chemoprevention of cancer. Cancer Res 45:1–8.

Wattenberg, L. W. (1992) Inhibition of carcinogenesis by minor dietary constituents. Cancer Res 52:2085S–2089S.

Zimmerman, H. J. and Maddrey, W. C. (1995) Acetaminophen (paracetamol) hepatotoxicity with regular intake of alcohol: Analysis of instances of therapeutic misadventure. Hepatology 22:767–773.

RECOMMENDED READINGS

Halliwell, B., Murcia, M. A., Chirico, S. and Aruoma, O. I. (1995) Free radicals and antioxidants in food and in vivo: What they do and how they work. Crit Rev Food Sci Nutr 35:7–20.

Steinmetz, K. A. and Potter, J. D. (1991) Vegetables, fruit, and cancer. II. Mechanisms. Cancer Causes Control 2:427–442.

CHAPTER 41

◆ ◆

Nutrition, Lipids, and Cardiovascular Disease

Henry N. Ginsberg, M.D., and Wahida Karmally, M.S., R.D.

OUTLINE

COMMON ABBREVIATIONS

ASCVD (atherosclerotic cardiovascular disease)*
CAD (coronary artery disease)*
CHD (coronary heart disease)*
HDL (high density lipoproteins)
IDL (intermediate density lipoproteins)
LDL (low density lipoproteins)
VLDL (very low density lipoproteins)

---

*ASCVD, CAD, and CHD are used interchangeably.

ATHEROSCLEROTIC CARDIOVASCULAR DISEASE

Atherosclerotic cardiovascular disease is the number one cause of death in Western nations and is rapidly becoming a prominent cause of death in economically "underdeveloped" countries as well. It was recognized more than 100 years ago that the atherosclerotic lesion was laden with lipids. In 1908, Ignatowski first showed that rabbits fed meat, dairy, and egg products developed lesions resembling human atherosclerosis (Ignatowski, 1908). Anitschkow and Chalatow (1913) followed soon after with proof that dietary cholesterol was the key nutrient responsible for hypercholesterolemia and atherosclerosis in this animal model. Following these groundbreaking investigations, numerous epidemiological studies of diet, nutrition, and atherosclerotic cardiovascular disease have generated an enormous database linking diets high in saturated fat and cholesterol to human diseases (U. S. Department of Health and Human Services, 1988; National Research Council, 1989). These observational studies were paralleled by the rapid development of the field of lipid and lipoprotein metabolism, with studies stretching from human dietary investigations to studies of diet and atherosclerosis in transgenic and "knockout" mouse models of human dyslipidemia. The epidemiological and basic studies were followed by intervention trials, culminating in two studies in which changes in diet alone were associated with less progression of coronary artery disease and fewer coronary events (Ornish et al., 1990; Watts et al., 1992). The evidence linking diet and atherosclerotic disease, with a particular focus on effects of diet on lipid and lipoprotein metabolism, is reviewed in this chapter.

Pathophysiology of Atherosclerosis

Despite a rapidly growing base of knowledge regarding the cellular and molecular biology of the vessel wall, plasma lipids and lipoproteins still occupy the central and key role in our understanding of atherogenesis. Present concepts concerning the development of the atherosclerotic lesion and a brief overview of lipoprotein transport are summarized in this chapter. Detailed reviews of the pathology and cell biology of atherosclerosis are available (Ross, 1995; Steinberg et al., 1989).

Plasma cholesteryl esters and triacylglycerols, two classes of hydrophobic neutral lipids, are transported through the plasma in the core of lipoprotein particles, as discussed in Chapters 7 and 14. The surface of the lipoprotein consists of amphipathic molecules, including free cholesterol, phospholipids, and apoproteins. There are two major classes of triacylglycerol-rich lipoproteins: chylomicrons and very low density lipoproteins (VLDL). Chylomicrons are assembled in the small intestine and carry dietary triacylglycerols and cholesterol, whereas VLDL are assembled in the liver and transport mainly endogenously derived core lipids. In the plasma, chylomicrons and VLDL lose their triacylglycerols after interacting with lipoprotein lipase at the vessel wall; they become, respectively, chylomicron remnants and VLDL remnants (also called IDL or intermediate density lipoproteins). Chylomicrons and VLDL also can be modified by the exchange of their core triacylglycerol for core cholesteryl ester from high density lipoproteins (HDL) and low density lipoproteins (LDL). Although the chylomicron remnant is, under normal conditions, almost quantitatively removed from plasma by the liver, VLDL remnants can be converted significantly to LDL in addition to being taken up by the liver. Once LDL are formed, they can be removed from plasma by LDL receptors.

The major protein on chylomicrons, VLDL, their remnants, and LDL is apoprotein B (apo B). The liver makes a full-length 540-kDa version of this polypeptide, which is necessary for both the initial secretion of VLDL into the blood stream and the removal of LDL via the LDL receptor. The intestine makes a shortened 210-kDa version of the protein as a result of mRNA editing: although this shorter protein is required for chylomicron secretion into the circulation, it lacks the receptor binding domain present in full-length apo B. All the apo B–containing lipoproteins are potentially atherogenic if their metabolism is not regulated properly. In contrast, HDL, which have a very different protein, apo A-I, as its major protein, are antiatherogenic under most conditions. (See Chapter 14 for a more detailed description of the assembly, secretion, and plasma metabolism of lipoproteins.)

The role of the apo B–containing lipoproteins is to transport exogenously and endogenously derived lipids to peripheral tissues: in the case of triacylglycerols, for energy utilization or storage; in the case of cholesterol, for steroidogenesis and cell membrane structural integrity. To carry out their role, lipoproteins must be able to move across the endothelial covering of blood vessels and reach the extracellular space. LDL is the predominant lipoprotein passing through the endothelial layer, but there is evidence that both chylomicron remnants and VLDL remnants can do so as well. Much of this transendothelial migration occurs in the capillaries, but some occurs in all vessels, including the large arteries. Present concepts of atherogenesis consider the passage of lipoproteins into the subendothelial space as the first critical step in the process. It appears that during a brief period of contact with the endothelial cell barrier, the lipoprotein may be "modified" (Steinberg et al., 1989). Modification may be in the form of oxidation of phospholipid, particularly phosphatidylcholine. Modified apo B–containing lipoproteins may be more liable to aggregate or to stick to extracellular matrix molecules in the subendothelial space. Alternatively, unmodified apo B lipoproteins may stick to matrix molecules in the subendothelial space, triggering interaction with overlying endothelial cells and subsequent modification of the lipoprotein. In either scheme, greater numbers of circulating lipoproteins will infiltrate the endothelium and be retained.

As illustrated in Figure 41–1, once modification/retention of apo B–containing lipoproteins occurs, signals to the endothelial cells result in synthesis and display of several cell adhesion molecules and of monocyte chemotactic proteins and in the secretion of monocyte colony-stimulating factor. Together, these molecules stimulate the formation, sequestering, and transmigration of circulating monocytes at the site of retained subendothelial lipoproteins (Gimbrone et al., 1995). Once the monocytes enter the subendothelial space, they are activated and transformed into macrophages. These macrophages further oxidize the retained lipoproteins, internalize them through one or more receptors, and develop into foam cells. They also secrete factors, such as transforming growth factor beta, which can stimulate smooth muscle cell proliferation and migration. Both the monocytes/macrophages and the activated smooth muscle cells begin to secrete extracellular matrix molecules as well. At this point, all the components of the advanced lesion are in place, and atherogenesis is well under way.

Lipoprotein (a) [Lp(a)] is composed of LDL with a second protein, apo(a), covalently linked to apo B. Apo(a) is a large protein with a highly variable size (200 to 700 kDa) that is synthesized in the liver. It is believed that apo(a) binds to LDL apo B in plasma. High plasma levels of Lp(a) have been linked in several studies to increased risk for atherosclerotic cardiovascular disease, and recent studies have suggested that certain diet components may affect Lp(a) levels (Berglund, 1995).

HDL, or the apo A-I–containing lipoproteins, appear to have protective effects against atherosclerosis. Two major hypotheses have been presented to explain the negative association of HDL cholesterol levels with atherosclerotic cardiovascular disease. First, a large body of data indicates a role for HDL in the reverse transport of cholesterol from tissues throughout the body back to the liver. Because the apo B–containing lipoproteins, particularly LDL, are thought to deliver several hundred milligrams of cholesterol to peripheral tissues daily, there must be some mechanism to balance that delivery system. HDL is thought to be the vehicle for such balance. Small, cholesterol-poor HDL particles (either spherical or disc-like) are good acceptors of free cholesterol from the extracellular surface of membranes. These HDL particles, enriched in free cholesterol, can be modified by the enzyme lecithin:cholesterol acyltransferase (LCAT); this enzyme esterifies the free cholesterol with a fatty acid (e.g., linoleate) from lecithin. The cholesteryl ester moves from the surface of the lipoprotein to the core (because of its hydrophobicity), allowing more free cholesterol to be adsorbed onto the surface. This process results in enlargement of the HDL particles. As HDL become enriched

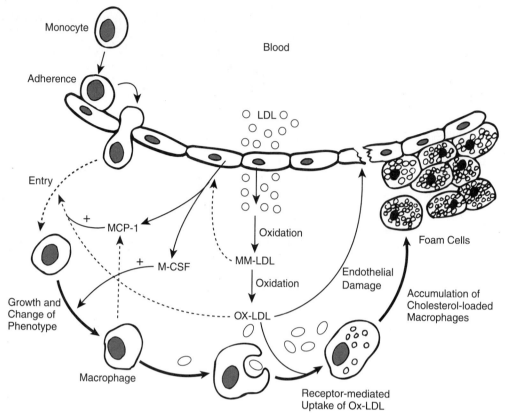

Figure 41-1. *Depiction of the early stages of atheroma formation, including LDL entry into the vessel wall, endothelial damage or dysfunction, LDL modification and oxidation, recruitment of monocytes into the vessel wall, and uptake of modified/oxidized LDL by monocyte-derived macrophages. MM-LDL, lightly oxidized LDL; OX-LDL, oxidized LDL; M-CSF, macrophage-colony stimulating factor; MCP-1, monocyte chemotactic protein. (From Steinberg, D. [1991] Antioxidants and atherosclerosis: A current assessment. Circulation 84:1420–1425.)*

in cholesteryl esters, they become significant vehicles for delivery of those esters to the liver, where the cholesterol can be converted to bile acids or excreted as biliary cholesterol. How this final step in the reverse cholesteryl transport pathway is achieved is unclear at this time: either the HDL delivers the cholesteryl esters via selective uptake or endocytosis of the entire HDL particle occurs. Recently, a potential receptor for selective delivery of HDL cholesteryl esters to hepatocytes and certain other cells, called scavenger receptor B1 (SRB1), was identified. Alternatively, HDL can transfer the cholesteryl esters to triacylglycerol-rich VLDL or chylomicrons via cholesteryl ester transfer protein (CETP). The latter transfer, which is bimolecular with a triacylglycerol going to HDL, can be followed by uptake of the chylomicron or VLDL remnant by the liver.

The second potential antiatherogenic activity of HDL relates to its role as an antioxidant and/or antiaggregant in the vessel wall. Much fewer data are available to support this activity. Of particular interest is the striking ability of human apo A-I to reduce atherosclerosis in mice lacking apo E, an apoprotein that is a key ligand for several hepatic receptors, including the LDL receptor. In this mouse model of severe hyperlipidemia and atherosclerosis, overexpression of the gene for apo A-I results in significant reductions in atherosclerosis despite very small increases in plasma HDL cholesterol levels. Additionally, it has been shown that apo A-I can directly protect LDL against oxidative modification in vitro. These recent reports support the finding of an antiatherogenic effect of apo A-I infusions into swine despite no measurable change in plasma HDL levels. This will be an exciting area of research to follow over the next few years.

Pathophysiology of Dyslipidemia

Despite the complexity of the atherosclerotic process and the multicomponent nature of the advanced lesion, a key initiator of atherogenesis appears to be the presence of increased amounts of retained and/or modified lipoproteins in the subendothelial space. The latter is a direct consequence of increased quantities of atherogenic lipoproteins in the circulation. It is, therefore, important to understand the pathophysiology of the various dyslipidemias. The more common types of hyperlipidemias and their clinical characteristics are summarized in Table 41–1.

Isolated Hypercholesterolemia. Elevated levels of fasting plasma total cholesterol are, in general, associated with increased concentrations of plasma LDL cholesterol, because LDL carries about 65% to 75% of total plasma cholesterol. If plasma triacylglycerol levels are markedly increased, VLDL cholesterol, which is usually 5% to 10% of total plasma cholesterol, may be high enough to elevate total plasma cholesterol concentrations even when LDL cholesterol levels are normal. VLDL cholesterol may be a major component of total cholesterol in dysbetalipoproteinemic subjects (with the apo E2/2 phenotype) as well. Finally, the rare individual with significantly elevated HDL cholesterol (>80 mg/100 mL) may appear to have moderately increased total plasma cholesterol.

Elevations of LDL cholesterol can result from single gene defects, polygenic disorders, and environmental effects on lipoprotein metabolism. Familial hypercholesterolemia (FH), which occurs in the heterozygous form in approximately 1 in 300 to 500 individuals, is associated with mutations in the gene for the LDL receptor (Brown and Goldstein, 1984). Plasma total and LDL cholesterol concentrations are increased at birth in FH subjects and remain so throughout life. In heterozygous FH adults, total cholesterol levels range from 300 to 500 mg/100 mL in the untreated state, and both tendon xanthomas (accumulations of

cholesteryl ester–filled macrophages over tendons, particularly the Achilles tendon) and premature atherosclerosis with coronary artery disease (CAD) are common. Plasma triacylglycerol concentrations are typically normal, whereas HDL cholesterol levels may be normal or reduced. Metabolic studies have demonstrated decreased fractional clearance of LDL apo B in subjects with FH, consistent with reduced numbers of LDL receptors, although increased production of LDL has also been observed. The latter may be the result of more efficient conversion of VLDL to LDL in the FH patients as a concomitant of reduced LDL receptor function and reduced VLDL remnant removal from plasma. On the other hand, increased assembly and secretion of VLDL (or denser apo B–containing lipoproteins) may be a concomitant of defective hepatic catabolism of circulating LDL. In any event, markedly elevated levels of LDL cholesterol are the hallmark of FH and are associated with increased risk for CAD in these patients. The homozygous form of FH occurs in 1 of 1 million individuals and is associated with plasma cholesterol levels > 500 mg/100 mL, large tendon and planar xanthomas, and very aggressive, premature CAD. These individuals almost always develop clinically significant CAD by early adulthood, often during adolescence.

Recently, a second single gene disorder that causes significant elevations of LDL cholesterol has been identified. A mutation in apo B, in the region of the protein associated with binding to the LDL receptor, has been linked to defective catabolism of LDL in vivo and to hypercholesterolemia. It is transmitted in an autosomal dominant fashion. Finally, subjects with familial combined hyperlipidemia, which is discussed later, can present with isolated elevations of LDL cholesterol (Goldstein et al., 1973).

Polygenic causes of hypercholesterolemia are much commoner than FH. In polygenic hypercholesterolemia, the environment plays a greater role in determining plasma LDL cholesterol concentrations. Most evidence indicates that both overproduction and reduced fractional catabolism of LDL play significant roles in the pathophysiology of this disorder. Both abnormal variables are probably affected

TABLE 41–1
Characteristics of Common Hyperlipidemias

Type	Plasma Lipid Levels	Lipoproteins	Clinical Signs
Isolated Hypercholesterolemia	**Heterozygotes**		
Familial hypercholesterolemia	Total cholesterol = 300–500 mg/100 mL	LDL	Usually develop xanthomas in adulthood and vascular disease at 30–50 y
	Homozygotes		
	Total cholesterol = 400–800 mg/100 mL	LDL	Usually develop xanthomas and vascular disease in childhood
Polygenic hypercholesterolemia	Total cholesterol = 225–350 mg/100 mL	LDL	Usually asymptomatic until vascular disease develops; no xanthomas
Isolated Hypertriglyceridemia			
Mild	Triacylglycerols = 250–750 mg/100 mL (plasma may be cloudy)	VLDL	Asymptomatic; may be associated with increased risk of vascular disease
Severe	Triacylglycerols > 750 mg/100 mL (plasma may be milky)	Chylomicrons, VLDL	May be asymptomatic; may be associated with pancreatitis, abdominal pain, hepatosplenomegaly
Hypertriglyceridemia and Hypercholesterolemia			
Combined hyperlipidemia	Triacylglycerols = 250–750 mg/100 mL	VLDL	Usually asymptomatic until vascular disease develops
	Total cholesterol = 250–500 mg/100 mL	LDL	Familial form (FCHL) may also present as isolated high triacylglycerols or as isolated high LDL cholesterol
Dysbetalipoproteinemia	Triacylglycerols = 250–500 mg/100 mL	VLDL, IDL	Usually asymptomatic until vascular disease develops; may have palmar or tuboeruptive xanthoma
	Total cholesterol = 250–500 mg/100 mL	VLDL, IDL LDL normal	
Low HDL Cholesterol			
Associated with hypertriglyceridemia	HDL = 20–35 mg/100 mL Total triacylglycerols > 250 mg/100 mL	HDL	Usually asymptomatic; may increase risk for vascular disease
Primary hypoalphalipoproteinemia	HDL = 5–25 mg/100 mL Total triacylglycerols < 250 mg/100 mL	HDL	Depending on etiology, may be asymptomatic; often associated with increased vascular disease

HDL, high density lipoproteins; IDL, intermediate density lipoproteins; LDL, low density lipoproteins; VLDL, very low density lipoproteins.

by dietary saturated fat and cholesterol consumption, by age, and by level of physical activity. Plasma total cholesterol levels are in the 250- to 350-mg/100 mL range. Plasma triacylglycerol and HDL cholesterol levels are usually normal. Tendon xanthomas are not present in these individuals. It is very likely that as genes related to regulation of cholesterol metabolism are identified, some of the polygenic forms of hypercholesterolemia will be found to be due to the interaction of two or more specific genes.

Hypertriglyceridemia. Elevated levels of fasting plasma triacylglycerols—in the range of 250 to 750 mg/100 mL—are generally associated with increased concentrations of VLDL triacylglycerols. When VLDL triacylglycerol levels are markedly elevated (regardless of etiology) or when lipoprotein lipase is either significantly reduced or totally deficient, chylomicron triacylglycerols may also be present, even after a 14-hour fast. Elevations in plasma triacylglycerols most often are associated with the synthesis and secretion of excessive quantities of VLDL triacylglycerol by the liver (Ginsberg et al., 1985). Hepatic triacylglycerol synthesis is regulated by substrate flow (particularly the availability of free fatty acids), by energy status (particularly the level of glycogen stores in the liver), and by hormonal status (particularly the balance between insulin and glucagon levels). Obesity, excessive consumption of simple sugars and saturated fats, inactivity, alcohol consumption, and glucose intolerance or diabetes mellitus commonly have been associated with hypertriglyceridemia. Although no single gene disorder associated with increased hepatic synthesis of triacylglycerols has been identified, some recent studies have suggested a link between abnormal bile acid metabolism and overproduction of triacylglycerols in some subjects with hypertriglyceridemia. It is believed that in this group of disorders, sometimes referred to as primary hypertriglyceridemia, only triacylglycerol synthesis is increased, and therefore the liver secretes a normal number of large, triacylglycerol-enriched VLDL particles. The secretion of a normal number of VLDL particles limits the rate of production of LDL particles, and these subjects may not be at increased risk for coincident elevations of LDL cholesterol. It should be noted, however, that subjects with familial combined hyperlipidemia, who will be described later, can present with isolated hypertriglyceridemia.

The degree of hypertriglyceridemia present in any individual will also depend on the quantity and activity of the two key triacylglycerol hydrolases, lipoprotein lipase and hepatic lipase. Most data suggest that lipoprotein lipase is normal in the majority of subjects with moderate hypertriglyceridemia (250 to 500 mg triacylglycerol/100 mL plasma), but lipoprotein lipase activity may be reduced in more severely affected individuals (>750 mg/100 mL). Several recent studies have suggested that heterozygosity for lipoprotein lipase deficiency, derived from specific mutations, occurs in about 5% to 10% of the hypertriglyceridemic population. Additionally, when VLDL triacylglycerol concentrations are markedly elevated (>1000 mg/100 mL), lipoprotein lipase may be saturated with substrate so that, in effect, the subject is relatively deficient in the enzyme during the postprandial period. Chylomicron triacylglycerols may then add to hypertriglyceridemia. If lipoprotein lipase is totally deficient, plasma triacylglycerol concentrations greater than 2000 mg/100 mL are commonly seen, with both chylomicrons and VLDL making significant contributions to the hyperlipidemic state. Hepatic lipase activity is frequently elevated in hypertriglyceridemic subjects, but the significance of this association is unclear; the high hepatic lipase activity may be relevant to the reduced HDL cholesterol levels found in this condition because hepatic lipase can hydrolyze HDL phospholipids and destabilize the HDL particle. Additionally, HDL can be elevated in subjects with a deficiency of hepatic lipase, a rare disorder in humans that results in defective final catabolism and/or abnormal remodeling of small VLDL and IDL.

Hypertriglyceridemia with Hypercholesterolemia. Hypertriglyceridemia can also occur in association with hypercholesterolemia in two phenotypes. In the first, called combined hyperlipidemia, both total plasma triacylglycerols and LDL cholesterol concentrations must, by definition, be greater than the 90th percentiles for age- and sex-matched controls (Goldstein et al., 1973). Although it is likely that a variety of combinations of regulatory defects in lipid metabolism account for a significant number of individuals with this phenotype, a familial form of combined hyperlipidemia (FCHL) has been identified in which probands (the initial case discovered within the family) may present with combined hyperlipidemia, with only hypertriglyceridemia, or with only elevated levels of LDL cholesterol. In the familial disorder, which appears to be transmitted as an autosomal dominant gene, the diagnosis must rest on the presentation, at some point in time, of combined hyperlipidema in the proband or, alternatively, the presence of various lipid phenotypes in first-degree family members, along with either isolated hypertriglyceridemia or an isolated elevation of LDL cholesterol in the proband. FCHL is not associated with abnormalities in LDL receptors. Thus, FCHL is not related to FH pathophysiologically.

From available studies, FCHL appears to be associated with secretion of increased numbers of VLDL particles (as determined by the flux of VLDL apo B) (Arad et al., 1990). Hence, individuals with FCHL will be predisposed to high levels of plasma VLDL triacylglycerols if, for any other reason (see earlier), they synthesize triacylglycerols at an increased rate. Once they have assembled and secreted increased numbers of large, triacylglycerol-rich VLDL, these individuals will attain varying levels of plasma triacylglycerols, dependent upon their ability to hydrolyze VLDL triacylglycerol (via lipoprotein lipase and, to a lesser degree, hepatic lipase). The ability to hydrolyze VLDL triacylglycerols will also regulate the generation of LDL in plasma. Thus, subjects with FCHL who have very high VLDL triacylglycerol concentrations might have normal or actually reduced numbers of LDL particles in the circulation and a normal LDL cholesterol concentration (if they are not able to catabolize VLDL efficiently). On the other hand, if individuals with FCHL are able to efficiently catabolize the increased numbers of VLDL particles that are entering their plasma, they will generate increased numbers of LDL particles and present with both hypertriglyceridemia and a high LDL cholesterol level. Finally, subjects with FCHL who are synthesizing only normal quantities of triacylglycerols, but secreting increased numbers of VLDL carrying normal triacylglycerol loads, will generate increased numbers of LDL particles and present with only elevated plasma LDL cholesterol concentrations. FCHL may occur in as many as 1 in 50 to 100 Americans; it is the most common familial lipid disorder found in survivors of myocardial infarction (Goldstein et al., 1973). Recent studies have demonstrated links between combined hyperlipidemia and insulin resistance (Reaven, 1988); the pathophysiological basis for this link is undefined presently.

The second disorder in which elevations of both plasma triacylglycerols and cholesterol can occur is dysbetalipoproteinemia. In this rare disorder affecting 1 in 10,000 people, mutations in the gene for apo E result in synthesis of defective forms of this apolipoprotein. Apparently, because apo E plays crucial roles in the catabolism of chylomicron and VLDL remnants (Mahley, 1988), subjects with defective apo E accumulate these cholesteryl ester–enriched remnant lipoproteins in their plasma. Hence, both VLDL triacylglycerol and VLDL cholesterol are elevated and chylomicron remnants are present in fasting plasma from dysbetalipoproteinemic subjects. LDL cholesterol levels are not elevated in this disorder. Of interest are the data indicating that 1 in 100 people are homozygous for the mutant apo E (the apo E2 isoform). Ninety-nine percent of these apo E2/2 subjects have normal plasma triacylglycerol and cholesterol levels; they also have reduced LDL cholesterol levels, possibly as a consequence of their inability to process VLDL normally. Thus, a second defect in lipid metabolism, not just the apo E2/2 genotype, must be present in the 1 in 10,000 individuals with the clinically relevant entity, dysbetalipoproteinemia.

Reduced HDL Cholesterol. Low concentrations of HDL cholesterol are most often seen in subjects with coexistent hypertriglyceridemia, although "primary hypoalphalipoproteinemia" has been identified in both individuals and families. The pathophysiological basis of reduced HDL cholesterol concentrations is not well defined and is probably quite complex (Horowitz et al., 1993; Tall, 1990). The relationship between hypertriglyceridemia and low HDL levels probably derives from (1) the cholesteryl ester transfer protein (CETP)–mediated transfer of cholesteryl ester from the core of HDL to VLDL, (2) the shift of surface components, particularly phospholipids and apolipoproteins C-II and C-III, from HDL to VLDL, and (3) the increased fractional catabolism of the cholesteryl ester–poor, surface-poor HDL that results from the first two processes. The complexity of the situation is highlighted, in most patients who present initially with hypertriglyceridemia and low HDL cholesterol concentrations, by the failure of HDL levels to normalize when fasting plasma triacylglycerols are significantly reduced.

Primary hypoalphalipoproteinemia refers to the state in which HDL cholesterol concentrations are markedly reduced but plasma triacylglycerol concentrations are normal. Although this disorder certainly exists, many subjects who present with this phenotype have had hypertriglyceridemia in the past or have an older (or more obese) first-degree relative who has both low HDL and increased triacylglycerol levels. Hence, carefully conducted family studies and long-term follow-up may be necessary to identify individuals who truly have primary reductions in HDL cholesterol. The basis for such reductions is unknown except for extremely rare situations in which genetic mutations in the area of the apo A-I gene have been described. Other rare disorders in which HDL cholesterol is severely reduced include Tangier disease and lecithin:cholesterol acyltransferase (LCAT) deficiency.

Epidemiology of Atherosclerosis

General Overview. Extensive reviews of the epidemiology of atherosclerosis are available in both journals and textbooks (National Research Council, 1989). The 20th century has seen the near disappearance of several infectious diseases in Western societies and the explosion of chronic diseases, particularly atherosclerosis. In the early part of the century, the rising incidence of coronary heart disease (CHD) paralleled increased caloric intake, particularly intake of saturated fats. Natural experiments attest to the importance of these factors; during World War II the incidence of CHD fell dramatically in occupied countries. By contrast, after the war, Japanese men who migrated to Hawaii and then to California consumed increased quantities of saturated fats, had increases in their plasma cholesterol levels, and began to suffer more and more from CHD. In the United States, the switch from a farming to an industrial society, together with a switch from a high-carbohydrate to a high-fat diet paralleled our epidemic of CHD in the 1950s through 1970s. During the past decade, reductions in dietary consumption of fat have correlated with the reduction in coronary artery disease (CAD) observed in the United States (Expert Panel on Detection, Evaluation, and Treatment of High Blood Cholesterol in Adults, 1993).

Risk Factors for Atherosclerotic Cardiovascular Disease. Numerous, long-term prospective studies, including the Framingham Study, the Honolulu Heart Study, and the Chicago Gas and Electric Company Study, have provided unique data regarding the role of genetic and environmental factors that increase risk for developing atherosclerotic cardiovascular disease (ASCVD) (National Research Council, 1989). Hypertension, smoking, hypercholesterolemia, and diabetes are the major risk factors for CAD and stroke. A low level of HDL cholesterol is also an important risk factor. Although prevalence of individual risk factors may differ by race or gender, the major risk factors are usually of similar importance in whites and blacks and in men and women. Age has a major impact in women, with premenopausal women having lower total and LDL cholesterol levels and higher HDL cholesterol concentrations than postmenopausal women. Hormone replacement therapy lowers total and LDL cholesterol and raises HDL cholesterol. A list of major risk factors from the National Cholesterol Education Program report is shown in Table 41–2.

Lipids and Lipoproteins as Risk Factors. As described earlier in this chapter, disorders of lipoprotein metabolism can lead to alterations in plasma cholesterol and triacylglycerol levels, and these disorders are usually associated with increased risk of cardiovascular disease. The association of plasma total cholesterol with CAD is quite robust, but this association is confounded by the distribution of cholesterol among the lipoprotein classes. High total cholesterol levels in blood are usually paralleled by high plasma concentrations of LDL cholesterol, and LDL levels are strong indicators of risk for atherosclerosis. On the other hand, HDL cholesterol levels are inversely related to risk for CAD, and extremes in HDL cholesterol, either at the low or high end, can confound the relationship between total cholesterol and risk. The issue of plasma triacylglycerols as a risk factor has been controversial for many years (Hall, 1995). This controversy stems from an absence of triacylglycerols in vessel wall lesions, the close inverse relationship between triacylglycerols and HDL cholesterol, and the lack of strong

NUTRITION INSIGHT

Risk Factors for Vascular Disease

Classic independent risk factors for cardiovascular disease include hypercholesterolemia, smoking, and hypertension. Over the past decade, numerous studies have demonstrated than an elevated plasma total homocysteine level is also a strong and independent risk factor for vascular disease. Results of a recent multicenter case-control study that involved 19 centers in 9 European countries and that included both men and women and all types of atherosclerotic vascular disease (cardiac, cerebral, and peripheral) demonstrated this relationship between homocysteine and vascular disease (Graham et al., 1997; Boers, 1997). When the relationship between plasma total homocysteine level and the risk of all categories of atherosclerotic vascular disease was considered, subjects with plasma total homocysteine levels in the top quintile had a risk that was double that of all other subjects combined (relative risk, or the ratio between the two risks, was ~2). When the top 10% of the fasting plasma total homocysteine distribution was compared with the lowest 10%, the relative risk was 3 instead of 2. The level of risk associated with hyperhomocysteinemia was equivalent to that associated with hypercholesterolemia or smoking, whereas hypertension was associated with a higher excess risk.

The relationships between smoking or fasting plasma cholesterol level and vascular disease are continuous; risk increases as the number of cigarettes smoked daily or the plasma cholesterol concentration increases. Similarly, a dose-response relationship is observed between plasma total homocysteine level and risk of vascular disease. Interactions of plasma homocysteine level and risk of vascular disease. Interactions of plasma homocysteine with other risk factors were also observed in the European multicenter study; an increased fasting homocysteine level showed a more-than-multiplicative effect on risk in smokers and in subjects with hypertension.

Benefits of smoking cessation, cholesterol reduction, and antihypertensive treatment in reducing risk of cardiovascular disease events have been well documented. Demonstration of the benefits of reductions of plasma homocysteine levels, possibly by administration of B vitamins (folate, vitamin B_6, and vitamin B_{12}), in reducing risk of vascular disease is currently being evaluated.

---

evidence that triacylglycerols are independent predictors of disease. The cholesterol transported in VLDL with triacylglycerols based on animal and cell studies can accumulate in arterial wall macrophages, and thus, elevated triacylglycerol levels may be a marker of increased delivery of non-LDL cholesterol to lesion sites.

The observation that HDL cholesterol levels are inversely related to CAD has led to numerous studies of HDL subclasses in an effort to identify the "truly antiatherogenic" type of HDL. HDL_2 (density of 1.063 to 1.12 g/mL) and HDL_3 (density of 1.12 to 1.21 g/mL) were the first major subclasses studied. Although several studies have indicated that only the larger, more cholesteryl ester–enriched HDL_2 is protective, other investigators have failed to see a difference between the two types of HDL (Silverman et al., 1993; Wilson et al., 1991). More recently, studies

in which HDL was subdivided according to apoprotein composition have raised the possibility that particles with apo A-I but not apo A-II are antiatherogenic, whereas particles with both apoproteins A-I and A-II are not; this work remains controversial (Lagrost et al., 1995).

Investigators studying LDL have also looked closely at heterogeneity in LDL. Small, dense LDL, which are commonly found in individuals with higher triacylglycerol and lower HDL cholesterol levels, have been proposed as the "more" atherogenic LDL (Austin et al., 1990). It is possible, based on studies showing greater penetration into the artery wall or increased predisposition for oxidative modification, that small, dense LDL are more atherogenic than "normal" LDL. On the other hand, patients with familial hypercholesterolemia have large, cholesteryl ester–enriched LDL that seem to be quite atherogenic.

TABLE 41-2
Risk Status* Based on Presence of CHD Risk Factors Other than LDL Cholesterol

Positive Risk Factors

Age:
  Men: ≥ 45 years
  Women: ≥ 55 years, or premature menopause
    without estrogen replacement therapy
Family history of premature CHD (definite myocardial
  infarction or sudden death before 55 years of age in
  father or other male first-degree relative, or before
  65 years of age in mother or other female first-
  degree relative)
Current cigarette smoking
Hypertension (≥ 140/90 mm Hg,† or on
  antihypertensive medication)
Low HDL cholesterol (≤ 35 mg/100 mL†)
Diabetes mellitus

Negative Risk Factor‡

High HDL cholesterol (≥ 60 mg/100 mL)

---

*High risk, defined as a net of two or more CHD risk factors, leads to more vigorous intervention. Age (defined differently for men and for women) is treated as a risk factor because rates of CHD are higher in elderly than in young people and higher in men than in women of the same age. Obesity is not listed as a risk factor because it operates through other risk factors that are included (hypertension, hyperlipidemia, decreased HDL cholesterol, and diabetes mellitus), but it should be considered a target for intervention. Physical inactivity is similarly not listed as a risk factor, but it too should be considered a target for intervention, and physical activity is recommended as desirable for everyone.

†Confirmed by measurements on several occasions.

‡If the HDL cholesterol level is > 60 mg/100 mL, subtract one risk factor (because high HDL cholesterol levels decrease CHD risk).

From Expert Panel on Detection, Evaluation, and Treatment of High Blood Cholesterol in Adults (1993) Summary of the second report of the National Cholesterol Education Program (NCEP) expert panel on detection, evaluation, and treatment of high blood cholesterol in adults (Adult Treatment Panel II). JAMA 269:3015-3023.

Finally, it cannot be overlooked that all the studies concerned with lipids, lipoproteins, and risk for CAD have used fasting blood samples for determination of lipid and lipoprotein levels. In recent years, increased interest in the postprandial period has led to a number of reports that link postprandial triacylglycerol levels to CAD (Patsch et al., 1992). This link may have its pathophysiological basis in the accumulation of atherogenic chylomicron remnants, the concomitant fall in HDL cholesterol, and/or the production of smaller, denser LDL during the postprandial period. Further studies, particularly ones focused on the effects of diet on postprandial lipoprotein metabolism, are needed.

EFFECTS OF DIET ON PLASMA LIPIDS AND LIPOPROTEINS

The amount and type of fatty acids in dietary fat, the dietary cholesterol level, as well as the caloric content and macronutrient composition of the diet, can influence the composition, concentration, and metabolism of plasma lipoproteins.

Dietary Fat and Fatty Acids

Dietary fatty acids are often divided into three major classes: saturated, monounsaturated, and polyunsaturated, and the ratio (by weight) of polyunsaturated fatty acids to saturated fatty acids is referred to as the P:S ratio. The major fatty acids found in dietary triacylglycerols (fats and oils) are listed in Table 41-3.

A number of studies have been used, alone and together, to generate equations that predict the changes in total and lipoprotein cholesterol that will occur in response to changes in intake of dietary fatty acids and cholesterol. These equations are given in Table 41-4.

Effects of Saturated Fatty Acids on Plasma Total and LDL Cholesterol Concentrations.

The classic studies of Keys et al. (1965) and Hegsted et al. (1965) demonstrated clearly

TABLE 41-3
The Major Dietary Fatty Acids by Class

Saturated Fatty Acids

  Lauric acid (12:0)
  Myristic acid (14:0)
  Palmitic acid (16:0)
  Stearic acid (18:0)

Monounsaturated Fatty Acids

  Oleic acid (18:1n-9)
  trans 16:1n-9 and *trans* 18:1n-9

Polyunsaturated Fatty Acids

  Omega 6
  Linoleic acid (18:2n-6)
  Omega 3
  α-Linolenic acid (18:3n-3)
  Eicosapentaenoic acid (20:5n-3)
  Docosahexaenoic acid (22:6n-3)

TABLE 41–4

Predictive Equations for Estimating Changes in Plasma Cholesterol and Lipoprotein Cholesterol in Response to Dietary Fatty Acids and Cholesterol*

(A) Keys Equation

$$\Delta TC = 1.35(2\Delta S - \Delta P) + 1.52\Delta Z$$

(B) Hegsted Equation

$$\Delta TC = 2.16\Delta S - 1.65\Delta P + 0.067\Delta C - 0.53$$

(C) Mensink and Katan Equations

$$\Delta TC = 1.51\Delta S - 0.12\Delta M - 0.60\Delta P$$
$$\Delta LDL\text{-}C = 1.28\Delta S - 0.24\Delta M - 0.55\Delta P$$
$$\Delta HDL\text{-}C = 0.47\Delta S + 0.34\Delta M + 0.28\Delta P$$

(D) Yu Equations

$$\Delta TC = 2.02\Delta 12\text{:}0\text{--}16\text{:}0 - 0.03\Delta 18\text{:}0 - 0.48\Delta M - 0.96\Delta P$$
$$\Delta LDL\text{-}C = 1.46\Delta 12\text{:}0\text{--}16\text{:}0 + 0.07\Delta 18\text{:}0 - 0.69\Delta M - 0.96\Delta P$$
$$\Delta HDL\text{-}C = 0.62\Delta 12\text{:}0\text{--}16\text{:}0 - 0.06\Delta 18\text{:}0 + 0.39\Delta M + 0.24\Delta P$$

*Where ΔTC, $\Delta LDL\text{-}C$, and $\Delta HDL\text{-}C$ = changes in plasma total, LDL, and HDL cholesterol in mg/100 mL; ΔS = change in percentage of daily energy from saturated fatty acids; ΔM = change in percentage of daily energy from monounsaturated fatty acids; ΔP = change in percentage of daily energy from polyunsaturated fatty acids; ΔZ = change in the square root of dietary cholesterol in mg/1000 kcal; ΔC = change in dietary cholesterol in mg/day (Hegsted).

Equations are from the following sources:

(A) Keys, A., Anderson, J. T. and Grande, F. (1965) Serum cholesterol response to changes in the diet. IV. Particular saturated fatty acids in the diet. Metabolism 14:776–787.

(B) Hegsted, D. M., McGandy, R. B., Myers, M. L. and Stare, F. J. (1965) Quantitative effects of dietary fat on serum cholesterol in man. Am J Clin Nutr 17:281–295.

(C) Mensink, R. P. and Katan, M. B. (1992) Effect of dietary fatty acids on serum lipids and lipoproteins. Arterioscler Thromb 12:911–919.

(D) Yu, S., Derr, J., Etherton, T. D. and Kris-Etherton, P. M. (1995) Plasma cholesterol–predictive equations demonstrate that stearic acid is neutral and monounsaturated fatty acids are hypocholesterolemic. Am J Clin Nutr 61:1129–1139.

that increases in the percent of calories from saturated fat are associated with increases in total plasma cholesterol levels. Substitution of saturated fat for polyunsaturated or monounsaturated fat or carbohydrates will raise total plasma cholesterol levels. Although numerous studies (Mensink and Katan, 1992; Yu et al., 1995) have been carried out since these original investigations, the regression coefficients proposed by Hegsted et al. (1965) and Keys et al. (1965) have generally stood the test of time. The response in total cholesterol is mirrored by changes in LDL cholesterol and apo B levels and is similar in men and women, older and younger individuals, pre-

and postmenopausal women, and whites and blacks (Ginsberg et al., 1998). Children also respond to changes in dietary saturated fat intake with the predicted changes in total and LDL cholesterol levels.

The mechanisms by which saturated fatty acids raise LDL cholesterol levels have been investigated intensely (Woollett et al., 1992a, 1992b). In a variety of animal models, downregulation of LDL receptors, coupled with increased production of cholesterol-carrying lipoproteins by the liver, accounts for the rise in plasma LDL levels. In hepatocytes from rats fed saturated fat, LDL receptor mRNA levels are depressed; similar effects have been observed in other rodents and in nonhuman primates. Less is known about the mechanisms underlying increased production of lipoprotein cholesterol; data concerning effects of intracellular cholesterol on apo B secretion are conflicting.

Several studies of the effects of saturated fats on human lipoprotein metabolism have been conducted. In a study of normal and hypercholesterolemic men, Turner et al. (1981) found that high-fat diets with very low P:S ratios were associated with increased rates of production and slightly reduced rates of clearance of LDL apo B compared with diets with very high P:S ratios. Shepherd et al. (1980) found that similar diets altered LDL clearance rates in normal subjects. Cortese et al. (1983) fed high-fat diets with varying P:S ratios to hyperlipidemic men; they observed that saturated fats increased both the number of VLDL secreted by the liver and the conversion of VLDL to LDL.

In the same series of studies from which Keys et al. (1965) and Hegsted et al. (1965) generated regression coefficients for saturated fats, coefficients were estimated for each of the individual saturated fatty acids from C12 through C18. In the succeeding years, interest in the individual saturated fatty acids increased intermittently; recently interest has peaked once again, in part because of technological advances that allow production of specific fatty acid blends that may be used in food production.

Palmitic (C16:0), myristic (C14:0), and lauric (C12:0) acids all seem to be hypercholesteremic compared with monounsaturated fatty acids (i.e., oleic acid), but the relative potency of these three individual saturated fatty acids in raising plasma cholesterol is not certain. They all seem to act by suppressing receptor-dependent LDL cholesterol clearance from the circulation and by increasing VLDL cholesterol secretion by the liver.

In the original studies by Keys et al. (1965) and Hegsted et al. (1965), contrasting effects of lauric acid (C12:0) were indicated; Keys assigned lauric acid a coefficient equal to that of palmitic acid and myristic acid, whereas Hegsted found it to have only a mild cholesterol-raising effect. More recent studies have not resolved the cholesterol-raising of lauric acid relative to palmitic acid but suggest that lauric acid does have an LDL cholesterol-raising effect compared with monounsaturated fatty acids (i.e., oleic acid) and a more or less equivalent LDL cholesterol-raising effect as compared with that of palmitic acid.

Data from both Keys et al. (1965) and Hegsted et al. (1965) suggested that myristic acid (C14:0) may be four to six times more cholesterolemic than palmitic acid. In a recent trial (Welty et al., 1995), the effect of myristic acid was tested on a large group of volunteers. Compared with both palmitic and oleic acids, myristic acid significantly raised both total and LDL cholesterol levels. Myristic acid was about 1.5 times as cholesterol-raising as was palmitic acid. Furthermore, several other investigators have reported that palmitic acid (C16:0) was less hypercholesterolemic than a combination of lauric acid and myristic acid when substituted for lauric plus myristic acid over a range of 5% to 18% of energy intake (Sundaram, 1994). However, there are also reports of no increase in total and LDL cholesterol when myristic acid was substituted for palmitic acid, and the cholesterol-raising effects of myristic acid relative to the other major saturated fatty acids remain in question.

Both the studies of Keys et al. (1965) and Hegsted et al. (1965) assigned a neutral role to stearic acid (C18:0), and this has been confirmed by more recent studies (Bonanome and Gandy, 1988). It must be pointed out, however, that relative to polyunsaturated fatty acids such as linoleic acid, stearic acid raises total cholesterol and LDL cholesterol. Recently, Yu et al. (1995) developed a new regression equation based on 18 studies that reported data on stearic and other fatty acids. In that equation, stearic acid was found to be neutral. The lack of a cholesterol-raising effect of stearic acid is due, in part, to its desaturation to oleic acid shortly after absorption as well as its higher incorporation into phosphatidylcholine (versus triacylglycerol and cholesteryl esters) compared with palmitic acid.

Effects of Polyunsaturated Fatty Acid on Plasma Total and LDL Cholesterol Concentrations. Human feeding studies in the early 1950s suggested that polyunsaturated fats had unique properties in that they reduced plasma cholesterol concentrations. Keys et al. (1965) and Hegsted et al. (1965) both estimated negative regression coefficients for this class of fatty acids. Although the reductions in total cholesterol that occurred when diets high in polyunsaturated fats were fed were confounded in many studies by concomitant reductions in HDL cholesterol (Mensink and Katan, 1992), LDL cholesterol levels fell as well. Indeed, the reductions in LDL levels appear to be not only a response to replacement of saturates by polyunsaturates in many studies, but also a direct result of some activity of polyunsaturated fatty acids. Meta-analysis of a number of well-controlled diet studies in humans have confirmed a direct LDL-lowering effect of an increase in the amount of polyunsaturated fatty acids in the diet, but this effect is not as potent as that obtained by reducing the amount of saturated fat in the diet (Mensink et al., 1992; Yu et al., 1995). This effect may be difficult to observe in single studies in which modest increases in dietary polyunsaturates are achieved. Additionally, polyunsaturates may be potent only when they are added to diets initially lacking or extremely low in this class of fats: Hayes (1992) suggested that 5% of calories from polyunsaturated fatty acids represents the upper end of the dose-response curve for the LDL cholesterol-lowering effect. The mechanisms for LDL lowering by consumption of diets high in polyunsaturates are the opposite of those demonstrated for saturates: increased LDL receptor function and reduced lipoprotein-cholesterol secretion from the liver.

Effects of Monounsaturated Fatty Acids and *trans* Fatty Acids on Plasma Total and LDL Cholesterol Concentrations. There has been much recent interest in the effects of monounsaturated fatty acids because of the low rates of atherosclerotic cardiovascular disease in the Mediterranean area where diets are high in fat but the fat is mainly olive oil. In the studies by Keys et al. (1965) and Hegsted et al. (1965), monounsaturated fats, specifically oleic acid, were found to have negligible independent cholesterol-lowering effects. This was accepted as a fact until the mid-1980s, when other investigators demonstrated that monounsaturates could lower total and LDL cholesterol in subjects fed diets in which monounsaturated fatty acids replaced saturated fatty acids. Ginsberg et al. (1990), in a study with young, healthy men, found that replacing 7% of calories from carbohydrates with oleic acid in an otherwise American Heart Association (AHA) Step 1 diet did not result in lower plasma total or LDL cholesterol. This finding is in accord with the predictive regression coefficient based on a meta-analysis of the effects of fatty acids published by Mensink and Katan (1992), although Yu et al. (1995) recently developed a predictive equation in which monounsaturates were given a small cholesterol-lowering value. Although replacement of saturated fat with monounsaturated fat has a cholesterol-lowering effect, the addition of a moderate amount of oleic acid to the diet (in the range of 5% to 10% of total calories as a replacement for carbohydrate calories) is unlikely to have a discernible effect on total or LDL cholesterol. Other monounsaturates, such as palmitoleic acid, are found in very low amounts in typical American diets; palmitoleic acid levels are higher in diets high in many types of nuts.

A unique, but commercially important, monounsaturated fatty acid is the *trans* isomer of C18:1n–9, elaidic acid. This fatty acid results from the commercial process to partially hydrogenate linoleic acid in the production of margarines. Early work by Mattson et al. (1975) in the 1960s led to the belief that elaidic acid acted like the *cis* isomer of oleic acid; it had no effect on plasma cholesterol concentrations. However, work published a few years later suggested a slight cholesterol-

raising effect of *trans* fatty acids. Finally, in 1990, Katan and colleagues (Mensink and Katan, 1990) published the first of a series of papers indicating that *trans* fatty acids might behave more like saturated fatty acids. LDL levels increased in a dose-response manner when dietary oleic acid was replaced by moderate to large amounts of elaidic acid (5% to 20% of total calories). HDL levels fell and Lp(a) levels increased on the high elaidic acid diet. These findings for LDL have been confirmed in other studies (Judd et al., 1994; Nestel et al., 1992), whereas the fall in HDL was observed in some (Judd et al., 1994; Lichtenstein et al., 1993) but not all studies (Nestel et al., 1992). Additionally, an increase in Lp(a) was not seen in the study by Lichtenstein et al. (1993), although it was observed by Nestel et al. (1992). The relevance of these findings to the American diet is unclear because the average intake of *trans* fatty acids is estimated at 2% to 4% of calories, which is appreciably lower than the intake of saturated fatty acids. On the other hand, some epidemiological data indicate a negative effect of *trans* fatty acid intake on morbidity and mortality. Estimates of the average intake of *trans* fatty acids from various food sources are listed in Table 41–5.

Effects of Fatty Acids on HDL Cholesterol Concentration. In their early studies, Keys et al. (1965) and Hegsted et al. (1965) examined only total plasma cholesterol levels on different diets. Indeed, it wasn't until the late 1970s, after the rediscovery of the importance of HDL cholesterol as a protective factor for CAD, that studies of the effects of dietary fatty acids on HDL cholesterol began to be conducted. In many of the early studies, large quantities of polyunsaturated fatty acids (up to 20% to 30% of total calories) were used to replace saturated and monounsaturated fatty acids; these studies demonstrated reductions in HDL cholesterol concentrations (along with lowering of LDL cholesterol levels). In the studies by Mattson and Grundy (1985) in which monounsaturated fatty acids were compared with polyunsaturated fatty acids as replacements for saturated fats, the "high poly" diets were associated with much lower HDL cholesterol levels than were the "high mono" diets.

TABLE 41–5
Estimated Average Daily Intake of Total Fat and trans Fat from Primary Food Sources of trans Fatty Acids*†

Food Source	Total Fat‡ (g/day)	trans Fat (g/day)
Vegetable		
Bread, commercial	4.0	0.3
Fried foods§	3.9	0.8
Cakes and related baked goods	2.9	0.3
Savory snacks	2.3	0.3
Margarine, stick‖	1.7	0.5
Margarine, soft and spreads‖	1.2	0.2
Cookies	1.2	0.2
Crackers	0.5	0.1
Household shortening‖	0.4	0.1
Animal		
Milk	5.5	0.2
Ground beef	3.4	0.1
Butter	1.3	0.1

*Values are 3-day averages from the U.S. Department of Agriculture (USDA) Continuing Surveys of Food Intakes by Individuals, 1989–1990 and 1990–1991.

†*Trans* composition data adapted from Nutrient Data Bank Bulletin Board (USDA/Agricultural Research Service, Riverdale, MD).

‡Total fat intake = 69 g/day; total energy intake = 7.355 MJ/day (1758 kcal/day).

§Home and food service combined.

‖Intake of these foods does not include use as ingredients in foods already listed in table.

LDL cholesterol concentrations were similar in the two diets. In several studies (Dreon et al., 1990; Wardlaw and Snook, 1990) in which smaller quantities of polyunsaturated fatty acids were added to an AHA Step 1 diet as replacement for saturated or monounsaturated fat, a smaller HDL lowering was observed (Ginsberg et al., 1994a).

A more systematic look at the effects of each class of fatty acids on HDL cholesterol levels can be achieved using the meta-analysis approach. In reports by Mensink and Katan (1992) and Yu et al. (1995), saturated, polyunsaturated, and monounsaturated fatty acids were all shown actually to have HDL cholesterol-raising effects. However, the relative potency of these fatty acid classes in raising HDL cholesterol was saturated > monounsaturated > > polyunsaturated. Thus, if monounsaturates are used as a replacement for saturates, a very slight reduction in HDL would result (monounsaturates raise HDL slightly less than saturates): this reduction would likely be statistically insignificant in most of the studies with small sample sizes. If polyunsaturates are used to replace saturates, the fall in HDL cholesterol would be greater because polyunsaturates raise HDL only about 40% as much as saturates; this effect has been statistically significant in most reported studies. This scheme makes it clear why replacement of total fat (of any fatty acid distribution) with carbohydrate (which is neutral regarding HDL cholesterol) results in significant reductions in HDL cholesterol levels: all fats raise the plasma HDL concentration.

Three human studies have addressed the mechanisms by which HDL falls during consumption of diets with different total fat contents. Blum et al. (1977) first studied HDL apo A-I metabolism in subjects consuming a diet very high in carbohydrate (80% of total calories) and low in fat (5% of total calories) or high in fat (40% of total calories) with typical carbohydrate content (40% of total calories). These investigators demonstrated that the fall in plasma concentrations of HDL cholesterol and apo A-I was associated with increased fractional clearance of apo A-I in individuals consuming the lower fat diets. Brinton et al. (1990) performed a similar experiment several years later in which they fed subjects diets in which fat provided 40% or 10% of total calories. They found that the fall in HDL cholesterol levels in subjects on the low-fat diet was associated mainly with reduced apo A-I production, although they also found that fractional clearance of apo A-I was higher in subjects fed the low-fat diet than in subjects fed the high-fat diet. Shepherd et al. (1978) compared diets with very high and very low polyunsaturated to saturated fat ratios and found that the lower HDL levels observed in subjects eating the high polyunsaturated fat diet were associated with significantly reduced rates of apo A-I appearance in plasma. Summarizing these studies, the consistent theme that emerges is that all fatty acids somehow increase secretion of apo A-I from the liver and/or the intestine, and that saturates stimulate apo A-I secretion more than polyunsaturates. Monounsaturates seem to be similar to saturates in their effect on apo A-I secretion. Replacing fatty acids with carbohydrates will result in a decrease in apo A-I secretion and also may result in increased fractional clearance of apo A-I, both of which will lead to lower plasma levels of this protein. Altered levels of apo A-I will result, under most conditions, in altered plasma concentrations of HDL cholesterol. (The relationship of apo A-I to HDL cholesterol is described in detail in Chapter 14.)

Effects of Fatty Acids on Triacylglycerol Concentrations. In general, saturated fatty acids increase plasma triacylglycerol levels moderately whereas polyunsaturated fatty acids reduce them to a similar degree. Exceptions to the moderate effects of fatty acids on plasma triacylglycerol are those effects observed when large amounts of ω3 fatty acids (4 to 8 g/day) are consumed (Harris et al., 1990). This class of fatty acids includes α-linolenic acid (18:3), eicosapentaenoic acid (EPA; 20:5), and docosahexaenoic acid (DHA; 22:6). Soybean and canola oils are good sources of α-linolenic acid, and EPA and DHA are found mainly in the fat tissue of cold-water fish. Consumption of large quantities of salmon oil was shown to significantly reduce the secretion of VLDL from liver in normal and hypertriglyceridemic humans. Omega-3 fatty acids also reduce postprandial triacylglycerol levels. EPA and DHA can increase the intracellular degradation of nascent apo B in cultured liver cells. Capsules of concentrated ω3 fatty acids have been used to treat patients with severe hypertriglyceridemia.

Effects of Fatty Acids on Lp(a) Levels. Lp(a) is a subclass of LDL that contains apo(a) in addition to apo B. Some, but not all, epidemiological studies have indicated increased risk for ASCVD as Lp(a) increases. Although some studies have suggested that greater than 90% of the variability in Lp(a) levels appears to be genetically determined, recent studies have found that increases in plasma Lp(a) levels occur in normal and dyslipidemic individuals when saturated fatty acids are decreased in the diet, with either replacement of dietary calories by carbohydrate or monounsaturated fat (Ginsberg et al., 1998). Lp(a) concentrations were not altered by changes in dietary saturated fats or cholesterol in several previous studies (Berglund,

1995). In contrast, Lp(a) levels did rise in the majority of studies in which *trans* fatty acids were increased (Mensink and Katan, 1990; Nestel et al., 1992; Lichtenstein et al., 1993). Further studies will be needed to investigate and confirm the mechanisms underlying these effects of fatty acids on Lp(a) concentrations in plasma.

Dietary Cholesterol

The role of dietary cholesterol in the development of both hypercholesterolemia and atherosclerosis has been the focus of many investigations over the past century. The studies by Ignatowski (1908) and later by Anitschkow and Chalatow (1913) indicated the importance of dietary cholesterol, and their work in rabbits has been supported by many studies in other animal models and by human dietary and epidemiological investigations (Stamler and Shekelle, 1988). However, although many continue to support the view that dietary cholesterol is the major atherogenic nutrient in the diet, other investigators have come to opposite conclusions after reviewing numerous human feeding studies. This controversy has been evident in the changing prominence of dietary cholesterol in the American Heart Association (AHA) Diet Statements published every several years (Chait et al., 1993; Grundy et al., 1989).

One reason for this controversy is that experimental animals may not be appropriate models. Clearly, humans do not respond to dietary cholesterol with the marked increases in plasma cholesterol observed in rabbits. Even rodent species, which are resistant to atherosclerosis, respond to dietary cholesterol and fat with larger increases in lipid levels than do humans. Another problem with the animal studies is that the amounts of cholesterol fed in most early studies were much beyond the highest intakes reported in humans. More recently, however, diets with modest increases in cholesterol content have been shown to significantly increase plasma cholesterol in nonhuman primates, with concomitant development of atherosclerosis.

Many studies of the effects of dietary cholesterol on plasma cholesterol levels in humans have been published during the past several decades. However, many were of poor quality, with little control over nutrient intake other than cholesterol. Several excellent studies deserve review. First, as always, the classic studies of Keys et al. (1965) and Hegsted et al. (1965) provided us with regression coefficients for the effects of dietary cholesterol on plasma total cholesterol levels. These coefficients suggested that for each 100 mg of dietary cholesterol added per day, plasma cholesterol would rise between 3 mg/100 mL (Keys et al., 1965) and 6 mg/100 mL (Hegsted et al., 1965). Hegsted et al. (1993), in a later review of more experiments, lowered their estimate of the effect of dietary cholesterol to be in line with that of Keys et al. (1965). Ginsberg carried out two very well controlled studies in healthy young men (1994b) and women (1995). Dietary cholesterol ranged from about 125 mg/day to 750 mg/day and was added to a National Cholesterol Education Program (NCEP) Step 1 diet. Several levels of cholesterol were fed, allowing for regression analysis of the results, as shown in Figure 41–2. For each addition of 1 egg (about 200 mg of cholesterol), LDL cholesterol increased about 3 to 4 mg/100 mL. This change was statistically significant, but obviously modest,

particularly in the setting of baseline LDL cholesterol levels of about 100 mg/100 mL. The changes observed amounted to about 60% of the original estimate of response reported by Keys et al. (1965). HDL cholesterol tended to increase in the men and significantly increased in the women (1 mg/100 mL for each egg added to the diet) (Ginsberg et al., 1994b, 1995).

Human metabolic studies of the effects of dietary cholesterol on lipoprotein production and degradation have added to our knowledge of the mechanism underlying effects on plasma levels. Dietary cholesterol does not seem, within the range of typical intakes, to affect VLDL production by the liver, but increased secretion of IDL directly into the circulation has been observed in a small group of subjects fed very high levels of cholesterol. Several studies of 3-hydroxy-3-methylglutaryl (HMG) CoA reductase inhibitors, which reduce endogenous cholesterol synthesis, have demonstrated reduced secretion of VLDL in vivo. Thus, the effects of dietary cholesterol on VLDL assembly and secretion remain incompletely characterized.

A number of studies have focused on the effects of dietary cholesterol on LDL metabo-

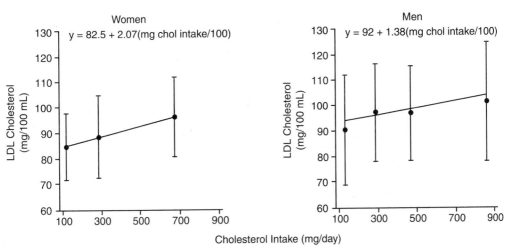

Figure 41–2. Response of plasma LDL cholesterol concentrations to increases in dietary cholesterol intake. Diets containing various amounts of cholesterol (provided by eggs) were consumed for 8 weeks with a washout period between diets. Individual points are means ± SD for 13 women or 20 men. The regression lines are the means of the individual regression lines for each of the 13 women or 20 men. (From Ginsberg, N. H., Karmally, W., Siddiqui, M., Holleran, S., Tall, A. R., Rumsey, S. C., Deckelbaum, R. J., Blaner, W. S., and Ramakrishnan, R. [1994] A dose-response study of the effects of dietary cholesterol on fasting and postprandial lipid and lipoprotein metabolism in healthy young men. Arterioscler Thromb 14:576–586; and Ginsberg, H. N., Karmally, W., Siddiqui, M., Holleran, S., Tall, A. R., Blaner, W. S., and Ramakrishnan, R. [1995] Increases in dietary cholesterol are associated with modest increases in both LDL and HDL cholesterol in healthy young women. Arterioscler Thromb Vasc Biol 15:169–178.)

lism. Ginsberg et al. (1981) determined LDL apo B turnover in 5 healthy men on diets containing 300 and 1200 mg of cholesterol/day. Both diets contained 40% of calories as fat, with a P:S ratio of 0.4. The three-fold increase in dietary cholesterol had no effect on LDL production or fractional clearance, and LDL cholesterol levels did not change. In a similar study by Packard et al. (1983), an eight-fold increase in dietary cholesterol (1800 mg/day compared with 200 mg/day) on top of a diet containing 40% of calories as fat, with a P:S ratio of 0.2, increased plasma cholesterol levels, and this was associated with both increased LDL production and decreased fractional removal of LDL. The differences in results in these two studies may have been related to the greater absolute cholesterol load or lower P:S ratio in the study by Packard et al. (1983).

Dietary Carbohydrates

Dietary recommendations to lower total fat intake include increasing dietary carbohydrate intake, because favorable plasma lipid and lipoprotein levels have been reported for populations and individuals whose habitual diet is high in carbohydrates. However, there is concern over reports of a decrease in HDL cholesterol and an elevation of plasma triacylglycerols with high carbohydrate consumption. Populations who eat high-carbohydrate diets have low plasma HDL cholesterol levels and low CHD rates. Plasma triacylglycerol levels are not significantly elevated in these populations, possibly because obesity is rare. Another issue currently being studied is whether it is advisable to recommend high-carbohydrate diets to individuals with insulin resistance and diabetes (Garg et al., 1994), who may have high plasma triacylglycerol and low HDL cholesterol levels. The concern is that high-carbohydrate diets may exacerbate the risk for heart disease. In a well-controlled multicenter study (Lefevre et al., 1997), small differences in plasma HDL cholesterol and triacylglycerol levels were observed in men and women fed diets higher in carbohydrate or higher in monounsaturated fatty acids; the diet higher in carbohydrate (lower in monounsaturated fatty acids) was associated with slightly lower HDL cholesterol and slightly higher triacylglycerol levels.

Dietary Fiber

Studies have shown that only water-soluble fiber plays a role in lipoprotein metabolism in humans. The soluble fiber content of oats, barley, guar gum, beans, and psyllium seeds is of interest in relation of CAD. A meta-analysis of 20 studies (Ripsin et al., 1992) found that intake of oat products reduces serum cholesterol levels. The lipid-lowering effect was dose-related and was most significant in individuals with the highest initial cholesterol levels. A daily intake of approximately 3 g of soluble fiber from oats has been reported to reduce serum cholesterol levels by 5.6 mg/100 mL (Davidson, 1991). The hypocholesterolemic effects of oats depend on the bran, which contains β-glucan, a water-soluble fiber. Controlled trials with psyllium have shown that a daily intake of 5.1 to 10.4 g of psyllium can lower total cholesterol levels by 4.8% to 14.8% and LDL cholesterol levels by 5.7% to 20.2% within 6 to 16 weeks and is tolerated well (Anderson et al., 1988; Levin et al., 1990; Sprecher et al., 1993). Although they have other beneficial effects, insoluble fibers in wheat and vegetables do not appear to reduce serum cholesterol levels. The mechanisms by which dietary fiber affects plasma lipid levels have not been established, but the major hypotheses are summarized in Chapter 8.

Dietary Protein

In the 1950's, population studies indicated that people who ate large amounts of soy protein had lower rates of atherosclerosis. Soy protein has been shown to lower serum cholesterol levels in animals and in hypercholesterolemic individuals when compared with casein and beef proteins. In a meta-analysis of 38 studies, which included data from 730 human subjects, Anderson et al. (1995) reported a 12.9% reduction in LDL cholesterol, a 2.4% rise in HDL, and a 10.5% reduction in triacylglycerols when the average intake of soy protein was 47 g per day. Of the studies included in this meta-analysis, 21 used isolated soy protein, 14 studies used textured soy protein, and 3 studies used a combination of the two types of protein. Four of the studies were in children and thirty-four were in adults. The mechanism underlying these responses to soy protein is not clear. Soy protein may affect cholesterol absorption, bile acid absorption, the insulin-glucagon ratio, serum thyroxine levels, and hepatic LDL receptor activity. It is also believed that the soy isoflavone termed genistein, a molecule that resembles estradiol, may play a role in cholesterol metabolism.

Proteins differ in amino acid composition, and this may affect cardiovascular risk. A chronic dietary supplement of L-arginine in animals has been shown to decrease platelet aggregation and the adhesiveness of the aortic endothelium for monocytes; to prevent the intimal thickening of coronary arteries; and to reverse endothelial dysfunction. These effects appear to be due to the metabolism of L-arginine to nitric oxide, whose many biological roles recently have been reviewed (Loscalzo, 1995). L-Arginine also has been shown to improve endothelial dysfunction of both coronary microvasculature and epicardial coronary arteries in cardiac transplant recipients. Platelet aggregation in hypercholesterolemic individuals is also reduced by L-arginine supplements. These findings are intriguing because L-arginine availability should not be rate limiting for nitric oxide synthesis under most dietary conditions. Arginine, which is generally higher in plant proteins, appears to have a hypocholesterolemic effect, whereas lysine and methionine, amino acids generally higher in animal proteins, appear to raise plasma cholesterol concentrations.

Energy

The states of overweight (body mass index greater than 25 kg/m²) or obesity (body mass index greater than 30 kg/m²) are the result of caloric intake in excess of energy expenditure. The association between obesity and an increased risk for cardiovascular disease is well established for both women and men (Donahue et al., 1987; Manson et al., 1990). Within a given range of body mass index, abdominal obesity also is a significant and independent predictor of coronary heart disease and is associated with insulin resistance, hypertension, and hyperlipidemia. Even levels of body fat that are average for the American population, and not labeled as overweight, increase the risk of elevated plasma lipid concentrations, glucose intolerance, and high blood pressure. The leanest individuals have a lower risk of CHD than those with average degrees of adiposity, suggesting that weight reduction may also benefit individuals who are not overtly overweight. A meta-analysis of 70 studies indicated that weight reduction was associated with significant decreases in total, LDL, and VLDL cholesterol levels, decreases in plasma triacylglycerol concentration, and increases in HDL cholesterol level (Dattilo and Kris-Etherton, 1992).

Alcohol

Epidemiological studies have shown a reverse trend between low to moderate alcohol consumption (less than 40 g/day of pure ethanol for men and less than 30 g/day for women) and coronary heart disease in both men and women (Kannel, 1988). This protective effect has been associated with an increased concentration of plasma HDL cholesterol as well as increased levels of HDL apoproteins A-I, A-II, and A-IV. Among the major subclasses of HDL, HDL_2 and HDL_3 are both increased by alcohol consumption. Reduced platelet aggregation and blood coagulation and increased fibrinolytic activity are all associated with alcohol consumption; these may be looked upon as possible additional underlying mechanisms for the cardioprotective effect of alcohol. These observations have led some physicians to recommend daily consumption of moderate amounts of alcohol: this translates into 1 5-ounce glass of wine, 12 ounces of beer, or 1.5 ounces of distilled spirits per day for women and no more than twice that for men.

This recommendation continues to be controversial because the data on alcohol are difficult to assess for lack of enough controlled human studies and because of a lack of clarity in the description of "moderate" and "heavy" drinking in relation to the pathophysiology of atherosclerosis. Excessive ethanol consumption can result in alcoholic cardiomyopathy. In addition, regular alcohol consumption raises blood pressure and contributes significantly to the prevalence of hypertension (Beilin and Puddey, 1993). Finally, although moderate drinking appears to have benefits, including an inverse correlation with CHD risk, any possible benefits must be balanced against risks. The risks include stroke, motor vehicle accidents, cancer, birth defects, and dangerous interactions with drugs. In addition, when people do not adhere to recommendations for low to moderate intake, both social and health problems will increase.

A potential metabolic risk derives from the observation that alcohol, given in moderate amounts, increases hepatic synthesis of VLDL. Similar responses are not seen with isocaloric intake of supplemental calories in the form of either carbohydrates or fats. Plasma triacylglycerol levels can be elevated for several hours up to several days in fasting individuals after alcohol ingestion (Ginsberg et al., 1974). HDL cholesterol levels, as noted, are increased modestly by alcohol, so the alcohol-induced hypertriglyceridemia is the exception to the rule that higher triacylglycerols are associated with lower HDL cholesterol levels. Low or subnormal levels of LDL cholesterol have been consistently found in chronic alcoholics. One possible explanation is that VLDL is less readily converted to LDL in alcoholics. Alternatively, excessive alcohol intake is usually associated with malnutrition and weight loss, and these may result in lower LDL levels.

DIET, BLOOD LIPIDS, AND ATHEROSCLEROSIS

Dietary Lipids

The 20th century has seen the continuous growth of a base of information supporting a significant role for diet in the atherogenic process. Following the groung-breaking studies in rabbits by Ignatowski (1908) and Anitschkow and Chalatow (1913), scientists were able to observe and record the "natural" experiment associated with World War II in which the incidence of CHD fell in occupied countries (Malmros, 1980). The similar patterns of association between increases in dietary fat intake and CAD seen in Japanese men migrating to Hawaii and the mainland United States (Kato et al., 1973) and in all Americans between 1950 and 1970 provided strong evidence for the link between diet and heart disease. At the same time, Keys et al. (1986), utilizing epidemiological approaches to support their clinical diet studies, reported the Seven Countries study that showed remarkable relationships between dietary saturated fatty acid intake and heart disease mortality.

Cohort studies such as the Ireland-Boston Heart Study and the Western Electric Study have added further support for hypotheses linking dietary saturated fatty acid and/or cholesterol to CAD. A detailed review of these data is provided in the Diet and Health report of the National Research Council (1989) and the Surgeon General's Report (U. S. Department of Health and Human Services, 1988). Probably the most convincing data derive from the clinical trials that have been carried out using only dietary interventions. In the early study of Dayton et al. (1968), higher amounts of polyunsaturates in the diet were associated with lower CHD events in an elderly population. The Finnish Mental Hospital Study (Miettinen et al., 1983) demonstrated reduced CHD in men and women receiving lower dietary saturated fat and cholesterol. More recently, the Oslo Heart Study (Hjermann et al., 1986) found that men given diets high in polyunsaturated and low in saturated fatty acids had fewer fatal and nonfatal CHD events. Both the Lifestyle Heart Trial (Ornish et al., 1990) and the STARS trial (Watts et al., 1992) showed less progression or even regression of coronary atherosclerosis in men treated with lower fat and cholesterol diets. The STARS trial also demonstrated fewer CHD events in the treated group compared with untreated men.

Overall, the link between dietary saturated fatty acids and CAD is clear and convincing. Similar, but less convincing, data are available for dietary cholesterol. The association between these dietary factors and atherosclerosis is almost certainly based on their effects on plasma lipid and lipoproteins, but separate effects on thrombogenic factors must be considered as well (Miller, 1995).

Antioxidants

The concept that oxidatively modified LDL is proatherogenic and exists in vivo is supported by a growing body of data. Supplementation of diets with nutrients that can act as antioxidants (e.g., ascorbic acid, α-tocopherol, and β-carotene) has been shown to inhibit the progression of atherosclerosis in animals. At present, clinical trial data are not sufficient to make recommendations regarding the use of antioxidant supplements to reduce the risk of CAD in humans (Jha et al., 1995).

A significant inverse relationship was found between plasma vitamin C and CAD in epidemiological studies (Gey et al., 1987). Ascorbate concentrations were also found to be lower in the aortas of people with atherosclerosis, diabetes, and CAD compared with unaffected control subjects. Ascorbate levels were also lower in smokers than in nonsmokers. It has been hypothesized that low concentrations of ascorbate in the arterial wall may predispose LDL to oxidation and that the greater levels of oxidized LDL promote atherogenesis.

Alpha-tocopherol is the predominant lipophilic antioxidant in plasma membranes and tissue and is the most abundant antioxidant in LDL. On average there are 6 molecules of α-tocopherol per LDL particle; they can function as antioxidants by trapping free radicals. Low plasma levels of α-tocopherol were inversely correlated with CAD in a cross-sectional study and with angina pectoris in a case-control study (Gey et al., 1991; Riemersma et al., 1991). In prospective studies (Stampfer et al., 1992b), α-tocopherol supplementation appeared to reduce the risk of coronary events in both men and women. In a randomized placebo-controlled study in men, the LDL oxidation kinetics in a group supplemented with 800 IU of α-tocopherol were similar to those in the group that received combined supplementation with 1.0 g of ascorbate, 30 mg of β-carotene, and 800 IU of α-tocopherol; there was a 40% decrease in the LDL oxidation rate after 3 months of α-tocopherol or combined supplementation.

Beta-carotene has been shown to be a powerful antioxidant. It is carried predominantly in the LDL particle. The antioxidant effects of β-carotene are most potent at low partial pressures of oxygen. Beta-carotene has been shown to inhibit oxidation of LDL and Lp(a) (Jialal et al., 1991). Smokers have lower LDL β-carotene levels relative to nonsmokers. The Physicians' Health Study, however, did not demonstrate benefit from β-carotene supplementation (Hennekens et al., 1996).

Completed randomized trials suggest that none of these antioxidants beneficially affects total mortality or mortality from cardiovascular disease (Hennekens et al., 1996; Omenn et al., 1996). The epidemiological data, however, suggest that high intakes of vitamin E from diet or supplementation that are sustained for 2 or more years are associated with a reduced risk for fatal or nonfatal cardiovascular disease. Use of β-carotene or vitamin C was less clearly associated with a reduced risk. (The antioxidant and other known functions of vitamin C, vitamin E, and β-carotene are discussed in Chapters 23, 25 and 26.)

Nutrient Intake Deficiency Associated with Homocysteinemia

Elevated levels of total homocysteine in the blood stream have been associated with an increased risk of cardiovascular disease (van Poppel et al., 1994). Recent clinical studies have linked moderate hyperhomocysteinemia to peripheral vascular, cerebrovascular, and coronary heart disease. A prospective study of male physicians indicated that plasma total homocysteine concentrations of 17 μmol/L, or 12% above the upper limit of normal, were associated with a three- to four-fold increase in the risk of acute myocardial infarction (Stampfer et al., 1992a). A high plasma homocysteine concentration and low levels of folate and vitamin B_6, through their role in homocysteine metabolism, were also associated with an increased risk of extracranial carotid artery stenosis. The effect of homocysteine is independent of the established risk factors such as hyperlipidemia and hypertension. An elevated homocysteine level may reflect inadequate availability of folate, vitamin B_6, or vitamin B_{12}. Supplementation with these vitamins, particularly folic acid, may normalize plasma homo-cysteine levels. (See Chapters 11 and 21 for further discussions of homocysteine and B vitamins.)

Iron

Iron overload on the myocardium as a poten-tial risk for coronary heart disease was indi-cated in animal experiments in which iron overload increased myocardial damage caused by anoxia and reperfusion. A role for iron in promoting oxidation of LDL cholesterol and atherosclerosis has been proposed, but convincing data are lacking. A prospective study in Finland (Salonen et al., 1992) showed a two-fold increase in acute myocardial in-farction among men with serum ferritin levels above 200 μg/L. In contrast, a study with American physicians (Stampfer et al., 1993) and a cohort study of Icelandic men and women (Jonsson et al., 1991) showed no asso-ciation between serum levels of ferritin or iron and the risk of myocardial infarction. Serum total iron-binding capacity was inversely cor-related with the risk of myocardial infarction (Jonsson et al., 1991). Increased risk for myo-cardial infarction has also been directly corre-lated with high serum iron concentrations (Morrison et al., 1994) but not associated with serum transferrin saturation levels (Sempos et al., 1994). In summary, the data presently available for a link between iron and CHD are inconsistent and do not justify changes in food fortification policy or dietary recommen-dations. (For more information about iron, see Chapter 31.)

Selenium

Selenium is an integral part of the antioxidant enzyme glutathione peroxidase and has been studied in relation to CHD. A reduced plasma selenium level has been associated with an increased risk of cardiovascular disease and death in some studies (Salonen et al., 1982). Other studies, however, did not show this asso-ciation (Salonen, 1987). Whereas high intake levels of selenium may not be protective, a low intake of selenium could be a risk factor. However, in a cross-sectional study of random population samples of apparently healthy mid-

dle-aged men in four European countries, se-lenium levels did not correlate with the re-ported rates of CHD (Riemesma et al., 1990). (More information about selenium can be found in Chapter 34.)

Chromium

Trials in humans showed that chromium ele-vated serum HDL and lowered total serum cholesterol levels (Anonymous, 1983; Roe-back et al., 1991). Men receiving β-adrenergic blocking agents (commonly used antihyper-tensive drugs that tend to lower HDL choles-terol) were given three daily doses of 200 μg of chromium or a placebo for 8 weeks; men treated with chromium had an increase in serum HDL cholesterol levels of 5.8 mg/100 mL. In this randomized, double-blind, pla-cebo-controlled study, no significant changes were seen in LDL or triacylglycerol levels (Roeback et al., 1991). In a study of 28 moder-ately obese, non–insulin-dependent diabetics, supplements of chromium picolinate for 2 months lowered plasma triacylglycerol levels by 17% (Lee and Reasner, 1994). In the Ameri-can population, chromium intake from self-selected meals can be as low as 25 μg/day. (Chromium and its nutritional significance are discussed in Chapter 36.)

DIETARY TREATMENT OF HYPERCHOLESTEROLEMIA

It is clear that efforts to optimize plasma lipid and lipoprotein levels and reduce the risk for CHD should start with diet modification. In general, diet modification should focus on

1. Reducing the intake of saturated fatty acids,
2. Reducing caloric intake in excess of energy requirements, and
3. Reducing the intake of dietary choles-terol.

Lowering intake of saturated fat and choles-terol should clearly be the most important focus of any nutritional treatment for hyper-cholesterolemia. For most people with ele-vated plasma cholesterol levels, dietary changes aimed at lowering saturated fat and cholesterol intake will be the only intervention required to lower serum cholesterol levels and thereby lower risk for CAD (Expert Panel on Detection, Evaluation, and Treatment of High Blood Cholesterol in Adults, 1993). The degree to which an individual's blood cholesterol level drops after initiation of diet therapy depends on the eating pattern before diet modification is initiated and the inherent degree of responsiveness. Individuals exhibit great biological variability. Usually patients with high cholesterol levels experience the greatest reductions in total and LDL cholesterol.

The NCEP has recommended a two-step approach (Table 41–6) to lower plasma total cholesterol concentrations by progressively reducing intakes of saturated fatty acids and cholesterol and to promote weight loss in overweight patients by reducing total caloric intake. The NCEP Step 1 diet, which is similar to the guidelines recommended by the AHA, is a population-based approach for lowering blood cholesterol. The recommendations include a total fat intake of 30% or less of total calories; an intake of saturated fat of 8% to 10% of calories; an intake of polyunsaturated fat up to 10% of calories; and an intake of 10% to 15% of calories as monounsaturates. Cholesterol intake should be less than 300 mg/day. Dietary treatment should be aimed at achieving and maintaining a healthy body weight and eating patterns via a permanent change in eating behavior. The NCEP Step 1 diet should be followed for a minimum of 3 months to allow time for a maximal response. The Step 1 diet should reduce plasma cholesterol levels about 10% from baseline, depending on previous diet pattern and inherent characteristics of responsiveness.

If the goal of therapy is not achieved with the Step 1 diet, the recommendation is to progress to the Step 2 diet. Advancement to the Step 2 diet may achieve a further 5% drop in plasma total cholesterol. There is significant individual variability in responsiveness, however, and the range of reduction in plasma cholesterol is from 0% to 25%. The NCEP Step 2 diet (see Table 41–6) calls for further reducing the saturated fat intake to less than 7% of calories and cholesterol intake to less than 200 mg/day.

Both the Step 1 and Step 2 diets recommend that patients achieve and maintain ideal body weight. Implementation of the Step 2 diet may require intensive nutritional counseling by a registered dietitian in order to lower the saturated fat and cholesterol content of the diet without jeopardizing food palatability and acceptability. The total fat intake, however, can be maintained at 30% of calories. This allows the individual to use sources of monounsaturated fatty acids (olive oil and canola [low erucic acid rapeseed] oil) or polyunsaturated fatty acids (corn and safflower oils) as a replacement for the additional removal of saturated fats.

The major contributors to saturated fatty

TABLE 41–6

The NCEP Two-Step Approach to Treat Hypercholesterolemia

Nutrient	Recommended Intake	
	Step 1 Diet	*Step 2 Diet*
Total fat	Less than 30% of total calories	Less than 30% of total calories
Saturated fatty acids	Less than 10% of total calories	Less than 7% of total calories
Polyunsaturated fatty acids	Up to 10% of total calories	Up to 10% of total calories
Monounsaturated fatty acids	10%–15% of total calories	10%–15% of total calories
Carbohydrates	50%–60% of total calories	50%–60% of total calories
Protein	10%–20% of total calories	10%–20% of total calories
Cholesterol	Less than 300 mg/day	Less than 200 mg/day
Total calories	To achieve and maintain desirable weight	To achieve and maintain desirable weight

Expert Panel on Detection, Evaluation, and Treatment of High Blood Cholesterol in Adults (1993), Summary of the second report of the National Cholesterol Education Program (NCEP) expert panel on detection, evaluation, and treatment of high blood cholesterol in adults (Adult Treatment Panel II). JAMA 269:3015–3023.

acid intake are higher fat red meats (especially hamburger), veal, lamb, pork, processed meat products, poultry with skin, and whole milk and dairy products. Fats that have a high percentage of saturated fat are solid at room temperature and are used in commercial preparation of cakes, pastries, cereals, and granola. The "nondairy" creamers and dairy substitutes for whipped cream and sour cream, which may be labeled as containing "no cholesterol" because they are derived from plants, are usually made with highly saturated coconut or palm oil or hydrogenated vegetable oil. These vegetable fats are frequently used commercially because they are inexpensive and resist oxidation, which extends their shelf life.

The polyunsaturated fatty acids are composed of two major categories—the ω6 and ω3 fatty acids (see Chapter 15). The main ω6 fatty acid found in dietary fats is linoleic acid (18:2), which is present in large amounts in safflower, sunflower, soybean, and corn oils. The oils in most cold-water fish are major sources of the very long-chain ω3 fatty acids: eicosapentaenoic acid (EPA) and docosahexaenoic acid (DHA). As noted earlier, these fatty acids are effective in lowering triacylglycerol levels when fed in large amounts. They have not been shown to be helpful in lowering LDL cholesterol levels and, therefore, are not recommended for the treatment of hypercholesterolemia. However, both high-fat fish (such as salmon, mackerel, and bluefish) that are rich in ω3 fatty acids and low-fat fish (such as sole, flounder, cod, and halibut) should be included in the diet plan because they are good sources of protein and useful substitutes for meat and cheese that are high in saturated fatty acids.

Monounsaturated fatty acids account for 50% or more of the fatty acids in a few vegetable oils. Olive oil and canola oil are such sources of monounsaturated fatty acids, primarily oleic acid. Monounsaturated fats should make up 10% to 15% of calories. The current American diet supplies as much oleic acid as is recommended, but the oleic acid is usually derived from animal fats that are also high in saturates. When the intake of animal fat is decreased, vegetable oil and nuts can be included in the meal plan to increase monounsaturated fat intake.

Dietary cholesterol is supplied only by animal foods. The organ meats (brain, liver, kidney, and sweetbread) are very rich sources of cholesterol. Meat (both muscle and fat) contains cholesterol. There is no significant difference in the cholesterol content of beef, lamb, pork, chicken, or turkey. Fish (except some shellfish such as shrimp) are slightly lower in cholesterol than meat or poultry.

The intake of protein that is recommended for the Step 1 or 2 diet is 10% to 20% of total calories. This is consistent with the guidelines of 15% of calories as protein that is used for the general population. To meet the Recommended Dietary Allowance for protein (0.8 g/kg body weight per day), individuals with lower caloric intakes may need closer to 20% of total calories as protein, whereas those with higher caloric intakes may meet their protein requirements with only 10% of total calories as protein. The sources of protein should include a variety of low-fat animal foods and plant foods such as legumes and grains. The amount of lean animal foods should be limited to a maximum of 5 to 6 oz per day, because high-protein foods are usually associated with high-fat content; exceptions are egg whites and isolated soy protein and casein supplements. The high-protein diets used in some fad diet/weight reduction programs can have significant adverse effects on serum cholesterol levels because of the simultaneous increase in saturated fat and cholesterol intake.

The carbohydrate content of the Step 1 or 2 diet should be approximately 55% of the total calories. The recommendation is to eat more foods containing complex carbohydrates and less refined and prepared foods containing high amounts of simple sugars (e.g., sucrose), because sources of complex carbohydrates (starch and dietary fiber) tend to be rich in other nutrients as well.

Dietary fiber is composed mainly of nondigestible complex carbohydrates. Whole wheat, whole grain cereals (caution: granolas that are made with animal fat and/or vegetable shortenings are high in saturated fatty acids), corn, and vegetables are good sources. The more insoluble types of dietary fiber may protect and help in the treatment of diseases of the intestinal tract (i.e., constipation, diverticulosis, hemorrhoids, and cancer of the colon and rectum). The more soluble types of fiber have been shown to lower LDL cholesterol, help control diabetes by slowing absorption of glucose, and aid in appetite control by creating satiety. Good sources of soluble fiber are oatmeal, oat bran, legumes containing gums such as β-glucans (e.g., dried peas and beans), psyllium seeds, and some fruits that contain pectin (e.g., grapefruit and apples).

Effects of dietary fiber per se on plasma cholesterol levels are difficult to evaluate because a diet rich in dietary fiber is also likely to be lower in fat and calories. Nevertheless, adding soluble fiber–containing foods to the diet could be a valuable adjunct to a low-saturated fat, low-cholesterol diet. Because eating large quantities of fiber can cause gastrointestinal side effects, it is important to add fiber-rich foods slowly to the diet to allow the gastrointestinal tract to adjust to the increased fiber load. It is also important to optimize the fluid intake when high-fiber diets are consumed because fluid is needed for the fecal bulking of the fiber.

REFERENCES

Anderson, J. W., Johnstone, B. M. and Cook-Newell, M. E. (1995) Meta-analysis of the effects of soy protein intake on serum lipids. N Eng J Med 333:276–282.

Anderson J. W., Zettwoch, N., Feldman, T., Tietyen-Clark, J. and Oeltgen, P. (1988) Cholesterol-lowering effects of psyllium hydrophilic mucilloid for hypercholesterolemic men. Arch Intern Med 148:292–296.

Anitschkow, N. and Chalatow, S. (1913) Ueber experimentelle Cholesterinsteatose and ihre Bedeutung fur die Entstehung einiger pathologischer Prozesse. Zentralbl Allg Pathol Anat 24:1–9.

Anonymous (1983) Chromium status and serum lipids. Nutr Rev 41:307–310.

Arad, Y., Ramakrishnan, R. and Ginsberg H. N. (1990) Lovastatin therapy reduces low density lipoprotein apo B levels in subjects with combined hyperlipidemia by reducing the production of apo B–containing lipoproteins: Implications for the pathophysiology of apo B production. J Lipid Res 31:567–582.

Austin, M. A., King M. C., Vranizan, K. M. and Krauss, R. M. (1990) Atherogenic lipoprotein phenotype. A proposed genetic marker for coronary heart disease risk. Circulation 82:495–506.

Beilin, L. J. and Puddey, I. B. (1993) Alcohol, hypertension and cardiovascular disease—implications for management (review). Clin Exp Hypertens 15:1157–1170.

Berglund, L. (1995) Diet and drug therapy for lipoprotein (a). Curr Opin Lipidol 6:48–56.

Blum, C. B., Levy, R., Eisenberg, S., Hall, M., Goebel, R.

H. and Berman, M. (1977) High density lipoprotein metabolism in man. J Clin Invest 60:795–807.

Boers, G. H. J. (1997) The case of mild hyperhomocysteinaemia as a risk factor. J Inherit Metab 20:301–306.

Bonanome, A. and Grundy, S. M. (1988) Effect of dietary stearic acid on plasma cholesterol and lipoprotein levels. N Engl J Med 318:1244–1248.

Brinton, E. A., Eisenberg, S. and Breslow, J. L. (1990) A low-fat diet decreases high density lipoprotein (HDL) cholesterol levels by decreasing HDL apolipoprotein transport rates. J Clin Invest 85:144–151.

Brown, M. S. and Goldstein, J. L. (1984) How LDL receptors influence cholesterol and atherosclerosis. Sci Am 251:58–66.

Chait, A., Brunzell, J. D., Denke, M. A., Eisenberg, D., Ernst, N. D., Franklin, F. A., Jr., Ginsberg, H., Kotchen, T. A., Kuller, L., Mullis, R. M., Nichaman, M. Z., Nicolosi, R. J., Schaefer, E. J., Stone, N. J., and Weidman, W. H. (1993) Rationale of the diet-heart statement of the American Heart Association: Report of the Nutrition Committee. Circulation 88:3008–3029.

Cortese, C., Levy, Y., Janus, E. D., Turner, P. R., Rao, S. N., Miller, N. E. and Lewis, B. (1983) Modes of action of lipid-lowering diets in man: Studies of apolipoprotein B kinetics in relation to fat consumption and dietary fatty acid composition. Eur J Clin Invest 13:79–85.

Dattilo, A. M. and Kris-Etherton, P. M. (1992) Effects of weight reduction on blood lipids and lipoproteins: A meta-analysis. Am J Clin Nutr 56:320–328.

Davidson, M. H., Dugan, L. D., Burns, J. H., Bova, J., Story, K. and Drennan, K. B. (1991) The hypocholesterolemic effects of beta-glucan in oatmeal and oatbran. A dose-controlled study. JAMA 265:1833–1839.

Dayton, S., Pearce, M. L., Goldman, H., Harnish, A., Plotkin, D., Shickman, M., Winfield, M., Zager, A. and Dixon, W. (1968) Controlled trial of a diet high in unsaturated fat for prevention of atherosclerotic complications. Lancet 2:1060–1062.

Donahue, R. P., Abbot, R. D. and Bloom, E. (1987) Central obesity and coronary heart disease in men. Lancet 1:821–824.

Dreon, D. M., Vranizan K. M., Krauss, R. M., Austin, M. A. and Wood, P. D. (1990) The effects of polyunsaturated fat vs. monounsaturated fat on plasma lipoproteins. JAMA 263:2462–2466.

Expert Panel on Detection, Evaluation, and Treatment of High Blood Cholesterol in Adults (1993) Summary of the second report of the National Cholesterol Education Program (NCEP) expert panel on detection, evaluation, and treatment of high blood cholesterol in adults (Adult Treatment Panel II). JAMA 269:3015–3023.

Garg, A., Bantle, J. P., Henry, R. R., Coulston, A. M., Griver, K. A., Raatz, S. K., Brinkley, L., Chen, I., Grundy, S. M., Huet, B. A. and Reaven, G. M. (1994) Effects of varying carbohydrate content of diet in patients with non-insulin-dependent diabetes mellitus. JAMA 271:1421–1428.

Gey, K. F., Brubacher, G. B. and Stahelin, H. B. (1987) Plasma levels of antioxidant vitamins in relation to ischemic heart disease and cancer. Am J Clin Nutr 45:1368–1377.

Gey, K. F., Puska, P., Jordan, P. and Moser, U. K. (1991) Inverse correlation between vitamin E and mortality from ischemic heart disease in cross-cultural epidemiology. Am J Clin Nutr 53:326S–334S.

Gimbrone, M., Jr., Cybulsky, I., Kume, N., Collins, T. and Resnick, N. (1995) Vascular endothelium. An integrator of pathophysiological stimuli in atherogenesis. Ann N Y Acad Sci 748:122–132.

Ginsberg, H. N., Barr, S. L., Karmally, W., Gilbert, A., Decklebaum, R., Kaplan, K., Ramakrishnan, R., Halloran, S. and Dell, R. (1990) Reduction of plasma cholesterol levels in normal men on an American Heart Association Step 1 diet or a Step 1 diet with added monounsaturated fat. N Engl J Med 322:574–579.

Ginsberg, H. N., Karmally, W., Barr, S. L., Johnson, C., Holleran, S. and Ramakrishnan, R. (1994a) Effects of increasing dietary polyunsaturated fatty acids within the guidelines of the AHA Step 1 diet on plasma lipid and lipoprotein levels in normal males. Arterioscler Thromb 14:892–901.

Ginsberg, H. N., Karmally, W., Siddiqui, M., Holleran, S., Tall, A. R., Blaner, W. S. and Ramakrishnan, R. (1995) Increases in dietary cholesterol are associated with modest increases in both low density and high density lipoprotein cholesterol in healthy young women. Arterioscler Thromb 15:169–178.

Ginsberg, H. N., Karmally, W., Siddiqui, M., Holleran, S., Tall, A. R., Rumsey, S. C., Deckelbaum, R. J., Blaner, W. S. and Ramakrishnan, R. (1994b) A dose-response study of the effects of dietary cholesterol on fasting and postprandial lipid and lipoprotein metabolism in healthy young men. Arterioscler Thromb 14:576–586.

Ginsberg, H. N. Kris-Etherton, P., Dennis, M. B., Elmer, P. J., Ershow, A., Lefevre, M., Pearson, T., Roheim, P., Ramakrishnan, R., Reed, R., Stewart, K., Stewart, P., Phillips, K. and Anderson, N. (1998) Effects of reducing dietary saturated fatty acids on plasma lipids and lipoproteins in healthy subjects: DELTA protocol-1. Arterioscler Thromb Vasc Biol 18:441–449.

Ginsberg, H. N., Le, N. A. and Gibson, J. C. (1985) Regulation of the production and catabolism of plasma low density lipoproteins in hypertriglyceridemic subjects. Effect of weight loss. J Clin Invest 75:614–623.

Ginsberg, H., Le, N. A., Mays, C., Gibson, J. and Brown, W. V. (1981) Lipoprotein metabolism in non-responders to increased dietary cholesterol. Arteriosclerosis 1:463–470.

Ginsberg, H., Olefsky, J., Farquhar, J. and Reaven, G. (1974) Moderate ethanol ingestion and plasma triglyceride levels. Ann Intern Med 80:143–149.

Goldstein, J. L., Schrott, H. G., Hazzard, W. R., Bierman, E. L. and Motulsky, A. G. (1973) Hyperlipidemia in coronary heart disease. II. Genetic analysis of lipid levels in 176 families and delineation of a new inherited disorder, combined hyperlipidemia. J Clin Invest 52:1544–1568.

Graham, I. M., Daly, L. E., Refsum, H. M., Robinson, K., Brattstrom, L. E., Ueland, P. M., et al. (1997) Plasma homocysteine as a risk factor for vascular disease: The European Concerted Action Project. JAMA 277:1775–1781.

Grundy, S. M., Brown, W. V., Dietschy, J. M., Ginsberg, H., Goodnight, S., Howard, B., La Rosa, J. C. and McGill, H. C. (1989) AHA conference report on cholesterol basis for dietary treatment. Circulation 80:729–734.

Hall, W. H. (1995) Triglyceride, high density lipoprotein, and coronary heart disease. NIH Consensus Development Panel on Triglyceride, High-Density Lipoprotein, and Coronary Heart Disease, February 26–28, 1992. JAMA 269:505–510.

Harris, W. S., Connor, W. E., Illingworth, D. R., Rothrock, D. W. and Foster, D. M. (1990) Effects of fish oil on VLDL triglyceride kinetics in humans. J Lipid Res 31:1549–1558.

Hayes, K. C. (1992) Dietary fatty acid thresholds and cholesterolemia. FASEB J 6:2600–2607.

Hegsted, D. M., Ausman, L. M., Johnson, J. A. and Dallal, G. E. (1993) Dietary fat and serum lipids: An evaluation of the experimental data. Am J Clin Nutr 57:875–883.

Hegsted, D. M., McGandy, R. B., Myers, M. L. and Stare, F. J. (1965) Quantitative effects of dietary fat on serum cholesterol in man. Am J Clin Nutr 17:218–295.

Hennekens, C. H., Buring, J. E., Manson, J. E., Stampfer, M., Rosner, B., Cook, N. R. Belanger, C., LaMotte, F., Gaziano, J. M., Ridker, P. M., Willet, W. and Peto, R. (1996) Lack of effect of long-term supplementation with beta carotene on the incidence of malignant neoplasms and cardiovascular disease. N Engl J Med 334:1145–1149.

Hjermann, I., Holme, I. and Leren, P. (1986) Oslo study diet and antismoking trial. Results after 102 months. Am J Med 80:7–11.

Horowitz, B. S., Goldberg, I. J., Merab, J., Vanni, T., Ramakrishnan, R. and Ginsberg, H. N. (1993) Increased plasma and renal clearance of an exchangeable pool of apolipoprotein A-I in subjects with low levels of high density lipoprotein cholesterol. J Clin Invest 91:1743–1752.

Ignatowski, A. I. (1908) Influence of animal food on the organism of rabbits. Izv Imp Voyenno-Med Akad Peter 16:154–176.

Jha, P., Flather, M., Lonn, E., Farkouh, M. and Yusuf, S. (1995) The antioxidant vitamins and cardiovascular disease. A critical review of epidemiologic and clinical trial data. Ann Intern Med 123:860–872.

Jialal, I., Norkus, E., Cristol, I. and Grundy, S. M. (1991) Beta carotene inhibits the oxidative modifications of low-density lipoprotein. Biochim Biophys Acta 1086:134–138.

Jonsson, J. J., Johannesson, G. M., Sigfusson, N., Magnusson, V., Thjodleifsson, B. and Magnusson, S. (1991) Prevalence of iron deficiency and iron overload in the adult Icelandic population. J Clin Epidemiol 44:1289–1297.

Judd, J. T., Clevidence, B. A., Muesing, R. A., Wittes, J., Sunkin, M. E. and Podczasy, J. J. (1994) Dietary *trans* fatty acids: Effects on plasma lipids and lipoproteins of healthy men and women. Am J Clin Nutr 59:861–868.

Kannel, W. B. (1988) Alcohol and cardiovascular disease. Proc Nutr Soc 47:99–110.

Kato, H., Tillotson, J. and Nichaman, M. Z. (1973) Epidemiologic studies of coronary heart disease and stroke in Japanese men living in Japan, Hawaii, and California. Am J Epidemiol 97:373–385.

Keys, A., Anderson, J. T. and Grande, F. (1965) Serum cholesterol response to changes in the diet. IV. Particular saturated fatty acids in the diet. Metabolism 14:776–787.

Keys, A., Menotti, A., Kavonen, M. J., Aravanis, C., Blackburn, H., Buzina, R., Djordjevic, B. S., Dontas, A. S., Fidanza, F. and Keys, M. H. (1986) The diet and 15-year death rate in the Seven Countries study. Am J Epidemiol 124:903–915.

Lagrost, L., Dengremont, C., Athias, A., deGeitere, C., Fruchart, J. C., Lallemant, C., Gambert, P. and Castro, G. (1995) Modulation of cholesterol efflux from Fu5AH hepatoma cells by the apolipoprotein content of high density lipoprotein particles. Particles containing various proportions of apolipoproteins A-I and A-II. J Biol Chem 170:13004–13009.

Lee, N. A. and Reasner, C. A. (1994) Beneficial effect of chromium supplementation on serum triglyceride levels in NIDDM. Diabetes Care 17:1449–1452.

Lefevre, M., Ginsberg, H. N., Kris-Etherton, P., Elmer, P. J., Stewart, P. W., Ershow, A., Pearson, T. A., Roheim, P. S., Ramakrishnan, R., Derr, J., Gordon, D. J. and Reed, R. (1997) Apo E genotype does not predict lipid response to changes in dietary saturated fatty acids in a heterogeneous normolipidemic population. Arterioscler Thromb Vasc Biol 17:2914–2923.

Levin, E. G., Miller, V. T., Muesing, R. A., Stoy, D. B., Balm, T. K. and LaRosa, J. C. (1990) Comparison of psyllium hydrophilic mucilloid and cellulose as adjuncts to a prudent diet in the treatment of mild to moderate hypercholesterolemia. Arch Intern Med 150:1822–1827.

Lichtenstein, A. H., Ausman, L. M., Carrasco, W., Jenner, J. L., Ordovas, J. M. and Schaefer, E. J. (1993) Hydrogenation impairs the hypolipidemic effect of corn oil in humans. Hydrogenation, *trans* fatty acids, and plasma lipids. Arterioscler Thromb 13:154–161.

Loscalzo, J. (1995) Nitric oxide and vascular disease. N Engl J Med 333:251–253.

Mahley, R. W. (1988) Apolipoprotein E: Cholesterol transport protein with expanding role in cell biology. Science 240:622–630.

Malmros, H. (1980) Diet, lipids and atherosclerosis. Acta Med Scand 207:207–214.

Manson, J. E., Colditz, G. A. and Stampfer, M. J. (1990) A prospective study of obesity and risk of coronary heart disease in women. N Engl J Med 322:882–889.

Mattson, F. H. and Grundy, S. M. (1985) Comparison of effects of dietary saturated, monounsaturated, and polyunsaturated fatty acids on plasma lipids and lipoproteins in man. J Lipid Res 26:194–202.

Mattson, F. H., Hollenbach, E. J. and Kligman, A. M. (1975) Effect of hydrogenated fat on the plasma cholesterol and triglyceride levels of man. Am J Clin Nutr 28:726–731.

Mensink, R. P. and Katan, M. B. (1990) Effect of dietary *trans* fatty acids on high-density and low-density lipoprotein cholesterol levels in healthy subjects. N Engl J Med 323:439–445.

Mensink, R. P. and Katan, M. B. (1992) Effect of dietary fatty acids on serum lipids and lipoproteins. Arterioscler Throm 12:911–919.

Miettinen, M., Turpeinen, O., Karvonen, M. J., Pekkarinen, M., Paavilainen, E. and Elosuo, R. (1983) Dietary prevention of coronary heart disease in women: The Finnish mental hospital study. Int J Epidemiol 12:17–25.

Miller, G. J. (1995) Lipoproteins and thrombosis: Effects of lipid lowering. Curr Opin Lipidol 6:38–42.

Morrison, H. I., Semenciw, R. M., Mao, Y. and Wigle, D. T. (1994) Serum iron and risk of fatal acute myocardial infarction. Epidemiology 5:243–246.

National Research Council, Food and Nutrition Board (1989) Diet and Health: Implications for Reducing Chronic Disease Risk. National Academy Press, Washington, D.C.

Nestel, P., Noakes, M., Belling, B., McArthur, R., Clifton, P., Janus, E. and Abbey, M. (1992) Plasma lipoprotein lipid and lp(a) changes with substitution of elaidic acid for oleic acid in the diet. J Lipid Res 33:1029–1036.

Omenn, G. S., Goodman, G. E., Thornquist, M. D., Balmes, J., Cullen, M. R., Glass, A., Koegh, J. P., Meyskens, F. L., Valanis, B., Williams, J. H., Barnhart, S. and Hammar, S. (1996) Effects of a combination of beta carotene and vitamin A on lung cancer and cardiovascular disease. N Engl J Med 334:1150–1155.

Ornish, D., Brown, S. E., Scherwitz, L. W., Billings, J. H., Armstrong, W. T., Ports, T. A., McLanahan, S. M., Kirkeeide, R. L., Brand, R. J. and Gould, K. L. (1990) Can lifestyle changes reverse coronary heart disease? The Lifestyle Heart Trial. Lancet 336:129–133.

Parkard, C. J., McKinney, L., Carr, K. and Shepherd, J. (1983) Cholesterol feeding increases low density lipoprotein synthesis. J Clin Invest 72:45–51.

Patsch, J. R., Miesenbock, G., Hopferwieser, T., Muhl-

berger, V., Knapp, E., Dunn, J. K., Gotto, J. R. and Patsch W. (1992) Relation of triglyceride metabolism and coronary artery disease: Studies in the postprandial state. Arterioscler Thromb 12:1336–1345.

Reaven, G. M. (1988) Role of insulin resistance in human disease. Diabetes 37:1595–1607.

Riemersma, R. A., Oliver, M., Elton, R. A., Alfthan, G., Vartianinen, E., Salo, M., Rubba, P., Mancici, M., Georgi, H., Vuilleumier, J. P. and Gey, K. F. (1990) Plasma antioxidants and coronary heart disease: Vitamins C, E, and selenium. Eur J Clin Nutr 44:143–150.

Ripsin, C. M., Keenan, J. M., Jacobs, D. R., Jr., Elmer, P. J., Welch, R. R., Van Horn, L., Liu, K., Turnbull, W. H., Thye, F. W., Kestin, M., Hegsted, M., Davidson, D. M., Davidson, M. H., Dugan, L. D., Denmark-Wahnefried, W. and Beling, S. (1992) Oat products and lipid lowering: A meta-analysis. JAMA 267:3317–3325.

Roeback, J. R., Jr., Hia, K. M., Chambless, L. E. and Fletcher, R. H. (1991) Effects of chromium supplementation on serum high-density lipoprotein cholesterol levels in men taking beta-blockers: A randomized, controlled trial. Ann Intern Med 115:917–924.

Ross, R. (1995) Cell biology of atherosclerosis. Annu Rev Physiol 57:791–804.

Salonen, J. T. (1987) Selenium in ischaemic heart disease. Int J Epidemiol 16:323–328.

Salonen, J. T., Alfthan, G. and Huttunen, J. K. E. (1982) Association between cardiovascular death and myocardial infarction and serum selenium in a matched-pair longitudinal study. Lancet 2:175–179.

Salonen, J. T., Nyyssonen, K., Korpela, H., Tuomilehto, J., Seppanen, R. and Salonen, R. (1992) High stored iron levels are associated with excess risk of myocardial infarction in eastern Finnish men. Circulation 86:1036–1037.

Sempos, C. T., Looker, A. C., Gillum, R. F. and Makuc, D. M. (1994) Body iron stores and the risk of coronary heart disease. N Engl J Med 330:1152–1154.

Shepherd, J., Parkard, C. J., Grundy, S. M., Yeshurun, D., Gotto, J. R. and Taunton, O. D. (1980) Effects of saturated and polyunsaturated fat diets on the chemical composition and metabolism of low density lipoproteins in man. J Lipid Res 21:91–98.

Silverman, D. I., Ginsberg, G. S. and Pasternak, R. C. (1993) HDL subfractions. Am J Med 94:636–645.

Sprecher, D. L., Harris, B. V., Goldberg, A. C., Anderson, E. C., Bayuk, L. M., Russell, B. S., Crone, D. S., Quinn, C., Bateman, J., Kuzmak, B. R. and Allgood, L. D. (1993) Efficacy of psyllium in reducing serum cholesterol levels in hypercholesterolemic patients on high- or low-fat diets. Ann Intern Med 119:545–554.

Stamler, J. and Shekelle, R. (1988) Dietary cholesterol and human coronary heart disease. Arch Pathol Lab Med 112:1032–1040.

Stampfer, M. J., Grodstein, F., Rosenberg, I., Willett, W. and Hennekens, C. (1993) A prospective study of plasma ferritin and risk of myocardial infarction in U.S. physicians. Circulation 87:688.

Stampfer, M. J., Malinow, M. R. and Willett, W. C. E. (1992a) A prospective study of plasma homocyst(e)ine and risk of myocardial infarction in U.S. physicians. JAMA 268:877–881.

Stampfer, M. J., Manson, J. A. E., Colditz, G. A., Speizer, F. E., Willett, W. C. and Hennekens, C. H. (1992b) A prospective study of vitamin E supplementation and risk of coronary disease in women. Circulation 86:l463.

Steinberg, D., Parthasarathy S., Carew, T. E., Khoo, J. C. and Witztum, J. L. (1989) Beyond cholesterol: Modifications of low density lipoprotein that increase its atherogenicity. N Engl J Med 320:915–924.

Sundaram, K. E. (1994) Dietary palmitic acid results in lower serum cholesterol than does lauric and myristic acid combination in normolipidemic humans. Am J Clin Nutr 59:841–846.

Tall, A. R. (1990) Plasma high density lipoproteins. Metabolism and relationship to atherogenesis. J Clin Invest 86:379–384.

Turner, J. D., Le, N.-A. and Brown, W. V. (1981) Effect of changing dietary fat saturation on low density lipoprotein metabolism in man. Am J Physiol 241:E57–E63.

United States Department of Health and Human Services, Public Health Service (1988) The Surgeon General's Printing Office, Washington, D.C.

van Poppel, G., Kardinaal, A., Princen, H. and Kok, F. J. (1994) Antioxidants and coronary heart disease. Ann Med 26:429–434.

Wardlaw, G. M. and Snook, J. T. (1990) Effect of diets high in butter, corn oil, or high-oleic acid sunflower oil on serum lipids and apolipoproteins in men. Am J Clin Nutr 51:815–821.

Watts, G. F., Lewis, B., Brunt, J. N., Lewis, E. S., Coltart, D. J., Smith, L. D., Mann, J. I. and Swan, A. V. (1992) Effects on coronary artery disease of lipid-lowering diet, or diet plus cholestyramine, in the St. Thomas' Atherosclerosis Regression Study (STARS). Lancet 339:1241–1242.

Welty, T. K., Lee, E. T., Yeh, J., Cowan, L. D., Go, O., Fabsitz, R. R., Le, N. A., Oopik, A. J., Robbins, D. C. and Howard B. V. (1995) Cardiovascular disease risk factors among American Indians. The Strong Heart Study. Am J Epidemiol 142:269–287.

Wilson, H. M., Patel, J. C. and Skinner, E. R. (1991) The distribution of HDL in coronary disease. Biochem Soc Trans 18:1175–1176.

Woollett, L. A., Spady, D. K. and Dietschy, J. M. (1992a) Saturated and unsaturated fatty acids independently regulate low density lipoprotein receptor activity and production rate. J Lipid Res 33:77–88.

Woollett, L. A., Spady, D. K. and Dietschy, J. M. (1992b) Regulatory effects of the saturated fatty acids 6:0 through 18:0 on hepatic low density lipoprotein receptor activity in the hamster. J Clin Invest 89:1133–1141.

Yu, S., Derr, J., Etherton, T. D. and Kris-Etherton, P. M. (1995) Plasma cholesterol-predictive equations demonstrate that stearic acid is neutral and monounsaturated fatty acids are hypocholesterolemic. Am J Clin Nutr 61:1129–1139.

RECOMMENDED READINGS

Expert Panel on Detection, Evaluation, and Treatment of High Blood Cholesterol in Adults (1993) Summary of the Second Report of the National Cholesterol Education Program (NCEP) expert panel on detection, evaluation, and treatment of high blood cholesterol in adults (Adult Treatment Panel II). JAMA 269:3015–3023.

Karmally, W. and Ginsberg, H. N. (1991) Dietary treatment of hypercholesterolemia. In: Drug Treatment of Hyperlipidemia (Rifkind, B. M., ed.). Marcel Dekker, New York.

Kris-Etherton, P. and Burns, J. (1998) Cardiovascular Nutrition: Strategies and Tools for Disease Management and Prevention. American Dietetic Association, Chicago.

National Research Council, Food and Nutrition Board (1989) Diet and Health: Implications for Reducing Chronic Disease Risk. National Academy Press, Washington, D.C.

CHAPTER **42**

◆ ◆

Translating Biochemical and Physiological Requirements into Practice

Christina Stark, M.S., R.D., C.N.

C O M M O N   A B B R E V I A T I O N S

AI (Adequate Intake)
DRI (Dietary Reference Intake)
DRV (Daily Reference Value)
EAR (Estimated Average Requirement)
RDA (Recommended Dietary Allowance)
RDI (Reference Daily Intake)
UL (Tolerable Upper Intake Level)

FOOD AS A SOURCE OF NUTRIENTS

When people sit down to a meal, they eat food, not nutrients. Most people don't think about the individual nutrients they are consuming, but instead focus on the flavor, texture, and aroma of the food. Although consumers do indicate that nutrition is an important factor when making food selections, other factors such as taste, cost, and convenience may outweigh any nutritional considerations. The challenge is to translate the biochemical and physiological requirements for food into practical guidelines so that people can make healthful food choices. Simply knowing nutrient requirements does not ensure that someone will consume an adequate diet.

Food is also made up of more than just nutrients. Some of these non-nutritive components, often referred to as phytochemicals in plant foods, may have important implications in terms of their health benefits. For example, soybeans contain a type of plant estrogen that may provide some of the protective effects of natural estrogens. Other plant compounds, such as allyl sulfides in onions and garlic, are also being studied for their anticancer and cholesterol-lowering properties (American Dietetic Association, 1995). Researchers are actively investigating the health benefits and risks of these naturally occurring substances, which are found in commonly consumed fruits, vegetables, and grains, as well as in less frequently consumed foods such as licorice and green tea. Understanding the importance of both nutritive and non-nutritive components in foods is critical to providing sound dietary advice.

This chapter explores various types of dietary recommendations, ranging from those focused on specific nutrients to those based on entire food groups. In the United States, these include the Recommended Dietary Allowances and the Dietary Reference Intakes, the Dietary Guidelines for Americans, and the Food Guide Pyramid. Many other countries, including Canada, Australia, New Zealand, India, Japan, those in Latin America, and most in Europe, have developed their own sets of recommended dietary intakes and/or dietary guidelines and goals (World Health Organiza-

tion, 1990). Both professionals and consumers can use these recommendations and guidelines in the promotion and selection of a healthful diet.

RECOMMENDED DIETARY ALLOWANCES AND DIETARY REFERENCE INTAKES

Definitions

In the United States, the Recommended Dietary Allowances (RDAs) have been the standards for measuring nutritional adequacy since 1941. A new term, Dietary Reference Intakes (DRIs), was introduced in 1997 (Institute of Medicine, 1997). DRIs refer to four different reference values that can be used for planning and assessing diets of individuals and groups. The DRIs were developed to address some of the limitations of having only a single set of reference values—the former RDAs. "DRIs" is not merely a new term; the establishment of DRIs represents a new approach supported by a growing understanding that different types of reference values are needed to apply dietary recommendations to individuals and groups.

The DRIs, which will eventually replace all the former RDAs, are being released as a series of seven reports. The first report contains DRIs for nutrients related to bone health and other body functions: calcium, phosphorus, magnesium, vitamin D, and fluoride (Institute of Medicine, 1997). The second report covers the B vitamins (Institute of Medicine, 1998). The other five reports, to be released in stages over several years, will cover antioxidants (e.g., vitamins C and E, selenium); macronutrients (e.g., protein, fat, carbohydrates); trace elements (e.g., iron, zinc); electrolytes and water; and other food components (e.g., fiber, phytoestrogens).

The DRIs consist of the following reference values: Estimated Average Requirement (EAR), Recommended Dietary Allowance (RDA), Adequate Intake (AI), and Tolerable Upper Intake Level (UL). The scientific data for developing DRIs consist of clinical trials; dose-response, balance, depletion/repletion, prospective observation, and case-control

NUTRITION INSIGHT

Phytochemicals and Functional Foods

Phytochemicals (phyto = plant) are non-nutritive substances naturally found in foods, such as fruits, vegetables, and grains, that have potential health benefits. Although hundreds of phytochemicals have already been identified (e.g., allyl sulfides in garlic and onions; lignans in flax and soybeans; isoflavones in soybeans; saponins in legumes; indoles and isothiocyanates in cruciferous vegetables), many remain undiscovered.

Functional foods are defined as any modified foods or food ingredients that may provide health benefits beyond the traditional nutrients they contain (American Dietetic Association, 1995). These foods may be modified to increase the content of certain nutrients or non-nutrient phytochemicals. Related terms that are sometimes used interchangeably with the term functional foods include designer foods and nutraceuticals. Techniques used to enhance the health-promoting components in foods include genetic engineering (for example, lycopene-rich tomatoes), plant breeding (high β-carotene carrots), food processing (oat bran cereal), and food fortification (calcium-enriched orange juice).

Consumer awareness of phytochemicals has increased, and there is public interest in consuming more phytochemical-rich foods and functional foods as a way to improve health.

Thinking Critically

1. What are the advantages and disadvantages of seeking out phytochemical-rich foods and functional foods as a way to improve health? How does this approach compare with taking supplements?

studies; and clinical observations in humans. The EARs, RDAs, AIs, and ULs refer to average daily intakes over 1 or more weeks. The Institute of Medicine's Food and Nutrition Board describes each value in the following way (Institute of Medicine, 1997, 1998):

Estimated Average Requirement (EAR): A nutrient intake value that is estimated to meet the requirement of half the healthy individuals in a group. This figure is to be used as the basis for developing the RDA and is to be used by nutrition policy makers in the evaluation of the adequacy of nutrient intakes of the group and for planning how much the group should consume.

Recommended Dietary Allowance (RDA): The average daily dietary intake level that is sufficient to meet the nutrient requirement of nearly all (97% to 98%) healthy individuals in a group. The RDA should be used in guiding individuals to achieve adequate nutrient intake aimed at decreasing the risk of chronic disease. It is based on an estimate of the average requirement plus an increase to ac-

count for the variation within a particular group.

Adequate Intake (AI): A value based on observed or experimentally determined approximations of nutrient intake by a group (or groups) of healthy people—used when an RDA cannot be determined. Individuals should use the AI as a goal for intake of nutrients for which no RDA exists. The AI is derived through experimental or observational data that show a mean intake that appears to sustain a desired indicator of health, such as calcium retention in bone for most members of a population group. For example, AIs have been set for infants through 1 year of age using the average observed nutrient intake of populations of breast-fed infants as the standard.

Tolerable Upper Intake Level (UL): The highest level of daily nutrient intake that is likely to pose no risk of adverse health effects to almost all individuals in the general population. As intake increases above the UL, the risk of adverse effects increases. This figure is not intended to be a recommended level of intake, and there is no established benefit for individuals to consume nutrients at levels above the RDA or AI. For most nutrients, this figure refers to total intakes from food, fortified food, and nutrient supplements.

In contrast, the former RDAs were defined as "the levels of intake of essential nutrients that, on the basis of scientific knowledge, are judged by the Food and Nutrition Board of the National Research Council to be adequate to meet the known nutrient needs of practically all healthy persons" (National Research Council, 1989a). Key aspects of the definition are that the former RDAs are only defined for essential nutrients, the amounts are adequate, and the RDAs meet the needs of healthy persons. They are not intended for those with special nutritional needs.

In the new DRIs, which represent a new paradigm, "three of the reference values are defined by a specific indicator of nutrient adequacy, which may relate to the reduction of the risk of chronic disease or disorders; the fourth is defined by a specific indicator of excess where one is available. In the former paradigm, the indicator of adequacy was usu-

ally limited to a classical deficiency state" (Institute of Medicine, 1997). Figure 42–1 shows how the four DRI values relate to the risks of either inadequacy or adverse effects. Like the former RDAs, the new DRIs apply to the healthy general population.

The former RDAs were developed specifically for the United States. The new DRIs provide for the first time one set of reference values for 12 life stage groups for the United States and Canada. Similar sets of recommendations, typically called recommended dietary intakes, exist for other countries. In addition, a World Health Organization study group has summarized recommended dietary intakes for energy, protein, vitamin A, folate, vitamin B_{12}, vitamin C, vitamin D, iron, and zinc (World Health Organization, 1990). A separate Food and Agriculture Organization/World Health Organization (FAO/WHO) expert group, recognizing the increased amount of international trade, has defined a single Nutrition Reference Value for 15 nutrients solely for labeling purposes (Astier-Dumas, 1990).

The use of professional judgment and interpretation to set an RDA, DRI, or other recommended intake is illustrated by the range

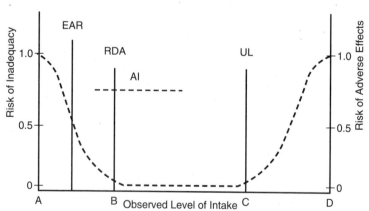

Figure 42–1. Dietary Reference Intakes (DRIs). This figure shows that the Estimated Average Requirement (EAR) is the intake at which the risk of inadequacy is 0.5 (50%). The Recommended Dietary Allowance (RDA) is the intake at which the risk of inadequacy is very small—only 0.02 to 0.03 (2% to 3%). The Adequate Intake (AI) does not bear a consistent relationship to the EAR or the RDA because it is set without being able to estimate the requirement. At intakes between the RDA and the Tolerable Upper Intake Level (UL), the risks of inadequacy and of adverse effects are both close to 0. The UL is the highest level of daily nutrient intake that is likely to pose no risks of adverse health effects to almost all individuals in the general population. At intakes above the UL, the risk of adverse effects increases. A dashed line is used because the actual shape of the curve has not been determined experimentally. The distances between points A and B, B and C, and C and D may differ much more than is depicted in this figure. (From Institute of Medicine, Food and Nutrition Board [1998] Dietary Reference Intakes: Thiamin, Riboflavin, Niacin, Vitamin B_6, Folate, Vitamin B_{12}, Pantothenic Acid, Biotin, and Choline. National Academy Press, Washington, D.C.)

of values for some nutrients in existing sets of standards in different countries. FAO/WHO did an analysis of the ranges of values for recommended dietary intakes around the world, based on the mean for active male adults. The ratios of the highest value to the lowest value were found to range from 1.3:1 for energy (3200 kcal/2450 kcal) to 50.0:1 for vitamin K (1.5 mg/0.03 mg) (Helsing, 1990). Other ratios included 2.5:1 for calcium, 2.8:1 for vitamin A, 4.6:1 for iron, and 8.6:1 for copper. Although the differences are due in part to biology, much of the difference can be explained by the different approaches used in setting the standards.

Criteria for Setting Dietary Recommendations

The first edition of the *Recommended Dietary Allowances,* published by the National Academy of Sciences in 1943, provided recommended intakes for energy and nine essential nutrients. The RDAs have been revised periodically based on new scientific knowledge and interpretations. The tenth edition was published in 1989 and provided values for 19 nutrients for 18 age/sex categories. With each revision there have been changes in the numbers of nutrients considered and the levels recommended, but the basic philosophy has been to define RDAs as levels sufficient to cover individual variations and provide a margin of safety above minimum requirements (Institute of Medicine, 1994).

In 1993, the National Academy of Sciences' Food and Nutrition Board held a national conference to discuss the future of the RDAs (Institute of Medicine, 1994). Based on that conference, the Food and Nutrition Board concluded that (1) there is sufficient new knowledge about certain vitamins and minerals and energy to support a review of the 1989 RDAs, (2) the concept of reduction in risk of chronic disease should be considered in the formulation of future RDAs, and (3) a new format for the RDAs should be considered seriously.

The first conclusion has been the basic justification for previous revisions of the RDAs. The second conclusion represents a major shift in how the RDAs are conceptualized. For example, the relationship between calcium and osteoporosis or the role of folic acid in cardiovascular disease will now be considered in setting new values. The Committee on the Scientific Evaluation of Dietary Reference Intakes of the Food and Nutrition Board addressed the third conclusion by deciding that the 1989 RDAs should be replaced in their entirety by the new DRIs.

Other countries with recommended dietary intakes are also struggling with how to define their levels—should they use a minimalist amount that prevents deficiency disease in all healthy people, an intermediate amount that allows for a large margin of safety, or a level that supports optimal nutrition? For example, when setting their Recommended Dietary Intake for vitamin C, Australia considered four criteria: (1) the amount to prevent scurvy, (2) the amount to provide tissue saturation, (3) the amount to maximize absorption of nonheme iron, and (4) the amount that may minimize risk of gastric cancer. The final recommended dietary intake was based on the amount required to prevent scurvy in smokers and to provide "reasonable" stores in most people but not to ensure tissue saturation (Truswell, 1990).

How RDAs and DRIs Are Used

The former RDAs are meant to be applied to groups of people, namely "practically all healthy people," and not any single individual. In fact, except for energy, the levels are set higher than the requirements of most individuals to account for the wide range of individual variation. Even so, the RDAs often have been inappropriately interpreted as the amounts of essential nutrients a healthy *individual* needs over time. Over the years, the RDAs have also been used for several other purposes, including establishing nutrient standards for food assistance programs such as the National School Lunch Program and School Breakfast Program, evaluating dietary survey data, designing nutrition education programs, developing and fortifying food products, and setting standards for food labels (Institute of Medicine, 1994).

The DRIs were purposely developed to address some of these inappropriate applica-

NUTRITION INSIGHT

Food Fortification with Folic Acid

As the former RDAs are being revised into Dietary Reference Intakes (DRIs), the role a nutrient plays in providing optimal health, rather than just preventing a deficiency disease, is being considered. For example, folate's role in reducing the risk of cardiovascular disease or preventing certain birth defects was considered in setting the DRIs for folate. The folate intake of women of child-bearing age is of concern, and the RDA for folate for this subgroup was increased to reflect new research.

Simply changing an RDA value, however, does not mean people will change their consumption of that nutrient. Another strategy for ensuring that a population group meets their need for a specific nutrient is to fortify certain foods. Earlier in this century, American manufacturers started fortifying salt with iodine, milk with vitamin D, and white bread with thiamin, niacin, riboflavin, and iron. Based on studies of folic acid and birth defects, the U. S. Public Health Service recommended in 1992 that all women of child-bearing age consume 0.4 mg of folic acid daily to reduce their risk of giving birth to children with neural tube defects. (The 1989 RDA for women was 0.18 mg; the 1998 RDA for women is 0.4 mg.) The Food and Drug Administration issued a regulation in 1996, which stated that, as of 1998, American manufacturers will be required to fortify certain grain products with folic acid in an effort to reduce the risk of neural tube birth defects (U. S. Department of Health and Human Services, 1996a). These products include most enriched breads, flours, corn meals, pastas, and rice. Required fortification levels range from 0.43 to 1.4 mg per pound of product.

The fortification levels chosen were designed to keep total daily intake of folic acid below 1 mg; intakes higher than that may mask symptoms of pernicious anemia, a form of vitamin B_{12} deficiency that primarily affects older people. Some have suggested that foods fortified with folic acid should also be fortified with vitamin B_{12} in order to address this concern. Food fortification policies must take into account how increased consumption of one nutrient may affect other nutrients. Policy makers must also determine whether the fortified foods are likely to be consumed by the target audience (e.g., women of child-bearing age) and whether that level is safe for other populations (e.g, elderly people).

tions of the former RDAs. In general, the newly defined RDAs should be used by individuals as a target intake, but these values are of limited use in assessing the adequacy of an individual's nutrient intake. AIs can be used as a target value for individuals if no RDAs exist. EARs are particularly useful for both evaluating and planning nutrient intakes of groups. Table 42–1 summarizes some of the suggested uses of DRIs, with the most widespread being dietary planning and assessment. A more thorough explanation on how to use various DRIs will be addressed in a separate report from the Institute of Medicine to be issued in the future.

Limitations of RDAs and DRIs

The former RDAs have several characteristics that limit their usefulness. Historically, RDAs

have not been established for several nutrients that are known to have important health consequences, such as carbohydrates, fat, saturated fatty acids, cholesterol, and fiber. Intakes of these nutrients can affect the risk of some chronic diseases, such as heart disease and certain cancers. Using the former RDAs as a goal ensures only that adequate amounts of proteins and most vitamins and minerals are consumed; they cannot be used, for example, to measure whether a diet is excessively high in fat.

The former RDAs and the new DRIs are also not a practical guide for use by consumers in selecting a healthful diet. The RDAs/DRIs focus on specific nutrients, whereas people make food selections based on individual foods and food groups. Dietary advice for consumers needs to focus on recommended food selections in the context of the total diet.

TABLE 42–1
Uses of Dietary Reference Intakes for Healthy Individuals and Groups

Type of Use	For the Individual	For a Group
Planning	**RDA:** aim for this intake. **AI:** use as a guide for intake.	**EAR:** use in conjunction with a measure of variability of the group's intake to set goals for the mean intake of a specific population. **AI:** since an EAR is unavailable, use as a basis for the formulation of tentative goals for the mean intake by a population. **UL:** use to ensure that goals for the mean intakes of specific population groups do not place individuals within the group at risk of overconsumption.
Assessment	**EAR:** use to examine the possibility of inadequacy; evaluation of true status requires clinical, biochemical, and/or anthropometric data. **UL:** use to examine the possibility of overconsumption; evaluation of true status requires clinical, biochemical, and/or anthropometric data.	**EAR:** use in the assessment of the prevalence of inadequate intakes within a group.

EAR = Estimated Average Requirement; RDA = Recommended Dietary Allowance; AI = Adequate Intake; UL = Tolerable Upper Intake Level

From Institute of Medicine, Food and Nutrition Board (1998) Dietary Reference Intakes: Thiamin, Riboflavin, Niacin, Vitamin B_6, Folate, Vitamin B_{12}, Pantothenic Acid, Biotin, and Choline. National Academy Press, Washington, D.C.

DIETARY ADVICE—GOALS AND GUIDELINES

Development of Dietary Guidelines

As the relationship between diet and health has become clearer, a new type of dietary advice has emerged in the form of dietary goals and guidelines. Unlike the RDAs, which focus on obtaining adequate amounts of essential nutrients, these guidelines emphasize the need to increase or decrease consumption of those food components that have been shown to affect the risk of certain chronic diseases. Another difference is that RDAs/DRIs state the amounts (weights) of intake recommended on a daily basis for various nutrients with no indication of whether typical intake is high or low, whereas dietary guidelines start with the estimated national diet and express desired changes, generally in terms of what percentage of total energy should come from the energy-producing nutrients.

In the United States, this shift in focus from obtaining adequate intakes to minimizing excessive intakes began in 1977 when a United States Senate Select Committee on Nutrition and Human Needs issued a set of recommendations known as the *Dietary Goals for the United States* (United States Senate, 1977). These goals provided quantitative recommendations on the amounts of complex carbohydrates, sugar, fat, saturated fat, cholesterol, and sodium that should be consumed. The Dietary Goals were controversial, in part because the diet plans developed to meet the goals were so different from the food patterns of typical Americans, particularly in terms of protein intake. Some scientists were also uncomfortable with the goals because they felt the evidence was insufficient to support such specific recommendations.

Subsequently, a new publication, *Nutrition and Your Health: Dietary Guidelines for Americans*, was jointly issued in 1980 by the United States Department of Agriculture (USDA) and the Department of Health, Education, and Welfare (now Health and Human Services). This publication was revised in 1985, 1990, and 1995 (U.S. Department of Agriculture and U. S. Department of Health and Human Services, 1995). The 1995 revision was the first one to be mandated by the government as a result of the National Nutrition Monitoring and Related Research Act, which requires the Secretaries of Agriculture and Health and Human Services to review and jointly issue the Guidelines every 5 years (Davis and Saltos, 1996). The 1995 guidelines are shown in Table 42–2. Although the Guidelines are similar in format to the seven recommendations of the original Dietary Goals, the Dietary Guidelines are notable for the absence of any specific numbers in any guideline, although quantitative information is included in the text of the supporting publication.

Sources of Dietary Guidelines

Like the RDAs, the Dietary Guidelines for Americans are intended for *healthy* Americans, in this case those age 2 years and older. The Guidelines are not intended for younger children and infants, whose dietary needs differ.

The Dietary Guidelines for Americans form the base of federal nutrition policy in the United States, but they are not the only set of dietary advice. Other agencies, organizations, and countries have also issued dietary goals or guidelines. In the United States, two authoritative reviews on the relationship between diet and health were published in the late 1980s. *The Surgeon General's Report on Nutrition and Health,* issued in 1988, contains advice similar to the Dietary Guidelines but also includes advice about fluoride, calcium, and iron intake (U. S. Department of Health and Human Services, 1988). In 1989, the Com-

mittee on Diet and Health of the National Academy of Sciences issued *Diet and Health: Implications for Reducing Chronic Disease Risk* (National Research Council, 1989b). This publication provides quantitative targets for intake of fat, saturated fat, cholesterol, sodium, and alcohol and a recommended number of servings of fruits and vegetables and complex carbohydrates, as well as more general advice for the intake of energy, protein, calcium, fluoride, and dietary supplements. Dietary goals are also included in the United States Department of Health and Human Services report *Healthy People 2000: National Health Promotion and Disease Prevention Objectives,* which identifies 300 specific health objectives in 22 priority areas including nutrition (U. S. Department of Health and Human Services, 1991). Specific risk reduction objectives target decreasing fat, decreasing sodium, increasing complex carbohydrates and fiber, increasing calcium, increasing breast-feeding, and decreasing iron deficiency.

Various health organizations and expert panels have also issued dietary guidelines, often to reduce the risk of a specific disease. For example, guidelines from the American Heart Association and the American Cancer Society are aimed at reducing the risk of heart disease and cancer, respectively. In addition, many countries around the world have issued dietary guidelines targeted to either the general population or specifically to high-risk groups (World Health Organization, 1990).

FOOD GUIDES

Development of Food Guides

The Dietary Guidelines are written for the general public, but there is still a need for more specific food-related advice if the guidelines are to be implemented. Advising someone to eat less fat, especially saturated fat, does no good if the person does not know which foods are sources of fat. Likewise, the Guidelines recommend choosing a diet with "plenty" of grain products, vegetables, and fruits, but if a person eats two servings of vegetables and fruits a day, how will he or she know if that amount is "plenty?" Food guides are designed

---

TABLE 42–2
Dietary Guidelines for Americans

- Eat a variety of foods
- Balance the food you eat with physical activity—maintain or improve your weight
- Choose a diet with plenty of grain products, vegetables, and fruits
- Choose a diet low in fat, saturated fat, and cholesterol
- Choose a diet moderate in sugars
- Choose a diet moderate in salt and sodium
- If you drink alcoholic beverages, do so in moderation

From U. S. Department of Agriculture/U. S. Department of Health and Human Services (1995) Nutrition and Your Health: Dietary Guidelines for Americans, 4th ed. USDA Home and Garden Bulletin No. 232. U. S. Government Printing Office, Washington, D. C.

to translate recommendations on nutrient intake into recommendations on food intake.

Over the years, the United States government has published various food guides (U. S. Department of Agriculture, 1993). The first federal food guide, based on five food groups, was issued in 1916. The five groups (namely milk and meat, cereals, vegetables and fruits, fats and fatty foods, and sugars and sugary foods) were chosen based on the knowledge at that time of food composition and nutritional needs. During the Depression in the 1930s, there was an increased need for advice on how to select foods economically, so family food plans were developed to serve as buying guides. These food plans still exist today, adjusted for inflation, and serve as the basis for food stamp allotments.

In 1943 a food guide known as the "Basic Seven" was issued; this food guide recommended a certain number of daily servings from each of seven food groups. This guide was simplified and modified in 1956 to what has become known as the "Basic Four." The Basic Four defined daily serving sizes and recommended a 2-2-4-4 pattern. This meant two servings from the milk and milk products group; two servings from the meat, fish, poultry, eggs, dry beans, and nuts group; four servings from the fruit and vegetable group; and four servings from the grain products group. The Basic Four guide was meant to represent a foundation diet that would supply a major portion of the RDAs for nutrients, but only part of the energy needs. It was expected that people would eat additional foods to fulfill their needs for additional energy and nutrients.

Because the Basic Four and previous food guides were developed in the context of preventing deficiency diseases, the primary focus was on getting enough nutrients from a variety of foods. This advice complemented USDA's goal of promoting the consumption of various agricultural products.

In 1979, following the publication of the Dietary Goals, the USDA published the *Hassle-Free Guide to a Better Diet*. This food guide included the same foundation diet as recommended in the Basic Four, but identified a fifth group of fats, sweets, and alcohol for which moderation was advised. This was a significant change from previous food guides, as the government had now identified a food group for which there was no recommended number of daily servings. Instead, consumers were simply being urged to eat sparingly from this group.

After publication of the *Hassle-Free Guide*, the first edition of the Dietary Guidelines was issued, and it became clear that a new food guide was needed to help consumers translate the advice in the Guidelines into actual food choices. In developing the new food guide, USDA first identified several philosophical goals for the guide: it should promote overall health, focus on the total diet, be useful to the target audience, and allow flexibility. Five steps were then used to develop the actual guide (U. S. Department of Agriculture, 1993).

The first step was the establishment of nutritional goals. The RDAs were used to establish the goals for protein, vitamins, and minerals, whereas the Dietary Guidelines were used to establish goals for other food components such as fat, cholesterol, and sodium. The second step was the definition of food groups. Foods were placed into groups based on their nutrient content, as well as how they were typically used in meals and where they had been placed in previous food guides. Subgroups were also identified to provide additional focus on important nutrients. For example, the bread group contains a subgroup emphasizing whole grains, and the vegetable group contains a subgroup emphasizing dark green vegetables.

The third step was the assignment of serving sizes. Decisions about serving size were based on several factors, including the typical serving sizes reported in food consumption surveys, the ease at which the serving size could be multiplied or divided to represent actual consumption, the nutrient content of the food (for example, calcium content was considered when determining serving sizes for dairy foods), as well as the serving sizes traditionally used in nutrition education materials. The fourth step was the determination of nutrient profiles for each food group and subgroup. This represented the average amount of nutrients and other food components provided by a serving from each group. These values were based on the most fre-

TABLE 42–3
Food Guide Sample Patterns at Three Caloric Levels

	Pattern A	Pattern B	Pattern C
Approximate kilocalories	1600	2200	2800
Bread Group (servings)	6	9	11
Vegetable Group (servings)	3	4	5
Fruit Group (servings)	2	3	4
Milk Group (servings)	2–3*	2–3*	2–3*
Meat Group (total ounces)	5	6	7
Total fat (grams)	53	73	93
Total added sugars (teaspoons)	6	12	18

*Women who are pregnant or breast-feeding, teenagers, and young adults to age 24 years need three servings.

From U. S. Department of Agriculture, Human Nutrition Information Service (1993) USDA's Food Guide: Background and Development. USDA Miscellaneous Publication No. 1514. U. S. Government Printing Office, Washington, D. C.

from the major food groups were determined based on what was needed to meet the recommended intakes for protein, vitamins, and minerals. Because the recommendations vary based on age and gender, the numbers of servings are expressed as ranges. USDA suggests that the lowest number of servings is appropriate for many sedentary women and some older adults, whereas the higher number of servings is appropriate for teenage boys, active men, and some very active women. The difference in energy needs also allows for a range in the amount of fat and added sugars that can be included in the diet. Table 42–3 shows sample patterns at three levels of caloric intake. Assuming a 25- to 50-year-old woman selects foods according to Pattern A, the percentage contributions of various food groups to meeting her RDA for selected nutrients is shown in Figure 42–2.

This new food guide was published in several USDA publications released in the mid-1980s and was also included in the third edition of the Dietary Guidelines published in 1990. Despite the release of a new food guide, many consumers and even some professionals still assumed USDA was using the Basic Four food guide. To improve the visibility and usefulness of the new food guide, the Food

quently consumed foods within a group as determined by food consumption surveys.

The fifth and final step was the determination of the numbers of servings. This decision had to balance the concerns about adequacy versus excess. Numbers of servings

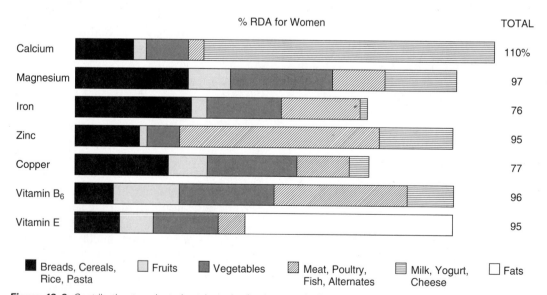

Figure 42–2. Contribution to selected nutrients by food groups in Pattern A (1600 kcal), women 25 to 50 years of age. Values are based on 1989 RDAs. (From U. S. Department of Agriculture, Human Nutrition Information Service [1993] USDA's Food Guide: Background and Development. USDA Miscellaneous Publication No. 1514. U. S. Government Printing Office, Washington, D. C.).

Guide Pyramid was developed as a graphic representation of the guide.

The challenge in developing a graphic was to find a way to represent visually the three key concepts of the new food guide: variety, proportionality, and moderation. These concepts needed to be conveyed in a way that was understandable and memorable. At a glance consumers needed to see that foods should be selected from a variety of groups, that more servings should come from some groups than others, and that some groups contained more fats and sugars than others. After considerable testing using focus groups, individual interviews, and other forms of market research, a pyramid with food pictures and fat and sugar symbols was chosen as the most effective graphic for communicating the key concepts (Fig. 42–3). USDA released the graphic and a consumer brochure, *The Food Guide Pyramid,* in 1992 (U.S. Department of Agriculture, 1992). Since its release, the Food Guide Pyramid has been widely used in nutrition education materials by both the public and private sectors.

Limitations of Food Guides

Despite the extensive research that went into its development, the Food Guide Pyramid is limited in its usefulness. As is true with all food guides, the adequacy of the diet still depends upon the food choices within food groups. Within each food group, foods vary in nutrient density (nutrients provided per kilocalorie). A poor diet could be selected consisting primarily of foods with low nutrient density that still satisfies the number of servings from each food group recommended by the Pyramid.

Another limitation of the Food Guide Pyramid is that foods representative of diverse cultures are not pictured. To address this limitation, nutrition educators have adapted the Pyramid to feature different foods so it can be used by culturally diverse audiences, such as Mexican Americans or Southeast Asians (Achterberg et al., 1994).

FOOD LABELS

Nutrition Information on Food Labels

The Food Guide Pyramid is only one tool to help Americans implement the Dietary Guidelines; food labels are another tool. Many consumers make food choices at the point of purchase, typically in a grocery store. The food label, which includes the "Nutrition

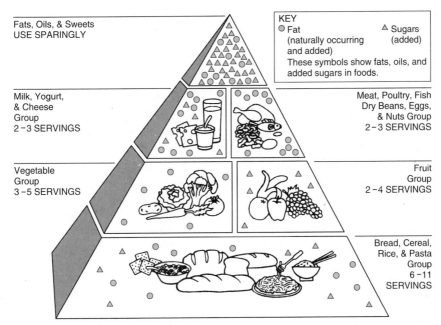

Figure 42–3. *The Food Guide Pyramid; a guide to daily food choices. (Source: U. S. Department of Agriculture and U. S. Department of Health and Human Services.)*

Facts" panel, provides consumers with information about the ingredients and nutrients contained in individual foods. This information can be used to compare products and to assess how a particular food fits into the context of the total diet.

Nutrition information has only recently been required on most packaged foods, although the government has been involved in the regulation of food labels since 1906 with the passage of the Federal Food and Drugs Act and the Federal Meat Inspection Act (U. S. Department of Health and Human Services, 1993b). These laws gave the federal government the authority to regulate the safety and quality of food. The 1906 Federal Food and Drugs Act was replaced in 1938 with the Federal Food, Drug and Cosmetic Act, which prohibited any labeling that was false or misleading. In 1973, the Food and Drug Administration (FDA) issued regulations that required nutrition labeling on any food that made a claim about its nutritional properties or that contained any added nutrients. Nutrition information appeared on other foods as well, but it was done on a voluntary basis.

Following the publication of the *Surgeon General's Report on Nutrition and Health* (U. S. Department of Health and Human Services, 1988) and the National Research Council's *Diet and Health* report (National Research Council, 1989b), the FDA and the USDA's Food Safety and Inspection Service (which regulates meat and poultry products) asked the Food and Nutrition Board of the National Research Council to come up with recommendations on how to improve food labels so they could be used to select healthful diets. Based on these and other recommendations, the FDA proposed new food labeling regulations in 1990, which would require, among other things, mandatory nutrition labeling on most foods and standard rules for the use of health claims. In the same year, the Nutrition Labeling and Education Act (1990) was passed, which also required several changes in the food label, including mandatory nutrition labeling.

The FDA issued the final regulations implementing the Nutrition Labeling and Education Act in 1993 (U. S. Department of Health and Human Services, 1993a). Although not required to do so by law, USDA's Food Safety and Inspection Service also issued new regulations at the same time mandating nutrition labeling on processed meat and poultry products and providing for voluntary nutrition information for raw meat and poultry products. These regulations went into effect in May, 1994, for most foods and in July, 1994, for meat and poultry products.

The new labeling regulations not only require that nutrition information be provided for more foods than in the past, but also the required information has been modified to reflect current concerns about diet and health. In addition to information on total Calories (kilocalories), protein, carbohydrate, and fat, which was required on the former food label, information on calories from fat and the amounts of saturated fat, cholesterol, and dietary fiber are now also required as part of the new Nutrition Facts panel (Fig. 42–4). The former label also required information on vitamin A, vitamin C, thiamin, riboflavin, niacin, calcium, and iron. The new food label makes the listing of thiamin, riboflavin, and niacin optional because there is less concern about getting adequate amounts of these three vitamins than in the past. Other values that are optional include Calories (kilocalories) from saturated fat and the amounts of polyunsaturated fat, monounsaturated fat, potassium, soluble fiber, insoluble fiber, sugar alcohol, β-carotene, and other essential vitamins and minerals.

Daily Values on Food Labels

As required by law, the nutrition information on the food label must be presented in a way that enables consumers to put the information into the context of the total daily diet. To meet this objective, nutrients are listed in terms of the percentage of Daily Value they provide. The Daily Values are based on two sets of reference values for nutrients: the Daily Reference Values (DRVs) and the Reference Daily Intakes (RDIs).

The DRVs were developed for nutrients, such as fat, carbohydrate, cholesterol, and fiber, for which no previous standards existed. The DRVs for the energy-providing nutrients are calculated based on the caloric content

Nutrition Facts

Serving Size ½ cup (114g)
Servings Per Container 4

Amount Per Serving

Calories 90   Calories from Fat 30

% Daily Value*

Total Fat 3g	**5%**
Saturated Fat 0g	**0%**
Cholesterol 0mg	**0%**
Sodium 300mg	**13%**
Total Carbohydrate 13g	**4%**
Dietary Fiber 3g	**12%**
Sugars 3g	
Protein 3g	

Vitamin A	80%	•	Vitamin C	60%
Calcium	4%	•	Iron	4%

* Percent Daily Values are based on a 2,000 calorie diet. Your daily values may be higher or lower depending on your calorie needs:

	Calories	2,000	2,500
Total Fat	Less than	65g	80g
Sat Fat	Less than	20g	25g
Cholesterol	Less than	300mg	300mg
Sodium	Less than	2,400mg	2,400mg
Total Carbohydrate		300g	375g
Fiber		25g	30g

Calories per gram:
Fat 9   •   Carbohydrate 4   •   Protein 4

Figure 42–4. Required format for nutrition information on food labels: The Nutrition Facts Panel. (From Food and Drug Administration [1993] How to Read the New Food Label. DHHS Publication No. [FDA] 93-2260. U. S. Government Printing Office, Washington, D. C.)

of the daily diet, which for labeling purposes was chosen as 2000 kcal (Table 42–4). RDIs, which replaced the term U. S. Recommended Daily Allowances (U. S. RDA), provide reference values for certain vitamins and minerals. The term Daily Value, which encompasses both DRVs and RDIs, is used on current food labels. The terms RDI and Daily Value were chosen, in part, to eliminate the use of the term U. S. RDA, which was easily confused with the term RDA.

U. S. RDAs were the standard chosen in 1973 as a reference for the previous food label. The U. S. RDAs, which consisted of a single value for each nutrient to simplify their use on a food label, were based on the RDAs, which consist of several values for each nutrient based on age and gender. The FDA used the 1968 RDAs as a basis for the U. S. RDAs and, in most cases, simply chose the highest figure from the age/sex categories to cover those with the greatest need. Other standards

TABLE 42–4
Daily Reference Values (DRVs)*

Food Component	DRV
Fat	65 g
Saturated fatty acids	20 g
Cholesterol	300 mg
Total carbohydrate	300 g
Fiber	25 g
Sodium	2400 mg
Potassium	3500 mg
Protein†	50 g

*Based on 2000 kcal a day for adults and children over 4 years only.

†DRV for protein does not apply to certain populations; Reference Daily Intake (RDI) for protein has been established for these groups: children 1 to 4 years: 16 g; infants under 1 year: 14 g; pregnant women: 60 g; nursing mothers: 65 g.

From U. S. Department of Health and Human Services, Food and Drug Administration (1993b) Focus on Food Labeling. FDA Consumer Special Report. DHHS Publication No. (FDA) 93-2262. U. S. Government Printing Office, Washington, D. C.

have been proposed for the RDIs, such as selecting the average, rather than the highest, value from the 1989 RDAs. To date, none of these proposals has been adopted, and the values used for food labeling purposes have not been updated; the current RDIs are the same values as the former U. S. RDAs (Table 42–5).

Serving Sizes on Food Labels

The nutrition information on a food label is based on a specified serving size. In the past, food manufacturers determined the serving size; under the current labeling regulations, serving sizes are more uniform and reflect the amount of that food customarily eaten at one time. The serving size does not necessarily represent the amount any given individual eats. Someone who eats more or less than the specified serving size of a given food will need to adjust the nutrition information accordingly.

The uniformity in serving sizes makes it easier for consumers to compare nutritional qualities of similar products than in the past. It also provides a consistent reference for nutrient content claims, such as "low fat" and "high fiber." The 1993 food labeling regulations provide standardized definitions for certain terms (U. S. Department of Health and Human Services, 1993a). For example, a "low-fat" food

must have 3 g or less of fat per serving, a "fat-free" food must have less than 0.5 g of fat per serving, a "low-sodium" food must have 140 mg or less of sodium per serving, and a "high-fiber" food must have 5 g or more of fiber per serving.

Health Claims on Food Labels

In addition to nutrient claims, food labels may also carry certain health claims. These are claims that link the consumption of a food or nutrient with the prevention or reduction in risk of a certain disease. For years, health claims were explicitly prohibited by federal regulations because any claim that a substance could affect the course of a disease was considered equivalent to a drug claim. That meant a food carrying a health claim on the label could be considered an unapproved new drug and technically could be seized. As the relationship between diet and disease became more established, the FDA modified

TABLE 42–5
Reference Daily Intakes (RDIs)*

Nutrient	Amount
Vitamin A	5000 IU
Vitamin C	60 mg
Thiamin	1.5 mg
Riboflavin	1.7 mg
Niacin	20 mg
Calcium	1.0 g
Iron	18 mg
Vitamin D	400 IU
Vitamin E	30 IU
Vitamin B_6	2.0 mg
Folic acid	0.4 mg
Vitamin B_{12}	6 µg
Phosphorus	1.0 g
Iodine	150 µg
Magnesium	400 mg
Zinc	15 mg
Copper	2 mg
Biotin	0.3 mg
Pantothenic acid	10 mg

*Based on The National Academy of Sciences' 1968 Recommended Dietary Allowances.

To convert IU (International Units) to units currently used, 1 IU of vitamin A = 0.30 µg of retinol equivalent, 1 IU of vitamin D = 0.025 µg of vitamin D_3, and 1 IU of vitamin E = 0.67 mg of α-tocopherol equivalents.

From U. S. Department of Health and Human Services, Food and Drug Administration (1993b) Focus on Food Labeling. FDA Consumer Special Report. DHHS Publication No. (FDA) 93-2262. U. S. Government Printing Office, Washington, D. C.

its policy, as reflected in the 1993 regulations that allow specific health claims on food packages under certain conditions (U. S. Department of Health and Human Services, 1993a). One condition is that the health claim must be based on significant scientific agreement by qualified experts.

As of August, 1999, federal regulations allow claims for the following diet-disease relationships:

- calcium and osteoporosis
- sodium and hypertension
- dietary saturated fat and cholesterol and coronary heart disease
- dietary fat and cancer
- fiber-containing grain products, fruits, and vegetables and cancer
- fruits, vegetables and grain products that contain fiber, particularly soluble fiber, and coronary heart disease
- fruits and vegetables and cancer
- folic acid and neural tube defects
- sugar alcohols and dental caries
- soluble fiber from whole oats and coronary heart disease
- soluble fiber from psyllium seed husk and coronary heart disease

The first seven health claims in the preceding list were authorized in the 1993 labeling regulations, but the ones for folic acid and neural tube defects and for sugar alcohols and dental caries were authorized by two separate regulations in 1996, the one for oat fiber and coronary heart disease in 1997, and the one for psyllium fiber and coronary heart disease in 1998 (U. S. Department of Health and Human Services, 1996b, 1996c, 1997, 1998). As new scientific evidence becomes available, the FDA will consider authorizing additional health claims.

Labeling of Dietary Supplements

The Nutrition Labeling and Education Act of 1990 was originally intended to apply to both foods and dietary supplements, including vitamins, minerals, amino acids, herbs, and similar products. Controversy over the proposed rules on health claims affecting supplements led to the Dietary Supplement Act of 1992, which exempted dietary supplements from

any new labeling requirements for 1 year to allow for further discussion (Dietary Supplement Act, 1992). Eventually the FDA issued regulations on January 4, 1994, stating that dietary supplements have to provide the same basic nutrition information as is found on labels of other foods (U. S. Department of Health and Human Services, 1994). These regulations also state that health claims on supplements are subject to the same approval process as is required for health claims on conventional food.

Additional legislation in the form of the Dietary Supplement Health and Education Act of 1994 became law in October, 1994 (Dietary Supplement Health and Education Act, 1994). This act defines "dietary supplement" and allows manufacturers to make claims about a product's ability to affect the structure or function of the body or to affect a person's general well-being. Unlike health claims, these "structure and function" claims do not need to be authorized in advance by the FDA, although a manufacturer is required to notify the FDA about the statement no later than 30 days after the product is first marketed. The act also allows the FDA to remove unsafe supplements from the market, but it puts the burden of proof on the government to demonstrate that a supplement or its ingredient is unsafe. This policy is significantly different from the standards required of food additive and drug manufacturers, who must demonstrate the safety of their products *before* new products are allowed on the market.

REFERENCES

Achterberg C., McDonnell, E. and Bagby, R. (1994) How to put the Food Guide Pyramid into practice. J Am Diet Assoc 94:1030–1035.

American Dietetic Association (1995) Position of the American Dietetic Association: Phytochemicals and functional foods. J Am Diet Assoc 95:493–496.

Astier-Dumas, M. (1990) RDI in Codex Alimentarius. Eur J Clin Nutr 44 (Suppl 2):31–32.

Davis, C. A. and Saltos, E. A. (1996) The Dietary Guidelines for Americans—Past, present, future. Fam Economics Nutr Rev 9:4–13.

Dietary Supplement Act of 1992, Public Law 102-571. 102nd Congress, 2nd session. October 29, 1992.

Dietary Supplement Health and Education Act of 1994, Public Law 103-417, 103rd Congress, 2nd session. October 25, 1994.

Helsing E. (1990) Problems in the process of formulating an RDI. Eur J Clin Nutr 44 (Suppl 2):33–36.

Institute of Medicine, Food and Nutrition Board (1994)

How Should the Recommended Dietary Allowances Be Revised? National Academy Press, Washington, D. C.

Institute of Medicine, Food and Nutrition Board (1997) Dietary Reference Intakes: Calcium, Phosphorus, Magnesium, Vitamin D, and Fluoride. National Academy Press, Washington, D. C.

Institute of Medicine, Food and Nutrition Board (1998) Dietary Reference Intakes: Thiamin, Riboflavin, Niacin, Vitamin B_6, Folate, Vitamin B_{12}, Pantothenic Acid, Biotin, and Choline. National Academy Press, Washington, D. C.

National Research Council, Food and Nutrition Board (1989a) Recommended Dietary Allowances, 10th ed. National Academy Press, Washington, D. C.

National Research Council, Food and Nutrition Board (1989b) Diet and Health: Implications for Reducing Chronic Disease Risk. National Academy Press, Washington, D. C.

Nutrition Labeling and Education Act of 1990, Public Law 101-535, 101st Congress, 2nd session. November 8, 1990.

Truswell, A. S. (1990) The philosophy behind Recommended Dietary Intakes: Can they be harmonized? Eur J Clin Nutr 44 (Suppl 2):3–11.

United States Department of Agriculture (1992) The Food Guide Pyramid. USDA Home and Garden Bulletin 252. U. S. Government Printing Office, Washington, D. C.

United States Department of Agriculture, Human Nutrition Information Service (1993) USDA's Food Guide: Background and Development. USDA Miscellaneous Publication No. 1514. U. S. Government Printing Office, Washington, D. C.

United States Department of Agriculture and United States Department of Health and Human Services (1995) Nutrition and Your Health: Dietary Guidelines for Americans, 4th ed. USDA Home and Garden Bulletin No. 232. U. S. Government Printing Office, Washington, D. C.

United States Department of Health and Human Services, Food and Drug Administration (1993a). Food labeling; General provisions; Nutrition labeling; Label format; Nutrient content claims; Health claims; Ingredient labeling; State and local requirements and exemptions; Final rules. Fed Reg 58:2066–2941.

United States Department of Health and Human Services, Food and Drug Administration (1993b) Focus on Food Labeling. FDA Consumer Special Report. DHHS Publication No. (FDA) 93-2262. U. S. Government Printing Office, Washington, D. C.

United States Department of Health and Human Services, Food and Drug Administration (1994) Dietary supplements; Establishment of date of application. Fed Reg 61:350–437.

United States Department of Health and Human Services, Food and Drug Administration (1996a) Food Standards: Amendment of standards of identity for enriched grain products to require addition of folic acid. Fed Reg 61:8781–8797.

United States Department of Health and Human Services, Food and Drug Administration (1996b) Food labeling:

Health claims and label statements; Folate and neural tube defects. Fed Reg 61:8752–8781.

United States Department of Health and Human Services, Food and Drug Administration (1996c) Food labeling: Health claims; Sugar alcohols and dental caries. Fed Reg 61:43433–43447.

United States Department of Health and Human Services, Food and Drug Administration (1997) Food labeling: Health claims; Oats and coronary heart disease. Fed Reg 62:3564–3601.

United States Department of Health and Human Services, Food and Drug Administration (1998) Food labeling: Health claims; Soluble fiber from certain foods and coronary heart disease. Fed Reg 63:8103–8121.

United States Department of Health and Human Services, Public Health Service (1988) The Surgeon General's Report on Nutrition and Health. DHHS Publication No. (PHS) 88-50210. U. S. Government Printing Office, Washington, D. C.

United States Department of Health and Human Services, Public Health Service (1991) Healthy People 2000: National Health Promotion and Disease Prevention Objectives. DHHS Publication No. (PHS) 91-50213. U. S. Government Printing Office, Washington, D. C.

United States Senate Select Committee on Nutrition and Human Needs (1977) Dietary Goals for the United States, 2nd ed. U. S. Government Printing Office, Washington, D. C.

World Health Organization (1990) Diet, Nutrition, and the Prevention of Chronic Diseases. WHO Technical Report Series No. 797. Geneva, Switzerland.

RECOMMENDED READINGS

Institute of Medicine, Food and Nutrition Board (1991) Improving America's Diet and Health: From Recommendations to Action (Thomas, P. R., ed.). National Academy Press, Washington, D. C.

Sutton, S. J., Layden, W. and Haven, J. (1996) Dietary Guidance and Nutrition Promotion: USDA's Renewed Vision of Nutrition Education. Fam Economics Nutr Rev 9(2):14–21.

United States Department of Agriculture, Agricultural Research Service, Dietary Guidelines Advisory Committee (1995) Report of the Dietary Guidelines Advisory Committee on the Dietary Guidelines for Americans, 1995: To the Secretary of Health and Human Services and the Secretary of Agriculture. National Technical Information Service, Springfield, Virginia.

United States Department of Agriculture, Center for Nutrition Policy and Promotion (1994) Using Food Labels to Follow the Dietary Guidelines for Americans: A Reference. Agriculture Information Bulletin No. 704. National Technical Information Service, Springfield, Virginia.

Yates, A. A., Schlicker, S. A. and Suitor, C. W. (1998) Dietary Reference Intakes: The new basis for recommendations for calcium and related nutrients, B vitamins, and choline. J Am Diet Assoc 98:699–706.

Index

◆ ◆

Note: Page numbers in *italics* refer to illustrations; page numbers followed by b refer to boxed material, and those followed by t refer to tables.